AF900312

Mediastinal Pathology

Neda Kalhor • Cesar Moran

Mediastinal Pathology

Springer

Neda Kalhor
Department of Pathology
The University of Texas MD
Anderson Cancer Center
Houston, TX
USA

Cesar Moran
Department of Pathology
The University of Texas MD
Anderson Cancer Center
Houston, TX
USA

ISBN 978-3-319-98979-2 ISBN 978-3-319-98980-8 (eBook)
https://doi.org/10.1007/978-3-319-98980-8

© Springer Nature Switzerland AG 2019
This work is subject to copyright. All rights are reserved by the Publisher, whether the whole or part of the material is concerned, specifically the rights of translation, reprinting, reuse of illustrations, recitation, broadcasting, reproduction on microfilms or in any other physical way, and transmission or information storage and retrieval, electronic adaptation, computer software, or by similar or dissimilar methodology now known or hereafter developed.
The use of general descriptive names, registered names, trademarks, service marks, etc. in this publication does not imply, even in the absence of a specific statement, that such names are exempt from the relevant protective laws and regulations and therefore free for general use.
The publisher, the authors, and the editors are safe to assume that the advice and information in this book are believed to be true and accurate at the date of publication. Neither the publisher nor the authors or the editors give a warranty, express or implied, with respect to the material contained herein or for any errors or omissions that may have been made. The publisher remains neutral with regard to jurisdictional claims in published maps and institutional affiliations.

This Springer imprint is published by the registered company Springer Nature Switzerland AG
The registered company address is: Gewerbestrasse 11, 6330 Cham, Switzerland

Preface

The mediastinum offers a wealth of pathology that is not limited to specific conditions. In the past, the mediastinum has been referred to as *Pandora's Box*, due to the different tumoral conditions that may appear in this thoracic area. It is of interest to highlight that the normal thymus itself has been a very mysterious gland in past decades, and we are still learning about it. Controversy has also existed in the past regarding the biologic behavior of the most common tumors seen in this area.

This textbook offers the collective experience of the authors and provides a practical approach to the diagnosis of the diverse tumors that can be seen in the mediastinum. Over the years during which we have practiced thoracic pathology, not only have we accrued the knowledge to approach this type of pathology but we also have looked into new ways to provide the best possible information so that patients afflicted with mediastinal tumors can be properly treated by their respective physicians. It is also important to highlight that, over the years, there have been different points of view regarding nomenclature and best way to predict clinical behavior in some of these tumors. In those particular areas, we are providing not only a historical perspective of what has been done in the past but also our own assessment of those changes. Nevertheless, we have tried to maintain a balance in the discussion, but inevitably we have stated our own personal approach. For the most part, the approach in this textbook is on daily practice, as pathologists are confronted with this type of pathology daily. In some areas, it is inevitable that current practice calls for ancillary tests, including immunohistochemistry and molecular techniques.

We are fortunate and indebted to Brett W. Carter, MD, and Edith M. Marom, MD, for their chapter on diagnostic imaging of mediastinal tumors. This subject is highly important in the assessment of any mediastinal tumor. In addition, we are also fortunate to have Larry R. Kaiser, MD, providing his views and sharing his wealth of experience as a thoracic surgeon in his chapter on the surgical approach to mediastinal tumors.

We consider that this textbook should be useful not only to general surgical pathologists or thoracic surgical pathologists but also to thoracic surgeons, radiologists, and oncologist, who are called upon to care of patients with mediastinal tumors. Finally, we hope that, by providing our experience with mediastinal pathology, all of us involved in the treatment and assessment of patients with mediastinal tumors can improve our daily communication in the interest of advancing patient care.

Houston, TX, USA — Neda Kalhor, MD
Houston, TX, USA — Cesar Moran, MD

Contents

Contributors

Brett W. Carter, MD The University of Texas MD Anderson Cancer Center, Department of Diagnostic Radiology, Houston, TX, USA

Larry R. Kaiser, MD Temple University Health System, Philadelphia, PA, USA

Lewis Katz School of Medicine, Temple University, Philadelphia, PA, USA

Health Sciences, Temple University, Philadelphia, PA, USA

Edith M. Marom, MD The Tel Aviv University, Sackler School of Medicine, Department of Diagnostic Imaging, Tel Aviv, Israel

Thoracic Imaging Section, The Chaim Sheba Medical Center, Department of Diagnostic Radiology, Ramat Gan, Israel

1 The Thymus: Practical Anatomy and Histology

Introduction

We have known about a structure in the mediastinal region that has been named the *thymus* for the last 2000 years, and yet we are still learning about it [1–4]. Interestingly, the issue of the name of this anatomical structure is still somewhat unsettled. Possible theories to account for its name include that it is derived from a plant with a similar name or from the Greek word *soul.* Several great scholars of antiquity including Ephesus and Galen de Pergamum were aware of this particular anatomical structure. Da Capri and Vesalio in the fourteenth century contributed to our understanding of the thymus by their work in anatomy, while other scholars during this period also contributed, predominantly to our understanding of the gross anatomy of the thymus. Even though great observations were made – such as the observation that the thymus is larger in the young than in the adult – for the most part, however, the thymus remained a mystery. An important development that allowed progress in our understanding of the thymus was the use of the optical microscope. Although for some time the progress seemed to have been negligible, toward the seventeenth century the concept was presented that the thymus was part of the lymphatic system. Regarding this issue, it was Hassall who in the middle of the eighteenth century presented his work on the microscopic anatomy of the thymus and described the differences between the thymus and lymphatic structures. Unfortunately, also in the eighteenth century and to some extent in early nineteenth century, some previous theories regarding the role of the thymus in certain pathological states were also revived. Concepts such as *thymic asthma* and *status thymolymphaticus* and its association with thymic death regained some acceptance, which unfortunately led to some controversial forms of therapy such as radiation exposure. Such concepts were taken for valid until approximately the mid part of the nineteenth century, when the use of radiation was completely refuted. In more recent decades, with the advent of thoracic surgery, diagnostic imaging, light microscopy, immunohistochemistry, and molecular biology, we have gained a wealth of knowledge regarding the thymus. However, we consider that there is still more to learn and to correlate with different tumoral conditions that have been described affecting the thymus.

Indeed, we have had 2000 years of knowledge regarding a structure that is more prominent in childhood than in adulthood, but yet, some of the most common tumors related to the gland occur in the adult patient population. It is very likely that the last word has not yet been written on the thymus, and as we progress in our knowledge of the thymus, much more is likely to be discovered. The attempt in this chapter is not to rewrite the abundant embryologic, anatomic, physiologic, and histologic characteristics of the thymus. On the contrary, our goal is to provide the diagnostic surgical pathologist with a practical guide to the most important aspects regarding this mysterious gland, so that such knowledge can be used in the diagnosis of the many conditions that may affect the thymus. More in-depth information regarding embryology, anatomy, physiology, and histology of the thymus can be easily encountered in dedicated textbooks on those disciplines.

Embryology and Anatomy

Current views regarding the embryology of the thymus have changed previous concepts about the thymus. Traditionally, it has been believed that the thymus derives from the endoderm of the third pharyngeal pouch on both sides. More recently, it has been stated that it is possible that the thymic epithelium derives from both endoderm and ectoderm of the third and fourth pharyngeal pouches. Even though the thymus seems to be differentiated by the 17th week, the differentiation of cortex and medulla of the thymus occurs in embryos of about 40 mm in length, while by the 10th week approximately 95% of the cells present are T-lymphocytes.

The anatomy of the gland is probably best observed in childhood when the thymus is larger. Normally, the thymus lies in the anterior mediastinum (Fig. 1.1). It has two upper horns (right and left) and extends into the neck area where

© Springer Nature Switzerland AG 2019
N. Kalhor, C. Moran, *Mediastinal Pathology*, https://doi.org/10.1007/978-3-319-98980-8_1

the upper horns of the thymus may make contact with the lower poles of the thyroid gland. Downward, the thymus extends to the fourth or fifth costal cartilage. The anterior portion of the thymus is related to the sternum, while the posterior aspect is related to the upper pericardium, aortic arch, left brachiocephalic vein, and the front and sides of the trachea. The lateral aspects of the thymus are related to the mediastinal pleura, lungs, and phrenic nerve. The thymus receives its blood supply from the internal thoracic artery and the superior thyroid artery, while its drainage is conducted by the inferior thyroid, internal thoracic, and left brachiocephalic veins. The weight of the thymus changes with age. In normal conditions in newborns, the thymus weighs approximately 10–15 grs. (Fig. 1.2a, b); at puberty, it weighs in at 30–40 grs. at its peak; in adults after involutions, it weighs approximately 10 grs., and the gross appearance of the gland may be that of adipose tissue (Fig. 1.3). At the functional level, the thymus is known for producing some hormones and peptides, most notably thymic humoral factor (THF), thymulin, thymopoietin, and thymosins, which have immune properties [5, 6].

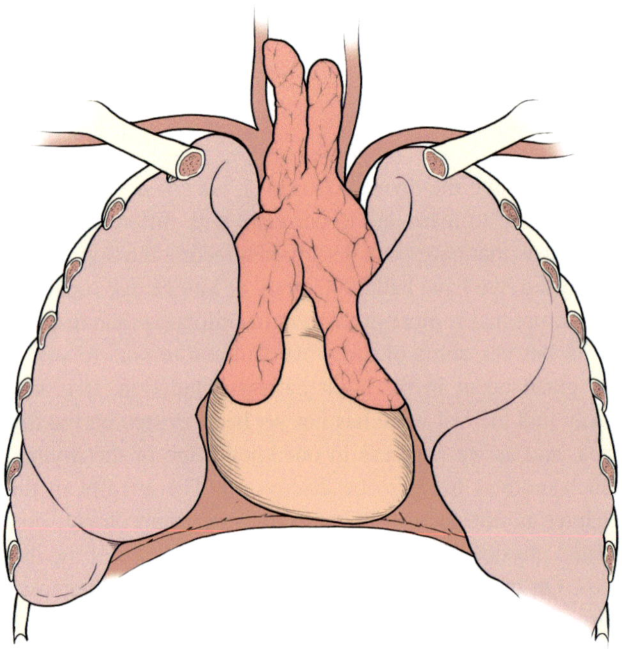

Fig. 1.1 Schematic view of the normal structures within the thoracic cavity. The thymus has two horns, the heart is behind, and the lungs are at the sides. (Copyright © 2016 with permission from Dr. Kalhor and Moran)

Histological Aspects

The schematic view of the normal thymus is depicted in Fig. 1.4. By light microscopy, the thymus appears as a lobulated structure in which each lobule has two basic components: the cortex and the medulla. Each one of these components of the thymic lobule is composed of lymphocytes (thymocytes), which are more prominent in the cortex than in the medulla, and epithelial cells (epitheliocytes), which are more prominent in the medulla than in the cortex [5, 7–10] (Figs. 1.5, 1.6, 1.7, 1.8, 1.9, and 1.10).

Thymic Lymphocytes (Thymocytes)

Thymic lymphocytes (thymocytes) represent approximately 90% of the total weight of the thymus, and, during their mat-

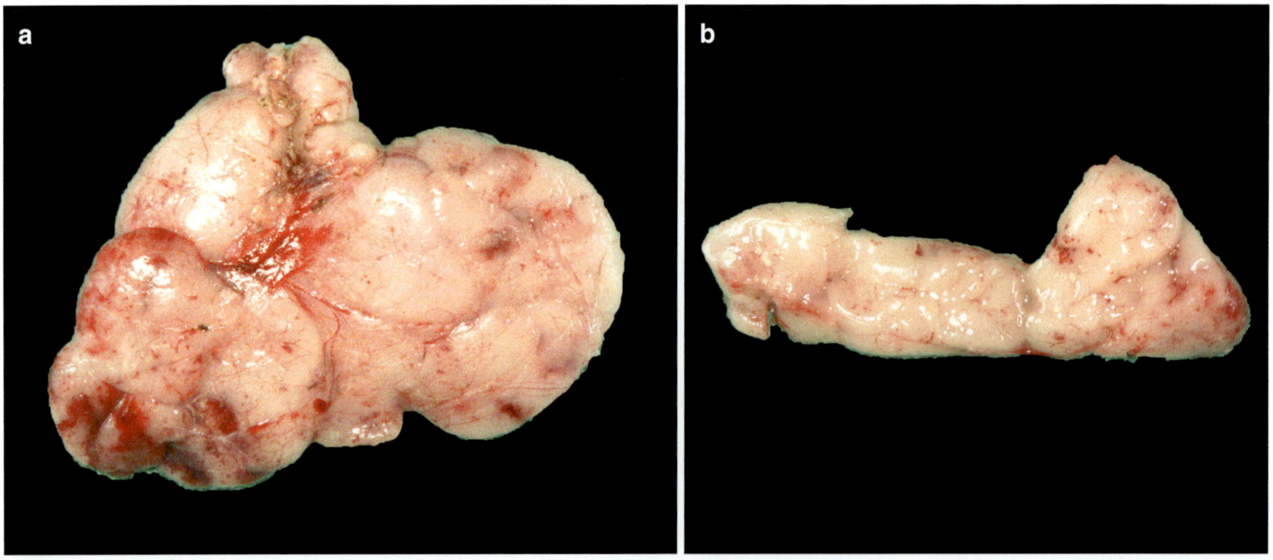

Fig. 1.2 (**a**) Normal thymus of a 2-month-old child with a more solid appearance. (**b**) Cut section the same thymus showing a more "fleshy" appearance. (**a**, **b**: Courtesy of Norma Quintanilla, MD – Texas Childrens Hospital, Houston)

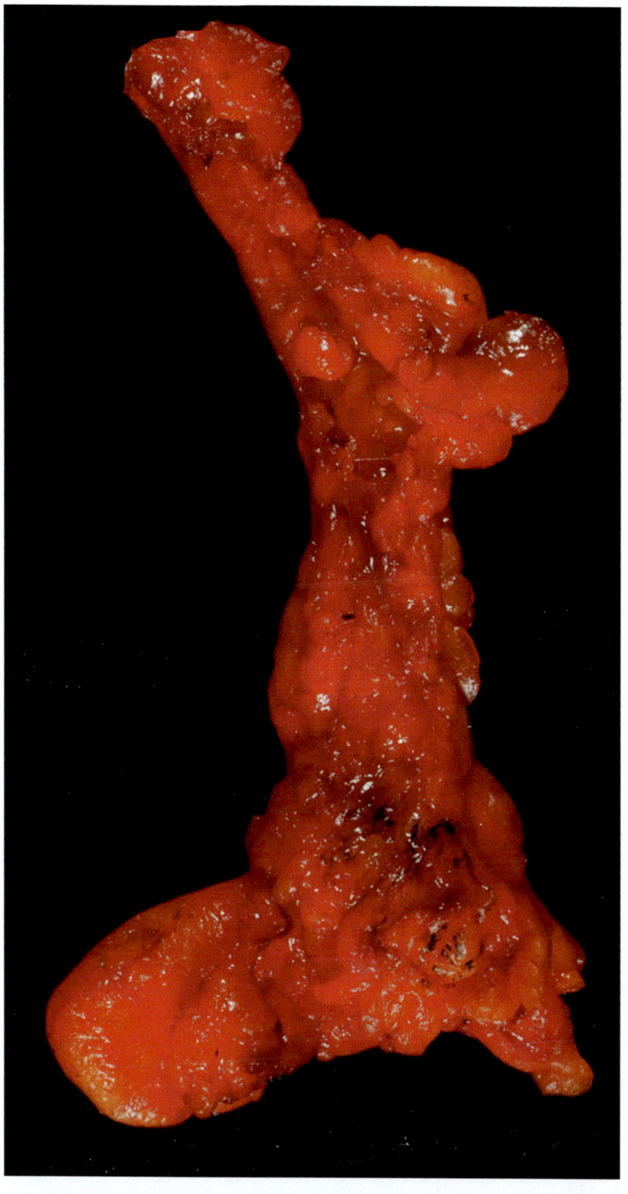

Fig. 1.3 Thymus of an adult individual showing more adipose tissue

uration, the thymocytes move from the deep cortex in the direction of the medulla. Figure 1.4 depicts the maturation process that the thymocytes undergo in the thymus. During this process of maturation and depending upon how strict one can be with this process, thymocytes could be divided into either three or four different types:

1. *Subcapsular thymocytes*: these are large blast cells, and they are double-negative CD4 and CD8. Also, these thymic blasts are CD3 negative. These large thymic blasts represent approximately 5% of the thymocytes.
2. *Cortical thymocytes*: these are smaller cells that may represent approximately 80–90% of the thymocytes. These cortical thymocytes are double-positive cells CD4 and CD8 positive and also CD3 positive.
3. *Medullary thymocytes*: these medullary thymocytes represent approximately 10–15% of the thymocytes and can be subdivided into two types of cells:
   (a) Single-positive medullary thymocytes, which can be positive for either CD4 or CD8
   (b) Immunocompetent single-positive medullary thymocytes, which are activated T-cells

Thymic Epithelial Cells (Epitheliocytes)

These cells are distributed in the thymus in different proportions. Epitheliocytes can be divided either into four or five different categories:

1. Subcapsular cortical (type 1).
2. Inner cortical (types 2–3): these cells are also known as thymic nursing cells (TNC).
3. Medullary (types 4–5).
4. Cells of Hassall's corpuscles: the Hassall's corpuscles are characterized by a concentric pattern of keratinization, and they are restricted to the medullary portion of the thymus. Hassall's corpuscles show a wide variety of changes depending not only on the age of the thymus but also on the different conditions that may affect the thymus pathologically (Figs. 1.11, 1.12, 1.13, 1.14, and 1.15).

Other Cellular Components of the Thymus

Even though most of the cellular component of the thymus is composed of thymocytes of T-cell lineage and epithelial cells, there are other cells in the thymus that are important and should be recognized:

1. *B-lymphocytes*: usually they present in the thymus in the form of germinal centers. However, they may appear singly admixed with T-cells and epithelial cells. Germinal centers may be seen normally in the thymuses of children and adolescents. It is possible that the origin of these germinal centers in a structure that is predominantly formed by T-cells is from preexisting perivascular B-cells. Needless to say, the presence of germinal centers is more commonly seen in pathological conditions such as myasthenia gravis and thymic hyperplasia, among others. However, it is important to mention that B-lymphocytes may also be seen clustering around Hassall's corpuscles, which have been suggested to be the cells that may give rise to thymic MALT lymphomas.

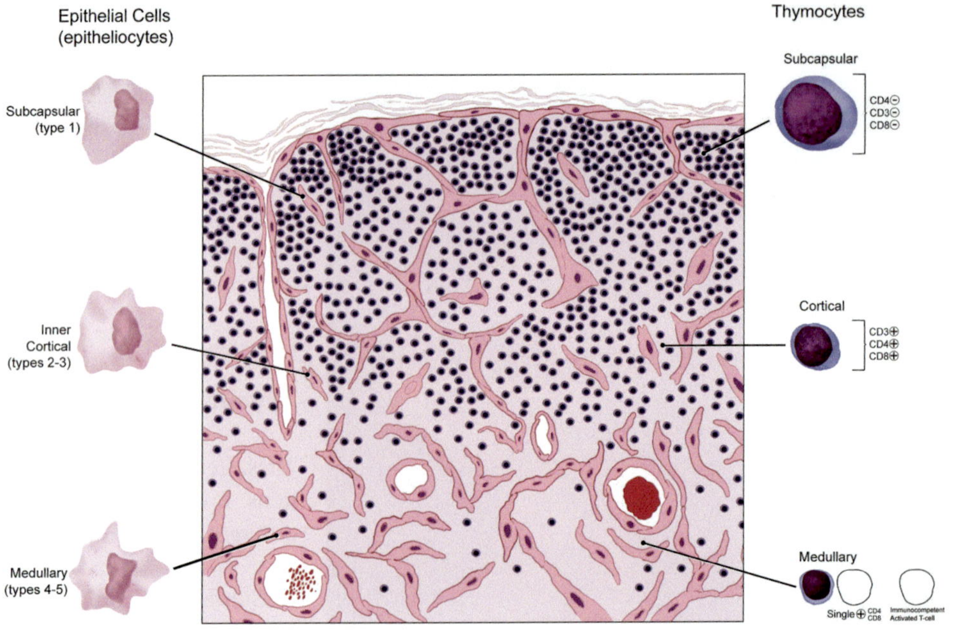

Fig. 1.4 Schematic view of a normal thymus showing the two main cells: thymocytes and epitheliocytes. (Copyright © 2016 with permission from Dr. Kalhor and Moran)

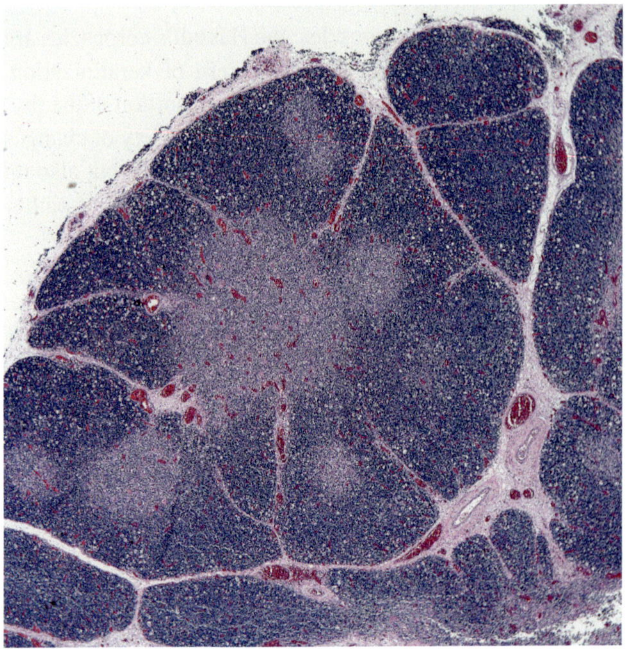

Fig. 1.5 Low power histological section of a normal thymus in a child under 1 year of age, showing a well-demarcated cortex and medulla

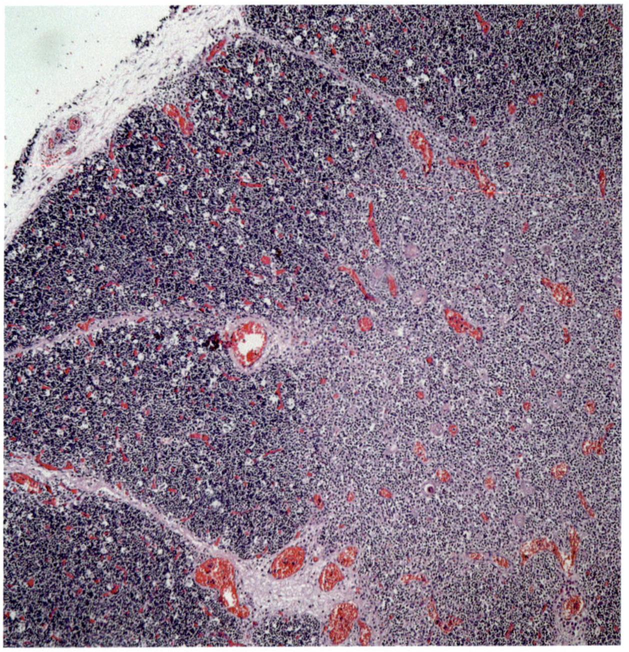

Fig. 1.6 Intermediate power view of a normal thymus showing well-defined cortex and medulla. Note the presence of Hassall's corpuscles

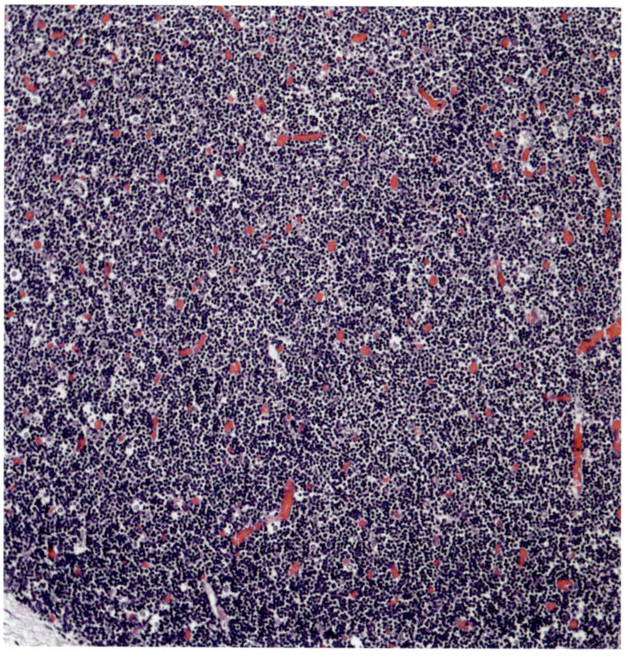

Fig. 1.7 High power view of the normal cortex of the thymus showing predominance of lymphocytes

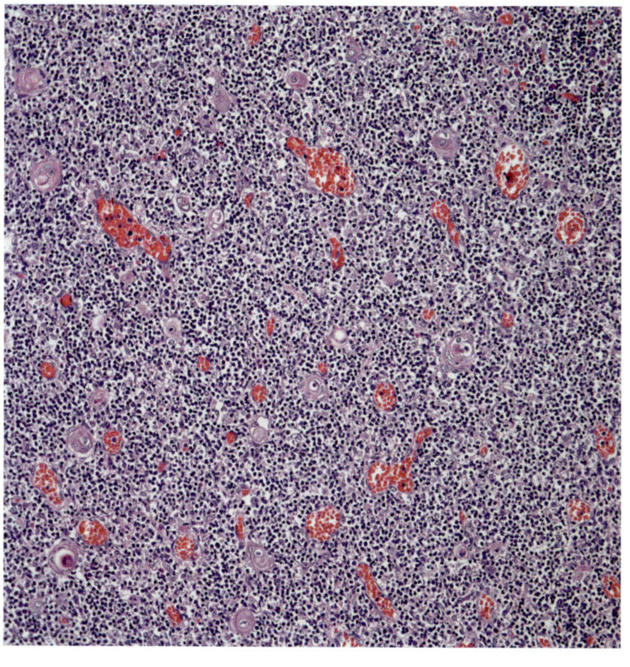

Fig. 1.8 High power view of the thymic medulla showing lymphocytes. However, epithelial cells are easily identified

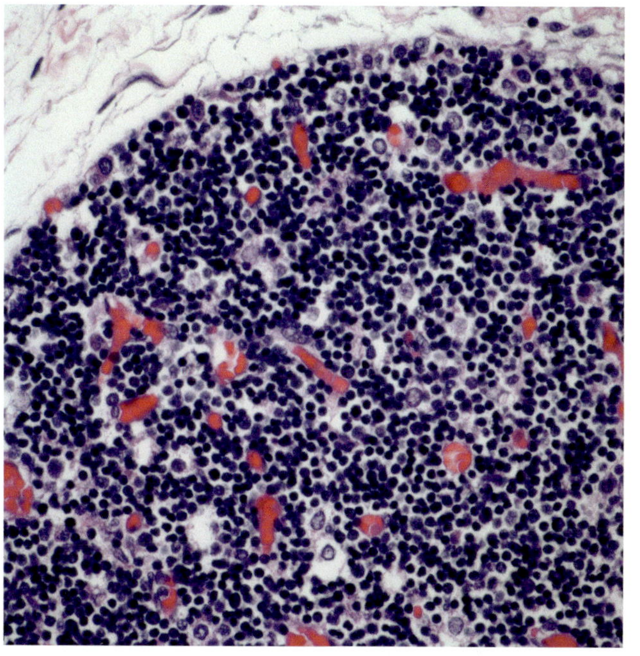

Fig. 1.9 High power view of the subcapsular cortex showing more atypical lymphoid cells

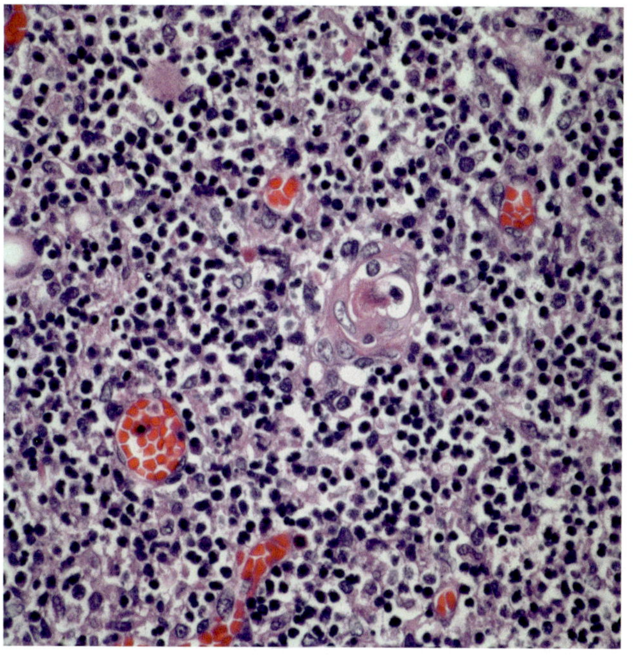

Fig. 1.10 High power view of the thymic medulla showing a Hassall's corpuscle surrounded by lymphocytes and epithelial cells

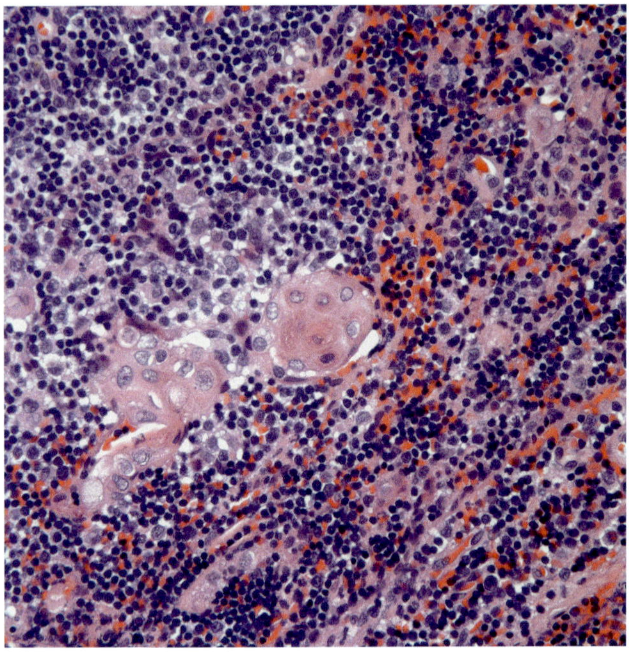

Fig. 1.11 Small Hassall's corpuscle with early keratinization and surrounded by lymphocytes

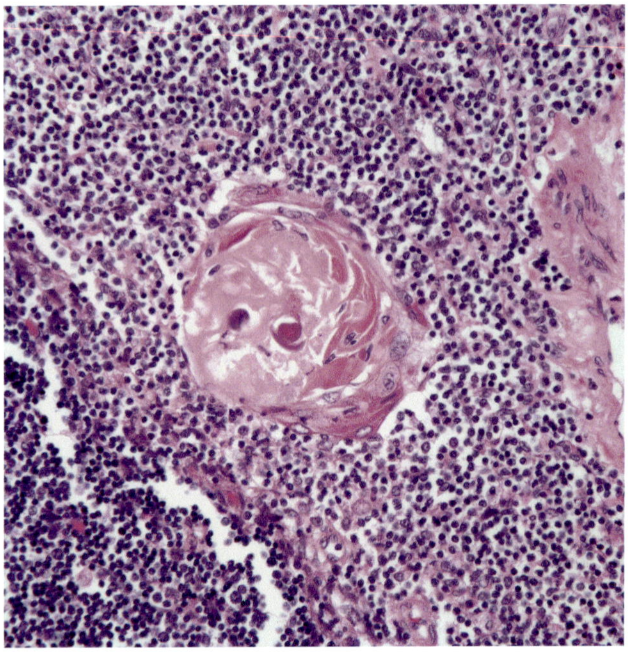

Fig. 1.12 Hassall's corpuscle with keratinization surrounded by epithelial cells and lymphocytes

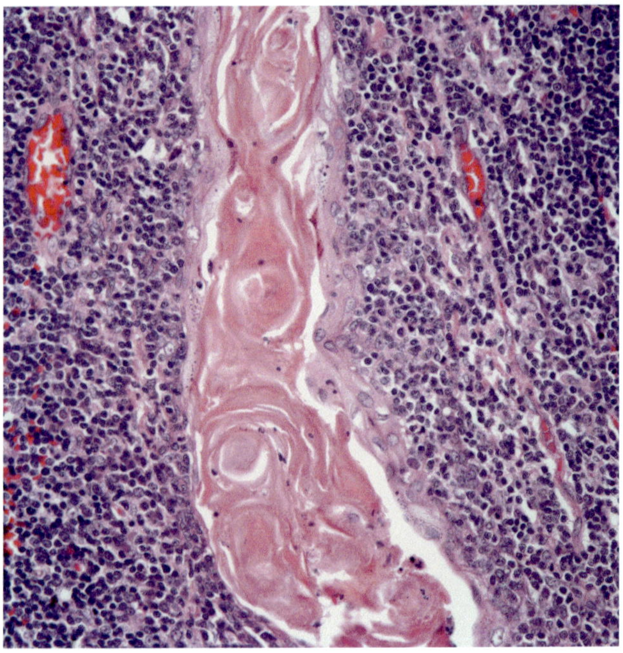

Fig. 1.13 Elongated Hassall's corpuscle with extensive keratinization

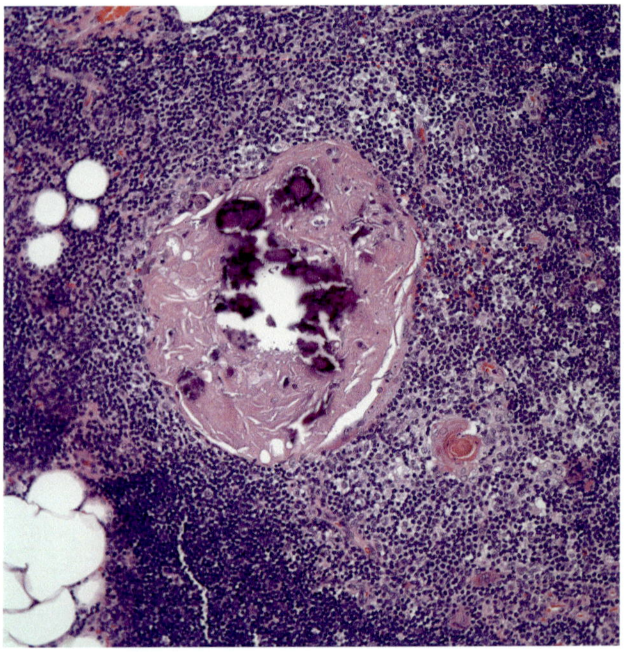

Fig. 1.14 Hassall's corpuscle with calcification

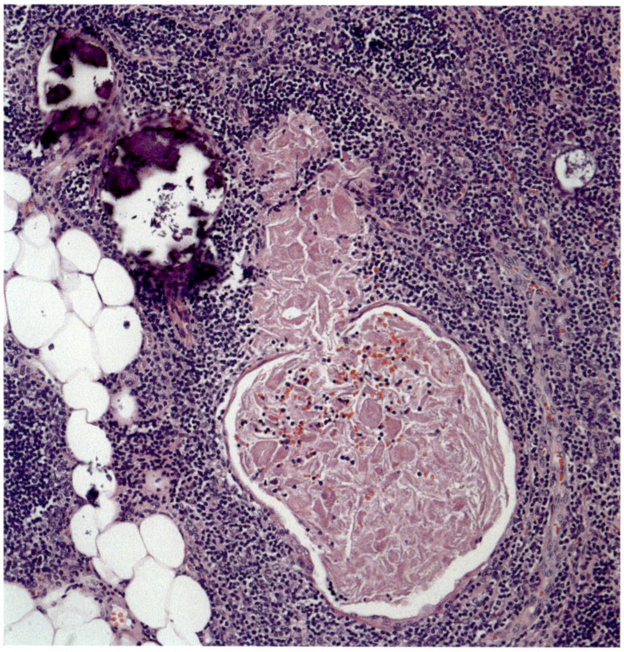

Fig. 1.15 Hassall's corpuscles showing calcification and keratinization

2. *Thymic macrophages*: these mononuclear cells are predominantly in the corticomedullary junction, where they phagocytize differentiating thymocytes.
3. *Interdigitating reticulum cells*: these cells are mainly located in the medulla.
4. *Langerhans cells*: these cells are also present in the medulla.
5. *Eosinophils*: these cells are more common in the connective tissue septa, and they are more commonly seen in thymuses of children.
6. *Mast cells*: these are also found in the connective tissue septa around vessels.
7. *Plasma cells*: they are not common in the thymus, and, when present, they are usually found in connective tissue septa and rarely in the medulla.
8. *Neuroendocrine cells*: these cells may represent a small component of the cellularity of the thymus.
9. *Myoid cells*: they may be located in the thymic medulla. These cells appear to be more conspicuous in pathological conditions such as myasthenia gravis and thymic hyperplasia. However, neoplasms showing extensive myoid component have been described.
10. *Germ cells*: these cells may also form a small component of the cellularity of the thymus.
11. *Sebaceous glands*: these glands rarely can be seen in the normal thymus, and it has been suggested that their occurrence may be related to the ectodermal distribution of the developing thymus.

Connective Tissue

The connective tissue present in the normal thymus contains vessels, fibrous tissue, nerves, and adipose tissue.

Thymic Involution

This process takes place as the individual becomes older, and possibly starts at puberty. Morphologically, one can identify such changes in the thymocyte population and the separation between the corticomedullary junction. Although this process is closely linked to age, in early involution, one may see the presence of decrease number of cortical thymocytes while in more advance stages, the thymic gland is virtually replaced by adipose tissue with only scattered islands of thymic epithelium or clusters of epithelial cells with or without scattered Hassall's corpuscles. The clusters of epithelial cells may be formed almost exclusively of spindle cells without lymphocytes. In some cases, the extensive areas of adipose tissue may be intermixed with connective tissue and strands of remnants of thymic epithelium. On the other hand, some thymic remnants are formed almost exclusively of lymphocytes, mimicking lymph nodes. However, in the periphery of these lymphoid remnants it is possible to identify some epithelial cells (Figs. 1.16, 1.17, and 1.18).

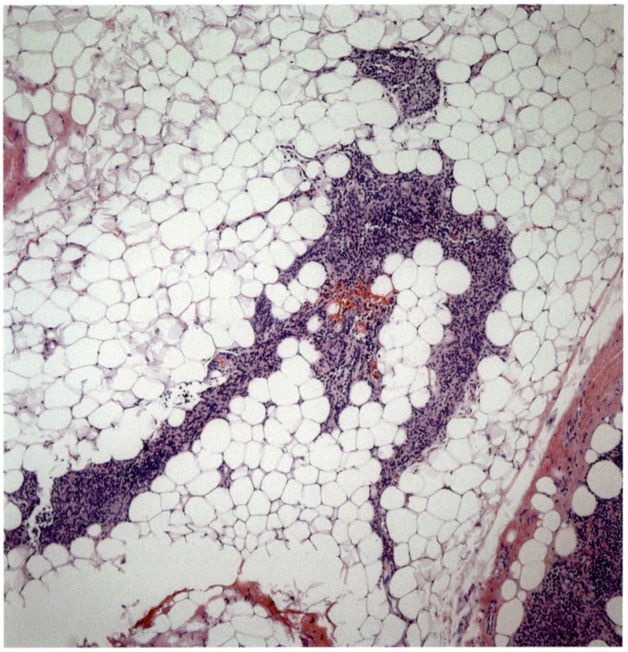

Fig. 1.16 Thymus with involution changes. Note the presence of abundant adipose tissue

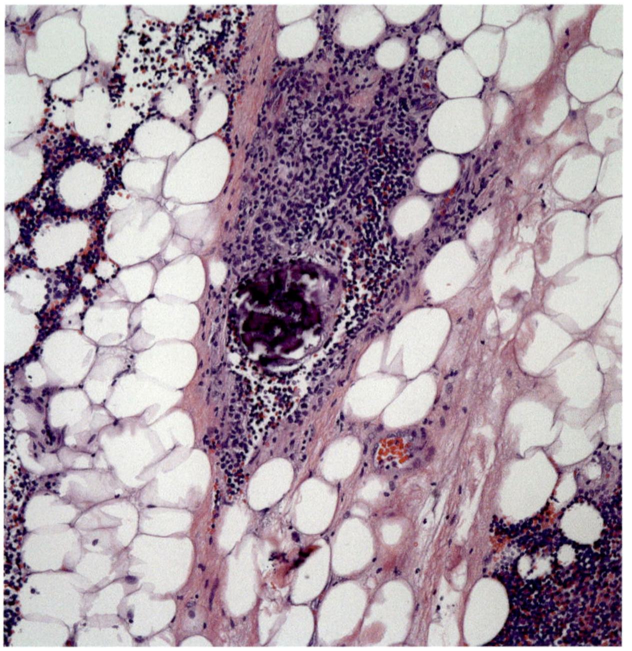

Fig. 1.18 Thymus with involution changes showing a calcified Hassall's corpuscle

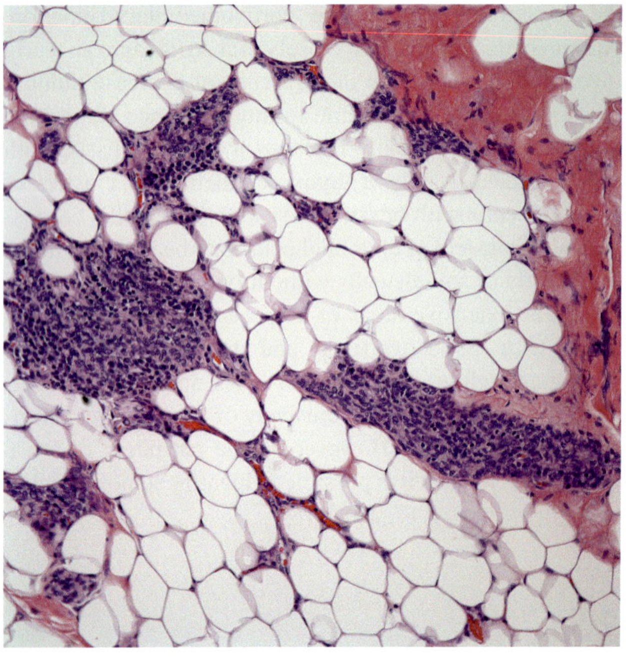

Fig. 1.17 Thymus with involution changes showing focal areas of residual thymic epithelium

Immunohistochemical Aspects

Although there are no large series on the immunohistochemical profile of the normal thymus, there are reports in which those studies have been performed by comparing the normal thymus to other thymic tumors, namely, thymomas and thymic carcinomas. Besides the conventional keratins and B- and T-cell markers, for instance, Cimpean [11] reported the expression of thymic epithelial cells for SOX2. According to the authors, the epithelial cells of the cortex and corticomedullary junction expressed SOX2. Wu and colleagues [12] evaluated the presence of p63 and X-linked inhibitor of apoptosis protein (XIAP) in thymic hyperplasia and thymoma, finding that p63 is consistently positive in nonneoplastic thymic epithelium, while XIAP expression was essentially negative in nonneoplastic thymus. Dotto and colleagues [13] also reported that p63 is positive in normal thymus. Chan and colleagues [14] evaluated the expression of MIC2 (O13) in normal thymus and showed that almost all lymphocytes in the cortex and fewer lymphocytes in the medulla express MIC2. Pescarmona and coworkers [15] evaluated the expression of nerve growth factor (NGF) and epidermal growth factor (EGF) in normal thymuses and identified that EGF is expressed in the subcapsular, cortical, and medullary epithelial cells, while the NFG was expressed only in the subcapsular and medullary epithelial cells. In our experience, we have observed normal thymus staining for pan-keratin, keratin 5/6, p40 (scattered cells), CD10 (scattered cells), common leukocyte antigen (CD45), CD20, S-100 protein, CD1a, CD8, CD4, Tdt, and CD23 in different proportion and intensity and in different components of the thymus, either cortex, medulla, or both (Figs. 1.19, 1.20, 1.21, 1.22, 1.23, 1.24, 1.25, 1.26, 1.27, 1.28, 1.29, and 1.30).

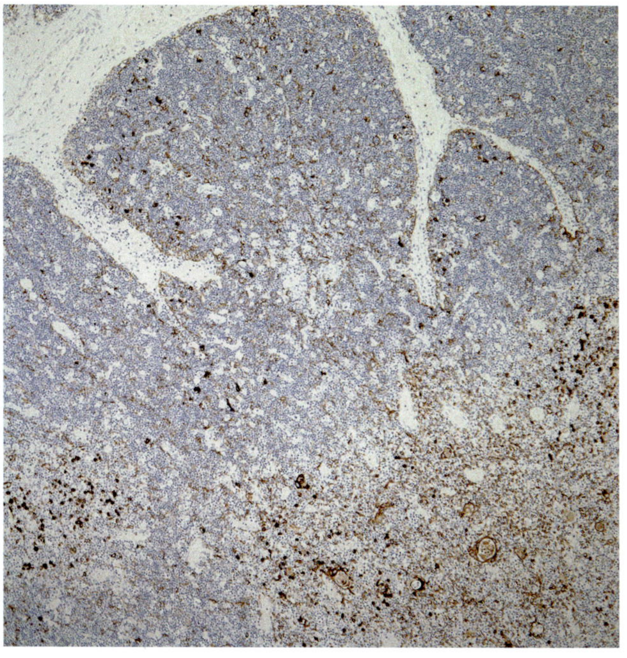

Fig. 1.19 Immunohistochemical stain for pan-keratin shows positive staining in the cortical and medullary epithelial cells. However, there is more in the medullary component

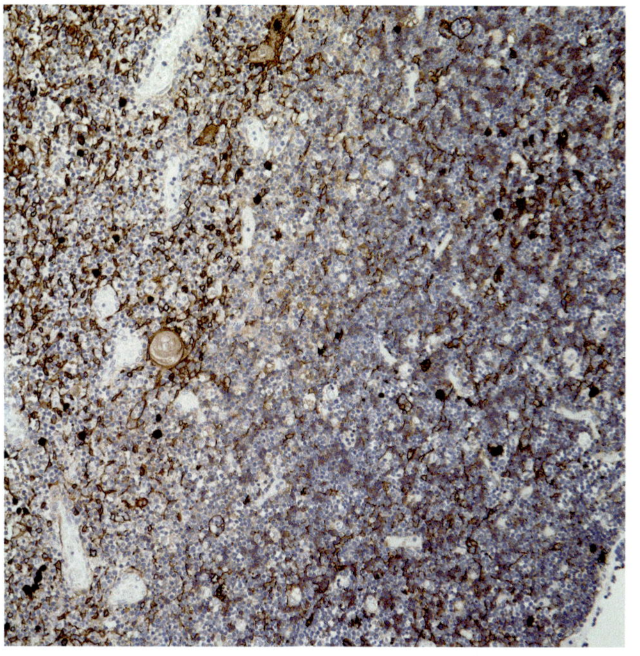

Fig. 1.20 Immunohistochemical stain for keratin 5/6 shows similar pattern as pan-keratin with staining of the epithelial cells of the cortex and medulla

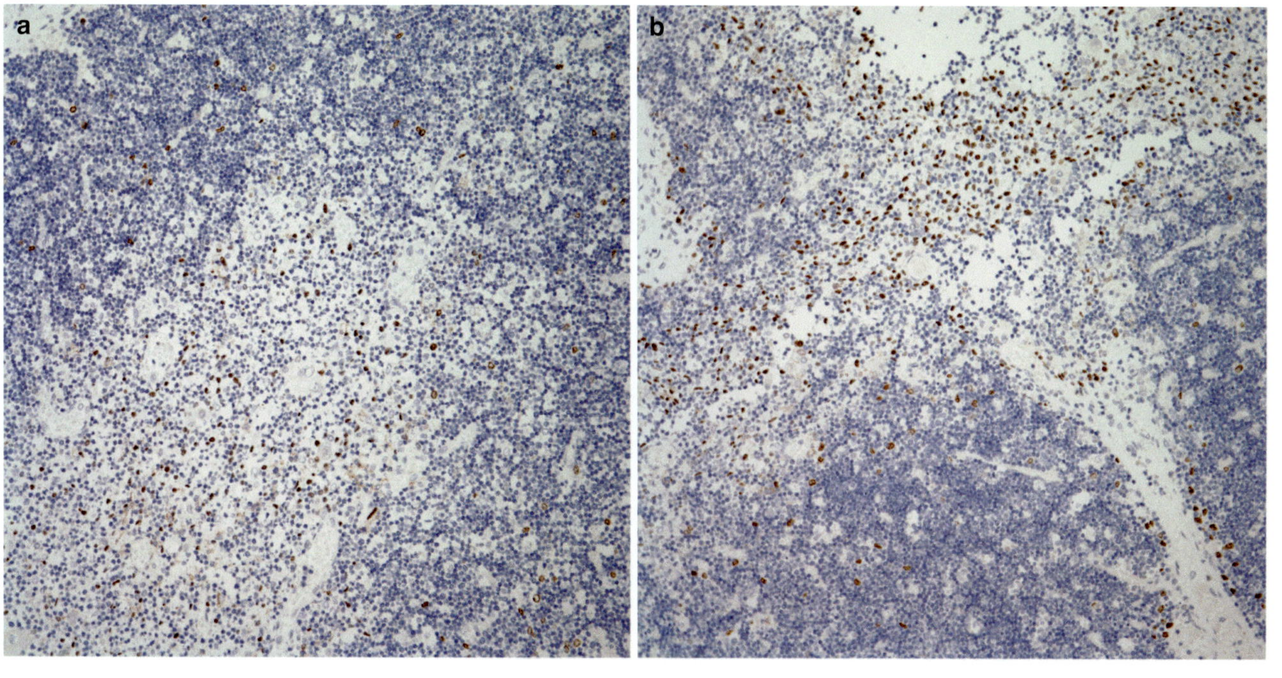

Fig. 1.21 (**a**) Immunohistochemical stain for p40 shows scattered positive epithelial cells in the cortex. More positive epithelial cells are in the medulla. (**b**) Higher magnification showing p40 staining more epithelial cells in the medulla

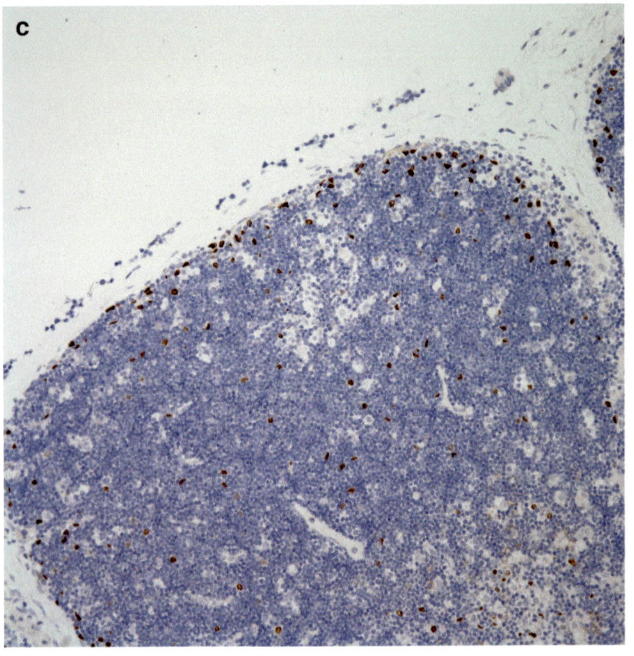

Fig. 1.21 (continued) (**c**) p40 stains only scattered epithelial cells in the cortex. However, many epithelial cells are in the subcapsular area

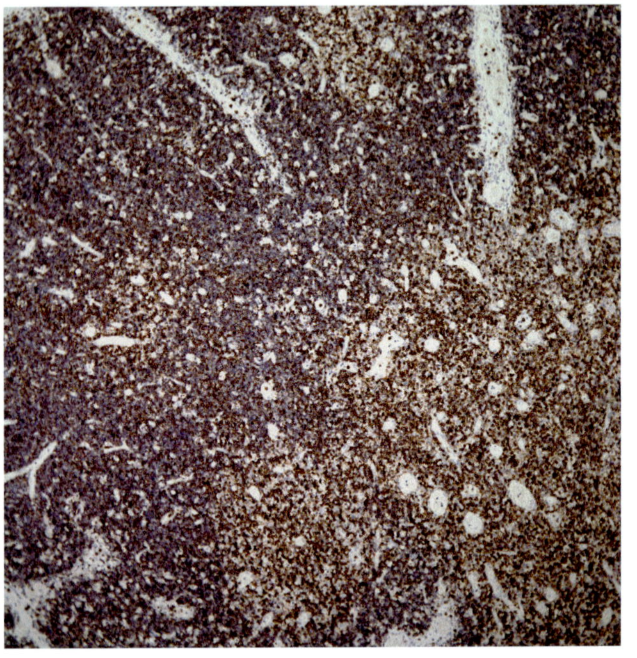

Fig. 1.23 Leukocyte common antigen shows positive staining in both cortical and medullary thymocytes

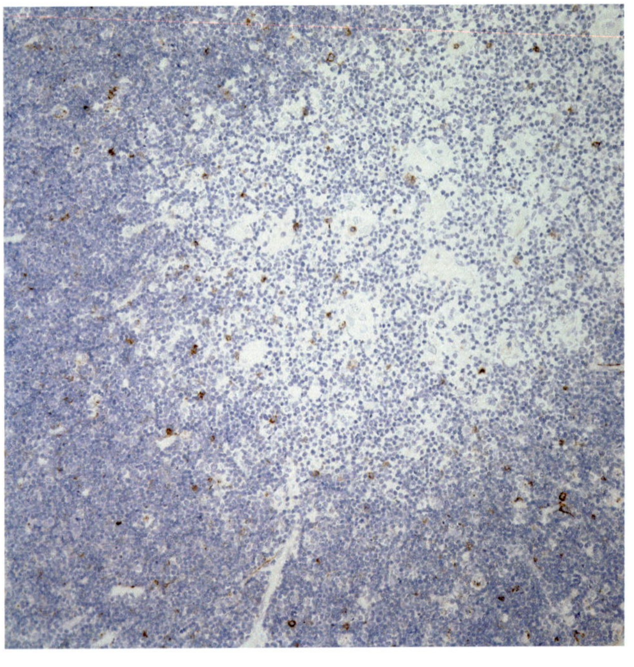

Fig. 1.22 CD10 immunostain shows scattered positive epithelial cells in the cortex and medulla

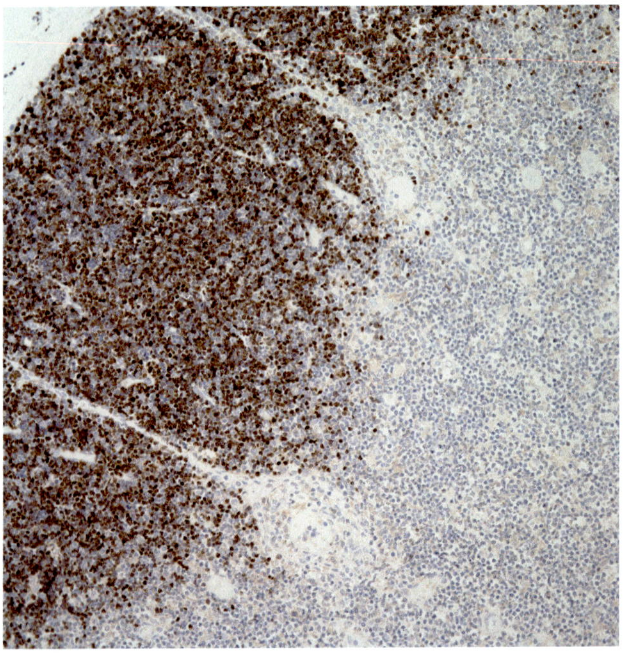

Fig. 1.24 Tdt immunostain shows positive staining in the cortical thymocytes

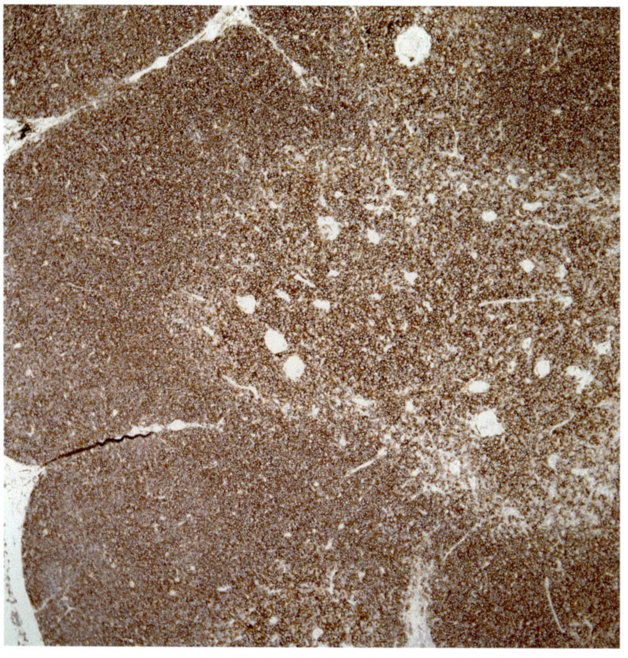

Fig. 1.25 CD4 immunostain shows positive staining of thymocytes in the cortex and medulla

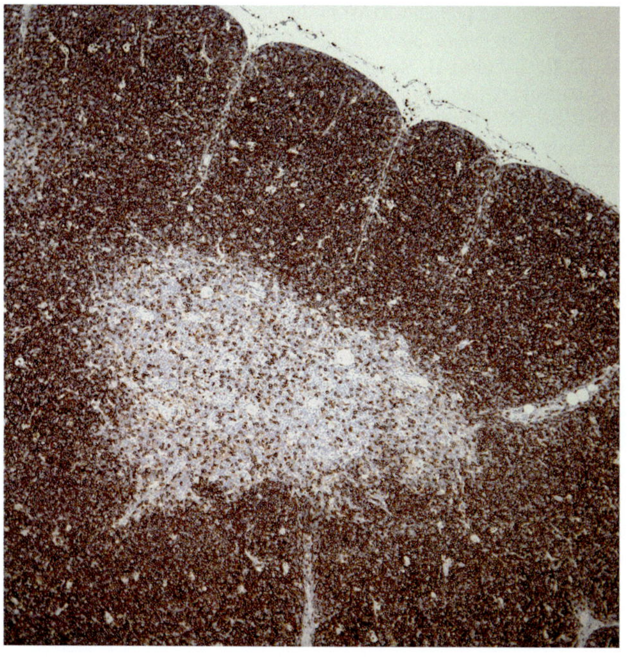

Fig. 1.26 CD8 shows predominantly positive staining of cortical thymocytes

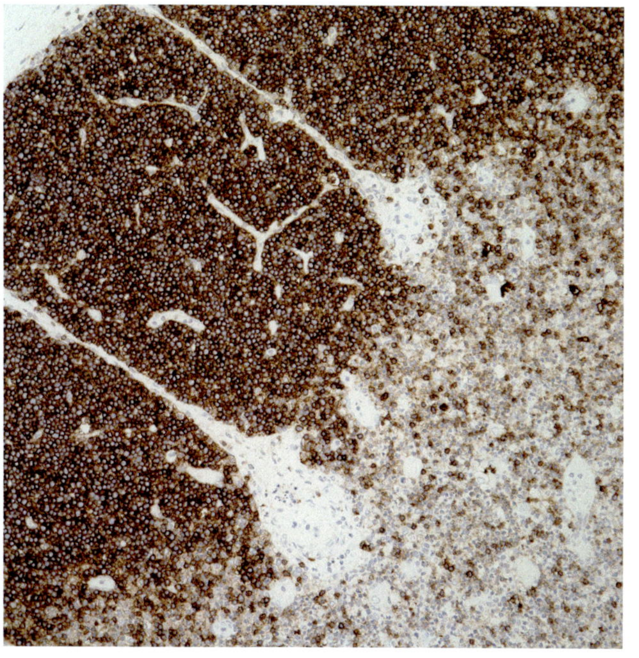

Fig. 1.27 CD1a shows predominantly positive staining of cortical thymocytes

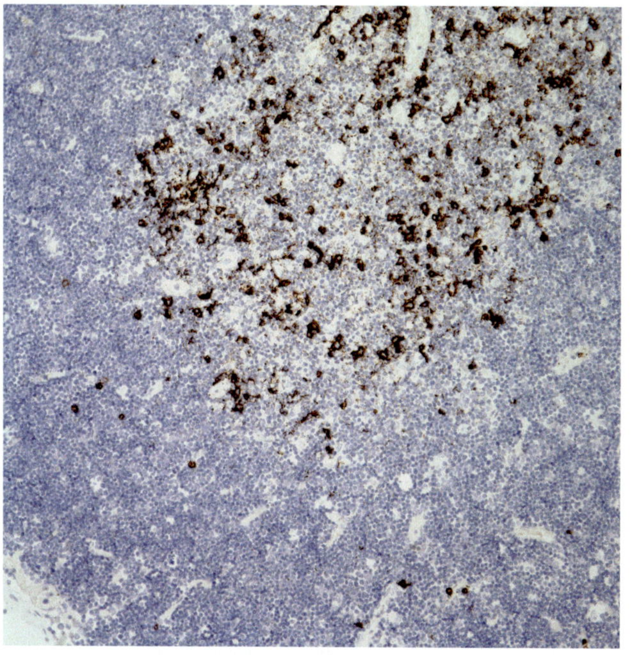

Fig. 1.28 CD20 shows scattered positive medullary thymocytes

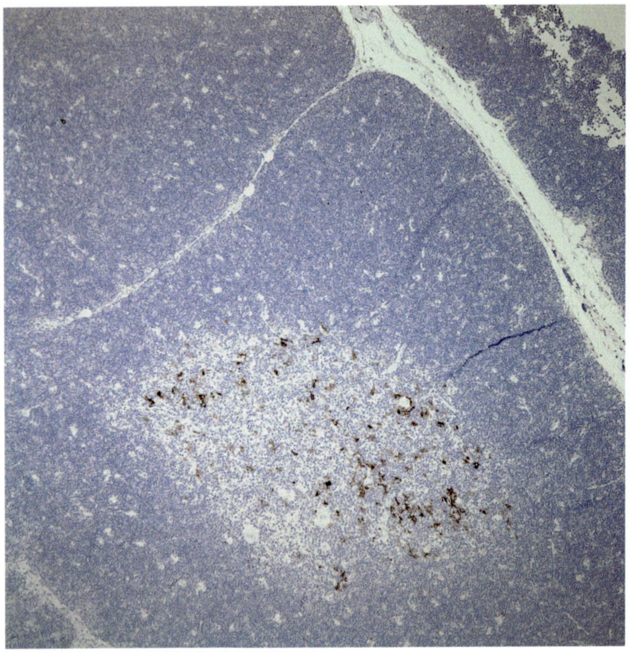

Fig. 1.29 CD23 shows scattered positive staining cells in the thymic medulla

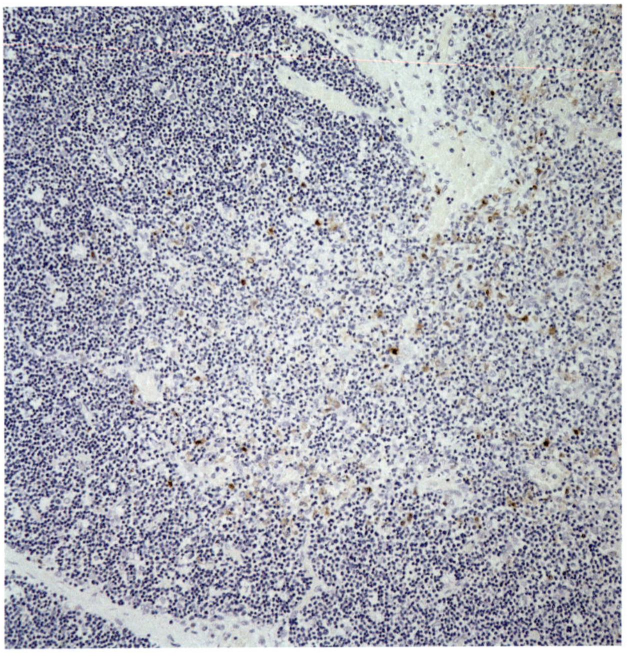

Fig. 1.30 S-100 protein shows positive scattered cells in the thymic medulla

References

1. Kirschner PA. The history of surgery of the thymus gland. Chest Surg Clin N Am. 2000;10:153–65.
2. Jacobs MT, Frush DP, Donnelly LF. The right place and the wrong time: historical perspective of the relation of the thymus gland and pediatric radiology. Radiology. 1999;210:11–6.
3. Miller J. the discovery of thymus function and thymus-derived lymphocytes. Immunol Rev. 2002;185:7–14.
4. Lavini C. Chapter 1: The thymus from Antiquity to the present day: the history of a mysterious gland. In: Lavini C, Moran CA, Morandi U, Schoenhuber R, editors. Thymus Gland Pathology. Milan: Springer; 2008.
5. Palumbo C. Chapter 2: Embryology and Anatomy of the thymus gland. In: Lavini C, Moran CA, Morandi U, Schoenhuber R, editors. Thymus Gland Pathology. Milan: Springer; 2008.
6. Kendal MD, Johnson HR, Singh J. The weight of the human thymus gland at necropsy. J Anat. 1980;131:483–97.
7. Suster S, Rosai J. Histology of the normal thymus. Am J Surg Pathol. 1990;14:284–303.
8. Henry K. Mucin secretion and striated muscle in the human thymus. Lancet. 1966;1:183–5.
9. Wolf M, Rosai J, Wright DH. Sebaceous glands within the thymus: report of three cases. Hum Pathol. 1984;15:341–3.
10. Isaacson PG, Norton AJ, Addis BJ. The human thymus contains a novel population of B-lymphocytes. Lancet. 1987;2:1488–92.
11. Cimpean A, Encina S, Raica M, Ribatti D. SOX2 gene expression in normal human thymus and thymoma. Clin Exp Med. 2011;11:251–4.
12. Wu M, Sun K, Gil J, Gan L, Burstein DE. Immunohistochemical detection of p63 and XIAP in thymic hyperplasia and thymomas. Am J Clin Pathol. 2009;131:689–93.
13. Dotto J, Pelosi G, Rosai J. Expression of p63 in thymomas and normal thymus. Am J Clin Pathol. 2007;127:415–20.
14. Chan JKC, Tsang WYW, Seneviratne S, Pau MY. The MIC2 antibody O13. Practical application for the study of thymic epithelial tumors. Am J Surg Pathol. 1995;19:1115–23.
15. Pescarmona E, Pisacane A, Pignatelli E, Baroni CD. Expression of epidermal and nerve growth factor receptors in human thymus and thymomas. Histopathology. 1993;23:39–44.

Imaging of Mediastinal Tumors

2

Introduction

Mediastinal masses include a wide variety of histopathologic entities of neoplastic, congenital, vascular, and lymphatic origin. As mediastinal lesions are relatively uncommon, many radiologists, pathologists, and other healthcare providers will only encounter many of these abnormalities infrequently. Imaging plays a critical role in the identification and assessment of mediastinal lesions, enabling formulation of a focused differential diagnosis and ultimately guiding further clinical management. In some instances, imaging features of mediastinal masses may be identified on cross-sectional imaging techniques such as computed tomography and magnetic resonance imaging that suggest a specific diagnosis. In other cases, a combination of imaging, pathological, and clinical information is necessary to narrow the differential diagnosis and guide management. In this chapter, we present the imaging features of key mediastinal lesions that radiologists and other healthcare providers will likely encounter in clinical practice.

Classification of Mediastinal Compartments

Identifying the specific compartment from which a mediastinal mass originates can be extremely useful in narrowing the differential diagnosis. Numerous classification systems have been devised and utilized by anatomists, clinicians, and radiologists. The existing radiology schemas represent arbitrary divisions of the chest based primarily on the lateral chest radiograph that are nonanatomical. A classification system based on cross-sectional imaging is needed as the identification and evaluation of mediastinal masses and formulation of treatment strategies are typically determined by findings on computed tomography (CT) or magnetic resonance (MR) imaging (not by chest radiography). A modern definition of mediastinal compartments based on cross-sectional imaging has been developed by the International Thymic Malignancy Interest Group (ITMIG) [1, 2]. This schema builds upon work performed by radiologists associated with the Japanese Association for Research on the Thymus (JART) [3]. In the ITMIG classification system, a three-compartment model is defined and includes defining prevascular, visceral, and paravertebral compartments with specific boundaries and structures included (Fig. 2.1a–d; Table 2.1).

The boundaries of the prevascular mediastinal compartment include (1) superiorly, the thoracic inlet; (2) inferiorly, the diaphragm; (3) anteriorly, the sternum; (4) laterally, the parietal mediastinal pleura; and (5) posteriorly, the anterior aspect of the pericardium as it wraps around in a curvilinear fashion. The major contents of the prevascular mediastinum include the thymus, fat, lymph nodes, and the left brachiocephalic vein, and the most common abnormalities originating in the prevascular compartment include thymic masses (cysts, hyperplasia, and thymic epithelial neoplasms), germ cell neoplasms, lymphoma, metastatic lymphadenopathy, and intrathoracic goiter.

The boundaries of the visceral mediastinal compartment include (1) superiorly, the thoracic inlet; (2) inferiorly, the diaphragm; (3) anteriorly, posterior boundaries of the prevascular compartment; and (4) posteriorly, a vertical line connecting a point on the thoracic vertebral bodies 1 cm posterior to the anterior margin of the spine (referred to as the visceral-paravertebral compartment boundary line). The major contents of the visceral compartment fall into vascular (including the heart, superior vena cava, ascending thoracic aorta, aortic arch, and descending thoracic aorta, intrapericardial pulmonary arteries, and the thoracic duct) and nonvascular (including the trachea, carina, esophagus, and lymph nodes) structures. In the ITMIG mode, all structures within the pericardium are included in the visceral mediastinal compartment. The most common lesions originating in this compartment include lymphadenopathy (due to lymphoma or metastatic disease), foregut duplication cysts, tracheal lesions, and esophageal neoplasms as well as abnormalities of the heart, pericardium, and great vessels.

The boundaries of the paravertebral mediastinal compartment include (1) superiorly, the thoracic inlet; (2) inferiorly, the diaphragm; (3) anteriorly, posterior boundaries of the visceral compartment; and (4) posterolaterally, a vertical line along the posterior margin of the chest wall at the lateral aspect of the transverse processes. The major

© Springer Nature Switzerland AG 2019
N. Kalhor, C. Moran, *Mediastinal Pathology*, https://doi.org/10.1007/978-3-319-98980-8_2

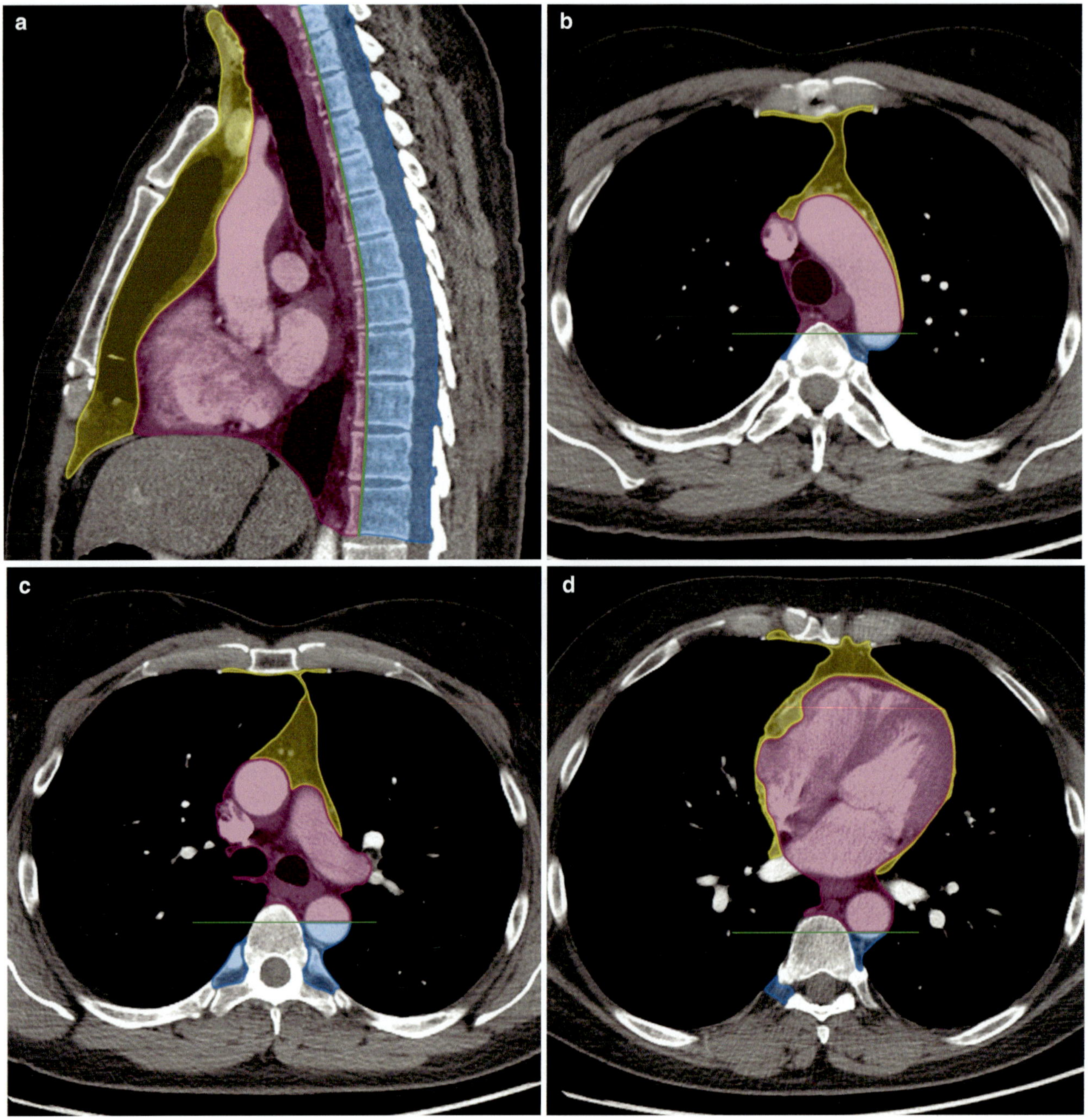

Fig. 2.1 ITMIG definition of mediastinal compartments. Sagittal reformatted CT image (**a**) and axial CT images at the levels of the aortic arch (**b**), left pulmonary artery (**c**), and left atrium (**d**) demonstrate the classification scheme. Note that the prevascular compartment (yellow) wraps around the heart and pericardium, which are located in the visceral compartment (purple). Blue, paravertebral compartment; green line, visceral-paravertebral compartment boundary line

Table 2.1 ITMIG definition of mediastinal compartments

Compartment	Boundaries	Major contents
Prevascular	*Superior*: thoracic inlet *Inferior*: diaphragm *Anterior*: sternum *Lateral*: parietal (mediastinal) pleural reflections; lateral margin of the bilateral internal thoracic arteries and veins and superior and inferior pulmonary veins *Posterior*: anterior to the pericardium, along the anterior margin of the superior vena cava, ascending aorta, and the lateral rim of the aortic arch, superior and inferior pulmonary veins	Thymus Fat Lymph nodes Left brachiocephalic vein
Visceral	*Superior*: thoracic inlet *Inferior*: diaphragm *Anterior*: posterior boundaries of the prevascular compartment *Posterior*: a vertical line connecting a point on each thoracic vertebral body at 1 cm posterior to its anterior margin	Nonvascular: trachea, main bronchi, esophagus, lymph nodes Vascular: heart, ascending thoracic aorta, aortic arch, and descending thoracic aorta, superior vena cava, intrapericardial pulmonary arteries, thoracic duct
Paravertebral	*Superior*: thoracic inlet *Inferior*: diaphragm *Anterior*: posterior boundaries of the visceral compartment *Posterolateral*: vertical line against the posterior margin of the chest wall at the lateral margin of the transverse process of the thoracic spine	Paravertebral soft tissues

contents of this compartment include the thoracic spine and paravertebral soft tissues, and most abnormalities in this region are neurogenic neoplasms arising from the dorsal root ganglia/neurons adjacent to the intervertebral foramina and other lesions related to infection and trauma.

General Considerations

Slightly more than half of all mediastinal masses arise from the prevascular/anterior compartment, whereas one fourth each are identified in the visceral/middle and paravertebral/posterior mediastinal compartments [4–13]. The prevalence of mediastinal tumors is difficult to establish for multiple reasons, such as the use of different radiologic and/or clinical classification systems to define the mediastinal compartments and the variable inclusion of nonneoplastic lesions such as thymic, pericardial, and foregut duplication cysts and various types of lymphoma between different studies. Despite these limitations, several studies have shown that the most common prevascular/anterior mediastinal masses include the following entities: thymic malignancy (35%), lymphoma (25% overall; 13% Hodgkin's lymphoma or HL and 12% non-Hodgkin's lymphoma or NHL), thyroid and other endocrine neoplasms (15%), benign teratoma (10%), malignant germ cell tumors (10% overall; 3% seminoma and 7% non-seminomatous germ cell tumor or NSGCT), and benign thymic cysts (5%) [4, 7, 9].

Role of Imaging

Due to the widespread use and availability of chest radiography, this modality may be the first to demonstrate mediastinal abnormalities in the clinical setting. Small lesions may not be visible, whereas large abnormalities may appear as an extra soft tissue mass or opacity. Primary mediastinal tumors are usually focal, unilateral lesions that abut the mediastinum and preclude radiographic visualization of the medial border of the mass lesion. Such neoplasms typically displace the normal mediastinal interfaces and manifest as mediastinal contour abnormalities. Once a lesion has been identified on chest radiography, cross-sectional imaging techniques such as computed tomography (CT) and magnetic resonance (MR) imaging are used to characterize the abnormality, generate a focused differential diagnosis, and guide further management. CT with intravenous (IV) contrast has traditionally been the imaging modality of choice for the evaluation and characterization of mediastinal tumors and other masses. In one study evaluating 127 anterior mediastinal masses, investigators demonstrated that CT was equal or superior to MR imaging in diagnosing specific lesions, except for thymic cysts which were better seen on MR imaging [14]. In fact, MR imaging is the most useful imaging modality for evaluating a suspected cystic mediastinal mass, as it is superior to CT in distinguishing cystic from solid lesions (such as thymic cysts from thymic neoplasms) and discerning cystic and/or necrotic components within solid masses [15]. Chemical shift imaging can be used to differentiate thymic hyperplasia from thymic epithelial neoplasms and other malignancies [16, 17]. Unenhanced MR imaging may also be performed to characterize mediastinal lesions in patients who are unable to undergo contrast-enhanced CT due to renal failure or severe allergy to IV contrast. 18F-fluorodeoxyglucose (FDG) positron-emission tomography (PET)/CT is not routinely performed to evaluate mediastinal masses but may be employed for staging, assessing response, and evaluating for disease recurrence once a diagnosis has been established. FDG PET/CT imaging of mediastinal abnormalities can be misleading, as normal and hyperplastic thymus and infectious and inflammatory lesions in the mediastinum may be FDG avid [13].

Imaging Approach to Mediastinal Lesions

In many cases, the presence of certain findings on cross-sectional imaging may suggest a specific diagnosis on imaging alone. For example, characteristics such as hyperdense and enhancing lesions that communicate with the thyroid gland, intralesional fat, cystic components, and regions of soft tissue density may be used to narrow the differential diagnosis. On the other hand, calcification cannot be used to discriminate between benign and malignant mediastinal lesions [13, 18]. In other instances, a combination of imaging, pathological, and clinical information/context can help narrow the differential diagnosis and guide further management.

Fat-Containing Lesions

Teratoma

The presence of intralesional fat on CT (with Hounsfield units measuring between −40 and − 120) in a heterogeneous mass in the prevascular mediastinum likely represents a mature (or benign) teratoma (Fig. 2.2). These germ cell neoplasms classically demonstrate a combination of fat, fluid, calcification (including bone- and toothlike structures), and soft tissue elements [18, 19] (Fig. 2.2). Approximately 50% of mature teratomas contain intralesional fat [18]. Fat-fluid levels are highly specific for mature teratoma, but this is a much less common presentation [20]. Young patients are typically affected.

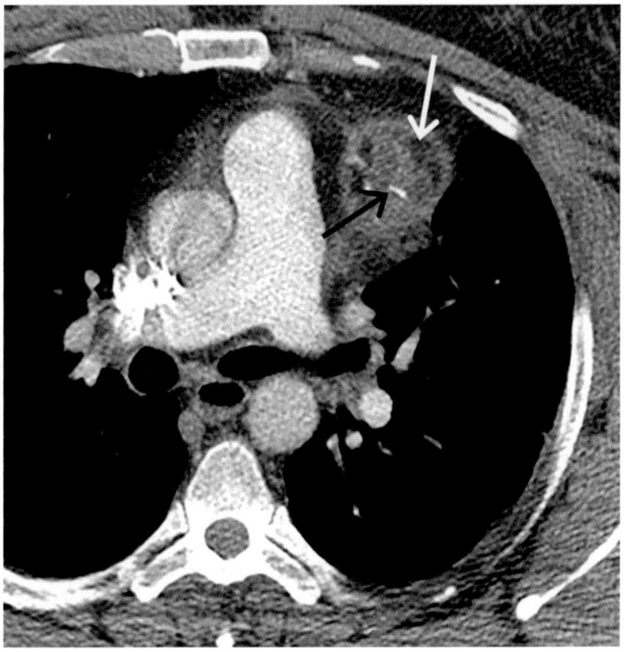

Fig. 2.2 Contrast-enhanced axial CT of a 33-year-old man demonstrates a left prevascular mediastinal mass composed of macroscopic fat (white arrow), calcification, (black arrow), and fluid. Surgical resection was performed due to severe chest pain, and pathology revealed benign teratoma. When a complex mass containing various amounts of fat, fluid, calcification, and soft tissue is present in the prevascular mediastinum, the most likely diagnosis is a benign teratoma

Thymolipoma

A large fat-containing mass in the prevascular mediastinum or one of the cardiophrenic angles on CT may represent a thymolipoma, a benign encapsulated lesion that usually contains 50–85% fat and a small amount of solid tissue and fibrous septa. These lesions may be very large at presentation with an average size of 20 cm. Direct connection with the thymus may be identified on imaging and is confirmatory [19, 21, 22]. Most patents are asymptomatic at presentation; however, associated with myasthenia gravis, Graves' disease, and hematological disorders have been reported [22]. Overall, thymolipoma represents <5% of prevascular mediastinal lesions [13].

Lipoma and Liposarcoma

Other mediastinal neoplasms with intralesional fat are less common and include entities such as lipoma and liposarcoma. Lipomas represent 2% of all primary mediastinal neoplasms and appear as encapsulated lesions composed primarily of fat with a small amount of soft tissue and vessels [23]. Liposarcomas are more aggressive malignancies that tend to have imaging features such as increased soft tissue components, local invasion, lymphadenopathy, and metastatic disease [23, 24].

Cystic Lesions

Thymic Cyst

Thymic cyst should be considered when a homogeneous and round, oval, or saccular lesion is present in the prevascular mediastinal compartment near the thymic bed. Thymic cysts typically manifest with fluid attenuation on CT (Hounsfield units between 0 and 20) (Fig. 2.3a, b). However, thymic cysts may contain regions of high attenuation due to hemorrhage, infection, or proteinaceous components, making differentiation between solid and cystic lesions/components difficult. In this scenario, MR imaging can be performed, which can differentiate cystic lesions with no soft tissue nodules or internal septations (such as unilocular thymic cysts) and those that demonstrate soft tissue components (representing either multilocular thymic cysts or cystic thymoma). Cystic thymoma should be strongly considered when symptoms related to myasthenia gravis or other paraneoplastic syndrome are also present, particularly in the setting of a combination of cystic and solid components [13, 25] (Fig. 2.4).

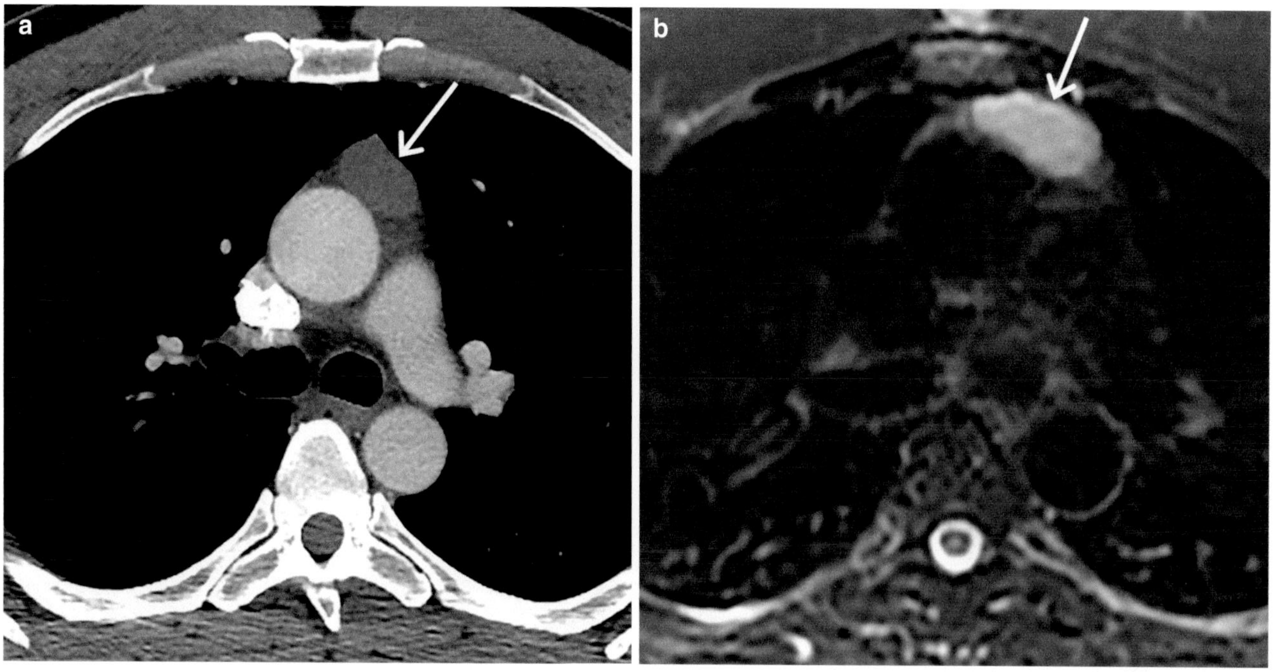

Fig. 2.3 Unilocular thymic cyst in a 43-year-old man. (**a**) Contrast-enhanced axial CT shows a well-circumscribed, fluid/water attenuation mass (arrow) in the prevascular mediastinum. MR imaging was subsequently performed to evaluate for internal soft tissue components. (**b**) T2-weighted MR imaging of the same patient demonstrate a purely cystic lesion (arrow) with no evidence of enhancing soft tissue components. Cystic lesions with no soft tissue nodules or internal septations on MR imaging can reliably be diagnosed as unilocular thymic cysts or cystic teratomas

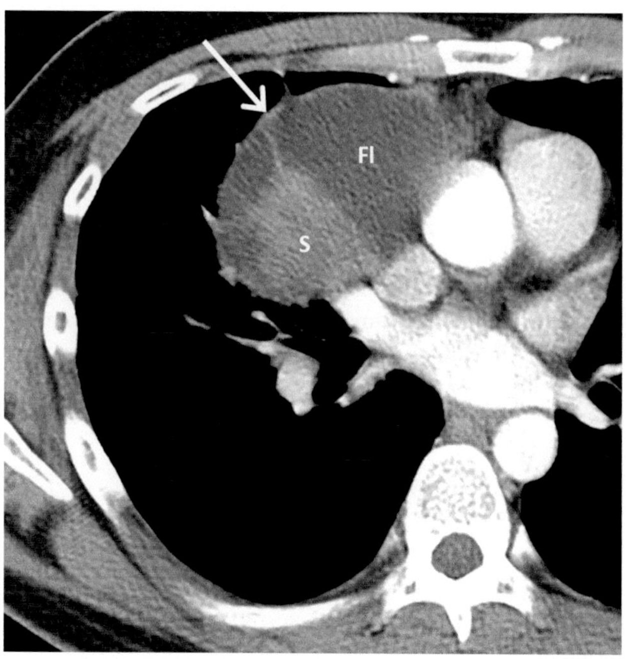

Fig. 2.4 Contrast-enhanced axial CT of a 37-year-old man with clinical symptoms of myasthenia gravis demonstrates a heterogeneous mass (arrow) in the right prevascular mediastinum with solid (S) and fluid (Fl) components. In this patient, cystic thymoma was strongly suspected and confirmed at CT-guided biopsy

Teratoma

Many mediastinal teratomas demonstrate a combination of fat, calcification, fluid, and soft tissue; however, mature cystic teratomas manifest as predominantly cystic lesions on CT (Fig. 2.5). Cystic teratomas most commonly arise from the prevascular mediastinum, with only 3–8% occurring in the paravertebral mediastinum [18].

Pericardial Cyst

Pericardial cysts are benign lesions comprised of connective tissue and a single layer of mesothelial cells, a small percentage of which may demonstrate a visible communication with the pericardial sac on imaging [26]. A homogeneous, low-density lesion measuring fluid attenuation with a thin or imperceptible wall in one of the cardiophrenic angles on CT can be confidently diagnosed as a pericardial cyst [26, 27] (Fig. 2.6).

Bronchogenic Cyst

Bronchogenic cysts are benign, may arise from any mediastinal compartment, but are most commonly identified near the carina in the visceral mediastinal compartment.

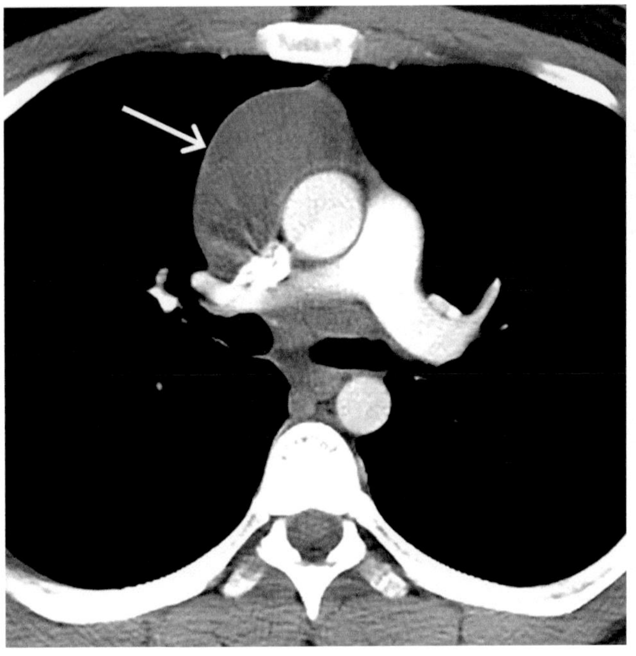

Fig. 2.5 Contrast-enhanced axial CT of a 19-year-old woman shows a homogeneous, fluid attenuation mass (arrow) in the right prevascular mediastinum. MR imaging (not shown) was subsequently performed to evaluate for internal soft tissue components and revealed a purely cystic lesion. Based on this imaging appearance alone, the differential diagnosis would include a unilocular thymic cyst or cystic teratoma; the latter was demonstrated at the time of surgical resection

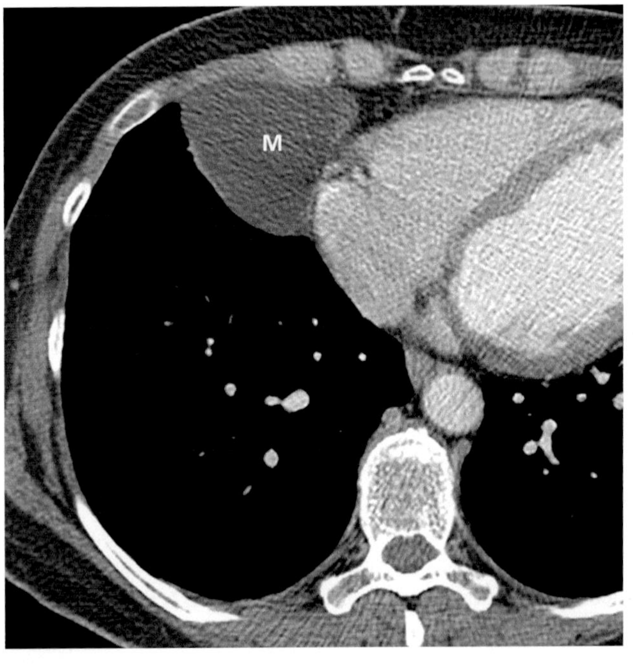

Fig. 2.6 Contrast-enhanced axial CT of a 50-year-old man shows a well-defined, homogeneous, fluid/water attenuation mass (M) in the right cardiophrenic sulcus. These findings are pathognomonic for a pericardial cyst, and no further evaluation is necessary

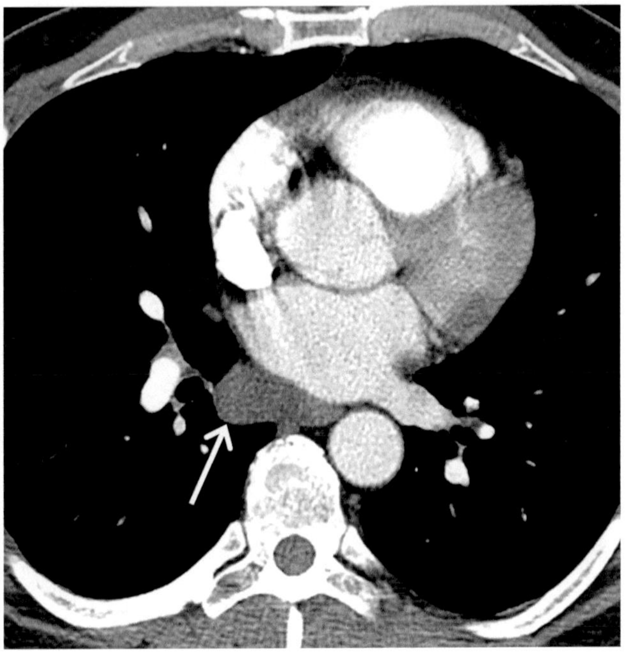

Fig. 2.7 Contrast-enhanced axial CT of a 55-year-old man demonstrates a mass (arrow) arising from the subcarinal region of the visceral compartment, consistent with a bronchogenic cyst. Although most bronchogenic cysts demonstrate homogeneous fluid/water attenuation, regions of internal high attenuation may be present when complicated by hemorrhage or infection or when proteinaceous components are present. When this happens, MR imaging can differentiate these high attenuation regions of fluid from soft tissue

Bronchogenic cysts manifest as solitary masses in smooth, round, or elliptical shapes with thin imperceptible walls on CT (Fig. 2.7). Most lesions demonstrate homogeneous low density, although regions of internal high density may be present when complicated by hemorrhage or infection or when proteinaceous components are present [26, 28]. Other imaging findings such as internal foci of air, suggestive of secondary infection and communication with the airways, calcification, and fluid-fluid levels have been reported [29]. Thin peripheral enhancement of the cyst wall may be present following the administration of IV contrast, but no internal enhancement of the cyst components should be present.

Esophageal Duplication Cyst

Esophageal duplication cysts are congenital lesions classified as foregut cysts of either bronchogenic or neurenteric origin, most of which arise from the visceral compartment adjacent to the esophagus [30]. On CT, esophageal duplication cysts manifest as spherical, unilocular masses of water attenuation on CT [31, 32]. Similar to other cysts in the mediastinum, esophageal duplication cysts complicated by hemorrhage or infection or those containing internal proteinaceous components may demonstrate regions of high density. In such a scenario, MR imaging can be performed for further evaluation. Peripheral enhancement of the cyst wall may be present following the administration of IV contrast, but no internal enhancement of the cyst components should be present.

Meningocele

An intrathoracic meningocele is anomalous herniation of the leptomeninges through a defect in an intervertebral foramen or vertebral body and is frequently associated with neurofibromatosis [26]. Intrathoracic meningoceles arise from the paravertebral compartment and appear as well-defined, homogeneous, low-attenuation lesions [26]. Associated enlargement of the intervertebral foramina, vertebral and/or rib anomalies, and scoliosis may be present.

Soft Tissue Lesions

Thyroid Goiter

A heterogeneous mass in the prevascular mediastinum, that is, intrinsically hyperdense, enhances, following the administration of IV contrast, and demonstrates continuity with the cervical thyroid gland which is consistent with a mediastinal goiter (Fig. 2.8a, b). Most lesions demonstrate high attenuation on unenhanced CT with Hounsfield units measuring 70–85 due to the presence of iodine, although internal regions of low attenuation within goiters representing cystic changes and calcification may also be present. Following the administration of IV contrast, prolonged and sustained enhancement is usually present. Not all mediastinal goiters demonstrate connection to the thyroid gland. However, when they are separate, these lesions often demonstrate similar imaging features. When there is loss of distinct mediastinal fascial planes or associated cervical or mediastinal lymphadenopathy is present, thyroid malignancy should be suspected [13, 33].

Thymic Epithelial Neoplasms

Thymic epithelial neoplasms are a group of neoplasms arising from the thymus that includes thymoma, thymic carcinoma, and thymic neuroendocrine tumors. A thymoma should be suspected when a homogeneous or slightly heterogeneous prevascular mediastinal mass is present on CT in men and women older than age 40 (Fig. 2.9). The diagnosis is supported by the presence of clinical symptoms of myasthenia gravis or other paraneoplastic syndrome such as pure red cell aplasia/Diamond-Blackfan syndrome or hypogammaglobulinemia [34]. Pleural and/or pericardial spread may be identified in advanced disease; however, lymphadenopathy is usually absent. In contrast, when a large prevascular mediastinal mass with imaging features such as heterogeneity, local

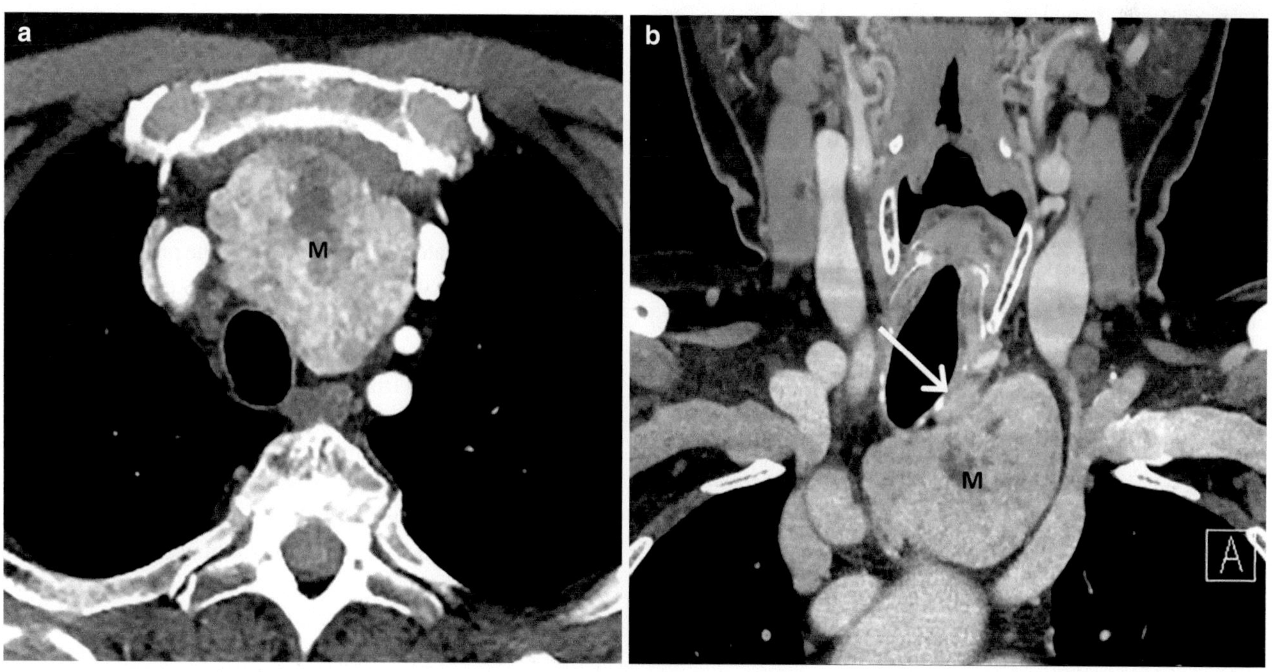

Fig. 2.8 Thyroid goiter in a 75-year-old man. (**a**) Contrast-enhanced axial CT shows an enhancing mass (M) in the prevascular mediastinum. (**b**) Coronal reformatted CT of the same patient demonstrates continuity of the mediastinal mass (M) with the thyroid gland (arrow). These imaging findings are pathognomonic for a thyroid goiter

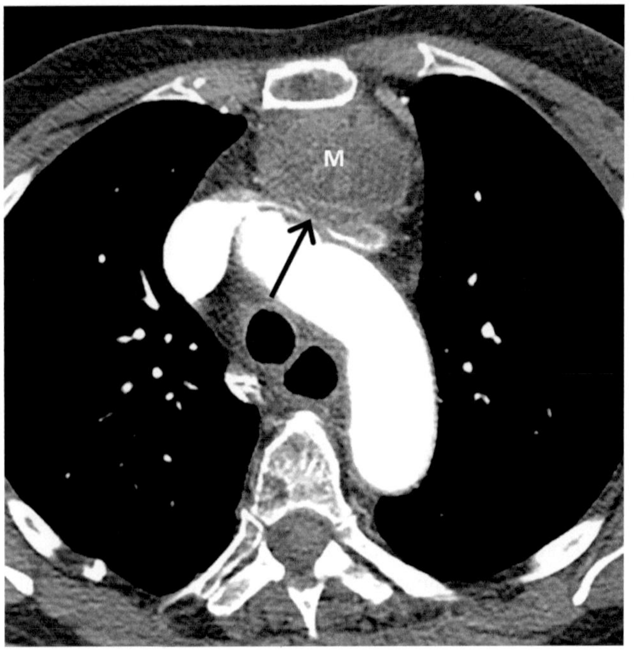

Fig. 2.9 Contrast-enhanced axial CT of a 50-year-old woman presenting with symptoms of myasthenia gravis demonstrates a heterogeneous mass (M) in the prevascular mediastinum invading the left brachiocephalic vein (arrow). The combination of clinical and imaging findings was highly suggestive of a thymoma, which was confirmed by CT-guided core needle biopsy

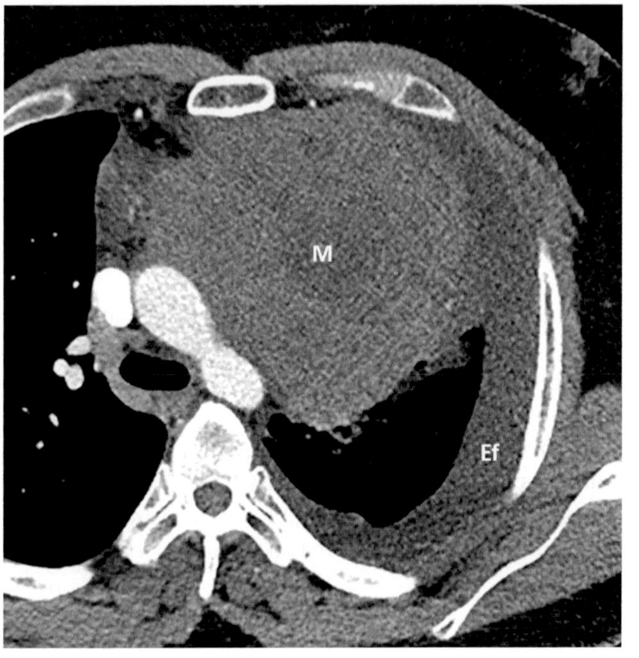

Fig. 2.11 Contrast-enhanced axial CT of a 52-year-old man shows a large and heterogeneous left prevascular mediastinal mass (M) with a left pleural effusion (Ef) due to pleural metastasis. CT-guided core needle biopsy revealed thymic carcinoid. In contrast to thymoma, features such as heterogeneity, local invasion, lymphadenopathy, and pleural effusion are more commonly seen with thymic epithelial neoplasms other than thymoma such as thymic carcinoma and thymic carcinoid

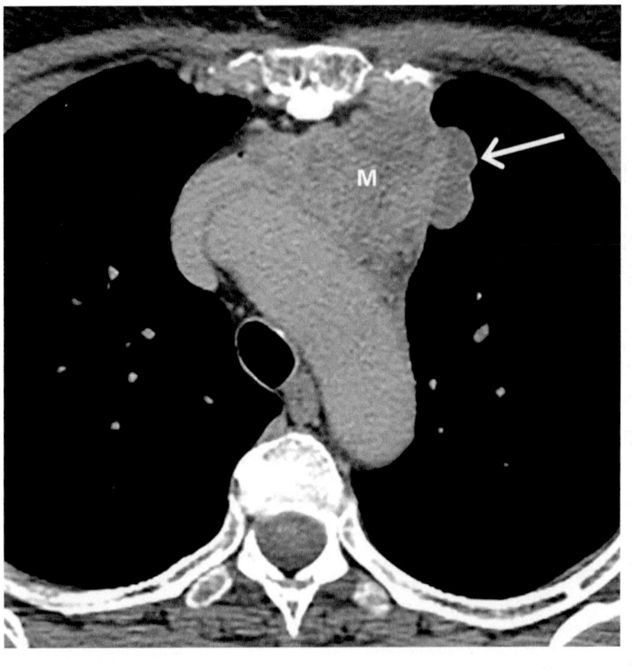

Fig. 2.10 Axial CT of a 78-year-old woman shows a heterogeneous prevascular mediastinal mass (M) with invasion of the left upper lobe (arrow). CT-guided core needle biopsy revealed thymic carcinoma. In contrast to thymoma, features such as heterogeneity, local invasion, lymphadenopathy, and pleural effusion are more commonly seen with thymic epithelial neoplasms other than thymoma such as thymic carcinoma and thymic carcinoid

invasion, lymphadenopathy, and pleural effusion is present on CT, other tumors such as thymic carcinoma and thymic carcinoid should be considered [35] (Figs. 2.10 and 2.11).

Lymphoma

Lymphoma should be considered when mediastinal lymphadenopathy or a lobulated soft tissue mass in the prevascular mediastinum is present on CT. The diagnosis is supported by the presence of associated lymphadenopathy in the lower neck or axillae, although this may not be present. Lymphoma may be difficult to distinguish from other etiologies of mediastinal soft tissue masses; however, some types demonstrate infiltrative behavior. When such findings are present on CT in the setting of "B" symptoms such as fever, weight loss, and night sweats, lymphoma should be strongly suspected (Fig. 2.12). Core needle biopsy combined with aspiration for flow cytometry or surgical biopsy is typically performed. After establishing the diagnosis, FDG PET/CT is the imaging modality of choice for staging, restaging, and assessing for treatment response and recurrence (Fig. 2.13a, b). FDG PET/CT is better than CT at identifying involved lymph nodes, with a sensitivity of 94% and a specificity of 100%, respectively, compared with 88%

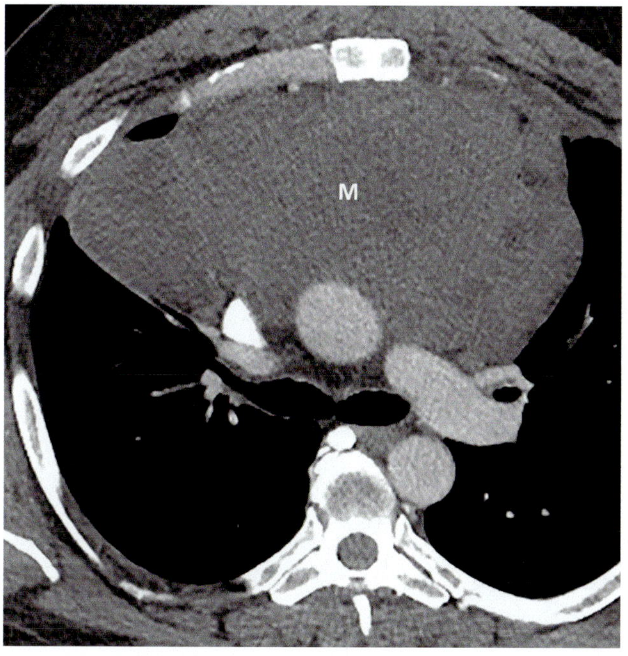

Fig. 2.12 Contrast-enhanced axial CT of a 39-year-old woman with "B" symptoms including fever, night sweats, and weight loss shows a large and heterogeneous prevascular mass (M). CT-guided core and fine needle aspiration biopsies revealed Hodgkin's lymphoma

and 86% for CT [36]. The sensitivity and specificity of FDG PET/CT in demonstrating organ involvement are 88% and 100%, respectively, compared with 50% and 90% for CT [36].

Non-teratomatous Germ Cell Tumors

Germ cell tumors (GCTs) account for 10–15% of prevascular mediastinal masses in adults and 25% in children [17]; only 3% of mediastinal GCTs arise from the paravertebral compartment [37]. Young men are most commonly affected [38]. Mediastinal GCTs are frequently divided into seminomas and NSGCTs, the latter of which include yolk sac, endodermal sinus, and mixed germ cell tumors, embryonal carcinomas, and choriocarcinomas.

Seminoma should be considered when a large, lobular homogeneous prevascular mediastinal mass is identified on CT in a young man 10–39 years of age [39] (Fig. 2.14). Pulmonary metastases are common but pleural effusions are rare [13]. Approximately 10% of mediastinal seminomas are associated with slightly elevated serum β-HCG; however, α-FP is typically normal [40, 41]; serum lactate dehydrogenase levels are usually elevated [41, 42]. NSGCT should be considered when a heterogeneous prevascular mediastinal mass is present with lung metastases on CT in patients younger than 40 years of age [18, 43] (Fig. 2.15). Markedly elevated serum α-FP or β-HCG levels are present in 90% of NSGCTs [40, 41, 44, 45].

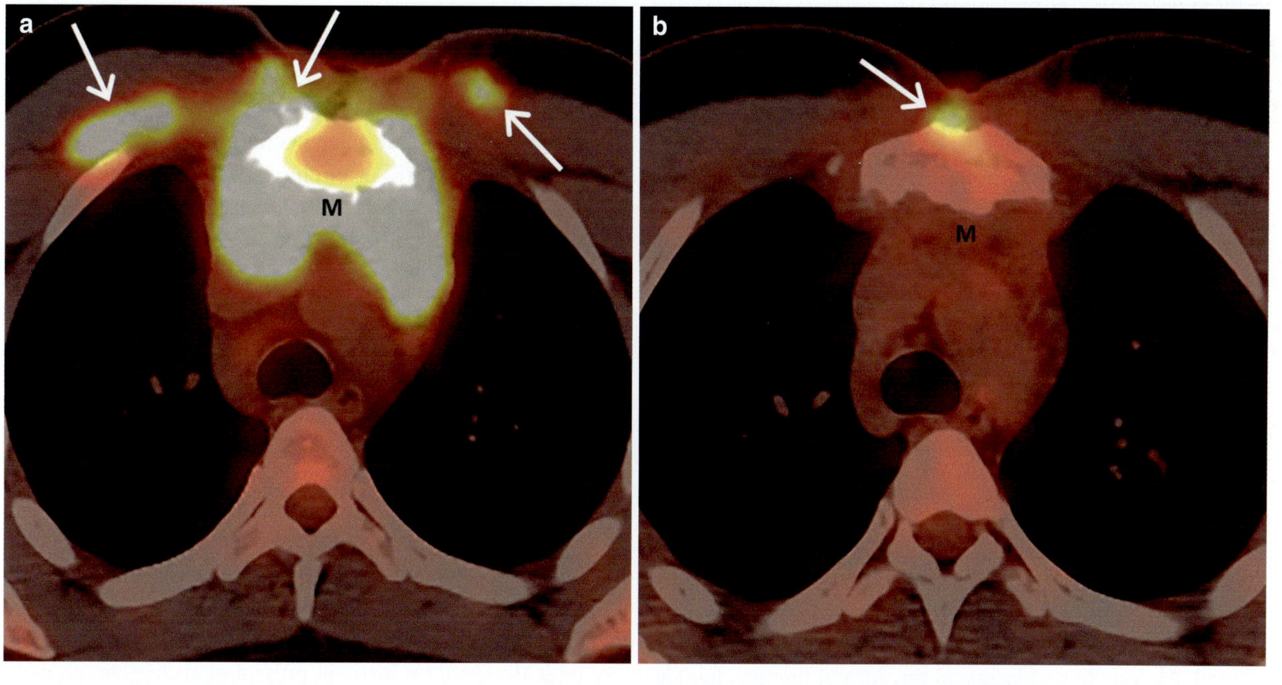

Fig. 2.13 Large B cell lymphoma in a 37-year-old man. (**a**) Fused axial FDG PET/CT at baseline demonstrates an FDG-avid prevascular mediastinal mass (M) that invades the anterior chest wall (arrows). (**b**) Fused axial FDG PET/CT following chemotherapy shows marked interval decrease in the size and FDG uptake of the mass (M) with only a small focus of increased FDG uptake (arrow) remaining in the anterior chest wall

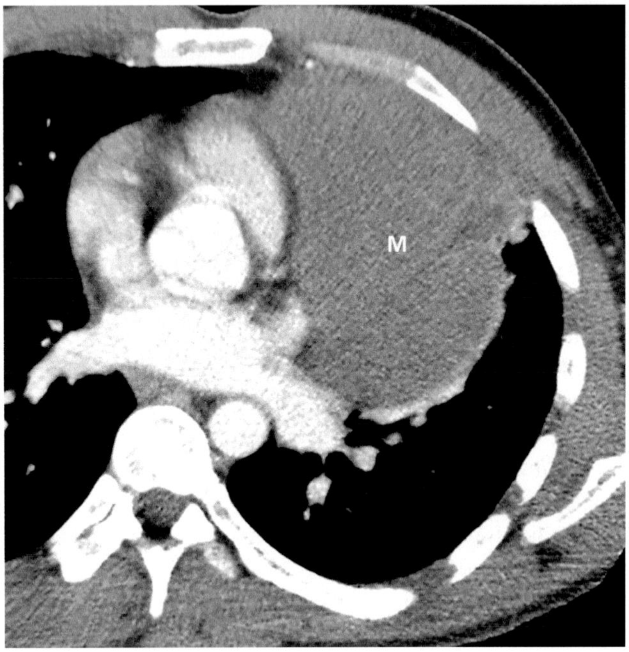

Fig. 2.14 Contrast-enhanced axial CT of a 25-year-old man presenting with chest pain demonstrates a large soft tissue mass (M) in the prevascular mediastinum. Serum levels of β-HCG and LDG were elevated, suggesting a primary mediastinal seminoma, which was confirmed at surgical resection

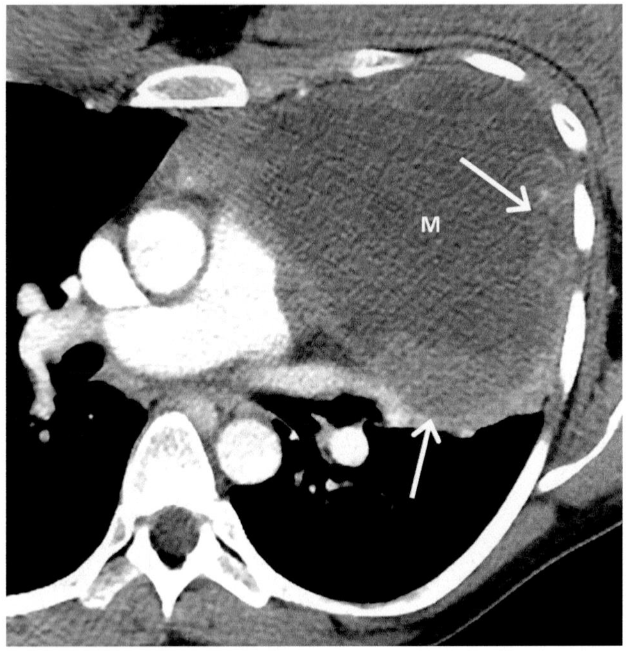

Fig. 2.15 Contrast-enhanced axial CT of a 32-year-old man shows a large, heterogeneous prevascular mediastinal mass (M) with central necrosis and peripheral enhancing soft tissue (arrows). Markedly elevated serum α-FP levels were present, suggesting NSGCT, which was confirmed with CT-guided core needle biopsy

Thymic Hyperplasia

Normal thymic tissue is typically seen in young patients and decreases with advancing age. By 40 years of age, the thymus is replaced by fat in most individuals. Thymic hyperplasia should be considered in the setting of uniform enlargement of the thymus in young patients or when soft tissue is present in the thymic bed that is similar in configuration to the normal thymus on CT. Patients who have been treated with chemotherapy, radiation therapy, or corticosteroids have experienced stresses such as burns or injuries, or those who have disorders such as myasthenia gravis, hyperthyroidism, collagen vascular diseases, or human immunodeficiency virus (HIV) infection, thymic hyperplasia should be considered when a low-density mass is present in the prevascular mediastinal compartment or there is diffuse, symmetric enlargement of the thymus on CT. Intralesional fat may be present but is uncommon. In cases in which the imaging appearance is not straightforward and the soft tissue in the thymic bed is nodular or bulky on CT, short interval follow-up imaging (~3 months) or chemical shift MR imaging with in-phase and out-of-phase gradient echo imaging can be performed. Thymic hyperplasia and the normal thymus demonstrate loss of signal on out-of-phase MR imaging sequences due to the suppression of microscopic fat interspersed between nonneoplastic thymus, whereas thymic epithelial neoplasms, lymphoma, and other malignancies do not suppress on out-of-phase MR imaging sequences (Fig. 2.16a–c).

Esophageal Neoplasms

Esophageal cancer and other neoplasms should be considered when asymmetric or circumferential thickening of the esophageal wall or a focal soft tissue mass associated with the esophagus is identified in the visceral compartment on CT [46]. The most common types of esophageal cancer include squamous cell carcinoma and adenocarcinoma. Definitive diagnosis requires histologic sampling, typically obtained through endoscopic ultrasound-guided biopsy.

Neurogenic Neoplasms

Neurogenic tumors represent the most common type of paravertebral mediastinal mass and account for 20% and 35% of all mediastinal tumors in adults and children, respectively [47]. Most neurogenic neoplasms are benign, and patients are typically asymptomatic at presentation. In general, neurogenic neoplasms can be classified as peripheral nerve sheath neoplasms, sympathetic ganglion tumors, and paragangliomas.

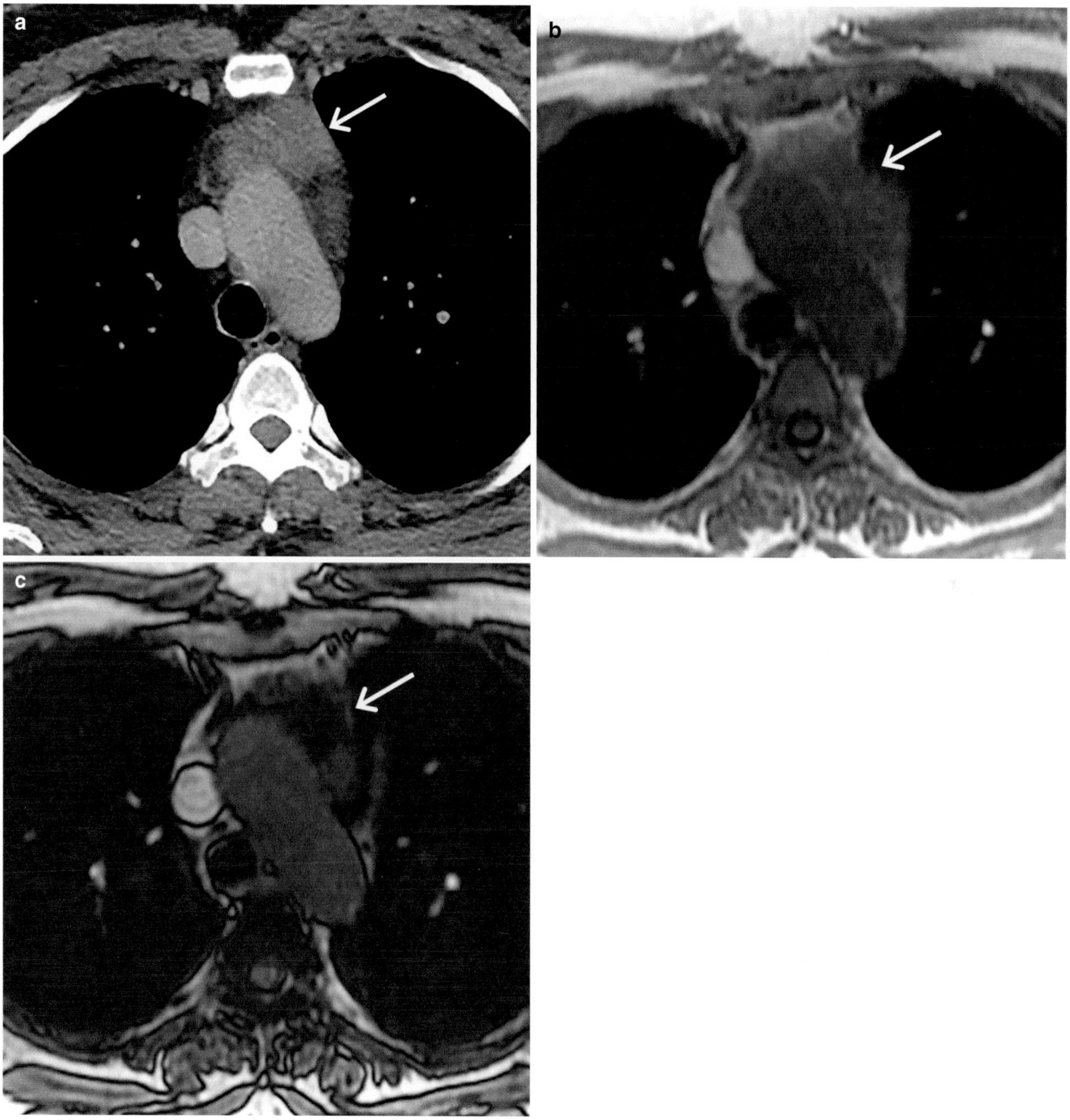

Fig. 2.16 Thymic hyperplasia in a 38-year-old woman. (**a**) Contrast-enhanced axial CT demonstrates a soft tissue mass (arrow) in the prevascular mediastinum that is non-specific and could be malignant or benign in etiology. (**b**, **c**) Axial T1-weighted in-phase (**b**) and out-of-phase (**c**) MR imaging of the same patient shows uniform high signal (arrow, **b**) on the in-phase sequence but complete loss of signal (arrow, **c**) on the out-of-phase sequence, confirming the presence of microscopic fat interspersed between hyperplastic thymic tissue

Peripheral nerve sheath tumors represent most neurogenic neoplasms of mediastinal origin, typically schwannomas and neurofibromas that arise from the paravertebral mediastinum in a "dumbbell" or "hourglass" configuration due to extension through the adjacent intervertebral foramen and spinal canal (Fig. 2.17). Internal hemorrhage and cystic changes may result in heterogeneity and are more commonly seen in schwannomas than neurofibromas [47]. MR imaging is superior to CT at demonstrating extension through the intervertebral foramen and/or spinal canal (Fig. 2.18a–c). Malignant transformation of a neurofibroma to a malignant peripheral nerve sheath tumor should be suspected when the former increases in size and/or neurological symptoms develop, particularly in patients with neurofibromatosis type 1 [48]. Sympathetic ganglion neoplasms include ganglioneuromas, ganglioneuroblastomas, and neuroblastomas. Compared to peripheral nerve sheath tumors and other sympathetic ganglion neoplasms, neuroblastomas are highly aggressive lesions that tend to metastasize early and manifest as heterogeneous masses with regions of internal hemorrhage, cystic degeneration, necrosis, or calcification on imaging [48].

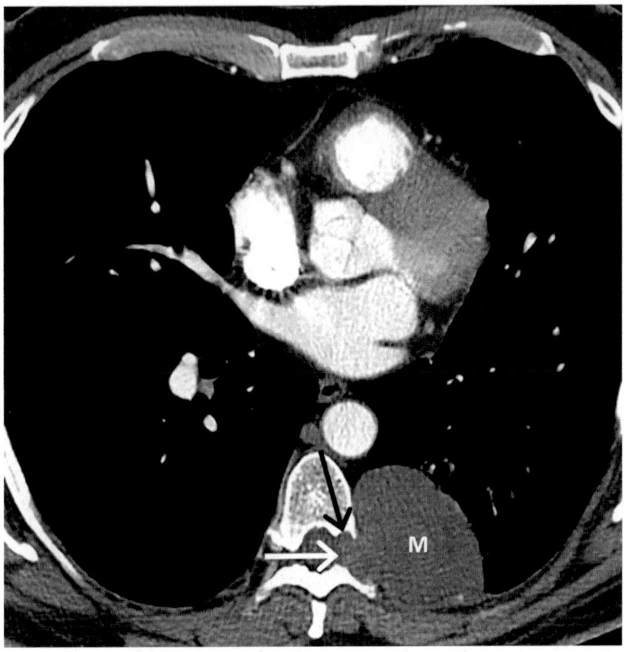

Fig. 2.17 Contrast-enhanced axial CT of a 59-year-old man presenting with back pain demonstrates a well-circumscribed mass (M) arising from the left paravertebral mediastinum. The mass extends through the adjacent intervertebral foramen (white arrow). There is sharply demarcated benign-appearing bone remodeling (black arrow) of the bone adjacent to this slowly growing benign tumor. Surgical resection was performed because of the patient's symptomatology, and pathology revealed a benign schwannoma

Miscellaneous Lesions

Paraspinal Abscess

Paraspinal abscess represents phlegmon surrounding a peripherally enhancing fluid collection and usually results from direct extension of adjacent infection, transcutaneous infection of deep tissue, and hematogenous spread from distant sites. Intravenous drug use and immunocompromised states predispose to paraspinal infections. Paraspinal abscess appears as an amorphous, ill-defined soft tissue lesion in the paravertebral region and low-density intramuscular fluid collections with or without internal foci of gas on CT. Diffuse or peripheral enhancement may be present following the administration of IV contrast. In the setting of paraspinal abscess due to tuberculosis infection, partial or complete calcification may be present. Associated abnormalities include destruction of the vertebral body endplates and spinal deformities.

Extramedullary Hematopoiesis

Extramedullary hematopoiesis represents a proliferation of hematopoietic cells outside of the bone marrow in the setting of failing marrow hematopoiesis and may be associated with disease processes such as myelofibrosis, β-thalassemia, hereditary spherocytosis, hemolytic anemia, and sickle cell anemia. Although most patients are asymptomatic, cord compression may rarely complicate intraspinal involvement. On CT, extramedullary hematopoiesis manifests as well-defined soft tissue masses in the paravertebral region along the costovertebral junctions (Fig. 2.19). Most lesions are composed of soft tissue;

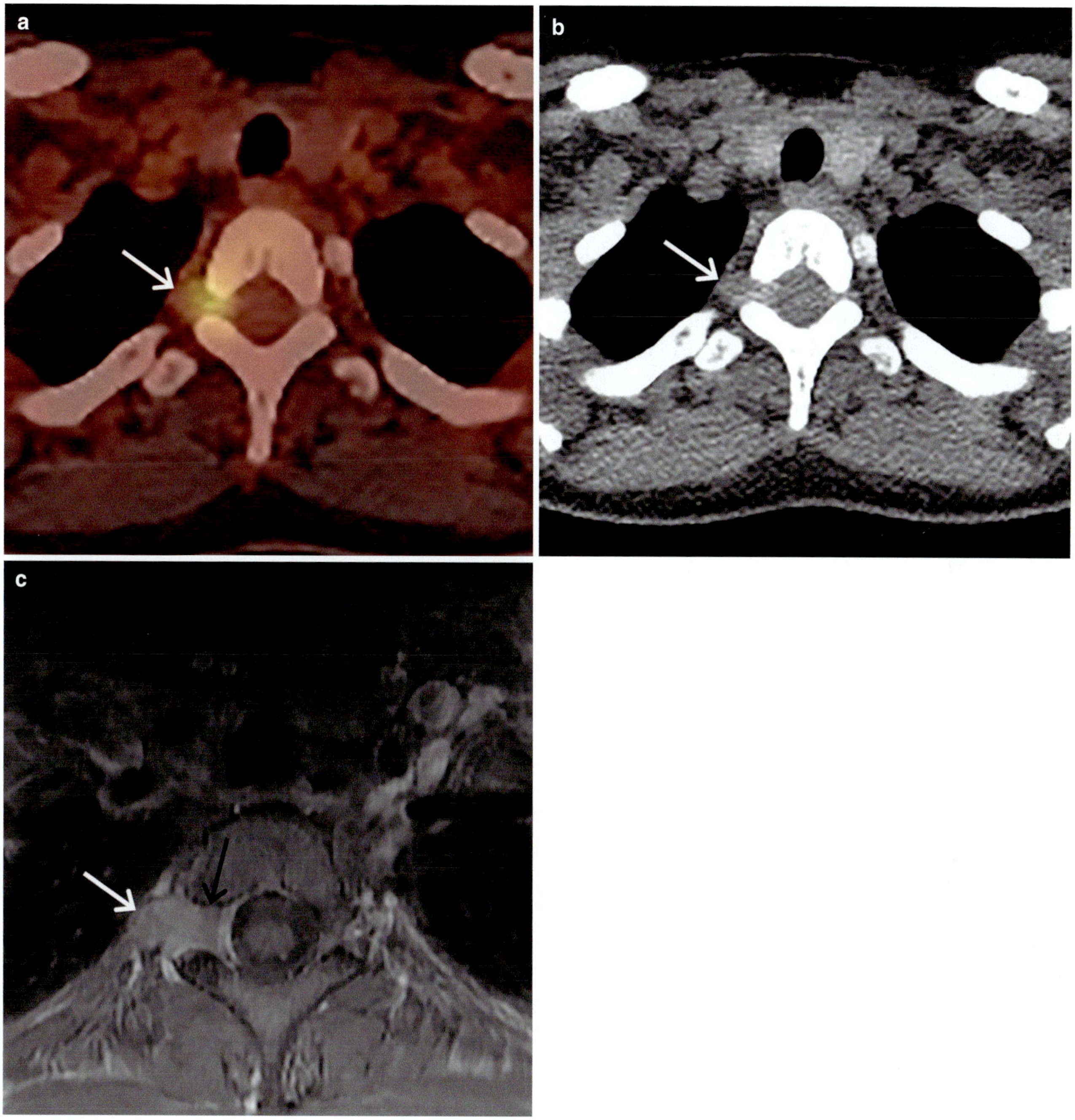

Fig. 2.18 Neurofibroma in a 26-year-old woman with neurofibromatosis type 1. (**a**, **b**) Fused axial FDG PET/CT (**a**) demonstrates focal increased FDG uptake (arrow, **a**) in the right paravertebral mediastinum in the upper mediastinum with a correlative soft tissue focus on unenhanced CT (arrow, **b**). (**c**). Axial contrast-enhanced T1-weighted image of the same patient demonstrates an enhancing lesion extending into the right intervertebral foramen and spinal canal consistent with a neurogenic neoplasm, in this case a neurofibroma

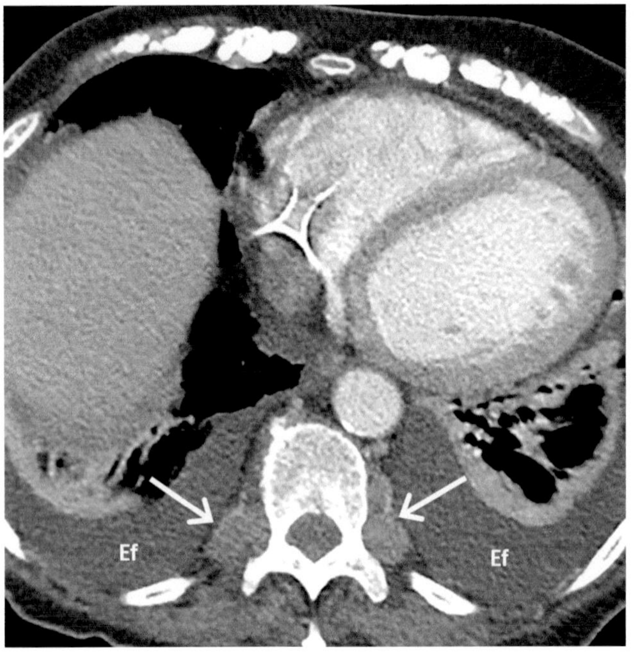

Fig. 2.19 Contrast-enhanced axial CT of a 71-year-old woman with myelofibrosis and extramedullary hematopoiesis demonstrates enhancing paravertebral masses (arrows) and bilateral pleural effusions (Ef). On CT, extramedullary hematopoiesis manifests as well-defined soft tissue masses in the paravertebral region along the costovertebral junctions, as in this case

however, internal regions of internal fat density may be seen in burned-out lesions. Mild or heterogeneous contrast enhancement may be seen following the administration of IV contrast. MR imaging is superior to CT in showing the presence and extent of intraspinal extension.

Conclusions

In the evaluation of mediastinal lesions, specific imaging findings may be present that enable the diagnosis by imaging findings alone. However, other lesions exhibit inconclusive imaging features, and a combination of imaging, pathological, and clinical information is necessary to establish the diagnosis. The approach outlined in this chapter can facilitate a streamlined discussion and further evaluation of patients presenting with these abnormalities.

References

1. Carter BW, Tomiyama N, Bhora FY, Rosado de Christenson ML, Nakajima J, Boiselle PM, et al. A modern definition of mediastinal compartments. J Thorac Oncol. 2014;9(9 Suppl 2):S97–101.
2. Carter BW, Benveniste MF, Madan R, Godoy MC, de Groot PM, Truong MT, Rosado-de-Christenson ML, Marom EM. ITMIG classification of mediastinal compartments and multidisciplinary approach to mediastinal masses. Radiographics. 2017;37(2):413–36.
3. Fujimoto K, Hara M, Tomiyama N, Kusumoto M, Sakai F, Fujii Y. Proposal for a new mediastinal compartment classification of transverse plane images according to the Japanese Association for Research on the Thymus (JART) General Rules for the Study of Mediastinal Tumors. Oncol Rep. 2014;31:565–72.
4. Davis RD Jr, Oldham HN Jr, Sabiston DC Jr. Primary cysts and neoplasms of the mediastinum: recent changes in clinical presentation, methods of diagnosis, management, and results. Ann Thorac Surg. 1987;44:229–37.
5. Levasseur P, Kaswin R, Rojas-Miranda A, N'guimbous JF, Merlier M, Le Brigand H. Apropos of a series of 742 operated patients. Nouv Press Med. 1976;5:2857–9.
6. Cohen AJ, Thompson L, Edwards FH, Bellamy RF. Primary cysts and tumors of the mediastinum. Ann Thorac Surg. 1991;51:378–84; discussion 385.
7. Rubush JL, Gardner IR, Boyd WC, Ehrenhaft JL. Mediastinal tumors. Review of 186 cases. J Thorac Cardiovasc Surg. 1973;65:216–22.
8. Wychulis AR, Payne WS, Clagett OT, Woolner LB. Surgical treatment of mediastinal tumors: a 40 year experience. J Thorac Cardiovasc Surg. 1971;62:379–92.
9. Mullen B, Richardson JD. Primary anterior mediastinal tumors in children and adults. Ann Thorac Surg. 1986;42:338–45.
10. Takeda S, Miyoshi S, Minami M, Ohta M, Minami M, Okumura M, et al. Clinical spectrum of primary mediastinal tumors: a comparison of adult and pediatric populations (Abstract). Chest. 2000;118:206S.
11. Whooley BP, Urschel JD, Antkowiak JG, Takita H. Primary tumors of the mediastinum. J Surg Oncol. 1999;70:95–9.
12. Azarow KS, Pearl RH, Zurcher R, Edwards FH, Cohen AJ. Primary mediastinal masses. A comparison of adult and pediatric populations. J Thorac Cardiovasc Surg. 1993;106:67–72.
13. Carter BW, Okumura M, Detterbeck FC, Marom EM. Approaching the patient with an anterior mediastinal mass: a guide for radiologists. J Thorac Oncol. 2014;9(9 Suppl 2):S110–8.13.
14. Tomiyama N, Honda O, Tsubamoto M, Inoue A, Sumikawa H, Kuriyama K, et al. Anterior mediastinal tumors: diagnostic accuracy of CT and MRI. Eur J Radiol. 2009;69:280–8.
15. Ackman JB, Wu CC. MRI of the thymus. AJR Am J Roentgenol. 2011;197:W15–20.
16. Inaoka T, Takahashi K, Mineta M, Yamada T, Shuke N, Okizaki A, et al. Thymic hyperplasia and thymus gland tumors: differentiation with chemical shift MR imaging. Radiology. 2007;243:869–76.
17. Takahashi K, Al-Janabi NJ. Computed tomography and magnetic resonance imaging of mediastinal tumors. J Magn Reson Imaging. 2010;32:1325–39.
18. Rosado-de-Christenson ML, Templeton PA, Moran CA. From the archives of the AFIP. Mediastinal germ cell tumors: radiologic and pathologic correlation. Radiographics. 1992;12:1013–30.
19. Molinari F, Bankier AA, Eisenberg RL. Fat-containing lesions in adult thoracic imaging. AJR Am J Roentgenol. 2011;197:W795–813.
20. Wright C. Germ cell tumors of the mediastinum. In: Pearson F, Cooper J, Deslauriers J, Ginsberg RJ, Hiebert C, Patterson G, Urschel H, editors. Thoracic Surgery. New York: Churchill Livingstone; 2002. p. 1711–9.
21. Gaerte SC, Meyer CA, Winer-Muram HT, Tarver RD, Conces DJ Jr. Fat-containing lesions of the chest. Radiographics. 2002;22:S61–78.
22. Nishino M, Ashiku SK, Kocher ON, Thurer RL, Boiselle PM, Hatabu H. The thymus: a comprehensive review. Radiographics. 2006;26:335–48.
23. Munden RF, Nesbitt JC, Kemp BL, Chasen MH, Whitman GJ. Primary liposarcoma of the mediastinum. AJR Am J Roentgenol. 2000;175:1340.

24. Hahn HP, Fletcher CD. Primary mediastinal liposarcoma: clinicopathologic analysis of 24 cases. Am J Surg Pathol. 2007;31:1868–74.
25. Choi YW, McAdams HP, Jeon SC, Hong EK, Kim YH, Im JG, et al. Idiopathic multilocular thymic cyst: CT features with clinical and histopathologic correlation. AJR Am J Roentgenol. 2001;177:881–5.
26. Jeung MY, Gasser B, Gangi A, Bogorin A, Charneau D, Wihlm JM, et al. Imaging of cystic masses of the mediastinum. Radiographics. 2002;22:S79–93.
27. Feigin DS, Fenoglio JJ, McAllister HA, Madewell JE. Pericardial cysts. A radiologic-pathologic correlation and review. Radiology. 1977;125:15–20.
28. Mendelson DS, Rose JS, Efremidis SC, Kirschner PA, Cohen BA. Bronchogenic cysts with high CT numbers. AJR Am J Roentgenol. 1983;140:463–5.
29. Yernault JC, Kuhn G, Dumortier P, Rocmans P, Ketelbant P, De Vuyst P. "Solid" mediastinal bronchogenic cyst: mineralogic analysis. AJR Am J Roentgenol. 1986;146:73–4.
30. Fitch SJ, Tonkin IL, Tonkin AK. Imaging of foregut duplication cysts. Radiographics. 1986;6:189–201.
31. Kuhlman JE, Fishman EK, Wang KP, Siegelman SS. Esophageal duplication cyst: CT and transesophageal needle aspiration. AJR Am J Roentgenol. 1985;145:531–2.
32. LeBlanc J, Guttentag AR, Shepard JA, McLoud TC. Imaging of mediastinal foregut cysts. Can Assoc Radiol J. 1994;45:381–6.
33. Naidich DP, Webb WR, Muller NL, Krinsky GA, Zerhouni EA, Siegelman SS. Mediastinum. In: Computed tomography and magnetic resonance of the thorax. 3rd ed. Philadelphia: Lippincott Williams and Wilkins; 1999. p. 82–3.
34. Benveniste MF, Rosado-de-Christenson ML, Sabloff BS, Moran CA, Swisher SG, Marom EM. Role of imaging in the diagnosis, staging, and treatment of thymoma. Radiographics. 2011;31:1847–61; discussion 1861.
35. Rosado-de-Christenson ML, Strollo DC, Marom EM. Imaging of thymic epithelial neoplasms. Hematol Oncol Clin North Am. 2008;22(3):409–31.
36. Schaefer NG, Hany TF, Taverna C, Seifert B, Stumpe KD, von Schulthess GK, et al. Non-Hodgkin lymphoma and Hodgkin disease: coregistered FDG PET and CT at staging and restaging–do we need contrast-enhanced CT? Radiology. 2004;232:823–9.
37. Duwe BV, Sterman DH, Musani AI. Tumors of the mediastinum. Chest. 2005;128(4):2893–909.
38. Tian L, Liu LZ, Cui CY, Zhang WD, Kuang YL. CT findings of primary non-teratomatous germ cell tumors of the mediastinum--a report of 15 cases. Eur J Radiol. 2012;81(5):1057–61.
39. Strollo DC, Rosado-de-Christenson ML. Primary mediastinal malignant germ cell neoplasms: imaging features. Chest Surg Clin N Am. 2002;12:645–58.
40. Economou JS, Trump DL, Holmes EC, Eggleston JE. Management of primary germ cell tumors of the mediastinum. J Thorac Cardiovasc Surg. 1982;83:643–9.
41. Bokemeyer C, Nichols CR, Droz JP, Schmoll HJ, Horwich A, Gerl A, et al. Extragonadal germ cell tumors of the mediastinum and retroperitoneum: results from an international analysis. J Clin Oncol. 2002;20:1864–73.
42. Bukowski RM, Wolf M, Kulander BG, Montie J, Crawford ED, Blumenstein B. Alternating combination chemotherapy in patients with extragonadal germ cell tumors. A Southwest Oncology Group study. Cancer. 1993;71:2631–8.
43. Lee KS, Lm J-G, Han CH, Han MC, Kim C-W, Kim WS. Malignant primary germ cell tumors of the mediastinum: CT features. AJR. 1989;153:947–51.
44. Wright CD, Kesler KA, Nichols CR, Mahomed Y, Einhorn LH, Miller ME, et al. Primary mediastinal nonseminomatous germ cell tumors. Results of a multimodality approach. J Thorac Cardiovasc Surg. 1990;99:210–7.
45. Kesler KA, Rieger KM, Ganjoo KN, Sharma M, Fineberg NS, Einhorn LH, et al. Primary mediastinal nonseminomatous germ cell tumors: the influence of postchemotherapy pathology on long-term survival after surgery. J Thorac Cardiovasc Surg. 1999;118:692–700.
46. Hong SJ, Kim TJ, Nam KB, Lee IS, Yang HC, Cho S, et al. New TNM staging system for esophageal cancer: what chest radiologists need to know. Radiographics. 2014;34(6):1722–40.
47. Nakazono T, White CS, Yamasaki F, Yamaguchi K, Egashira R, Irie H, et al. MRI findings of mediastinal neurogenic tumors. AJR Am J Roentgenol. 2011;197:W643–52.
48. Juanpere S, Cañete N, Ortuño P, Martínez S, Sanchez G, Bernado L. A diagnostic approach to the mediastinal masses. Insights Imaging. 2013;4:29–52.

Surgical Approaches to the Mediastinum

3

Introduction

Contrary to the belief of many, the mediastinum actually can be defined by specific boundaries and landmarks. Basically, the mediastinum encompasses the region from the thoracic inlet to the diaphragm as the superior and inferior boundaries, the pleural reflections laterally, the sternum anteriorly and the spine posteriorly. Interestingly, a number of different anatomical classifications have been put forth to describe the various compartments of the mediastinum, but, from a surgical standpoint, it perhaps is easiest and most straightforward to use the terms superior, middle, anterior, and posterior (Fig. 3.1). When we think in terms of surgical pathology, essentially all entities can be fitted into one of these compartments. There have been a number of attempts to further define mediastinal compartments such as that of the Japanese Association for Research on the Thymus (JART) [1]. Their classification is based on axial computed tomographic (CT) images and, as noted above, proposes four compartments: superior, anterior (prevascular zone), middle (peri-tracheoesophageal zone), and posterior (paravertebral zone). A retrospective look at data collected from 445 pathologically proven lesions allowed them to validate their proposed classification. Thymic epithelial neoplasms, lymphomas, and a majority of germ cell tumors were classified within the anterior mediastinum. The majority of substernal goiters were located in the superior compartment, while the majority of masses found in the middle mediastinum were cysts specifically of bronchopulmonary foregut origin or pericardial. Neurogenic lesions comprised the majority of lesions found in the paravertebral (posterior) zone.

A mediastinal mass may be discovered when a patient presents with symptoms suggestive of pulmonary pathology – such as chest pain or cough – but many are found serendipitously when a CT scan is done for some other reason. A large anterior mediastinal mass often may be suggested by the finding of an additional soft tissue mass seen on plain chest radiograph especially on the lateral projection. The so-called silhouette sign, where there is a loss of a normal border of an intrathoracic structure, may be noted. Once an abnormality is noted or suspected on a chest radiograph, the definitive study is a CT scan that provides cross-sectional imaging that defines the location of the lesion as well as the size and additional characteristics that may be present. Magnetic resonance imaging (MRI) has not been found to add any additional information if the lesion is solid. However, MRI clearly is superior to CT in delineating a cystic from a solid lesion and should be obtained if there is suspicion that a lesion may be cystic [2]. The location of a mediastinal mass as defined by the CT scan aids greatly in the differential diagnosis of a particular lesion. As a rule, more than half of all mediastinal masses locate to the anterior mediastinum, and the majority of these are thymic in origin, whether epithelial or the more common lymphoma. One fourth of lesions are found in the middle mediastinum and another fourth in the posterior compartment. The superior mediastinum or peri-tracheobronchial location is where lymph node metastasis from pulmonary pathology is found and may be approached for definitive histologic characterization either by mediastinoscopy or, more commonly in the current era, by endoscopic bronchial ultrasound localization (EBUS) and needle aspiration. As noted above substernal goiters also localize to the superior mediastinum [3].

Surgical Approaches to the Anterior Mediastinum

The typical computed tomographic (CT) appearance of a lesion found in the anterior mediastinum is seen in Fig. 3.2. The approach chosen depends to a great extent on the appearance of the lesion and the suspected diagnosis. A large, invasive lesion should be distinguished from a well encapsulated lesion since this distinction determines whether completely resecting the lesion or simply proceeding to obtain a tissue sample for definitive diagnosis is the more prudent approach. Lesions occurring in the anterior mediastinum include, but are not limited to, lymphoma, thymoma, and other primary lesions of thymic origin including thymic carcinoma, germ cell tumors and teratoma, substernal goiter, parathyroid adenoma,

© Springer Nature Switzerland AG 2019
N. Kalhor, C. Moran, *Mediastinal Pathology*, https://doi.org/10.1007/978-3-319-98980-8_3

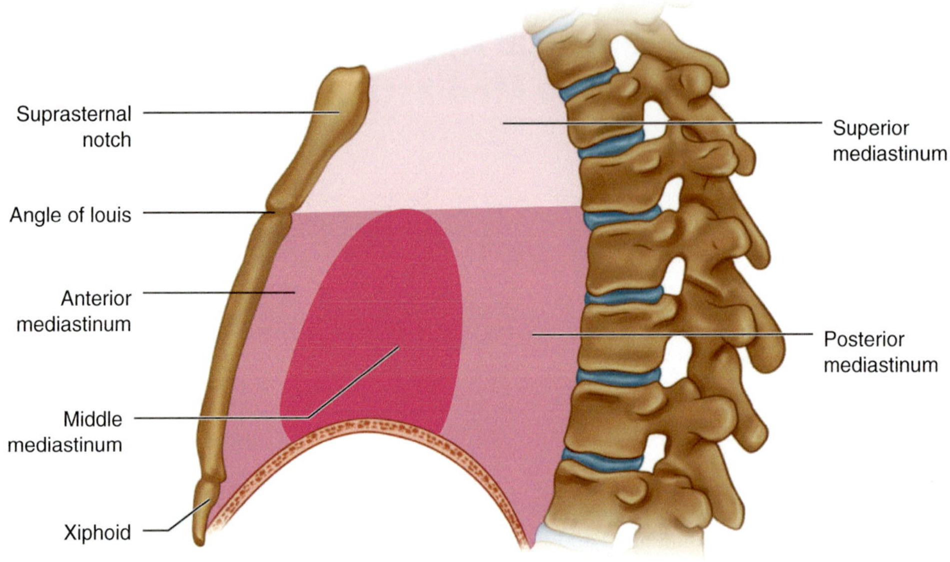

Fig. 3.1 Diagram showing the classical description of the compartments of the mediastinum

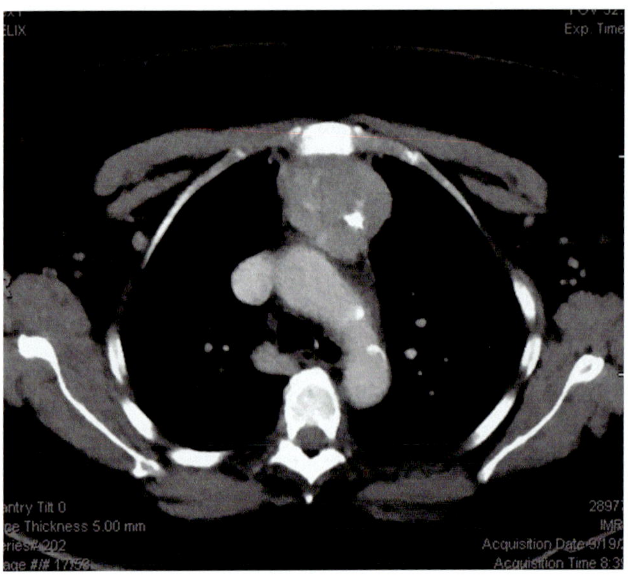

Fig. 3.2 CT scan of a thymoma. Note the location in the anterior mediastinum in close proximity to the aorta and superior vena cava

thymic cysts, and pericardial cysts. A large invasive lesion where lymphoma is suspected requires an approach that allows for a tissue sample to be obtained (Fig. 3.3). A core needle biopsy may yield sufficient tissue for complete phenotyping and genotyping of a lymphoma, but if more tissue is needed, a more invasive procedure is required. Lesions located in the anterior mediastinum are not accessible via mediastinoscopy as the reach of the mediastinoscope is limited to the superior mediastinum. The mediastinoscope is passed along the anterior aspect of the trachea posterior to the innominate artery and the aorta, allowing for sampling of lymph nodes in the paratracheal region as well as the subcarinal space.

The anterior mediastinum may be accessed via several approaches, with the one chosen based most commonly on the location of the lesion but using the least invasive approach. The most direct approach involves an anterior mediastinotomy either through the second intercostal space or excision of the second costal cartilage on the involved side (Fig. 3.4). With excision of the cartilage, it is possible and preferable to remain extrapleural in approaching the lesion, thus avoiding having to place a chest tube. Once the lesion is visualized, sufficient material is easily obtained to allow for a definitive pathologic diagnosis.

Alternatively, a video-assisted thoracoscopic approach (VATS) may be utilized to obtain tissue. This requires single lung ventilation to allow for the placement of a thoracoscope into the appropriate pleural space. Despite being characterized as "minimally invasive," this approach actually is the more invasive approach compared to the anterior mediastinotomy that allows one to remain extrapleural. It is recommended that a frozen section be performed on the specimen obtained to assure that diagnostic material is present. It is clearly preferable not to have to subject the patient to a repeat procedure if only on permanent section it is determined that inadequate material was obtained.

Thymoma

Tumors of the thymus gland account for approximately 50% of the epithelial lesions occurring in the anterior mediastinum [3]. The presentation of these lesions varies from the incidental discovery of a mass on a CT scan of the chest done for some other reason to symptoms caused by a variety of paraneoplastic syndromes, the most common one being myasthenia gravis. Other associated syndromes include pure red cell aplasia and Eaton-Lambert syndrome. Imaging studies demonstrate a spectrum of appearances as they can vary from a well encapsulated discrete lesion with no obvious evidence of invasion to a large clearly invasive mass (Fig. 3.5a, b). There have been a number of staging systems proposed for characterizing thymomas, but the one most commonly utilized is that of Masaoka [4]:

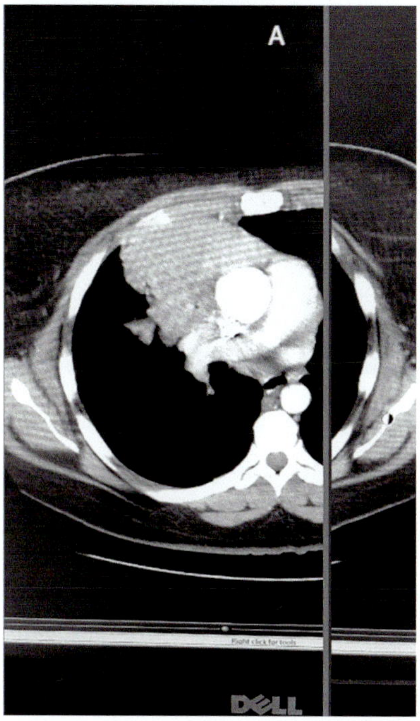

Fig. 3.3 A large, invasive anterior mediastinal mass characteristic of lymphoma. The appearance warrants a biopsy for histologic confirmation as well as obtaining tissue for further molecular and genetic characterization

Stage I: Macroscopically and microscopically completely encapsulated
Stage IIA: Microscopic transcapsular invasion
Stage IIB: Macrosopic invasion into surrounding fatty tissue or grossly adherent to but not through mediastinal pleura or pericardium
Stage III: Macroscopic invasion into neighboring organs, such as the pericardium, lung, great vessels)
Stage IVA: Pleural or pericardial dissemination
Stage IVB: Lymphogenous or hematogenous metastasis

This staging system has been clinically validated, and there is a direct correlation with prognosis. The World Health Organization (WHO) developed a histological classification system in 1999, with revisions in 2004 and later 2015 [5]. This system also correlates with prognosis both independently and when used alongside the Masaoka classification. Moran and colleagues looked at 250 cases of thymoma with an emphasis on the WHO histologic subtyping and found that more than 50% of tumors after subtyping fell into mixed categories, effectively diminishing the clinical impact of histologic subtyping over staging [6]. The authors propose a staging system that is statistically significant for both overall

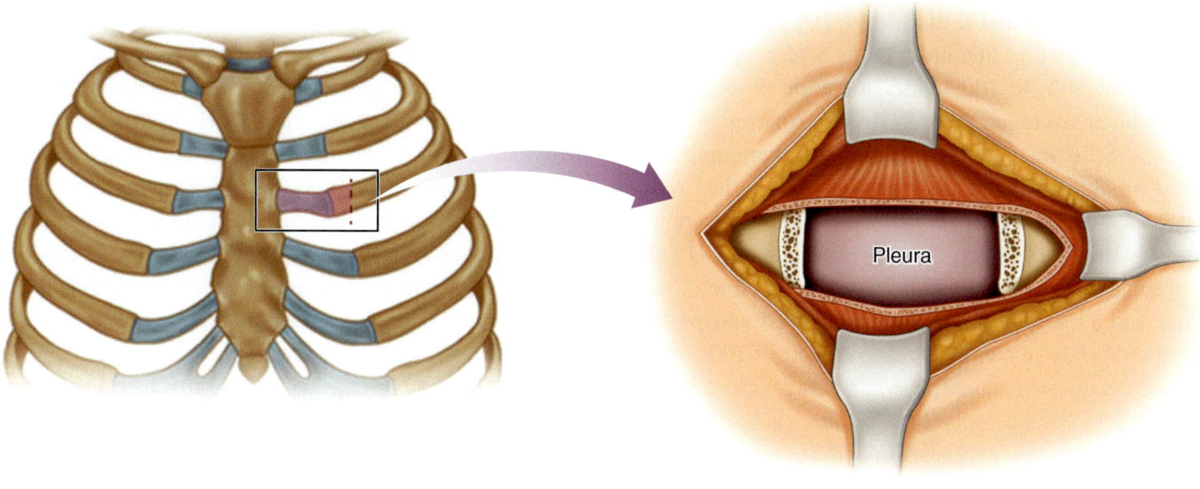

Fig. 3.4 Diagram showing the approach for a mediastinotomy with excision of the second costal cartilage to gain access and remain extrapleural

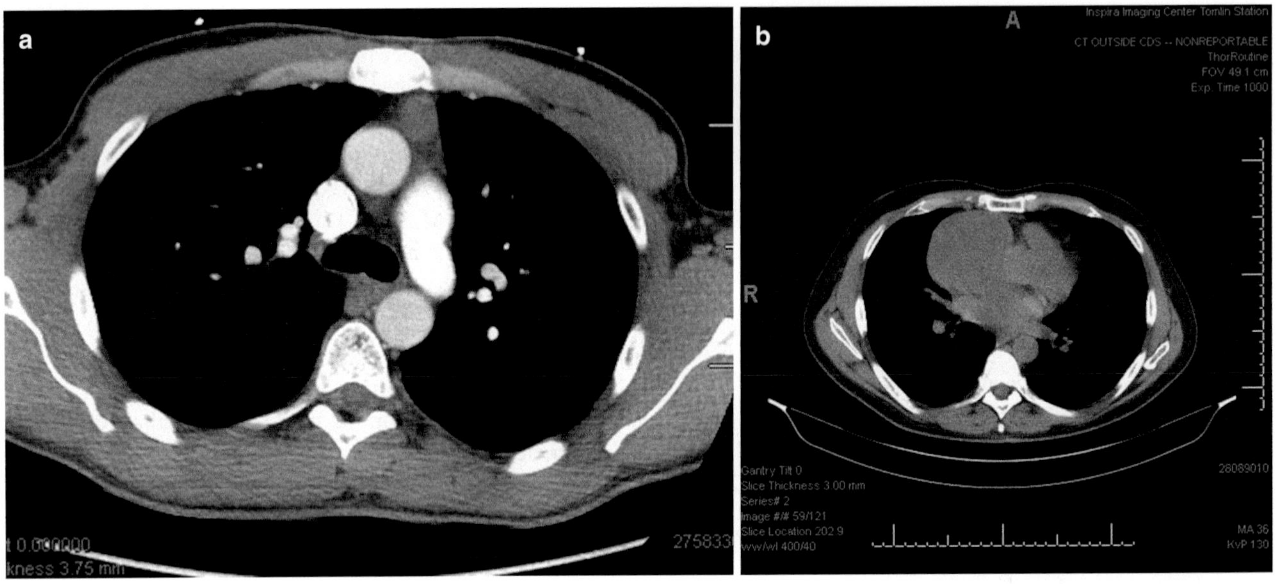

Fig. 3.5 (**a**) A small, well encapsulated thymoma that should be easily excised via a minimally invasive approach. (**b**) An invasive thymoma that warrants a multidisciplinary approach including resection

and recurrence-free survival and offers better stratification and improved histological definitions for proper staging [7].

Additionally, there has been a recent push to utilize the classic tumor-node-metastasis (TNM) classification with modifications provided by the International Thymic Malignancies Interest Group (ITMIG), among others, so it would be included in the 8th edition of the American Joint Committee on Cancer's *AJCC Cancer Staging Manual* [8]. This system has a number of similarities to the modified Masaoka classification especially as it relates to the T component in addition to including parts of the WHO classification.

Surgical resection remains the definitive treatment for thymoma with high overall and disease-free survival rates in patients with stage I and II disease [9, 10]. Detterbeck, in a review of the existing literature, notes 5-year survival rates ranging from 80% to 100% after resection of stage I thymoma, with an average rate of 91% [11]. An average 5-year survival of 80% was reported for stage II thymoma, with a higher variability in results among the series (range 42–100%). Average overall 10-year survival rates were 87% (range 75–100%) for stage I and 67% for stage II [12–15]. The average recurrence rate was 3% after resection of stage I tumor and 11% for stage II thymoma. Well-encapsulated stage I tumors have a complete resection rate of 100%, while complete resection of stage II lesions averages close to 90%, but depending on the report, these rates can vary widely. Despite the temptation to remove only the tumor itself, definitive treatment for thymomas should include a total thymectomy as there are at least anecdotal reports of the later appearance of myasthenia gravis when residual thymus is left behind [16, 17]. Wang reported significantly better survival at 5 years following complete thymectomy compared to tumor resection alone (92% vs 59%), although this difference did not hold up at 10 years [18]. Conversely, a more recent study showed no difference in survival between total thymectomy and tumor resection alone [19].

With more invasive lesions, specifically Masaoka stage III where there is tumor invasion of adjacent structures, definitive resection still is the treatment of choice with the recognition that a more radical procedure may be required [20–22]. Resection of the pericardium or a portion of lung presents no real additional challenge, but superior vena cava or innominate vein involvement produces some increased complexity. The innominate vein usually can be resected with impunity, but superior vena caval involvement requires reconstruction ideally with autogenous material preferably a spiral vein graft. Alternatively, prosthetic material can be used to reconstruct the superior vena cava [23]. Hemidiaphragm, if involved, also may be resected and reconstructed with a prosthetic patch usually polytetrafluoroethylene (PTFE). The key with these lesions is to accomplish a complete resection ideally with negative margins. Even in those cases where pleural involvement is present, it is reasonable to proceed with resection and pleurectomy in an attempt to remove all gross disease [24, 25]. In selected patients, pleuropneumonectomy also may be considered [24, 26]. Justification exists to proceed with these extended procedures recognizing if a complete resection is accomplished survival rates can approximate those achieved in stage I and II tumors [27]. In a study from the Massachusetts General Hospital, the overall survival for patients with stage III disease was 71% at 5 years and 54% at 10 years. For those patients where a complete resection could be accomplished, the 5- and 10-year survival was 86% and 69%, respectively. Alternatively, for those who had an incomplete resection, 5-year survival was 28% and only 14% at 10 years. Radiation therapy did not significantly alter survival following incomplete resection [28, 29].

It is illustrative here to briefly discuss the surgical approaches to the anterior mediastinum that are common for any lesion in this location whether thymoma, germ cell tumor or other. The standard operation has been the median sternotomy with total thymectomy and resection of the tumor. As noted above, any invaded structures are taken en bloc, and reconstruction is carried out as required. There are situations, depending on the location of the tumor, when a posterolateral thoracotomy may be the approach of choice, but the sternotomy allows access to both pleural reflections as well as nicely exposes the brachiocephalic vessels. In recent years, VATS has been used to resect smaller less invasive lesions, and very recently robotic approaches have been championed. The increased degrees of freedom allowed by the robotic arms facilitate the dissection [30, 31]. For small, well encapsulated lesions, a transcervical approach also has been used to resect the entire gland and the tumor [32–34].

Germ Cell Tumors

Primary mediastinal germ cell tumors are extremely rare and occur mostly in males. They represent only about 10% of all anterior mediastinal masses. They may present as mature teratomas with no malignant feature or seminomatous or non-seminomatous tumors [35]. A specific staging classification has been proposed for these tumors [36]. Mature teratomas, which account for 60–70% of all mediastinal germ cell tumors, are fascinating lesions characterized by mature elements from all three germinal layers, ectoderm, endoderm, and mesoderm, and thus may contain fat, cartilage, bone, teeth, and glandular epithelia (Fig. 3.6) [37, 38]. Imaging studies demonstrate most commonly a multilocular, well circumscribed partially cystic mass containing fluid and fat density and often calcifications [39]. The serum markers, beta-HCG and alpha-fetoprotein, usually are not elevated. Complete excision usually via median sternotomy is the definitive treatment for these lesions, but they need to be closely examined to assure the absence of any malignant elements [38, 40].

Primary mediastinal seminomatous germ cell tumors (PMSGCT) are seen most commonly between the ages of 20 and 40 years and present as a lobulated, homogenous mass [36, 41, 42]. Serum beta-HCG and alpha-fetoprotein usually are normal or very mildly elevated. Histologic confirmation is required and usually can be obtained with fine needle aspiration or with a VATS procedure. First-line treatment usually is systemic chemotherapy with radiation therapy if chemotherapy results in less than an optimal result. Surgical resection occasionally is recommended if residual tumor exists following first-line therapy [43, 44].

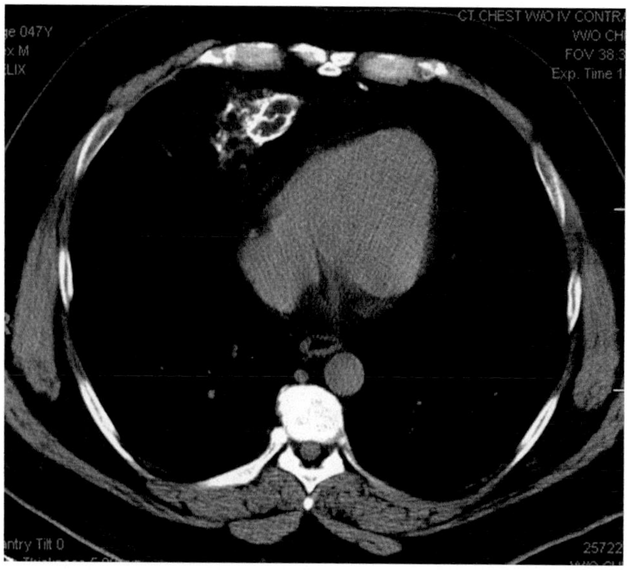

Fig. 3.6 Classic appearance of a mature teratoma. Note the significant calcification as well as the extensive fat density

Non-seminomatous primary mediastinal germ cell tumors may occur as choriocarcinoma or embryonal or yolk sac tumor. Not uncommonly, all three elements are found in one of these tumors [36]. They commonly present with chest pain or cough and usually when first seen already are large invasive masses. Serum markers are elevated in essentially all of these tumors with a few rare exceptions. If markers are elevated, a tissue diagnosis is not required as the patient is treated with platinum-based chemotherapy. These lesions have a poorer prognosis than those arising in either the testis or retroperitoneum, with an overall 5 y survival of approximately 50% compared with 80% for testis [45–49]. The role of surgical resection for these lesions remains somewhat controversial. Previously, the only indication for operation was residual tumor with negative serum markers. Now there are centers that recommend resection for residual tumor even with markers remaining elevated [50–52]. Median sternotomy is the most commonly employed approach to resect these lesions though VATS, and robotic-assisted techniques have their own adherents.

Parathyroid Adenomas

The inferior parathyroids originate from the third pharyngeal pouch and are those with the most variable location, since they may migrate with the thymus and parathyroid tissue can occur anywhere along this course. In a surgical series of 112 patients, inferior parathyroids were found in 60% of cases in a mediastinal location [53]. Less commonly are superior parathyroid glands found in aberrant locations as they arise from the fourth pharyngeal pouch. Patients suspected of having primary hyperparathyroidism usually have a localization study done to image the adenoma. Often, a minimal incision can be performed to remove a single parathyroid adenoma that has been localized to the neck. The rapid parathormone assay that can be performed while the patient is in the operating room to assure removal of the offending adenoma has greatly aided the parathyroid surgeon [54]. If an aberrant inferior gland is localized in the mediastinum, several approaches may be employed (Fig. 3.7). Some surgeons have simply removed as much thymus as they can through their standard incision. Others have employed a median sternotomy or VATS approach to remove the aberrant gland [55–57]. We have utilized a transcervical approach employing a specially made retractor that lifts the manubrium to allow visual access as we remove the thymus gland that contains the adenoma [58] (Fig. 3.8).

Surgical Approaches to the Posterior Mediastinum

The posterior mediastinum is bounded anteriorly by the posterior pericardium and extends posterior to the chest wall and laterally includes the costovertebral sulci. There are a number of structures within this compartment including the descending thoracic aorta, the inferior vena cave, the azygous vein, the sympathetic chain, the thoracic duct, the esophagus, and the intercostal nerves and nerve roots arising from vertebral foramina. The majority of lesions occurring within the posterior mediastinum are benign, and this fact significantly informs our choice of surgical approach. Lesions are classified as cystic or solid with the cystic lesions being part of the

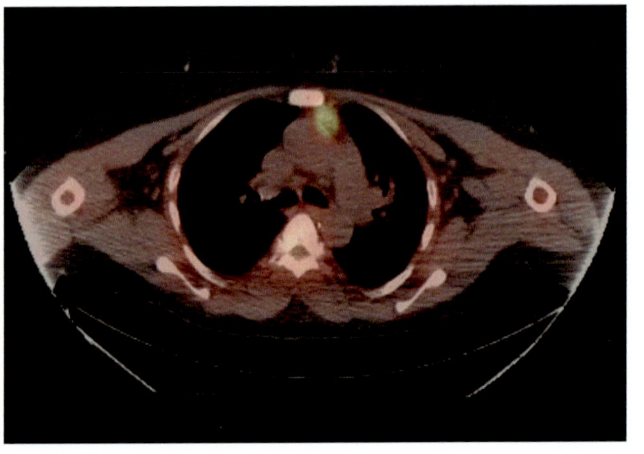

Fig. 3.7 Localization of a parathyroid adenoma in the anterior mediastinum in close proximity or within the thymus gland

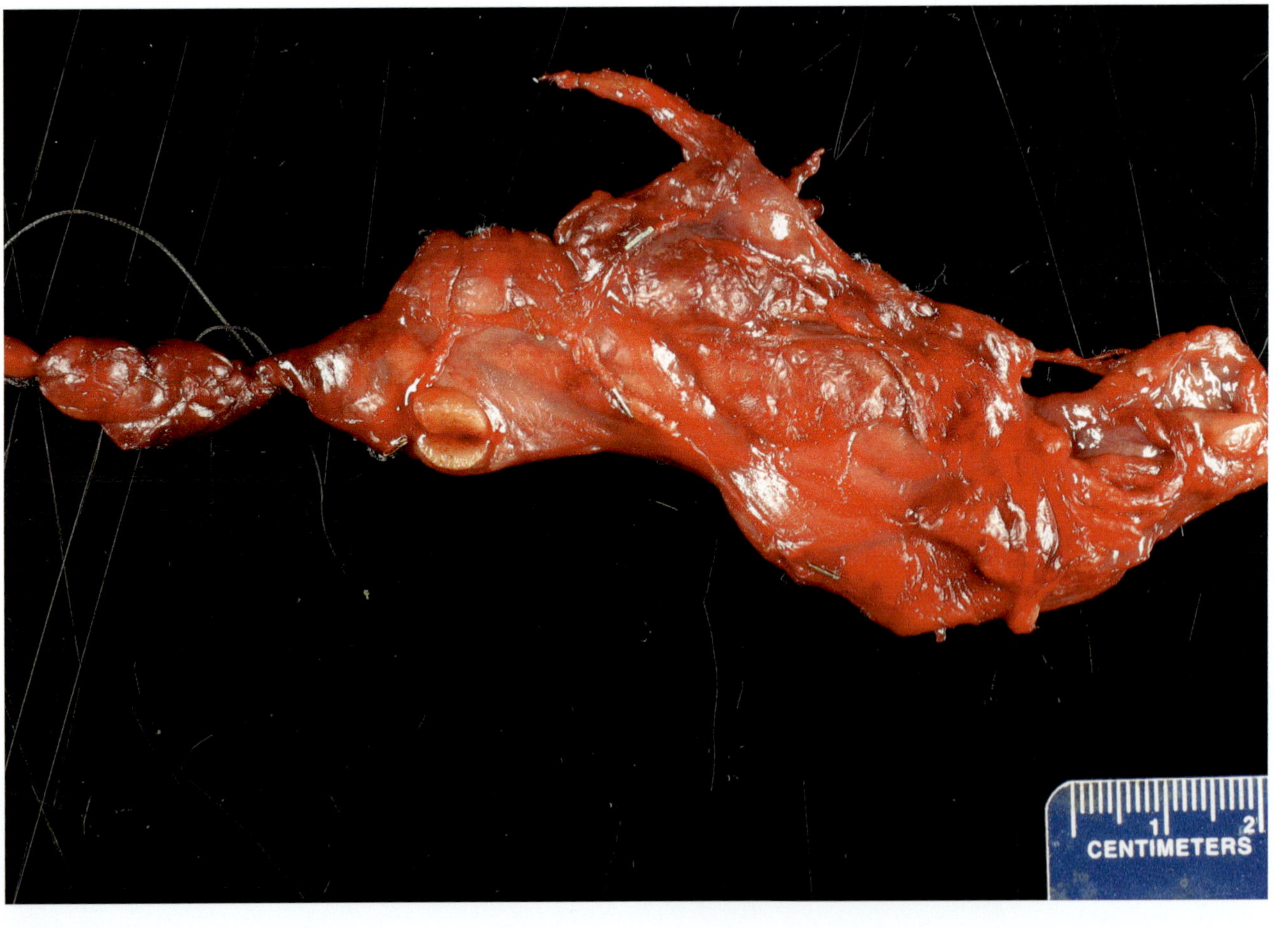

Fig. 3.8 Parathyroid adenoma within the resected thymus gland

spectrum of bronchopulmonary foregut abnormalities specifically either bronchogenic cysts or esophageal duplication cysts [59, 60]. These lesions rarely communicate with either the esophagus or bronchus, but ruling out either of those possibilities at times is critical. Solid lesions most commonly are either schwannomas, ganglioneuromas, or neurofibromas [61–63]. Occasionally, a pheochromocytoma or ganglioneuroma arises from random rests of mediastinal paraganglionic cells and may be hormonally active. A patient who presents with a posterior solid mediastinal mass and hypertension that is difficult to control should be screened with urinary catecholamine testing.

Cystic lesions if asymptomatic may be simply observed, though they can become symptomatic if they get infected. When infection occurs, it is extremely difficult to eradicate, and surgical excision is the treatment of choice (Fig. 3.9). Often, the patient is uncomfortable knowing there is a mass in their chest and wishes to have it excised. Bronchoscopy and esophagoscopy should be carried out to assure no communication prior to resection so as to plan the surgical approach. Most of these may be removed via a VATS approach and occasionally via mediastinoscopy [64, 65]. The entire cyst wall should be resected unless it is so adherent to an adjacent structure, in which case a portion of the cyst wall can remain [66]. Often, it is helpful to drain the lesion of what usually is thick mucoid material prior to dissecting out the wall, though I must admit it is very satisfying to be able to resect the entire cystic lesion intact as it makes for a very nice photograph. These lesions tend not to recur. Surprisingly, some of them may attain quite a large size prior to becoming symptomatic and may compress adjacent structures including the trachea or main stem bronchus.

The approach to solid lesions in the posterior mediastinum is similar to that utilized for cystic lesions. As previously noted, the majority of lesions occurring in the posterior mediastinum are benign. Schwannoma, or neurilemoma, is the most common tumor seen and occurs as a benign, encapsulated lesion in which the cellular architecture is structurally identical to the syncytium of Schwann cells (Fig. 3.10a, b) [61, 67, 68]. While the perineurium forms the capsule of the mass, the neoplastic cells proliferate within the endoneurium. These lesions may originate from either peripheral or sympathetic nerves and occasionally from cranial nerves. Most commonly, they are found as incidental findings on a CT scan done for some other reason as they, for the most part, essentially are asymptomatic [68]. Often, they are found immediately adjacent to a vertebral body closely aligned with a neural foramen (Fig. 3.11). Especially for larger lesions, it is critically important to obtain, in addition to the CT scan, an MRI to look specifically at the neural foramen to assure there is no tumor in the foramen or, more importantly, in the spinal canal [69]. These so-called dumbbell tumors need to be recognized preoperatively since the surgical management differs from that of a tumor without intraspinal extension [70].

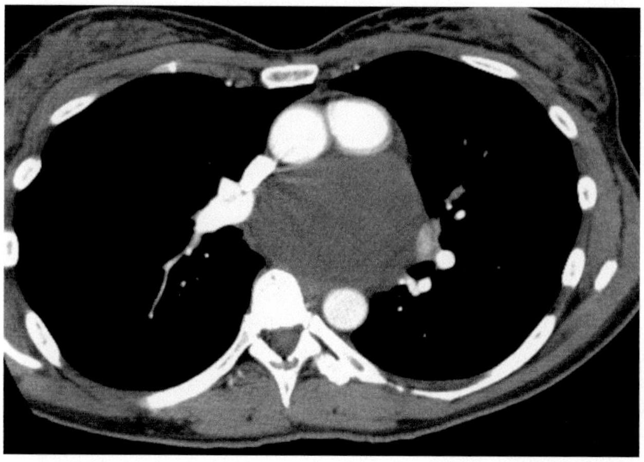

Fig. 3.9 A large bronchogenic cyst compressing major vasculature

A video-assisted thoracoscopic approach is the procedure of choice for these benign usually encapsulated lesions as long as there is no extension into the spinal canal [71]. Robotic-assisted approaches also are becoming increasingly utilized as the additional degrees of freedom afforded by the robotic arms facilitate dissection [72, 73]. Under one-lung ventilation, the videothoracoscope is inserted and the lesion visualized. Simply incising the overlying pleura allows for mobilization of the mass [74]. Depending upon from where the tumor has arisen, it may be necessary to put a clip on a nerve root as it exits the foramen. Securing the nerve root is critically important since the level of the extension of the dural sheath varies, and, if not secured, a spinal fluid leak may occur with significant consequences. The lesion usually just peels off the vertebral body or rib. For lesions with intraspinal extension, a combined approach usually with a neurosurgeon is indicated. Ideally, the intraspinal portion is accessed by the neurosurgeon through a posterior laminectomy approach and resected [70, 75, 76]. Then the patient is positioned for VATS, and the intrathoracic portion of the lesion is removed. If intraspinal extension is unrecognized and the tumor removed leaving part in the spinal canal, there is the likelihood of hemorrhage within the canal that could have dire neurological consequences if not dealt with expeditiously. The complete removal of benign posterior mediastinal schwannomas should result in cure with the risk of local recurrence very low.

As mentioned earlier, there are rare cases of malignant posterior mediastinal tumors, and, when suspected, it is best to approach these via open thoracotomy since they often are adherent to adjacent structures including the aorta [77, 78]. Malignant schwannomas account for approximately 1–2% of all neurogenic tumors occurring in the posterior mediastinum [61].

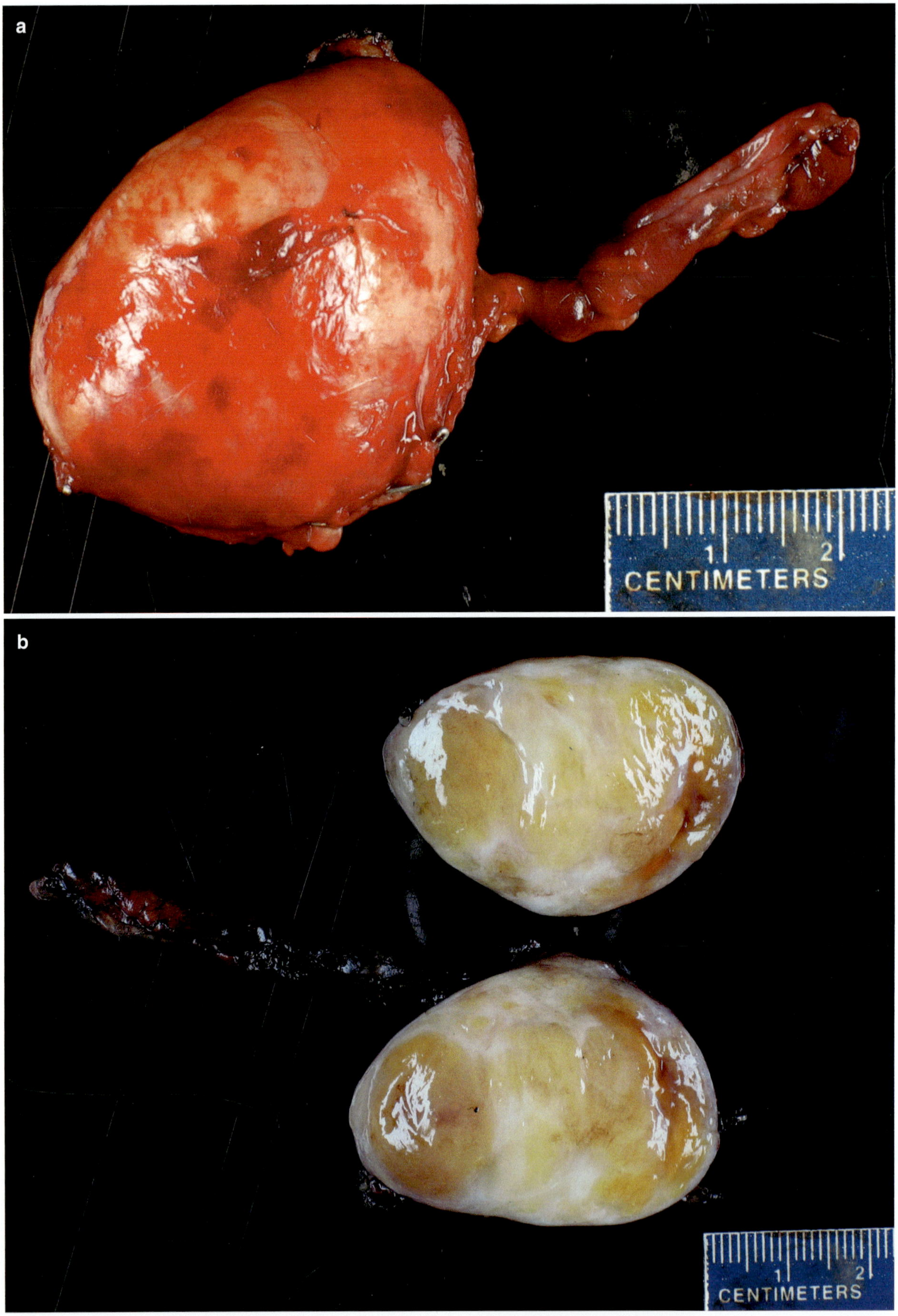

Fig. 3.10 (**a**) Benign schwannoma or neurilemmoma with the nerve root. (**b**) The appearance of the lesion bisected

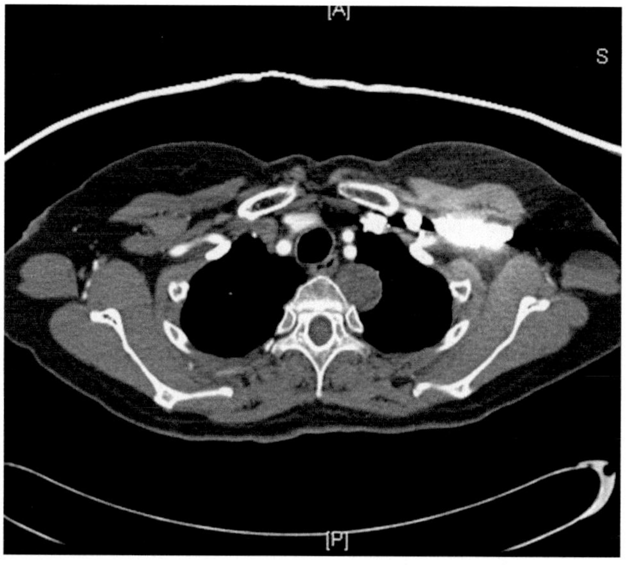

Fig. 3.11 CT scan of a paravertebral mass, classic for a benign schwannoma. This lesion is easily accessible with a VATS or robotic-assisted approach

Care must be taken to avoid the thoracic duct which lies on the vertebral bodies and, if injured, results in a chyle leak that can be devastating if left untreated. The intent is to achieve a complete resection of all gross disease. A suspected pheochromocytoma occurring in the posterior mediastinum requires pretreatment with the usual alpha blocker and potentially beta blockade as well. Ganglioneuroma, neuroblastoma, and ganglioneuroblastoma – tumors of sympathetic ganglion origin – occur almost exclusively in infants and young children, with the latter two lesions considered malignancies. Principles of resection remain the same for these lesions with the exception that the malignant lesions usually are treated with a chemotherapeutic regimen prior to any attempt at surgical resection.

Lesions of the mediastinum are among the more intriguing issues faced by thoracic surgeons. The decision as to whether to first obtain a tissue diagnosis as opposed to embarking on a complete resection can be challenging. It is safe to say no thoracic surgeon wants to complete a radical resection with a vascular reconstruction only to find out the offending lesion proved to be a lymphoma. Frozen section diagnosis can be unreliable for certain anterior mediastinal masses; thus, it often proves beneficial to wait for the permanent sections to be read. Some pathologists are perfectly comfortable with relying on the frozen section for a definitive diagnosis, thus allowing the surgeon to proceed with resection. Median sternotomy has been the mainstay approach to the mediastinum for many years, but with the advent of minimally invasive surgical techniques, that is rapidly changing. VATS and robotic-assisted approaches are applicable for many lesions, but larger, invasive lesions still require a sternotomy. The aim of any definitive operation for a mediastinal mass is a complete resection with negative resection margins, and thus the surgeon must be prepared to do whatever is necessary to accomplish that aim. That includes being prepared to take the innominate vein, resect a portion of the superior vena cava and reconstruct it, resect a portion of atrium or diaphragm, or remove a portion or an entire lung. The CT scan with coronal and sagittal reconstructions is helpful in planning the operative approach along with the judicious use of MRI scans, especially if there is a concern of vascular or nerve invasion. Great care must be taken in assessing posterior mediastinal lesions that lie in the costovertebral angle in proximity to neural foramina to assure lack of invasion into the spinal canal.

References

1. Fujimoto K, Hara M, Tomiyama N, Kusumoto M, Sakai F, Fujii Y. Proposal for a new mediastinal compartment classification of transverse plane images according to the Japanese Association for Research on the Thymus (JART) general rules for the study of mediastinal tumors. Oncol Rep. 2014;31:565–72.
2. Carter BW, Meinoshin O, Detterbeck FC, Marom EM. Approaching the patient with an anterior mediastinal mass: a guide for radiologists. J Thorac Oncol. 2014;9:S110–8.
3. Carter BW, Maron EM, Detterbeck FC. Approaching the patient with an anterior mediastinal mass: a guide for clinicians. J Thorac Oncol. 2014;9(suppl 2):S102–9.
4. Masaoka A, Monden Y, Nakahara K, Tanioka T. Follow-up study of thymomas with special reference to their clinical stages. Cancer. 1981;48:2485–92.
5. Marx A, Chan JKC, Coindre J-M, Detterbeck F, Girard N, Harris NL, et al. The 2015 World Health Organization classification of tumors of the Thymus: continuity and changes. J Thorac Oncol. 2015;10:1383–95.
6. Moran CA, Weissferdt A, Kalhor N, Solis LM, Behrens C, Wistuba II, et al. Thymomas I: a clinicopathologic correlation of 250 cases with emphasis on the World Health Organization schema. Am J Clin Pathol. 2012;137(3):444–50.
7. Moran CA, Walsh G, Suster S, Kaiser L. Thymomas II: a clnicopathologic correlation of 250 cases with a proposed staging system with emphasis on pathologic assessment. Am J Clin Pathol. 2012;137(3):451–61.
8. Detterbeck FC, Stratton K, Giroux D, Asamura H, Crowley J, Falkson C, et al. The IASLC/ITMIG Thymic epithelial tumors staging project: proposal for an evidence-based stage classification system for the forthcoming (8th) edition of the TNM classification of malignant tumor. J Thorac Oncol. 2014;9:S65–72.
9. Anile M, Diso D, Vitolo D, Rendina EA, Venuta F. Surgical treatment of early stage thymoma. Lung Cancer. 2010;70(1):116–7.
10. Venuta F, Anile M, Rendina EA, Vitolo D, de Giacomo T, Coloni GF. The value of transcapsular invasion in patients with thymoma. Arch Pathol Lab Med. 2009;133(9):1364–5.
11. Detterbeck F, Parsons AM. Thymic tumors: a review of current diagnosis, classification, and treatment. In: Thoracic and esophageal surgery. 3rd ed. Philadelphia: Elsevier; 2008. p. 1589–614.
12. Regnard J-F, Magdeleinat P, Dromer C, Dulmet E, de Montpreville V, Levi JF, et al. Prognostic factors and long-term results after thymoma resection: a series of 307 patients. J Thorac Cardiovasc Surg. 1996;112:376–84.

13. Maggi G, Casadio C, Cavallo A, Cianci R, Molinatti M, Ruffini E. Thymoma: results of 241 operated cases. Ann Thorac Surg. 1991;51:152–6.
14. Park MS, Chung KY, Kim KD, Yang WI, Chung JH, Kim YS, et al. Prognosis of thymic epithelial tumors according to the new World Health Organization histologic classification. Ann Thorac Surg. 2004;78:992–7. discussion 997–998.
15. Wilkins KB, Sheikh E, Green R, Patel M, George S, Takano M, et al. Clinical and pathologic predictors of survival in patients with thymoma. Ann Surg. 1999;230:562–74.
16. Crucitti F, Doglietto GB, Bellantone R, Perri V, Tommasini O, Tonali P. Effects of surgical treatment in thymoma with myasthenia gravis: our experience in 103 patients. J Surg Oncol. 1992;50:43–6.
17. Filosso PL, Venuta F, Oliaro A, Ruffini E, Ruffini E, Rendina EA, Margaritora S, et al. Thymoma and inter-relationships between clinical variables: a multi Centre study in 537 patients. Eur J Cardiothorac Surg. 2014;45(6):1020–7.
18. Wang LS, Huang MH, Lin TS, Huang BS, Chien KY. Malignant thymoma. Cancer. 1992;70:443–50.
19. Nakagawa K, Asamura H, Matsuno Y, Suzuki K, Kondo H, Maeshima A, et al. Thymoma: a clinicopathologic study based on the new World Health Organization classification. J Thorac Cardiovasc Surg. 2003;126:1134–40.
20. Kondo K. MondenY. Therapy for thymic epithelial tumors: a clinical study of 1,320 patients from Japan. Ann Thorac Surg. 2003;76(3):878–84.
21. Venuta F, Rendina EA, Kepletko W, Rocco G. Surgical management of stage III thymic tumors. Thorac Surg Clin. 2011;21:85–91.
22. D'Andrilli A, Venuta F, Rendina EA. Surgical approaches for invasive tumors of the anterior mediastinum. Thorac Surg Clin. 2010;20:265–84.
23. D'Andrilli A, De Cecco CN, Maurizi G, Muscogiuri G, Baldini R, David V, et al. Reconstruction of the superior vena cava by biologic conduit: assessment of long term patency by magnetic resonance imaging. Ann Thorac Surg. 2013;96:1039–45.
24. Ishikawa Y, Matsuguma H, Nakahara R, Suzuki H, Ui A, Kondo T, et al. Multimodality therapy for patients with invasive thymoma disseminated into the pleural cavity: the potential role of extrapleural pneumonectomy. Ann Thorac Surg. 2009;88:952–7.
25. Lucchi M, Davini F, Ricciardi R, Duranti L, Boldrini L, Palmiero G, et al. Management of pleural recurrence after curative resection oh thymoma. J Thorac Cardiovasc Surg. 2009;137:1185–9.
26. Wright CD. Pleuropneumonectomy for the treatment of Masaoka stage IVA thymoma. Ann Thorac Surg. 2006;82:1234–9.
27. Nakahara K, Ohno K, Hashimoto J, Maeda H, Miyoshi S, Sakurai M, et al. Thymoma: results with complete resection and adjuvant postoperative irradiation in 141 consecutive patients. J Thorac Cardiovasc Surg. 1988;95:1041–7.
28. Wright CD, Choi NC, Wain JC, Mathisen DJ, Lynch TJ, Fidias P. Induction chemoradiotherapy followed by resection for locally advanced Masaoka stage III and IVA thymic tumors. Ann Thorac Surg. 2008;85:385–9.
29. Myojin M, Choi NC, Wright CD, Wain JC, Harris N, Hug EB, et al. Stage III thymoma: pattern of failure after surgery and postoperative radiotherapy and its implication for future study. Int J Radiat Oncol Biol Phys. 2000;46(4):927–33.
30. Rueckert J, Swierzy M, Badakhshi H, Meisel A, Ismail M. Robotic-assisted thymectomy: surgical procedure and results. Thorac Cardiovasc Surg. 2015;63(3):194–200.
31. Limmer KK, Kernstine KH. Minimally invasive and robotic-assisted thymus resection. Thorac Surg Clin. 2011;21(1):69–83.
32. Donahoe L, Keshavjee S. Video-assisted transcervical thymectomy for myasthenia gravis. Ann Cardiothorac Surg. 2015;4(6):561–3.
33. Shrager JB. Extended transcervical thymectomy: the ultimate minimally invasive approach. Ann Thorac Surg. 2010;89(6):S2128–34.
34. Khicha SG, Kaiser LR, Shrager JB. Extended transcervical thymectomy in the treatment of myasthenia gravis. Ann N Y Acad Sci. 2008;1132:336–43.
35. Kesler KA. Germ cell tumors of the mediastinum. In: Pearson GF, et al., editors. Thoracic and esophageal surgery. 3rd ed. Philadelphia: Elsevier; 2008.
36. Moran CA, Suster S. Primary germ cell tumors of the mediastinum: I. Analysis of 322 cases with special emphasis on teratomatous lesions and a proposal for histopathologic classification and clinical staging. Cancer. 1997;80:681–90.
37. Allen MS. Benign mediastinal germ cell tumors. In: Wood DE, Thomas Jr CR, editors. Mediastinal tumors. Berlin: Springer-Verlag; 1995. p. 41–2.
38. Shintani H, Funaki S, Nakagiri T. Experience with thoracoscopic resection for mature teratoma: a retrospective analysis of 15 patients. Interact Cardiovasc Thorac Surg. 2013;16:441–4.
39. Nichols CR. Mediastinal germ cell tumors: clinical features and biologic correlates. Chest. 1991;99:472–9.
40. Peterson CM, Buckley C, Holley S, Menias CO. Teratomas: a multimodality review. Curr Probl Diagn Radiol. 2012;41(6):210–9.
41. Weidner N. Germ-cell tumors of the mediastinum. Semin Diagn Pathol. 1999;16:42–50.
42. Heitmiller RF, Marasco WJ. Primary mediastinal seminoma. In: Wood DE, Thomas Jr CR, editors. Mediastinal tumors. Berlin: Springer-Verlag; 1995. p. 49–54.
43. Rivera C, Arame A, Jougon J, Velly JF, Begueret H, Dahan M, et al. Prognostic factors in patients with primary mediastinal germ cell tumors, a surgical multicenter retrospective study. Interact Cardiovasc Thorac Surg. 2010;11(5):585–9.
44. Takeda S, Miyoshi S, Ohta M, Minami M, Masaoka A, Matsuda H. Primary germ cell tumors in the mediastinum: a 50-year experience at a single Japanese institution. Cancer. 2003;97(2):367–76.
45. Kesler K, Einhorn L. Multimodality treatment of germ cell tumors of the mediastinum. Thorac Surg Clin. 2009;19:63–9.
46. Rodney AJ, Tannir NM, Siefker-Radtke AO, Liu P, Walsh GL, Millikan RE, et al. Survival outcomes for men with mediastinal germ-cell tumors: The University of Texas M. D. Anderson Cancer Center experience. Urol Oncol. 2012;30(6):879–85.
47. Liu Y, Wang Z, Peng ZM, Yu Y. Management of the primary malignant mediastinal germ cell tumors: experience with 54 patients. Diagn Pathol. 2014;19(9):33–9.
48. Kesler K, Rieger K, Hammoud Z, Kruter LE, Perkins SM, Turrentine MW, et al. A 25-year single institution experience with surgery for primary mediastinal nonseminomatous germ cell tumors. Ann Thorac Surg. 2008;85:371–8.
49. Sarkaria IS, Bains MS, Sood S, Sima CS, Reuter VE, Flores RM, et al. Resection of primary mediastinal non-seminomatous germ cell tumors: a 28-year experience at Memorial Sloan-Kettering Cancer Center. J Thorac Oncol. 2011;6(7):1236–41.
50. Riggs SB, Burgess EF, Gaston KE, Merwarth CA, Raghavan D. Postchemotherapy surgery for germ cell tumors--what have we learned in 35 years? Oncologist. 2014;19(5):498–506.
51. Vuky J, Bains M, Bacik J, Higgins G, Bajorin DF, Mazumdar M, et al. Role of post chemotherapy adjunctive surgery in the management of patients with nonseminoma arising from the mediastinum. J Clin Oncol. 2001;19:682–8.
52. Hartmann JT, Nichols CR, Droz JP, Horwich A, Gerl A, Fossa SD, et al. Prognostic variables for response and outcome in patients with extragonadal germ-cell tumors. Ann Oncol. 2002;13(7):1017–28.
53. Wang C. Parathyroid reexploration: a clinical and pathologic study of 112 cases. Ann Surg. 1977;186:140.
54. Wang C, Gaz R, Moncure A. Mediastinal parathyroid exploration: a clinical and pathologic study of 47 cases. World J Surg. 1986;10:687.
55. Peeler BB, Martin WH, Sandler MP, Goldstein RE. Sestamibi parathyroid scanning and preoperative localization studies for patients

with recurrent/persistent hyperparathyroidism or significant comorbid conditions: development of an optimal localization strategy. Am Surg. 1997;63:37.

56. Onoda N, Ishikawa T, Yamada N, Okamura T, Tahara H, Inaba M, et al. Radioisotope-navigated video-assisted thoracoscopic operation for ectopic mediastinal parathyroid. Surgery. 2002;132:17–9.
57. Norton J, Schneider P, Brennan M. Median sternotomy in reoperations for primary hyperparathyroidism. World J Surg. 1985;9:807.
58. Smythe WR, Bavaria JE, Hall RA, Kline GM, Kaiser LR. Thoracoscopic removal of mediastinal parathyroid adenoma. Ann Thorac Surg. 1995;59:236–8.
59. Occhipinti H, Heidinger BH, Franquet E, Eisenber RL, Bankier AA. Imaging the posterior mediastinum: a multimodality approach. Diagn Interv Radiol. 2015;21(4):293–306.
60. Vargas D, Suby-Long T, Restrepo CS. Cystic lesions of the mediastinum. Semin Ultrasound CT MR. 2016;37(3):212–22.
61. Lee JY, Lee KS, Han J. Spectrum of neurogenic tumors in the thorax: CT and pathologic findings. J Comput Assist Tomogr. 1999;23(3):399–406.
62. Reeder LB. Neurogenic tumors of the mediastinum. Semin Thorac Cardiovasc Surg. 2000;12:261–7.
63. Bicakcioglu P, Demirag F, Yazicioglu A, Aydogdu K, Kaya S, Karaoglanoglu N. Intrathoracic neurogenic tumors. Thorac Cardiovasc Surg. 2014;62(2):147–52.
64. Liu R, Adler DG. Duplication cysts: diagnosis, management, and the role of endoscopic ultrasound. Endoscopic Ultrasound. 2014;3:152–60.
65. McAdams HP, Kirejczyk WM, Rosado-de-Christenson ML, Matsumoto S. Bronchogenic cyst: imaging features with clinical and histopathologic correlation. Radiology. 2000;217(2):441–6.
66. Jung HS, Kim DK, Lee GD, Sim HJ, Choi SH, Kim HR, et al. Video-assisted thoracic surgery for bronchogenic cysts: is this the surgical approach of choice? Interact Cardiovasc Thorac Surg. 2014;19(5):824–9.
67. Takeda S, Miyoshi S, Minami M, Matsuda H. Intrathoracic neurogenic tumors--50 years' experience in a Japanese institution. Eur J Cardiothorac Surg. 2004;26(4):807–12.
68. Cardillo G, Carleo F, Khalil MW, Carbone L, Treggiari S, Salvadori L, et al. Surgical treatment of benign neurogenic tumours of the mediastinum: a single institution report. Eur J Cardiothorac Surg. 2008;34(6):1210–4.
69. Pavlus JD, Carter BW, Tolley MD, Keung ES, Khorashadi L, Lichtenberg JP. Imaging of thoracic neurogenic tumors. AJR Am J Roentgenol. 2016;207(3):552–61.
70. Shadmehr MB, Gaissert HA, Wain JC, Moncure AC, Grillo HC, Borges LF, et al. The surgical approach to "dumbbell tumors" of the mediastinum. Ann Thorac Surg. 2003;76(5):1650–4.
71. Rakovich R, Deslauriers J. Video-assisted and minimally-invasive open chest surgery for the treatment of mediastinal tumors and masses. Vis Surg. 2017;3:25–37.
72. Pacchiarotti G, Wang MY, Kolcun JPG, Chang KH, Al Maaieh M, Reis VS, et al. Robotic paravertebral schwannoma resection at extreme locations of the thoracic cavity. Neurosurg Focus. 2017;42(5):E17.
73. Melfi F, Fanucchi O, Davini F, Viti A, Lucchi M, Ambrogi MC, et al. Ten-year experience of mediastinal robotic surgery in a single referral Centre. Eur J Cardiothorac Surg. 2012;41(4):847–51.
74. Li Y, Wang J. Experience of video-assisted thoracoscopic resection for posterior mediastinal neurogenic tumours: a retrospective analysis of 58 patients. ANZ J Surg. 2013;83(9):664–8.
75. Nam KH, Ahn HY, Cho JS, Kim YD, Choi BK, Han IH. One stage posterior minimal laminectomy and video-assisted Thoracoscopic surgery (VATS) for removal of thoracic dumbbell tumor. J Korean Neurosurg Soc. 2017;60(2):257–61.
76. Vallieres E, Findlay JM, Fraser RE. Combined microneurosurgical and thoracoscopic removal of neurogenic dumbbell tumors. Ann Thorac Surg. 1995;59:469–72.
77. Torres-Mora J, Dry S, Li X, Binder S, Amin M, Folpe AL. Malignant melanotic schwannian tumor: a clinicopathologic, immunohistochemical, and gene expression profiling study of 40 cases, with a proposal for the reclassification of "melanotic schwannoma.". Am J Surg Pathol. 2014;38(1):94–105.
78. Ortega P, Suster D, Falconieri G, Zambrano E, Moran CA, Morrison C, et al. Liposarcomas of the posterior mediastinum: clinicopathologic study of 18 cases. Mod Pathol. 2015;28(5):721–31.

Benign Tumors and Tumor-Like Conditions

4

Introduction

The tumors that this chapter encompasses represent a diverse group of lesions that do not necessarily have much in common as a group. Thus, the lesions will be grouped in many cases by the gross appearance and presentation and when possible by the main histopathological features. Needless to say, the lesions for the most part are unusual tumors in the mediastinal compartment, and in some instances, only a few cases have been described in the literature.

In order to facilitate their study, this chapter will discuss three separate types of tumors, which have been separated into three main categories:

1. Cystic tumors
2. Solid tumors and tumor-like conditions
3. Histiocytic tumors

Cystic Tumors

Cystic tumors in the mediastinum in general are rare, and in many instances, more common tumors in this region will present with cystic changes, which makes interpretation a challenge. Examples of such an occurrence would include cystic thymomas and thymic carcinomas as well as lymphomas, namely, Hodgkin lymphoma and MALT lymphoma. However, the descriptions of the lesions in this section will be exclusively those not associated with other malignant neoplasms, as those specific tumoral conditions have been discussed elsewhere in this text.

In general, the true incidence of mediastinal cysts is difficult to estimate, as in the majority of reports of cystic tumors, these lesions have been placed among other tumors, which although cystic belong to other group of tumors. For instance, the reports of mediastinal cysts commonly include germ cell tumors, namely, cystic teratomatous tumors and less common lymphoproliferative tumors.

In addition, as these cystic tumors are benign, their reports are less likely to occur unless the cyst has an unusual pathology associated with it, which in many cases would be an associated malignant neoplasm. In this section, to facilitate their study and also likely to reflect our daily practice, we have divided these cystic tumors into three different groups. In addition, in order to facilitate sub-categorization, they have been separated by the presence of cyst lining, which becomes an essential part of the proper interpretation of these cystic tumors. It is also important to highlight that in a number of cases, it is difficult to identify specific epithelium, which at times can make the interpretation of a specific cyst much more difficult, thus leaving the generic name of "benign foregut cyst." The lack of identification of specific cyst lining may be due to several reasons, including poor sampling. Thus, an emphasis will be placed on the proper identification of a cyst lining to adequately diagnose these tumors.

Based on the above explanation, we can separate these cystic tumors into these specific categories:

1. Foregut cysts
   (a) Bronchogenic cyst
   (b) Esophageal cyst
   (c) Enteric cyst
2. Mesothelial cysts
   (a) Pericardial cyst
   (b) Pleural cyst
3. Thymic cyst
   (a) Unilocular
   (b) Multilocular

Foregut Cysts

This type of cystic tumor appears to be the most common benign cyst in the mediastinum and specifically will include bronchogenic, esophageal, and enteric (neurenteric) cysts. All these cysts are the result of developmental

© Springer Nature Switzerland AG 2019
N. Kalhor, C. Moran, *Mediastinal Pathology*, https://doi.org/10.1007/978-3-319-98980-8_4

errors during early embryogenesis. It is approximately around the 26th day of gestation that the respiratory and esophageal elements start developing. Approximately in the 6th week, primitive lung buds begin to form; it is an embryological error in the budding that may give rise to bronchogenic cyst. Early embryological errors in the budding process may give rise to mediastinal cysts, while late errors in the development may give rise to peripheral and parenchymal cysts. Embryological errors in the development of the laryngotracheal diverticulum also may give rise to esophageal cysts.

In 1945, Laipply [1] reviewed the literature on cysts and cystic tumors of the mediastinum, dividing these cystic tumors into two main categories: congenital and acquired. Among the congenital types, the author included dermoid, epidermoid cysts, teratoma, and cystic lymphangioma among the classical foregut cysts. Regarding bronchogenic cysts (bronchial cysts), it is of interest that the authors provided an account of 34 cases reported in the literature up to 1944, 19 males and 14 females (2 unknown) ranging from one stillborn to patients over the age of 60-years. Clinically, symptoms of airway obstruction were identified in some patients, while in 16 of the 35 reported cases, the patients were asymptomatic. In two cases, the cysts were incidentally discovered during an autopsy procedure. In addition, the author included within the description of "gastroenteric cysts" gastric, enteric, and esophageal cysts. In Laipply's [1] review of the literature up to 1944, only 12 cases of mediastinal gastric cysts had been reported plus a couple of additional cases by the author, totaling 14 cases accounting for 8 males and 5 females (1 patient's gender was not provided), and all these patients were children of no more than 10 years. The symptoms of these patients were similar to other cystic mediastinal lesions and usually attributed to compression of adjacent structures including dyspnea, cyanosis, dysphagia, and hemoptysis. Regarding enteric cysts, the author noted that the reported cases in the literature up to 1944 were even less than other cysts with only 3 cases reported with an additional 2 probable cases. Three of these cases were in stillborn, and the two other cases were in children under 1 year of age. However, Schwarz and Williams [2] in 1942 reported 2 cases of what the authors described as thoracic gastric cysts and accounted for 12 previous cases with similar histological findings. It is possible that the discrepancy in the number of cases reported is due to the strict criteria of having mixed enteric and respiratory epithelium or more strict criteria of only gastric epithelium. In any case, Schwarz and Williams [2] divided these cystic tumors into functional and nonfunctional cysts, being that 5 of the 12 previously reported cases were in the category of functional cyst. All these functional cysts were described in children under 10 years of age except for one case in a 23 year old. Anatomically, all these cystic tumors were located in the posterior mediastinum. In 1946, Blades [3] reported cases treated at Army Thoracic Surgery Centers in the USA, and the author accounted for 109 patients who had been operated upon for mediastinal tumors during a period of approximately 3 years. The author noted that the cases included represented cases of individuals either with clinical symptoms or who had a mass discovered by chest films after entering active duty military service. The author included in this report 94 benign and 15 malignant tumors. Of those 94 benign tumors, 23 were bronchogenic cysts. This finding is of interest taking into account Laipply's review of the literature up to 1944, which accounted for only 34 cases recorded up to that time [1]. Clinically, the patients presented with cough and chest pain; however, in the majority of cases, the mass was discovered during a routine chest roentgenologic examination. In addition, only 1 out of 94 benign tumors corresponded to an esophageal cyst. In 1958, Richards and Reeves [4] presented a study of mediastinal cysts and tumors during a period of 25 years (1930–1955), reporting 14 cases in children from birth to 14 years of age. However, the authors only described three cases in detail corresponding to one enterogenous cyst, one bronchial cyst, and one intrapericardial teratoma. In 1963, Pachter and Lattes [5] presented their experience by reporting 20 cases of mediastinal cysts. The authors described cystic tumors consisting of eight bronchogenic cysts, three gastric cysts, four pericardial cysts, and four undesignated cysts. The bronchogenic cysts were identified in five women and three men ranging from 1 month to 66 years of age. Six of these tumors were located in the posterior mediastinum and ranged in size from 2 to 15 cm. Four patients were asymptomatic, and four patients presented with symptoms of chest pain and dyspnea. Interestingly, the authors noted that only in one of the bronchogenic cysts was the presence of cartilage identified, while one case had the classic unilocular architecture. On the other hand, all gastric cysts occurred in children under 1 year of age: two females and one male. One was asymptomatic, while two presented with melena, hematemesis, abdominal colic, and cyanosis. All these gastric cysts were located in the posterior mediastinum. Wychulis and colleagues [6] presented a 40-year experience with mediastinal tumors from a single institution over a period ranging from 1929 to 1968. All the cases reported in this study represented cases in which an exploratory thoracotomy had been performed, omitting any cases in which only a biopsy specimen was available for diagnosis. Based on these criteria, the authors identified 1064 patients ranging in age from infancy to the ninth decade of life, with approximately 8% of patients under 15 years of age. No gender predilection was identified. Although this report includes many tumoral conditions, the authors identified approximately 18% of these mediastinal tumors as "benign cysts." The authors grouped bronchogenic cysts, esophageal cysts, and gastric (intestinal) cysts under the designation of "enterogenous cysts." In this group, the author identified 83 cases (54 bronchogenic cysts, 27 esophageal cysts, and 2 gastric cysts) in 46 males and 37 females within the ages of 2 months and 64 years of age. The majority of these patients were asymptomatic. Important to mention is the fact that, in 17 cases, it was not possible to identify the cyst lining, and the cysts were labeled as "non-specific cysts." Oldham [7] also analyzed 330 patients with mediastinal tumors and cysts from two different institutions, encountering that 25% of these tumors corresponded to mediastinal cysts including pericardial, bronchogenic, enteric, and non-specific. The author further analyzed 1000 previously reported cases in the literature of mediastinal tumors and cysts, arriving at an estimated incidence of 21% for mediastinal cysts including pericardial, bronchogenic, enteric, and non-specific. In a report of 105 cases in patients less than 16 years of age, over a period ranging from 1935 to 1968, Whittaker and Lynn [8] identified only 12 cystic tumors corresponding to bronchogenic cysts and "alimentary tract duplications." Davis and colleagues [9] analyzed 400 consecutive patients with primary mediastinal lesions over a period from 1930 to 1986. The patients were 212 males and 188 females ranging in age from 7 days to 83 years of age. The authors identified 99 (25%) of patients with primary cystic lesions including 39 bronchogenic cysts, 11 enteric cysts, and 36 pericardial cysts. The authors concluded that primary cysts are the most common lesions in the middle mediastinum, 60% in their account; however, these cystic lesions included the benign cyst and also other mesenchymal lesions, lymphomas, and carcinomas. On the other hand, benign cysts including bronchogenic and enteric cysts occurred in their experience in about 34% of the cases. Reed and Sobonya [10] analyzed 86 foregut cysts in the thorax, identifying 75 cases in the mediastinum and 11 cases in intrapulmonary location. The 75 foregut cysts corresponded to 66 bronchogenic and 9 enteric cysts; 58 of the bronchogenic cysts were located in the anterior and 8 in the posterior mediastinum, while 8 of the 9 enteric cysts were located in the posterior mediastinum. Associated anomalies such as vertebral body anomalies were observed in the enteric cysts. From the radiological point of view, some reports have emphasized the imaging features of these cystic lesions [10–12]. Nakata and colleagues [11] reported seven patients with bronchogenic cysts in which computed tomography was available showing that the two cysts had homogeneous high-density areas, while four patients had low-density areas. All cases had similar water density masses on chest radiography. In a radiological-pathological correlation presented by Madewell and colleagues [12], the authors described a neurenteric cyst in the posterior mediastinum, which radiologically had a smooth surface and homogeneous density with no calcification or lucency. Reed and Sobonya [10] provided radiographic features for the 86 cases that they evaluated, showing that most of the cysts were solid and of homogeneous water density. Air was contained in four bronchogenic cysts and one enteric cyst; no calcifications were identified within the cysts, but peripheral calcifications occasionally occurred in both bronchogenic and enteric cysts.

More recent reviews on this topic have been presented in the literature [13–15]. In a general review of cystic lesions of the mediastinum, Wick [13] stated that bronchogenic cysts might occur at any age with no gender predilection; in the mediastinum, these cysts are usually asymptomatic and detected on routine chest films. Wick [13] also added that enteric cysts typically occur in children under 15 years of age and common symptoms would include dysphagia among others. The reviews provided by Wright and Petroze [14, 15] essentially reiterated similar findings as those of Wick and others.

Based on previous and current literature, surgical resection appears the treatment of choice for these cystic tumors, and complete surgical resection appears to be curative. In cases in which a fatal outcome has been documented, it appears that it may have been related to a postoperative outcome rather than to the malignant potential of the cystic lesion.

Pathological Features

Macroscopically, these cystic lesions are either unilocular or septated, and in general they are round to oval masses. Bronchogenic cysts may be composed of thin walls containing clear fluid and mucoid material, or they may have a solid appearance. The size of these tumors may also vary from a few centimeters to more than 10 cm in greatest dimension. Bronchogenic cysts may be attached to the carina or bronchus by a stalk. Also, enteric cysts may be unilocular or septated cystic lesions with thick walls and corrugated lining. The size of enteric cysts is similar to that of bronchogenic cysts.

Histologically, the identification of specific epithelium will aid in the specific designation for these cystic tumors.

Bronchogenic Cyst

Typically, they are lined by respiratory epithelium (ciliated pseudo stratified). However, in some cases, the ciliated epithelium may be absent. The walls of the cyst are composed of fibroconnective tissue, which may contain mucous glands, hyaline cartilage, and smooth muscle. Marked inflammatory reaction is not a feature of these cysts. Some cases have been described as not containing hyaline cartilage (Figs. 4.1, 4.2, 4.3, 4.4, and 4.5).

Enteric Cyst

Typically, these cysts will show intestinal epithelium, but more often the epithelium is gastric, which may contain all the gastric layers including mucosa, muscularis mucosae, submucosa, and serosa. The mucosa may show branching glands containing parietal and chief cells (Figs. 4.6, 4.7, 4.8, 4.9, 4.10, and 4.11).

Esophageal Cysts

Typically, these cysts will be lined by squamous type of epithelium. The cystic walls are composed of fibroconnective tissue, which in some instances may contain mucous glands and layers of smooth muscle. In some of the cases described in the literature, a mixed type of epithelium has been described showing squamous and respiratory epithelium (Fig. 4.12).

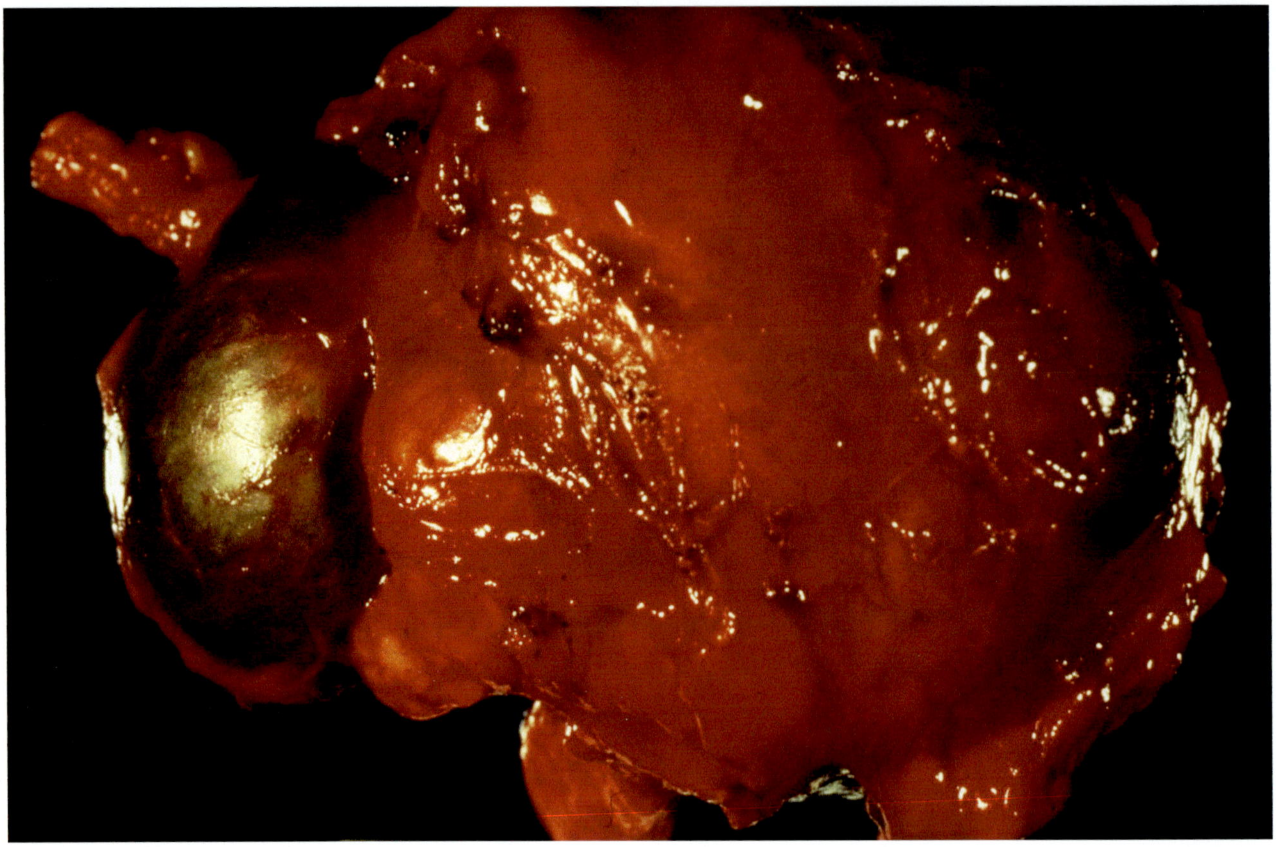

Fig. 4.1 Large bronchogenic cyst; note the well circumscription of the lesion

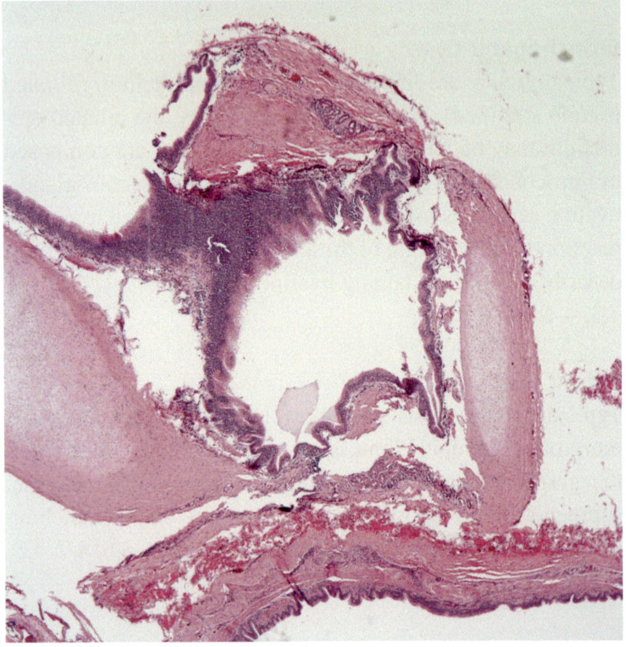

Fig. 4.2 Low power view of a bronchogenic cyst showing cystic structures and cartilage

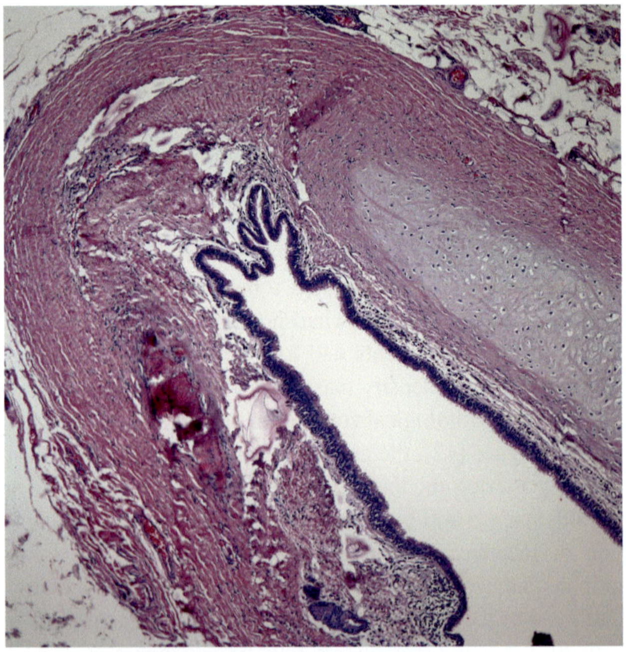

Fig. 4.3 Bronchogenic cyst showing respiratory type of epithelium lining and cartilage

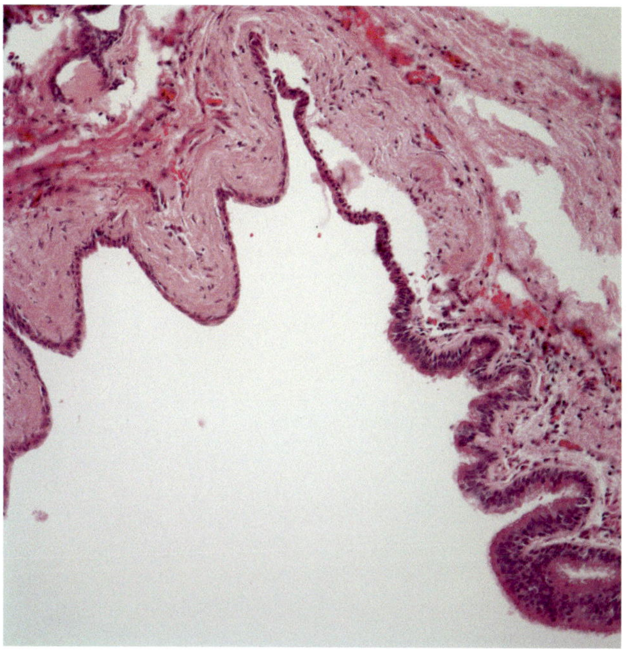

Fig. 4.4 Bronchogenic cyst showing transitional areas of respiratory epithelium and flatten cuboidal epithelium

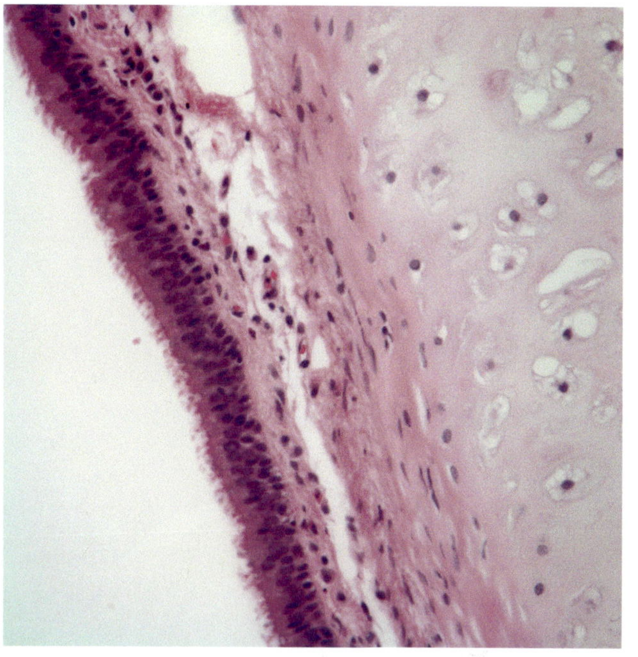

Fig. 4.5 Higher magnification of a bronchogenic cyst showing ciliated epithelium and cartilage

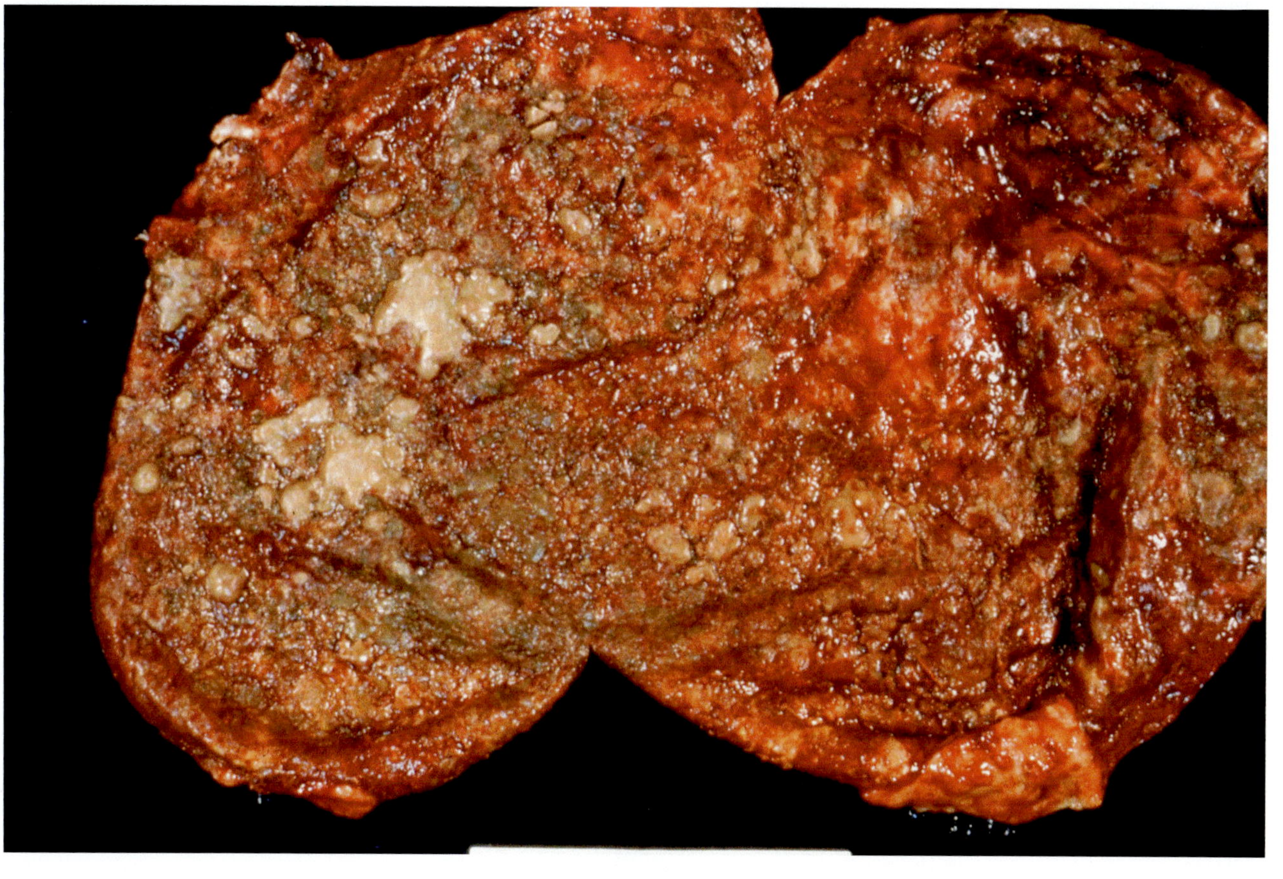

Fig. 4.6 Enteric cyst showing a corrugated surface

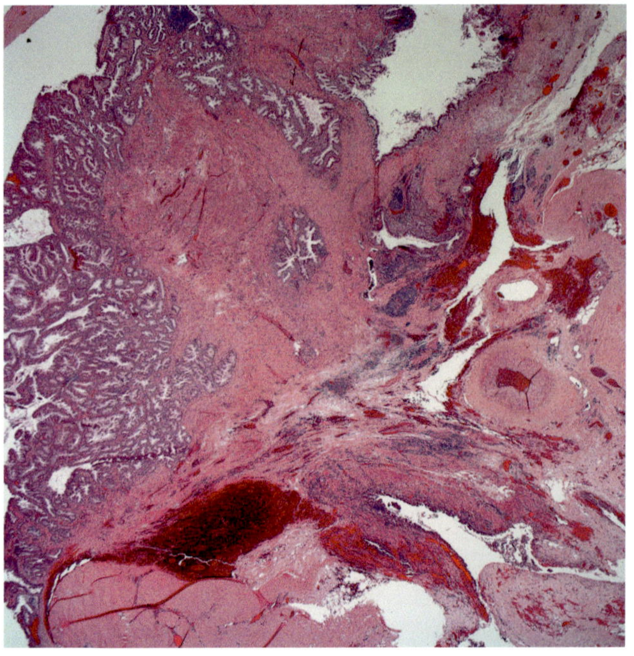

Fig. 4.7 Low power view of an enteric cyst showing cystic structures and enteric epithelium

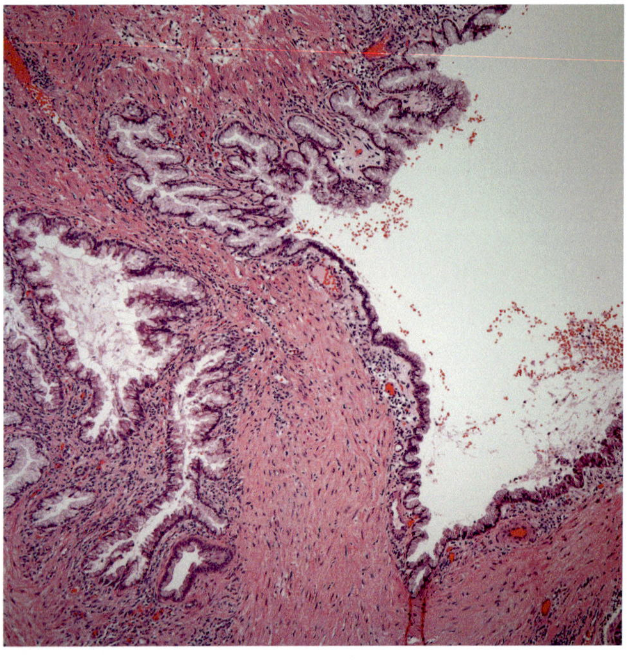

Fig. 4.8 Enteric cyst in which the cystic structures are lined by columnar epithelium

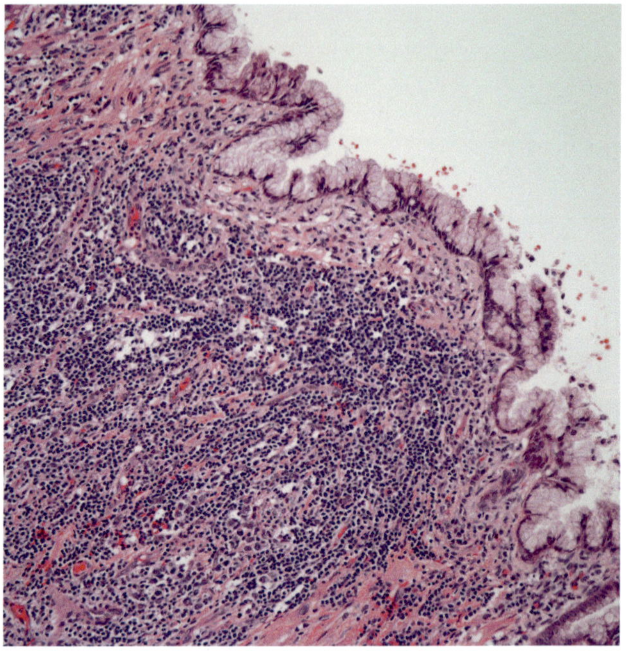

Fig. 4.9 Closer view of an enteric cyst showing columnar epithelium and inflammatory changes in the cystic wall

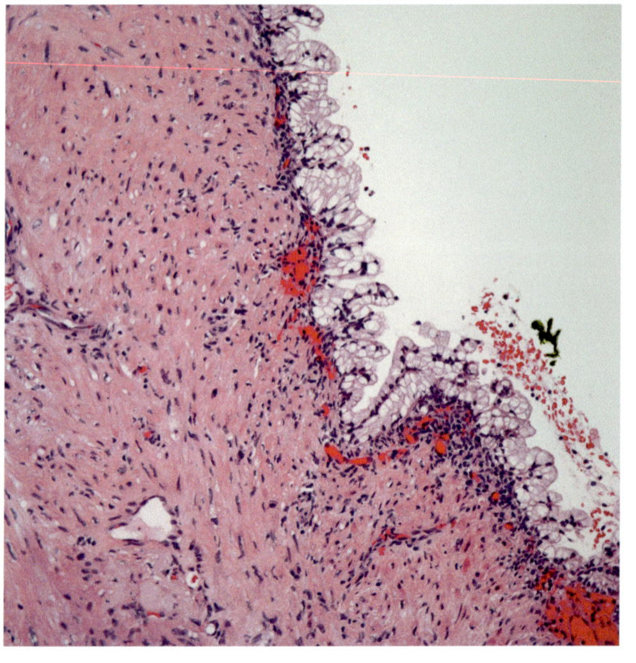

Fig. 4.10 Enteric cyst lined by columnar epithelium and absence of inflammatory reaction in the wall of the cyst

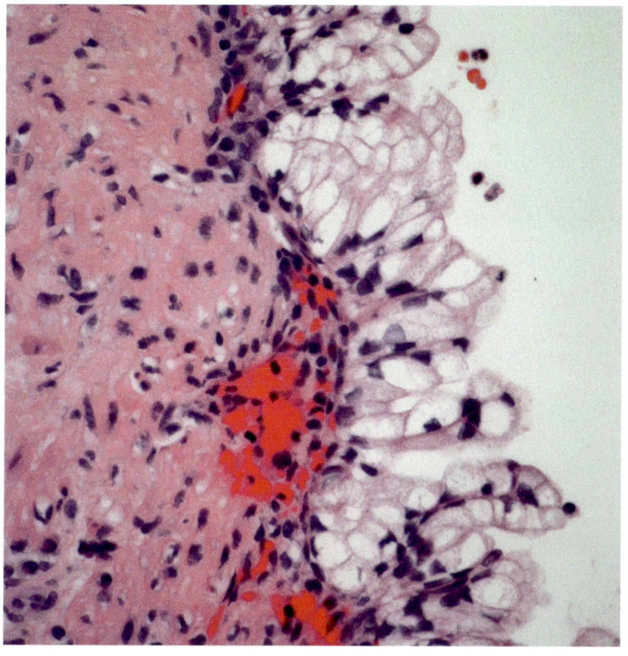

Fig. 4.11 Closer view of the lining of an enteric cysts showing columnar epithelium

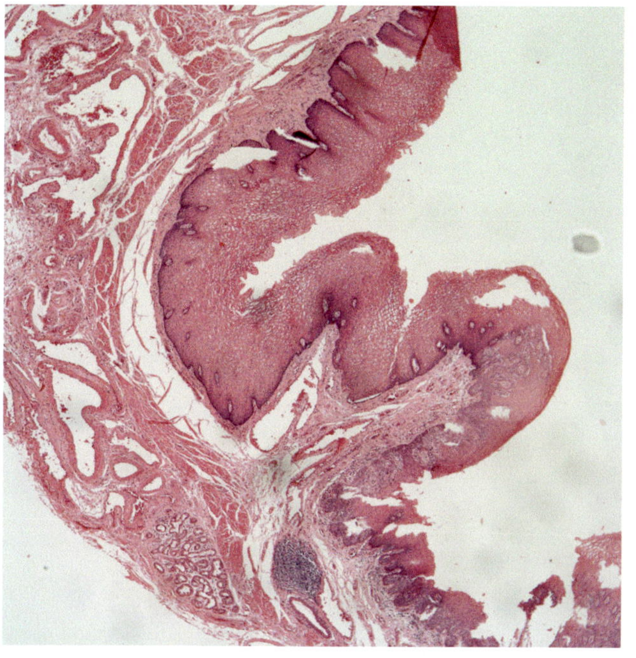

Fig. 4.12 Esophageal cyst showing squamous type of lining

Unclassified Foregut Cyst

This designation is left for a group of cystic tumors in which no specific type of lining is identified. Important to highlight is the need for proper sampling of these lesions in order to unequivocally state that there is no specific lining and not to classify them into the well-known groups.

Immunohistochemical Features

The use of immunohistochemical stains in the diagnosis of foregut cyst is limited and has little diagnostic value. The use of markers such as TTF-1, keratin, and CDX-2 would provide the results of the different types of epithelium whether that is respiratory or enteric. However, the use of these markers is not needed as one can easily identify those types of epitheliums, and the use of these markers has only academic value.

Mesothelial Cysts

This group of benign cysts predominantly occurs in the pericardium and in the pleura. In some instances, they are referred to as pleuropericardial cysts as they share the same type of lining. It is believed that pericardial cysts result from an anomalous development of the pericardium. In the review by Blades [3], the author described ten pericardial cysts in adult patients, all of them asymptomatic. However, in some cases, patients may present with symptoms of chest pain [16]. In the review by Pachter and Lattes [5], the authors stated that pericardial cyst was the second most common after bronchogenic cysts and accounted for four cases, three men and one woman between the ages of 36 and 64-years. The cysts are usually found in the cardiophrenic angle on the left side, adjacent to the pericardium, diaphragm, and anterior chest wall. In the review of mediastinal tumors and cysts by Oldham [7], the author identified 33 cases of pericardial cysts among 330 patients, while Davis and colleagues [9] identified 36 out of 400 consecutive patients over a period of 56 years. In a more specific study on pericardial cysts, Wychulis and colleagues [17] identified 72 patients: 38 women and 34 men between the ages of 17 and 73-years; however, the cysts were less common in patients under the age of 20. Clinically, 54 patients were asymptomatic, and the cysts were discovered incidentally during routine chest films. In 17 patients, symptoms of substernal and precordial pain and palpitations were present. In addition, there were no electrocardiographic abnormalities that could be attributed to the cysts. Anatomically, 53 cysts were located in the right side and 19 in the left, while 54 of the 72 cysts were located in the cardiophrenic angle. The cysts located more superiorly were adherent to the aortic arch and superior vena cava. Feigin and colleagues [18] reported the radiographic findings of 41 pericardial cysts, showing that one third of the patients had symptoms of chest pain, dyspnea, and persistent cough. In addition, the authors stated that in 35 cases the cyst was visualized as a round radiodensity touching both the hemidiaphragm and anterior chest wall. In 15 of 41 cysts, the cysts occurred in the left border of the heart. In six cases, the cysts were difficult to diagnose and were confused with other common tumors such as thymomas among others.

Complete surgical resection is the treatment of choice for these cystic tumors and appears to be curative.

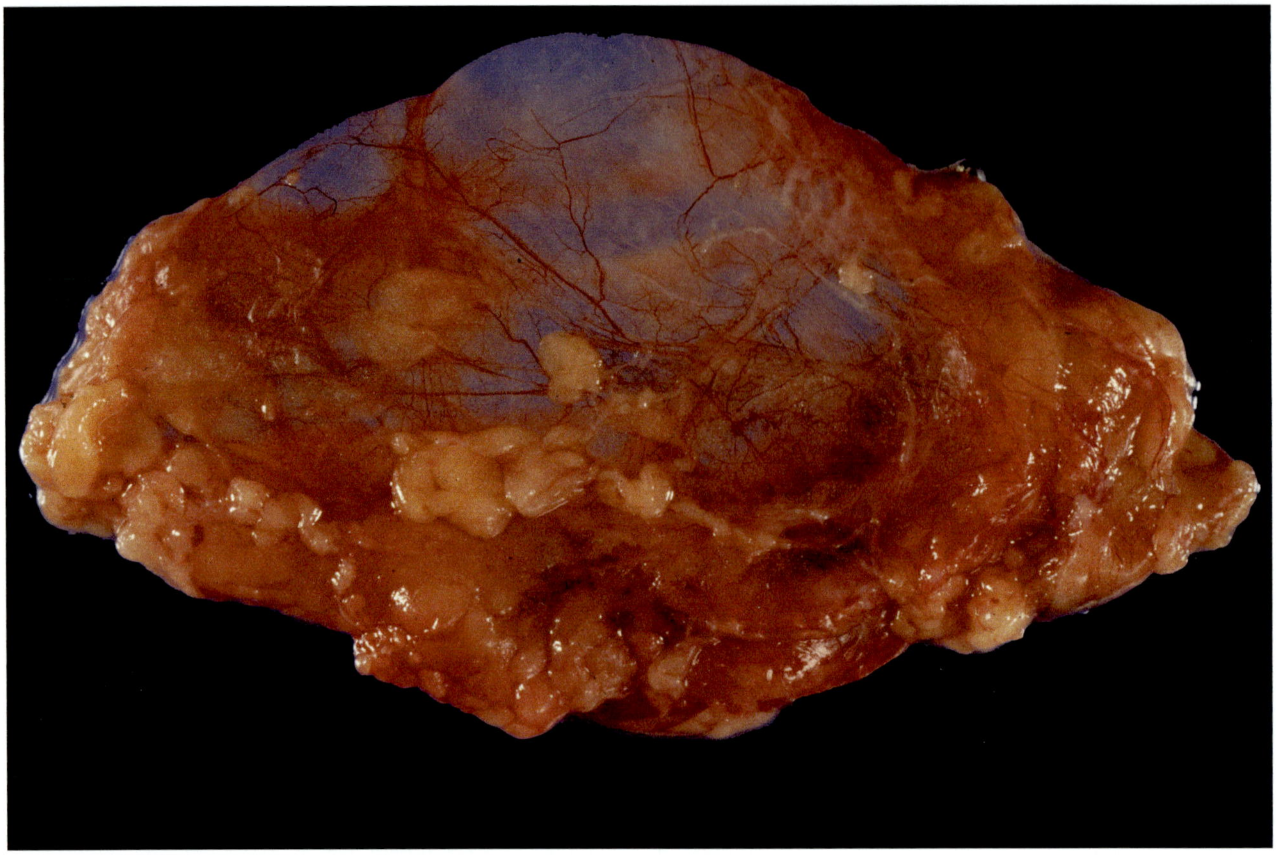

Fig. 4.13 Mesothelial cyst showing a unilocular cyst surrounded by adipose tissue

Pathological Features

Macroscopically, they are thin-walled cystic lesions, most of the time uniloculated (Fig. 4.13). However, unusual cases may show a multilobated appearance. In either case, the cysts may contain clear or yellowish fluid. In some cases, communication with the pericardial cavity has been observed. The size of these cysts is variable and may range from a few centimeters to more than 10 cm in greatest diameter.

Histologically, the wall of the cyst is composed of fibroconnective tissue lined by a single layer of mesothelium. The cyst walls rarely show marked inflammatory reaction (Figs. 4.14, 4.15, and 4.16).

The use of immunohistochemical stains including keratin 5/6 and calretinin may aid in the identification of the mesothelial lining.

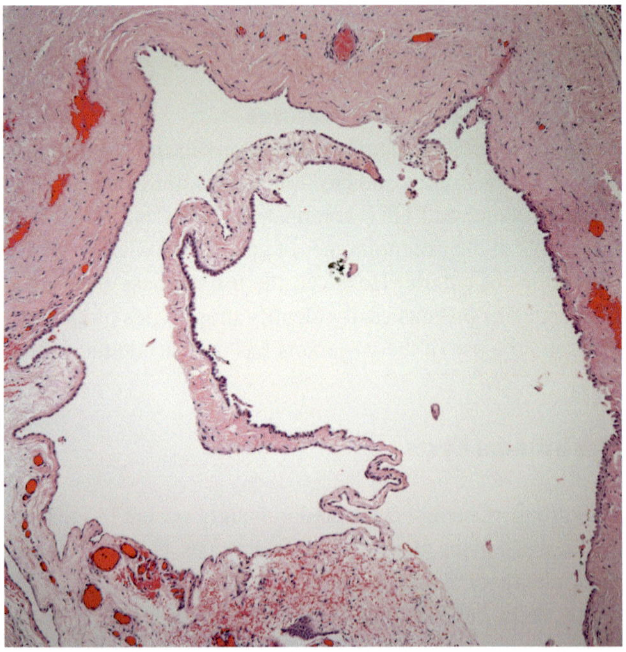

Fig. 4.14 Low power view of a mesothelial cyst showing a cystic structure lined by mesothelium

Thymic Cysts

Essentially, there are two types of thymic cysts that likely have different histogenesis. These two types include unilocular and multilocular thymic cysts. There have been several theories to account for the occurrence of these thymic cysts [19–22], mainly unilocular thymic cysts, including the persistence of remnants of the branchial cleft epithelium dragged downward with the thymus anlage, arising from the failure of the original thymic tubule to lose its lumen, further differentiation of the thymic cord into tubules, distension of Hassall's corpuscles, regressive changes in Hassall's corpus-

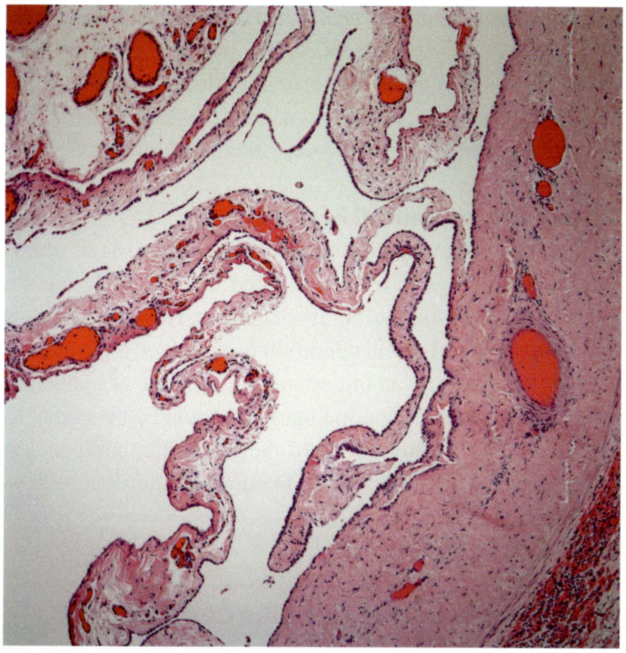

Fig. 4.15 Mesothelial cysts with several cystic structures lined by mesothelial lining

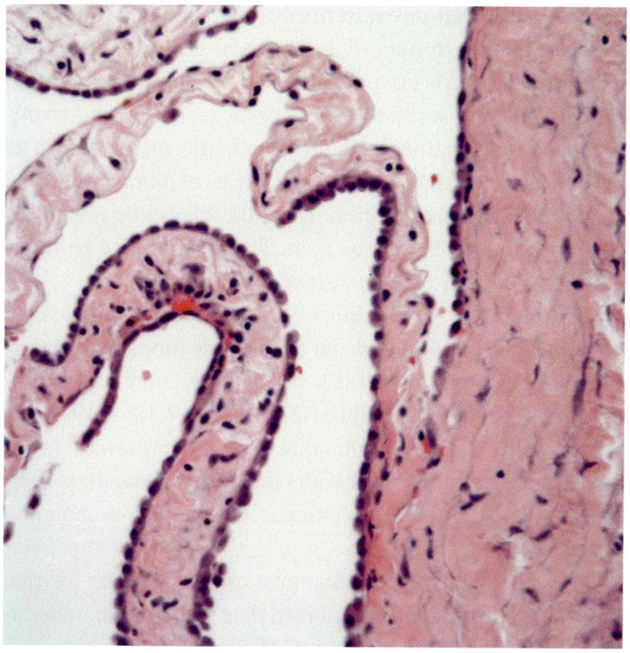

Fig. 4.16 Higher magnification of the mesothelial lining showing lack of atypia

cles, or necrosis of the medullary tissue, producing "sequestral cysts." However, it is believed that unilocular thymic cysts are congenital in nature [13, 15]. In the review by Pachter and Lattes [5], the authors stated that, up to 1959, only 23 cases of thymic cysts had been reported in the literature, and, of those, 19 were in the mediastinum. In addition, in their account of reporting 20 cases of mediastinal cysts, the authors found only one case of thymic cyst. According to their description, the thymic cyst belonged to the unilocular type. In the review by Wychulis and colleagues [6] encompassing 40 years of experience, the authors described 19 thymic cysts occurring in 10 females and 9 males ranging in age from 7 months to 79 years. Only two patients were younger than 30 years. Most of these patients were asymptomatic. According to the authors, 12 cysts were unilocular, while 7 cysts were multilocular thymic cysts. In this report, no specific details regarding these cysts were provided. In general, it is believed that unilocular thymic cysts represent congenital cysts, while multilocular thymic cysts represent acquired lesions. They can occur in any age group but appear to be more common between 20 and 50 years of age [13]. On the other hand, multilocular thymic cysts have been the focus of more specific reports. The largest series of multilocular thymic cysts is the one presented by Suster and Rosai [23] in which the authors studied 18 such cases and suggested that the features present in these cystic lesions argue in favor of this lesion perhaps being the result of cystic transformation of medullary duct epithelium-derived structures induced by an inflammatory process. The patients described included 15 men and 3 women between the ages of 15 and 76 years. The majority of patients were asymptomatic, and, upon imaging, the lesions were sharply demarcated from mediastinal fat and soft tissues. Patients with symptoms included such symptoms as chest pain and dyspnea. All the cysts were located in the anterior mediastinum, and surgical resection was performed in all. Important to highlight is that even though most patients with thymic cysts are asymptomatic, acute symptomatology such as cardiac tamponade has been reported [24]. Equally important to highlight is that contrary to unilocular thymic cysts or other mediastinal cysts, multilocular thymic cysts have the potential to recur. In the series of 18 cases reported by Suster and Rosai [23], the authors documented three cases in which the lesion had recurred; in one case, it had recurred numerous times. It is significant to call attention to the fact that the treatment modality in three patients was surgical resection followed by radiation therapy, while in one patient, it was surgical resection followed by chemotherapy. Although the majority of the cases described corresponded to a benign cystic tumor, in four cases an additional neoplasm was identified within the walls of the cysts: two thymomas and two basaloid carcinomas. In the remaining cases, surgical resection of the tumors was performed, which appears to be the treatment of choice for these patients.

Pathological Features

Unilocular thymic cyst as its name implies is generally a round to oval cystic tumor that ranges in size from 1 to more than 15 cm in greatest dimension. They are generally present with a smooth outer surface containing clear to yellowish fluid or in some cases hemorrhagic fluid. The internal surface of the cyst is usually smooth and shiny. The cystic wall is usually thin. On the contrary, multilocular thymic cysts appear to be well-circumscribed cystic tumors, which can measure from 3 to more than 15 cm in greatest dimension. The outer surface is tan-gray and focally hemorrhagic, soft to rubbery. The cut surface of these cystic lesions shows multiloculated cavities filled with turbid or hemorrhagic fluid. The cyst walls are usually thick, and areas of fibrosis may be seen. In some cases, adhesions to the pleura or other surrounding structures may be seen. This feature may be occasionally confused with metastatic disease.

Histologically, the features of the unilocular thymic cyst are rather straight forward and do not pose problems in interpretation. The cyst's wall can be lined by columnar, cuboidal, or squamous epithelium (Figs. 4.17, 4.18, 4.19, 4.20, and 4.21). However, the epithelial lining often shows skipped areas. In addition, the cyst walls may show cholesterol cleft granulomas, degenerating cellular debris, and granulation tissue.

The histopathological features of multilocular thymic cysts are somewhat more complex than those of the unilocular variant. In general, the gamut of changes that can be seen in multilocular thymic cysts includes not only the multiple cystic structures, which can be lined by cuboidal, squamous, or columnar epithelium, but also the presence of germinal centers, lymphoid hyperplasia, cholesterol cleft granulomas, remnant of residual thymic epithelium, and areas in which the inflammatory reaction may appear as invading adipose tissue. The presence of normal or dilated Hassall's corpuscles and areas of fibrosis with inflammatory reaction are commonly identified. Calcifications and hyalinization are seen in some cases (Figs. 4.22a, b, 4.23, 4.24, 4.25, 4.26, 4.27, 4.28, 4.29, 4.30, 4.31, 4.32, 4.33, and 4.34). One important feature that has been described and that may pose significant problems in interpretation is the presence of pseudoepitheliomatous hyperplasia. Suster and colleagues [25] reported the presence of this histological feature in six cases of multilocular thymic cysts characterized by the presence of exuberant proliferation of the cyst lining epithelium, which show atypical squamous cells with large hyperchromatic nuclei, prominent nucleoli, and scattered mitotic figures. The remaining features in these cases were those of multilocular thymic cysts. However, such findings do not appear to influence the outcome in these cystic tumors.

Differential Diagnosis

Contrary to other mediastinal cysts, which are relatively easy to interpret by identifying the lining epithelium, multilocular thymic cysts may pose some challenges in interpretation, either because of the lesions may show prominent lymphoid hyperplasia, which in the setting of a cystic tumor may be confused with a MALT lymphoma, or because of the presence of atypical squamous epithelium, which can be confused with a cystic squamous cell carcinoma. However, the most important issue to note in the diagnosis of multilocular thymic cyst is the generous sampling that must take place. It is not infrequent that malignant tumors, either primary or metastatic, have features similar to those of multilocular thymic cysts [26–34]. Therefore, it is imperative that a reasonable sampling takes place in order to not miss an associated malignancy.

Immunohistochemical Features

The use of immunohistochemistry in the diagnosis of multilocular thymic cysts is rather limited and basically has no value as a diagnostic tool for its diagnosis. However, in cases in which another tumoral condition is suspected to be associated, it then becomes an important tool. The use of epithelial, lymphoid, or neuroendocrine markers would be beneficial to rule out the possibility of any of the tumoral conditions that have been recorded to have the features of multilocular thymic cyst.

Solid Tumors and Tumor-Like Conditions

In this rather heterogeneous group of conditions, we have grouped several benign tumors as well as tumor-like conditions that, in any given time, clinically and radiologically can mimic a more common malignant mediastinal tumor. However, it is important to highlight that some of the entities that will be discussed in this section represent unusual tumoral entities. In view of their rarity, it is important to keep them in the differential diagnosis of mediastinal tumors. In addition, because of their rarity as a primary mediastinal tumor, they may be overlooked or misinterpreted. The conditions that will be presented in this section include:

- Sclerosing/fibrosing mediastinitis
- Thymic hyperplasia
- Adenomatoid tumor
- Glomus tumor
- Cholesteroloma
- Pecoma
- Sclerosing hemangioma

It is significant to note that these lesions have no association with each other and may present as a mediastinal tumors in a wide spectrum of clinical settings. Thus, each one of these entities will be discussed separately.

Sclerosing/Fibrosing Mediastinitis

The knowledge of a process characterized by fibrous proliferation has been known for quite some time. However, early reports on sclerosing mediastinitis seem to give credit to different individuals for the initial description of this process. Based on many publications on this subject, it is very

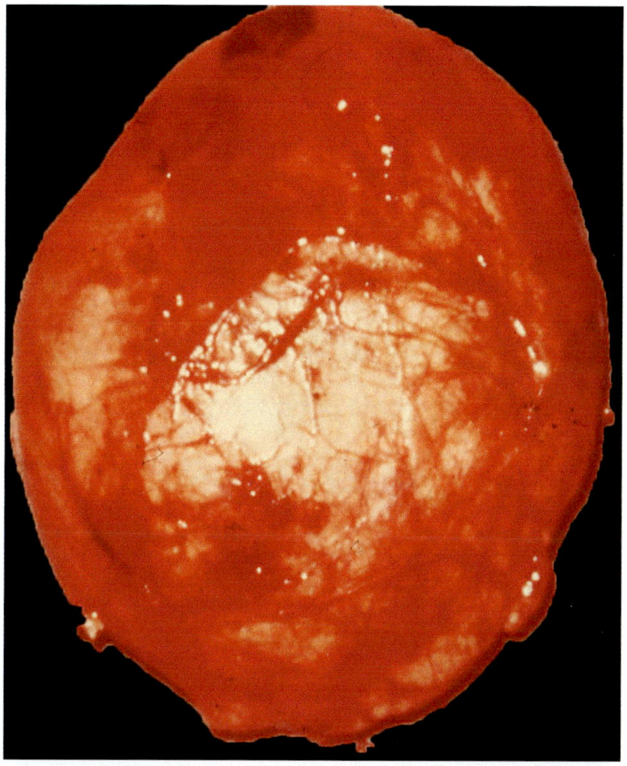

Fig. 4.17 Unilocular thymic cyst showing a single ovoid lesion

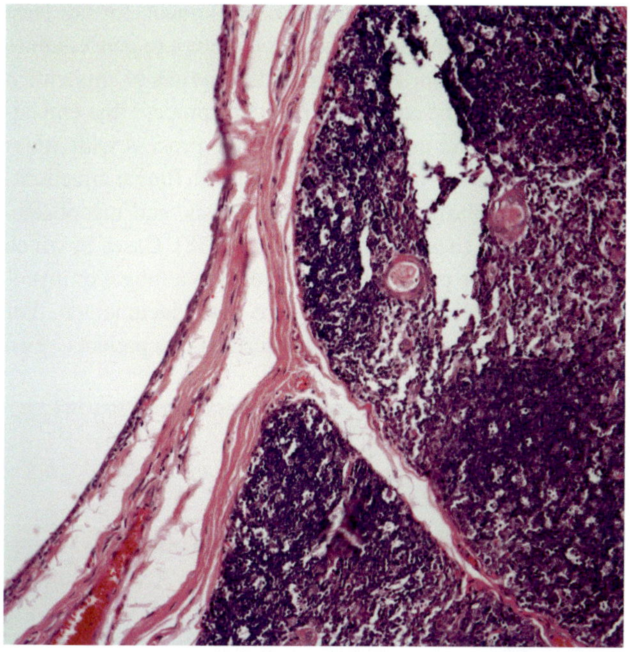

Fig. 4.19 Unilocular thymic cyst showing a cystic structure with adjacent thymus

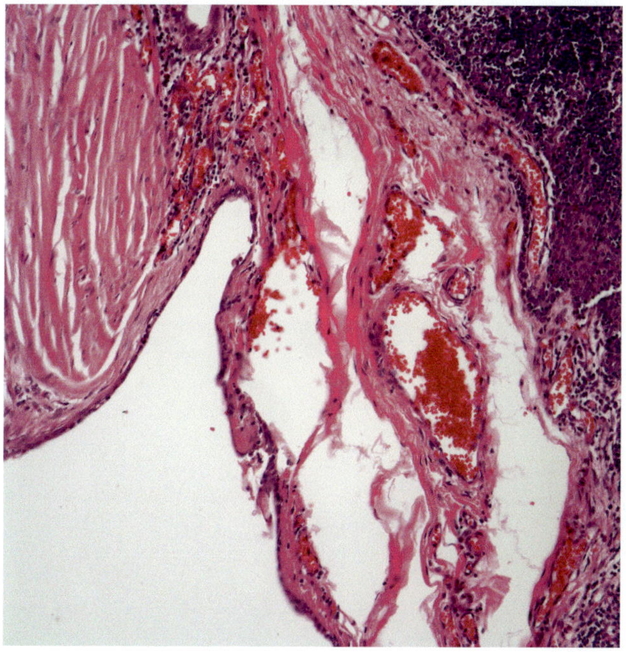

Fig. 4.18 Low power view of a unilocular thymic cyst showing a single cystic structures lined by flattened epithelium

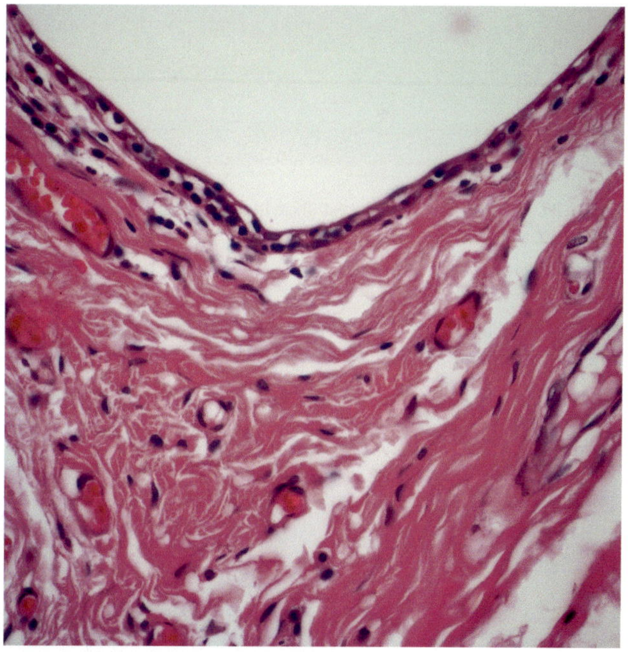

Fig. 4.20 Higher magnification of the lining of a unilocular thymic cyst showing flattened epithelium

likely that this condition has been known for at least 150 years. Nevertheless, we will not attempt to give credit to anyone in particular for the first description of this entity. However, since the early reports on this process, the emphasis was placed on the association of the process with infectious conditions commonly associated with fungal infections, such as histoplasmosis and blastomycosis, and mycobacterial infections such as tuberculosis [35–38]. Cases in which the origin of the process was not linked to a fungal or mycobacterial infection, however, were also documented. For instance, Lohman in 1948 [39] described five patients – two

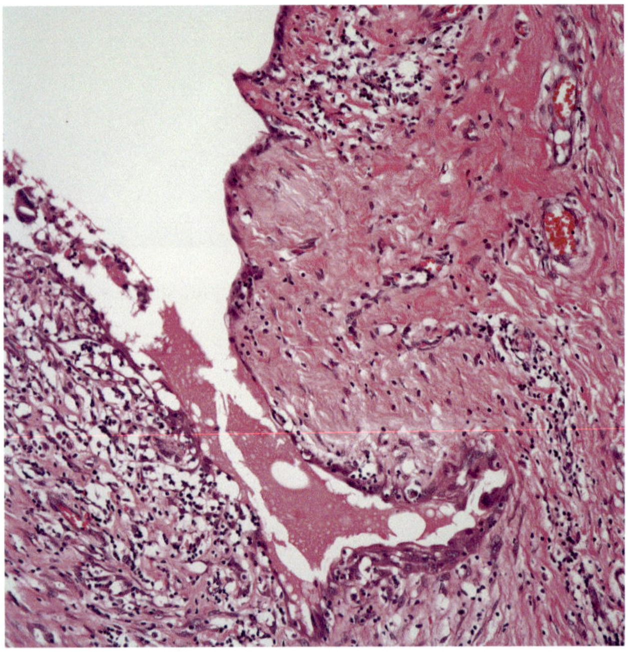

Fig. 4.21 Unilocular thymic cyst showing transitional areas of squamous and cuboidal type of epithelium

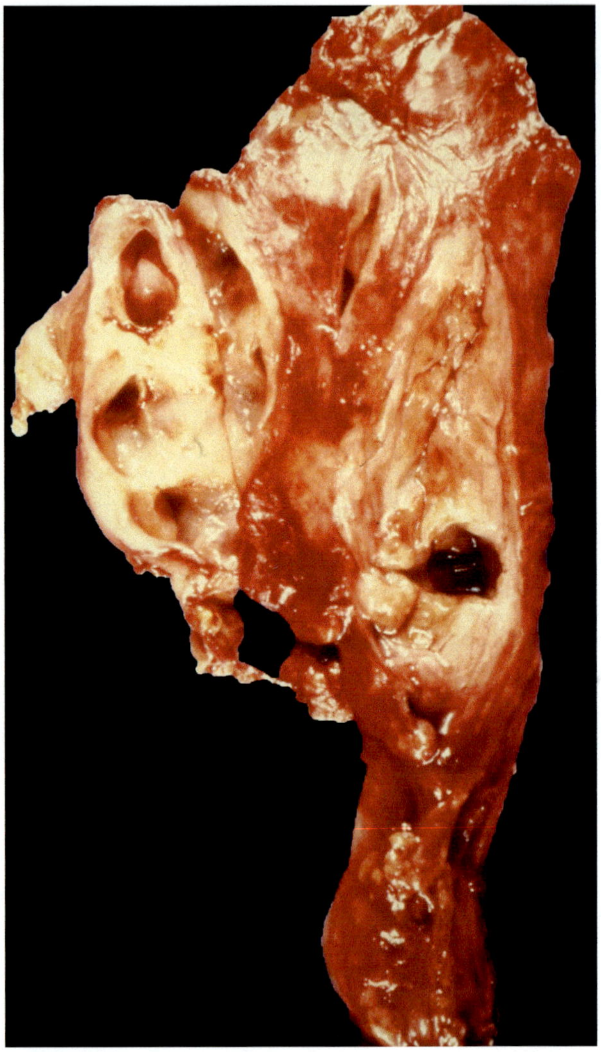

Fig. 4.23 Multilocular thymic cyst showing cystic structures and solid areas

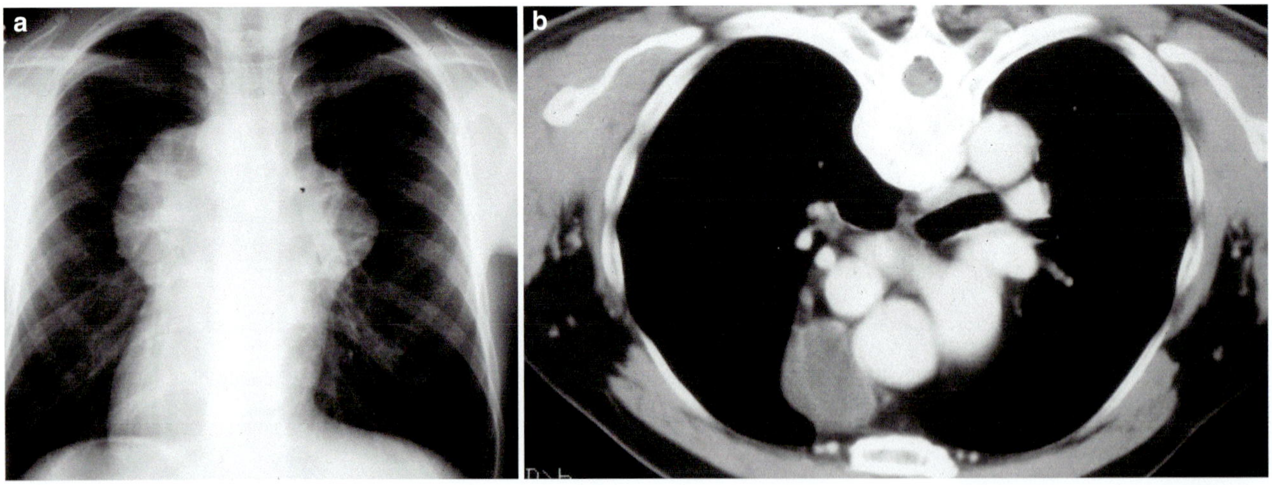

Fig. 4.22 (**a**) Plain chest imaging showing an anterior mediastinal mass; (**b**) computerized tomography showing a cystic mass in the anterior mediastinum

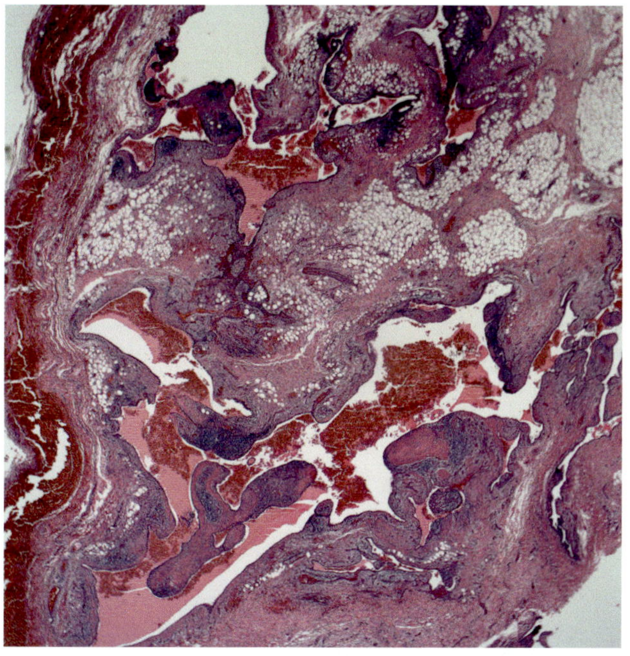

Fig. 4.24 Low power view of a multilocular thymic cysts. Note the several cystic structures of the lesion

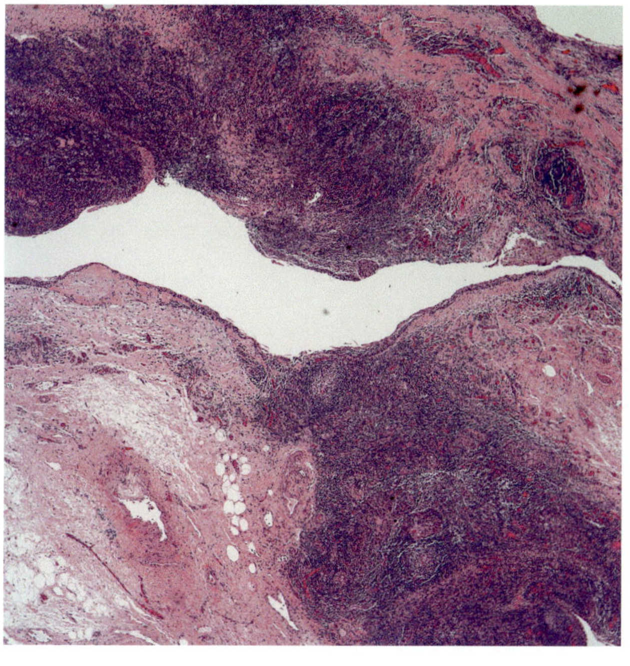

Fig. 4.25 Multilocular thymic cyst showing prominent inflammatory changes in the cystic wall

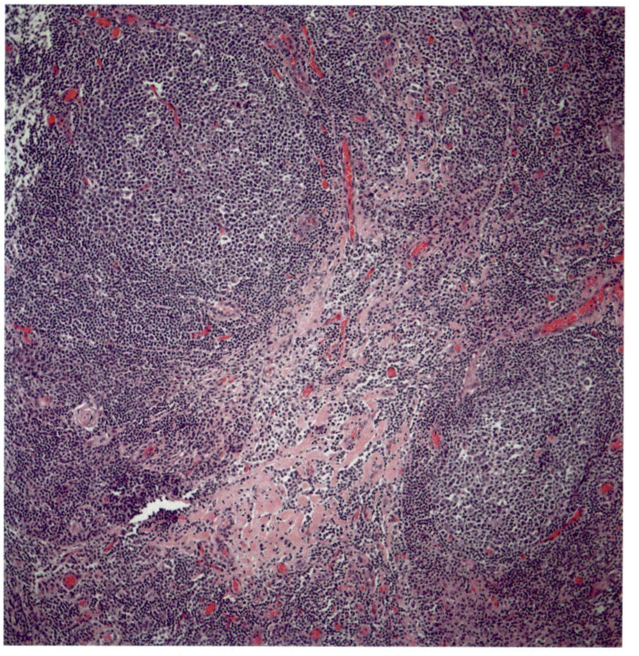

Fig. 4.26 Multilocular thymic cyst with adjacent follicular hyperplasia

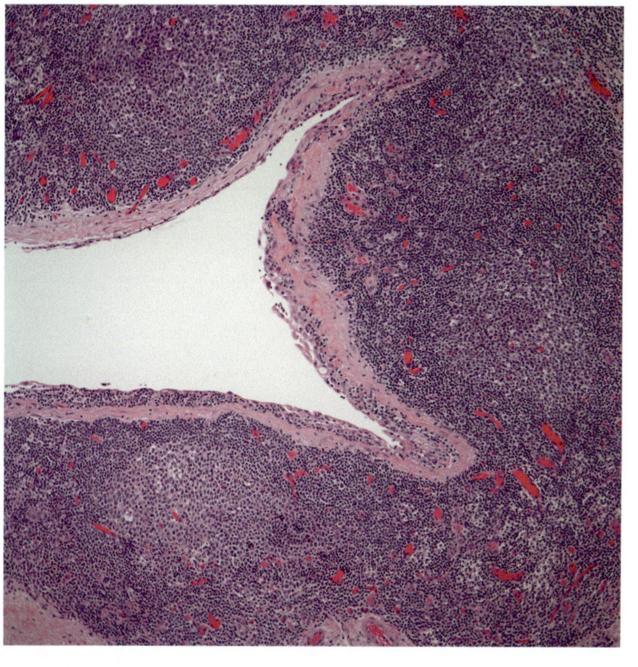

Fig. 4.27 Multilocular thymic cyst showing a cyst lined by a flattened epithelium and lymphoid hyperplasia of the cystic wall

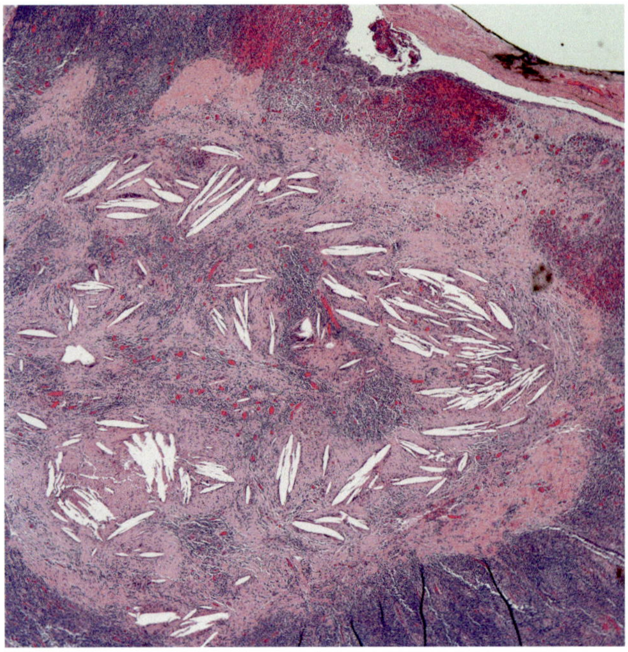

Fig. 4.28 Cholesterol cleft granuloma in the wall of a cyst in a multilocular thymic cyst

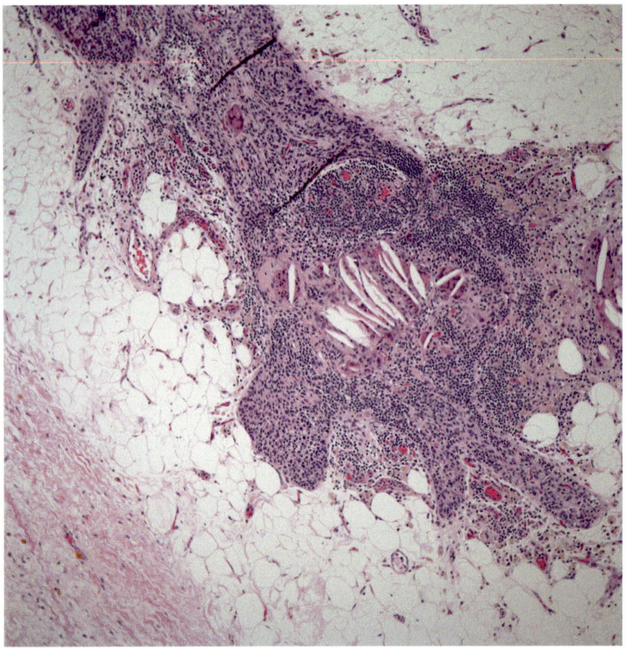

Fig. 4.29 Remnants of thymic epithelium in a multilocular thymic cyst

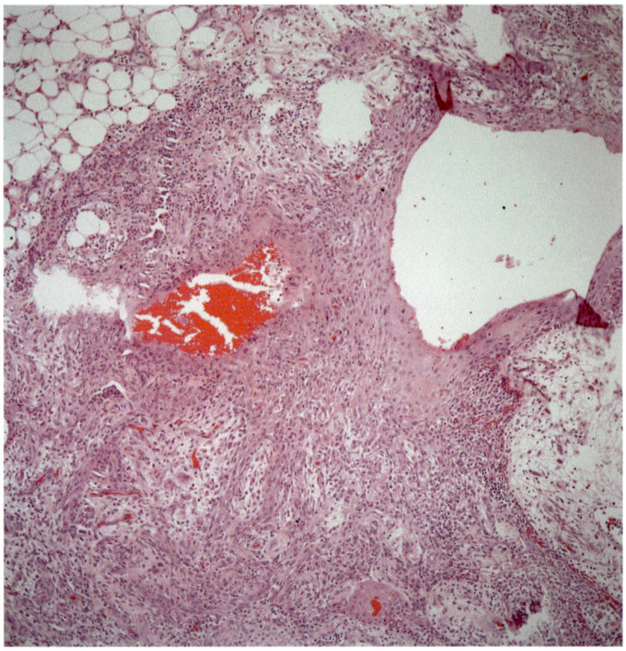

Fig. 4.30 Atypical pseudoepitheliomatous hyperplasia in a multilocular thymic cyst

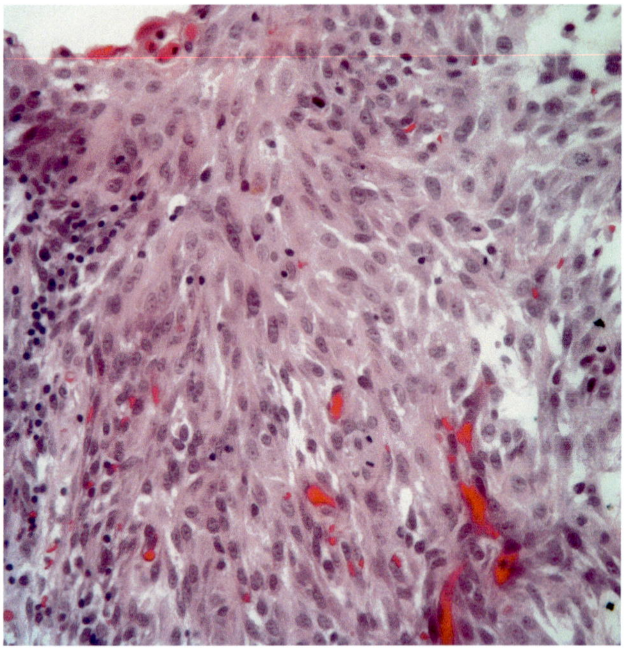

Fig. 4.31 Squamous epithelium with mild atypia; mitotic figures may be present

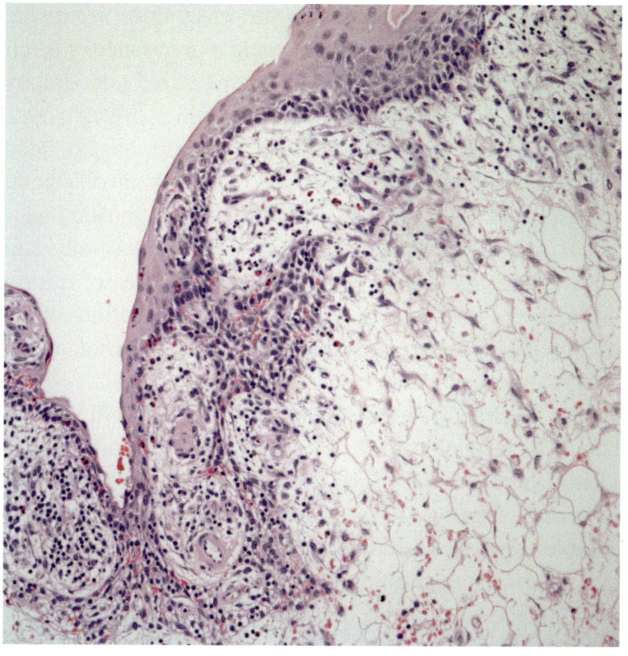

Fig. 4.32 Squamous epithelium without atypia lining the wall of a cyst in a multilocular thymic cyst

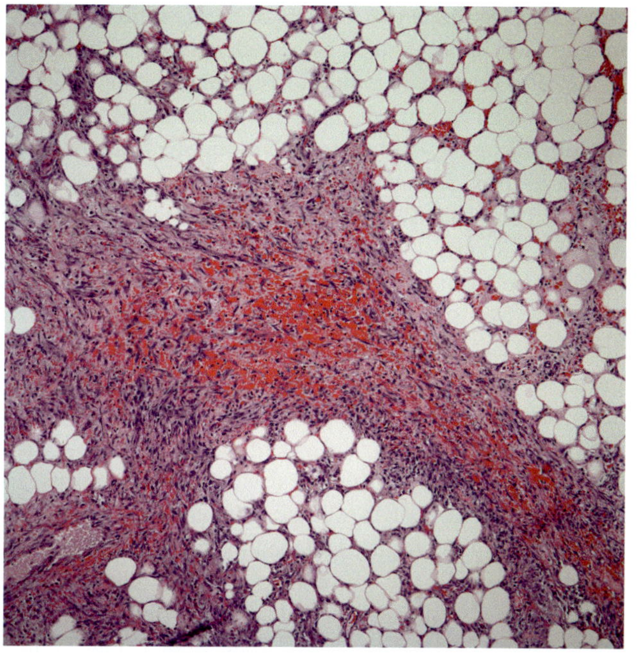

Fig. 4.34 Adhesions in a multilocular thymic cyst showing fibroblastic and inflammatory response

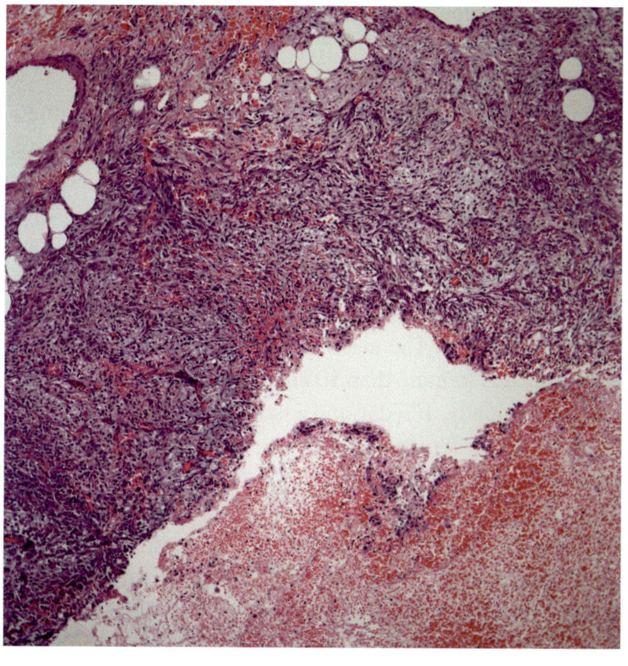

Fig. 4.33 Multilocular thymic cyst in which the lining is obliterated by extensive inflammatory reaction

men and three women between the ages of 27 and 65 years – who in the opinion of the author developed this process as a result of an acute trachea-bronchitis or pharyngitis. In 1968, Schowengerdt and associates [40] reviewed two decades of cases reported in the literature and added three cases of their own. In their review of 180 cases, the authors separated two types of cases into granulomatous mediastinitis and chronic fibrous mediastinitis. Based on that separation, the authors identified 27 cases of granulomatous mediastinitis (26%) and 64 cases of chronic fibrous mediastinitis (83%). The involvement of adjacent structures by the process appeared to be similar whether the etiology was infectious or not, as the process may involved the vena cava, esophagus, bronchi, pulmonary vein, artery, larynx, and thoracic inlet. Interestingly, the authors also provided information regarding the etiological agent in these two processes. In cases of granulomatous mediastinitis, histoplasma and mycobacterial infection accounted for the large majority of the cases. However, in those cases under the designation of chronic fibrous mediastinitis, two cases of histoplasma were also identified. Among the noninfectious etiologies, sarcoidosis and silicosis were mentioned as possibilities. Based on the lack of known etiology involved in the development of fibrous mediastinitis, the term "idiopathic" mediastinitis has also been used, which appeared to become the more common term as the incidence rose from 23% in 1934 to 65% in 1946 to 96% in 1969 [40]. However, it is also important to highlight that, in some cases in which no specific organism is associated with the process and is assumed to be "idiopathic," the histology still shows some giant cells, which would be somewhat suspicious for a possible infectious process in resolution. It is important to mention the association that has been reported of fibrous mediastinitis with concurrent retroperitoneal fibrosis [41]. Schowengerdt et al. [40]

concluded that these two variants of mediastinitis (granulomatous and fibrous) should be considered as manifestations of the same process. In terms of idiopathic fibrosing mediastinitis, several hypotheses have been mentioned regarding etiology including chronic infection, repeated trauma leading to fibrosis, inflammation in adipose tissue leading to fibrosis, iatrogenic as a result of adverse drug effect, and an immune response [42]. In a presentation of 30 cases of fibrosing/sclerosing lesions of the mediastinum, Flieder and associates [43] studied 17 men and 13 women between the ages of 10 and 64 years. However, according to the authors, the inclusion of cases in this study was for patients with negative serologic tests for *Blastomyces*, coccidioidin, histoplasma yeast, mycelium, and aspergillus as well as negative tissue cultures and histochemical stains for organisms. In addition, any case that showed granulomatous inflammation in tissue samples was not included in this particular study. Racial information was available in 29 patients, which showed that 11 males and 8 females were African-American, while 5 males and 5 females were Caucasian. Clinical information was available in 28 patients and included cough, shortness of breath, sore throat, chest pain, hemoptysis, fever, and weight loss. Five patients presented with facial swelling or prominent venous collaterals. Radiographically, all the lesions were located in the anterior mediastinum and demonstrated asymmetrical mediastinal widening. In addition, in some cases, the process also involved the hilum, paratracheal area, great vessels, trachea, carina, lung, pericardium, and thymus. In 19 patients in whom bronchoscopic findings were available, the presence of tracheal, carinal, and bronchial narrowing was documented.

More recently, Rossi and associates [44] have proposed a different approach in terms of classification/etiology of this entity. The authors have suggested two main categories for sclerosing mediastinitis: infectious and idiopathic. The infectious aspect of it has been well recognized for many years; however, the idiopathic sclerosing mediastinitis is the one that poses more problems for identifying its etiology. It is here were Rossi and associates [44] further divide this process: (a) isolated, (b) associated with other fibroinflammatory disorders (peritoneal fibrosis, sclerosing pancreatitis, etc.), and (c) associated with systemic autoimmune diseases. The isolated and the one associated with other fibroinflammatory disorders can be associated with IgG4. In the same line of thinking, Rossi and associates [45] also made the same claim for idiopathic retroperitoneal fibrosis and IgG4-related disease. Inoue and associates [46] documented a case of sclerosing mediastinitis in which the patient identified IgG4 plasma cells in the fibrous tissue and also a high serum level of IgG4. The patient was treated with steroid, and remission was observed after treatment. The authors stated that IgG4 level is a good selection indicator for steroid therapy in these patients.

Recent reports on the diagnostic imaging of sclerosing mediastinitis also have been presented. For instance, Worrell and associates [47] reviewed the computerized tomography of 12 cases, observing large masses averaging 5–9 cm, none of them showing calcifications. Five of these lesions extended to the neck, and all had vascular or airway involvement. Gorospe and associates [48] evaluated the diagnostic imaging of six patients with idiopathic fibrosing mediastinitis and the possible association with IgG4-related disease; raising awareness of the possible extrathoracic manifestations of the IgG4-related spectrum including sclerosing cholangitis, autoimmune pancreatitis, or retroperitoneal fibrosis.

The treatment for sclerosing mediastinitis will depend largely on its etiology. For cases in which a microorganism is identified, the use of proper antimicrobial agents will be the treatment of choice. In cases linked to the spectrum of IgG4 complex, the use of steroids may be considered. However, if the sclerosing mediastinitis occurs in association with an autoimmune process, then the treatment of the underlying condition should take precedence. In the idiopathic cases in which no etiology is identified, surgical resection of the mass should be the treatment of choice; however, it is important to highlight that complete surgical removal of the mass may not be possible in some cases, thus leaving the possibility of additional medical treatment post-surgery.

Pathological Features

The emphasis in this section will be placed on the noninfectious cases of this process. It is understood that if the etiology is an infectious organism, the possibilities may be quite broad.

Macroscopically, the mass is firm, tan-yellowish, bulbous, and gelatinous to gray-white. Hemorrhage and necrosis are not part of this process. The cut surface may be slightly lobulated and homogeneous. The mass may range in size from a couple of centimeters to more than 10 cm in greatest diameter.

Histologically, Flieder and associates [43] separated the histopathological features of fibrosing/sclerosing mediastinitis into three separate stages:

1. Lesions predominantly characterized by edematous fibromyxoid tissue composed of spindle cells and numerous inflammatory cells (Figs. 4.35, 4.36, and 4.37).
2. Lesions with thick, glassy bands of haphazardly arranged eosinophilic hyaline material encircling and infiltrating mediastinal structures. Scattered inflammatory cells may be seen in this stage (Figs. 4.38 and 4.39).
3. Obliterative lesions with extensions into mediastinal and pulmonary structures composed of acellular dense collagen with occasional lymphoid follicles (Figs. 4.40 and 4.41). Inflammatory cells are absent but dystrophic calcifications may be seen. This latter stage is the "classic" sclerosing mediastinitis.

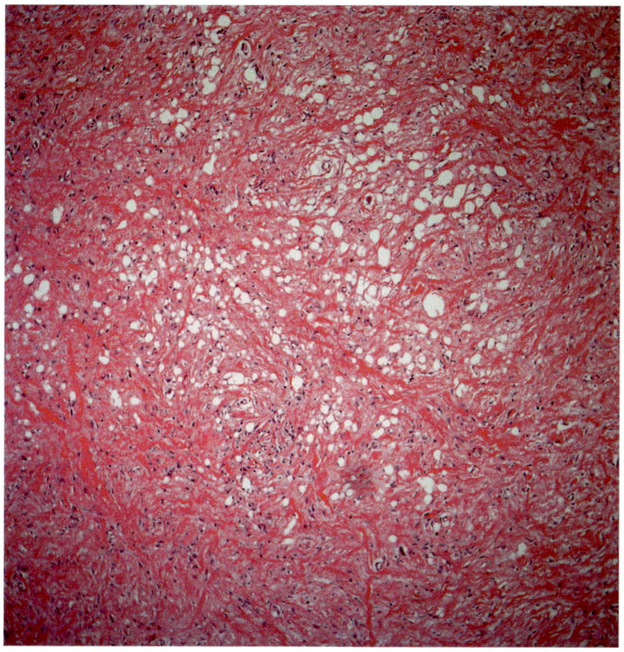

Fig. 4.35 Sclerosing mediastinitis showing a loose fibromyxoid stroma

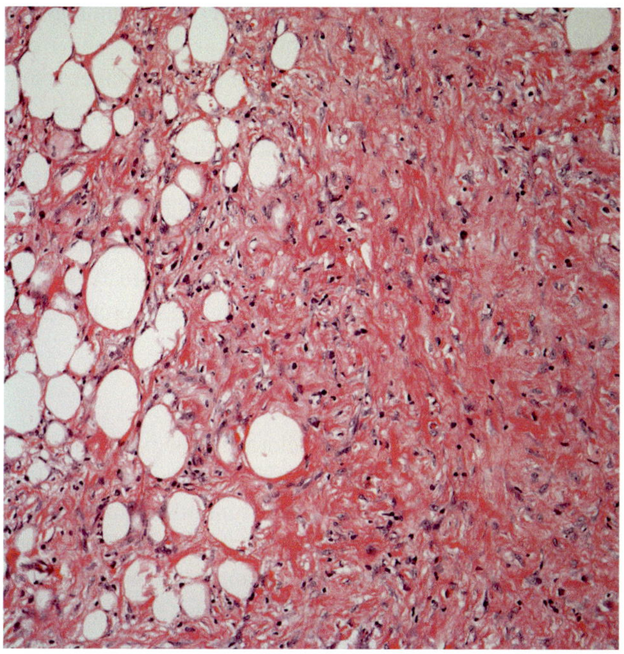

Fig. 4.36 Fibrous component showing spindle cells

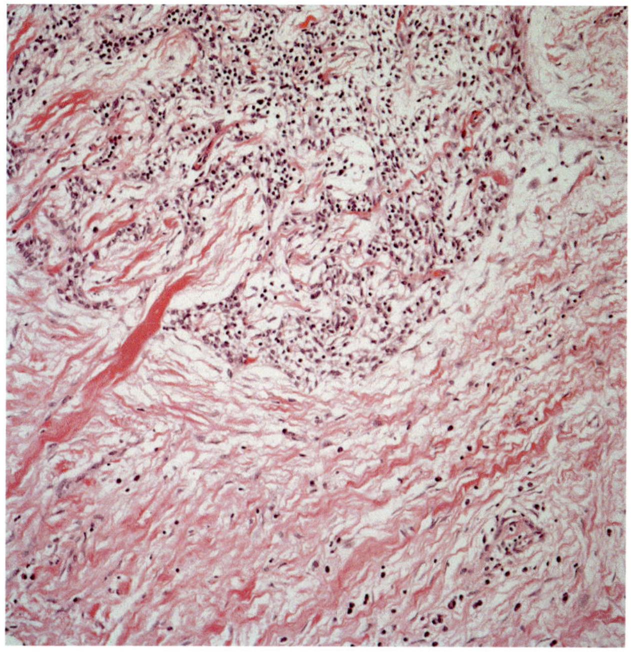

Fig. 4.37 Fibrous component and entrapped thymic epithelium

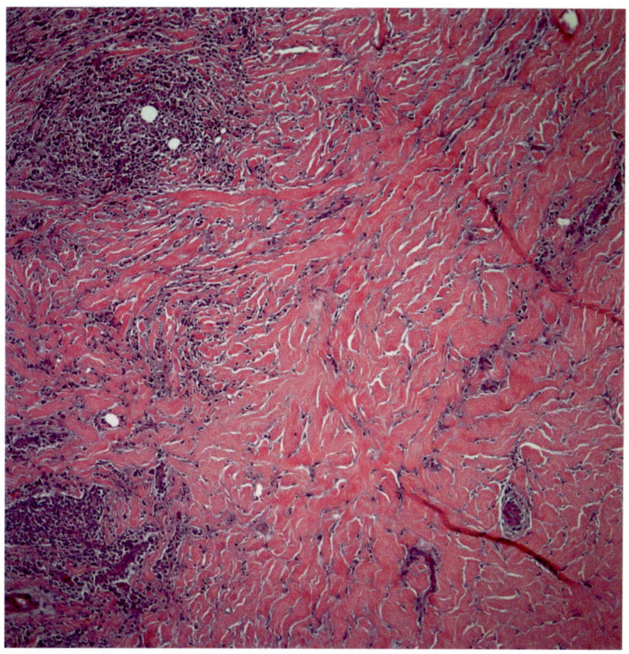

Fig. 4.38 Dense hyalinized tissue with areas of inflammatory reaction

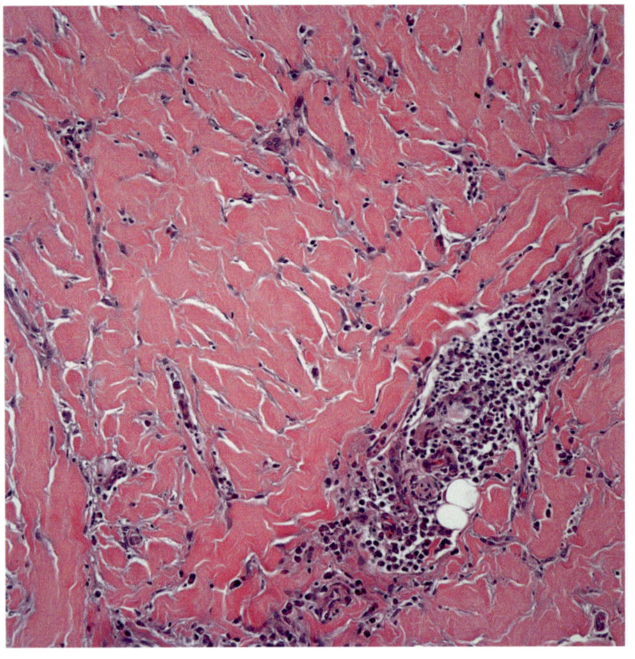

Fig. 4.39 Focal inflammatory area in a dense fibrous tissue

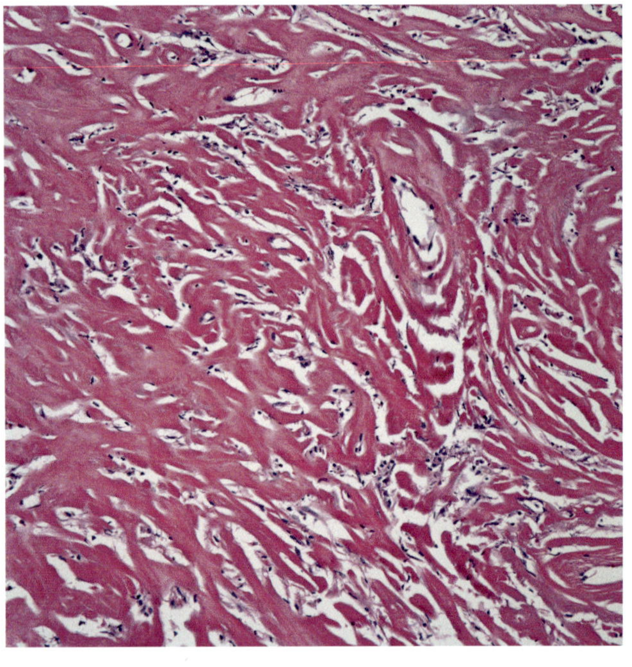

Fig. 4.40 Marked hyalinization in an obliterative type of sclerosing mediastinitis

Immunohistochemical Features

The use of immunohistochemical markers in the diagnosis of sclerosing mediastinitis is rather limited and likely will be used in the context of the stage of the process. For instance, in the cases reported by Flieder and associates [43], the authors stated that all the stages shared some common features. The lymphocytes showed positive staining with CD45, CD45RO, and CD3 with fewer cells staining for CD20, while the plasma cell component did not show any kappa or lambda chain restriction. In addition, other stains performed, including keratin, CD15, estrogen, and progesterone receptors, were negative. Important to highlight is that in the early stages of the process where the lesion may show more spindle cell component, smooth muscle actin and vimentin may show positive staining in these areas. However, S-100 protein and CD1a are negative. Vascular markers such as CD31, CD34, and D2-40 will stain the vessel proliferation commonly seen in this process.

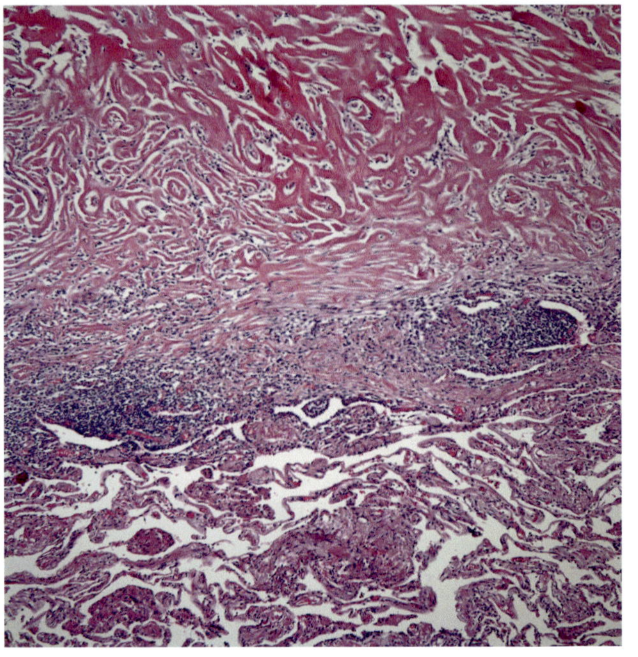

Fig. 4.41 Sclerosing mediastinitis involving peripheral lung parenchyma

Differential Diagnosis

Even though the diagnosis of sclerosing mediastinitis in its classic form does not represent a diagnostic challenge, it is important to separate this process from other tumoral conditions that may also show extensive areas of hyalinization. In this context, there are several tumoral conditions that may show extensive hyalinization, including lymphomas encompassing Hodgkin's and non-Hodgkin's, as well as thymoma and thymic carcinoma. However, there are other less common lesions that may mimic sclerosing mediastinitis such as solitary fibrous tumors of the mediastinum. If the material available is only a small mediastinoscopic biopsy, then the interpretation will become a challenge since one cannot unequivocally rule out some of the possibilities mentioned. When adequate tissue is available, then the use of immunohistochemical stains should provide valuable information to the proper interpretation of this process. In cases in which the possibility of lymphoma is considered, the use of B- and T-cell markers as well as CD30 and CD15 should help in the final interpretation. The use of keratin stains and STAT6 should aid in separating sclerosing mediastinitis from a thymic epithelial neoplasm or a solitary fibrous tumor. It is also important to highlight that sclerosing mediastinitis may extend into the pulmonary parenchyma and the material obtained for diagnosis may derive from a pulmonary biopsy. In this setting, it is important to properly correlate the imaging and determine that the process is predominantly in the mediastinal compartment and not in the lung. This is important as the entity known as "pulmonary hyalinizing granuloma" should be carefully considered and ruled out. Hyalinizing granuloma of the lung and sclerosing mediastinitis may share some histopathological features, and it may be a challenge to separate both only on histological grounds.

Thymic Hyperplasia

True thymic hyperplasia is a rare process that requires good clinical and radiological correlations, with special care on the age of the particular individual. One can define true thymic hyperplasia as an increase in the weight and size of the gland. However, the presence of the thymus by imaging can be detected normally in children ages 2 or 3; thus, the interpretation of true thymic hyperplasia should be considered very carefully in this age group. In adults, thymic hyperplasia may be associated with underlying conditions. Examples of it are classically represented by the changes observed in the thymus in patients with myasthenia gravis. However, to that effect, morphometric studies attempting to measure the size of germinal centers in non-thymomatous patients with myasthenia gravis have not shown a clear correlation between the number of germinal centers and the clinical improvement of these patients [49]. In 1978, Levine and Rosai [50] presented their views on thymic hyperplasia and neoplasia and stated that the weight of the thymus should always be compared with standard graph before being considered abnormal. The authors also added that the "hyperplasia" observed in myasthenic patients is actually related more to "follicular" or "germinal center" hyperplasia as the thymus itself is rarely enlarged. In addition, in order to explain the occurrence of germinal centers in the thymus, the authors advanced their own proposal, which essentially delves into the normal anatomy of the thymus. In this proposal, the thymus is divided into two separate zones: (1) the cortex and medulla and (2) a zone within the perivascular spaces of the thymus (extraparenchymal zone). It is in this latter zone where plasma cells and possibly B-lymphocytes may be encountered, which in turn may give rise to germinal centers. Of course, the authors clearly stated that such a proposal remained to be proven. In 1987, Hofmann and associates [51] presented their views on the issue of true thymic hyperplasia and stated that it can occur in three different forms: (1) de novo, without any associated underlying condition; (2) as a rebound phenomenon in recovery from severe stress and steroid treatment or associated with malignant tumors; and (3) in association with endocrine abnormalities such as sarcoid and Beckwith-Wiedemann syndrome. Important to note is that patients with thymic hyperplasia usually present with a mediastinal mass by imaging. Hofmann and associates [51] in a separate study on lymphofollicular thymic hyperplasia stated that the germinal centers observed in the thymus are essentially the same as those occurring in lymph nodes and that they originate in the interlobular septal space and displace the thymic parenchyma by extension. In a more recent report on thymic hyperplasia, Milka and associates [52] analyzed 13 such cases, over a 13-year period (1995–2008), identifying 9 cases of follicular thymic hyperplasia and 4 cases of "true" thymic hyperplasia in 9 women and 4 men. All patients with follicular thymic hyperplasia had a history of myasthenia gravis, while in the group of "true" thymic hyperplasia, three patients had received medical (drug) treatment for different conditions.

Clinically, the patients affected by thymic hyperplasia may present with different symptomatology or be completely asymptomatic, while others may present with respiratory distress [53]. However, it is important to take into consideration any possible underlying condition as well as any medical treatment. In that regard, the age of the patients may also affect their underlying condition and in general that may range from early adolescence to older than 40 years. Diagnostic imaging usually will demonstrate the presence of an anterior mediastinal mass, and, as would be expected, the differential diagnosis by imaging may include more common pathological entities such as thymoma. Surgical resection of the mediastinal mass is the treatment of choice and, of course, treatment of whatever underlying medical condition that may be associated.

Pathological Features

Macroscopically, since there may be an enlarged thymic gland, the resected specimen would show an ill-defined mass that may keep some of the normal anatomic features of the thymus. The mass may range in size from a few centimeters to more than 10 in greatest diameter. At the cut surface, it may show a lobular configuration and light tan color. Hemorrhage and necrosis are usually not seen in association with thymic hyperplasia. However, cystic changes may be present.

Histologically, the use of the term "true" thymic hyperplasia was designed to separate the thymic hyperplasia seen in patients without any associated condition from the patients with an underlying myasthenia gravis. Therefore, histologically, there are two types: follicular thymic hyperplasia encountered in the background of myasthenia gravis or any other autoimmune disease and "true" thymic hyperplasia.

True Thymic Hyperplasia

Its name implies an enlargement of the thymic gland preserving the normal structures of the gland. Thus, one would expect to clearly identify cortical and medullary compartments as well as the presence of Hassall's corpuscles. In this case, the size and weight of the gland are increased, but the histology is that of a normal thymus (Fig. 4.42).

Follicular Thymic Hyperplasia

As its name implies, the hallmark of this process is the presence of germinal centers haphazardly distributed in the thymus. However, their presence may or may not be associated with an increase in size and weight of the thymic gland (Fig. 4.43).

Immunohistochemical Studies

Although the histological features of both variants of thymic hyperplasia are easy to identify, the use of immunohistochemical markers would be of aid to identify the distribution of B- and T-cells within the tissue studied. In addition, the use of keratin will outline some residual thymic epithelium as well as Hassall's corpuscles.

Differential Diagnosis

In cases of "true" thymic hyperplasia, the main differential diagnosis will be a separation with a thymoma with medullary differentiation. However, the well-demarcated cortical and medullary areas in true thymic hyperplasia coupled with the gross features of the resected specimen should lead to a correct interpretation. The challenge is with a small biopsy; in such cases, an unequivocal diagnosis of one entity over the other is not possible, and the final diagnosis should be reserved after the surgical resection. In cases of follicular thymic hyperplasia, there are many neoplastic entities that may also show follicular hyperplasia, namely, germ cell tumors, thymomas, and lymphomas. Among the benign tumoral conditions are multilocular thymic cyst and thymic hyperplasia with LESA-like features. (These entities are discussed in different chapters throughout this text.)

Adenomatoid Tumor

The occurrence of this tumor in the mediastinal compartment is rare, and only a few cases have been reported in the literature [54–56]. Interestingly, the cases reported have been women over 50 years of age. Clinically, these patients have been either asymptomatic or presented with non-specific symptoms such as chest pain. Two of the tumors described have been in the anterior mediastinum and one in the posterior mediastinum in close proximity to the vertebra. Surgical resection appears to be the treatment of choice, and it is curative in these patients.

Pathological Features

Macroscopically, the tumors may be solid or cystic and can measure up to 6 cm in greatest diameter. The tumors appear

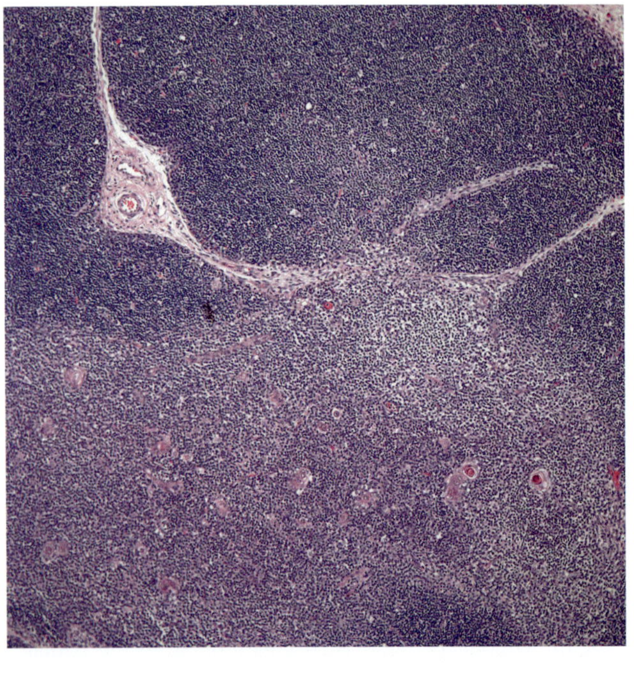

Fig. 4.42 True thymic hyperplasia showing distinct cortical and medullary areas

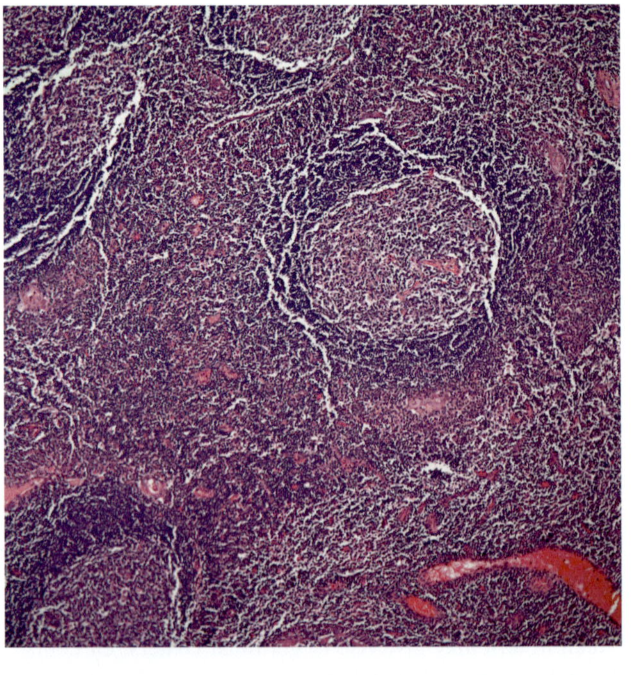

Fig. 4.43 Thymic follicular hyperplasia showing the presence of germinal centers

to be relatively well circumscribed but not encapsulated and light tan in color. Areas of hemorrhage and necrosis are not components of this tumor.

Histologically, the characteristics are those of adenomatoid tumors elsewhere, mainly the presence of an epithelioid cellular proliferation arranged in chords or nests embedded in a loose fibroconnective tissue. In some areas, the tumor cells may adopt signet ring cell morphology; however, mitotic activity and cellular atypia are usually absent (Figs. 4.44, 4.45, 4.46, 4.47, 4.48, and 4.49). In cases with cystic changes, the epithelioid cells may be hugging the walls of the cysts.

Immunohistochemical features of these tumors will be similar to those seen in mesothelial proliferations or mesothelioma. Namely, the presence of keratin 5/6, calretinin, WT-1, and keratin should show positive staining in the epithelioid cells, while CEA, B72.3, CD15, PAX-8, and MOC-31 are negative.

Differential Diagnosis

The three most important considerations include adenocarcinoma, mesothelioma, and thymoma. In this setting, the positive staining of the tumor for keratin 5/6 and calretinin while negative for CEA, MOC-31, and CD15 would exclude the possibility of adenocarcinoma. However, thymomas may show positive staining for keratin 5/6, and, in some cases, calretinin may show focal positive staining; one possible aid in these cases will be the use of T-cell markers including TdT to identify the presence of T-lymphocytes, which will be more closely associated in cases of thymoma. Of course, the histopathological features of both tumors are different and should suffice for a final interpretation. In cases of mesothelioma, once again from the purely immunohistochemical point of view, both tumors will show similar immunophenotype; however, good clinical and radiological correlations will lead to the correct interpretation. In some cases in which the distinction from mesothelioma becomes an issue, one can attempt to perform p16 molecular analysis by FISH, as adenomatoid tumors will show negative results, while mesotheliomas may show positive results in about 30–50% of the cases.

Glomus Tumor

This is another benign tumor that has a rare occurrence in the mediastinum. Most of what is described about the glomus tumor in the mediastinum has been through single case reports [57–61] or in general descriptions of glomus tumors in the thoracic cavity [62, 63]. The tumors appear to be more common in adult individuals and also more often in the anterior mediastinum, with no apparent gender predilection. It is also important to mention that the malignant counterpart of this tumor has also been described in the mediastinal location [64]. Clinically, the presence of non-specific symptoms such as dyspnea and chest pain may be present, while some patients may be completely asymptomatic. Surgical resection appears to be the treatment of choice for these patients, and it is curative.

Pathological Features

Macroscopically, these tumors are ill defined and soft, some tumors may be hemorrhagic. These tumors may range in size from 3 to 5 cm in greatest dimension.

Histologically, the features of mediastinal glomus tumors are similar to those in soft tissue (Figs. 4.50, 4.51, 4.52, and 4.53). However, in our experience, we observed five different growth patterns for these tumors: (1) dilatation of large vessels filled with blood and with only focal areas of more conventional tumor, (2) myxohyaline areas, (3) solid cellular proliferation mixed with dilated vascular spaces in a hemangiopericytic pattern, (4) solid cellular proliferation with discrete vascular spaces, and (5) hypocellular tumors with dilated vessels and cellular areas composed of cells with clear cytoplasm. In some tumors, it is common to find some of these growth patterns alternating with each other. The cellular proliferation in these tumors is essentially composed of medium size cells with round to oval nuclei and inconspicuous nucleoli. Cystic changes may occur in some tumors. Mitotic activity is absent in these tumors, and the occurrence of increase mitotic activity should alert for the possibility of glomangiosarcoma.

Immunohistochemical stains may aid in the diagnosis of glomus tumors, as these tumors show positive staining for smooth muscle actin and muscle-specific actin. Other markers including keratin, desmin, S-100 protein, HMB-45, neuroendocrine markers, CD34, and CD31 are negative. However, in a report on glomus tumors by Mravic and associates [65], the authors found that CD34 was positive in about 34% of the cases.

Molecular analyses in a few glomus tumors in soft tissues have shown a gene fusion involving MIRI 43 in band 5q32 with either NOTCH2 in Ip13 in GTI or NOTCH1 in 9q34 in GT2 [66].

Differential Diagnosis

Due to the rarity of this tumor in the mediastinal compartment, there are other tumors that should be considered in the differential diagnosis. In a mediastinoscopic biopsy, atypical thymoma would lead the entities to be considered; however, the use of immunohistochemical stains, mainly the use of broad-spectrum keratin and keratin 5/6, should lead to the correct interpretation, as glomus tumors are negative for these epithelial markers. Vascular tumors such angiosarcoma and epithelioid hemangioendothelioma also should be considered, and the staining for these tumors for CD34 and CD31 also will lead to the proper interpretation. Because of the positive staining for actin, these tumors should also be separated from a garden-variety leiomyoma.

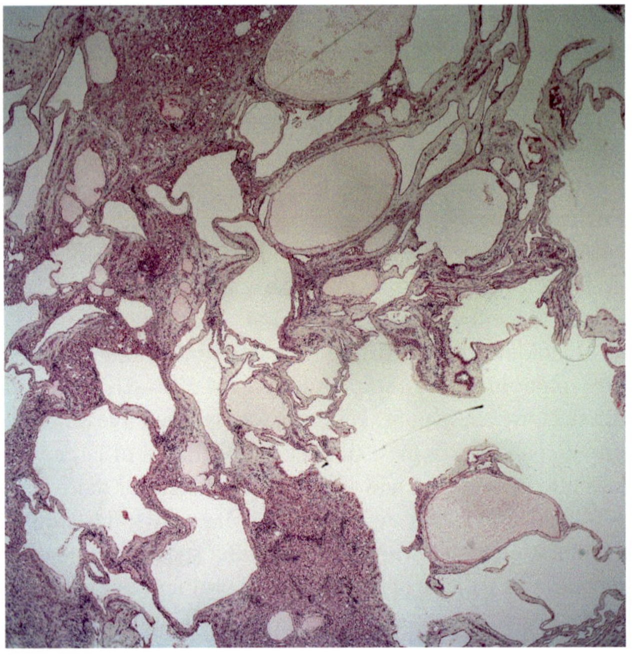

Fig. 4.44 Low power view of a thymic adenomatoid tumor; note the prominent cystic changes

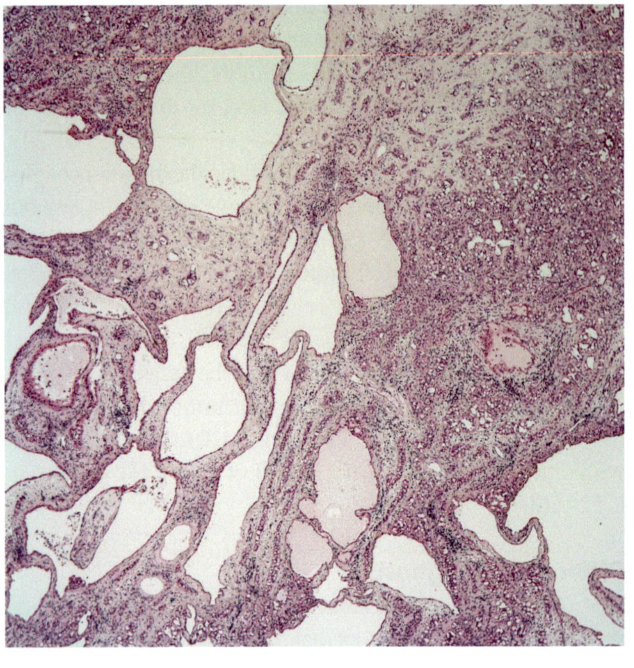

Fig. 4.45 Thymic adenomatoid tumor showing cystic and solid components

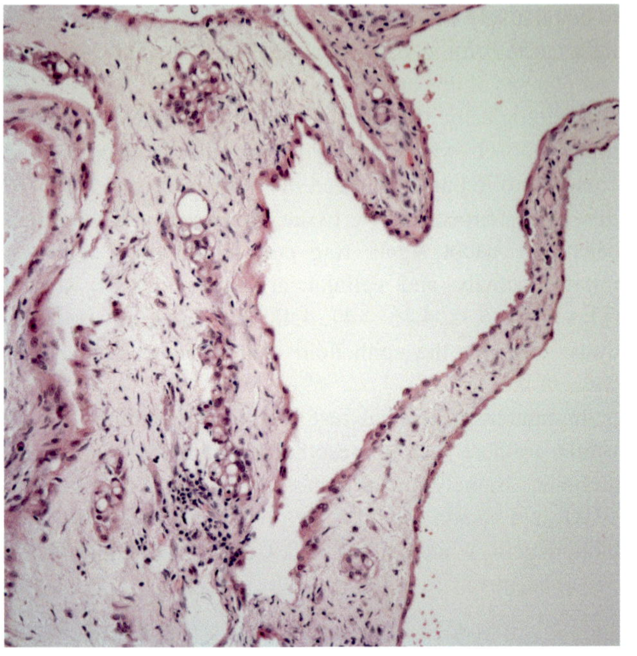

Fig. 4.46 Cystic changes in an adenomatoid tumor with only focal cellular areas in the wall of the cysts

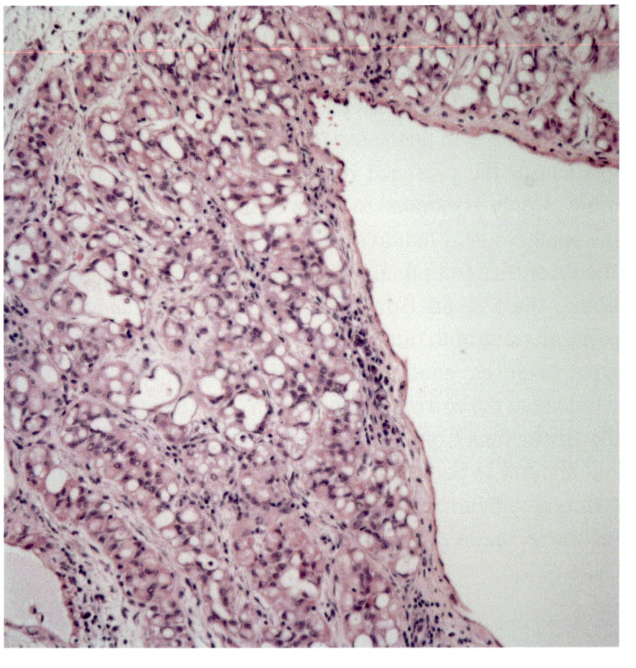

Fig. 4.47 Cystic changes in an adenomatoid tumor with adjacent solid component

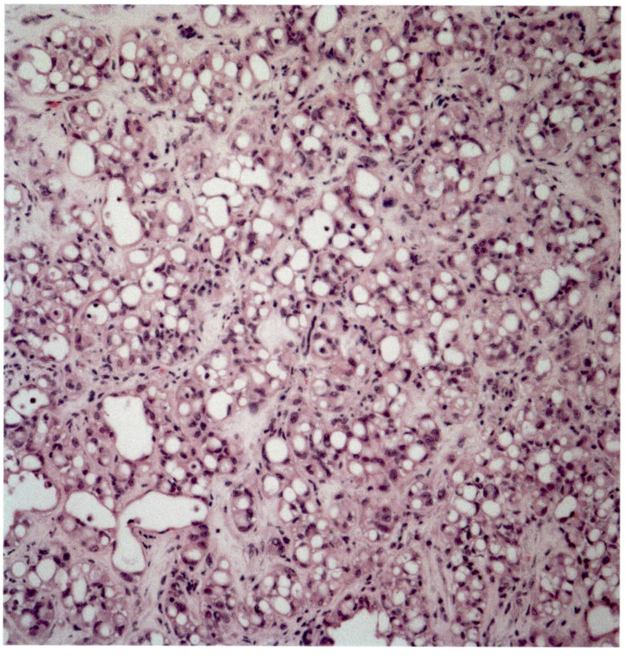

Fig. 4.48 Solid component of a thymic adenomatoid tumor showing cords and nest of tumor cells

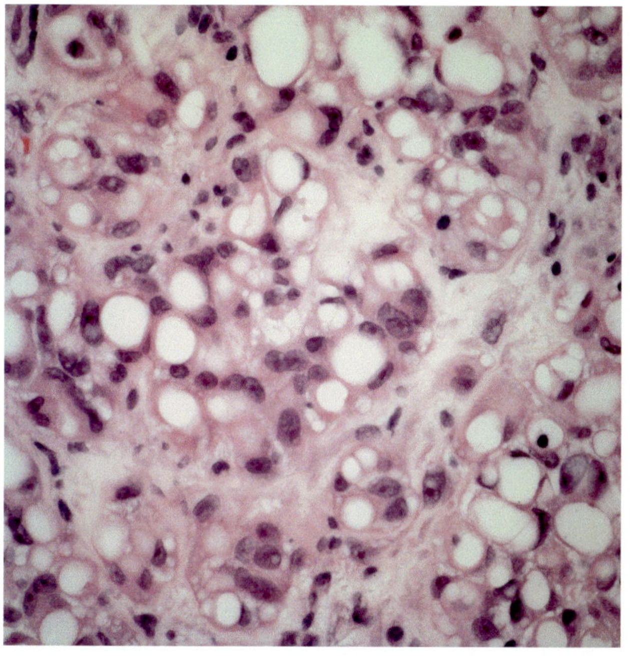

Fig. 4.49 Higher magnification of a thymic adenomatoid tumor showing cells with signet ring cell appearance

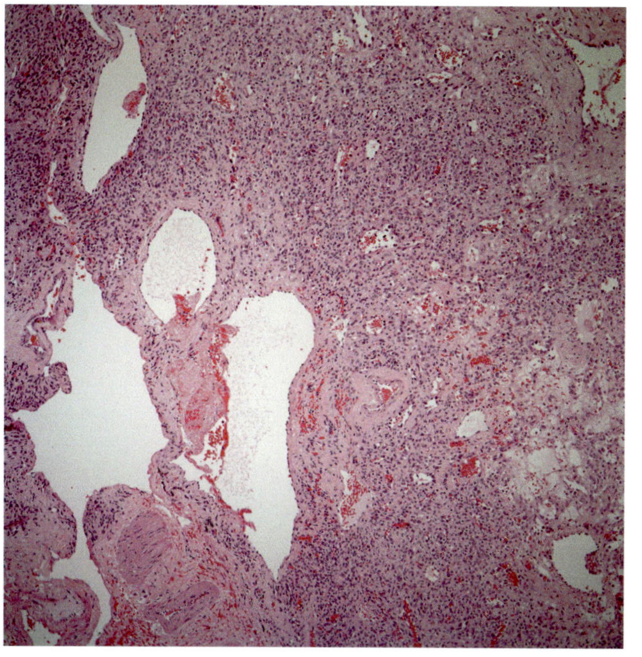

Fig. 4.50 Thymic glomus tumor showing cystic and solid changes

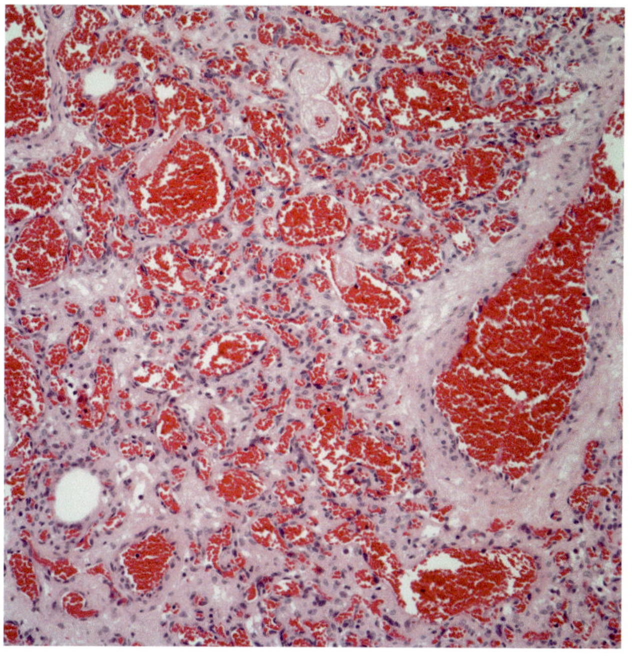

Fig. 4.51 Thymic glomus tumor showing areas mimicking a vascular tumor

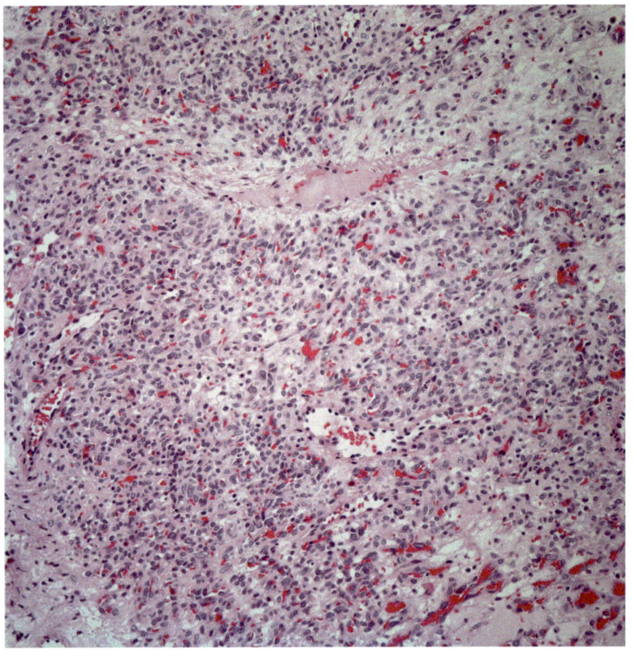

Fig. 4.52 Solid areas of a thymic glomus tumor showing sheets of tumor cells

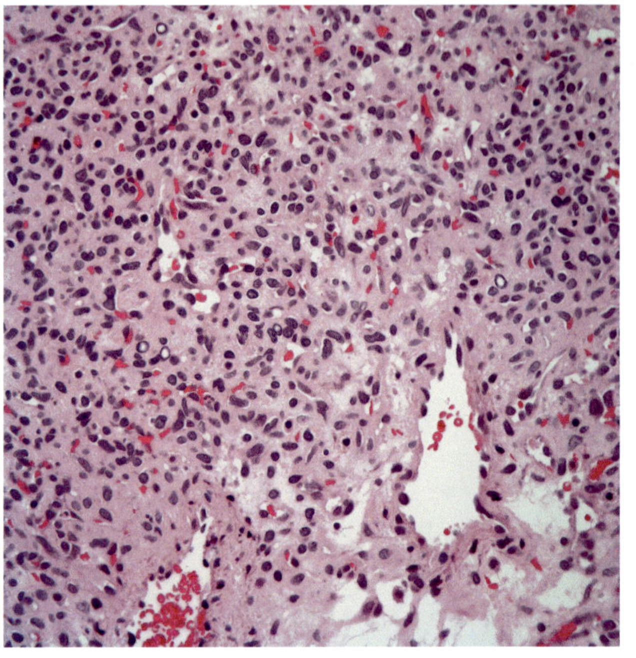

Fig. 4.53 Higher magnification of a thymic glomus tumor showing a homogeneous cellular proliferation of rather small cells; note the absence of mitotic activity or marked nuclear atypia

Cholesteroloma

This is also another benign tumoral condition of unusual occurrence in the mediastinal compartment. Although this process had been reported in the past, it was not until recently that a small series of four cases was presented in the literature under the designation of thymic cholesteroloma [67]. The four cases described are in four adult men between the ages of 58 and 71 years. Two of these lesions were discovered incidentally while these patients were being evaluated for different clinical conditions. Only one of the four patients described presented with symptoms of cough and dyspnea, and one was asymptomatic. Surgical resection of the lesion was performed, which appears to be the treatment of choice, and it is curative.

Pathological Features

The tumors appear to range in size from 2 to 6 cm in greatest dimension and are described as soft to rubbery lesions and well circumscribed but not encapsulated.

Histologically, the lesions at low power are characterized by showing a subtle nodular or alveolar architecture composed of nodules of varying sizes and exclusively of cholesterol cleft granulomata. Inflammatory cells are present but not very conspicuous and multinucleated giant cells are present. The nodules are separated by thick fibrovascular septa with minimal inflammatory reaction (Figs. 4.54 and 4.55). Remnants of thymic tissue are usually present.

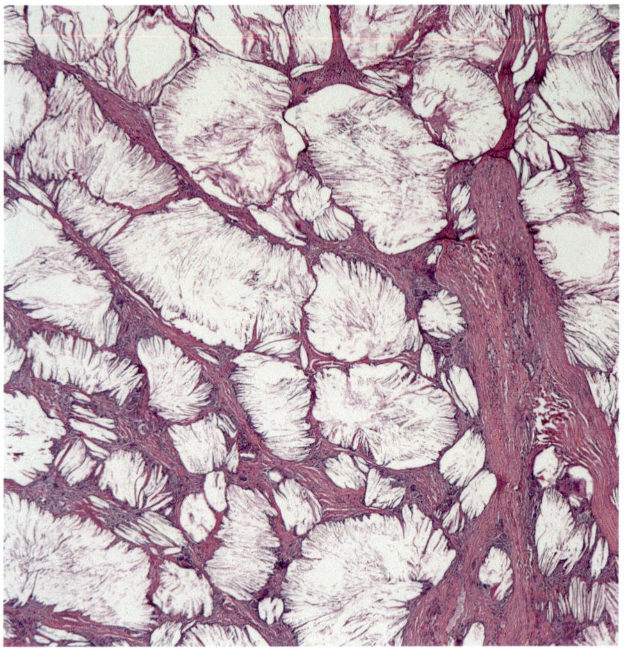

Fig. 4.54 Mediastinal cholesteroloma showing a lobular appearance

The use of immunohistochemical stains for the diagnosis of thymic cholesteroloma is not necessary.

Differential Diagnosis

The features of this lesion are so characteristic that it is unlikely that this lesion will be confused for another either

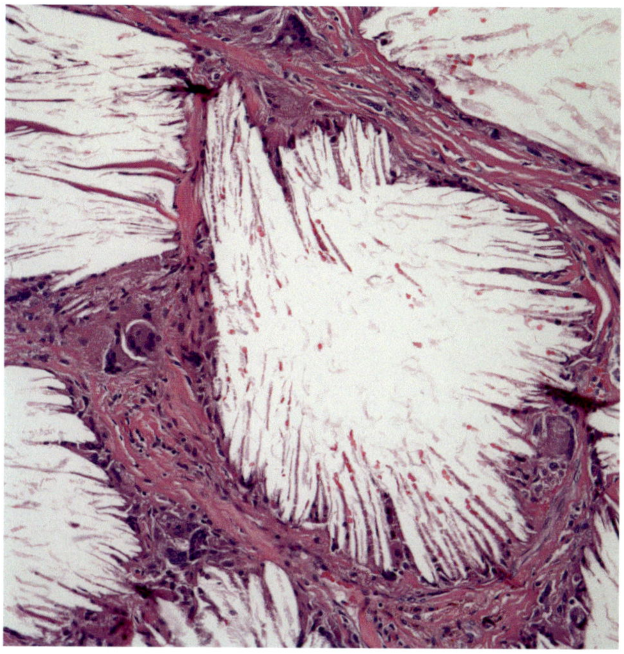

Fig. 4.55 Higher magnification of a cholesteroloma showing the typical cholesterol cleft granulomata

benign or malignant neoplasm; however, in a small mediastinoscopic biopsy, which likely will show the presence of cholesterol cleft granulomas, possible considerations include cystic teratoma and multilocular thymic cyst. In both of these tumoral conditions, cholesterol cleft granuloma may be present. An unequivocal diagnosis of thymic cholesteroloma can be best made after complete surgical resection.

Mediastinal Pecoma

The thoracic tumors that have been grouped within the perivascular epithelioid cell differentiation include clear cell "sugar" tumor, lymphangioleiomyomatosis, and angiomyolipoma [68]. Of those, as it has been described in other sections in this text, angiomyolipomas may occur in the mediastinal compartment. Clinically, some PEComas occur in the background of tuberous sclerosis complex, while some appear to occur in patients without that association. More specifically, clear cell "sugar" tumors are predominantly more common in the lung parenchyma. Only rare cases have been described in the mediastinal compartment. In the case reported by Liang and colleagues [69], a man 63 years of age was found to have an "opacity" involving the lung and mediastinum. Diagnostic imaging showed the mass involving both anatomic areas, and surgical resection was performed. After histopathological evaluation, the authors arrived at a final diagnosis of malignant epithelioid angioleiomyoma.

In our experience, we have seen a single case in which the tumor shows all the characteristics of a clear cell "sugar" tumor, and it occurred in an adult female patient without any association with tuberous sclerosis; the tumor was limited only to the anterior mediastinal compartment. This example represents what has been quoted as "extrapulmonary sugar tumor." Surgical resection appears to be the treatment of choice in these patients and likely is curative. However, in cases in which the tumor is linked to the tuberous sclerosis complex, the prognosis may be different.

Pathological Features

Macroscopically, these tumors may be soft and well circumscribed, measuring a few centimeters in diameter. Necrosis is not common, and focal areas of hemorrhage may be seen.

Histologically, the tumor is characterized by sheets or cords of medium size cells with clear cytoplasm, round to oval nuclei, and inconspicuous nucleoli. The cellular proliferation is admixed with delicate thin fibrous connective tissue and prominent ectatic blood vessels. The blood vessels are thickened, and the cellular proliferation is dispersed around the vessel without invading into the endothelial lining of the vessels. The cellular proliferation is fairly homogeneous, and there is no cellular atypia or mitotic activity (Figs. 4.56, 4.57, 4.58, and 4.59). Areas of hemorrhage or necrosis are not common. Focal areas of thymic rimming may be seen in cases involving the thymus.

Immunohistochemical stains may be of aid in the diagnosis of these unusual tumors as clear cell "sugar" tumor is commonly positive for CD34 and HMB-45 while negative for keratin, S-100 protein, desmin, and neuroendocrine markers.

PEComas as a family of tumors harbor TFE3 gene rearrangement and TSC2 mutations.

Differential Diagnosis

By far, the most important differential diagnosis for these tumors in the anterior mediastinum is to separate them from clear cell thymic carcinoma. In that setting, the use of keratin antibodies should lead to the correct interpretation. Some germ cell tumors may also show clear cell component, but usually germ cell tumors are more common in young male patients and also positive for keratin markers.

Sclerosing Hemangioma (Extrapulmonary Pneumocytoma)

Currently, this benign tumor is classified as pneumocytoma as it has been described exclusively in the lung parenchyma [70]. In our experience, we have observed two cases: one in a 21-year-old male with history of asthma and one in a 34-year-old female patient who presented with symptoms of chest pain and dyspnea. Diagnostic

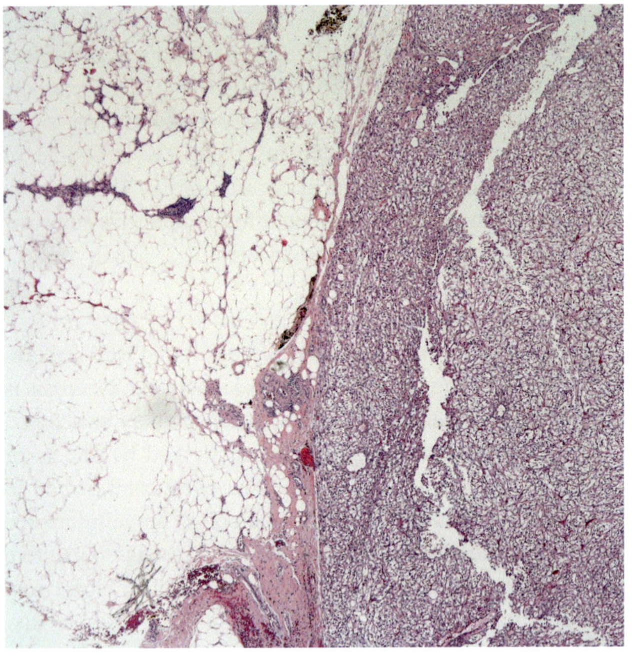

Fig. 4.56 Low power view of a mediastinal PEComa (extrapulmonary sugar tumor) showing a well-circumscribed tumor; note the presence of focal thymic tissue in the periphery

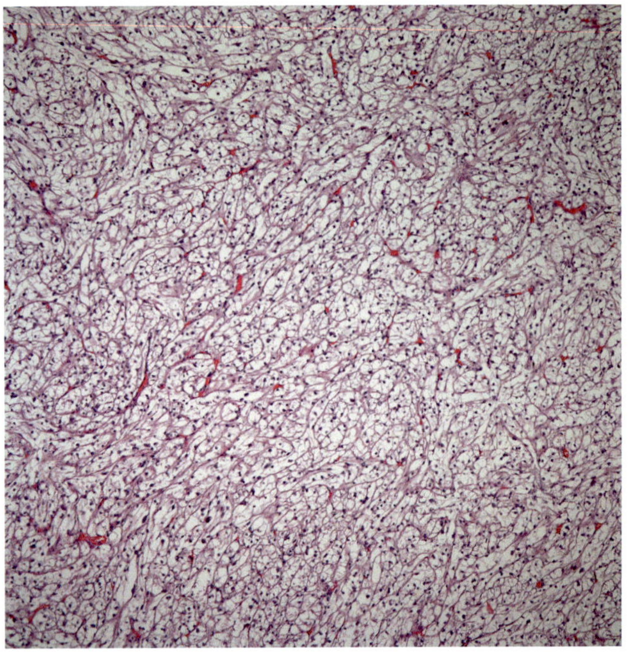

Fig. 4.57 Mediastinal PEComa showing sheets of clear cells

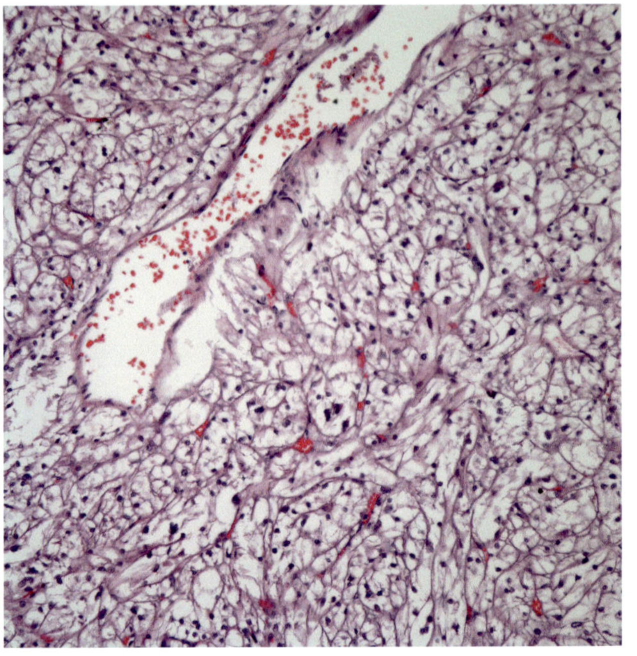

Fig. 4.58 Prominent ectatic vessels are commonly seen in extrapulmonary sugar tumor

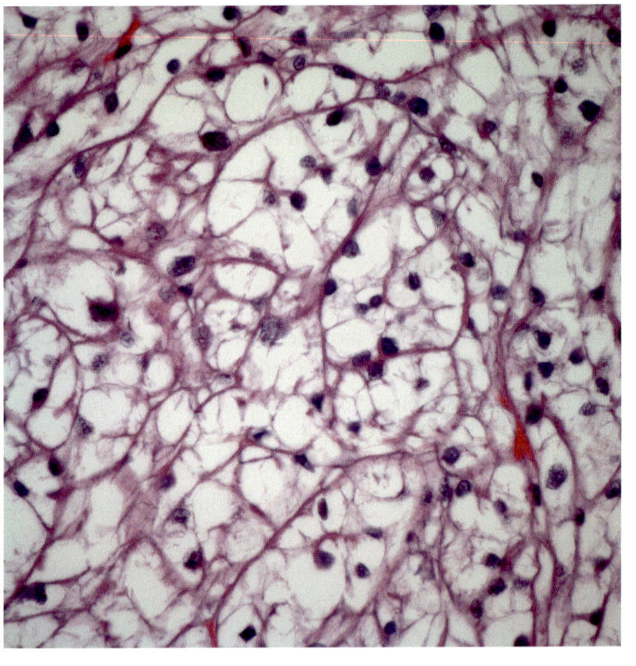

Fig. 4.59 Higher magnification of a PEComa (extrapulmonary sugar tumor) showing absence of cellular atypia and mitotic activity

imaging disclosed the presence of an anterior mediastinal mass in both patients without any pulmonary involvement. This occurrence appears to be highly unusual, and it is possible that the tumors occur in the background of ectopic pulmonary tissue. Surgical resection of the anterior mediastinal tumors was performed, and, during surgery, no lung involvement was identified. The treatment of choice in these cases may be surgical resection alone; however, as in the tumors occurring in the lung parenchyma, metastatic disease to lymph node may be present. Thus, it is advisable for tumors occurring in the mediastinum to procure lymph nodes for evaluation. For those tumors with the classic histology, surgical resection may be curative.

Pathological Features

Macroscopically, the tumors may range in size from 4 to 9 cm in greatest diameter. The tumors are well circumscribed, soft, and focally hemorrhagic. Necrosis is not a feature of these tumors.

Histologically, the tumors showed essentially the same features as those described in the lung parenchyma. The tumor is composed of a dual cellular proliferation: surface cells and stromal cells arranged in some areas with a pseudopapillary growth pattern. Dilated blood vessels filled with blood are present in some areas, while in other cases, the tumor may have a more solid appearance (Figs. 4.60, 4.61, 4.62, and 4.63). Areas of hyalinization often are present; however, frank necrosis is not a feature of this tumor. Focal areas showing calcifications may be present as well as focal areas composed of spindle cells or cells with clear cytoplasm. Mitotic activity and/or cellular atypia are unusual in these tumors.

Immunohistochemical stains may be of aid just as for those tumors in the lung parenchyma. Essentially, these tumors are positive for TTF-1, keratin 7, and broad-spectrum keratin, while other areas may also show positive staining for epithelial membrane antigen. Vascular markers such as CD31, CD34, Factor VIII, and Ulex are negative.

Differential Diagnosis

The diagnosis of sclerosing hemangioma in a biopsy is very challenging and can be even more challenging when the mass is in the mediastinum. Even in resected specimens of mediastinal tumors, the diagnosis should be made with care as the tumor may show features that may be shared with other more common tumors such as thymomas or mesotheliomas. In cases of thymomas, these tumors are generally positive for keratin 5/6, which sclerosing hemangioma is not. On the other hand, in cases of mesothelioma, similarly keratin 5/6 is positive which again will be most unusual in cases of sclerosing hemangioma. Other considerations include thymic adenocarcinoma; however, in these tumors, cytologic atypia and mitotic activity may lead to the correct interpretation.

Histiocytic Tumors

Contrary to the spectrum of this type of tumor in the lung parenchyma, the mediastinal involvement by these processes is rare and may be limited to only sporadic case reports of some of these histiocytic lesions. In the lung parenchyma, classically, the more common histiocytic tumors described include Langerhans cell histiocytosis, Erdheim-Chester disease, and Rosai-Dorfman disease; in the mediastinum, the two that appear to be relatively more common are Langerhans cell histiocytosis and Rosai-Dorfman disease. Therefore, the discussion of these lesions in this section will be limited to Langerhans cell histiocytosis and Rosai-Dorfman disease. However, it is important to mention that cases of Erdheim-Chester disease involving the mediastinal compartment have been described, although it appears that in those cases the process has been with involvement of different anatomic structures that include the mediastinum [71, 72].

Langerhans Cell Histiocytosis (LCH)

The thymic involvement of LCH is rare and has been the subject of several case reports with only small series of cases [73–77]. In many cases, the process is well known to affect other anatomic areas, while in some cases the process appears to have presented as a mediastinal involvement alone with possible congenital origin. Only some unusual cases appear to affect the thymic gland alone. Most of the cases described in the literature are in children of different ages. In a study of 1423 children less than 18 years of age from the French national cohort [77], the authors encountered 37 cases in which the prevalence of mediastinal involvement varied with the age at diagnosis: for patients 1 year old or less, such prevalence is approximately 7%, while for patients older than 5 years, such prevalence is less than 1%. In addition, the authors documented that in 13 patients (35%), the diagnosis was related to mediastinal involvement-related symptoms including respiratory distress, superior vena cava syndrome, cough, and polypnea. All the patients had multisystem disease, and 35 of 37 were treated with a steroid and vinblastine. Death occurred in five patients; however, the overall 5-year survival rate was 87%. The authors concluded that mediastinal involvement by LCH occurs mainly in children. Diagnostic imaging commonly shows thymus enlargement and calcifications. In a separate study in children but with emphasis on histological patterns of thymic involvement, Picarsic and colleagues [78] presented 9 cases of their own and reviewed the literature of an additional 23 cases, identifying 4 separate pathologic groups: (1) microscopic collections of hyperplastic LCH-like cells in incidental thymectomies of patients without LCH disease, (2) solitary LCH of the thymus with gland

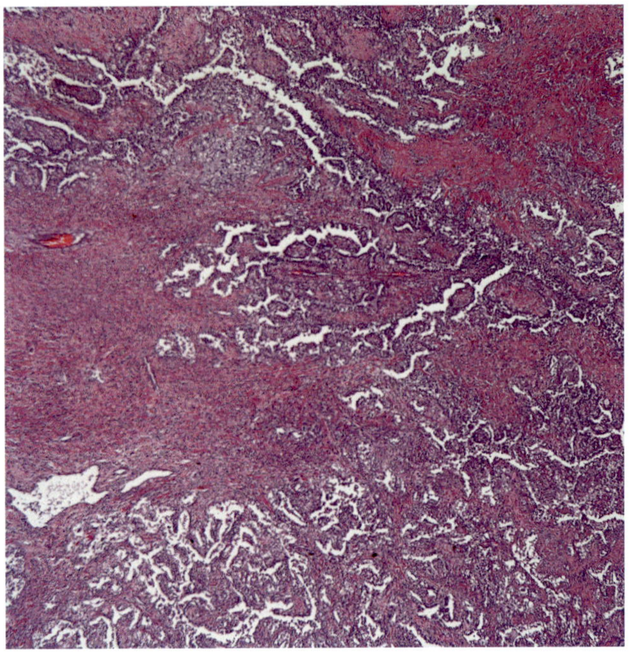

Fig. 4.60 Low power view of a mediastinal sclerosing hemangioma showing a papillary growth pattern with solid stromal component

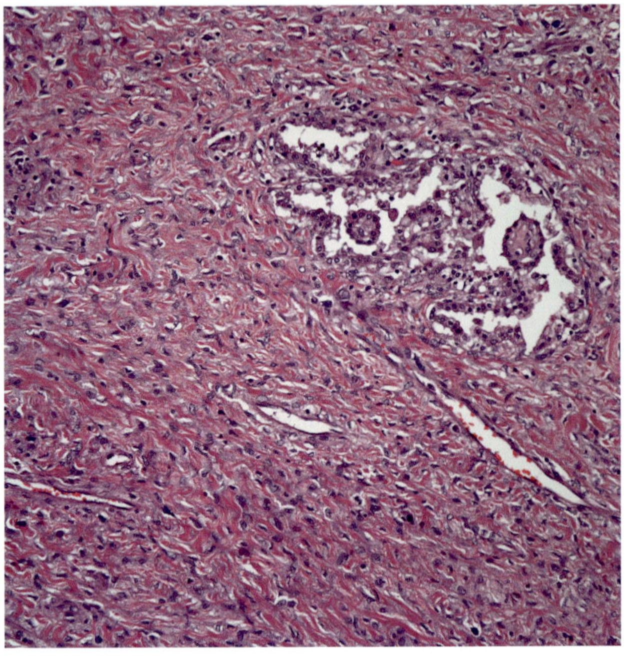

Fig. 4.62 Prominent stromal component in a mediastinal sclerosing hemangioma

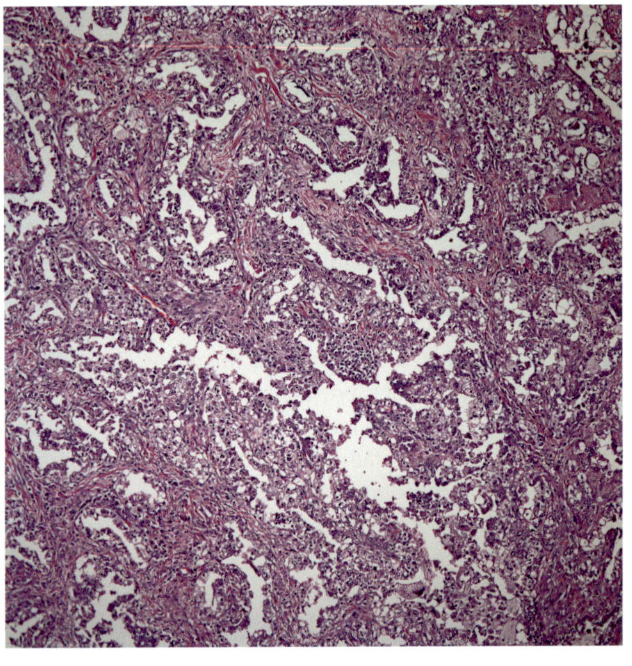

Fig. 4.61 Prominent glandular-like appearance of a mediastinal sclerosing hemangioma

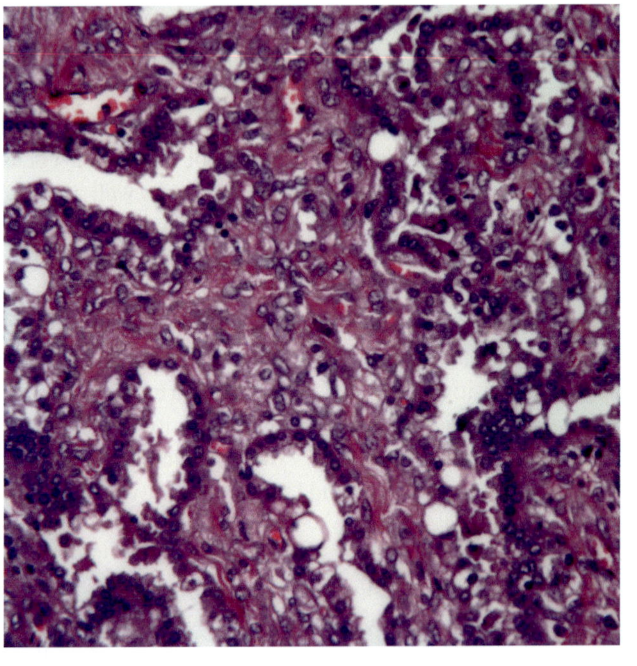

Fig. 4.63 Mediastinal sclerosing hemangioma showing two distinct cellular components

disruption, (3) variable thymic involvement in multisystemic LCH disease with either restricted pattern or diffuse thymic involvement, and (4) mixed histiocytic lesions with concurrent LCH and juvenile xanthogranuloma-like proliferation.

The treatment and prognosis in these patients are essentially based on the systemic nature of the disease. In patients in whom the LCH is found incidentally in a thymectomy, the patient likely will not receive any additional treatment, while those with systemic disease will be treated accordingly, and their prognosis is dependent on response to treatment.

Pathological Features

As it has been stated, in the descriptions of the thymic involvement by LCH, the macroscopic findings will also be related to the background in which thymectomy is performed. In cases in which there is no history of LCH and the patients get a thymic resection for an unrelated reason [79], it is most likely the thymus will not show any specific abnormality on gross examination. However, in cases in which there is a history of LCH with mediastinal involvement and in which the thymus may be involved in a diffuse fashion, it is likely that the gland not only may be enlarged but also may show some nodularity. Therefore, the gross evaluation of thymus is dependent on the background in which the gland is obtained.

Histologically, the low power view will show the presence of discrete nodules embedded in a background of lymphoid thymic stroma. The nodules are composed of medium size cells with round to oval nuclei and inconspicuous nucleoli. At higher magnification in some of the nuclei, it is possible to identify grooving of the nuclei. In some of these nodules, sprinkle eosinophils may be present. Necrosis and presence of multinucleated giant cells are rare in this pattern. In the diffuse pattern, the thymic lymphoid stroma seems to merge with the histiocytic proliferation; however, in this pattern, it is possible to observe focal areas of punctate necrosis and multinucleated giant cells (Figs. 4.64, 4.65, 4.66, and 4.67).

Immunohistochemical stain for S-100 protein and CD1a should help in the evaluation of these nodules. In some cases, the use of Langerin may also help.

Differential Diagnosis

In cases in which there is no history of LCH, the nodules in the thymus may be overlooked or interpreted as a normal component of the thymus, which, in addition, may have follicular hyperplasia. However, when the process is diffused in the thymus and the patient is suspected of a "histiocytosis," then the differential diagnosis would include some of the other histiocytic lesions including Rosa-Dorfman disease, Erdheim-Chester disease, and juvenile xantogranuloma. In this setting, some histopathological features coupled with some immunohistochemical support may lead to the correct interpretation. For instance, in cases of Rosai-Dorfman disease, the process commonly has numerous plasma cells, the histiocytes are large, and even though it is positive for S-100 protein, it is also negative for CD1a. In cases of Erdheim-Chester disease, the histiocytes are rather smaller in comparison to those in LCH, and the distribution of the process is somewhat different; the process is negative CD1a. Juvenile xanthogranulomatosis is a bit more difficult, taking into account that some cases of LCH may show some xantogranuloma-like areas; however, once again, the use of S-100 protein and CD1a should lead to the correct interpretation.

Rosai-Dorfman Disease (RDD)

Although RDD has been described almost in every organ system in the human body, this type of histiocytosis is of rare occurrence in the thymus, and it has been only rarely reported in the literature [80, 81]. In the case described by Wu and colleagues [80], a 42-year-old man also had a primary splenic diffuse large B-cell lymphoma, and possibly the thymectomy was performed for reasons other than RDD. However, it is important to note that reports of patients with primary mediastinal mass without previous history of RDD are lacking in the literature. We have been able to observe a couple of cases in which such presentation was obtained and in which diagnostic imaging revealed the presence of an anterior mediastinal mass which was resected under the impression of a tumoral conditions other than RDD. However, these types of cases are encountered only rarely in the general practice. Based on the available literature, it is difficult to determine what the natural course of RDD limited to the thymus is. However, it appears that surgical resection needs to be performed in these cases.

Pathological Features

In the cases that we have evaluated, the resected thymic mass has been soft, and the cyst measures approximately 4–5 cm in greatest diameter. It has been ill defined and not encapsulated.

Histologically, RDD is characterized by the presence of a histiocytic proliferation composed of large histiocytes with round nuclei and inconspicuous nucleoli. This histiocytic proliferation is accompanied by numerous plasma cells and lymphocytes. Emperipolesis can be identified in focal areas. Of interest, residual thymic tissue can be easily identified, and, toward the periphery, the thymus may show areas similar to those observed in a multilocular thymic cyst (Figs. 4.68, 4.69, 4.70, 4.71, and 4.72).

Immunohistochemical stains may be of aid in the diagnosis as the histiocytes are positive for S-100 protein and negative for CD1a.

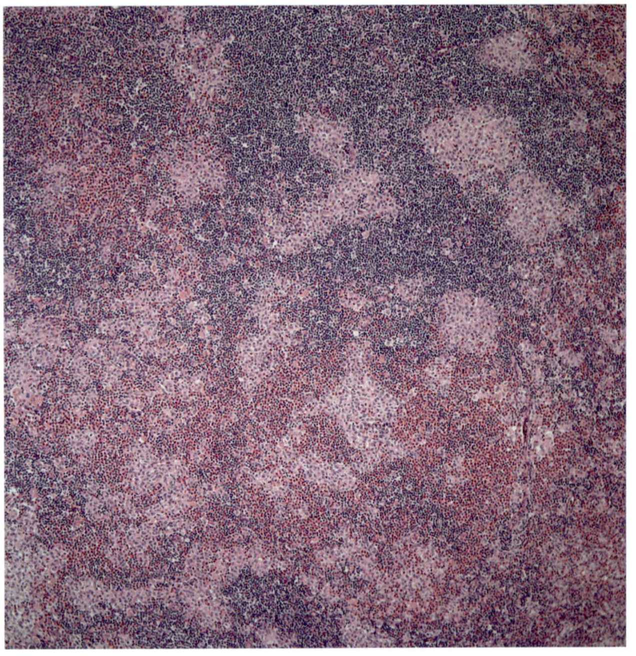

Fig. 4.64 Low power view of Langerhans cell histiocytosis involving the thymus

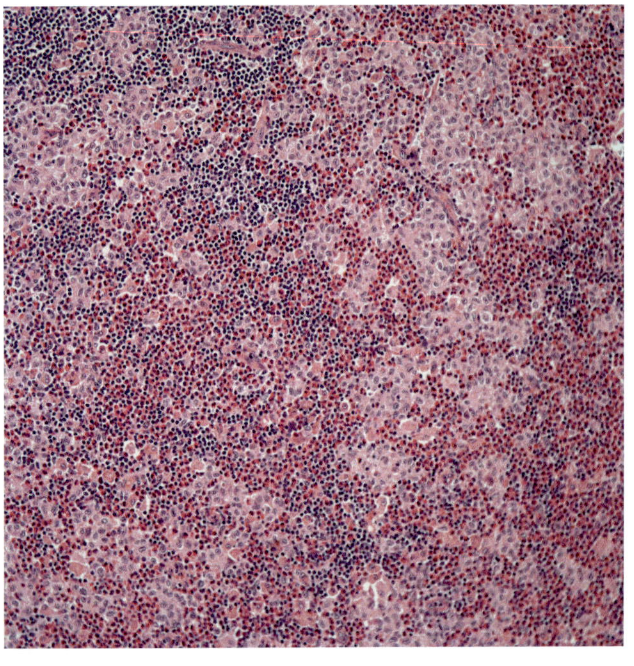

Fig. 4.65 Thymic Langerhans cell histiocytosis showing marked presence of eosinophils

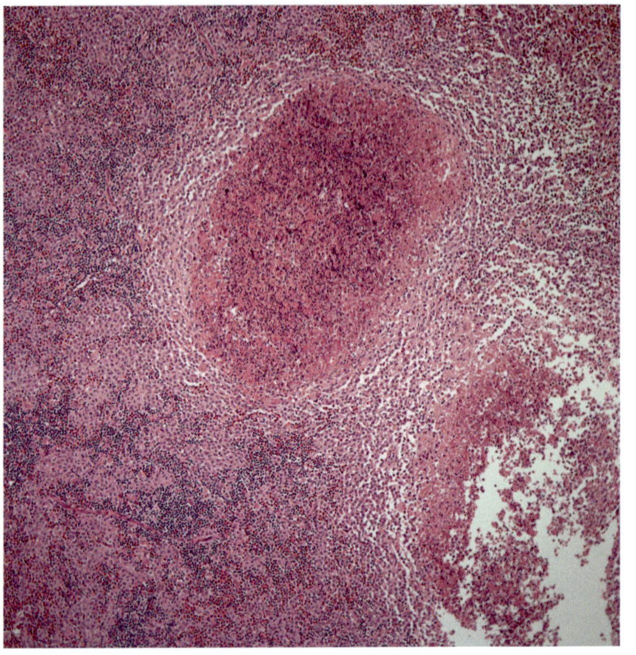

Fig. 4.66 Thymic Langerhans cell histiocytosis showing focal areas of necrosis

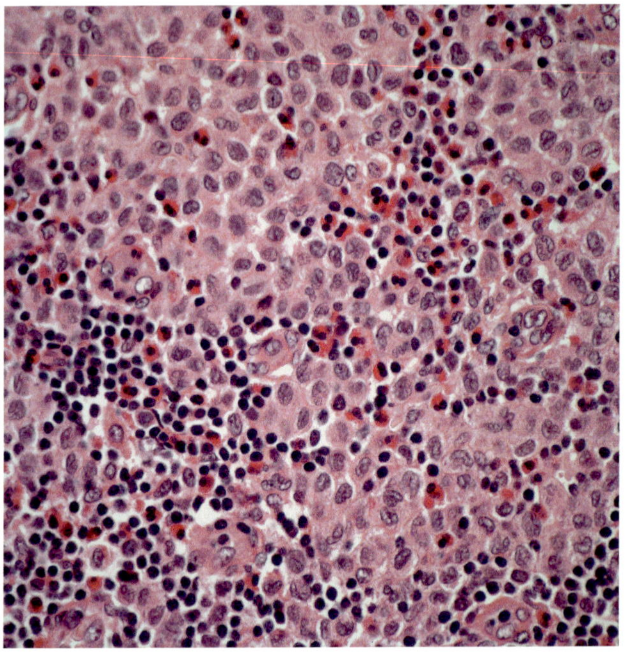

Fig. 4.67 High power view thymic Langerhans cell histiocytosis showing the classic features of the histiocytes

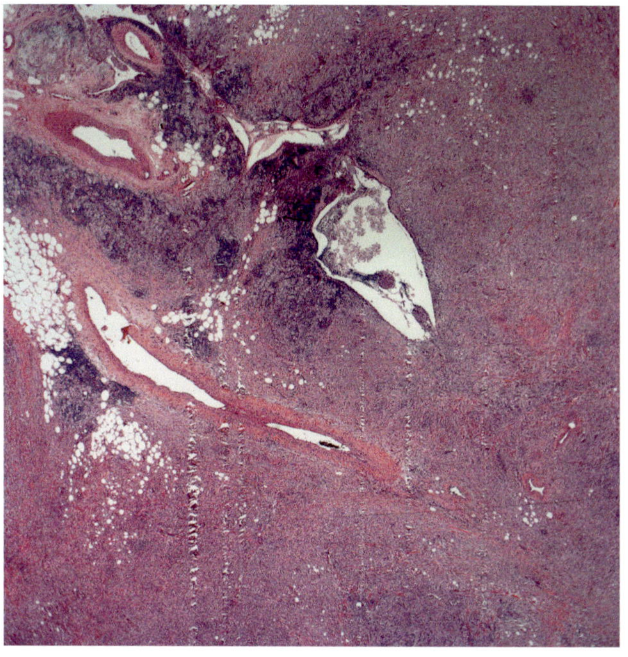

Fig. 4.68 Rosai-Dorfman disease involving the thymus; note the cystic thymic changes

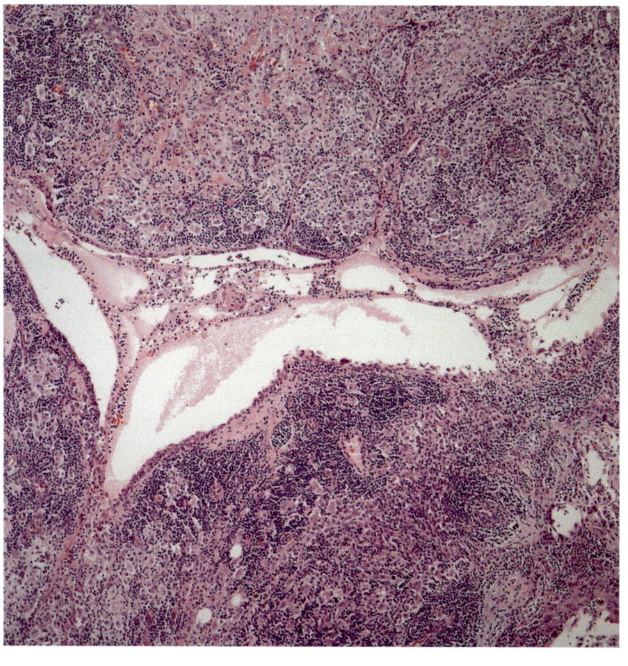

Fig. 4.69 Thymic cystic changes in Rosai-Dorfman disease of the thymus

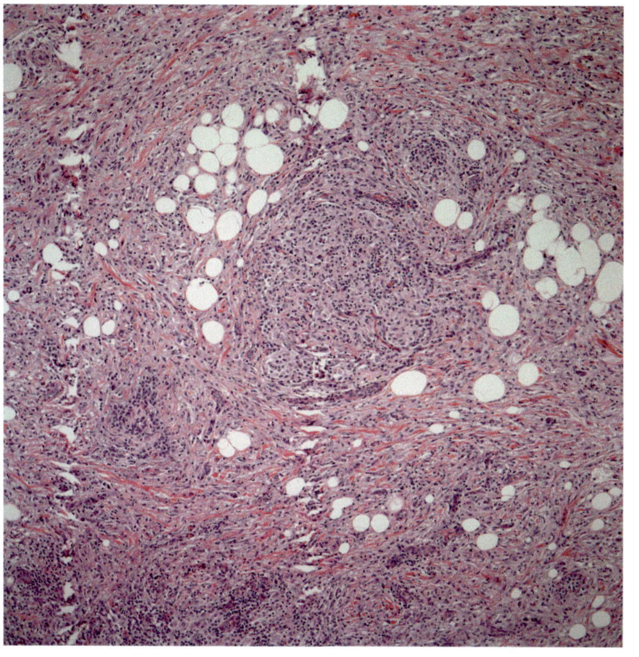

Fig. 4.70 Rosai-Dorfman disease involving thymic adipose tissue

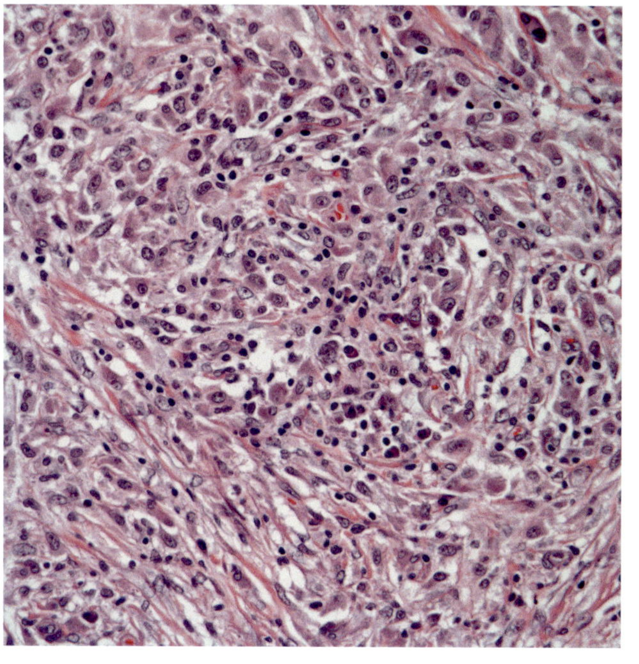

Fig. 4.71 Large histiocytes admixed with plasma cells in Rosai-Dorfman disease of the thymus

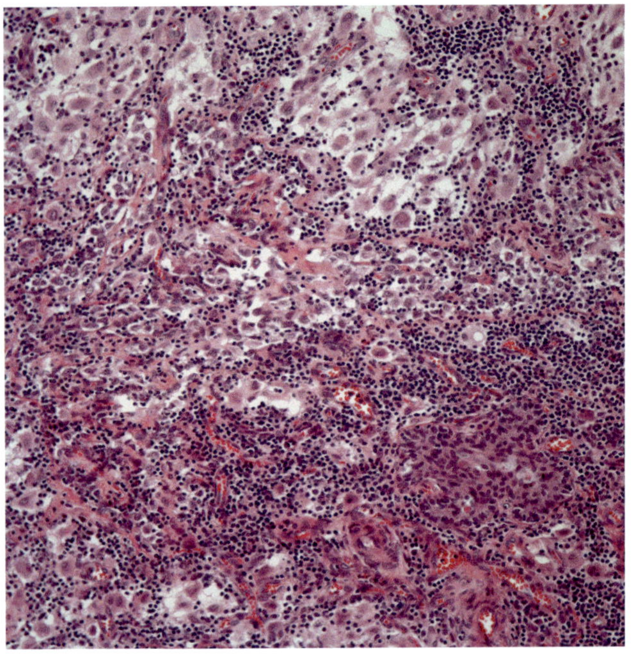

Fig. 4.72 Large histiocytes of Rosai-Dorfman disease admixed with thymic lymphocytes

Differential Diagnosis

RDD needs to be separated mainly from other histiocytic proliferations such as LCH. In this setting, RDD would show negative staining in the histiocytes for CD1a and also for Langerin. However, more importantly, in the mediastinal area where lymphomas are much more common than RDD, it is essential that RDD is separated from any lymphoproliferative process. A wider panel of immunohistochemical stains including B-and T-cell markers in addition to CD15 and CD30 would help in the proper interpretation of RDD or lymphoma.

References

1. Laipply TC. Cysts and cystic tumors of the mediastinum. Arch Pathol. 1945;39:153–61.
2. Schwarz H, Williams CS. Thoracic gastric cysts: report of two cases with review of the literature. J Thorac Surg. 1942;12:117–30.
3. Blades B. Mediastinal tumors. Report of cases treated at ARMY thoracic surgery centers. Ann Surg. 1946;123:749–65.
4. Richards GJ, Reeves RJ. Mediastinal tumors and cysts in children. Am J Dis Child. 1958;95:284–91.
5. Pachter MR, Lattes R. Mediastinal cysts: a clinicopathologic study of twenty cases. J Dis Chest. 1963;44:416–22.
6. Wychulis AR, Payne WS, Clagett OT, Woolner LB. Surgical treatment of mediastinal tumors: a 40 year experience. J Thorac Cardiovasc Surg. 1971;62:379–92.
7. Oldham HN. Mediastinal tumors and cysts. Ann Thorac Surg. 1971;11:246–75.
8. Whittaker LD, Lynn HB. Mediastinal tumors and cysts in the pediatric patient. Surg Clin North Am. 1973;53:893–904.
9. Davis RD, Oldham HN, Sabiston DC. Primary cysts and neoplasms of the mediastinum: recent changes in clinical presentation, methods of diagnosis, management, and results. Ann Thorac Surg. 1987;44:229–37.
10. Reed J, Sobonya RE. Morphologic analysis of foregut cysts in the thorax. Am J Roentgenol Radium Therapy, Nucl Med. 1974;120:851–60.
11. Nakata H, Nakayama C, Kimoto T, Nakayama T, Tsukamoto Y, Nobe T, et al. Computed tomography of mediastinal bronchogenic cysts. J Comput Assist Tomogr. 1982;6:733–8.
12. Madewell JE, Sobonya RE, Reed JC. RPC from the AFIP. Radiology. 1973;109:707–12.
13. Wick MR. Cystic lesions of the mediastinum. Sem Diag Pathol. 2005;22:241–53.
14. Wright CD. Mediastinal tumors and cysts in the pediatric population. Thorac Surg Clin. 2009;19:47–61.
15. Petroze R, ED MG. Pediatric Chest II: Benign tumors. Surg Clin N Am. 2012;92:645–58.
16. Pickhardt OC. Pleuro-diaphragmatic cyst. Ann Surg. 1934;99:814.
17. Wychulis AR, Connolly DC, McGoon DC. Pericardial cysts, tumors, and fat necrosis. J Thorac Cardiovasc Surg. 1971;62:294–300.
18. Feigin DS, Fenoglio JJ, McAllister HA, Madewell JE. Pericardial cysts: a radiologic-pathologic correlation and review. Radiology. 1977;125:15–20.
19. Smart J. A case of a large thymic cyst successfully removed from the anterior mediastinum. Br Med J. 1947;41:84.
20. Fridjohn MH. Cyst of the thymus in a newborn baby. Br Med J. 1934;2:553.
21. Speers FD. Thymic cysts. N Y Med Coll and Flower Hosp Bull. 1938;1:142.
22. Crellin JA, Pugh TF, Janton OH. Benign thymic cyst: a case report. Dis Chest. 1950;XVIII:154.
23. Suster S, Rosai J. Multilocular thymic cyst: an acquired reactive process. Study of 18 cases. Am J Surg Pathol. 1991;15:388–98.
24. Greipp PR, Gau GT, Dockerty MB, Westbrook P, Pluth JR. Thymic cyst presenting as an acute mediastinal mass. Chest. 1973;64:125.
25. Suster S, Barbuto D, Carlson G, Rosai J. Multilocular thymic cysts with pseudoepitheliomatous hyperplasia. Hum Pathol. 1991;22:455–60.
26. Moran CA, Suster S, El-Naggar A, Luna MA. Carcinomas arising in multilocular thymic cysts of the neck: a clinicopathological study of three cases. Histopathology. 2004;44:64–8.
27. Moran CA, Suster S. Mucoepidermoid carcinomas of the thymus. A clinicopathologic study of six cases. Am J Surg Pathol. 1995;19:826–34.
28. Hatori H. High-grade thymic carcinoma other than basaloid or mucoepidermoid type could be associated with multilocular thymic cyst: report of two cases. Histopathology. 2003;44:501–2.
29. Moran CA, Suster S. Mediastinal seminomas with prominent cystic changes: a clinicopathologic study of 10 cases. Am J Surg Pathol. 1995;19:1047–53.
30. Leong ASY, Brown JH. Malignant transformation in a thymic cyst. Am J Surg Pathol. 1984;8:471–5.
31. Weissferdt A, Moran CA. Primary MALT-type lymphoma of the thymus: a clinicopathological and Immunohistochemical study of six cases. Lung. 2011;189:461–6.
32. Weissferdt A, Kalhor N, Moran CA. Cystic well-differentiated squamous cell carcinoma of the thymus: a clinicopathological and Immunohistochemical study of six cases. Histopathology. 2016;68:333–8.
33. Moran CA, Suster S, Silva EG. Low-grade serous carcinoma of the ovary metastatic to the anterior mediastinum simulating multilocular thymic cysts: a clinicopathologic and Immunohistochemical study of 3 cases. Am J Surg Pathol. 2005;29:496–9.

34. Moran CA, Suster S. Cystic well-differentiated neuroendocrine carcinoma (carcnoid tumor): a clinicopathologic and Immunohistochemical study of two cases. Am J Clin Pathol. 2006;126:377–80.
35. Mathisen DJ, Grillo HC. Clinical manifestations of mediastinal fibrosis and histoplasmosis. Ann Thorac Surg. 1992;54:1053.
36. Langerstrom CF, Mitchell HG, Graham BS, Hammon JW. Chronic fibrosing mediastinitis and superior vena caval obstruction from blastomycosis. Ann Thorac Surg. 1992;54:764–5.
37. Goodwin RA, Nickell JA, De Prez RM. Mediastinal fibrosis complicating healed primary histoplasmosis and tuberculosis. Medicine (Blastimore). 1972;51:227–46.
38. Dines DR, Bernatz PE, Pairolero PC. Mediastinal granuloma and fibrosing mediastinitis. Chest. 1979;75:320–4.
39. Lohman AJ. Mediastinitis anterior chronica. Acta Med Scan. 1948;131(1):51–65. CXXXI, Fasc I.
40. Schowengerdt CG, Suyemoto R, Main FB. Granulomatous and fibrous mediastinitis. J Thorac Cardiovasc Surg. 1968;57:365–79.
41. Longmire WP, Goodwin WE, Buckberg GD. Management of sclerosing fibrosis of the mediastinal and retroperitoneal areas. Ann Surg. 1967;165:1013.
42. Light AM. Idiopathic fibrosis of mediastinum: a discussion of three cases and review of the literature. J Clin Pathol. 1978;31:78–88.
43. Flieder DB, Suster S, Moran CA. Idiopathic fibroinflammatory (fibrosing/sclerosing) lesions of the mediastinum: a study of 30 cases with emphasis on morphologic heterogeneity. Mod Pathol. 1999;12:257–64.
44. Rossi GM, Emmi G, Corradi D, Urban ML, Maritati F, Landini F, et al. Idopathic mediastinal fibrosis: a systemic immune-mediated disorder. A case series and review of the literature. Clin Rev Allerg Immunol. 2017;52(3):446–59.
45. Rossi GM, Rocco R, Buttini EA, Marvisi C, Vaglio A. Idiopathic retroperitoneal fibrosis and its overlap with IgG4-related disease. Intern Emerg Med. 2017;12:287–99.
46. Inoue M, Nose N, Nishikawa H, Takahashi M, Zen Y, Kawaguchi M. Successful treatment of sclerosing mediastinitis with high serum IgG4 level. Gen Thorac Cardiovasc Surg. 2007;55:431–3.
47. Worrell JA, Donnelly EF, Martin JB, Bastarache JA, Loyd JE. Computed tomography and the idiopathic form of proliferative fibrosing mediastinitis. J Thorac Imaging. 2007;22:235–40.
48. Gorospe L, Aya-Carbonero AM, Fernandez-Mendez MA, Arrieta P, Muñoz-Molina GM, Cabañero-Sánchez A, et al. Idopathic fibrosing mediastinitis: spectrum of imaging findings with emphasis on its association with IgG4-related disease. Clin Imaging. 2015;39:993–9.
49. Moran CA, Suster S, Gil J, Jagirdar J. Morphometric analysis of germinal centers in nonthymomatous patients with myasthenia gravis. Arch Pathol Lab Med. 1990;114:689–91.
50. Levine GD, Rosai J. Thymic hyperplasia and neoplasia: a review of current concepts. Hum Pathol. 1978;9:495–515.
51. Hofmann WJ, Moller P, Otto HF. Thymic hyperplasia. I. Ture thymic hyperplasia. Review of the literature. Klin Wochenschr. 1987;65:49–52.
52. Hofmann WJ, Moller P, Otto HF. Thymic hyperplasia. II. Lymphofollicular hyperplasia of the thymus. An immunohistologic study. Klin Wochenschr. 1987;65:53–60.
53. Ruco LP, Rosati S, Palmieri B, Pescarmona E, Rendina EA, Baroni CD. True thymic hyperplasia: a histological and Immunohistochemical study. Ann Thorac Surg. 1989;47:741–5.
54. Plaza JA, Domnguez F, Suster S. Cystic adenomatoid tumor of the mediastinum. Am J Surg Pathol. 2004;28:132–8.
55. Goto M, Uchiyama M, Kuwabara K. Adenomatoid tumor of the mediastinum. Gen Thorac Cardiovasc Surg. 2016;64:47–50.
56. Parekh V, Winokur T, Cerfolio RJ, Stevens TM. Posterior mediastinal adenomatoid tumor. A case report and review of the literature. Case Rep Pathol. 2016;2016:6898526. May. 2016;8:2016.
57. Jang SH, Cho HD, Lee JH, Lee HJ, Jung HY, Kim KJ, et al. Mediastinal glomus tumor: a case report and literature review. J Path and Transl Med. 2015;49:520–4.
58. Lee TJ, Reddy GP, Leung JWT, Gotway MD. Mediastinal glomangioma: CT and octreotride scintigraphy appearance and review of the literature. J Thorac Imaging. 2008;23:289–91.
59. Kanakis M, Rapti N, Chorti M, Lioulias A. Asymptomatic glomus tumor of the mediastinum. Case Rep Surg. 2015;5:631635.
60. Rychlik IJ, O'Donnell ME, Davey P, Meraud R, McGuigan J. Glomus tumor of the mediastinum. Asian Cardiovasc Thorac Ann. 2014;22:95–7.
61. Hirose T, Hasegawa T, Seki K, Yang P, Sano T, Morizumi H, et al. Atypical glomus tumor in the mediastinum: a case report with immunohistochemical and ultrastructural studies. Ultrastruct Pathol. 1996;20:451–6.
62. Gaetner EM, Steinberg DM, Huber M, Hayashi T, Tsuda N, Askin FB, et al. Pulmonary and mediastinal glomus tumors. Report of five cases including a pulmonary glomangiosarcoma: a clinicopathologic study with literature review. Am J Surg Pathol. 2000;24:1105–14.
63. Weissferdt A, Kalhor N, Moran CA. Intrathoracic glomus tumors and glomangiosarcomas: a clinicopathological and Immunohistochemical study of 14 cases with emphasis on anatomic distribution. Virch Arch. 2016;469:541–6.
64. Choi YJ, Yang KH, Gang SJ, Kim BK, Kim SM. Malignant glomus tumor originating in the superior mediastinum. An Immunohistochemical and ultrastructural study. J Korean Med Sci. 1991;2:157–63.
65. Mravic M, LaChaud G, Nguyen A, Scott MA, Dry SM, James AW. Clinical and histopathological diagnosis of glomus tumor: an institutional experience of 138 cases. Int J Surg Pathol. 2015;23(3):181–8.
66. Mosquera JM, Sboner A, Zhang L, Chen CL, Sung YS, Chen HW, et al. Novel MIRI 43-NOTCH fusions in benign and malignant glomus tumor. Genes Chromosomes Cancer. 2013;52:1075–87.
67. Weissferdt A, Kalhor N, Moran CA. Primary thymic cholesteroloma: a clinicopathological correlation of four cases of an unusual benign lesion. Virch Arch. 2015;467:609–11.
68. Thway K, Fisher C. Pecoma: morphology and genetics of a complex tumor family. Ann Diag Pathol. 2015;19:359–68.
69. Liang W, Xu S, Chen F. Malignant perivascular epithelioid cell neoplasm of the mediastinum and the lung: one case report. Medicine (Baltimore). 2015;94(22):e904.
70. Kalhor N, Staerkel GA, Moran CA. So-called sclerosing hemangioma of lung: current concept. Ann Diag Pathol. 2010;14:60–7.
71. Massaccesi C, Colella S, Fioretti F, D'Emilio V, Panella G, Primomo G, et al. An unusual thoracic localizations of Erdheim-Chester disease. Case Report Respir Med Case Rep. 2017;20:116–9.
72. Sioka C, Estrada-Veras J, Maric I, Gahl WA, Chen CC. FDG PET images in a patient with Erdheim-Chester disease. Clin Nucl Med. 2014;39:170–7.
73. Tekkesin F, Okur A, Derinkuyu BE, Akyürek N, Oğuz A, Karadeniz C, et al. Multisystem Langerhans cell histiocytosis with thymic involvement diagnosed with anterior mediastinal mass in a 2-month-old boy. Turk J Pediatr. 2016;58:424–8.
74. Kanamitsu K, Washio K, Oda M, Noda T, Oyama T, Tanimoto T, et al. Suspected early onset of congenital Langerhans cell histiocytosis involving ectopic cervical thymus and mediastinal thymus, simultaneously. Pediatr Blood Cancer. 2015;62:1491–2.
75. De Montjoye L, Dano H, Marot L, Tennstedt D, Brichard B, Van Eeckhout P, et al. Langerhans cell histiocytosis involving the skin and the thymus. Eur J Dermatol. 2015;25:82–3.
76. Oishi N, Kondo T, Mochizuki K, Inoue T, Kasai K, Nakazawa T, et al. Localized Langerhans cell histiocytosis of the thymus with BRAF V600 mutation: a case report with Immunohistochemical and genetic analysis. Hum Pathol. 2014;45:1302–5.

77. Ducassou S, Seyrig F, Thomas C, Lambilliotte A, Marec-Berard P, Berger C, et al. Thymus and mediastinal node involvement in childhood Langerhans cell histiocytosis: long-term follow up from the French national cohort. Pediatr Blood Cancer. 2013;60: 1759–65.
78. Picarsic J, Egeler RM, Chikwava K, Patterson K, Jaffe R. Histologic patterns of thymic involvement in Langerhans cell proliferations: a clinicopathologic study and review of the literature. Pediatr Dev Pathol. 2015;18:127–38.
79. Novak L, Castro CY, Listinsky CM. Multiple Langerhans cell nodules in an incidental thymectomy. Arch Pathol Lab Med. 2003;127:218–20.
80. Wu W, Cao L, Li Y, Yu X, Huang H, He J. Primary splenic diffuse large B-cell lymphoma in a patient with thymus Rosai-Dorfman disease. Am J Med Sci. 2012;344:155–9.
81. Lim R, Wittram C, Ferry JA, Shepard JA. FDG PET of Rosai-Dorfman disease of the thymus. AJR Am J Roentgenol. 2004;182:514.

Salivary Gland-Type Tumors

5

Introduction

Salivary gland-type tumors of the thymus represent a subgroup of tumors and a subject that for the most part has been ignored in the literature. The attention that salivary gland-type tumors in the thorax get is essentially due to those tumors that occur in the lung. Needless to say, the occurrence of this family of tumors in the lung [1–8] is by far much more common when compared to their counterpart in the thymus and pleura. As a matter of fact, it is not until recently that the focus on salivary gland-type tumors of the thymus has generated some interest [9]. However, it is important to mention that, contrary to salivary gland-type tumors of the lung, the spectrum of salivary gland-type tumors in the thymus is also more varied, as the tumors in this location will span from the unusual benign tumor to the most conventional malignant neoplasm. Therefore, in this chapter, the entire spectrum of this family of tumors will be discussed. In addition, because of the potential association of adenoid cystic carcinoma with basaloid carcinoma of the thymus [10], this latter entity has been included in this chapter for completeness. Important to highlight is that morphologically basaloid carcinoma of the thymus also may mimic similar tumors that occur in the salivary glands, thus the importance of adding basaloid carcinoma in the discussion of salivary gland-type tumors of the thymus.

The tumoral conditions that will be discussed in this chapter include benign tumors thymic hyperplasia with lymphoepithelial sialadenitis (LESA)-like features, sebaceous lymphadenoma, and mixed tumor (pleomorphic adenoma) as well as malignant tumors including mucoepidermoid carcinoma (MEC), epithelial-myoepithelial carcinoma, adenoid cystic carcinoma, and basaloid carcinoma.

Benign Tumors

Thymic Hyperplasia with Lymphoepithelial Sialadenitis (LESA)-Like Features

The description of this rather unusual type of benign salivary gland-type tumor of the thymus has been only recently recognized in the literature [11]. Weissferdt and Moran described four cases, two men and two women, between the ages of 37 and 53 years. In three of these patients, the mediastinal mass was identified during a routine chest radiograph, while in one patient the symptomatology was non-specific, and the patient was being followed for breast carcinoma. None of the patients had any history of any autoimmune disease including myasthenia gravis. Clinical follow-up in these patients showed the benign nature of the process. All the patients have their mediastinal tumors removed surgically.

In the description of this unusual benign LESA-like tumor, the authors argued that even though the prominent histology in LESA-like tumors is that of thymic hyperplasia, the clinical and morphological features are distinct enough to warrant a separation of LESA-like tumor from the conventional true thymic hyperplasia. In addition, the older age group for LESA-like tumor (average age 41) and the lack of any associated autoimmune process, which is a common feature in true thymic hyperplasia, seem to be unusual for LESA-like thymic tumor. Furthermore, the authors added that in the salivary glands LESA is considered an autoimmune lesion and is one of the defining components of Sjogren disease, thus the preferred designation of LESA-like tumor of the thymus.

© Springer Nature Switzerland AG 2019
N. Kalhor, C. Moran, *Mediastinal Pathology*, https://doi.org/10.1007/978-3-319-98980-8_5

Pathological Features

Grossly, the resected material was described as "enlarged and lobulated thymic gland" ranging in size from 11 to 21 cm in greatest dimension. The cut surface was fleshy and tan-yellow in color. Multiple nodules were identified measuring up to 4 cm in greatest dimension. Cystic areas were identified in one case, while necrosis and hemorrhage were not identified in any of the cases.

Histologically, the low power view shows lobulated solid and cystic cellular areas surrounded by mature adipose tissue. Some of the cystic structures are lined by squamous epithelium and filled with amorphous eosinophilic material with or without cholesterol clefts (Figs. 5.1, 5.2, and 5.3). High power view shows that the solid component is made up of dense lymphoid tissue with numerous lymphoid follicles with germinal centers (Figs. 5.4 and 5.5). Plasma cells are present in the interfollicular areas, and in some cases Russell bodies are identified. In addition, one prominent feature is the presence of thymic epithelium, which could be present in the form of clusters, nests, and islands of thymic epithelial cells. In some areas, the epithelium surrounds lymphoid follicles. Hassall corpuscles are numerous (Fig. 5.6), and some show cystic dilatation and calcification. Cholesterol cleft granulomas are also identified in these cases (Fig. 5.7). Areas of hemorrhage, necrosis, or cellular atypia with mitotic activity are not identified.

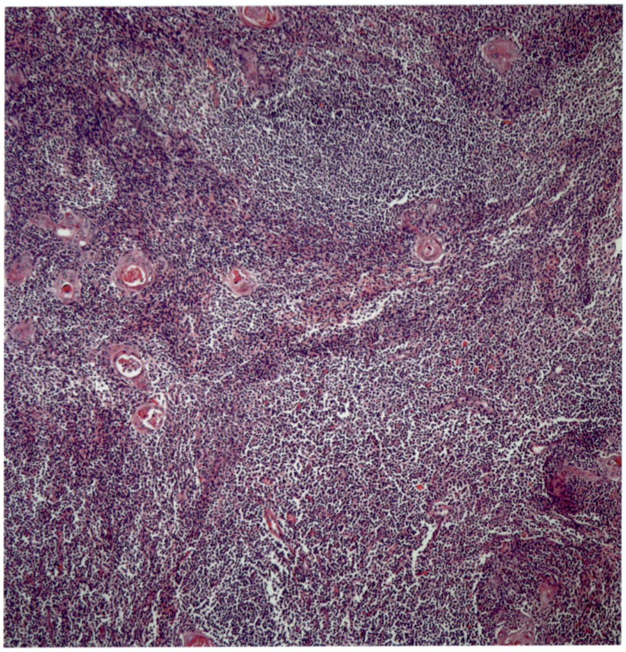

Fig. 5.2 Higher magnification showing strands of thymic epithelium and the prominent lymphoid component

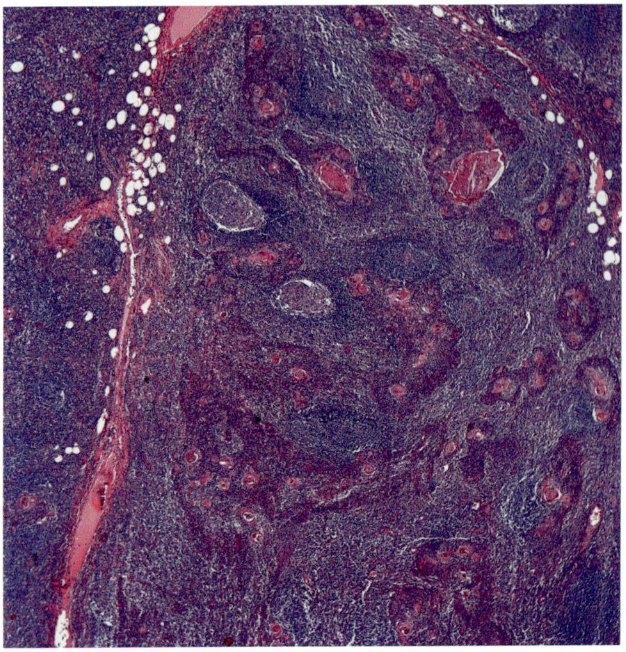

Fig. 5.1 LESA like thymic lesion showing the classic pattern of epithelial islands embedded in a lymphocytic stroma

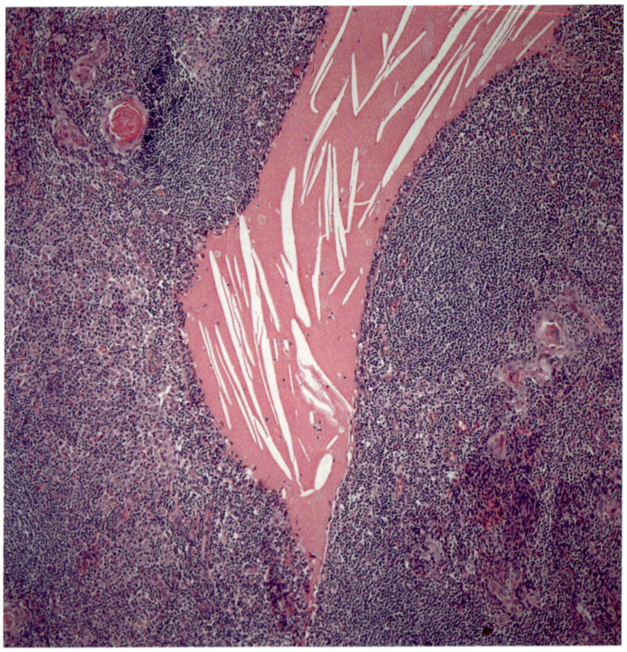

Fig. 5.3 LESA-like thymic lesion showing cystically dilated space filled with acellular material

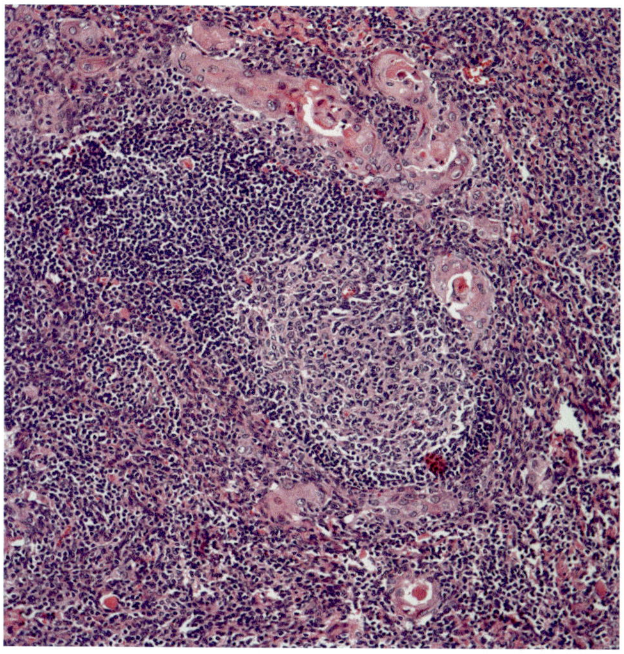

Fig. 5.4 LESA-like lesion of the thymus showing a not so conspicuous germinal center

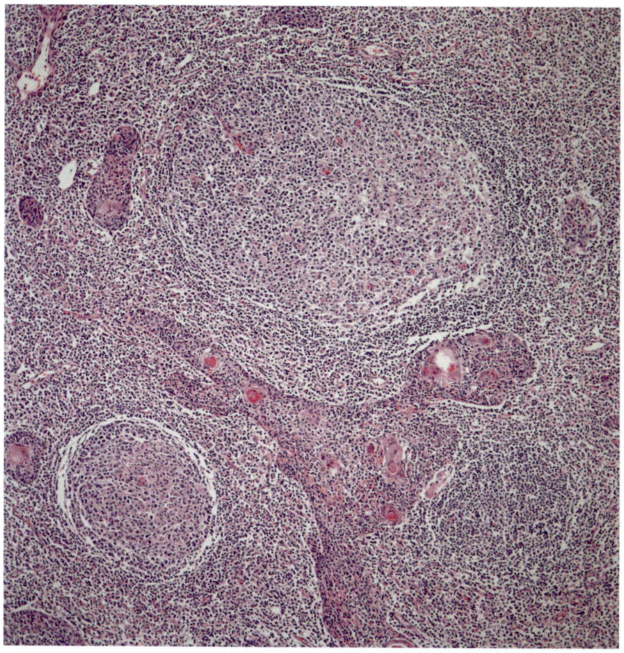

Fig. 5.5 LESA-like thymic lesion showing prominent germinal centers

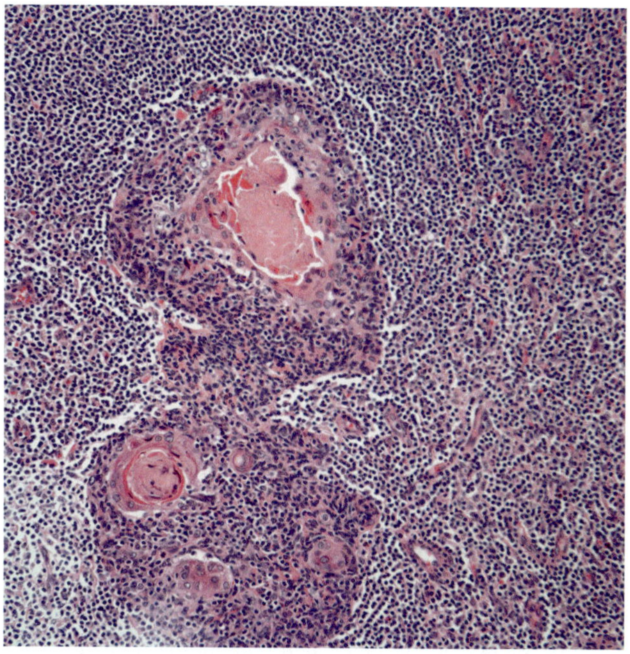

Fig. 5.6 LESA-like thymic lesion showing small nests of epithelial cells containing Hassall's corpuscles

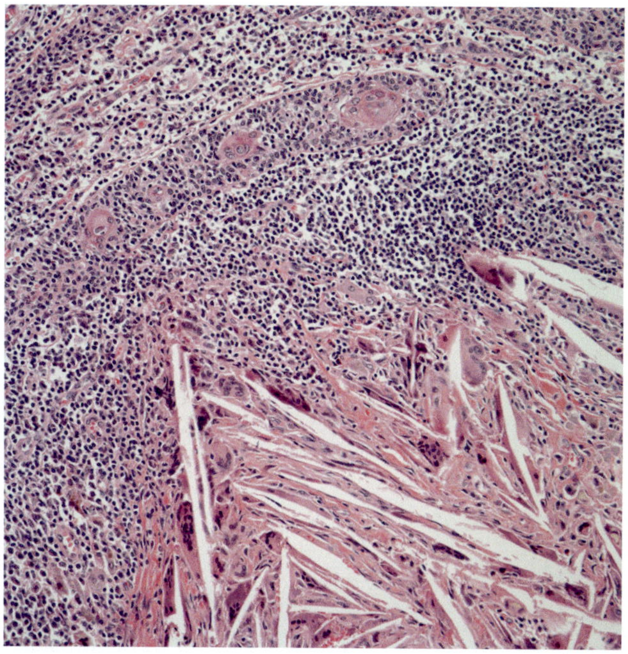

Fig. 5.7 LESA-like thymic lesion showing cholesterol cleft granuloma adjacent to a strand of thymic epithelium

Immunohistochemical and Molecular Features

As it would be expected in these types of lesions, the use of lymphoid and epithelial markers would be of aid in determining the exact components of these proliferations. CD20 would highlight the B-cell lymphocytic component (Fig. 5.8); CD3 would highlight T-lymphocytes in the interfollicular areas (Fig. 5.9). On the other hand, pancytokeratin would highlight the thymic epithelium and Hassall's corpuscles as well as the cystic lining (Fig. 5.10). The use of kappa and lambda chains to determine clonality would be another important aid in order to exclude the possibility of a malignant lymphoproliferative tumor, which in cases of LESA-like would show a polyclonal pattern.

Differential Diagnosis

By far the most common pitfall with these unusual tumors would be with thymoma and lymphoma, MALT type. In the former, lack of prominent lobulation and the presence of strands of thymic epithelium in a background of lymphoid hyperplasia would be unusual for thymoma. On the other hand, MALT lymphoma is another consideration; however, the absence of monoclonality by immunohistochemistry or

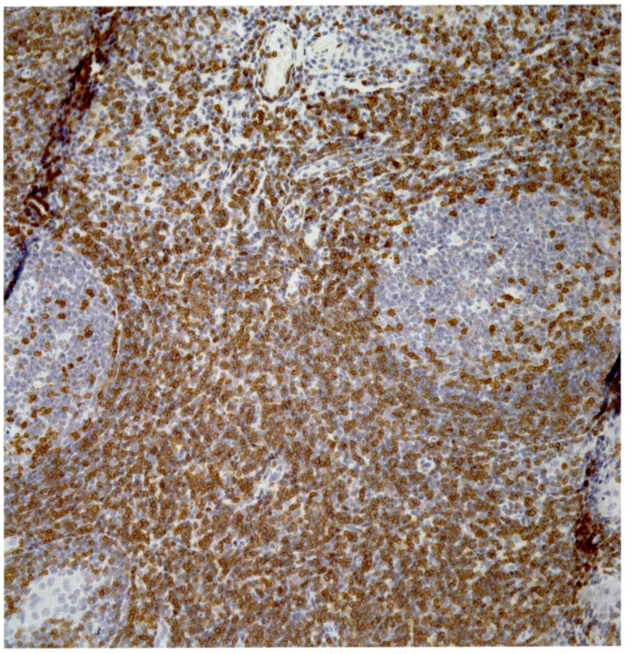

Fig. 5.9 CD3 immunohistochemical stain showing lymphocytes decorated predominantly in the interfollicular areas

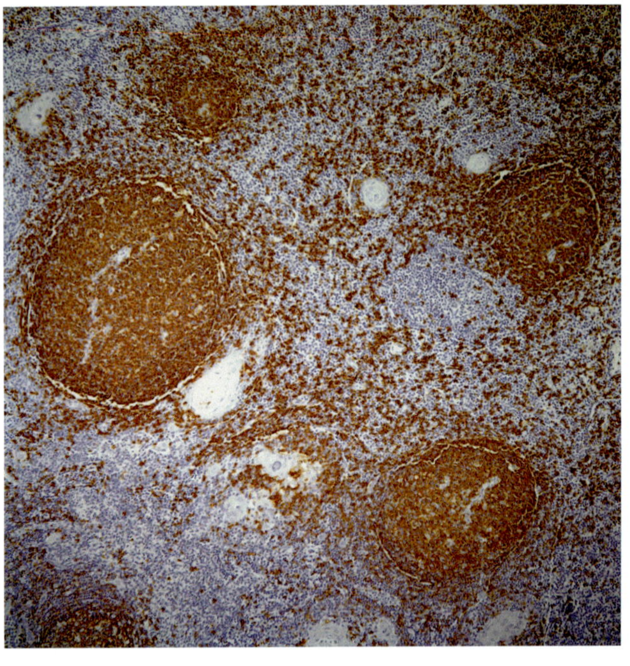

Fig. 5.8 CD20 immunohistochemical stain showing lymphocytes decorating predominantly the germinal centers

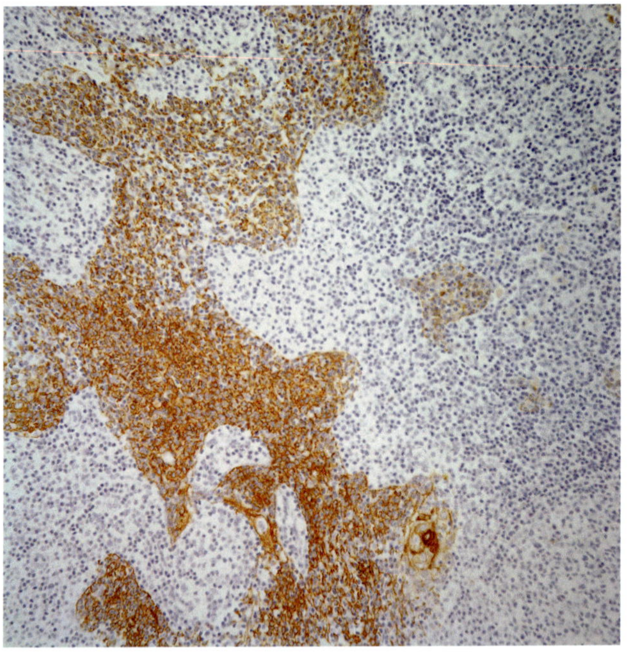

Fig. 5.10 Cytokeratin immunohistochemical stain decorating the residual thymic epithelium

flow cytometry plus the morphological findings of strands of thymic epithelium in a background of thymic hyperplasia will also be unusual for MALT lymphoma.

Perhaps the separation of LESA-like from true thymic hyperplasia may pose a more significant academic problem as both may share some histological features; however, the morphological features of LESA-like plus the clinical background may be used as an aid to properly separate these two lesions. Ultimately, both of those lesions would need complete surgical resection for proper classification. The use of mediastinoscopic biopsies in the diagnosis of these lesions may pose a significant problem in arriving at a specific diagnosis.

Sebaceous Lymphadenoma

This benign tumoral condition also represents an unusual salivary gland-type tumor of the thymus, which has been only recently described in the literature [12]. As its analogous tumor in the salivary gland, this tumor in the thymus is in the great majority of cases diagnosed only after complete surgical resection. Biopsy material from mediastinoscopic biopsies may prove to be a diagnostic challenge as the tumor may be easily confused with other more common tumoral conditions of the thymus. In the original description of this benign tumor, the authors described two patients, one being followed for breast carcinoma while the other patient was asymptomatic, and the mediastinal mass was discovered during a routine chest radiograph. In both patients there was evidence of an anterior mediastinal mass, which was surgical removed. Similar to the same tumors in the salivary gland, complete surgical resection appears to be the treatment of choice for this tumor in the thymus. None of the patients had a related autoimmune process including myasthenia gravis.

Pathological Features

Grossly, the tumors were described as irregular, light tan soft tissue with slight lobulation and focal cystic changes. Areas of necrosis and hemorrhage were not identified.

Histologically, the lesions are characterized by the presence of solid and cystic epithelial islands embedded in a prominent lymphoid background (Figs. 5.11, 5.12, and 5.13). The epithelial islands appear haphazardly distributed and forming small tubular structures with keratinization and in some areas with hyalinization (Fig. 5.14). In addition, groups of epithelial islands show medium-sized cells with clear cytoplasm, round to oval nuclei, and small to inconspicuous nucleoli, characteristic of sebaceous cells (Figs. 5.15 and 5.16). Cellular atypia and mitotic activity are not present. The lymphoid component is characterized by the presence of focal hyperplastic changes with formation of germinal centers.

Immunohistochemically, the use of epithelial markers such as pan-keratin or low molecular weight keratin CAM 5.2 may aid in identifying the epithelial component, while B- and T-cell markers will decorate the lymphoid component. In addition, the use of adipophilin may help in identifying the presence of sebaceous changes (Fig. 5.17).

Differential Diagnosis

The most important differential diagnosis would be with thymoma. However, in cases of thymoma, the lack of tumor lobulation at the microscopic level plus the presence of haphazard epithelial islands with scattered Hassall's corpuscles should raise some concerns about the possibility of thymoma. One other possibility is to dismiss the lesion as some type of follicular hyperplasia. In this setting, the presence of haphazard epithelial islands plus the presence of sebaceous differentiation should raise some doubts about this lesion being just follicular hyperplasia. The use of immunohistochemical stains

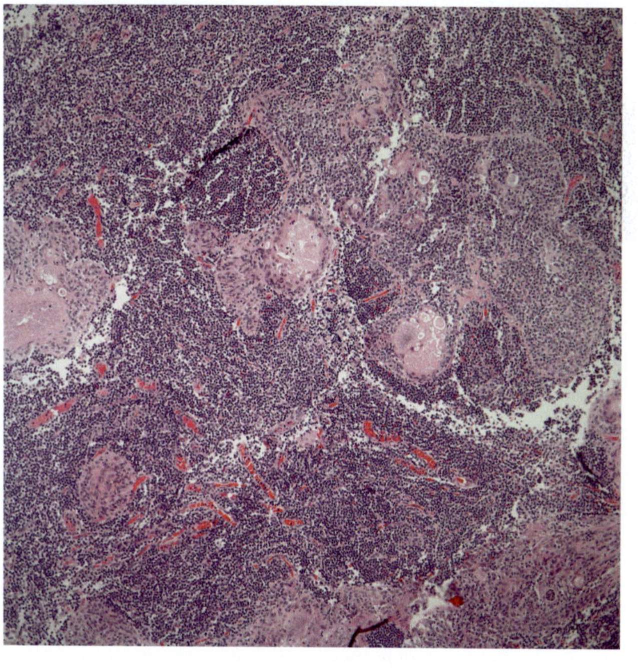

Fig. 5.11 Thymic sebaceous lymphadenoma showing tubular epithelial structures embedded in a lymphoid stroma

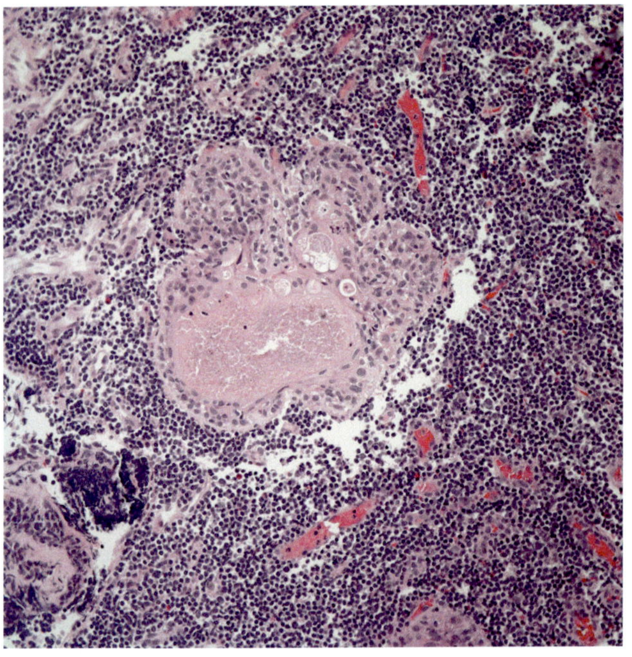

Fig. 5.12 Closer view of the epithelial islands showing some cells with vacuolated clear cytoplasm

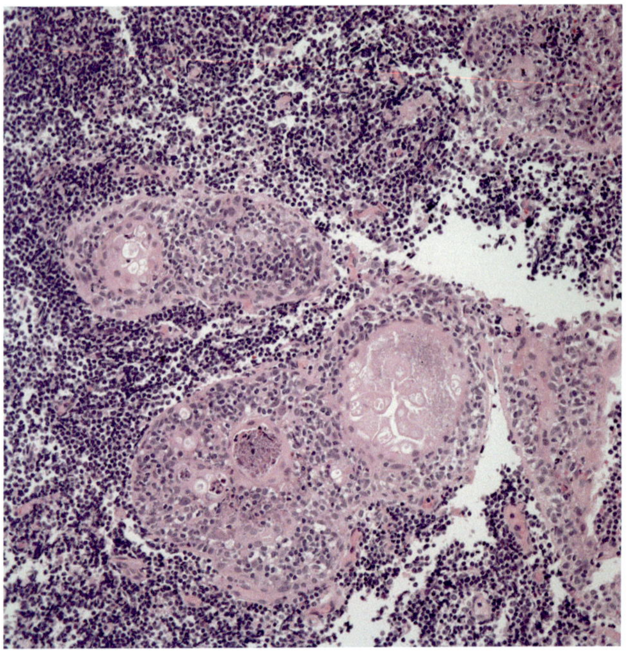

Fig. 5.13 Higher magnification at the adjacent cells in epithelial islands showing clear vacuolated cytoplasm

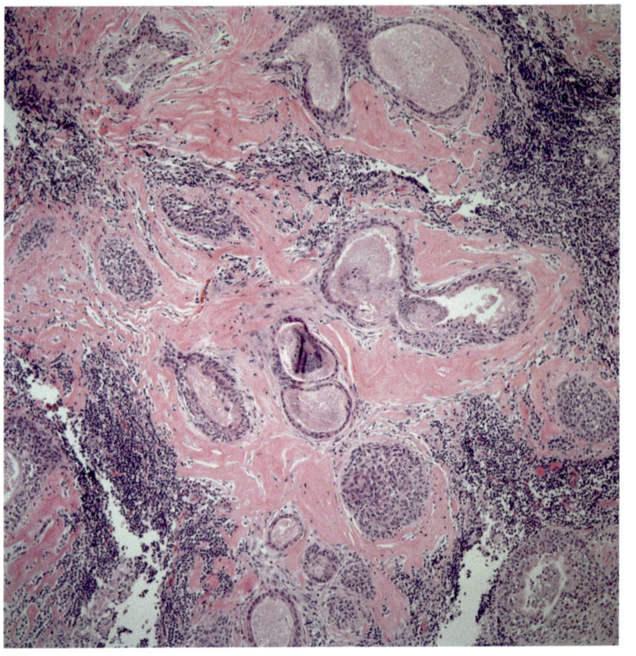

Fig. 5.14 Thymic sebaceous adenoma showing hyalinization and epithelial tubular structures

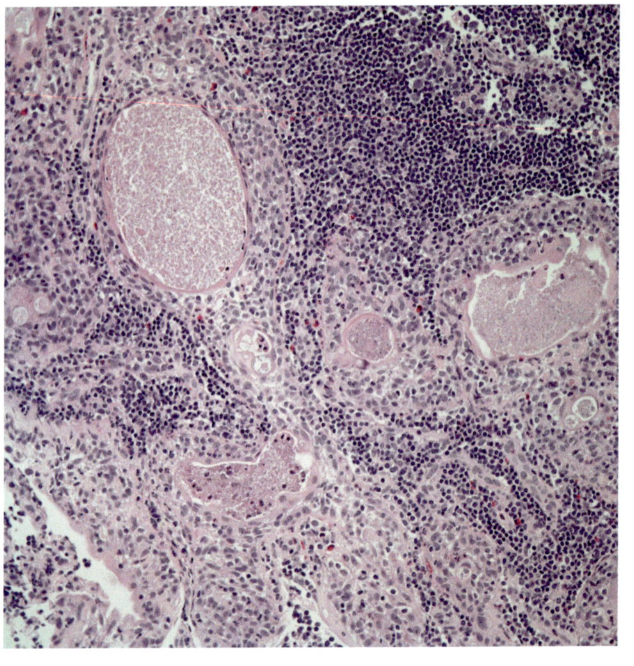

Fig. 5.15 Sebaceous lymphadenoma showing dilatation of Hassall's corpuscles and adjacent sebaceous cells

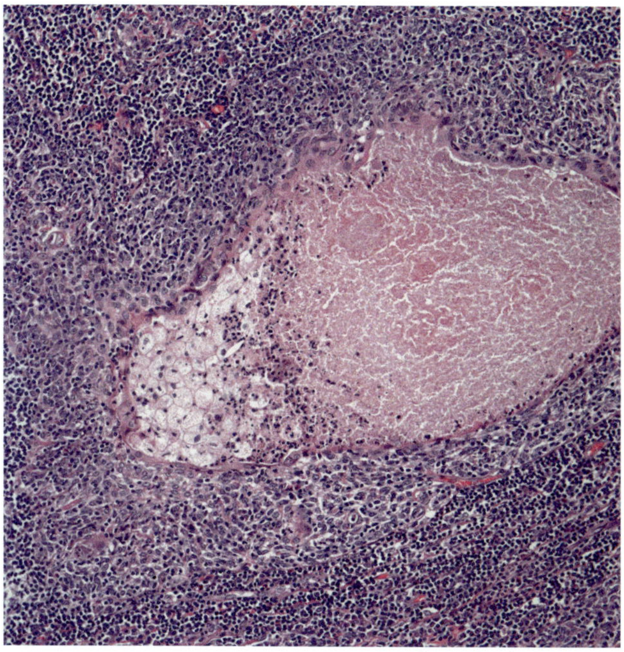

Fig. 5.16 Epithelial island showing at the tip sebaceous differentiation

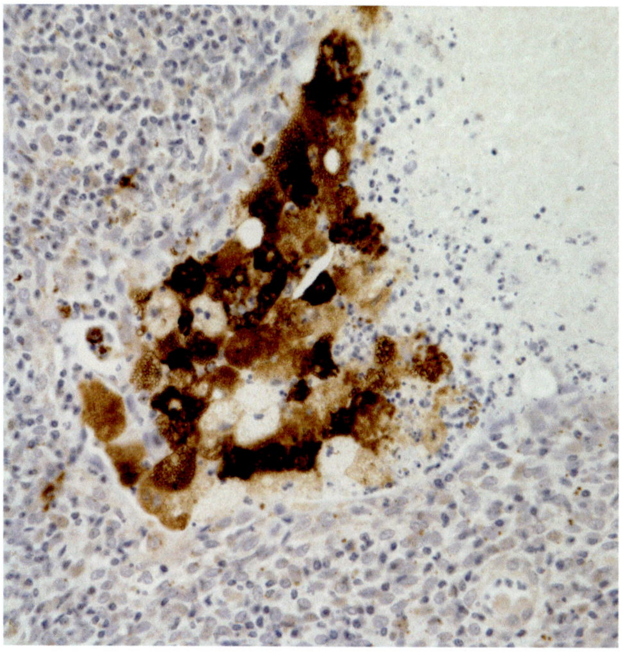

Fig. 5.17 Immunohistochemical stain for adipophilin showing strong positive reaction in the sebaceous cells

for epithelial and lymphoid markers has limited value in this context. The use of adipophilin needs to be considered.

Mixed Tumor (Pleomorphic Adenoma)

This is another salivary gland-type tumor that has been only rarely reported in the literature as primary in the mediastinum [13–15]. In 1952, Chen and Takana [13] described two patients with anterior mediastinal tumors and what the authors titled "mixed tumor with malignant hyperplasia." However, based on the descriptions provided, it is possible that the tumors reported may have represented teratomatous tumors and not necessarily "mixed tumor" in the sense of pleomorphic adenoma. In one of the cases, the description of anaplastic epithelium and the consideration of the authors of a pulmonary anlage tumor raise some doubts as to whether that particular tumor is indeed a "pleomorphic adenoma," and the possibility of a teratomatous lesion with malignant component may be more accurate. On the other hand, in the second case, the authors fully acknowledged that the tumor in question is a benign cystic teratoma.

Contrarily, Feigin and Lee described two cases of what the authors described as mixed tumor or pleomorphic adenoma of the mediastinum [14, 15]. In the case described by Feigin and colleagues [14], the patient is a 38-year-old asymptomatic man who was found to have a middle mediastinal mass by imaging, and surgical resection of the mass showed a 7 cm soft mucoid mass. Histologically, the tumor was composed of spindle and stellate cells embedded in a myxoid stroma admixed with focal epithelial elements in the form of nests, small glands, and trabeculae. No cellular atypia or mitotic activity was identified in this tumor. The case described by Lee and colleagues [15] is of a 54-year-old woman who presented with chest pain, and a CT scan showed the presence of a posterior mediastinal mass. Surgical resection showed a 6 cm well-defined, lobulated, gray/yellow mass with myxoid changes. The histological description of the tumor is similar to the case described by Feigin [14]. In both of these two cases, clinical follow-up showed no recurrence of the tumor.

Pathological Features

As it has been documented by the cases described, these tumors are usually well demarcated, soft, and lobulated with some cystic changes and with myxoid areas. The tumor generally lacks necrosis or hemorrhage. The size of the tumor may be more than 5 cm in greatest diameter.

Histologically, the tumor is composed of an epithelial component that may be in the form of small glands, nests, or trabeculae of cells without atypia or mitotic activity (Fig. 5.18). These epithelial aggregates are generally embedded in a myxoid stroma, which may show the presence of spindle or stellate cells without atypia or mitotic activity (Figs. 5.19 and 5.20).

Immunohistochemical studies are not really needed in order to confirm the diagnosis. However, epithelial markers such as pan-keratin will decorate the epithelial component, and, in some areas, S-100 protein and smooth muscle actin may also show positive staining. The stroma of the tumor is usually positive for vimentin and focally positive for smooth muscle actin.

Differential Diagnosis

The most important differential diagnosis is with a mature cystic teratoma of the mediastinum. In this setting the lack of the three germinal layers will help in separating these two tumors. However, it is important to highlight that in small mediastinoscopic biopsies, the separation of these two tumors may not be as simple and may pose significant problems in arriving at a specific diagnosis. The definitive diagnosis of mixed tumor is best made after complete surgical resection and proper sampling of the tumor. In the majority of cases, the gross appearance of the tumor also should provide a lead about the diagnosis.

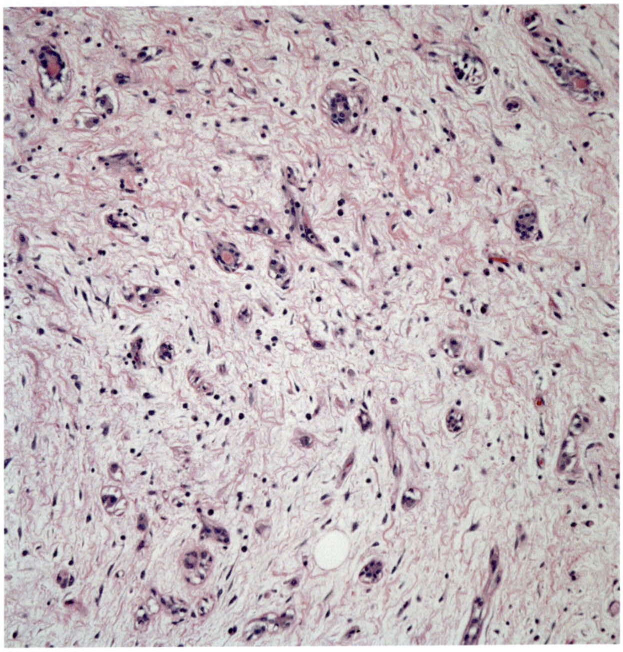

Fig. 5.19 Mixed tumor of the mediastinum showing predominantly fibroconnective tissue with small islands of epithelial cells

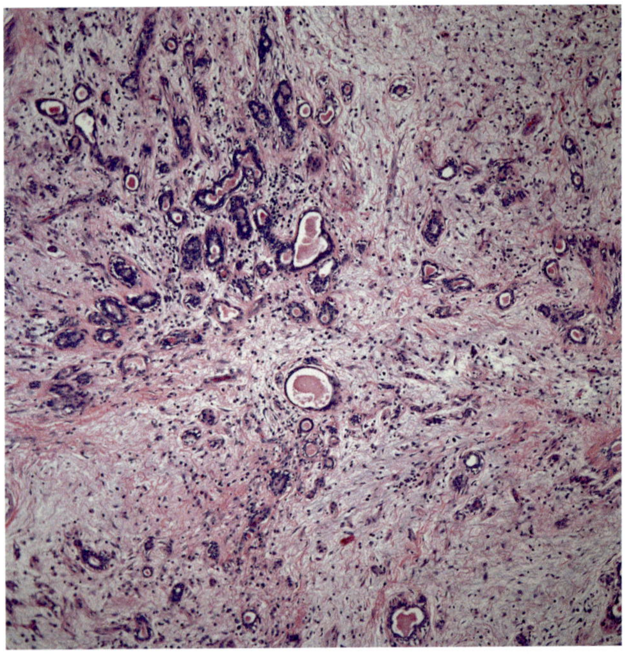

Fig. 5.18 Mixed tumor of the mediastinum showing tubular epithelial structures embedded in a loose fibroconnective tissue. Note the lack of atypia or mitotic activity

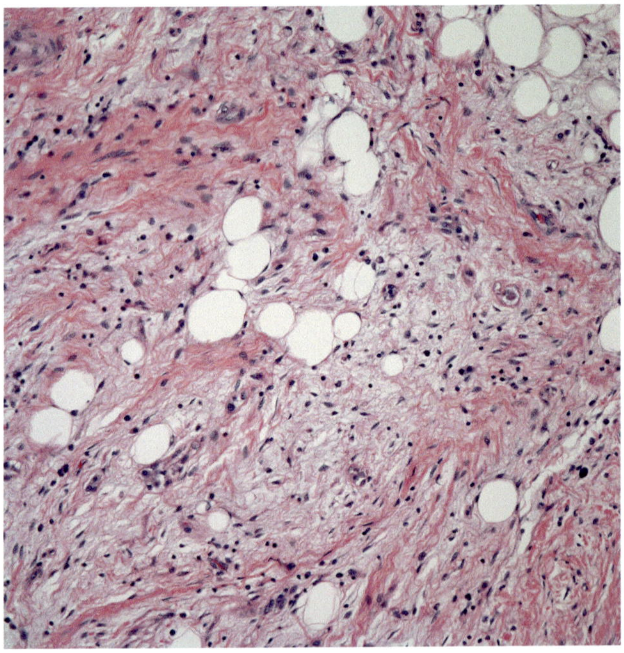

Fig. 5.20 Mediastinal mixed tumor showing fibroconnective tissue admixed with adipose tissue

Malignant Tumors

Mucoepidermoid Carcinoma (MEC)

MEC represents likely the most common salivary gland-type tumor in the thymus. However, despite the fact that it is the most commonly reported, thymic MEC remains an unusual primary tumor of the thymus. The credit for the first description of thymic MEC is given to Tanaka and colleagues [16], who in 1982 described a 43-year-old woman admitted to the hospital for systemic lupus erythematosus (SLE)-like symptoms and who on radiographic imaging showed the presence of an anterior mediastinal mass. The tumor appeared to be invading the pericardium; thus, total removal was not successful. The patient underwent irradiation, and, 6 years after initial diagnosis, the patient died. Autopsy was performed showing the presence of a large anterior mediastinal mass. Subsequent reports [17–20] on thymic MEC very much have mirrored the case reported by Tanaka [16]. The tumor does not seem to have a predilection for any particular gender, and the age of the patients has varied between 31 and 70 years. Clinically the patients have presented with symptoms of chest pain and dyspnea. Diagnostic thoracic imaging has shown the presence of an anterior mediastinal tumor. Even though there is no real association between thymic MEC and autoimmune disease including myasthenia gravis, Woo and colleagues [21] described a 47-year-old woman with an anterior mediastinal mass who after complete clinical evaluation was also diagnosed with myasthenia gravis while the anterior mediastinal mass was histologically a thymic MEC, low grade. It is also important to highlight that, although most cases of thymic MEC are tumors limited to the mediastinum, in the case described by Yasuda and colleagues [20], despite the low grade histology, the tumor appeared to be spreading in the pericardium and pleura. The patient received chemoradiation, and after 14 months the patient has remained disease-free. In a different case reported by Noda and colleagues [22], the authors described a 53-year-old man with an anterior mediastinal tumor, which histologically was considered low grade and according to the authors "Masaoka stage II and considered by the World Health Organization (WHO) type C thymic tumor." Based on that, the patient was treated with multimodality therapy including surgery, radiotherapy, and systemic chemotherapy. The patient died 7 years after initial diagnosis of tumor progression. Also Fuse and colleagues [23] described a single case of a 74-year-old man, who presented with chest pain and was found to have an anterior mediastinal tumor, which upon diagnostic imaging appeared to be invading into the subcutis through the sternum. Biopsy material examined was interpreted as high-grade mucoepidermoid carcinoma, which was followed by treatment with a combination of cisplatin and irinotecan. The patient died 6 months after initial diagnosis due to progressive disease.

Essentially there are only two small series of thymic MEC [24, 25]. One is a report of six cases belonging to two men and four women between the ages of 17 and 66 years (median age 34.5 years) [24]. The patients presented with non-specific symptoms including chest pain and dyspnea. Surgical resection was performed in five of these six patients, and, in those who had surgical resection of the tumor, the histology was that of a low-grade tumor. In one patient, mediastinoscopic biopsy was followed by radiation therapy, and, 2 years later, the patient died of tumor. In those patients with low-grade tumor in whom follow-up was available, the patients were disease-free between 1 and 3 years. The series reported by Nonaka and associates [25] involved ten patients between the ages of 8 and 84 years, six men and four women. Clinically some patients presented with non-specific symptoms of chest pain and weight loss. All tumors were located in the anterior mediastinum, and histologically eight cases were of low-grade histology, while two were of high-grade histology. Follow-up in these patients showed that those patients with tumors of high histology died 1 year after initial diagnosis, while those patients in whom the histology of the tumor was low grade and follow-up was available were disease-free. One important aspect of this report is the occurrence of a thymic MEC in an 8-year-old child, an occurrence that had not been previously reported. Unfortunately, even though the histology of the tumor was deemed to be of low grade, there was only an incisional biopsy; no known therapy was available, and the child was lost to follow-up.

Based on the available literature on thymic MEC, it is important to highlight that clinically these patients are more likely adults over 30 years of age who present with non-specific symptoms such as chest pain and dyspnea, while others are completely asymptomatic. Despite the fact that there are some cases that may occur in patients with autoimmune diseases such as myasthenia gravis, this occurrence may be more coincidental rather than factual. Diagnostic imaging is important to determine the presence of an anterior mediastinal tumor and also to determine the extent of disease; however, definitive diagnosis is accomplished by histological examination. The rationale to proceed with surgical resection or with any other mode of therapy such as radiation or chemotherapy will be based not only on the interpretation of low- or high-grade tumor but also on the imaging of limited disease to the mediastinum or dissemination of the disease to adjacent organs.

Pathological Features

Grossly, the majority of these tumors are described as solid and cystic tumoral lesions, which can measure more than 10 cm in greatest dimension. The proportion of solid and cystic areas varies from case to case, but in those with a prominent cystic component, the cysts will show the presence of mucoid material. In cases in which the tumor is limited to the mediastinal compartment, it is likely that no additional adjacent tissue will be present; however, in some cases suspicious for pleural or pericardial involvement, those structures may be attached to the main tumoral mass.

Histologically, the tumors are characterized by the presence of a mixture of epidermoid elements and mucus-secreting epithelial cells (so-called mucocytes) (Figs. 5.21, 5.22, 5.23, 5.24, 5.25, 5.26, 5.27, 5.28, and 5.29). The epidermoid component may vary from well-to-moderately-to-poorly differentiated. Those histological characteristics are based on the presence of cellular and nuclear atypia, mitotic activity with presence of atypical mitotic figures, areas of hemorrhage, and/or necrosis. In contrast, the mucus-secreting cells do not display any significant atypical features. The tumor in addition commonly displays the presence of multiple cystic structures that may be lined by either squamous epithelium or a low cuboidal attenuated epithelium. In some cases, one can observe the presence of cystic areas in which there is a transition between the normal squamous epithelium and the beginning of the epidermoid component of the mucoepidermoid carcinoma. In some cases, the epidermoid component may show extensive areas of clear cell component. In the uninvolved cystic structures, the cyst may show inflammatory changes or areas of hemorrhage. These tumoral areas may be separated by thin fibroconnective tissue or may be embedded in a lymphoid stroma, which may contain germinal centers or cholesterol cleft granulomas. In peripheral areas of the tumor, it is possible to identify strands of thymic epithelium or residual normal thymic tissue with Hassall's corpuscles. The presence of necrosis and hemorrhage in addition to the presence of an epidermoid component with nuclear atypia and mitotic activity should alert to the possibility of a high-grade tumor (Figs. 5.30, 5.31, and 5.32).

Histochemical, Immunohistochemical, and Molecular Features

Histochemically, the most important stain to perform is mucicarmine to highlight the mucus-secreting cells, which may be in close association with the epidermoid component. On the other hand, immunohistochemical stains may be limited to highlight the epidermoid component of the tumor, which essentially will stain like any other conventional squamous cell carcinoma, namely, by showing positive staining for pan-keratin, keratin 5/6, p63, and p40. Although the use of those immunohistochemical stains may aid in the diagnosis, it cannot differentiate the tumor from a conventional squamous cell carcinoma. Thus, the correct interpretation is one based on morphological findings.

Regarding molecular techniques, the literature is rather limited, and, although the association of extra thymic MEC and the t(11;19)(q21;p13) fusion has been described in many cases, there is not enough case material of thymic MEC with that information in order to better determine the rate of positivity. For instance, Roden and associates [26] reported two cases of thymic MEC with MAML2 rearrangement, while Prieto-Granada [27] reported a thymic MEC in which the rearrangement was negative.

Although it is important to correlate molecular findings with thymic MEC, one cannot lose track that the morphological characteristics of thymic MEC alone should be enough to make an unequivocal diagnosis of thymic MEC.

Differential Diagnosis

The most important and most difficult challenge will be the separation of mucoepidermoid carcinoma from a conventional squamous cell carcinoma. In mediastinoscopic biopsies, it could represent a real challenge, and one should look carefully for the presence of mucus-secreting cells (so-called mucocytes) either on morphological evaluation or by performing a mucicarmine histochemical stain. If that feature is present and identified, the diagnosis can be established. One other way would be to perform molecular studies for MAML2; however, as stated earlier, if the rearrangement is present, then it is in keeping with the diagnosis of MEC; however, negative rearrangement does not rule out the diagnosis of thymic MEC. The use of conventional immunohistochemical stains may prove to be limited as both MEC and squamous cell carcinomas may stain positively for keratin, keratin 5/6, p63, and p40. One other possibility that is commonly mentioned is the separation of MEC from adenosquamous carcinoma. In adenosquamous carcinoma, one must identify areas that otherwise would be in keeping with adenocarcinoma. Those areas are not a component of a thymic MEC. Thus, such diagnosis should really not be considered in the differential diagnosis of thymic MEC. Finally, in small biopsies, atypical thymoma may also present a challenge. In addition, the immunohistochemical profile of MEC and atypical thymoma may be similar; however, atypical thymoma would not show the presence of mucus-secreting cells admixed with the epidermoid component. Of course, in resected material, the diagnosis is made with more comfort. One important pitfall to recognize is the diagnosis in small biopsies of high-grade mucoepidermoid carcinoma, which can be easily interpreted as conventional squamous cell carcinoma unless there are more conventional areas of low-grade MEC.

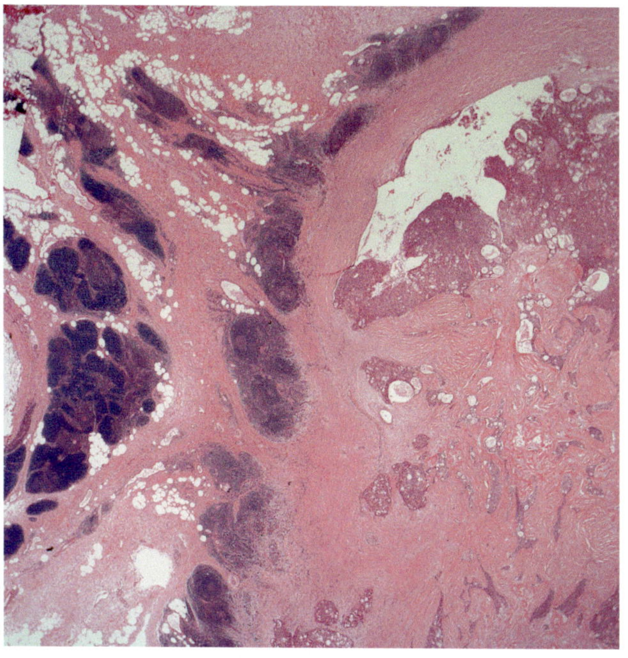

Fig. 5.21 Low-grade thymic MEC showing areas of adjacent thymic tissue in the periphery

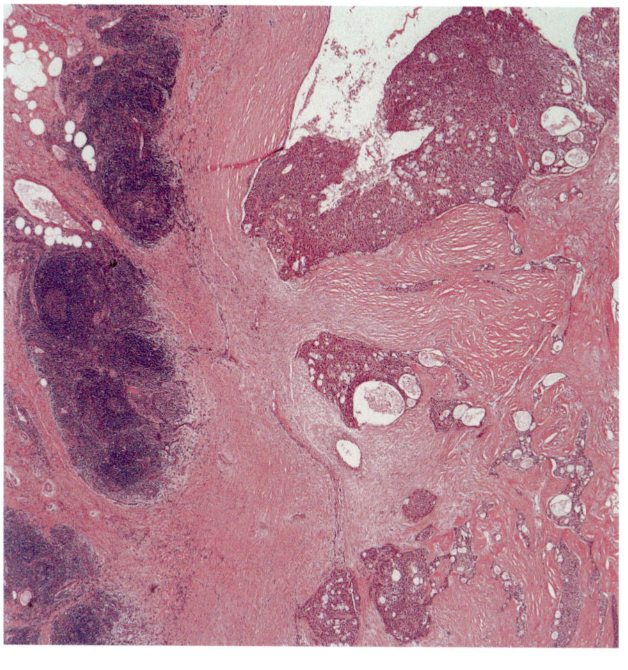

Fig. 5.22 Thymic MEC with prominent cystic changes

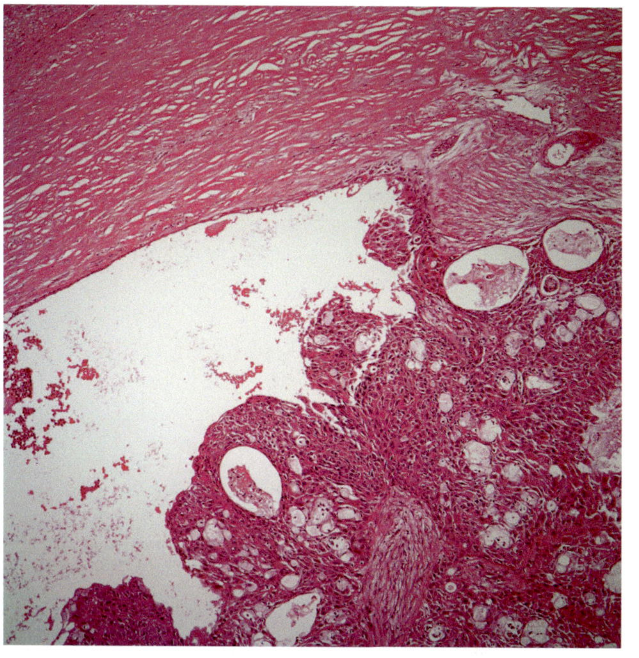

Fig. 5.23 Thymic MEC showing transitional areas between the non-neoplastic cystic lining with the neoplastic lining

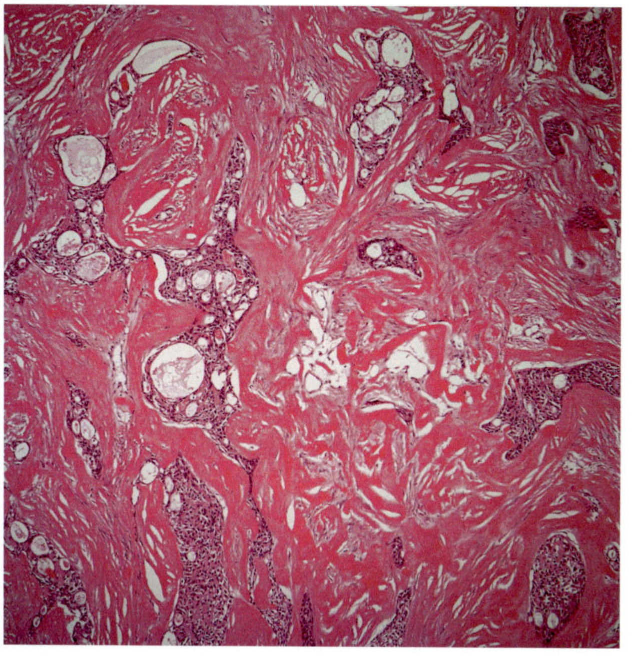

Fig. 5.24 Thymic MEC with extensive hyalinization

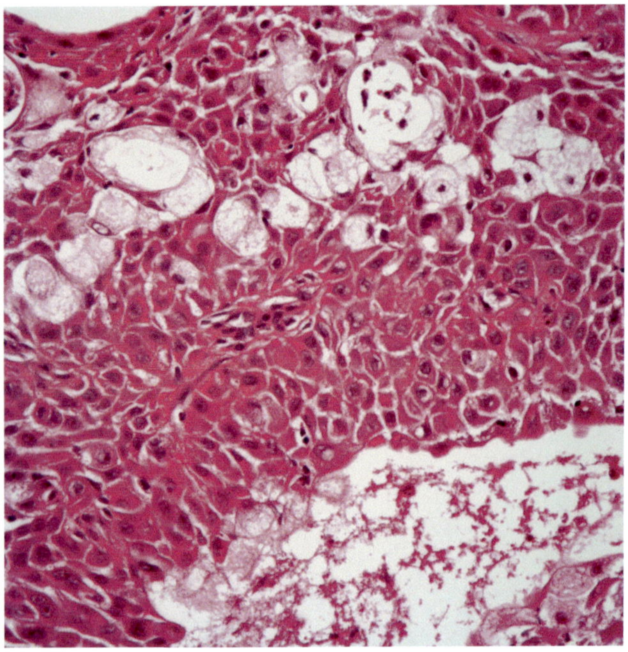

Fig. 5.25 Higher magnification of the epidermoid component admixed with mucus-producing cells (so-called mucocytes)

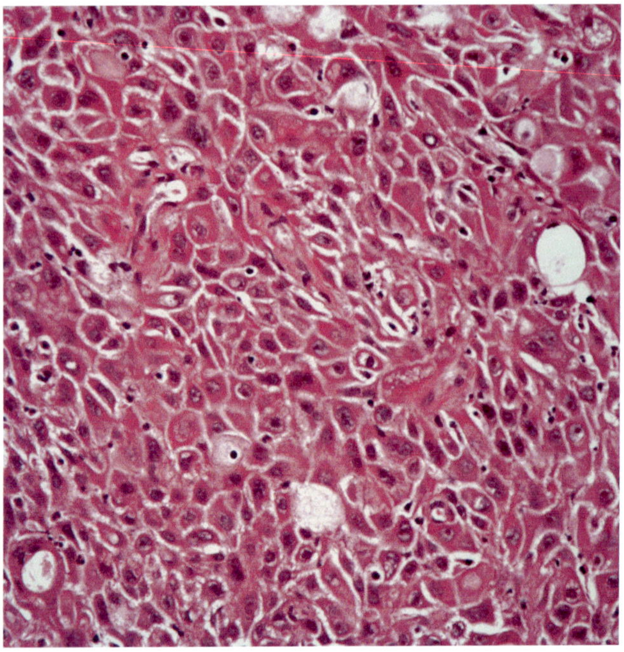

Fig. 5.26 Higher magnification of the epidermoid component showing lack of keratinization or mitotic activity

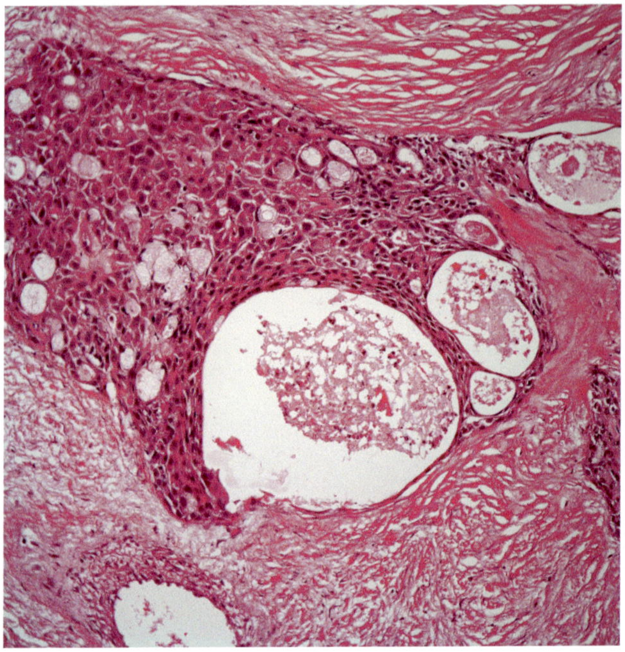

Fig. 5.27 Thymic MEC showing microcystic changes and the classic admixture of epidermoid and mucus-producing cells

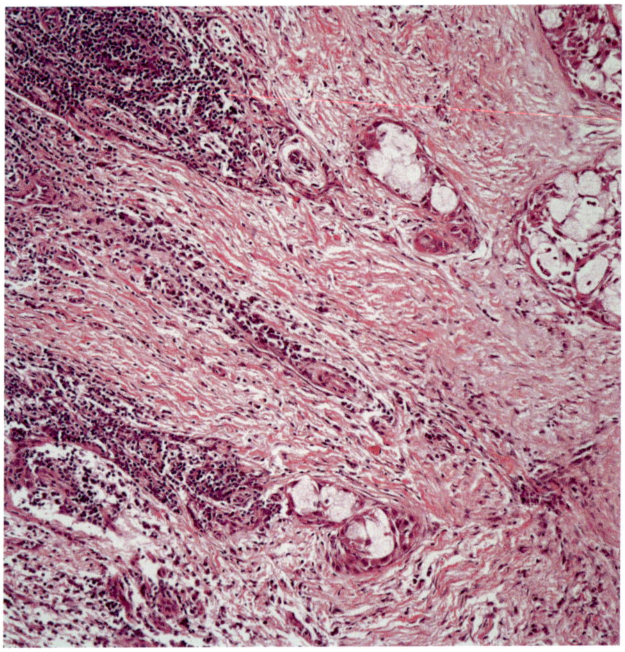

Fig. 5.28 Small islands of MEC merging with residual thymic tissue

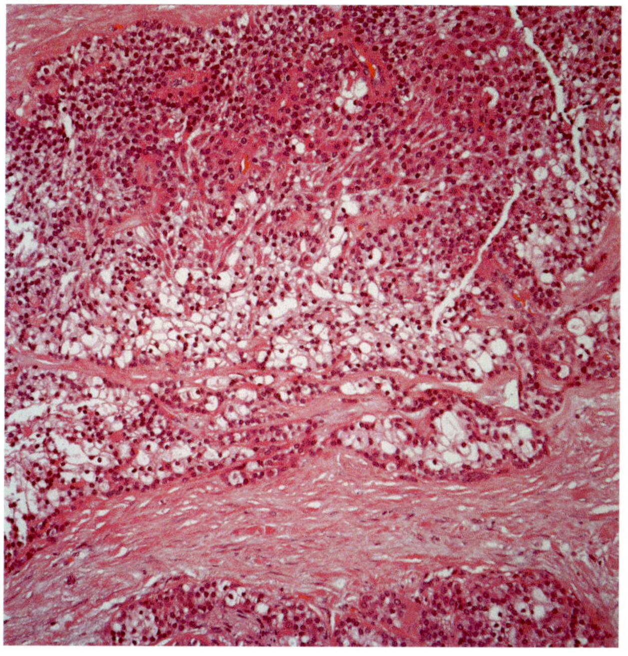

Fig. 5.29 Thymic MEC showing extensive areas of clear cell component

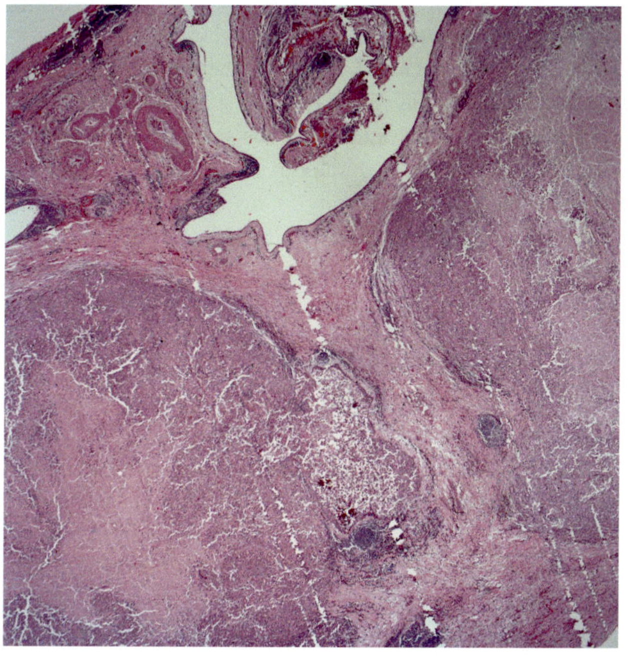

Fig. 5.30 High-grade thymic MEC showing extensive areas of necrosis

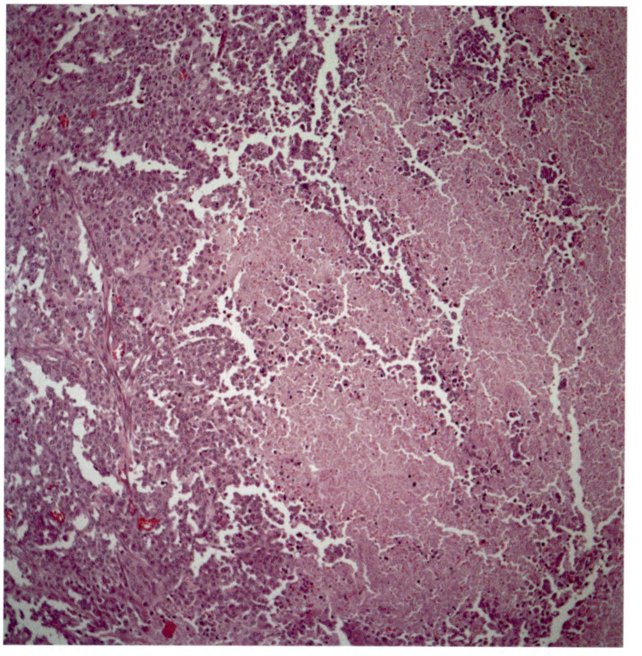

Fig. 5.31 High-grade thymic MEC showing areas of necrosis and increased cellularity

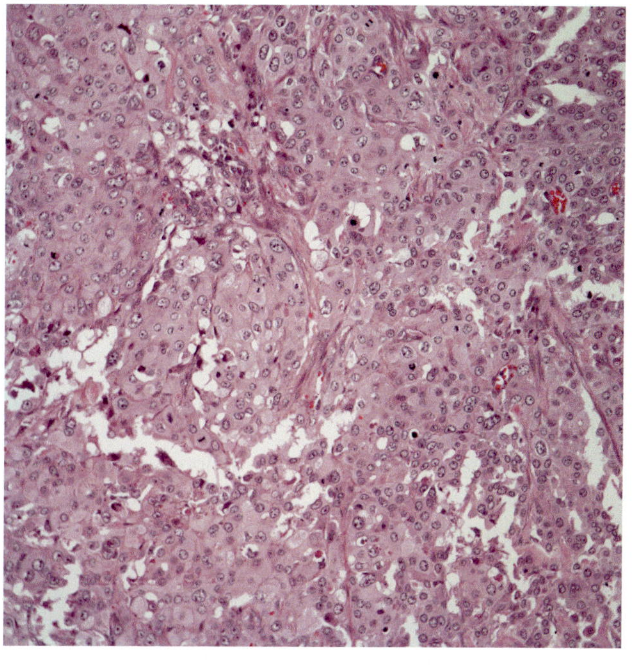

Fig. 5.32 High-grade MEC showing nuclear atypia and mitotic activity. Residual mucus-secreting cells are still present

Epithelial-Myoepithelial Carcinoma

This type of salivary gland tumor of the thymus is the most unusual of all as there is only a single case described in the literature [28]. The case reported is of a young man aged 25 years who presented with chest pain and dyspnea. Diagnostic imaging revealed the presence of an anterior mediastinal mass. Mediastinal biopsy was inconclusive, and the final diagnosis became apparent only after complete surgical resection. Even though the follow-up in the case was within 1 year and the patient was disease-free at that time, it is likely that the general behavior of these tumors is similar to those described in the salivary glands. However, it is important to recognize that this type of tumor appears to have ubiquitous distribution within the thoracic cavity; nevertheless, the tumor remains as rare when it occurs in the lung. Cases of epithelial-myoepithelial carcinomas of the lung have been reported to develop metastatic disease to lymph nodes, but cases of this tumor occurring primarily in the lung or thymus with widespread metastasis have not been described. It is possible that the treatment of choice when these tumors occur in the thymus is complete surgical resection and close follow-up.

Pathological Features

It is difficult to draw meaningful statements about the gross features of these tumors based on the current available literature. However, it is likely that these tumors may present as solid tumoral masses in the anterior mediastinum, which likely will be larger than 3 cm in greatest dimension. The cut surface may be light tan and homogeneous. Rarely, the tumor will show extensive areas of necrosis or hemorrhage. However, these features may be indistinguishable from other more common epithelial neoplasms of the thymic region, namely, thymoma.

The histological features of this tumor essentially recapitulate those seen in the salivary gland or in the lung. The low power view may be of a glandular type of tumor in which the glandular structures may be separated by discrete fibrocollagenous tissue (Figs. 5.33 and 5.34). However, the tumor characterizes for the presence of duct-like structures, tubules, or sheets of neoplastic cells. In the areas in which the tumor forms tubular structures, these tubules may show areas of an inner epithelial component and outer layers of clear cells representing the myoepithelial areas. In some areas the tumor may have a more solid appearance with sheets of neoplastic cells, some of them showing prominent clear cell features (Figs. 5.35 and 5.36). However, the tumor does not show marked nuclear atypia, mitotic activity, necrosis, or hemorrhage.

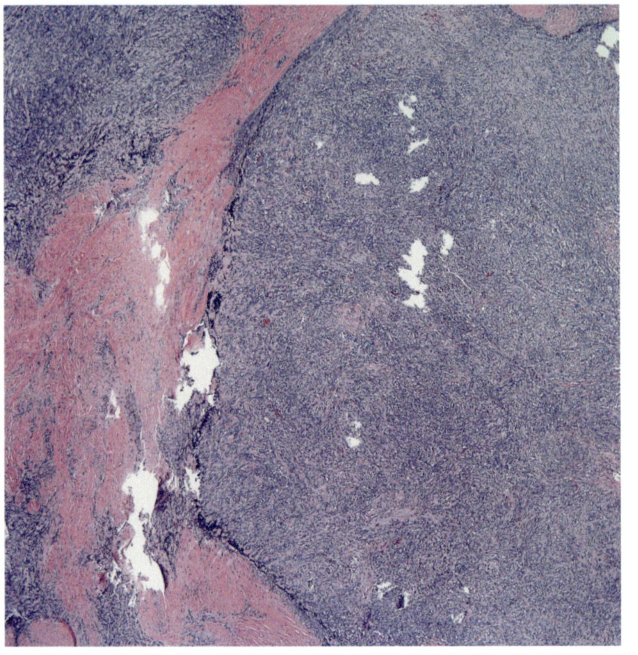

Fig. 5.33 Low power view of E-M carcinoma of the thymus showing a lobulated tumor

Immunohistochemical Features

Immunohistochemical stains may be helpful in the diagnosis, as the tumor may show positive staining for keratin or epithelial membrane antigen in the epithelial component, while S-100 protein and smooth muscle actin (Fig. 5.37) may show positive staining in the myoepithelial component of the tumor. Generally, keratin 5/6, p40, and p63, which are commonly expressed in thymoma or thymic carcinoma, are negative in epithelial-myoepithelial carcinoma.

Differential Diagnosis

The most important differential diagnosis would be with metastatic disease from an extrathymic origin. In this setting, a careful clinical history would be the most important clue in arriving at a more specific diagnosis.

Once the possibility of metastatic disease has been excluded, then important considerations would be with thymoma and thymic carcinoma. Thymoma is a very heterogeneous type of neoplasm that can show different growth patterns. However, if that is a consideration, the absence of staining for keratin 5/6 and the presence of positive staining in tumor cells for epithelial membrane antigen are features that are not shared by thymomas. In addition, the lack of a lymphoid component, which could also stain for T immature cells, would be unusual. In the setting of thymic carcinoma, the use of immunohistochemical markers such as keratin 5/6, p63, and p40 would be helpful as those markers are commonly expressed in thymic carcinoma.

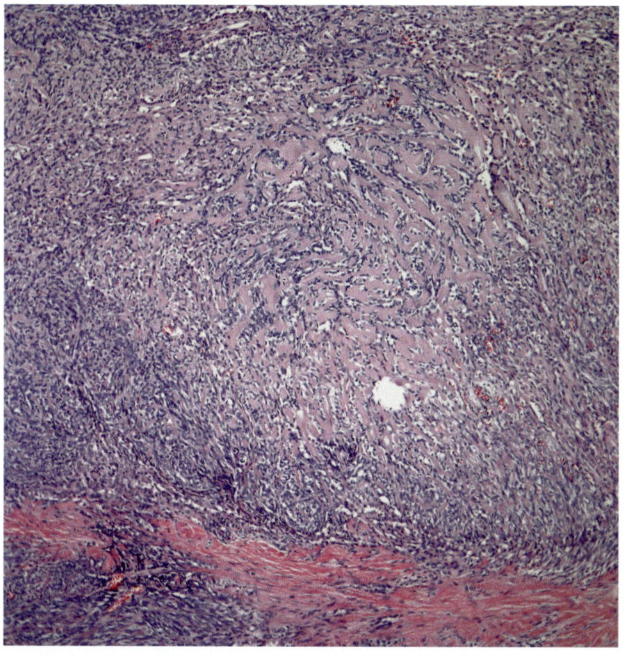

Fig. 5.34 Closer view at one of the lobules of tumor cells; the tumor shows a subtle glandular appearance

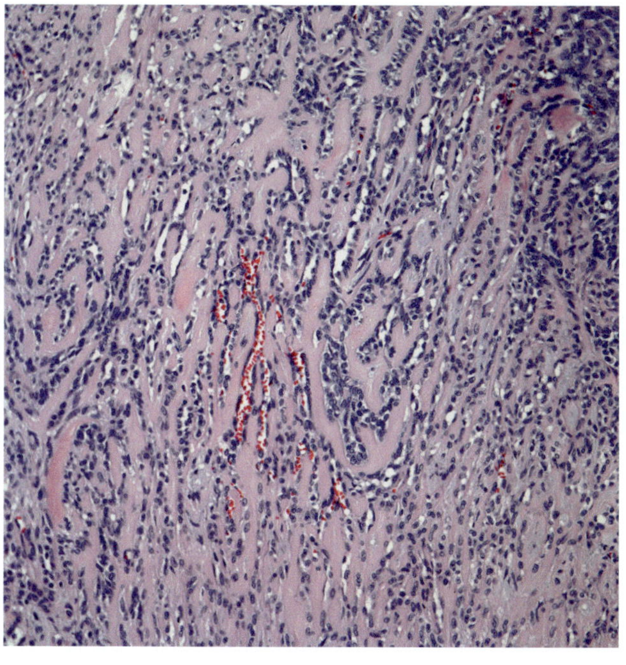

Fig. 5.35 Higher magnification showing collapsed glands with interspersed abundant basal membrane tissue. Note the presence of clear cells

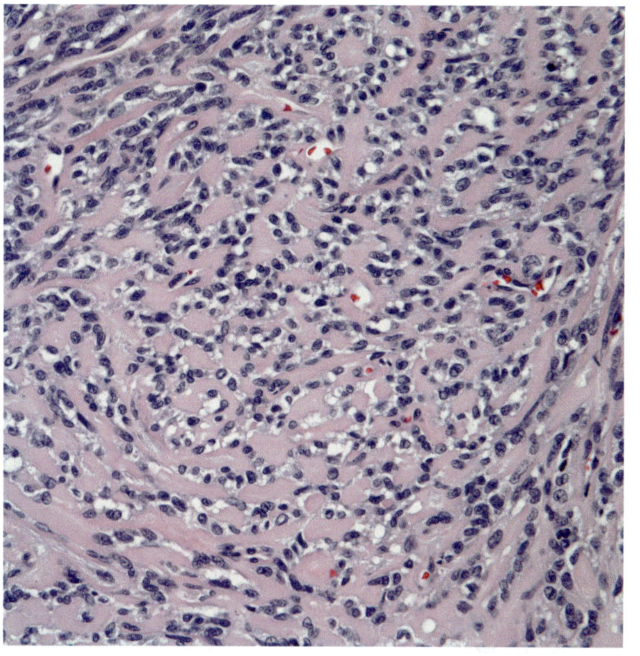

Fig. 5.36 In some areas the tumor may show a more solid proliferation; however, note the presence of delicate basal membrane and clear cells

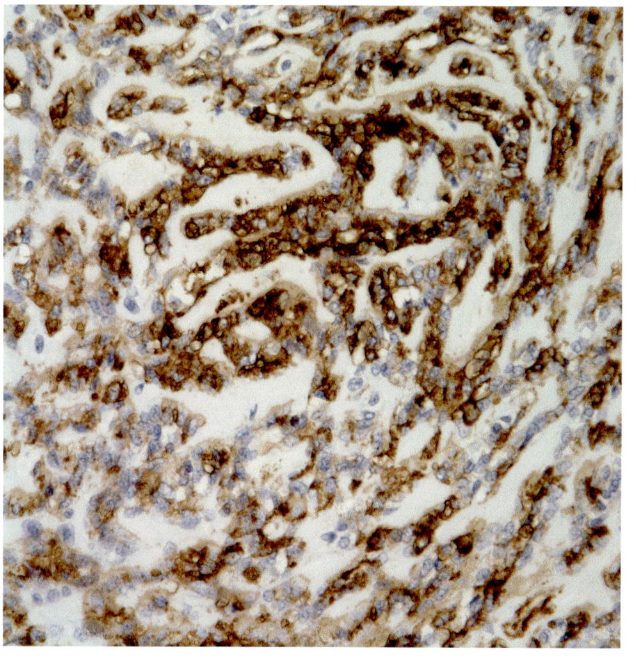

Fig. 5.37 Smooth muscle actin immunohistochemical stains shows numerous clear cells positive

Adenoid Cystic Carcinoma

This is another unusual primary thymic tumor that has been reported a few times in the literature [29–32]. In 2007, Di Tomasso and associates [29] reported four cases of a thymic tumor with adenoid cystic carcinoma-like features. The patients were older individuals between the ages of 63 and 77 years who were asymptomatic and with no evidence of previous tumor anywhere else except in the thymic area. These cases were interpreted as "a subtype of well differentiated thymic carcinoma of low-grade malignancy." Two patients were lost to follow-up, one patient died of a different cause, and one patient was alive 20 months after initial diagnosis. Banki and associates [30] reported a case in a 65-year-old woman who presented with weight loss, shortness of breath, and chest pain. The patient was initially thought to have a non-small cell lung carcinoma for which she received treatment. However, subsequent thoracotomy showed that the mass was originating from the right lobe of the thymus and interpreted as adenoid cystic carcinoma of the thymus. The patient was disease-free 2 years after initial diagnosis. One additional case of a thymic tumor with adenoid cystic carcinoma-like features was also described by Rampisela and associates [31] in a 47-year-old woman who presented with abdominal pain, and diagnostic imaging showed the presence of an anterior mediastinal mass. Surgical resection of the mass was performed followed by radiation therapy. Several years later, the patient was found to be alive. Contrary to those previously described cases, Kanzaki and associates [32] described a case in a 66-year-old man who presented with a cough and was found to have a mediastinal mass with bone and pulmonary metastases by imaging.

Pathological Features

Grossly, these tumors may range from a few centimeters to more than 10 cm in greatest dimension, are well demarcated, are tan to yellow in color, and have cystic changes on the surface. Areas of necrosis may be present.

Histologically, the tumors are characterized by a cylindromatous growth pattern composed of gland-like structures lined by two rows of medium-sized cells and angulated nuclei. These structures may contain a mucoid material within its lumen and be separated by thick fibrocollagenous tissue (Figs. 5.38a–c, 5.39a–c, and 5.40). Even though mitotic activity is not high, mitotic figures are present with mild to moderate nuclear atypia. In some areas the cells are forming small cluster of neoplastic cells and can be associated with areas of necrosis.

Histochemical, Immunohistochemical, and Molecular Features

Histochemical stains for periodic acid-Schiff and Alcian blue may help in identifying the intraluminal component. Immunohistochemical stains for keratin, CD5, S-100 protein, keratin 5/6, p63, keratin 19, 34βE12, MOC-31, CD10, p40, and MYB have been reported in some of the cases. In addition, in one case reported, the authors reported that two signals of the MYB gene per cell were detected by fluorescence in situ hybridization; however, no translocations or monosomy of the gene were detected.

Differential Diagnosis

In small biopsies adenoid cystic carcinoma can be easily confused with adenocarcinoma or another type of non-small cell carcinoma. Thus, it is not surprising that in some of the cases reported the final interpretation was not made until after complete surgical resection. Once the resection is available, the histology of the tumor, namely, the cylindromatous growth pattern, is so characteristic that the interpretation rarely would be difficult. However, in some circumstances, the tumor can mimic other types of thymic carcinoma or thymomas, mainly those tumors that show papillary component. The immunohistochemical staining pattern of the cases reported do not allow a confident separation of adenoid cystic carcinoma from a variant of conventional thymic carcinoma or thymoma. Thus, the final interpretation will rely heavily in the morphological evaluation of the tumor.

Basaloid Carcinoma

Thymic basaloid carcinoma of the thymus is an unusual tumor that has been reported only seldom in the literature, and more recently its relationship with a true salivary gland-type tumor, namely, adenoid cystic carcinoma, has been raised. Therefore, the tumor is discussed in this section even though there is no well-established proof that this tumor corresponds to the salivary gland anlage type of neoplasms. However, not only basaloid carcinomas of the thymus may show some adenoid cystic-like morphological features; basaloid tumors have also been described in the salivary glands.

In 1982, Snover and associates [33], in a description of eight cases of thymic carcinoma, stated that there are five distinctive morphological variants of thymic carcinoma, one of these variants being basaloid carcinoma. One of the eight cases described corresponded to a thymic basaloid

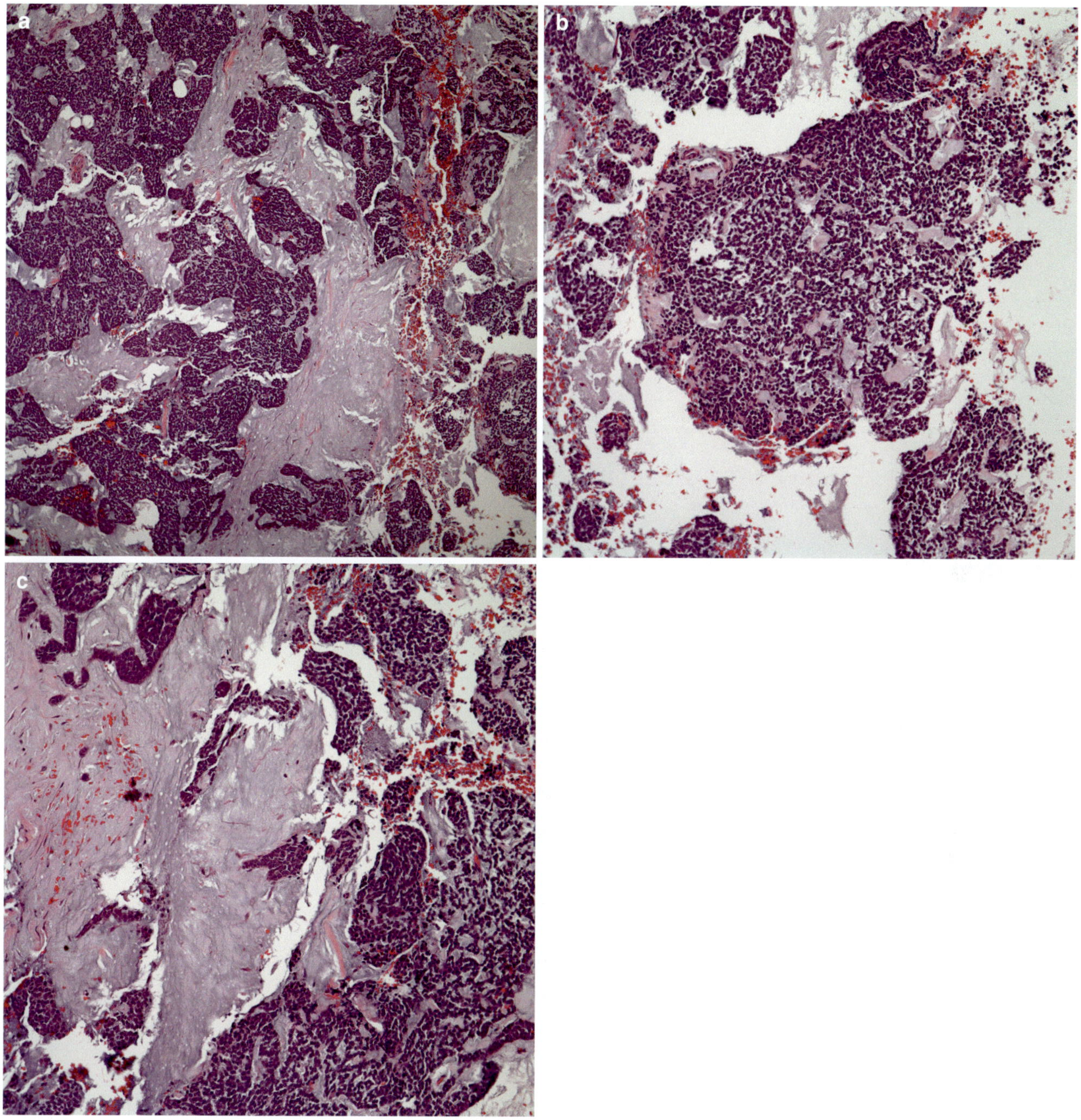

Fig. 5.38 (**a**) Low power view of a thymic adenoid cystic carcinoma showing neoplastic cells embedded in a mucoid background; (**b**) Adenoid cystic carcinoma showing focal gland-like formation; (**c**) Adenoid cystic carcinoma with extensive areas of mucoid material

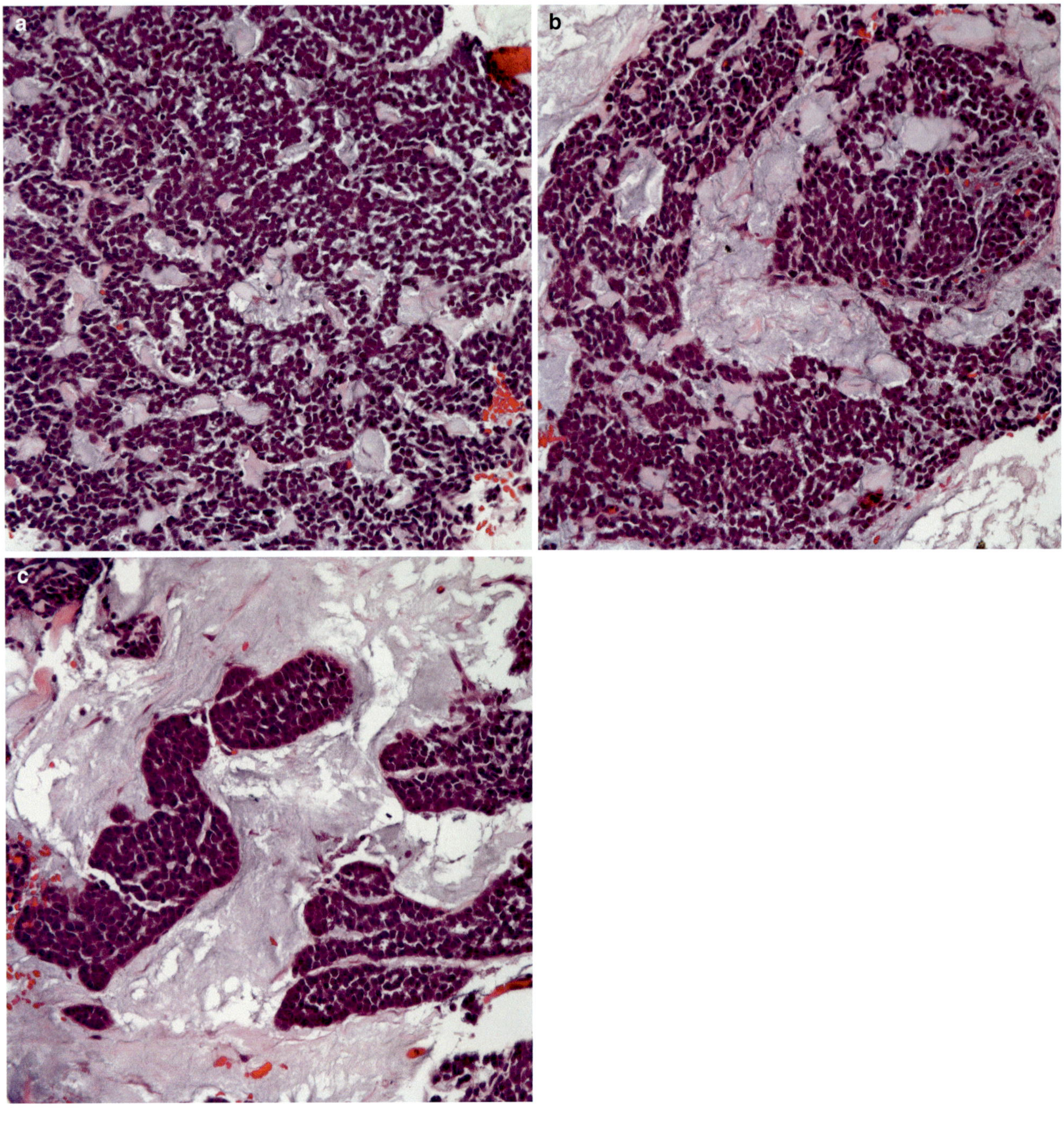

Fig. 5.39 (**a**) Adenoid cystic carcinoma showing tubular-like structures; (**b**) adenoid cystic carcinoma with a more solid component and only small gland-like structures; (**c**) extensive mucoid material with only islands of neoplastic cells

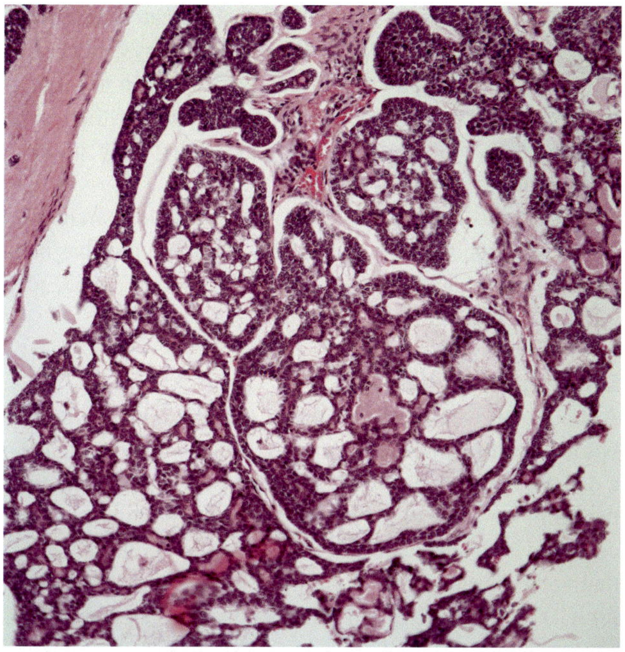

Fig. 5.40 Adenoid cystic carcinoma with more conventional characteristics

carcinoma, and the authors made an analogy to similar cutaneous tumors designated as basal cell carcinomas. Interestingly, in their histopathologic description, the tumor was noted to have gland-like spaces, which stained weakly for mucicarmine. In 1999, Ritter and Wick [34] in a review of primary carcinomas of the thymus gland also highlighted the histopathological features of these gland-like spaces containing stromal mucin, stating that those features produce a certain resemblance to adenoid cystic carcinoma. More recently, Brown and coworkers [10] described 12 cases of thymic basaloid carcinoma and addressed its relationship with adenoid cystic carcinoma. The authors presented an extensive discussion about basaloid carcinoma and basaloid squamous cell carcinoma of different organs systems, and, although, in the end, the authors concluded that basaloid carcinoma is perhaps best regarded as adenoid cystic carcinoma-like.

Important to highlight is the fact that basaloid carcinomas of the thymus are rare, with fewer than 30 cases reported in the literature, most of them in the form of case reports [35–41]. All these tumors have been described in adult individuals in a range of 40 to more than 70 years of age, with a male predominance for the tumor. Clinically, the patients may present with non-specific symptoms such as chest pain and dyspnea, while some patients may be completely asymptomatic, and the tumor is found during a routine chest image. Diagnostic imaging techniques such as plain film and chest CT scan are good modalities to determine the presence of an anterior mediastinal mass; however, histopathological analysis is the golden standard to determine the type of neoplasm. The largest series of thymic basaloid carcinomas is the one by Brown and coworkers [10] who presented 12 primary basaloid carcinoma of the thymus. The patients were ten men and two women between the ages of 34 and 77 years who presented with non-specific symptoms such as chest pain and dyspnea. This basic clinical information is similar to that described in previous case reports. However, this series of cases highlights something more important and that is the biologic behavior of these tumors. Basaloid carcinomas of the thymus have been initially regarded as low malignant potential; however, in Brown and coworkers' [10] series of cases, the authors stated that these tumors may follow a more aggressive behavior as 5 of their 12 patients described had died of the tumor in a period of 34 months and only 2 were alive and disease-free at 12 and 17 months. Whether there are some other features beyond the extent of the disease that can be correlated with clinical behavior remains to be determined. In that regard, take the case described by Sakakura and coworkers [40] of a 72-year-old man who was diagnosed with thymic basaloid carcinoma with pleural dissemination and who 1 year after surgery developed new pleural nodules; however, the patient remained alive 36 months later. A more aggressive neoplasm was also described by Matsuo and coworkers [38] in a 41-year-old woman who presented with thymic basaloid carcinoma with liver metastasis and who 1 year after initial surgery developed recurrent metastatic disease in the liver; however, the patient has remained alive 12 months after. These cases and those described by Brown and coworkers [10] highlight the fact that basaloid carcinoma, despite complete surgical resection, may follow an aggressive behavior. Tagawa and coworkers [42] documented a thymic basaloid carcinoma in a 61-year-old woman with what the authors described as distant metastases. On imaging, the patient appeared to have right hilar lymphadenopathy and a small nodule in the right lung. The patient was treated with S-1 plus cisplatin chemotherapy with concurrent radiation and after 11 months was disease-free. However, there are some drawbacks about this particular case: first, the initial diagnosis was established on a biopsy specimen, which, according to the illustration presented, indicated that the tumor could have been a different type of thymic carcinoma besides basaloid carcinoma; and second, the patient received treatment followed by resection of the mediastinal tumor, at which time not much residual carcinoma was found, once again casting doubts as to whether the neoplasm in question really corresponded to thymic basaloid carcinoma. It is well known that some squamous cell carcinoma of the thymus may actually show some palisading of the nuclei similar to that seen in basaloid carcinomas.

Based on the available literature, it is important to highlight that complete surgical resection is the treatment of choice for these tumors. Whether additional chemotherapy or radiation therapies are beneficial is difficult to unequivocally state as there are not enough cases reported in the literature to draw a meaningful conclusion. However, it is also important to highlight that thymic basaloid carcinoma, once thought to be a low-grade type of carcinoma, in some cases may follow a more aggressive behavior.

Pathological Features

Grossly, the tumors reported have been described as solid and cystic, or as predominantly cystic neoplasms that measured a few centimeters in diameter to more than 10 cm. In the cases described as cystic, the features may be indistinguishable from a true multilocular thymic cyst, while in those tumors with solid and cystic components, the tumor may be indistinguishable from cystic thymoma. Areas of hemorrhage and necrosis can be identified in some cases, namely, in the cystic areas of the tumor. Adhesions to the pericardium or pleura may be present.

Histologically, the hallmark of the tumor is the presence of a basaloid appearance (Fig. 5.41a, b) similar to that described in analogous cutaneous basal cell carcinomas, namely, the presence of peripheral palisading, which can have two distinct morphological growth patterns including a cystic appearance in which the tumor displays gland-like structures similar to those seen in adenoid cystic carcinoma and solid areas. Some of those cystic structures may contain an acellular material in their lumen and usually merge or are admixed with more solid component of the tumor, which can be arranged in small nests of tumor cells (Figs. 5.42a, b, 5.43a, b, and 5.44a, b). Focal squamous differentiation may be seen in some cases, while in others a spindle cell component has been observed. At higher magnification, the cells of basaloid carcinoma are small with inconspicuous nuclei and scant cytoplasm; mitotic activity is present, but it will be unusual to have makedly increased mitotic activity, as it usually ranged from 3–4 mitotic figures per 10 hpf. Necrosis in the form of comedonecrosis has been described in some cases. In a tumor in which the appearance is that of a cystic neoplasm, the tumor may have a predominant cystic component similar to that seen in a multilocular thymic cyst; in these cases it is possible to identify areas of transition between the nonneoplastic epithelium lining the cystic structures and the neoplastic epithelium of the basaloid thymic carcinoma. However, it is important to highlight that some basaloid carcinomas may be cystic without having multilocular thymic cyst-like areas. Although this is not an important discrimination to make, it is important only for academic purposes and for the identification of potential multilocular cysts that may undergo malignancy within its walls.

Immunohistochemical stains for basaloid carcinomas have been reported in the literature, and the tumor has been found to be positive for pan-cytokeratin, CD117, p63, p53, CD5, and collagen IV.

Differential Diagnosis

Although in a resected specimen the diagnosis of thymic basaloid carcinoma should not pose a problem, there may be a considerable challenge in small biopsies. In such cases, if the tumor shows a gland-like appearance, the tumor may be confused with adenoid cystic carcinoma. In addition, the fact that some basaloid carcinomas may show positive staining for CD117 may also add some confusion. However, true myoepithelial differentiation in thymic basaloid carcinoma has not been reported unequivocally. One other possibility in a small biopsy would be with atypical thymoma, as atypical thymomas are known to have areas of peripheral palisading. However, in atypical thymomas, the tumor may show some immature lymphocytes (Tdt-positive lymphocytes), which may be unusual in cases of basaloid carcinoma of the thymus. In a resected specimen with prominent cystic component similar to that seen in multilocular cyst (MTC), a benign cystic tumor will become the most important differential diagnosis or a multilocular thymic cyst with pseudoepitheliomatous hyperplasia. In such cases, the presence of basaloid areas of tumor cells would be more in keeping with the diagnosis of basaloid carcinoma. Perhaps the most important differential diagnosis is to separate true basaloid thymic carcinoma from basaloid squamous cell carcinoma of the thymus. It is very possible that these two conditions may behave differently, and careful analysis of these two tumors may be an important consideration in terms of treatment and clinical behavior. However, it is also important to highlight that the use of immunohistochemical stains may be limited as both tumors may show similar immunophenotype. Due to the rarity of these tumors, a more comprehensive study attempting to separate or unify these tumors is still pending.

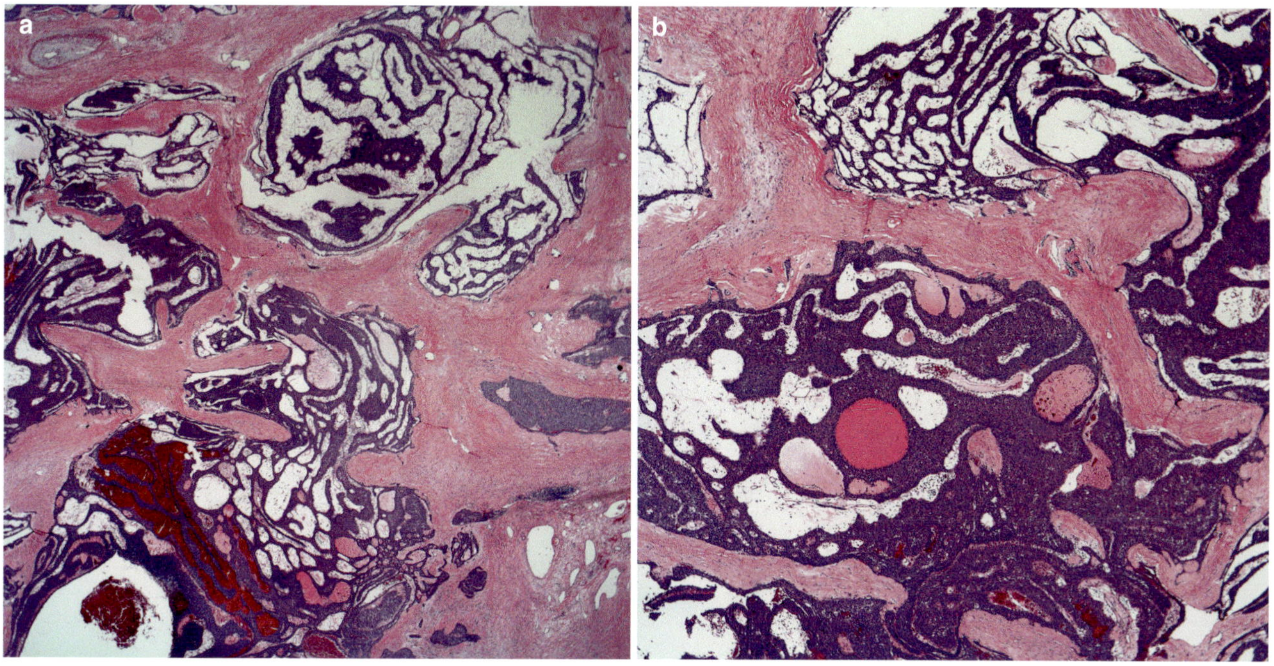

Fig. 5.41 (**a**) Low power view of a thymic basaloid carcinoma showing neoplastic cells separated by extensive fibrocollagenous strands; (**b**) Basaloid carcinoma showing thin and broad fronds of neoplastic cells

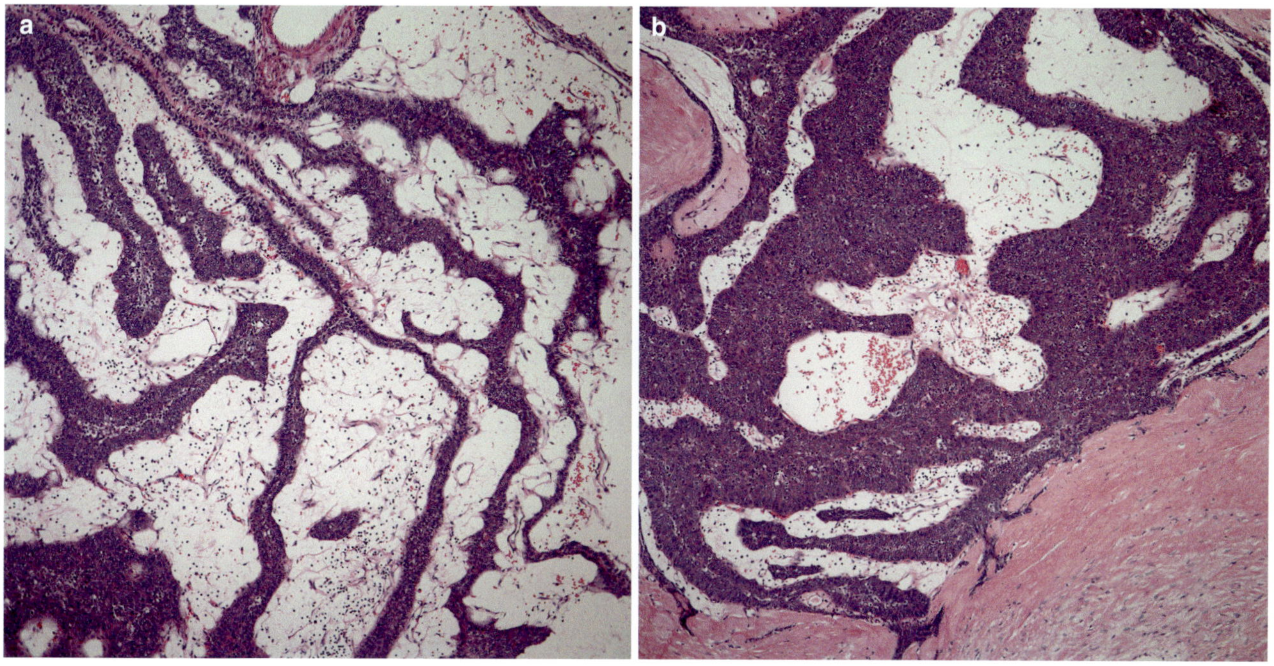

Fig. 5.42 (**a**) Thymic basaloid carcinoma showing thin strands of neoplastic cells; (**b**) Thymic basaloid carcinoma showing broad strands of neoplastic cells

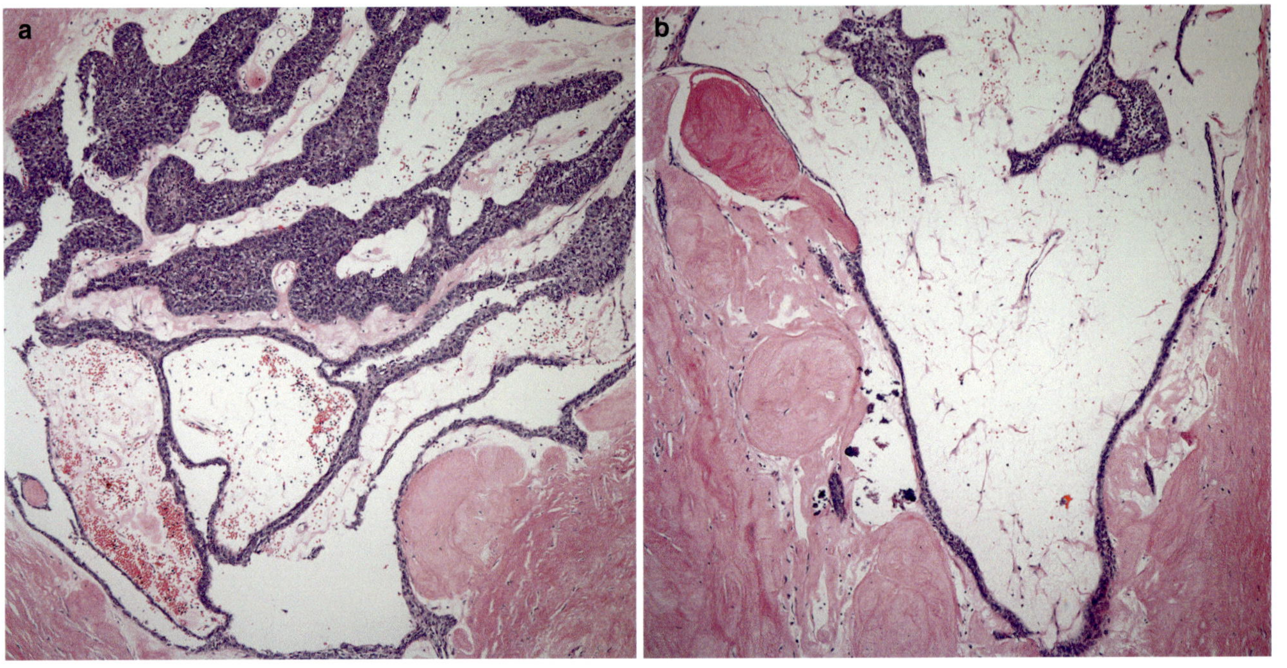

Fig. 5.43 (**a**) Thymic basaloid carcinoma showing a mixture of thin and broad strands of neoplastic cells; (**b**) Thymic basaloid carcinoma showing extensive presence of fibroconnective tissue and only small islands of neoplastic cells within a cystic-like structure

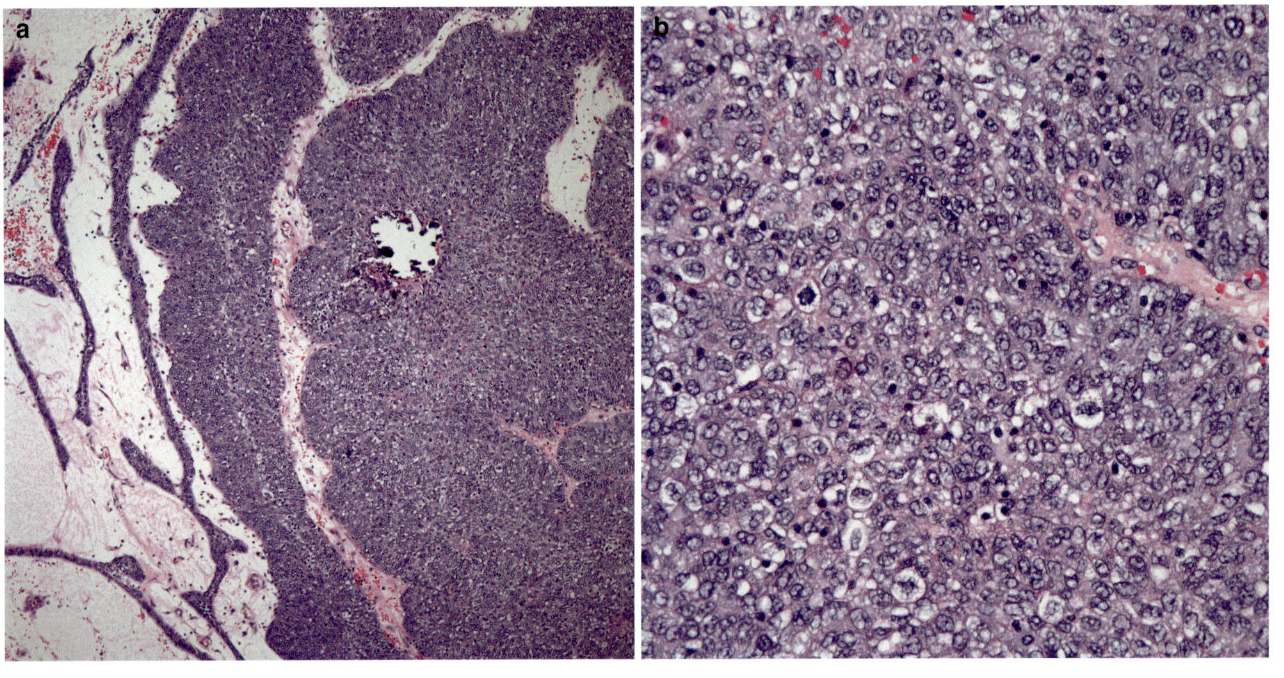

Fig. 5.44 (**a**) Thymic basaloid carcinoma showing thin strands of neoplastic cells adjacent to a more solid component; (**b**) Higher magnification of the solid component showing moderate nuclear atypia and scattered mitotic figures

References

1. Moran CA. Primary salivary gland-type tumors of the lung. Sem Diagn Pathol. 1995;12:106–22.
2. Hguyen CV, Suster S, Moran CA. Pulmonary epithelila-myoepithelial carcinoma: a clinicopathologic and immunohistochemical study of 5 cases. Hum Pathol. 2009;40:366–73.
3. Moran CA, Suster S, Askin FB, Koss MN. Benign and malignant salivary-gland type mixed tumors of the lung. Cancer. 1994;73:2481–90.
4. Moran CA, Suster S, Koss MN. Primary adenoid cystic carcinoma of the lung. A clinicopathologic and immunohistochemical study of 16 cases. Cancer. 1994;73:1390–7.
5. Moran CA, Suster S, Koss MN. Acinic cell carcinoma of the lung ("Fechner tumor"): a Clinicopathologic, immunohistochemical, and ultrastructural study of five cases. Am J Surg Pathol. 1992;16:1039–50.
6. Yousem SA, Hoccholzer L. Mucoepidermoid tumors of the lung. Cancer. 1987;60:1346–52.
7. England DM, Hochholzer L. Truly benign "bronchial adenoma" report of 10 cases of mucous gland adenoma with immunohistochemical and ulstratural findings. Am J Surg Pathol. 1995;19:887–99.
8. Falk N, Weissferdt A, Kalhor N, Moran CA. Primary salivary gland-type tumors: a review and update. Adv Anat Pathol. 2016;22:355–75.
9. Kalhor N, Weissferdt A, Moran CA. Primary salivary gland-type tumors of the thymus. Adv Anat Pathol. 2017;24(1):15–23.
10. Brown JG, Familiari U, Papotti M, Rosai J. Thymic basaloid carcinoma: a clinicopathologic study of 12 cases, with a general discussion of basaloid carcinoma and its relationship with adenoid cystic carcinoma. Am J Surg Pathol. 2009;33:1113–24.
11. Weissferdt A, Moran CA. Thymic hyperplasia with lymphoepithelial sialadenitis (LESA)-like features: a clinicopatholgoic and immunohistochemical study of 4 cases. Am J Clin Pathol. 2012;138:816–22.
12. Weissferdt A, Kalhor N, Moran CA. Sebaceous lymphadenoma of the thymus: a clinicopathologic and immunohistochemical study of two cases. Hum Pathol. 2016;56:189–93.
13. Chen WC, Tanaka N. On the mixed tumor of the mediastinum. Gann. 1952;43:415–7.
14. Feign GA, Robinson B, Marchevsky A. Mixed tumor of the mediastinum. Arch Path Lab Med. 1986;110:80–1.
15. Lee YK, Kim YH, Kim GY, Youn HC. Pleomorphic adenoma presenting with a mediastinal mass. Thoracic Cancer. 2014;5:89–92.
16. Tanaka M, Shimokawa R, Matsubara O, Aoki N, Kamiyama R, Kasuga T, et al. Mucoepidermoid carcinoma of the thymic region. Acta Pathol Jpn. 1982;32:703–12.
17. Brightman I, Moragan JA, Kunze WP, Sheppard MN. Primary mucoepidermoid carcinoma of the thymus – a rare cause of mediastinal tumour. Thorac Cardiovasc Surg. 1992;40:90–1.
18. Stefanou D, Goussia AC, Arkoumani E, Metafratzi ZM, Syminelakis S, Arkoumani E, et al. Mucoepidermoid carcinoma of the thymus: a case presentation and a literature review. Pathol Res Pract. 2004;200:567–73.
19. Kim GD, Kim HW, Oh JT, Jo H-J, Juhng S-K. Mucoepidermoid carcinoma of the thymus: a case report. J Korean Med Sci. 2004;19:601–3.
20. Yasuda M, Yasukawa T, Ozaki D, Yusa T. Mucoepidermoid carcinoma of the thymus. Jpn J Thorac Cardiovasc Surg. 2006;54:23–6.
21. Woo WL, Panagiotopoulos N, Gvinianidze L, Proctor I, Lawrence D. Primary mucoepidermoid carcinoma of the thymus presenting with myasthenia gravis. J Thorac Dis. 2014;6:E223–5.
22. Noda T, Higashiyama M, Oda K, Higaki N, Takami K, Okami J, et al. Mucoepidermoid carcinoma of the thymus treated by multimodality therapy: a case report. Ann Thorac Cardiovasc Surg. 2006;12:273–8.
23. Fuse ET, Kamimura M, Takeda Y, Kawaishi M, Kimura S, Niino H, et al. Response of a thymic mucoepidermoid carcinoma to combination chemotherapy with cisplatin and irinotecan: a case report. Lung Cancer. 2008;59:403–6.
24. Moran CA, Suster S. Mucoepidermoid carcinoma of the thymus: a clinicopathologic study of six cases. Am J Surg Pathol. 1995;19:826–34.
25. Nonaka D, Klimstra D, Rosai J. Thymic mucoepidermoid carcinoma: a clinicopathologic study of 10 cases and review of the literature. Am J Surg Pathol. 2004;28:1526–31.
26. Roden AC, Erickson-Johnson MR, Yi ES, Garcia JJ. Analysis of MALM2 rearrangement in mucoepidermoid carcinoma of the thymus. Hum Pathol. 2013;44:2799–805.
27. Prieto-Granada CN, Inagaki H, Mueller J. Thymic mucoepidermoid carcinoma: report of a case with CTRCI/3-MALM2 molecular studies. Int J Surg Pathol. 2015;23:277–83.
28. Weissferdt A, Kalhor N, Moran CA. Pleuromediastinal epithelial-myoepithelial carcinoma: a clinicopathologic and immunohistochemical study of two cases. Am J Clin Path. 2016;146(6):736–40.
29. Di Tommaso L, Kuhn E, Kurrer M, Zettl A, Marx A, Müller-Hermelink HK, et al. Thymic tumor with adenoid cystic carcinoma-like features: a clinicopathologic study of 4 cases. Am J Surg Pathol. 2007;31:1161–7.
30. Banki F, Khalil K, Kott MM, Cota AL. Adenoid cystic carcinoma of the thymus gland: a rare case. Ann Thorac Surg. 2010;90:e56–8.
31. Rampisela D, Zreik R, Donner LR. Thymic tumor with adenoid cystic carcinoma-like features: a study of a clinically favorable case followed for 9 years. Int J Surg Pathol. 2015;23:557–60.
32. Kanzaki R, Okura N, Kitahara N, Kitahara N, Okimura A, Kawahara K, et al. Thymic carcinoma with adenoid cystic carcinoma-like features with distant metastases. Ann Thorac Cardiovasc Surg. 2012;18:544–7.
33. Snover DC, Levine GD, Rosai J. Thymic carcinoma: five distinctive histological variants. Am J Surg Pathol. 1982;6:451–70.
34. Ritter JH, Wick MR. Primary carcinomas of the thymus gland. Sem Diag Pathol. 1999;16:18–31.
35. Lezzoni JC, Nass LB. Thymic basaloid carcinoma: a case report and review of the literature. Mod Pathol. 1996;9:21–5.
36. Kawashima O, Kamiyoshihara M, Sakata S, Kurihara T, Ishikawa S, Morishita Y. Basaloid carcinoma of the thymus. Ann Thorac Surg. 1999;68:1863–5.
37. Tanimura S, Tomoyasu H, Khono T, Matsushita H. Basaloid carcinoma originated from the wall of thymic cyst presenting as pericardial and thoracic effusion: report of a case. Kyobu geka. Jpn J Thorac Surg. 2002;55:571–5.
38. Matsuo T, Hayashida R, Kobayashi K, Tanaka Y, Ohtsuka S. Thymic basaloid carcinoma with hepatic metastasis. Ann Thorac Surg. 2002;74:579–82.
39. Morisaki Y, Takagi K, Sano S, Furuya T, Ishikawa M, Torigoe T, et al. Basaloid carcinoma of the thymus: report of a case. Surg Today. 2006;36:68–70.
40. Sakakura N, Tateyama H, Usami N, Yokoi K. Thymic basaloid carcinoma with pleural dissemination that developed after a curative resection: report of a case. Surg Today. 2010;40:1073–8.
41. Weissferdt A, Moran CA. Thymic carcinoma associated with multilocular thymic cyst: a clinicopathologic study of 7 cases. Am J Surg Pathol. 2011;35:1074–9.
42. Tagawa T, Ohta M, Kuwata T, Awaya H, Ishida T. S-1 plus cisplatin chemotherapy with concurrent radiation for thymic basaloid carcinoma. J Thorac Oncol. 2010;5:572–3.

6 Staging for Thymoma and Thymic Carcinoma

Introduction

The staging of thymomas – just as its classification – is a rather controversial topic as there is not a universally accepted staging system for these tumors. In addition, often one of the proposed staging systems presented for thymomas has been adapted for thymic carcinomas, which has obscured even more the issue of thymoma and thymic carcinoma. It is very important to highlight the issue that thymoma is not the benign counterpart of thymic carcinoma nor is thymic carcinoma the malignant counterpart of thymoma. Those two thymic epithelial tumors represent two different clinicopathological entities; unfortunately, there is a tendency by some to try to lump both of these tumors into one category, while in reality the clinical behavior and treatment for those two tumors are rather different.

It is interesting and important to highlight the issue that even in the early large series of thymomas, the authors did not present a staging system, and the focus in those series was more on the histological classification of thymomas. An example of this is the focus by Bernatz and colleagues [1] when addressing the issue of classification, stating "some prognostic significance could be gained through study of cell types," basically assessing the issue of separating these tumors by the percentage of cell types into predominantly lymphocytic, predominantly epithelial, mixed types, and spindle cell type. However, even though the authors did not present a formal staging system, they emphasized the issue that, in their experience, three fourths of these tumors are noninvasive. Nevertheless, the authors also identified that regardless of their specific cell type, such findings did not correlate with the invasiveness of the tumors, as all the cell types were seen to be noninvasive and invasive. The authors clearly stated that they found no differences between the histological features of invasive and noninvasive neoplasms. On the contrary, larger series of thymic carcinomas are few and also focused on the clinicopathological aspects of the tumor rather than on the staging [2]. More recently different reviews addressing not only the historical aspects of the different schemas but also addressing their pitfalls and shortcomings have been presented [3–5]. Also important to highlight is that, even in larger series of cases, the authors have decided to lump together thymomas and thymic carcinomas as well as neuroendocrine carcinoma [6].

In this chapter, we will analyze each one of the proposed staging systems for thymoma and thymic carcinoma. However, since we consider these two tumors to represent different clinicopathological entities, a distinction in the staging system will be discussed with the hope that not only will it help in daily practice when dealing with these tumors but also that it may provide better triaging of patients for treatment purposes.

Staging of Thymoma

Sometime after Bernatz and colleagues [1] presented their views regarding the histological classification of thymomas, once again these same authors [7] presented a study of 181 patients diagnosed with thymomas over a period of 20 years, from 1949 to 1969. This study emphasized "factors influencing prognosis." In this group of patients, the authors found that 44% had thymomas associated with myasthenia gravis, while 36% of the tumors were grossly invasive. The average age was 50 years; however, patients with myasthenia gravis were 13 years younger than those without such an association. In addition, no significant gender distribution was noted. Needless to say, patients with invasive tumors had poor survival, and the presence of invasion was more important than the association with myasthenia gravis. One important feature that the authors identified was that myasthenia in invasive tumors did not alter the prognosis, contrary to the presence of myasthenia in noninvasive tumors where it may shorten survival. Important to highlight is that all histological

© Springer Nature Switzerland AG 2019
N. Kalhor, C. Moran, *Mediastinal Pathology*, https://doi.org/10.1007/978-3-319-98980-8_6

types were identified among the invasive and noninvasive tumors. Similarly significant is that the presence of distant metastases was a rare event and was found in only 2 out of 181 patients, both cases with metastatic disease to the liver.

In 1979, Bergh and colleagues [8] presented a series of 43 patients with thymoma, corresponding to 20 women and 23 men between the ages of 17 and 73 years. All the thymomas were classified according to the Bernatz histological classification [1] into lymphocyte-rich, epithelial-rich, and mixed. The authors defined the three stages as follows:

- Stage I – Intact capsule or growth within the capsule
- Stage II – Pericapsular growth into the mediastinal fat
- Stage III – Invasive growth into the surrounding organs, intrathoracic metastases, or both

Based on this "staging system," the authors documented that tumor removal was possible in 25 patients in stages I or II and in 14/18 patients in stage III. Pleural metastases were observed in patients in stage III. It is of interest to highlight that, in this particular series of cases with the proposed staging system, the authors were able to identify only one patient with tumor relapse in stage II and five patients in stage III. In addition, the authors noted a "considerable" difference in survival between stages II and III and suggested not lumping these together. The authors also added that the association of superior vena cava syndrome appeared to be indicative of poor prognosis. However, the emphasis of this series of cases was on the accomplishment of complete surgical resection, as the authors noted low recurrence and high survival for stages I and II. Interestingly, the authors concluded that the diagnosis of thymoma might be questioned in patients with lymph node metastasis. In a separate report of 103 patients with thymoma, Wilkins and Castleman [9] staged the patients using the Bergh approach with "minor" modifications:

- Stage I – Intact capsule or growth within the capsule
- Stage II – Pericapsular growth into the mediastinal fat tissue or adjacent pleura or pericardium
- Stage III – Invasive growth into the surrounding organs, intrathoracic metastases, or both

It is obvious that the "minor" modifications took place in stage II, as the authors added involvement of pleura and pericardium. Even though there is not a specific explanation for the addition of two different structures to stage II, it is possible that such an argument is due to the survival noted by the authors in stages I and II, which documented only 1 of 18 patients in stage II who died due to complications of myasthenia gravis (MG). However, the authors also concluded that the presence of MG is not an adverse factor affecting survival. More interestingly, by 1991, Wilkins and associates [10] reported 85 cases of thymoma from 1972 to 1989, 32 of these patients with history of MG; however, in this report, the authors used the Masaoka staging schema, recommending that all patients to be followed for a minimum period of 10 years and that patients in Masaoka's stages II and III to receive postoperative radiotherapy. The authors also added that the presence of MG is no longer considered an adverse factor in survival.

In 1981 in a study of 96 cases of thymoma, Masaoka proposed what has been the most popular staging system for thymoma [11]. The emphasis in this staging system is on the macroscopic and microscopic aspects of the tumor. The proposed system is as follows:

- Stage I – Macroscopically completely encapsulated and microscopically no capsular invasion
- Stage II:
  1. Macroscopic invasion into the surrounding fatty tissue or mediastinal pleura
  2. Microscopic invasion into the capsule
- Stage III – Macroscopic invasion into the neighboring organ, i.e., the pericardium, great vessels, or lung
- Stage IVa – Pleural or pericardial dissemination
- Stage IVb – Lymphogenous or hematogenous metastasis

The patients were 56 men and 40 women between the ages of 8 months and 67 years. Histologically, all tumors were grouped according to the Bernatz classification [1], and all the different types were seen in the different staging systems proposed. Based on this proposed staging system, 50 patients were in stages I and II, while 46 patients were in stages III and IV. However, closer breakdown of the different stages shows that only 11 patients were in stages IVa and IVb, while 32 were in stage III, which accounts for 93 patients and not the 96 stated in the manuscript. However, the authors provided a 5-year survival rate of each clinical stage as follows: 92.6% for stage I, 85.7% for stage II, 69.6% for stage III, and 50% for stage IV. Interestingly, the authors point out that only 89 thoracotomies were evaluated at their center and that two patients refused the operation. Also important to highlight in this study is that all the histological subtypes of thymomas were seen in all the different stages proposed.

Based on this proposal for staging thymomas, there are several issues that deserve attention:

1. The authors observed a thymoma in an 8-month-old child. One would have to wonder if that in fact might have been a thymoma or a different thymic neoplasm.
2. Even though the manuscript states that the study contained 96 cases, in fact there were only 86 thoracotomies evaluated, and, as the authors point out, in at least two patients, surgical resection did not take place. Thus, one

would have to wonder about the "true staging" of those patients.

3. For stage I – What happens with tumors that may be "macroscopically" encapsulated but the microscopic evaluation reveals invasion?
4. How is it possible in stage II-1 to evaluate macroscopic invasion of the surrounding fat in a case that may be only "minimally invasive?"
5. For stage II-2, microscopic invasion into the capsule does not represent invasive thymoma.
6. For stage II-1 and stage IVa, regarding pleural involvement: there is a play of words, and one wonders what the authors meant exactly by "invasion" and/or "dissemination." One could easily move a patient from stage II-1 to stage IVa.
7. It is very likely that statistically there is not a significant difference between stage I and stage II. That is highly important for treatment purposes and possibly impacts long-term survival.

In 1994, Koga and associates [12] reviewed 79 thymomas and modified the previously proposed schema of Masaoka [10]. The modifications introduced by Koga and associates [11] are essentially in stage II of the Masaoka staging system. The system is as follows:

- *Original Masaoka*
- Stage II
  1. Macroscopic invasion into the surrounding fatty tissue or mediastinal pleura
  2. Microscopic invasion into the capsule
- *Koga's modifications*
- Stage II
  1. Microscopic transcapsular invasion
  2. Macroscopic invasion into the thymic or surrounding fatty tissue, or grossly adherent to but not breaking through the mediastinal pleura or pericardium

Even though in this review of Masaoka's schema the issue of transcapsular invasion is clarified, the authors technically introduced additional problems:

1. There are some thymomas that invade the thymic tissue, and yet the tumors are encapsulated, thus posing some problems for this stage.
2. Tumor "grossly adherent to the pleura but not breaking through it": Does this mean that if the tumor breaks through, it becomes stage III? If so, then stage III needs some modification. In addition, the tumor may be adherent to the pleura and/or pericardium as it is commonly seen but without actual invasion. Thus, there is no pleural invasion, which raises the issue of the actual significance of "grossly adherent."

In 1991, Pescarmona and associates [13] analyzed 83 patients with thymoma by age, sex, presence of MG, staging, and histological subtype. Important to mention in this study is that the authors used a different histological typing of tumors – cortical, medullary, and mixed. Based on their analysis, the authors concluded that age, sex, and presence of MG did not prove to represent significant prognostic factors. However, the authors stated that clinical stage and histological type had "significant" prognostic value. The patients evaluated corresponded to 44 women and 39 men ages 21–83 years. Histologically, 34 thymomas were cortical, 13 medullary, and 36 mixed. Clinically, using the Masaoka proposed schema [11], 23 patients were in stage I, 26 patients in stage II, 26 patients in stage III, and 8 patients in stage IV. It is of interest to note that none of the patients was further categorized in stages II-1, II-2, IVa, or IVb, and this raises the possibility that those features were either not important or ignored. The authors arrived at an important conclusion and that is that "medullary-type tumors are, in most cases, fully benign." Furthermore, the authors concluded that (1) stages I and II medullary-type and stage I mixed-type thymomas have an excellent prognosis; (2) stages I and II cortical-type thymoma and stages II and III mixed thymomas have an intermediate prognosis; and (3) stages III and IV cortical-type thymoma have the least favorable prognosis. It is of interest to highlight that the authors arrived at one important conclusion regarding the "benign" nature of "medullary thymoma" by having examined only 13 cases of this type of tumor, and, according to the authors, "most of those cases" were in stage I. Further studies of this particular type of thymoma have demonstrated that it is very likely that such an assumption is incorrect [14, 15]. Numerous other series of thymomas using the proposed Masaoka's schema for staging have been presented in the literature. Blumberg and coworkers [16], in a study from 1949 to 1993, retrospectively evaluated 118 patients with thymoma with the goal of determining independent factors to predict survival. The authors concluded that patients in stage I require no further therapy after complete surgical resection and that, for patients with invasive disease and large tumor, neoadjuvant therapy should be considered. Regnard and coworkers [17] presented their experience with 307 thymoma cases in which the authors observed that complete surgical resection should be taken into account in clinical-pathologic staging, as the authors observed that patients in Masaoka's stage III had a significantly higher survival rate if those patients had complete surgical resection of the tumor. In addition, the authors did not find any significant difference between patients who received postoperative radiation therapy and those who did not. Based on their findings, the authors proposed a modification to the Masaoka's schema in which most of the wording of the stages was essentially kept but the authors added the surgical resectability of the tumor: complete or incomplete resection. Safieddine and coworkers [18] presented their experience with 262 patients with the goal of determining prognostic factors for cure, recurrence, and long-term survival after surgical resection of thymoma. One interesting variable in this study is that the authors also used the histological schema proposed by the World Health Organization (WHO); however, the authors essentially concluded that complete surgical resection is associated with good prognosis while advanced staging is associated with poor prognosis. Demirci and coworkers [19], in a study of 47 patients with thymoma and thymic carcinoma using also the WHO histological schema for subtyping thymoma, concluded that the most important prognostic factor for overall survival was the extent of resection. Contrary to previous experiences reported by others with large series of cases, Cardillo and coworkers [20], in a report of 61 patients including 18 patients with thymic carcinoma, concluded that complete surgical resection, "Masaoka stage," induction chemotherapy, and histological WHO subtyping are independent predictors of survival in locally advanced thymoma/thymic carcinoma. Interestingly, more recently the International Thymic Malignancy Interest Group (ITMIG), stating that no official staging schema has been defined, introduced their own modification to an already "not so clear" Masaoka's schema. One of those "modifications" was to introduce an already known term: "minimally invasive." The remainder of the Masaoka schema was kept [21]. Even Dr. Masaoka himself has provided his own follow-up regarding his own staging schema [22]: in a review of 211 thymomas, Masaoka concluded that his staging schema remains a valuable prognostic factor. However, he also added that the combination of stages I and II and the separation of stage III into subgroups are not recommended, while, for patients in stage IVb, it is best to include positive lymph nodes. While some of his suggestions seem to be appropriate, combining his own proposed schema and mixing it with a TNM system does not seem appropriate but rather misleading.

In a departure from the Masaoka staging schema [11], Yamakawa in collaboration with Masaoka and others [23] presented a "tentative tumor-node-metastasis" classification of thymoma. The authors evaluated 207 patients with thymoma and stated that lymphogenous and hematogenous metastases were infrequent and that lymphogenous metastases were present in "few cases." However, the authors also concluded that TNM classification of thymomas had little advantage over conventional clinical staging. It is of interest, however, to highlight that the authors also evaluated the TNM system in 13 cases of thymic carcinoma and 6 cases of thymic carcinoid, stating that in these tumors, the TNM classification was more useful. Nevertheless, the authors advanced the following TNM schema:

- *T-factor*
  - T1 – macroscopically completely encapsulated and microscopically no capsular invasion
  - T2 – macroscopically adhesion or invasion into the surrounding fatty tissue or mediastinal pleura, or microscopic invasion into the capsule
  - T3 – invasion into neighboring organs, such as the pericardium, great vessels, and lung
  - T4 – pleural or pericardial dissemination
- *N-factor*
  - N0 – no lymph node metastasis
  - N1 – metastasis to anterior mediastinal lymph nodes
  - N2 – metastasis to intrathoracic lymph nodes except anterior mediastinal lymph nodes
  - N3 – metastasis to extrathoracic lymph nodes
- *M-factor*
  - M0 – no hematogenous metastasis
  - M1 – hematogenous metastasis

It is evident by the descriptions that the TNM proposal is based on the early definitions of Masaoka's schema with the same recurrent problems of "invasion into the capsule" and "invasion and dissemination in pleura or pericardium." Most puzzling about the definitions of the T-factor are the T1 and T2: how can a tumor be called T2 while it is both an encapsulated tumor (invasion into the capsule) and at the same time has macroscopic adhesion or macroscopic invasion into surrounding fatty tissue? The T2 definitions in this TNM schema are ambiguous at best if not plainly incorrect. In addition, the N-factor requires that the surgeon provides an extensive lymph node sampling, which has essentially been more recently found to likely be not correct.

Following this trend, Kondo [24], stating that system for all thymic epithelial tumors is desirable (including thymic carcinoma and carcinoid), also supported the TNM system. Kondo also added that the N and M factors influence the prognosis more than the T-factor. However, one has to wonder how is it that the author was able to properly address the proposed Yamakawa TNM schema [23] with the pitfall and shortcoming already mentioned, or, perhaps, as it was concluded by their own proponents of the TNM proposal, the system works better for thymic carcinoma and not very well for thymoma. Following the same concept of the TNM system, Bedini and coworkers [25] proposed their own interpretation of the TNM system, which the authors called the INT (Istituto Nazionale Tumori). Their INT system is as follows:

- T1 – no capsular invasion
- T2 – microscopic invasion into the capsule or extracapsular involvement limited to the surrounding fatty tissue or normal thymus
- T3 – direct invasion into the mediastinal pleura and/or anterior pericardium

- T4 – direct invasion into the neighboring organs, such as the sternum, great vessels, and lung; implants to the mediastinal pleura or pericardium, only if anterior to phrenic nerves
- N0 – no lymph node metastasis
- N1 – metastasis to anterior mediastinal lymph nodes
- N2 – metastasis to intrathoracic lymph nodes other than anterior mediastinal
- N3 – metastasis to prescalene or supraclavicular nodes
- M0 – no hematogenous metastasis
- M1a – implants to the pericardium or mediastinal pleura beyond the sites defined in the T4 category
- M1b – hematogenous metastasis to other sites or involvement of lymph nodal stations other than those described in the N categories

Regarding this proposal, the authors not only kept ambiguous terms such as invasion into the capsule or extracapsular involvement for the same stage, but they also added new ambiguous issues. For instance, similar definitions are provided for T4 and M1a with the caveat of "beyond the sites defined in the T4 category." What are those sites? Is there any other site besides the lung, great vessels, and possibly heart that were already mentioned in the T4? If the tumor goes below the diaphragm, then it will be M disease. Furthermore, even in the larger series of cases and in those which proposed the TNM system, it was stated that the number of cases that involve lymph nodes is not large; needless to say, the number of cases that involved supraclavicular lymph nodes must be exceedingly rare, if they exist at all, unless they are thymic carcinoma. If the latter is correct, then once again, it proves that the TNM system may work better for thymic carcinoma and not very well for thymoma. In 2004, Asamura and associates [26], with the thought in mind that thymoma needs a new staging system, launched a different spin of a modified Masaoka's schema and provided a staging system in which tumor size appears to be a conspicuous feature, namely, a tumor size of 10 cm. In addition, the authors [26] provided a breakdown of the stages into two different schemas. This proposal is as follows:

- Stage I – tumors without any invasion into other structures/organs regardless of capsular involvement
- Stage II:
  - Tumors smaller than 10 cm in diameter and involving only one neighboring structure/organ (Schema 1)
  - Tumors of all combinations of diameter and number of involved structures/organs other than those in stage III (Schema 2)
- Stage III:
  - Tumors of all combinations of diameter and number of involved structures/organs other than those in stage II (Schema 1)
  - Tumors 10 cm or more in diameter and involving two or more neighboring structures/organs
- Stage IV – tumors with pleural or pericardial dissemination (IVa) or lymphatic/vascular metastasis (IVb)

Several concerns can be raised about the approach of this Masaoka-modified system. Although according to conventional wisdom one can assume that a larger tumor is likely to become invasive, how is that the size of 10 cm became the "magic size?" The author correctly observed that stages I and II of Masaoka's schema provide similar clinical follow-up; thus, the authors cleverly merge those stages into one. Interestingly, their stage I includes encapsulated tumors and the minimally invasive neoplasm. Stage IV of Masaoka's schema is essentially untouched, while stages II and III include two different schemas based on tumor size and involvement of structures/organs. However, it is here where the "play" of staging and schemas becomes a puzzle. For instance, it is well known that tumor size and invasiveness do not correlate, and tumors of less than 10 cm can show the so-called drop metastasis (invasion into the diaphragm), thus following the Asamura-modified Masaoka's system; such a tumor can easily be staged II – schema 1. More important is the fact that, in this system, the authors mention structure/organs for stage II schema 2 and structure/organs for stage III schema 1 but do not specify what structures they mean. It is one thing to have invasion into the great vessels and quite another to have invasion into the pericardium. Also, the authors interject another "magic number" for structures involved: two or more. The number of variables included in this system interestingly has not been found statistically significant in any other series of cases. One important feature to highlight in this study is the fact that, out of the 152 cases presented, the authors did not find evidence of metastatic disease in lymph nodes in any of the cases.

More recently, the ITMIG has published a series of review manuscripts without the actual review of cases and has made several proposals regarding the use of a universal system for thymic epithelial tumors (thymoma and thymic carcinoma) following the TNM system. Interestingly, one of those proposals is incorporated in the 8th edition of the TNM classification of malignant tumors. One has to wonder how is that a system is applied that consistently by different series of cases has shown not to be appropriate to be staged. And yet the ITMIG is proposing to include it as the standard staging system for thymoma; this is clearly not the most scientific manner of adopting a system for any pathological condition [27–30]. Perhaps this is a similar story to the one about the subtyping of thymomas by the WHO, which was never conceived as a classification but merely as a "translator" of two different proposed schemas. One can easily identify two glaring problems with the ITMIG approach: (1) proposing a TNM system for thymoma which clearly has shown to be ineffective for these tumors and (2) attempting to use a TNM system for thymoma and thymic carcinoma, which even those who have published series of cases of thymic epithelial neoplasm have concluded as a system better suited for thymic carcinoma than thymoma. The most important conclusion that one can draw regarding the ITMIG proposal is that it is based on "some literature review" and not on actual comprehensive review of cases. It is important to highlight in this context an observation made by Wick [31] in a review of prognostic factors for thymic epithelial neoplasm, in which the author stated "the TNM substrata were created intuitively rather than being tied to a rigorous statistical modeling procedure… one must be skeptical of their soundness unless and until TNM systems for thymic tumors are tested systematically."

In a different study, Gamondes and associates [32] evaluated 65 patients with thymoma over a period of 17 years. The patients were 28 men and 37 women between the ages of 20 and 73 years. Fifty-four patients had a history of MG. However, contrary to previous studies using the Masaoka schema [11], this particular study focused on the French schema for thymic tumors, also known for its acronym GETT (Groupe d'Etudes des Tumeurs Thymiques), which is as follows:

- Stage I
  - A. Encapsulated, noninvasive. Total excision
  - B. Localized growth into the surrounding structures. Total excision
- Stage II
  - A. Invasive growth into the surrounding organs. Total excision
- Stage III
  - A. Invasive growth into surrounding organs. Incomplete excision
  - B. Invasive growth into the surrounding organs. Biopsy of the tumor
- Stage IV
  - A. Largely invading tumor cells with clavicular lymph nodes or pleural or pulmonary grafts
  - B. Hematogenous metastasis

From the description of the different stages, it is evident that this system is essentially based on "complete surgical resection of the tumor," which essentially could be used in a more abbreviated form and that is (A) complete surgical resection and (B) incomplete surgical resection or unresectable. For instance, that is exactly the difference between stage IB and stage IIA. On the other hand, for stage IVA, as it has been the experience of others, lymphogenous metastasis is rare, and also the presence of "pleural or pulmonary grafts" is rather ambiguous as it was in the Masaoka schema with pleural invasion and pleural dissemination, for two different stages. However, one essentially can shorten this staging system into complete resection and incomplete resection or unresectable, regardless of the anatomic structures involved. Based on this GETT system, the 65 cases evaluated [14] broke down as follows: 38 cases were in stage I, 6 in stage II, 13 in stage III, and 8 in stage IV. The mean survival for all patients was 70 months. Thus, the authors concluded that the prognosis of thymoma relates to total surgical resection and stage of the tumor, and it is not influenced by age, sex, tumor cell type, or the presence or absence of MG.

One of the most recent proposals exclusively for the staging of thymomas was a collaborative effort of a group of pathologists and surgeons based on a study of 250 thymomas [33]. The authors essentially separated patients into those with limited disease (limited to the mediastinal compartment without invasion into any adjacent structure) and patients with tumors with invasion. The goals of this staging system are not only to stratify patients who need only surgical resection as opposed to those who may need additional medical treatment but also to clearly determine which structures are involved so that the staging is more reproducible by anyone involved in the treatment of these patients. The study included only surgical resections in 120 men and 130 women between the ages of 13 and 92 years. The sizes of these tumors vary from 2 to 20 cm in diameter: 80% of the tumors were larger than 5 cm with an average size of 7 cm; however, tumor size did not correlate with invasiveness of the tumor. The staging system is as follows:

- Stage 0 – Encapsulated tumor. No evidence of tumor invasion into adjacent structures (Fig. 6.1a, b)
- Stage I – Invasive tumor that has breached the capsule of the tumor. The tumor is into the perithymic fat (Fig. 6.2a–c), but it is not compromising adjacent structures (pleura, pericardium, etc.).
- Stage II – Direct invasion
  - IIA
    - Innominate vein
    - Mediastinal pleura
    - Lung (Fig. 6.3a, b)
  - IIB
    - Pericardium (Fig. 6.4a, b)
  - IIC
    - Great vessels (aorta, superior vena cava) (Fig. 6.5a, b)
    - Heart
- Stage III – Metastatic disease
  - IIIA – Intrathoracic structures
    - Diaphragm (so-called drop metastases) (Fig. 6.6a, b)
    - Lymph nodes
  - IIIB – Extrathoracic (Fig. 6.6c, d)

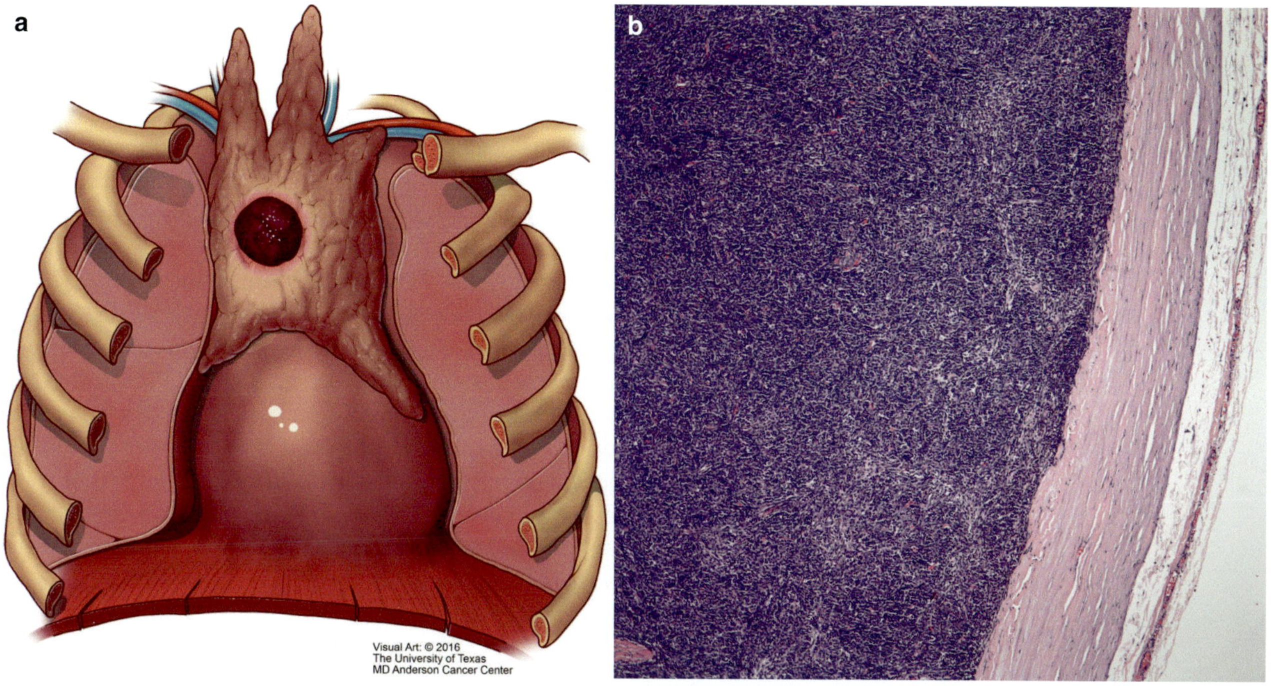

Fig. 6.1 (**a**, **b**) Stage 0. (**a**) Graphical illustration of an encapsulated thymoma. (**b**) Histological section of an encapsulated thymoma. (**a**: Copyright © 2016 with permission from Dr. Kalhor and Moran)

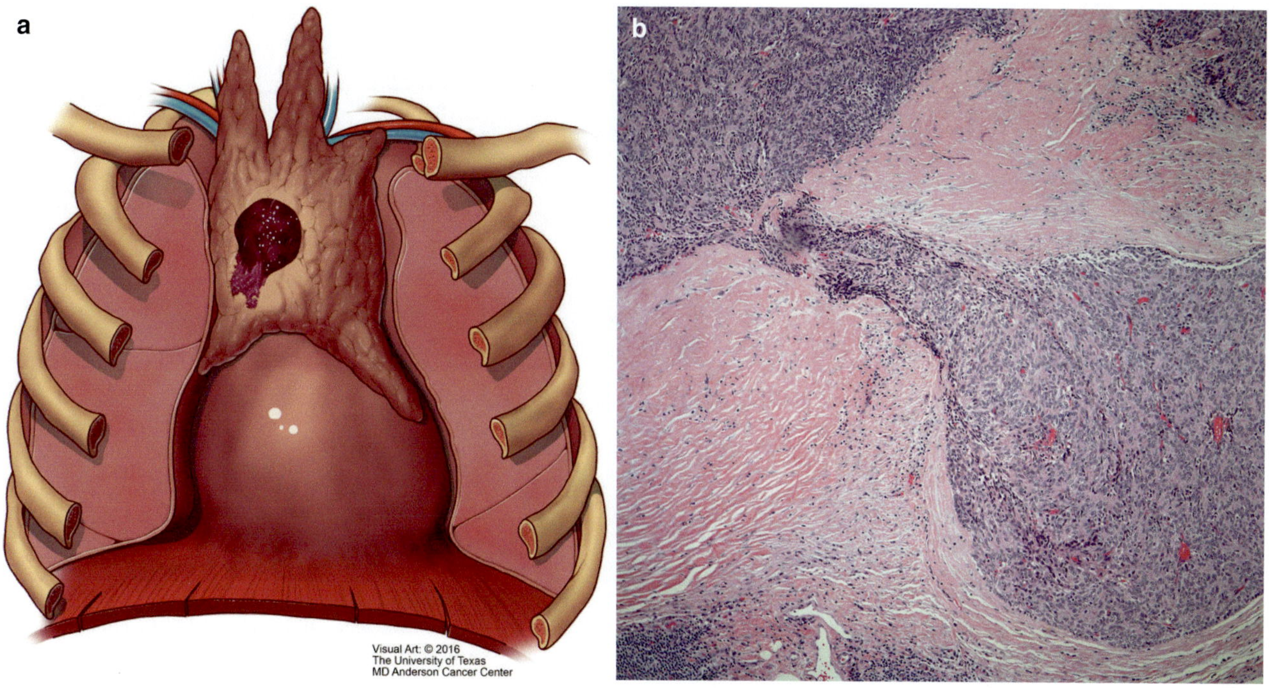

Fig. 6.2 (**a**–**c**) Stage I. (**a**) Graphical illustration of a minimally invasive thymoma. (**b**) Thymoma has breached the capsule. (**a**: Copyright © 2016 with permission from Dr. Kalhor and Moran)

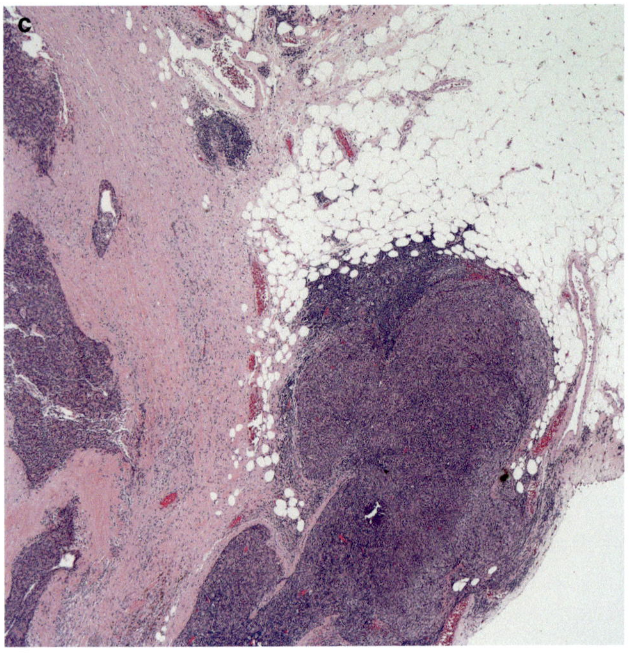

Fig. 6.2 (continued) (**c**) Thymoma is invading the perithymic adipose tissue

In this study, of 250 cases, the authors observed statistically significant overall survival curves with a p-value of 0.044, while the recurrence-free survival p-value was 0.015. The important message of this staging system is to lower down the number of patients who by the fact that they have invasive disease will be inevitably treated as such with possible radiation therapy. The staging system's goal is to make the determination that, in some cases, even though the tumor is invasive (limited disease), the patients may be treated with surgical resection alone. In addition, this staging system places the pathologist in more direct control of proper staging by documenting the structures involved. Needless to say, the schema provides histological definitions of what is to be diagnosed as pleural or pericardial invasion. More recently, in a multi-institutional effort to clarify not only histological classification but also staging for thymomas, Weissferdt and associates [34] reported 1470 thymoma cases in which the authors found statistically significant correlation using this particular schema.

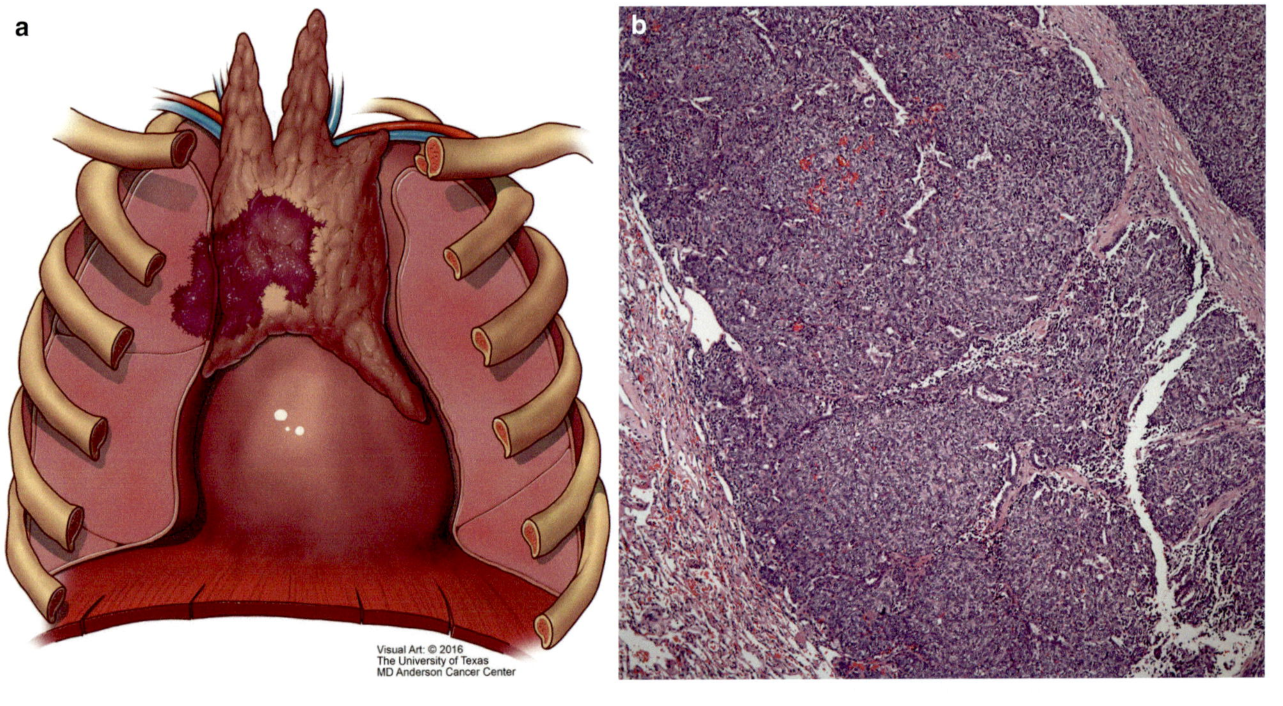

Fig. 6.3 (**a**, **b**) Stage IIA. (**a**) Graphical illustration of a thymoma with direct invasion of the pleura and lung. (**b**) Histological section of an invasive thymoma going through the visceral pleura into the lung parenchyma (**a**: Copyright © 2016 with permission from Dr. Kalhor and Moran)

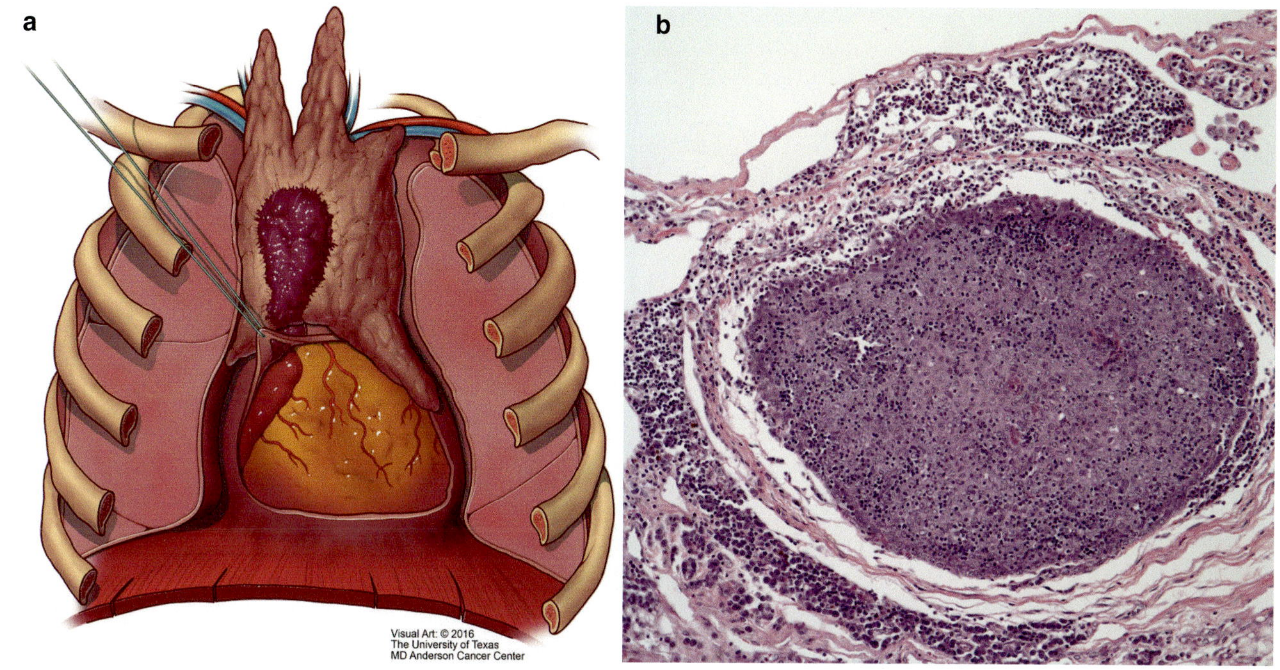

Fig. 6.4 (**a**, **b**) Stage IIB. (**a**) Graphical illustration of a pericardial invasion of a thymoma. (**b**) Histological section of a thymoma invading the pericardium (**a**: Copyright © 2016 with permission from Dr. Kalhor and Moran)

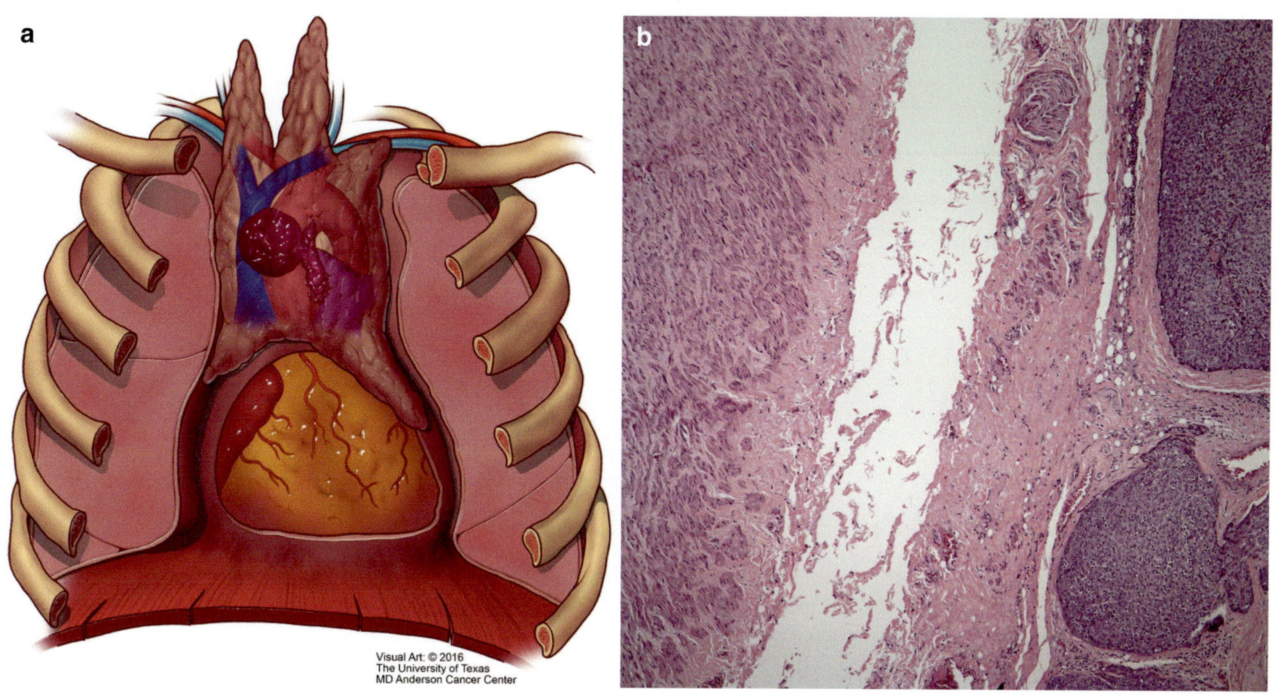

Fig. 6.5 (**a**, **b**) Stage IIC. (**a**) Graphical illustration of a thymoma invading the great vessels. (**b**) Histological section of a thymoma adjacent to the wall of a great vessel. (**a**: Copyright © 2016 with permission from Dr. Kalhor and Moran)

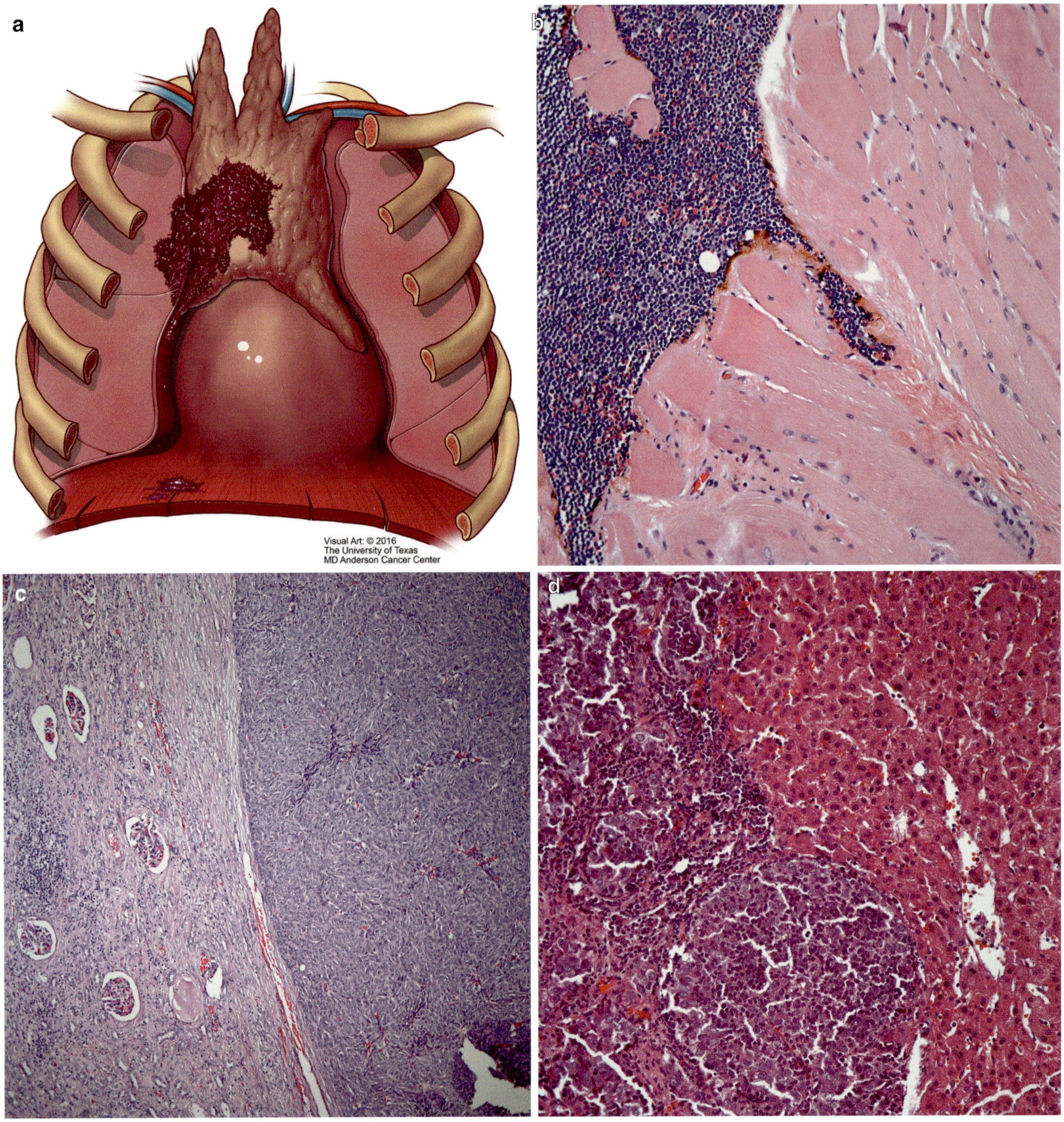

Fig. 6.6 (**a**–**d**) Stages IIIA (**a** and **b**) and IIIB (**c** and **d**). (**a**) Graphical illustration of a thymoma showing diaphragmatic invasion, so-called drop metastasis. (**b**) Histological section of a thymoma infiltrating the skeletal muscle of the diaphragm. (**c**) Metastatic spindle cell thymoma to the kidney. (**d**) Metastatic thymoma to the liver (**a**: Copyright © 2016 with permission from Dr. Kalhor and Moran)

Staging of Thymic Carcinoma

Contrary to the several publications on the staging of thymomas, a specific staging system for thymic carcinoma has been essentially nonexistent. Part of this problem is that the approach taken for thymic epithelial neoplasms (thymoma and thymic carcinoma) has been that of "one size fits all," and little attention has been placed to addressing different problems with the diagnosis, treatment, and staging of thymic carcinoma. In addition, one important fact to recognize is that thymic carcinoma is not a common neoplasm, and it is an entity that requires unequivocal pathological-radiological correlation. Regarding thymic carcinoma, it has been stated that it corresponds to a poorly defined group of lesions that have as a common denominator a primary location in the anterior mediastinum without evidence of a similar tumor elsewhere [35]. Therefore, even though the histology may not represent a problem in diagnosis, it is the specific anatomic location that cannot be determined by histological evaluation alone in the great majority of cases. As stated above, even in the larger series of thymic carcinomas presented [2], the issue of staging has been for the most part not properly addressed or staged-based on the staging system designed for thymomas.

Using the TNM approach for thymomas, Yamakawa and associates [23] stated that such an approach appears to be more useful for thymic carcinoma and thymic carcinoids than for thymoma. The most important issue with this study is that not only was it designed for thymomas (207 cases) but also that the number of cases of thymic carcinoma and thymic carcinoid was limited to 19 cases in total. In 1999, Blumberg and associates [36] evaluated 43 cases of thymic carcinoma and observed that the overall survival was 65% at 5 years and 35% at 10 years, while the overall recurrence was 65% at 5 years and 75% at 10 years. In addition, the authors did not observe any correlation with age, gender, tumor size, or Masaoka staging. One important feature that the authors correlated with survival was innominate vein invasion. The authors concluded, based on their analysis of the 43 cases, that Masaoka's staging system does not appear to predict outcome for patients with thymic carcinoma. Tseng and associates [37] presented a similar experience in a study of 38 cases of thymic carcinoma over a period from 1988 to 2002. The authors observed a median survival of 81 months and a median recurrence of 52 months after a follow-up ranging from 15 months to 10 years. Based on this experience, the authors concluded that the prognosis of thymic carcinoma appears to be mainly dependent on tumor invasion of the great vessels and also added that Masaoka's staging could not predict prognosis. Interestingly, the authors also stated that nodal metastasis (perithymic or paratracheal) was relatively rare and that nodal status did not influence prognosis.

Tsuchiya and associates [38] presented a more formal TNM staging for thymic carcinoma, recognizing the need to separate thymoma from thymic carcinoma, which essentially modified or readapted the previously presented TNM staging proposal of Yamakawa [23] (see the previous description of this system). Basically, the proposal of Tsuchiya and associates [38] defines groups as follows:

- Stage I – T1 or T2 N0 M0
- Stage II – T1 or T2 N1 M0
- Stage III – T3 N0 or N1 M0
- Stage IV – (a) T4 N0 or N1 M0, (b) any T N2 M0, or (c) any T, any N M1

Although this proposal addresses important issues such as the presence of lymph node metastasis, there are several shortcomings with this study: (1) the number of cases presented (19 cases) is hardly a large enough study, even with uncommon tumors, to propose a rather cumbersome staging system when it comes to lymph node sampling, (2) there is no statistically significant difference presented by the authors to support their proposal, (3) the T descriptions are at best ambiguous and not clearly stated, and (4) the requirement of extensive lymph node sampling is not only clinically unsupported but also statistically not proven to be significant.

Lee and associates [39], in a report of 60 patients (42 men and 18 women over a period of 20 years from 1986 to 2005) with thymic carcinoma, staged all the patients following Masaoka's schema of thymoma. Based on that schema, they identified that the 5-year survival rate after complete resection was 85% and that those patients did significantly better than those with incomplete surgical resection or nonsurgical treatment. This finding led the authors to conclude that the most important factor for disease control and long-term survival of patients with thymic carcinoma is complete surgical resection of early Masaoka stage. A few issues are worth mentioning regarding this particular study: (1) the authors decided to include in this study what appears to be bona fide thymic carcinoma and also cases of neuroendocrine carcinoma (possibly carcinoid and atypical carcinoid); (2) despite the fact that the authors mention that anterior mediastinal lymph nodes were obtained, there is no mention whether those were positive or negative; in either case, such findings should have been correlated with the outcome; and (3) the authors provide their own definition of "complete resection" as follows:

- R0 resection – macroscopically and microscopically total resection of the tumor
- R1 resection – microscopically incomplete resection (pleural seeding, completely resected is considered R1)
- R2 resection – macroscopically incomplete resection

This type of redefinition of complete surgical resections raised a different issue regarding the Masaoka staging system. For instance, pleural seeding, which likely represents what Masaoka defined as pleural "dissemination," is a late stage in Masaoka's schema, which, if viewed in a different way, can lead to a different interpretation of this R0, R1, and R2 resection: R0 for encapsulated tumors or minimally invasive neoplasms and R1/R2 for everything else. However, as it has been the experience of others, the lymph node issue is not defined and clearly not addressed in this schema. Essentially, the findings of Lee and associates [38] are in agreement with the majority of views regarding thymic epithelial neoplasms (thymoma/thymic carcinoma) and that complete surgical resection of the tumor is the most important predictor of prognosis. Also in support of the Masaoka staging system, Hosaka and associates [40] presented a series of 21 patients (15 men and 6 women) with thymic carcinoma. The spin of this study is to highlight that histologic grade and Masaoka stage predict prognosis in patients with thymic carcinoma. The authors presented 14 cases of squamous cell carcinoma, 2 of adenocarcinoma, 2 of atypical carcinoid, and 2 of undifferentiated carcinoma. Fourteen patients had complete surgical resection, and the 5-year survival rate in those patients was 66.8%. Based on those findings, the authors concluded that patients with early Masaoka stage and low or intermediate histologic grade had favorable prognoses. Important to highlight in this study are the following: (1) the authors state that "systematic lymph node dissection was not routine," thus leaving the unknown factor of possible nodal invasion, despite the fact that the authors documented a case of "recurrence" in a mediastinal lymph node; (2) even though the authors raised the valid issue of histological grade, it is also known that the occurrence of thymic adenocarcinoma is very uncommon; (3) just like other series of cases, this study also includes neuroendocrine neoplasms; and (4) the number of cases of higher-grade histology are too few to properly assess the impact of histology and outcome in a more comprehensive statistical manner. It is possible that the suggestion in this manuscript is that higher-grade tumors have increased tendencies to be in late stages; however, if that is the hypothesis, then the total number of cases – whether low-, intermediate-, or high-grade histology – is definitely not adequate to make such an assessment. It is very possible that only cases of intermediate histology are represented by the cases of neuroendocrine neoplasms, which have been shown to have a different survival rate (see the Chap. 9), rather than by the conventional cases of thymic carcinoma, which traditionally have been divided into low- and high-grade neoplasms.

Park and associates [41], raising the issue of the importance of lymph node dissection in cases of thymic carcinoma, presented a series of 37 patients who had complete surgical resection of thymic carcinoma. The patients were divided into four groups: (1) no lymph node dissection Nx = 8 cases, (2) limited dissection N0 = 13 cases, (3) extensive dissection N0b = 10 cases, and (4) node metastasis N1 = 6 cases. In those six patients with lymph node metastasis, the lymph nodes were either anterior mediastinal or intrathoracic. Based on this experience, the authors concluded that extensive lymph node dissection of more than ten lymph nodes is required to predict prognosis accurately and added that anterior mediastinal and paratracheal lymph nodes should be dissected in thymic carcinoma. Interestingly, despite the fact that the authors acknowledge the role of lymph nodes as predictor of survival in patients with thymic carcinoma, the actual staging of the patients presented in this study was the Masaoka staging system of thymomas with the caveat of lymph node sampling, once more raising concerns whether the best staging system is the one presented for thymoma or a TNM approach. In that regard, Viti and associates [42] reviewed the extensive literature on the topic of lymph node metastasis and lymphadenectomy in thymic carcinoma and carcinoids and concluded that the surgical approach for thymic carcinoma should include a form of lymphadenectomy to allow nodal staging.

Based on the existing literature, in 2012 we presented a series of 65 thymic carcinomas [43], of which in 33 cases, lymph node sampling was available [44]. The proposed staging system for thymic carcinoma, contrary to the one for thymoma, clearly states the need for the use of a TNM system and suggests abandoning the Masaoka schema for this particular tumor. Our schema is a three-tier system as follows:

- T1 – tumor limited to thymic gland (Fig. 6.7a–c)
- T2 – tumor invading the visceral pleura, lung, pericardium, great vessels, chest wall, or diaphragm (Fig. 6.8a–c)
- T3 – direct extrathoracic tumor extension, beyond the thoracic inlet (consisting of the manubrium, the first thoracic vertebra, and the first ribs and their cartilages) or diaphragm
- N0 – no lymph node metastasis
- N1 – lymph node to intrathoracic lymph nodes
- M0 – no distant metastasis
- M1 – distant metastasis (indirect tumor spread, including metastasis to extrathoracic lymph nodes) (Fig. 6.9a, b)

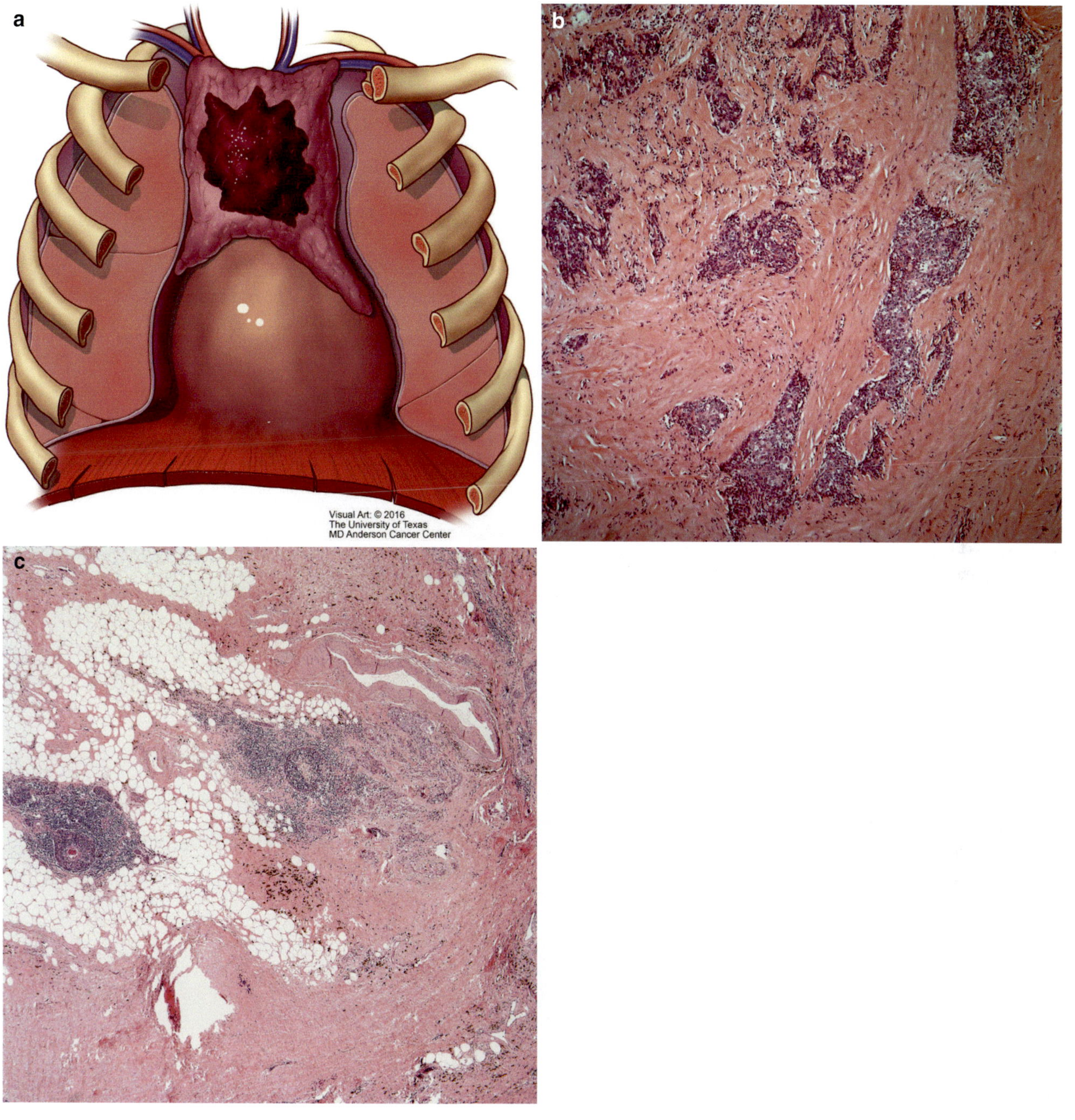

Fig. 6.7 (**a**–**c**) T1 thymic carcinoma. (**a**) Graphical illustration of the tumor is limited to the thymus gland in the anterior mediastinum. (**b**) Histological illustration of a thymic carcinoma; note the loss of organotypical features. (**c**) Tumor is limited to the thymic gland; note small remnants of the thymic tissue (**a**: Copyright © 2016 with permission from Dr. Kalhor and Moran)

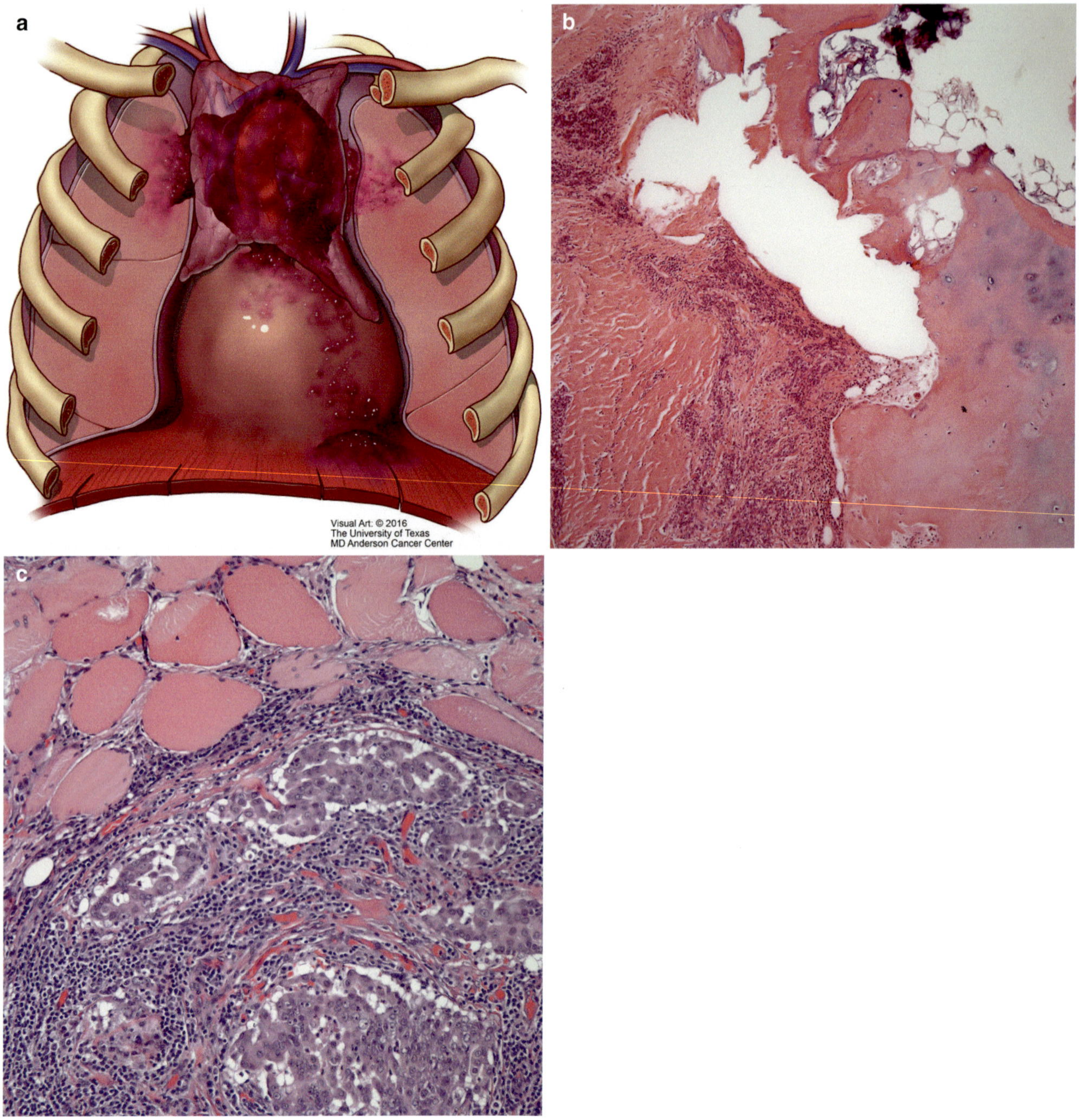

Fig. 6.8 (**a**–**c**) T2 thymic carcinoma. (**a**) Graphical illustration of the different routes that thymic carcinoma may invade. (**b**) Thymic carcinoma invading the cartilage of a rib. (**c**) Thymic carcinoma infiltrating the diaphragm (**a**: Copyright © 2016 with permission from Dr. Kalhor and Moran)

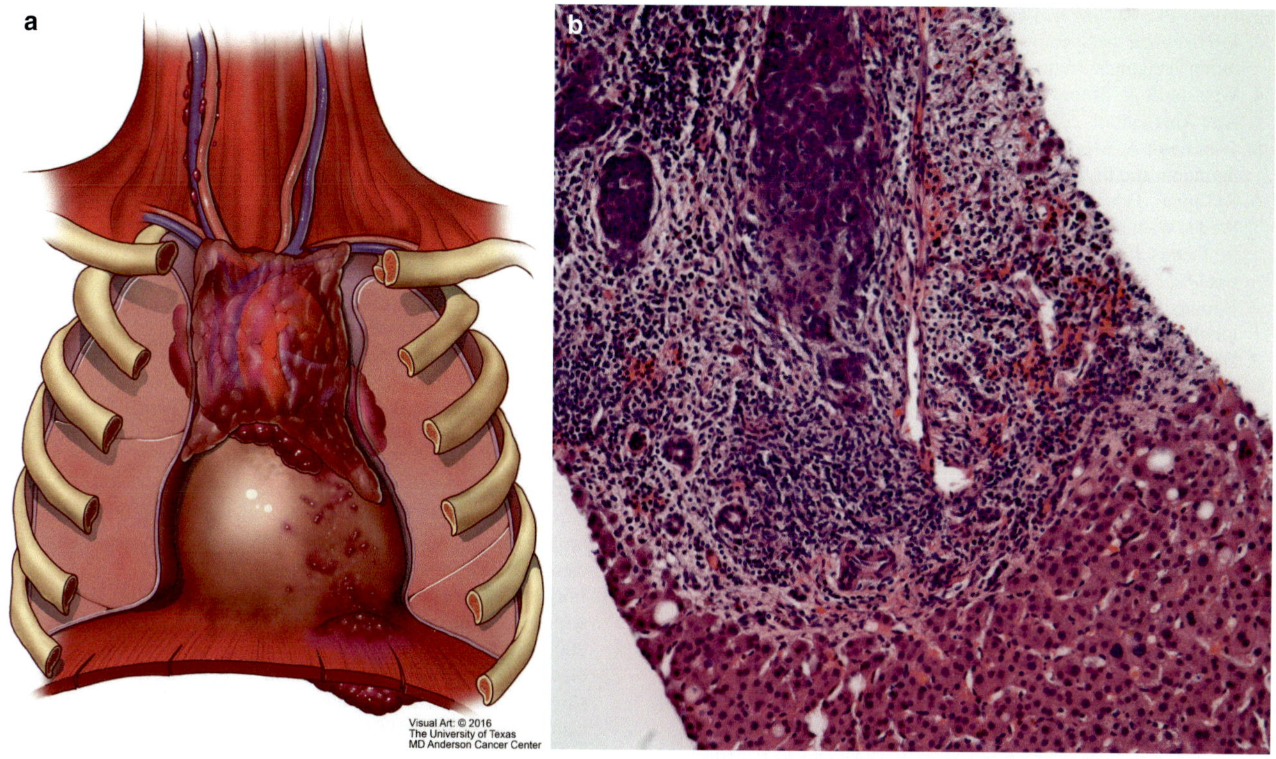

Fig. 6.9 (**a**, **b**) M1 thymic carcinoma. (**a**) Graphical illustration of M disease in thymic carcinoma either beyond the thoracic inlet or below the diaphragm. (**b**) Liver biopsy with metastatic thymic carcinoma (**a**: Copyright © 2016 with permission from Dr. Kalhor and Moran)

Based on this TNM system, the staging groups are as follows:

- Stage I – T1N0M0
- Stage II – T2N0M0
- Stage III – T3N0M0
  - Any T, N1, M0
  - Any T, any N, M1

Based on this study, we encountered 7 patients in stage I, 11 patients in stage II, and 15 patients in stage III. In addition, it was documented that 27 of the 33 patients had received additional therapy besides the surgical resection, while two patients were documented to have received no additional therapy besides the surgical resection. The clinical follow-up information ranged from 1 to 128 months, identifying 19 patients alive over a period of 3 to 126 months after diagnosis, while 14 patients had died of the tumor. Of the 19 patients who were found to be alived, 6 were in stage I, 7 were in stage II, and 6 were in stage III. On the other hand, of the 14 patients who had died, 1 was in stage I, 4 were in stage II, and 9 were in stage III. This information was correlated using the Masaoka and Tsuchiya proposal, and we encountered no statistically significant correlation by those two proposals when used as proposed. Correlations can be observed by combining different proposed staging categories, which essentially make those proposals unworkable. On the contrary, when analyzed using our proposed staging system, we obtained clear and significant correlation. One important difference in our opinion is the lymph node involvement by tumor, which in our opinion should be regarded as stage III regardless of the location of the lymph node.

Summary

It is highly advisable that the staging of thymoma and the staging for thymic carcinoma be separated as the two tumors represent two different clinicopathological entities. In one tumor, thymoma, the tumor should be staged according to the extent of tumor invasion, while in thymic carcinoma, a TNM approach should be followed to properly predict prognosis in these patients. Based on our experience, the two systems proposed by us [33, 44] are the ones that we suggest for staging thymoma and thymic carcinoma.

References

1. Bernatz PE, Harrison EG, Claggett OT. Thymoma: a clinicopathologic study. J Thorac Cardiovasc Surg. 1961;42:424–4444.
2. Suster S, Rosai J. Thymic carcinoma: a clinicopathologic study of 60 cases. Cancer. 1991;67:1025–32.

3. Filoso PL, Ruffini E, Lausi PO, Lucchi M, Oliaro A, Detterbeck F. Historical perspectives: the evolution of the thymic epithelial tumors staging system. Lung Cancer. 2014;83:126–32.
4. Weissferdt A, Moran CA. Staging of primary mediastinal tumors. Adv Anat Pathol. 2013;20:1–9.
5. Weissferdt A, Moran CA. Staging of thymic epithelial neoplasms: thymoma and thymic carcinoma. Pathol Res Pract. 2015;211:2–11.
6. Ruffini E, Detterbeck F, van Raemdonck D, Rocco G, Thomas P, Weder W, et al. Tumours of the thymus: a cohort study of prognostic factors from the European Society of Thoracic Surgeons database. Eur J Cardiothoracic Surg. 2014;46(3):361–8.
7. Bernatz PE, Khonsari S, Harrison EG, Taylor WF. Thymoma: factors influencing prognosis. Surg Clin N Am. 1973;53:885–92.
8. Bergh NP, Gatzinsky P, Larsson S, Lundin P, Ridell B. Tumors of the thymus and thymic region: I. Clinicopathological studies on thymomas. Ann Thorac Surg. 1978;25:91–8.
9. Wilkins EW, Castleman B. Thymoma: a continuing survey at the Massachusetts General Hospital. Ann Thorac Surg. 1979;28:252–6.
10. Wilkins EW, Grillo HC, Scannell JG, Moncure AC, Mathisen DJ. Role of staging in prognosis and management of thymoma. Ann Thorac Surg. 1991;51:888–92.
11. Masaoka A, Monden Y, Nakahara K, Tanioka T. Follow-up study of thymomas with special reference to their clinical stages. Cancer. 1981;48:2485–92.
12. Koga K, Matsuno Y, Noguchi M, Mukai K, Asamura H, Goya T, et al. A review of 79 thymomas: modifications of staging system and reappraisal of conventional division into invasive and non-invasive thymoma. Pathol Int. 1994;44:359–67.
13. Pescarmona E, Rendina EA, Venuta F, D'Arcangelo E, Pagani M, Ricci C, et al. Analysis of prognostic factors and clinicopathological staging of thymoma. Ann Thorac Surg. 1990;50:534–8.
14. Weissferdt A, Carlos Hernandez J, Kalhor N, Moran C. Spindle Cell Thymomas: an Immunohistochemical Study of 30 Cases. Appl Immunohistochem Mol Morphol: AIMM. 2011;19:329–35.
15. Moran CA, Kalhor N, Suster S. Invasive spindle cell Thymomas (WHO type a): a Clinicopathologic correlation of 41 cases. Am J Clin Pathol. 2010;134(5):793–8.
16. Blumberg D, Port JL, Weksler B, Delgado R, Rosai J, Bains MS, et al. Thymoma: a multivariate analysis of factors predicting survival. Ann Thorac Surg. 1995;60:908–14.
17. Regnard JF, Magdeleinat P, Dromer C, Dulmet E, de Montpreville V, Levi JF, et al. Prognostic factors and long-term results after thymoma resection: a series of 307 patients. J Thorac Cardiovasc Surg. 1996;112:376–84.
18. Safieddine N, Liu G, Cuningham K, Ming T, Hwang D, Brade A, et al. Prognostic factors for cure, recurrence and long-term survival after surgical resection of thymoma. J Thorac Oncol. 2014;9:1018–22.
19. Demirci S, Turhan K, Ozsan N, Yalman D, Cakan A, Cok G, et al. Prognostic factors for survival in patients with thymic epithelial tumors. Thorac Cardiov Surg. 2011;59:153–7.
20. Cardillo G, Carleo F, Giunti R, Lopergolo MG, Salvadori L, De Massimi AR, et al. Predictors of survival in patients with locally advanced thymoma and thymic carcinoma (Masaoka stages III and IVa). Eur J Cardiothorac Surg. 2010;37:819–23.
21. Detterbeck FC, Nicholson AG, Kondo K, Van Schil P, Moran C, et al. The Masaoka-Koga stage classification for thymic malignancies. Clarification and definition of terms. J Throac Oncol. 2011;6:S1710–6.
22. Masaoka A. Staging system of thymoma. J Thorac Oncol. 2010;5:S304–12.
23. Yamakawa Y, Masaoka A, Hashimoto T, Niwa H, Mizuno T, Fujii Y, et al. A tentative tumor – node – metastasis classification of thymoma. Cancer. 1991;68:1984–7.
24. Kondo K. Tumor-Node metastasis staging system for thymic epithelial tumors. J Thorac Oncol. 2010;5:S352–6.
25. Bedini AV, Andreani SM, Tavecchio L, Fabbri A, Giardini R, Camerini T, et al. Proposal of a novel system for the staging of thymic epithelial tumors. Ann Thorac Surg. 2005;80:1994–2001.
26. Asamura H, Nakagawa K, Matsuno Y, Suzuki K, Watanabe SI, Tsuchiya R, et al. Thymoma needs a new staging system. Interact Cardiovasc Thorac Surg. 2004;3:163–7.
27. Kondo K, van Schil P, Detterbeck FC, Okumura M, Stratton K, Giroux D, et al. The IALSC/ITMIG thymic epithelial tumors staging project: proposals for the N and M components for the forthcoming (8th) edition of the TNM classification of malignant tumors. JTO. 2014;9:S81–7.
28. Bhora FY, Chen DJ, Detterbeck FC, Asamura H, Falkson C, Filosso PL, et al. The ITMIG/IASLC thymic epithelial tumors staging project: a proposed lymph node map for thymic epithelial tumors in the forthcoming 8th edition of the TNM classification of malignant tumors. JTO. 2014;9:S88–96.
29. Nicholson AG, Detterbeck FC, Marino M, Kim J, Stratton K, Giroux D, et al. The IASLC/ITMIG thymic epithelial tumors staging project: proposals for the T component for the forthcoming (8th) edition of the TNM classification of malignant tumors. JTO. 2014;9:S73–80.
30. Detterbeck FC, Asdamura H, Crowley J, Falkson C, Giaccone G, Giroux D, et al. The IASLC/ITMIG thymic malignancies staging project: development of a stage classification for thymic malignancies. JTO. 2013;8:1467–73.
31. Wick MR. Prognostic factors for thymic epithelial neoplasms, with emphasis on tumor staging. Hematol Oncol Clin N Am. 2008;22:527–42.
32. Gamondes JP, Balawi A, Greenland T, et al. Seventeen years of surgical treatment of thymoma: factors influencing survival. Eur J Cardiopthorac Surg. 1991;5:124–31.
33. Moran CA, Walsh G, Suster S, Kaiser L. Thymoma II: a clinicopathologic correlation of 250 cases with a proposed staging system with emphasis on pathologic assessment. Am J Clin Pathol. 2012;137:451–61.
34. Weissferdt A, Kalhor N, Bishop J, Jang SJ, Ro J, Petersson F, et al. Thymoma: a clinicopathologic correlation of 1470 cases. Hum Pathol. 2018;73:7–15.
35. Moran CA, Suster S. Thymic carcinoma: current concepts and histologic features. Hematol Oncol Clin N Am. 2008;22:393–407.
36. Blumberg D, Burt ME, Bains MS, Downey RJ, Martini N, Rusch V, et al. Thymic carcinoma: current staging does not predict prognosis. J Thorac Cardiovasc Surg. 1998;115:303–8.
37. Tseng YL, Wang ST, Wu MH, Lin MY, Lai WW, Cheng FF. Thymic carcinoma: involvement of great vessels indicates poor prognosis. Ann Thorac Surg. 2003;76:1041–5.
38. Tsuchiya R, Koga K, Matsumo Y, Mukai K, Shimosato Y. Thymic carcinoma: proposal for pathological TNM and staging. Pathol Inte. 1994;44:505–12.
39. Lee CY, Bae MK, Park IK, Kim DJ, Lee JG, Chung KY. Early Masaoka stage and complete resection is important for prognosis of thymic carcinoma: a 20-year experience at a single institution. Eur J Cardiothorac Surg. 2009;36:159–63.
40. Hosaka Y, Tsuchida M, Toyabe S, Umezu H, Eimoto T, Hayashi J. Masaoka stage and histologic grade predict prognosis in patients with thymic carcinoma. Ann Thorac Surg. 2010;89:912–7.
41. Park IK, Kim YT, Jeon JH, Kim HS, Hwang Y, Seong YW, et al. Importance of lymph node dissection in thymic carcinoma. Ann Thorac Surg. 2013;96:1025–32.
42. Viti A, Bertolaccini L, Terzi A. What is the role on lymph nodal metastases and lymphadenectomy in the surgical treatment and prognosis of thymic carcinomas and carcinoids? Interact Cardiovasc Thorac Surg. 2014;19:1054–8.
43. Weissferdt A, Moran CA. Thymic carcinoma, part 1: a clinicopathologic and Immunohistochemical study of 65 cases. Am J Clin Pathol. 2012;138:103–14.
44. Weissferdt A, Moran CA. Thymic carcinoma, part 2: a clinicopathologic correlation of 33 cases with a proposed staging system. Am J Clin Pathol. 2012;138:115–21.

Thymoma

7

Introduction

Thymomas are epithelial neoplasms of the thymic epithelium. They represent the most common epithelial tumor in the mediastinum, and they often occur in the anterior aspect of the mediastinal compartment. The nomenclature, classification, staging, and numerous other details related to these tumors are often at the center of controversy and disagreement. However, in general terms, thymomas are tumors of unusual occurrence that collecting a reasonable number to generate meaningful information is difficult. If to that fact, we add the differences in opinion regarding the diagnosis of these tumors, then it should not be difficult to understand that collecting a large series of cases of these tumors is a difficult task.

Most of the controversy dates back to early publications on this tumor, which over the years have perpetuated this controversy. In 1955, the first series of fascicles by the Armed Forces Institute of Pathology (AFIP) included a specific fascicle on "Tumors of the Thymus Gland," whose author (Dr. Castleman) listed in the section on thymoma the following synonyms and related terms: benign lymphocytic lymphoma, carcinoma, epithelioma, lymphoepithelioma, lymphosarcoma, malignant thymoma, mixed tumor, myxosarcoma, perithelioma, and reticulum cell sarcoma [1]. In addition, the fascicle has a different entry on "malignancy of thymoma" and the description listed is that of a tumor that spreads outside of the mediastinal compartment. Basically, the message of this fascicle is that there are two types of thymomas: benign (encapsulated) and malignant (invasive). Interestingly, the author of the fascicle is clear in his opinion regarding the heterogeneity of thymomas. Twenty years later, in 1975, the AFIP published the second series of fascicles, and this time the authorship was given to Drs. Rosai and Levine, who, in the section on thymoma, also listed as synonyms and related terms similar entities as the previous fascicle [2]. However, the authors also stated that those terms appear to be misnomers and that their use should be discouraged. The authors also emphasized the heterogeneity of these tumors and stated that the natural history of these tumors is that of a slow-growing tumor; furthermore, they described the two most important prognostic determinants: the gross findings – specifically whether the tumor is encapsulated or invasive – and the presence of myasthenia gravis. It was not until 1995, the 3rd series of AFIP fascicles, authored by Shimosato and Mukai, that there appear to be clear entries for thymoma and thymic carcinoma, which is a departure from the previous grouping of these tumors [3]. Essentially, over the last 50 years, we have seen the concept of thymoma evolve in many different directions, and it is likely this process will continue. However, it is important to highlight that thymomas do not represent the benign counterpart of thymic carcinoma, nor is thymic carcinoma the malignant counterpart of thymoma. In our opinion, all thymomas are potentially malignant neoplasms, which, if diagnosed and operated upon in early stages, clearly follow a more protracted course. Furthermore, it appears to be a continuum process of differentiation of the thymic epithelium which could explain the differences between these two tumoral conditions.

In this chapter, we will not discuss the staging of these tumors, and the reader should consult the chapter in this text on staging, which specifically addresses the staging of thymoma and thymic carcinoma. This chapter will be devoted to:

- Epidemiological aspects
- Etiological aspects
- Clinical aspects:
  - Special associations
  - Histological classification and clinical studies

© Springer Nature Switzerland AG 2019
N. Kalhor, C. Moran, *Mediastinal Pathology*, https://doi.org/10.1007/978-3-319-98980-8_7

- Pathological aspects:
  - Anatomical orientation of the specimen
  - Sampling issues
  - Gross features
  - Histological features
  - Immunohistochemical aspects
  - Molecular aspects

Epidemiological Aspects

Epidemiological studies on thymomas are just as rare as the tumor itself. Since thymoma may be associated with a wide spectrum of clinical conditions, it is often difficult to determine its true incidence and prevalence. In 2003, Engels and Pfeiffer [4] attempted to evaluate the incidence of thymoma. The authors used population-based cancer incidence data collected by the National Cancer Institute's Surveillance, Epidemiology, and End Results (SEER) program. For the primary analysis corresponding to the years 1973–1998, data were obtained from the registries of nine cities in the USA. At this point, it is important to highlight that, as the authors noted, SEER collects data only on "malignant thymoma." Therefore, these particular data are very likely to be contaminated due to few different reasons: (1) during 1973–1998, it is likely that many cases that were diagnosed as "malignant thymoma" were in fact thymic carcinomas; (2) this study probably includes only cases deemed to be "malignant," most likely invasive thymomas; and (3) since it is often believed that encapsulated thymomas are benign, it is likely that those cases were not accounted in this study. In any case, the data were classified by gender, age, racial background, and the presence of malignancies following the diagnosis of thymoma. The data from the 9 cities provided 849 cases of "malignant thymoma," which is approximately 0.15 per 100,000 person-years. The mean age was 56 years, and only 11% of cases occurred before the age of 35 years. In addition, the authors noted that the incidence increases until the age 77 and then decreases. The overall incidence appeared to be higher in men than in women: 0.16 vs 0.13 per 100,000 person-years. Regarding racial background, thymomas in white individuals accounted for 0.12 per 100,000 person-years, black individuals 0.20 per 100,000 person-years, and "other" races 0.29 per 100,000 person-years. Also, the authors noted an overall elevated cancer risk among thymoma patients. In 2012, Siesling and colleagues [5] evaluated the incidence and prevalence of what the authors called "rare thoracic cancers" – including tumors from the trachea, thymus, and mesothelioma – under the RARECARE data from the EUROCARE, with a mean population covered of about 162 million, which is approximately 39% of the population of the 21 countries participating in the RARECARE. The study included the database from 1978 to 2002 in 89 population-based cancer registries and accounted for 17,688 cases of "rare thoracic cancer." Interestingly, for the thymus, the authors appear to have included "malignant thymoma" and thymic carcinoma. Once again, it raises the possibility that some cases of encapsulated thymomas may have been deemed to represent benign tumors and therefore were not collected in this study. The authors also stated that 2.4% of the cases were registered based on death certificate only, which accounted for 1.6% of thymic epithelial tumors; 92% of the epithelial tumors of the thymus were microscopically verified, and 6.3% were censored before 5 years. The incidence of epithelial tumors of the thymus was calculated at 1.7 per million per year, and "malignant thymomas" were the most common: 1.4 per million per year. Also, Engels [6], in a more specific approach to the epidemiology of thymoma and associated malignancies, stated that thymoma patients have elevated risk for developing B-cell non-Hodgkin lymphoma and possibly soft tissue sarcomas. In addition, the author noted the higher incidence of thymomas among Asian and Pacific Islanders in the USA. Interestingly, the breakdown provided is as follows: non-Hispanic - white 0.10; non-Hispanic - black 0.18; Hispanic 0.08; and Asian/Pacific Islander, 0.25, all per 100,000 person-years.

Based on what is available regarding the incidence and prevalence of thymoma, it is clear that it is difficult to estimate with certainty the true incidence and prevalence, as the cases that are included in databases are "biased" towards including only cases that are believed to be "malignant," likely leaving the majority of thymomas out of the statistics, since the majority of thymomas are probably encapsulated. Therefore, the quoted incidence of thymomas is likely to represent the incidence of "invasive thymomas" and not the incidence of thymomas in general.

Etiological Aspects

Even though it is well recognized that thymomas originate from the thymic epithelium, it remains an enigma as to whether the thymic epithelium corresponds to one type of cell, or multiple types of cells, or even other structures that can give rise to thymomas. To that extent, many controversial issues over the years have been generated regarding the normal thymus. For instance, the origin of Hassall's corpuscles has been the subject of different interpretations; these include aggregates of medullary epithelial cells, complex tubular structures, derivatives from entodermal pharyngeal pouch, and/or originating from the ectoderm of the third pharyngeal branchial clefts. In 1981, Shier [7] conducted a comparative study including fetal thymus, thymuses from young adults, thymic cysts, and thymomas. The author concluded that his findings were in keeping with those of Schambacher, who considered that the thymus is composed of two different types of epithelium: reticular epithelium and medullary duct epithelium. In addition, the author stated that his findings indicated a slightly different embryologic origin of the medullary duct epithelium, namely, from the uppermost part of the pharyngeal pouch. Interestingly, the author noted that, in order to determine the relative frequency of the presence of differentiated structures in thymoma, one should study multiple sections from different areas, which is something highly important that over the years we have emphasized, and that is critical in tissue sampling in the diagnosis of thymoma. More important is the light microscopic description provided for the "reticular epithelial cells," which can be regular, polygonal, and spindly, while the medullary duct epithelium is recognized by its formation of ducts, cysts, or tubules of different shapes and sizes. The author concluded that "thymomas are complex epitheliomas with diversified reticular-epithelial and medullary duct differentiation." In more recent years, the use of immunohistochemical techniques and molecular biology has allowed some investigators to further analyze thymuses and thymomas with a different perspective. Zhou and colleagues [8] investigated genetic abnormalities in thymic epithelial tumors, which, according to the authors, belong to different types of thymoma. The authors concluded that karyotypic instability plays a role in the development of some thymomas (spindle cell type and mixed cellularity [WHO type A and B2]) and thymic carcinoma. Manley and Blackburn [9] have provided a different perspective regarding the organogenesis of the thymus and have suggested the possibility of a single endodermal origin to account for the non-hematopoietic cells of the thymus. The authors argue that the origins and relationships of the constituent cell types of any mature organ can only be identified via lineage analysis (the use of experimental methods to trace the embryonic origins of the cells that contribute to organ formation), and that histological analysis of cells and tissue morphology or gene expression/marker studies alone are not sufficient to determine lineage, as these methods rely on properties of cells that can change during embryonic development. Interestingly, the authors also stated that it is not clear yet what induces the initial formation of the primordium from the third pharyngeal pouch. In addition, several of the pathways that have been implicated in the thymus development and/or thymocyte differentiation have not been linked to the initiation of organogenesis. Also, the authors argue that, even though neural crest cells play an important role in early thymus organogenesis, the function of thymic mesenchyme remains controversial. Furthermore, it is argued that hematopoietic cells are not required for thymus organogenesis or thymic epithelial cell differentiation. Hale [10], in a review on the histologic and molecular assessment of human thymus, also stated that understanding age-related changes is important in the evaluation of patients with diseases affecting the thymus. The authors stated that while thymic volume and weight remain relatively constant, the portion of the thymus containing thymic epithelium and participating in production of new T-cells decreases progressively with age. However, thymopoiesis continues in normal human adults into at least the eighth decade of life. Unfortunately, the biology of these tumors (thymomas) often becomes entangled with histology and staging. An example of this is covered in a review presented by Cheney [11] on the biologic spectrum of thymic epithelial neoplasm, in which the author described the behavioral spectrum as ranging from "entirely benign" to highly aggressive, and added that such a spectrum is explained by thymic organogenesis. Although the concept of organogenesis has been floating around for decades and seems to be reasonable, Manley and Blackburn [9] have pointed out that there are still several issues that need to be sorted out regarding thymic organogenesis. Indeed, many thymomas recapitulate the morphological features of normal thymus; however, as pointed out by Suster [12], this results in an organ whose "normal" histological appearance can vary widely depending on the age of the patient. It becomes evident that, even though by light microscopy one can observe similarities between thymus and thymomas, beyond that realm one can only speculate on possible mechanisms of organogenesis that may be implicated in the development of these tumors. Nevertheless, over the years, we have conceptualized and addressed the issue of thymic epithelial neoplasms as being part of a continuous spectrum of differentiation that ranges from well to moderately to poorly differentiated neoplasms: thymoma – atypical thymoma – thymic carcinoma [13]. Such a hypothesis can be best illustrated by tumors that either show higher-grade histology after recurrences or tumors within the same tumor that show areas of thymoma and thymic carcinoma [14, 15]. Such progression is depicted in Fig. 7.1 in which we have attempted to provide an approximate degree of differentiation that could take place in thymomas using as a platform normal or involuted thymus.

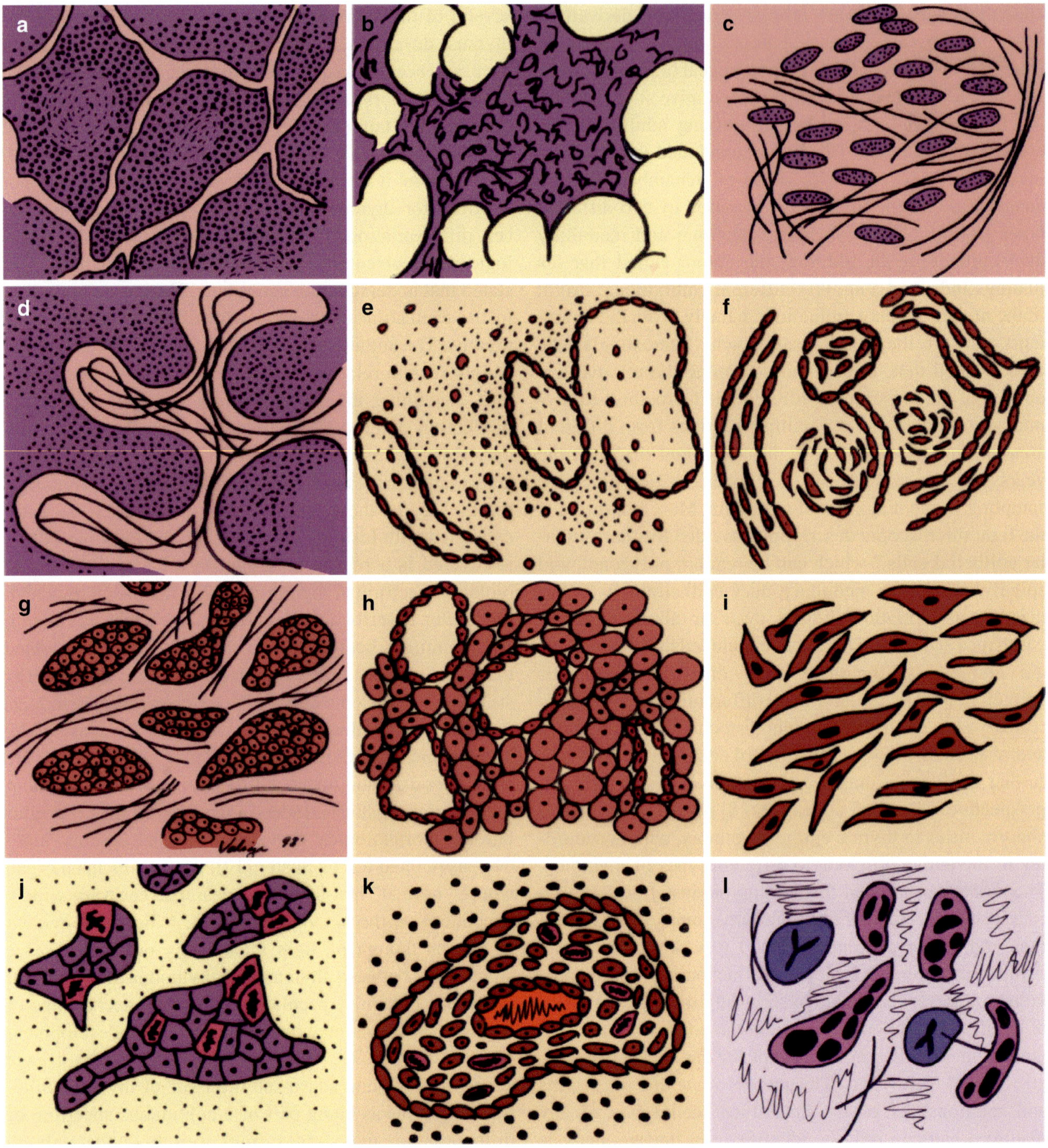

Fig. 7.1 From left to right and top to bottom. (Copyright © Drs.Kalhor and Moran)

Thymus in a child (A)	Thymus in the adult (B)	Involutional changes (C)
L-R thymoma (D)	Mixed cell thymoma (E)	Spindle cell thymoma (F)
Atypical thymoma – preservation of organotypical features (G)	Atypical thymoma – perivascular spaces (H)	Atypical spindle cell (I)
Thymic carcinoma – loss of organotypical features (J)	Thymic carcinoma – inflammatory reaction (K)	Thymic carcinoma – cellular atypia and mitotic activity in epithelial cells (L)

Clinical Features

Common Clinical Associations

The association of thymoma with many medical conditions, whether autoimmune or others, is well known and extensive [16–27]. Table 7.1 depicts some common medical conditions that over the years have been associated with thymoma. However, myasthenia gravis is the medical condition that appears to have the closest association with thymoma. Traditionally, it has been stated that about 10–15% of patients with myasthenia gravis (MG) have an associated thymoma. It has also been stated that 40% of patients with thymoma have one or more paraneoplastic autoimmune conditions, 20–25% of that being MG. In general terms, MG is an autoimmune disease producing autoantibodies against the nicotinic acetylcholine receptor. MG appears to affect women more than men. The etiology of MG is still unknown, but it could be iatrogenic due to D-penicillamine and alpha-interferon and also due to bone marrow transplantation. In addition, to the many medical conditions, thymomas have also been associated with other neoplasms of either epithelial or lymphoid origin. In a recent retrospective clinicopathological analysis [28] of 187 thymic malignancies including thymomas, thymic carcinomas, and neuroendocrine carcinomas, the authors encountered immunological abnormalities in 21.8% of the thymoma group. Secondary malignancies were present in 13.3% of these patients. We recently reported a series of more than 14 hundred cases in which pertinent clinical information was obtained in 807 patients showing that MG was the most common association with 17%, while several other autoimmune conditions accounted for 3.8%. Interestingly, other neoplastic processes were seen in about 6.8% of the patients [29]. Based on the available literature, it is safe to state that the percentage of thymoma patients associated with MG is somewhere between 15% and 20%. Nevertheless, there is a meaningful group of patients, approximately 10%, who may have another associated condition, whether autoimmune, neoplastic, or other. Therefore, it would be prudent that newly diagnosed patients with thymoma also be screened for other medical and neoplastic conditions.

Table 7.1 Clinical and neoplastic diseases associated with thymoma[a]

Autoimmune, non-autoimmune diseases, and syndromes
Myasthenia gravis
Sjogren syndrome
Pemphigus vulgaris
Guillain-Barre syndrome
Polymyalgia rheumatic
Lupus erythematosus
Polymyositis
Hashimoto thyroiditis
Rheumatoid arthritis
Limbic encephalitis
Neuromyotonia
Stiff person syndrome
Myotonic dystrophy
Mixed connective tissue diseases
Myocarditis
Graft-versus-host disease
Hypogammaglobulinemia
Pure red cell aplasia
Intestinal pseudo-obstruction
Paroxysmal nocturnal hematuria
Acrokeratosis
Lichen planus
Conjunctivitis
Cancer-associated retinopathy
Glomerulonephritis
Thalassemia
Neoplastic diseases of different organ systems
Thyroid carcinoma
Cholangiocarcinoma
Breast carcinoma
Lung carcinoma
Gastrointestinal carcinoma (gastric, esophagus, colon)
Hepatic carcinoma
Genitourinary carcinoma (kidney, prostate, bladder)
Endometrial carcinoma
CNS malignancies
Malignant lymphoproliferative disorders (lymphoma, myeloma)

[a]Although we have attempted to include all possible conditions that have been associated with thymomas, it is possible that some of them may have been missed

On the other hand, it is also possible that somewhere around 50% of the thymoma patients may not present with any specific symptoms such as those associated with the medical conditions previously described, and the symptoms may be non-specific and related to the size of the tumor, which may be compressing adjacent structures, and elicit symptoms of chest pain, dyspnea, cough, general malaise, etc. It is also important to highlight that often patients may be completely asymptomatic and the mediastinal tumor is discovered during routine chest films.

Histological Classifications and Clinical Studies

Since the beginning of the nineteenth century, thymic tumors started to be seen as a complex group of tumors that because of the location became the center of misconceptions. In a report of five cases of thymoma, Reid and Marcus [30] in 1948 quoted a dissertation by Grandhomme at the University of Heidelberg, who in 1900 applied the term "thymoma" to all malignant tumors of the thymus. In addition, the authors quoted Ewing's opinion that tumors of the thymus have resisted attempts at interpretation and classification. Due to this initial misconception regarding the nature of these tumors, the term "thymoma" was invariably used for any tumor technically arising from the mediastinal compartment, thus, the diversity of early classifications. It is obvious that many cases regarded as malignant thymomas then clearly belong today in a different group of tumors. Nevertheless, these views regarding thymic tumors provide the background demonstrating the difficulty in understanding, classifying, and designating proper nomenclature for these thymic epithelial tumors over the years. The cleansing of the literature is still an ongoing process that even today represents an unfinished work. Essentially, in the first part of the nineteenth century, the reports of thymoma and "malignant thymoma" were available mainly in the form of short series of cases or individual case reports. It is more important to highlight that, prior to 1961, there were at least nine different schemas regarding the histological classification of thymomas [31–41]. Unfortunately, some of these different schemas included tumors that were not of epithelial origin (such as leukemia and lymphoma), while others included sarcomas. In some schemas, the tumors were divided by the presence of myasthenia gravis, while in others germ cell tumors were also included. Essentially, prior to 1961, it is obvious that the diagnosis of thymomas was not restricted to tumors of epithelial origin but rather to tumors that originated from the thymic area. The diagnosis was driven by location and not by histology.

In 1961, Bernatz and colleagues [42] published one of the largest series on thymoma by collecting 138 cases from a single institution; these included 96 surgical resections from which 3–4 histological sections were available for interpretation. The remaining of the cases were biopsy specimens. More important is the fact that the authors carefully excluded other conditions that over the years have also been called thymoma; these included lymphomas, seminomas, Hodgkin lymphoma, teratomas, and other metastatic malignancies. In addition, the authors did not include other thymic lesions that could also be interpreted as thymomas; those included thymolipomas, thymic cysts, and thymic hyperplasia. This publication in essence set in motion not only more strict criteria for tumors that should be called thymomas but also a classification system that even today has an excellent morphological approach. The authors proposed morphological criteria for the histological classification of thymomas was based on the relative presence of lymphocytes and epithelial cells within the tumor. Thus, the authors proposed dividing thymomas into:

- Lymphocytic (30% of their cases)
- Epithelial (16% of their cases)
- Mixed (reticulo-epithelial) (30% of their cases)
- Spindle (24% of their cases)

In addition, the authors separated these histologies and correlated them with the gross appearance of the tumor, dividing them into five different groups: (1) tumors of 5 cm or less, (2) tumors more than 5 cm, (3) cystic, (4) multiple or diffuse, and (5) invasive. The proportion of the different histologies was as follows: 30 cases were lymphocytic, 19 were epithelial, 36 were mixed, and 29 were spindle. Interestingly, cases in which the tumors were more than 5 cm were in the spindle cell category.

It is important to note that the authors did not clarify the issue of "malignant thymoma," although possibly they were leaning more toward the concept of "invasive thymomas." Of the 138 patients in this series, 64 (46%) had associated myasthenia gravis. Follow-up information in this series of cases showed that 76.9% of these patients survived 3 years, 63.2% survived 5 years, and 50% survived 10 years. The authors also noted that thymomas rarely metastasized to distant organs, and most of the time thymomas have local extension into intrathoracic organs. In addition, the authors observed that in 23 patients in which the tumor was unresectable, the survival was of nearly 2 years. In 1962, Lattes [43] also reviewed the subject of thymoma and other tumors of the thymus and reported on 107 cases. The problem with this series of cases is that it includes cases of seminoma, Hodgkin lymphoma, and possibly other lymphomas, leaving probably only 92 cases of actual thymomas. Therefore, it is difficult to properly address the issue of "thymomas," as the survival is addressed in terms of myasthenic and nonmyasthenic patients, treated and non-treated patients, and other medical conditions associated and separated by histology. In addition, the subject of "malignant thymoma" is not clearly addressed. On this latter subject, Mottet in 1964 [44] published a single case report of a 32-year-old man with a thymic tumor that the author interpreted as "malignant thymoma." Autopsy findings in this particular case show tumor spreading to the liver, lungs, vena cava, thoracic wall, and meninges. Interestingly, judging by the illustration provided in this report, it is possible that the thymic tumor represents a thymoma with mixed histological features including lymphocytes rich, mixed lymphocytic and epithelial, and predominantly epithelial. Similar cases of an aggressive nature were also described by Rachmaninoff and Fentress [45] and by Minkowitz and colleagues [46], who described a 43- and a 37-year-old woman, respectively, with what the authors interpreted as thymoma with metastasis outside of the thoracic cavity. Interestingly, judging the histological description and some of the illustrations presented, one can argue of the possibility of "thymic carcinoma" rather than thymoma or the possibility of combined tumors thymoma/thymic carcinoma. Also, Rosen and colleagues [47] described a single case of a 74-year-old man who presented with an anterior mediastinal tumor that spread into the lung parenchyma. The interpretation by the author was that of "metastatic thymoma presenting as a solitary pulmonary nodule"; however, the authors described that at thoracotomy other nodules were identified in the lung and that the initial "pulmonary nodule" was peripheral. Similar interpretation was also provided in a description of a single case report by Gravanis [48], who described a 54-year-old woman in whom the tumor involved the superior vena cava, pericardium, and lung. Both of these cases raise the possibility not of metastatic disease but rather of invasive disease. It is important to highlight that the early publications of single case reports appear to be directed by the concept that thymomas, like any other tumor, are not benign neoplasms but can invade and metastasize outside the thoracic cavity, a concept that was not accepted just then. On that subject, another important publication is the one by Fechner [49], who reported four cases of what the author called "recurrence of noninvasive thymomas." This concept is highly important in three different ways: (1) the possible recurrence of what has been considered a "benign thymoma," (2) the malignant potential of all thymomas, and (3) the statement that recurrence of thymomas usually is in the form of pleural implants. This latter view has only been addressed more recently by addressing the staging system; for the most part, it has been ignored by those who have addressed the staging of thymomas, and it is a feature that we have commonly observed in our practice. The four cases described by Fechner [49] were in two men and two women between the ages of 25 and 51 years. The initial tumors in the four patients described were noninvasive neoplasms, and recurrence took place after a period ranging from 2 to 9 years. As the author stated in this report, such occurrence is rare and may account for no more than 2% of the cases; however, it clearly defines that thymomas cannot be regarded a "benign" tumors just because they are encapsulated. On the other hand, some authors were interested in further defining the epithelial nature of these tumors by ultrastructural analysis of the cell, which, in Toker's report of two cases [50], identified not only the lymphocytic population but also the presence of cytoplasmic fibers and desmosomes, which characterizes the epithelial nature of these tumors. Similarly, Levine and Bensch [51] reported the ultrastructural findings of a spindle cell thymoma in which the authors demonstrated the epithelial nature of the tumor.

In the 1970s, a few additional advances were made in terms of refining the diagnosis of thymomas. Bernatz and colleagues [52] reported their experience with the survival of 181 patients who had surgery for thymoma. It is possible that some cases in this series may have been reported previously in 1961 by the same authors [42]. The cases were separated into four groups following the classification schema previously presented by the authors: 44% of the patients had a history of MG, and 36% of the tumors were invasive. No gender difference was identified, and the average age was 50 years. Survival analysis in this group of patients showed that after 15 years, only 12.5% of the patients with invasive tumors were alive, while 47% of patients with noninvasive tumors were alive. Only 2 out of the 181 patients had metastatic disease to distant organs (liver). Of the 66 tumors in which invasiveness was observed, the authors identified all types of histological variants, which were also associated with either invasion or encapsulation. Interestingly, the authors noted that spindle cell thymomas tend to be localized and slow growing, rarely associated with myasthenia gravis, and with good prognosis. However, in this series of 181 cases, 40 cases were considered to have spindle cell morphology, and 7 of those cases were invasive tumors, which would account for approximately 17.5% of this type. In 1974, Jain and Frable [53] reported a series of 32 cases of thymoma under the heading "Analysis of Benign and Malignant Criteria." The authors stated that features associated with benign thymomas include nodularity and encapsulation, while "malignant thymoma" tumors lose the nodularity and have infiltrative margins. Also, the authors stated that degeneration and necrosis are more common in malignant thymoma. In terms of mitotic activity, the authors stated that "malignant thymomas" have 0–6 mitotic figures per high-power field. Of the 32 cases presented, 16 cases were coded as "malignant." Interestingly, as the authors sort the thymomas by cell type, they identified that only three cases had spindle cell morphology and the tumors were encapsulated. Although the authors did not present a survival curve on these cases, they stated that follow-up in 14 patients with "malignant thymoma" showed that 12 had died after a period of 0–5 years (average 16 months), 1 patient with recurrent tumor, and 1died in the postoperative period. However, it is not clear from this report if patients died due to tumor or due to something else. In 1976, Salyer and Eggleston [54] reported on 65 patients with thymoma in which the authors stated unequivocally that the most significant prognostic feature is the presence or absence of capsular integrity. In addition, the authors clearly stated that the histologic type of thymoma has no value in predicting prognosis. Follow-up information on 42 of 49 cases was available for at least 3 years. More important is the observation by the authors that the tumor per se may not be regarded as "the" cause of death but rather that there are other contributing factors such as inanition or increased susceptibility to infection. In 25 cases, the tumor was associated with MG. Regarding the histology of these tumors, the authors stated that due to the well-known variation of patterns and cell predominance within a given tumor, the classification of these tumors is rather subjective. Furthermore, the authors added that, in terms of histological assessment of thymomas, it requires the examination of multiple sections and highlighted the arbitrary nature of categories. In addition, the authors stated that invasive growth cannot be predicted by histologic type as it occurs in all types. In terms of survival, the authors divided the patients into two categories: those with an associated syndrome such as MG or other and those without any particular syndrome. In those with an associated syndrome, the 5-year survival rate was 30%, while in the group without an associated syndrome, the survival at 5 years was 61%. Based on such information, it is logical to consider that the survival of patients with thymoma is affected by the presence of an associated medical condition in addition to the invasiveness of the tumor or lack of it. In 1977, LeGolvan and Abell [55] reported 46 patients with thymoma in which the authors did not find gender predilection; 16 patients had associated MG, 25% of patients were asymptomatic, and 20% of patients had other endocrine abnormalities, and 20 thymomas were reported as infiltrative. The overall survival at 5 years was 67%, while the authors noted that 17% of the patients died as a result of recurrent and infiltrative thymoma, and 18% of patients died due to unrelated causes to the thymoma. The authors concluded that histological classification of the tumors was of little value in predicting final outcome and that the prognosis of these tumors is more closely related to the invasiveness of the neoplasm. Bergh and colleagues [56] reported a similar number of cases (43 patients) and not only provided a schema for staging thymomas (see the chapter in this text on staging) but also concluded that surgical-pathological staging is of high importance in therapeutic decisions, stressing the importance of total thymectomy. It is of interest to note that, in Bergh's experience, tumors that were encapsulated or tumors that infiltrated the perithymic adipose tissue had no deaths and no complications, although the authors documented a recurrence at 8 years postsurgical resection. Wilkins and Castleman [57] reported 103 patients with thymoma, 56 associated with MG. Of the 103 thymomas, 37 were invasive tumors and 66 encapsulated. The overall survival of these patients was 64% at 5 years and 54% at 10 years. When the tumors were divided by invasiveness or encapsulation, the survival rate was 55% at 5 years and 40% at 10 years for invasive tumors, while 75% and 67% at 5 and 10 years for encapsulated tumor. More importantly, the authors concluded that MG is not an adverse factor for prognosis, while invasiveness of the tumor affects long-term survival, and the 10-year cumulative survival of patients in whom complete removal of the tumor is accomplished is about 68%. At the same time, further ultrastructural studies to demonstrate the epithelial nature of these tumors were also carried out [58, 59]. Important to mention is that as experience was being accumulated with these tumors and their diagnosis became more specific, different treatment options also were being considered [60, 61]. Shellito and colleagues [60] reported a single case of an invasive thymoma with response to oral corticosteroids, while Boston [61] reported two cases of invasive thymoma treated with chemotherapy.

In 1981, Masaoka and colleagues [62] reported 96 cases of thymoma (three patients were excluded from the final evaluation) which were used for their initial staging schema (see the chapter in this text on staging). In this study, the authors estimated the 5-year survival rate of patients with total resection at 88.9% and the non-radically treated group at 44.4%, while the overall survival rate at 5 years was estimated at 74.1% and at 10 years at 57.1%. Recurrence after total resection was observed in 6 of 69 patients, while about 50% of patients treated with subtotal resection survived more than 5 years with postoperative radiation therapy. Verley and colleagues [63] compared the clinical stages, histological features, and survival of 200 cases encompassing more than 27 years of experience at a single institution. The authors identified a hundred patients with associated MG and 14 others with other autoimmune diseases, which the authors concluded did not have an adverse effect in the survival of these patients. Interestingly, contrary to other publications, the authors also identified that invasiveness often parallels histologic typing and added that that both appeared to be two distinct parameters to predict prognosis. However, the histological types used in this study grouped the spindle cell types and the oval cell types together, separated those from the "lymphocyte-rich," and included two other variants, "differentiated and undifferentiated." Judging from the illustrations provided in this publication, it is possible that some of the tumors included as differentiated and undifferentiated may have represented "thymic carcinomas." Based on the grouping of histological subtypes used in this study, it is difficult to determine whether the authors' conclusions regarding a possible association between histology and invasiveness of the tumors are reproducible. Even though their schema for staging thymomas varies somewhat from what Masaoka had already presented, still the tumors were divided by encapsulation and invasion. The survival rate for the group with encapsulated tumors was 85% and 80% at 5 and 10 years, respectively, while for the invasive tumors, it was estimated to be at 50% and 35% at 5 and 10 years, respectively. Up to 1985, most of the clinicopathological studies presented on thymomas included surgically resected material and often the histological classification of thymomas presented by Bernatz and colleagues [42], and the overwhelming majority of reports clearly separated thymomas into those which were invasive and those which were encapsulated.

In 1985, Marino and Muller-Hermelink [64] reported 58 thymomas and 13 thymic carcinomas encompassing a 16-year experience and, based on that experience, formulated their histological classification. Important to highlight regarding this histological classification is that contrary to previous reports on these tumors in which the material used for the formulation of a classification system was based on surgical resections, the Marino-Muller-Hermelink study and proposal for histological classification was based only on biopsy material. At this juncture, it is critical to hark back to previous statements by Salyer and Eggleston [54], who stated that, due to the heterogeneity of thymomas, multiple histological sections are needed for proper evaluation. Nevertheless, despite such warnings by previous reports of cases presented in the literature with more material available for review, Marino and Muller-Hermelink, with only minute fragments of tissue, presented the so-called histogenetic classification system, which, according to the authors, was based on the normal histological features of the normal thymus. Thus,

- Cortical thymoma
- Medullary thymoma

- Mixed type of thymoma (**the** presence of medullary and cortical components)

At this point, it is important to clarify the terms applied in this classification and the corresponding analogous terms used in previous classification, namely, that of Bernatz and coauthors [42]:

M-H classification, no. of cases	Bernatz et al. classification, no. of cases
• Cortical thymoma – 25 biopsies →	• Lymphocyte-rich – 41 surgical resections
• Cortical thymoma →	• Mixed – 41 surgical resections
• Medullary thymoma –3 biopsies →	• Spindle cell thymoma – 33 surgical resections
• Mixed thymoma – 21 biopsies →	• N/A

One important observation regarding this proposal is the statement made by the authors that "medullary" thymomas (spindle cell thymomas) were benign. Such statement with the evaluation of only three small biopsies is unparalleled in modern surgical pathology even for 1985. Needless to say, one also has to wonder how is that mixed histologies could have been properly evaluated with a small biopsy, which raises the possibility that such histological interpretation may also have been not entirely accurate.

Even though this report is detailed in terms of the histological classification proposed, there are no data on survival. The main drawback of this report is the difficulty to unequivocally state which cases were possibly encapsulated as only biopsy material was evaluated. Also, the absence of what Bernatz [42] referred to as "epithelial thymoma" deserves highlighting. Such a definition would arrive in a different publication but under a different term and interpretation. In 1992, Kirchner and coauthors [65] reported what the authors interpreted as "well-differentiated thymic carcinoma." The authors presented 26 cases characterized by a predominance of epithelial cells, low mitotic rate, "epidermoid differentiation," slight moderate atypia, and constant presence of inter-epithelial immature cortical thymocytes, lobular growth, and formation of epithelial palisades around perivascular spaces. This description is somewhat similar to cases described as epithelial-rich thymomas. More interesting is the fact that the authors also documented that 77% of the patients had an associated MG. This classification proposal now stands as follow:

M-H classification	Bernatz et al. classification
Well-differentiated thymic carcinoma	Epithelial-rich thymoma

In addition, Muller-Hermelink and coauthors [66] followed the new histological classification with an immunohistochemical study of 12 thymomas using monoclonal antibodies. The authors concluded that cortical thymomas and areas of mixed thymoma showed staining for the non-squamous-type keratin 35βH11, while medullary thymoma showed staining for squamous-type keratin 34βE12-IV/82. In 1989, Kirchner and coauthors [67] presented a study of 95 cases from the same institution as the original "histogenetic classification." However, the authors detailed their classification system by stressing that thymomas are related to the structural components of normal thymus and, based on that concept, divided the thymomas as follows:

- Medullary
- Mixed
- Predominantly cortical
- Cortical
- Well-differentiated thymic carcinoma

Based on this publication, it is important to highlight a few issues. The section of material and methods glaringly shows no details about what had been examined; it is possible that, coming from the same institution, the same material may have been used. However, the authors merely made the statement "adequate tissue sections." It is difficult to determined what "adequate" may have meant. However, such information is of utmost importance, as the authors arrived to very specific conclusion: (1) medullary and mixed thymomas are always benign tumors, and (2) predominantly cortical, cortical, and well-differentiated thymic carcinomas are low-grade malignant tumors. Once again, this report likely included the same three medullary thymomas already published by the same authors, which also represented biopsy specimens. It is highly important to mention a few points:

1. The basis for this so-called histogenetic classification assumes a proper allocation of cortical epithelial cells for cortical thymomas and medullary cells for medullary thymoma.
2. Still using biopsy material, the authors are making unequivocal correlations of histology and clinical behavior.
3. By making the unequivocal correlation of histology and clinical behavior, the authors are stating that the prognosis of a thymoma can be unequivocally determined with a small biopsy.
4. It is rather "reckless" that, with the evaluation of only three cases (likely biopsies), the authors or any practicing pathologist can make the determination of "benign tumor." Even if one adds the 16 cases referred to as "mixed thymoma," that still would make the series total 19 cases, which renders this interpretation at best premature if not flat-out incorrect.

On the issue of the "histogenetic classification," the same authors, Kirchner and Muller-Hermelink [68], in a manuscript titled "New approaches to the diagnosis of thymic epithelial tumors," documented a study of their own with 25 such tumors (6 well-differentiated thymic carcinoma, 6 cortical thymomas, 8 predominantly cortical, and 5 mixed thymomas) in which the author used different monoclonal antibodies. The authors concluded that "the different histological tumor types cannot be defined." Therefore, the presence or absence of reactivity does not allow for clear immunohistochemical differentiation between the different tumor types. Furthermore, "the immunophenotypes of the epithelial neoplastic cells cannot be strictly correlated to the immunophenotypes of different epithelial cells in the normal thymus." This particular study conducted by the authors of the so-called "histogenetic classification" clearly debunks their own classification. In addition, to this particular study by the authors of the "histogenetic classification," Giraud and coauthors [69] also conducted a study using different hormones, antigenic markers for cortical and subcapsular/medullary thymic areas, and tumor-associated antigens. The authors concluded that their results did not correspond to the histological classification of cortical and medullary thymoma, and also that their results did not support the theory of different embryologic origins for cortical and medullary thymoma. On the other hand, at the morphological level, Dawson and coauthors [70] conducted a study of thymomas, attempting to assess consistency in the classification of thymoma and applying this "histogenetic classification." The study was conducted by three pathologists who were able to categorize only 26 of the 74 thymomas; they concluded that the classification of thymoma into cortical, medullary, or mixed pattern is difficult to apply and that surgical staging remains the better guide to prognosis. The overall survival rate observed in this group of cases was 78% at 5 years. More interesting is to highlight that the authors reported a worse prognosis for those tumors with mixed histology, contrary to the reports by those who proposed the "histogenetic classification," which is something to be expected as in this study 63 of the 74 cases reported represented surgical resections and not biopsy specimens. In a different attempt to use the "histogenetic classification," Pan and coauthors [71] evaluated 112 thymomas and concluded that not only does staging remain the most important factor affecting outcome but also that subclassification of cortical thymomas into organoid thymoma, conventional thymoma, and well-differentiated thymic carcinoma does not correlate with clinical behavior. In this report, 50 cases were encapsulated, and 62 were invasive in different stages; survival rates of those patients with encapsulated tumors were 94% and 87% at 5 and 10 years, respectively, while those patients in stage IV (Masaoka staging) were 41% and 22% at 5 and 10 years, respectively. Another attempt to correlate the histogenetic classification and correlate with clinical behavior was performed by Kornstein and coauthors [72], who evaluated 100 thymomas of which 48 were invasive tumors. The authors concluded that the "histogenetic classification," although conceptually attractive, is no more advantageous than the traditional classification proposed by Bernatz [42].

Just as it would be expected, having a new proposal for the classification of thymomas also "inspired" the publication of new series of cases in support of the attractive "histogenetic classification." Pescarmona and coauthors [73], in a report of 20 cases of what the authors designated as "microscopic thymoma" and based on the histological assessment of the microscopic thymomas, stated that their observations provide morphological evidence for a possible multifocal origin of thymoma from distinct epithelial clones present in the different topographic areas of the human thymus. It is important to highlight that the surgical resections of the thymuses in this study were performed because of the clinical presence of MG, and that the "microscopic thymomas" measured in size 0.2–0.4 mm. Again, Pescarmona and coauthors [74] presented a different study of 80 cases of thymoma in which the authors compared the "histogenetic classification" with what the authors referred to as the "Salyer-Eggleston classification." The authors concluded that the "histogenetic classification" correlated with age, surgical stage, and prognosis. Here, it is important to highlight that the initial premise of the histogenetic classification was the same as that stated by the proponents of such a classification: to provide by histological means the prognosis of thymoma patients. However, now in a different spin, Pescarmona and coauthors [74] attempted to correlate the "histogenetic classification" to surgical stage. Therefore, this study, which is supposed to support the "histogenetic classification," truly represents an exercise in a correlation between surgical stage and prognosis. Indeed, the authors documented that certain histological variants are in different stages; however, this point had already been amply represented in 1973 by Bernatz and coauthors [52] in a study of 181 cases in which the authors observed that all histological variants can be either encapsulated or invasive. The authors [74] observed that medullary thymomas had a survival rate of 100% at 5, 10, and 20 years, while cortical thymomas had a survival rate of 52% at 5 years and 45% at 10 and 20 years. Closer analysis of this series of cases shows that the authors were able to study only 11 cases of medullary thymomas (spindle cell thymoma); 9 of those cases were encapsulated, and 2 cases were stage II of Masaoka staging system (minimally invasive tumors). This casts some serious doubt about the conclusions drawn by the authors. Other groups of authors [75] from the same institution published 74 cases of thymoma (possibly included in this study are cases that were used for different publications, namely, in reference 74). In this study, the authors classified thymomas according to the "histogenetic classification," and the same number of medullary thymomas (spindle cell thymoma) reported in a similar publication by the same group of authors was used in this study: nine cases. The conclusions are very similar to their report of 80 cases [74], and the same drawback can be stated about this study. Concluding that medullary thymomas (spindle cell thymomas) are benign by analyzing nine cases is at best inaccurate. Ho and associates [76] also presented a study of 87 cases and classified the tumors according to the proposed "histogenetic classification." The authors also covered 15 cases of thymic carcinomas, including a group of tumors that the authors considered unclassified tumors. Therefore, the real number of thymomas is 72 cases, and the authors stated that "cortical thymomas" are more frequently associated with advanced stage. However, as the authors clearly stated in this report, 43 of the 72 thymomas were encapsulated leaving only 29 cases of invasive thymomas, which, for statistical purposes, is not an adequate number from which to draw any conclusion regarding histological subtypes and survival or staging. In addition, there are other drawbacks to this study:

1. Once again the number of medullary thymomas (spindle cell thymomas) is only nine cases;
2. The authors compared the survival rate of thymomas to that of thymic carcinomas, and, in order to come up with a higher number of cases, "medullary thymomas" are grouped together with "mixed thymomas." However, by grouping these cases as such, they also documented 2 of 21 cases as invasive tumors in Masaoka's stages II and III, which, for all practical purposes, is insufficient for a meaningful statistical analysis of invasive tumors
3. As the survival curve is presented with a follow-up of 66 cases including thymic carcinomas, the authors draw lines for the different histological groups. However, it is important to highlight that not only was the survival curve drawn from the staging of the tumor and not necessarily from the histological subgrouping of the thymoma category, but also the inclusion of thymic carcinomas in this curve obscures the real meaning of the thymoma category.

Tan and Sng [77], also in support of the "histogenetic classification," reported on 60 cases of "thymoma," including 12 cases of the so-called well-differentiated thymic carcinoma and 5 cases of otherwise thymic carcinomas. Therefore, the real number of thymoma cases is 55 and not 60 as the manuscript claims. The authors concluded that the "histogenetic classification" has predictive utility and represents a major step in the understanding of the biology of the thymic epithelial tumors. Already one conclusion becomes somewhat inaccurate as the authors of the "histogenetic classification" themselves had already stated 6 years earlier that "the immunophenotypes of the epithelial neoplastic cells cannot be strictly correlated to the immunophenotypes of different epithelial cells in the normal thymus [68]." In addition, the authors of this manuscript, once again departing from the premise that histologic subtyping predict prognosis, use Masaoka staging system to correlate their findings. Worse than in previous publications, the authors were able to document only three cases of "medullary thymoma" (spindle cell thymoma), two of which were encapsulated, therefore once again casting serious doubt on the validity of their conclusions. It is only logical to assume that if in a group of tumors there are only three representing a particular variant, the great majority would be among other variants and likely in different stages as well. Nevertheless, the authors documented a follow-up in 54 patients with a mean duration of 29.6 months, in which 9 patients had died. Also, Close [78], in collaboration with the authors of the "histogenetic classification," evaluated 51 thymic epithelial neoplasms; as it would be expected, the conclusion was that of high reproducibility. However, it is important to highlight that the section of materials and methods is rather obscure in terms of specifically stating the numbers of biopsies, surgical specimens, and autopsies. More significant is to emphasize that once again the number of "medullary thymomas" (spindle cell type) and "mixed thymomas" is minimal, with only five cases in total (three spindle cell type), and, even after a different analysis by the authors of the "histogenetic classification," the number went up to seven cases. Whether those cases represented biopsy specimens is not clarified. Kuo and Lo [79], in support of the "histogenetic classification," evaluated 71 thymoma cases concluded that "cortical thymoma" should be regarded as a potentially malignant tumor, while "medullary thymomas" are benign. Interestingly, the authors stated that the mixed categories of thymomas also have the potential for invasiveness, which is the opposite view of the original "histogenetic classification." Once again, the same issue is highlighted: the number of cases coded as "medullary thymoma" (spindle cell type) was only 7, and all of them were encapsulated. Even though most of what had been reported in support of the "histogenetic classification" had taken place mainly in Asia, support for the histogenetic classification gained the support of the Massachusetts General Hospital. The first of two publications [80, 81] came from essentially the same group. In this first publication in 1993 [80], the authors evaluated 122 cases of thymic epithelial tumors, which included 6 thymic carcinomas. Important to highlight from this study are (1) the authors did not find any correlation between epithelial cell morphology and antigen expression; (2) of the 122 cases, only 8 corresponded to "medullary thymomas"; (3) all "medullary thymomas" (spindle cell type) were either encapsulated (5 cases) or identified invading through the capsule (3 cases); and (4) a total of 68 thymomas were invasive and 48 encapsulated. In a second publication by essentially the same group [81], the authors reported a study of 116 thymomas and assessed the effect of histologic classification and other factors including stage, size of the tumor, lymphoid hyperplasia, MG, age, sex, and treatment on the survival of these patients; at least 6 of these cases were thymic carcinomas. The same 6 cases of thymic carcinoma are also included in this report, and, contrary to the previous report of 122 cases, which also included the same 6 thymic carcinomas, now the number of thymomas has been reduced in number. Nevertheless, the authors concluded that the "histogenetic classification" has prognostic significance, independent of tumor stage. They also added that medullary thymomas were benign tumors with no risk of recurrence even when capsular invasion was present. Now let us analyze this report with some more detail: (1) the number of cases of "medullary thymoma" (spindle cell type) continues to be the same as in the already-published study by the same authors: only eight cases; (2) in the previous publication, these "medullary thymomas" were labeled as encapsulated or invading through the capsule; now it appears that five of these "medullary thymomas" were encapsulated and three cases were stage IIa and IIb (likely minimally invasive tumors). In addition, now 50 of the tumors studied represented encapsulated thymomas, thus, leaving 60 cases of invasive tumors. The tumors coded as "well-differentiated thymic carcinomas" recurred more often and earlier than other subtypes. Therefore, based on this experience, the authors further concluded that "adjuvant therapy appears unnecessary for medullary and mixed thymomas, even when they are invasive." The actual freedom from relapse for patients with "well-differentiated thymic carcinoma" was 58% at 5 years and 46% at 10 years, while it was 100% for other subtypes, respectively. The larger and most important question to ask based on this report is: If the survival rate for all other subtypes of thymomas is 100 at 5 and 10 years, respectively, except for the "well-differentiated thymic carcinoma" (atypical thymoma), then what is the need for a subclassification of thymomas? What the authors have clearly defined in this study is that any subtyping of thymoma has little value in the prognosis of these patients, and that the type that is more important to recognize is this so-called well-differentiated thymic carcinoma (atypical thymoma) that happens to have been described as an invasive tumor in all the cases presented in this series of cases.

However, others follow the most conventional approach. For instance, Hofmann and associates [82] reported 98 thymomas in which the authors correlated clinical manifestations and gross and histologic pathological findings. In this report, 52% of thymomas were encapsulated, 26% were invasive, and 3% were thymic carcinomas. The authors followed the conventional Bernatz [42] histological classification. Even though the authors documented 52 thymomas as encapsulated tumors, in 18 cases, the capsular status could not be determined. Important to note is the observation of the histological evaluation in which the authors stated that in an individual thymoma, various cellular differentiations may be present, as the authors documented that in 20% of their cases, the tumor may show mixed histologies. No survival data were presented by the authors regarding these 98 cases. Maggi and associates [83] also reported 169 cases of thymoma with more emphasis on the surgical treatment over 28 years. The authors identified 73% of the patients with associated MG and followed a schema somewhat different from other staging schemas available at that time. The authors separated thymomas into three categories: non-invasive, intrathymic, and invasive. It is possible that those tumors referred to as "intrathymic" may represent tumors which we often referred to as "minimally invasive tumors." Based on such a schema, 106 cases were considered noninvasive, with possibly 63 cases as invasive tumors. The overall survival rate at 5, 10, and 15 years was estimated to be 84%, 79%, and 65%, respectively. The authors also noted that a shorter survival rate was observed between invasive and noninvasive tumors, that being at 65% versus 85%, respectively, at 5 years. Lewis and associates [84] also reported their experience with 283 thymoma cases in 147 women and 136 men between the ages of 16 and 90 years (mean: 52 years). Clinically, 46% had MG and 10% other paraneoplastic syndromes. In 32% of the cases, the tumors were locally invasive at operation, 6% with lung or pleural involvement. Intrathoracic recurrence occurred in 15% of the patients who had total excision, 3% developed distant metastasis, 13% died of tumor, and 16% died due to MG. The overall survival rate was estimated at 67% and 53% at 5 and 10 years, respectively. The authors concluded that poor prognostic factors include larger tumors size, local invasion, metastasis at initial operation, and predominantly epithelial tumors. In addition, the authors stated that thymomas rarely metastasize outside of the thoracic cavity. Three additional statements deserve highlighting: (1) the authors of this report made the suggestion to discard the term "malignant thymoma" in order to avoid confusion with thymic carcinoma; (2) the authors stated that thymic epithelial neoplasms may be viewed as a spectrum encompassing thymoma and thymic carcinoma; and (3) they described a group of cases with high proportion of epithelial cells demonstrating variable degrees of cytologic atypia, which may be difficult to classify and would be expected to behave in an "intermediate manner." The authors most likely were referring to atypical thymomas.

Meanwhile, others have attempted to correlate survival rate with not only histological pattern but also with proliferative activity. Pich and associates [85] reported 60 cases of thymoma, which were analyzed by DNA flow cytometry and argyrophilic nucleolar organizer regions (AgNORs). The authors concluded that proliferative activity evaluated by AgNORs is the best predictor for long-term survival. Also emphasizing complete resection and adjuvant postoperative irradiation, Nakahara and associates [86] reported their experience with 141 patients; interestingly, the authors encountered that tumors in which there was breaching of the capsule by the tumor and those which were considered encapsulated fair very much the same, with survival rates of 100% at 5 years and 94.7 at 10 years. Deaths occur in patients after 15 years postsurgical resection, and the authors did not find any statistical significance between survival rate and histologic subtyping of thymomas. The authors concluded that complete surgical resection followed by postoperative radiation therapy results in a "benign" postoperative course, regardless of the stage and histologic type. Meanwhile, case reports of metastasis from thymomas to sites outside of the thoracic cavity were also documented [87, 88].

As experience was being accumulated with the different publications presented on thymoma cases, the literature regarding treatment options for these patients was growing. In that regard, some authors have stated that separating thymomas into encapsulated and invasive according to surgical and gross findings appears to be insufficient for the clinical assessment of the malignancy and prognosis, and they considered that the histology of the thymomas can predict the clinical course [89]. However, other publications have considered the encapsulation or invasion of the tumor sufficient information for possible additional treatment with either radiation therapy or chemotherapy [90–93]. In 1988, Curran and associates [94] reported their experience with 103 cases of thymoma and the role of mediastinal irradiation following complete or incomplete surgical resection. Of the 103 thymomas, 43 tumors were encapsulated, and only 3 patients had "thoracic dissemination or metastases." The 5-year actual survival rate was estimated at 67%, while the relapse-free survival rate was estimated at 100% for encapsulated tumor and 69% and 53%, respectively, for late stages. The authors concluded that total resection alone appears to be inadequate therapy resulting in high local failure with poor salvage therapy results. Although very informative regarding additional treatment for thymoma patients, this report does not have detailed histological features of the tumors. On the other hand, Godell and associates [95], in a report of 22 thymoma cases, concluded that combination chemotherapy is effective in the first-line postsurgical treatment of incomplete resected thymoma and also in the treatment of local or metastatic relapses after radiation.

Unfortunately, it is also important to highlight that, despite progress made on the issue of terminology regarding the usage of "malignant thymoma," some series of cases were presented using specifically the terminology of malignant thymoma. Park and associates [96] presented a series of "malignant thymomas" (most likely invasive thymomas) in which the authors emphasized the potential benefit of chemotherapy in these patients. Also, Wang and associates [97] reported on 61 patients with tumors under the designation of "malignant thymoma" (most likely invasive thymomas) in whom resection was performed in 55.7% of the patients. The authors concluded that factors that may affect prognosis include resectability, tumor staging, MG, postoperative irradiation, or chemotherapy. The overall cumulative survival was 59% and 34% at 5 and 10 years, respectively.

It is important to highlight that there are other proposals for the classification of thymomas. Monden and associates [98] evaluated 15 fetal thymuses and 100 thymomas, correlated them with ultrastructural findings, and, based on such comparison, divided thymomas as follows:

- Well-differentiated
  - *Mature or immature Hassall's bodies*
- Moderately differentiated
  - *Polygonal cell*
  - *Clear cell*
  - *Spindle cell*
- Poorly differentiated
  - *Polygonal and spindle cells*
- Undifferentiated
  - *Clear cytoplasm, solid pattern, no lymphocytes*

It is apparent from this classification that the undifferentiated thymoma and likely the poorly differentiated thymoma represent different variants of thymic carcinoma. Regarding the well and moderately differentiated tumors, it is difficult to assume specific categories.

Levine and Rosai in 1978 [99] classified thymomas as follows:

- Benign thymoma (encapsulated)
- Malignant thymoma
  - *Type I: with no or minimal cytologic atypia*
    - *Locally invasive*
    - *With true lymphatic or hematogenous spread*
  - *Type II: with cytologically malignant (thymic carcinoma)*

There are obvious drawbacks with this proposal: (1) some encapsulated thymomas are known to recur; (2) the issue of malignant thymoma has for decades obscured the classification of these tumors, as that terminology truly represents a different neoplasm: thymic carcinoma.

Also, Kuo [100], in a study of 9 thymuses and 34 thymomas analyzed by immunohistochemistry with cytokeratin profiles, presented a classification approach:

- Spindle cell thymoma
- Small polygonal cell thymoma
- Mixed thymoma

- Organoid thymoma
- Large polygonal cell thymoma
- Squamoid thymoma

This particular proposal not only has an inadequate number of cases but also stresses immunohistochemistry as a route to proper classification. Needless to say, the comparison with staging is also lacking.

At this juncture, based on the available literature, it is important to highlight that there was a relative confusion regarding the classification of thymomas. In 1995 [101], we highlighted several issues regarding the histological classification of thymoma, which reflected some of the opinions expressed by different authors in different clinicopathological correlations.

It is possible that, because of many discrepancies in the histological classification of thymomas, the World Health Organization (WHO) proposed developing an "official" classification system." What was the reasoning behind this proposal? Why at this point in time? Who was behind such proposal? The answers to these questions are difficult to determine. What we can say for sure is that, for a tumor that affects probably less than 1 per 100,000 people, it was given quite a bit of attention all of a sudden. Nevertheless, a group of "experts" was assembled to shed some light in the thymoma argument, and this group of individuals came up with a system of letters and numbers in 1999 [102]:

- Thymoma, type A (spindle, medullary)
- Thymoma, type AB (mixed)
- Thymoma type B1 (lymphocyte-rich, lymphocytic, predominantly cortical, organoid)
- Thymoma B2 type (cortical)
- Thymoma B3 (epithelial, atypical, squamoid, well-differentiated thymic carcinoma)
- Thymoma type C (thymic carcinoma)

Unfortunately, very few people read the most important component of the 1999 WHO publication [102]. Let us rescue some important statements:

1. "...the terminology chosen here is non-committal, one based on a combination of letter and numbers."
2. "It is not proposed as a new classification, but mainly to facilitate comparison among the many terms and classification schemes that have been offered over the years."

Based on this approach, one can only conclude that the letters and numbers really represent a translation of previous classifications schemas, mainly of the one proposed by Bernatz and the so-called histogenetic classification. However, such comparison may be at best uneven. The Bernatz classification was based on surgical resections and had a morphological approach; on the contrary, the Marino-Muller-Hermelink classification proposal was based on 45 biopsies from which the authors not only designated cell of origin for these tumors (which was not proven in later studies by the same authors) but also assigned clinical behavior. Keep in mind that the number of biopsies in the original proposal in which the authors claimed that medullary thymomas are benign represented the total experience of three biopsy specimens. As a matter of fact, in all the subsequent studies in support of this "histogenetic classification," the number of cases of medullary thymomas" has been in single digits. The larger question here is: How is it possible that a non-proven and questionable classification was taken so seriously by the WHO? In addition, the letters and numbers could have been easily substituted for names of cities, lakes, or any other structure, and the result would have been exactly the same.: a translator. Nevertheless, the WHO Blue Book [102] was published, but there are also important issues that were not discussed therein:

- Sampling: the heterogeneity of these tumors is well known, and it would have been appropriate for the "experts" to shed some light on that issue.
- A meaningful discussion on staging is absent. Interestingly, one statement made in the introduction of the Blue Book is:
  - ".... the importance of evaluating thymic epithelial neoplasms on the basis of their presence and degree of invasiveness (using staging criteria)."
- According to this translation, these tumors are always either A or B, which is far from the reality of these tumors when properly sampled.

In 1999, we proposed a classification system with a novel conceptual approach, and divided thymic epithelial neoplasms into three more specific tumors [103]:

- Thymoma
- Atypical thymoma
- Thymic carcinoma

The basic premise of this conceptual approach is the determination of cytologic degree of atypia and the identification of organotypical features of thymic differentiation, which may allow for more accurate classification of these tumors. However, we also emphasized that staging of the tumor provides a more reliable prognosis of these tumors rather than the histological categorization. This approach, compared to previous classification, is as follows:

Bernatz	Histogenetic	Suster-Moran
Spindle cell	*Medullary thymoma*	*Thymoma*
Mixed (lymphoepithelial)	*Predominantly cortical*	*Thymoma*
Lymphocyte rich	*Cortical thymoma*	*Thymoma*
Predominantly epithelial	*Well-differentiated thymic carcinoma*	*Atypical thymoma*

As it would be expected, this different approach to the concept of thymoma was received with some animosity by some who had previously endorsed the "histogenetic classification" [104], and, among some of the issues raised, we detail a few:

- No data was presented to support this proposal.
  - In time, such data have been abundantly published in the literature, not with biopsy specimens but in large scale with hundreds of cases and more recently with more than a thousand cases [29, 105, 106]. The data not only question the WHO schema but flat out clarifies the incorrect statement by the authors that "medullary thymomas" are always benign and does not deserve additional treatment even when invasive.
- One other issue raised was that because one of us (CAM) had participated in the WHO committee on the histological typing of tumors, it would not be optimal to suggest a totally new proposal.
  - It is obvious that both authors of this condemnation did not read the preface of the Blue Book, which states the following:
    "… modifications are almost certain to be needed …. It necessarily represents a view from which some pathologists may wish to dissent."

Others took a more objective and open-minded approach [107], while our response to the strongly worded letter [107] included the following [108]:

1. Unbeknownst to the authors of this letter [104], the manuscript that they cited had been a personal invitation from the editor of AJCP to shed some light on the issue of thymoma, at the same time that the authors of that review were working on a particular study involving several hundreds of cases.
2. The stated premise of the author of the letter is that all "medullary thymomas" are benign and that even when they are invasive they do not deserve treatment. We consider that such assumptions are at best wrong if not flat-out reckless.
   (a) Once again, in time our assessment of that type of thymoma has been proven in large series of cases [105, 106]
3. We took as more disturbing the implication that presenting our ideas (for that matter anybody's ideas) should be done only with the blessing of any given organization or group of individuals.
   (a) This particular issue has remained disturbing when it comes to thoracic pathology in general, as any ideas contradicting the WHO authors are not accepted in what appears to be a high-jacking of thoracic pathology by a group who consider themselves the "elite" of thoracic pathologists.

Into 2000, we started to highlight some of the problems with the current classification systems. Something that has been relatively obscure in the literature of thymoma is the issue of sampling. Sampling goes to the heart of the issue of histological classification, taking into account that one classification system was based on surgical resections [42], while the "histogenetic classification" was based only on biopsy samples [64]. An important question arises: in a tumor that is well known for its heterogeneity, does the sampling of the tumor play a role in the final classification of the thymoma? The obvious answer would be that it does. However, up to now, there are only a few larger studies which have addressed perhaps the most important issue surrounding the histological classification of thymomas. So we attempted to clarify this issue by evaluating 630 surgical resections of thymomas [109]. We encountered that a cut-off number of five sections appears to provide a difference in subgrouping thymomas and concluded that histopathologic classification of thymomas has limited practical relevance for the assessment of prognosis in cases with limited biopsy material. Furthermore, proper evaluation of histology and aggressive potential in thymoma should be based on ample sampling and assessment of capsular integrity. If, on the other hand, we want to keep uniformity in the histological classification of thymomas, then it would more appropriate if the WHO would recommend not to take many sections of these tumors, which will lead to uniformity. However, that would be reckless, and if that recommendation does not exist, and if more than 50% of these tumors will show mixed histologies, then what is the importance of the WHO schema? Thus, the more practical approach is that of the categorization of thymoma, atypical thymoma, and thymic carcinoma.

As it would be expected, the WHO's schema of letters and numbers was received by the community of pathologists exactly the opposite of the way intended: as a "new classification." Therefore, different publications now have addressed the importance of the WHO classification, not realizing that what they were describing was a mere substitution for names from previous classifications. Chen in association with the proponents of the "histogenetic classification" [110] reported 200 cases from China and stated that the "WHO classification" predicts prognosis. Interestingly, one of the authors of this manuscript was a participant in the initial committee for the typing of thymic tumors, and knew full well that the WHO schema does not represent a "new classification"; however, for this publication such detail was ignored. In any case, the authors [110] grouped their cases according to the WHO schema of letters and numbers; interestingly, only 8 of the 200 cases belong to the type A (spindle cell/medullary thymoma). The results obtained by the authors of this study are truly "impressive," as the authors obtained a perfect clockwise survival curve among the different types of thymoma: type A ⇒ type AB ⇒ type B1 ⇒ B2 ⇒type B3 ⇒type C (thymic carcinoma). A few years later, this particular study would be used in the 2004 publication of WHO as the "poster child" for how much improved the "classification of thymomas" had become. Nakagawa and associates [111] presented their experience with a report of 130 thymoma patients whose message was that the "WHO classification" correlates with clinical stage; also of interest is that out of 130 cases, only 18 were type A (spindle/medullary), and 15 of those cases were either encapsulated or minimally invasive tumors. In Okamura and associates' clinical study [112], of 273 patients, once again the same number of type A thymoma resurfaces with 18 cases of this variant. Nevertheless, the authors concluded that the "WHO classification" may be helpful in clinical practice for the assessment and treatment of patients with thymoma.

Two important and highly unusual issues with all these new manuscripts in support of the letters and numbers are that not one of them mentions the type of material examined and, worse, the number of sections available for review, features that clearly affect subtyping. In addition, all the cases appear to be placed in specific slots (type A, B1, etc.) without cases that show mixed histologies; those findings cast significant doubt as to the correct appraisal of these tumors. More disturbing is the fact that, since the publication of the WHO letters and numbers became available, only a few manuscripts contradicting such views have appeared, and the WHO members have taken special interest in casting them aside.

In 2004, the World Health Organization released the new version of Tumours of the Lung Pleura, Thymus, and Heart [113]. Here it is important to highlight the following:

- All the members of the initial 1999 committee are absent except for one of the editors.
- In an almost coup d'etat, the schema of letters and numbers that was not intended for a new classification now has become the official classification of the WHO.
- The grading of malignancy is presented as follows:
  - Type A and AB – generally benign tumors
  - Type B1 – low-grade malignant tumors, 10-year survival 90%
  - Type B2 – greater degree of malignancy
  - Type B3 – in advance stages shows poor prognosis
- The authors of this new version of the WHO nicely illustrated their study of 200 cases from China and presented the survival curves of that study [110].
- At this point, it is essential to properly analyze those statements:

1. Type A and AB thymomas without any further analysis are considered benign tumors. Up to 2004, the literature on spindle cell thymoma (type A) had been poor, and the authors of the WHO Book have had the experience of evaluating only a handful of those tumors.
2. If type B1 is a low-grade tumor with a survival at 10 years of 90%, then what is the purpose of separating that tumor from the spindle cell thymoma? Actually, the authors have contributed to the notion that both of them are just thymomas and that separation between A and B1 is artificial.
3. What is the meaning of "greater degree of malignancy for type B2? Related to what? If it is against B1 type, then could it be 11%? 15%? One can only wonder. As we have suggested before, perhaps A, B1, and B2 should just simply be classified as thymomas.
4. Type B3 in advanced stages shows poor prognosis. Here the authors became confused with their own terminology. Are they evaluating "grade of malignancy" or staging? The authors conveniently switched to "staging" for type B3. Once again, if A, B1, and B2 are similar and B3 is somewhat different, perhaps the authors just prove the notion of the categorization: thymoma–atypical thymoma–thymic carcinoma.
5. The most disturbing aspect, perhaps, and what has become a pattern for the authors of the WHO publications on thoracic tumors, is the blatant disregard for publications that contradict their views, even when they come from solid clinicopathological correlations. That pattern of "selective amnesia" has become obvious in later publications by this reputable entity. The authors interestingly did not include two important publications that had become available only 2 years before the 2004 publication of the WHO document.

   (a) Chalabreysse and associates [114] from Lyon, France, reported 90 thymic epithelial tumors and followed the schema of letters and numbers; 56% of the tumors were invasive, and 67% of the patients underwent total resection. The authors did not observe a significant difference in prognosis for types A and B, suggesting that those types of thymoma should be regarded as a morphologic continuum rather than distinct histological variants.

   (b) Rieker and associates [115] from the University of Heidelberg presented a study of 218 cases and evaluated these cases using the Bernatz and the schema of letter and numbers of the WHO. The authors observed a good interobserver agreement between WHO and Bernatz. However, the authors stated that when subgroups were added (B1, B2, etc.), the agreement was not as good. The authors finally concluded that further simplification and subclassification into three subgroups led to classes with good discriminative power in respect of survival. Their overall survival curve showed similar outcomes for thymomas A, B1, and B2. Also a "very good" interobserver agreement was observed in the simplified classification. The authors stated:

> ".... Our results are in favor of a classification that permits accurate allocation of these neoplasms to simple and reproducible diagnostic categories, as proposed by Suster and Moran" [103]

Kim and associates [116] presented a study of 108 cases – 50 encapsulated and 58 invasive tumors – and observed that the histological subtype closely correlated with the Masaoka staging. The tumor-related survival was estimated to be 88% and 77.9% at 5 and 10 years, respectively. In addition, they noted that B3 tumors (atypical thymoma) had an intermediate prognostic ranking. The authors concluded that Masaoka stage is the most important determinant of survival in surgically resected cases of thymoma, and further stated that interobserver agreement needs improvement. From this study, one can observe two important issues: (1) the authors properly identified the WHO as a schema and not as a classification system, and (2) their results seem to be more in keeping with the concept of thymoma–atypical thymoma–thymic carcinoma. Also, Kim and associates [117] retrospectively reviewed 100 patients who underwent thymectomy for WHO type B thymoma, concluding that tumor recurrence was significantly associated with advanced Masaoka stage regardless of the WHO subtype of B thymoma. In support of the WHO schema, Rena and colleagues [118] reported 178 thymomas: 112 tumors were encapsulated, while 66 were invasive with an estimated disease-free survival of 94% for stage I and 66% for stage III at 10 years. The authors concluded that the Masaoka staging system, WHO classification, and complete resection were significant independent prognostic factors. Similar findings were obtained in a study of 249 cases from China by Su and colleagues [119], who concluded that the Masaoka stage was the most important prognostic factor.

In order to bring some clarity to the issue of type A thymoma (spindle cell/medullary thymoma) and to demonstrate that histologic subtyping of thymoma does not correlate with encapsulation or invasion, we undertook a review of 210 invasive thymomas in which appropriate sampling was undertaken: a minimum of 5 sections per tumor, as this is our standard [106]. Of the 210 invasive thymomas, we identified 41 cases (19.5%) of pure spindle cell (WHO type A) in which the tumor not only spread outside of the capsule but also invaded other structures such as the pleura, lung, thyroid, and skeletal muscle of the diaphragm. Following that particular study, we evaluated 250 thymoma cases, once again with a minimum of five sections per tumor, in order to evaluate the reproducibility of the WHO schema [105–120]. In our study, we encountered 21.6% of spindle cell thymomas (WHO type A) and 9.2% of atypical thymoma (WHO type B3), while the remaining were in the various types of thymomas (WHO B1 and B2). More important is that more than 50% of the thymomas became mixed histologies when appropriate sampling was observed, therefore diluting the relevance of the subtyping for these tumors. In addition, when we analyzed the survival of these patients based on the histologic type, whether the tumors were separated by groups of A and AB against B1, B2, and B3 or when separated by A, AB, and B1 against B2 and B3, no statistical significance was observed. It simply does not correlate. Therefore, not only does the WHO schema not correlate with survival when appropriate samples of the different types of thymomas are available for study, but the WHO schema also does not correlate with the staging of thymomas; therefore, leaving a subtyping of tumors that, although attractive, has no clinical relevance. Based on our observations in this study, we proceeded to propose a staging system (see chapter on staging) which represents a collaborative work between thoracic surgeons and thoracic pathologists, and which clearly identifies who will benefit from surgery alone and who may need additional therapy [120]. The proposed staging system essentially divides patients between those with limited disease (stages 0 and 1) and patients with more widespread disease (stages 2 and 3). Meanwhile, others were kinder in their appraisal of the WHO schema. Zucalli and colleagues [121] evaluated 129 thymomas in which 4 pathologists independently classified those tumors according to the WHO schema; the result was only a "moderate agreement." It is important to highlight that, in this study, two representative hematoxylin-eosin (H&E) sections were available for evaluation, which goes exactly to the core of the problem. If four pathologists have only moderate agreement with only two H&E sections, what is to be expected if one has at least five? In a large study on thymomas, Guerra and colleagues [122] reported on a multi-institutional study and encountered 750 cases, 676 with complete surgical resection. The authors compared the WHO schema against what the authors called the "collapsed scheme" (merging types A, AB, and B1/B2), which is Suster-Moran's approach (thymoma – atypical thymoma – thymic carcinoma). The authors observed an overall survival and cumulative incidence of recurrence for all cases of 91% and 0.11, respectively. The authors concluded that the WHO schema shows lack of clinical significance in influencing prognosis, while the "collapsed scheme" revealed fair stratification of risk to relapses and better correlation with patients' clinical characteristics.

What is more amusing is that, in order to "solidify" the WHO schema, a study of 72 selected cases by 18 pathologists was conducted by some of the members of the WHO [123]. The issue should not have been about the diagnosis of thymomas; the issue should have been that when ample sampling is done on these tumors, the WHO schema losses clinical relevance, and there is no correlation between the WHO schema and stage of the tumor. More interesting to see in this publication is the "convincing effect" on authors who in the past have expressed serious concerns about the WHO schema. It becomes obvious that by adding those authors to this publication, suddenly the WHO schema will gain the credibility that it badly needed.

In 2014, the last version of the WHO classification of tumors of the lung, pleura, thymus, and heart was released [124]. As was expected, despite the abundant literature on the fact that the WHO schema has questionable clinical relevance, the authors – mainly the same individuals from 2004 – once again made official a schema that was not intended as a new classification. More interesting in this publication is the 10-year overall survival rates that are given to the different types of thymoma: A, 100%; B1, 85–100%; B2, 70–90%; and B3, 50–70%. Does it look very familiar? Yes, it does: that is exactly what the Suster-Moran stratification of thymomas means: thymoma (types A, AB, B1, and B2)-atypical thymoma (type B3). This 2014 WHO schema for thymomas is clearly a repetition of the same errors of 2004 and once again illustrates the blatant disregard for publications that contradict the status quo.

However, once again to correct misconceptions and egregious disregard for clinicopathological series that contradict the WHO schema, a more convincing series of cases needed to be assembled. A newly formed Thymic International Group representing practicing pathologists and thoracic surgeons from 14 institutions in 11 countries assembled what constitutes the largest series of thymomas up to now: 1470 resected specimens [29]. The cases were stratified using the Suster-Moran histological system [103], and the staging system proposed by Moran-Walsh-Suster-Kaiser [120]. Clinical follow-up data were obtained in 1339 patients with a mean of 69.2 months (over 5 years). All cases of thymoma (A, AB, B1, B2) represented 87.3% of the cases (1284 cases) (193 cases were pure spindle cell type), and atypical thymoma represented 12.7% of the cases (186 cases). Statistical analysis of this group of 1339 cases in whom clinical follow-up was available showed the Suster-Moran histological classification statistically significant, with a p value for cumulative survival probability of $p = 0.038$. In addition, when the clinical information available was statistically correlated with the Moran's staging system, it shows $p = 0.001$. Therefore, now on a large scale with an excess of a thousand cases, not only is the Suster-Moran's histological schema shown to be clinically significant, but also the staging system is easily reproducible by pathologists, and carries statistically significant prognosis (Figs. 7.2 and 7.3).

It is also important to highlight the occurrence of thymomas in the pediatric age group. There have been only a few reports on this particular topic due to the rarity of such

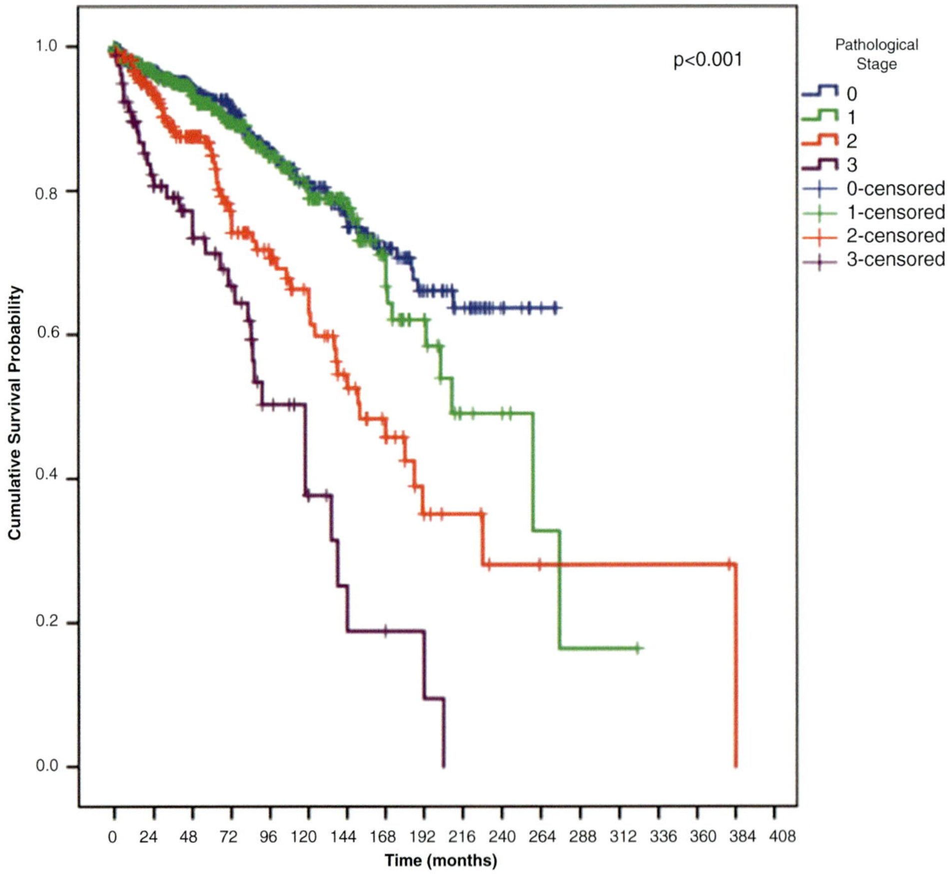

Fig. 7.2 Kaplan-Meier statistical analysis of pathological staging of thymoma and the Moran's proposed pathological stage, showing statistical significance $p = 0.001$. (Used with permission from Moran [29])

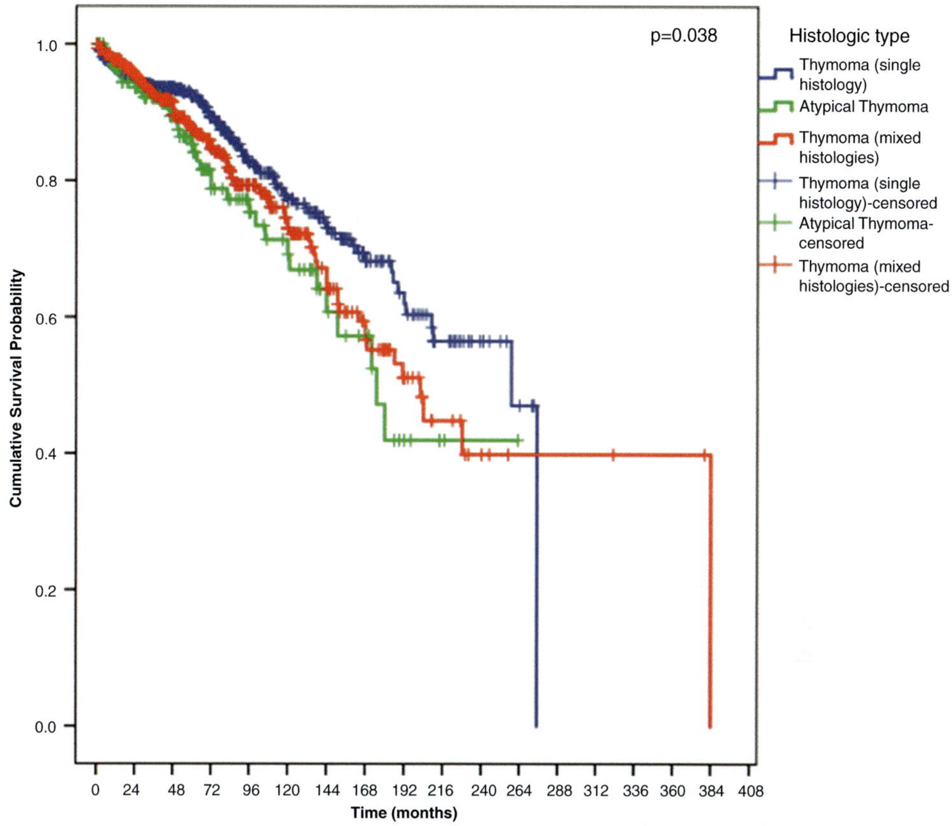

Fig. 7.3 Kaplan-Meier statistical analysis of histological type against cumulative survival probability showing statistical significance $p = 0.038$. (Used with permission from Moran [29])

occurrence. Ramon y Cajal and Suster [125] reported ten cases of thymic epithelial neoplasm in children under 16 years of age (ranging from 1 to 16 years); seven of these tumors were coded as thymomas with similar histological features as those in the adult population. Also, similar to the adult population, some of those tumors were encapsulated, while others were invasive. It is only logical to believe that the outcome in these children will depend on the invasiveness of the tumor at the time of diagnosis. Pescarmona and colleagues [126] reported five thymomas in children ages 11–15 years. All the cases in this report were of encapsulated thymomas, and the follow-up reported no recurrences or metastasis.

Regarding the treatment of thymomas, over the last 20 years, a similar trend has been observed, which mainly involves the additional treatment of radiation therapy or chemotherapy for patients with advanced stage thymoma. The results of these types of treatments are fairly similar [127–134]. It is very possible that the decision regarding additional treatment options for advanced thymomas is based on the stage of the tumor and the surgical resectability, rather than the histological features of the tumor, which brings us to the concept of WHO/Histogenetic classification of tumors; once a tumor is invasive, the treatment options are based on staging regardless of how the cells look, whether spindle or round. Regarding the use of neoadjuvant chemotherapy (cyclophosphamide, doxorubicin, cisplatin, and prednisone) and the impact on histopathological assessment of thymomas, we have observed that such treatment appears to affect more those thymomas with lymphocytic component than other histologies [135]. However, the histological changes observed – namely, necrosis, cystic changes, hemorrhage, calcification, cholesterol cleft granulomas, and histiocytic proliferation – may also be seen in thymomas with no prior treatment.

Pathological Aspects

Anatomical Orientation and Sampling

Even though a great deal of emphasis is placed on diagnostic accuracy for thymomas, little information is available in terms of anatomical orientation of the specimen and sampling of the tumor.

We have carefully analyzed the issue of orientation and have come to understand that once the specimen is transferred to the pathology gross room, if the specimen has not been properly oriented by the surgical team in the operating room, very likely the pathologist will have difficulty in orienting the specimen. The pathologist then will likely take what is the most appropriate action, and that is to ink the surgical borders of the tumor. However, even though that type of practice is helpful in providing pathological information regarding complete surgical removal of the tumor, if the tumor is invasive and the tumor is present at the ink border of resection, it becomes important to know which border is the one that is compromised. It is important to highlight that if the surgical team or the team who eventually will make the decision about additional therapy for the patient is not interested in which surgical border is compromised, then there is no need for special orientation of the specimen. However, we have found that often such information is important for the thoracic surgery team. Therefore, over the years, we have emphasized with our colleagues that proper marking be made to the specimen in order to properly sample the areas of importance. In certain circumstances, the pathologist should participate in the surgical orientation of the specimen. We consider that such practice is highly important and such communication needs to be established, which in turn may alleviate any problematic issues once the case is sampled (Figs. 7.4, 7.5, 7.6, 7.7, 7.8, 7.9, 7.10, 7.11, 7.12, 7.13 and 7.14a, b).

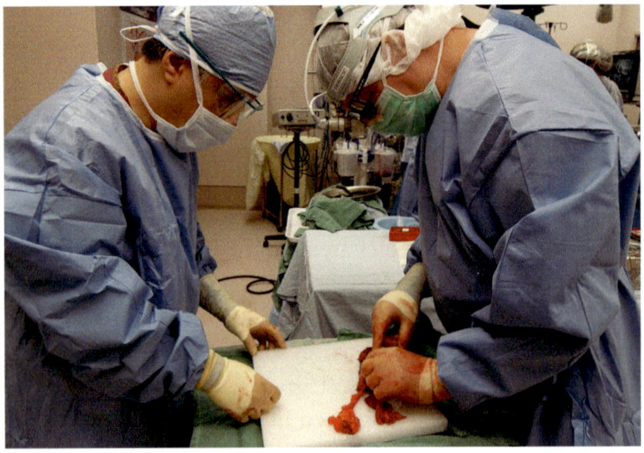

Fig. 7.4 Thoracic surgeon and pathologist properly orienting the specimen before the specimen leaves the operating room (Dr. Garret Walsh and one of us)

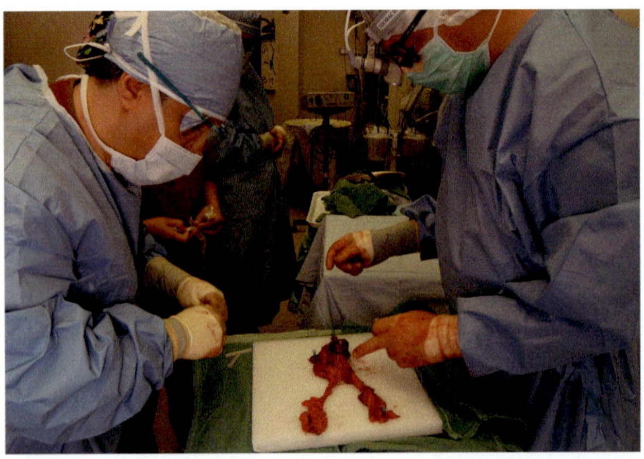

Fig. 7.5 The specimen is pinned down providing specific orientation

Once the specimen is oriented, we proceed to ink the specimen and, using different ink colors, identify specific anatomical structures of interest not only to the surgeon but

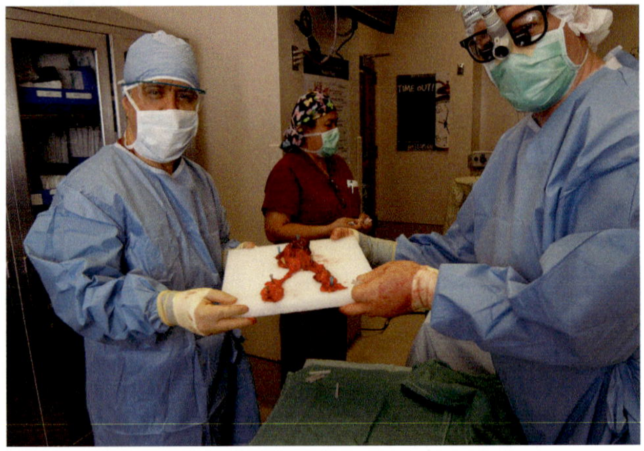

Fig. 7.6 Specimen is finally oriented and pinned down, ready to go to the pathology gross room

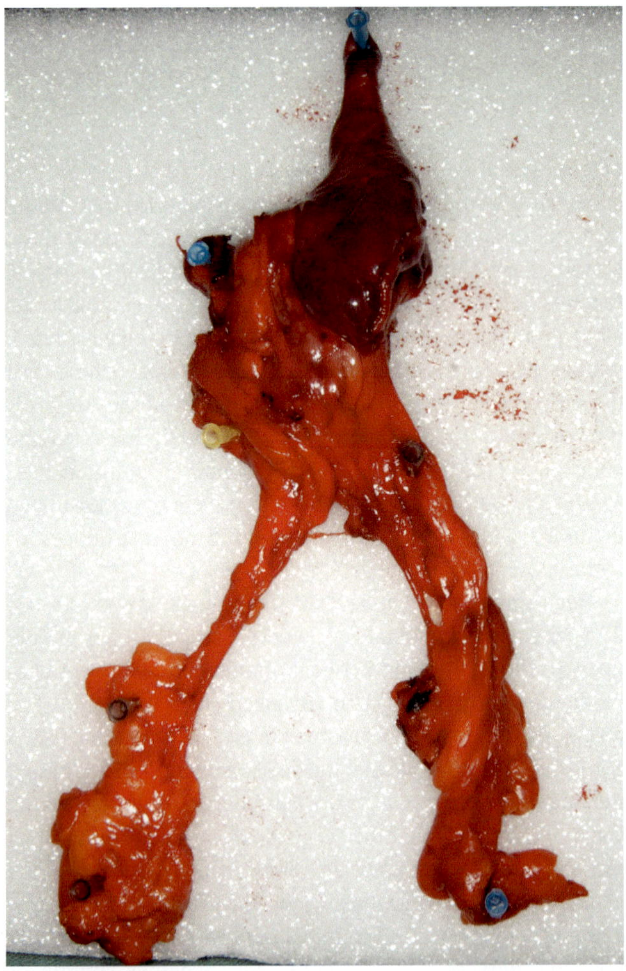

Fig. 7.7 The thymectomy specimen is received in the pathology gross room properly oriented

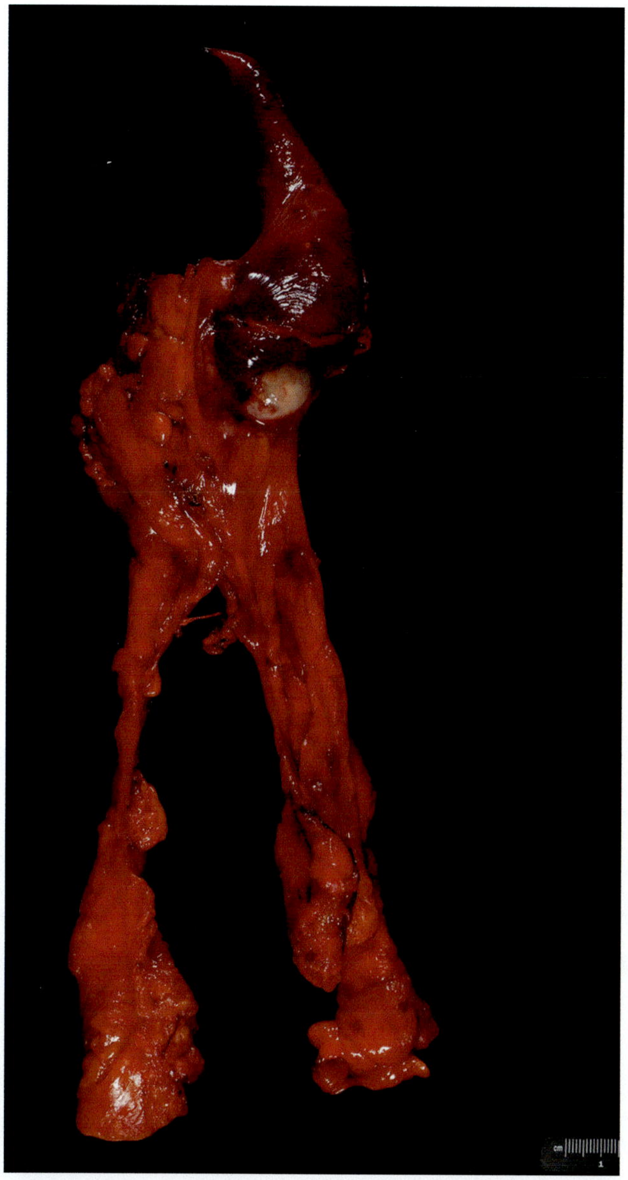

Fig. 7.8 The same case as Fig. 7.7. Now the specimen is grossly evaluated for invasiveness by the pathologist to determine which structures may be involved. In this particular case, the invasiveness of the tumor is obvious

also to the pathologist. Once the ink is applied, then we proceed to sample the specimen, preserving normal anatomic distribution and taking sections perpendicular to the capsule and perpendicular to the ink borders, paying special attention to the adjacent structures that may be available, or placing special attention on sampling the tumor in a manner that will help to easily determine whether the tumor is encapsulated or invasive (Figs. 7.15a, b, 7.16 and 7.17). In addition, depending on the size of the tumor, we sample at least one section per centimeter of tumor for tumors that are large enough. However, in tumors that are small, we submit the entire tumor for evaluation. This particular sampling not only is helpful in the final histological classification of the tumor but also diminishes the risk of any possibility of invasive areas in a given tumor [109, 120]. Needless to say, detailed gross description of the tumor is important; just as the tumor shows heterogeneous histology, so do gross features. Careful attention should be placed on the circumscription of the tumor. However, a common error that we have identified is the gross description in which the tumor is flat out called "encapsulated" only to later discover that under microscopic evaluation, the tumor has transcapsular invasion. Therefore, the ideal description for cases in which one suspects encapsulation is the use of a word such as circumscribed, well-defined, or other words that connote the possible noninvasive nature of the tumor. On the other hand, if one sees macroscopic evidence of tumor invasion in adjacent organs, not only it is important to describe the tumors as such, but also appropriate sampling needs to be performed. The gross description of the tumor is not to be taken lightly; it is important in the final evaluation of these tumors.

Gross Features

The macroscopic features that may be encountered in cases of thymoma are varied and need special attention. In general, the tumor may be small, only a couple of centimeter in

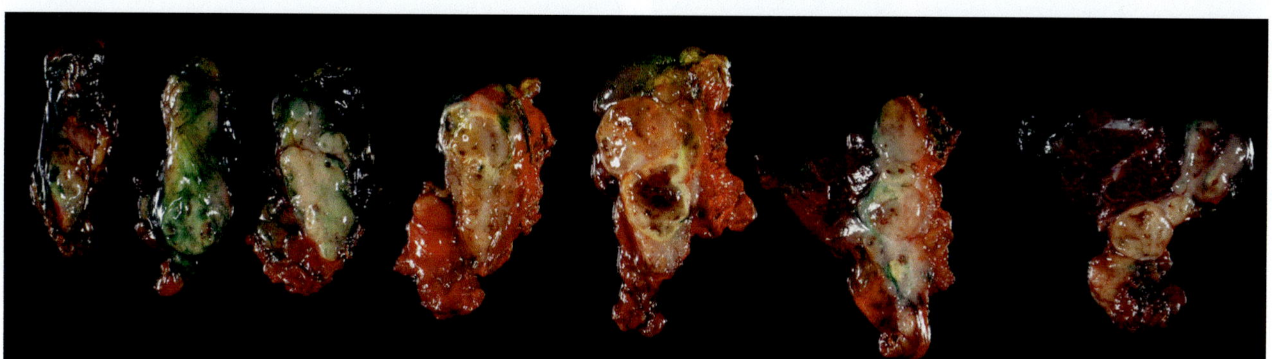

Fig. 7.9 The specimen is properly inked and sectioned preserving as much as possible its anatomical landmarks

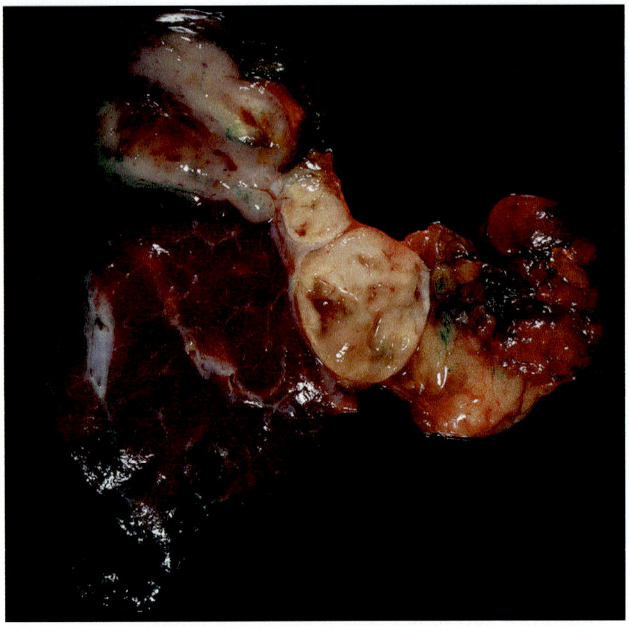

Fig. 7.10 Closer view at one of the cross sections of the specimen showing its infiltrative features

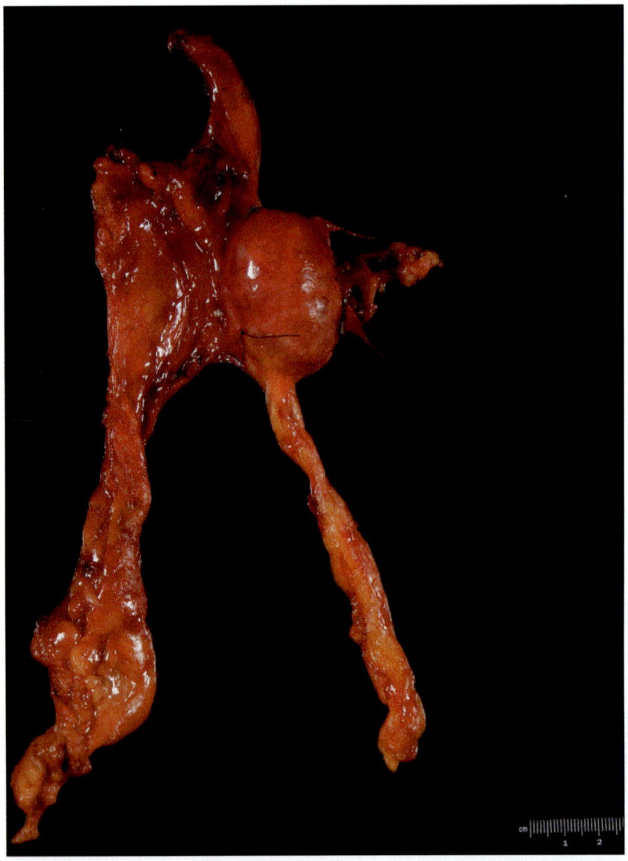

Fig. 7.11 Thymectomy specimen in which the tumor comes to the gross pathology room already oriented with specific markings; a double stitch is easily identifiable

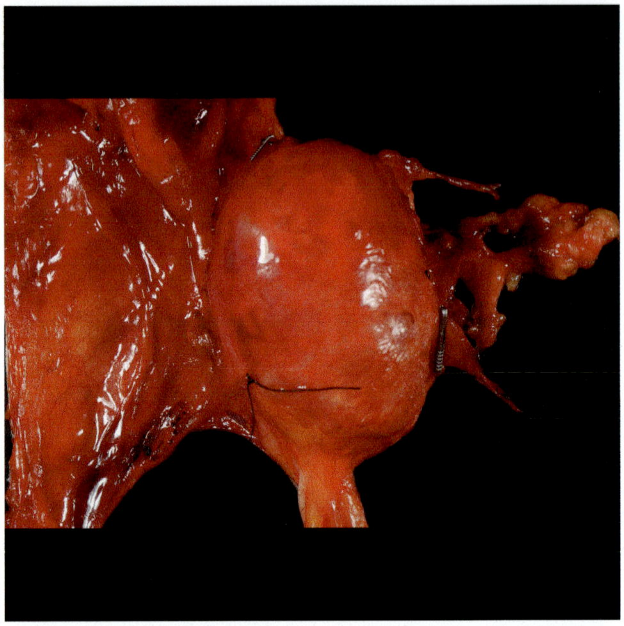

Fig. 7.12 Different aspects of the same specimen showing a long metal staple that provides further orientation of the specimen

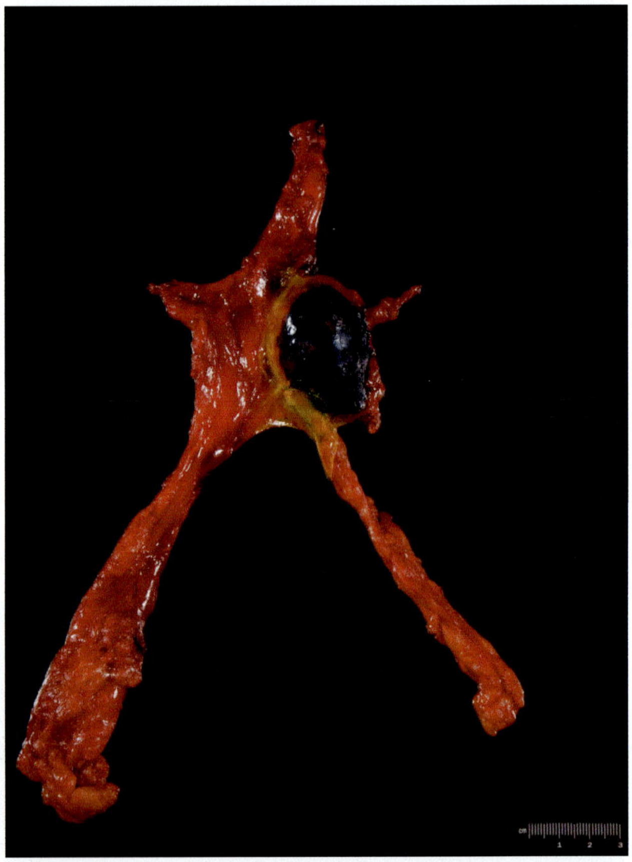

Fig. 7.13 Once in the pathology gross rooms, the pathologist follows the specific marking for orientation and inked those markings with different colors of ink. Note that the surgeon's markings are still with the specimen

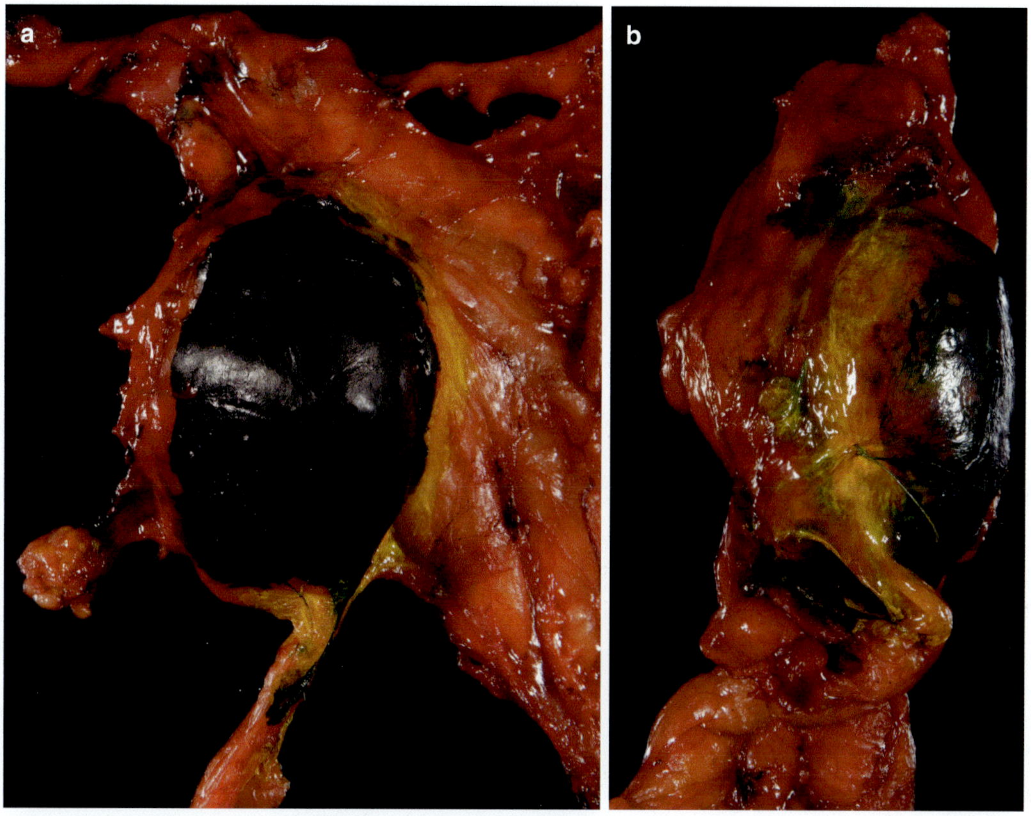

Fig. 7.14 (**a**) Closer view at the specimen showing black and yellow ink. (**b**) Still the markings are not removed from the specimen

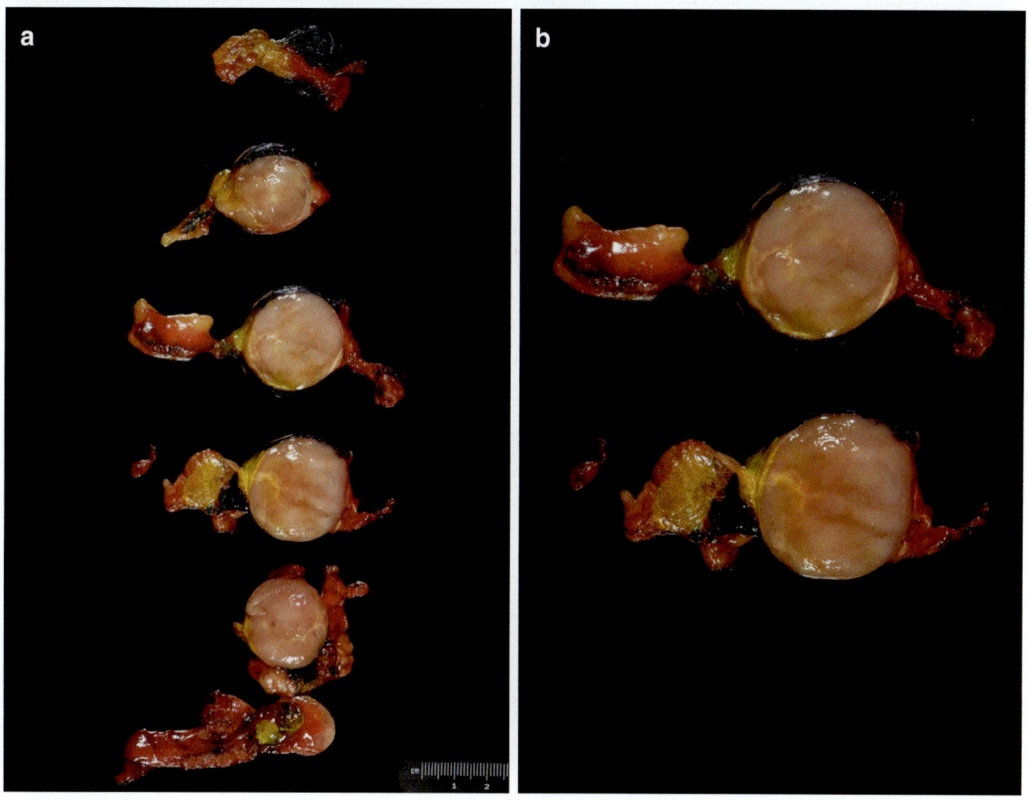

Fig. 7.15 (**a**) The specimen is serially sectioned in order to preserve its anatomical orientation and also to determine what sections will eventually be important to evaluate by microscopic examination. (**b**) Closer view of a couple of the cross sections of this thymoma

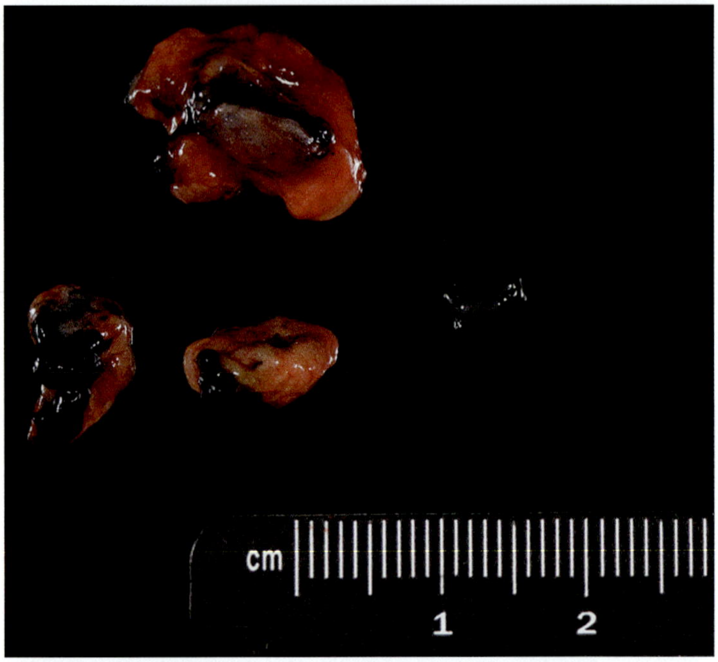

Fig. 7.16 We also advise that lymph nodes be removed at the time of surgery to properly document metastatic disease, and those are submitted separately and designated according to the anatomical station from where they were removed

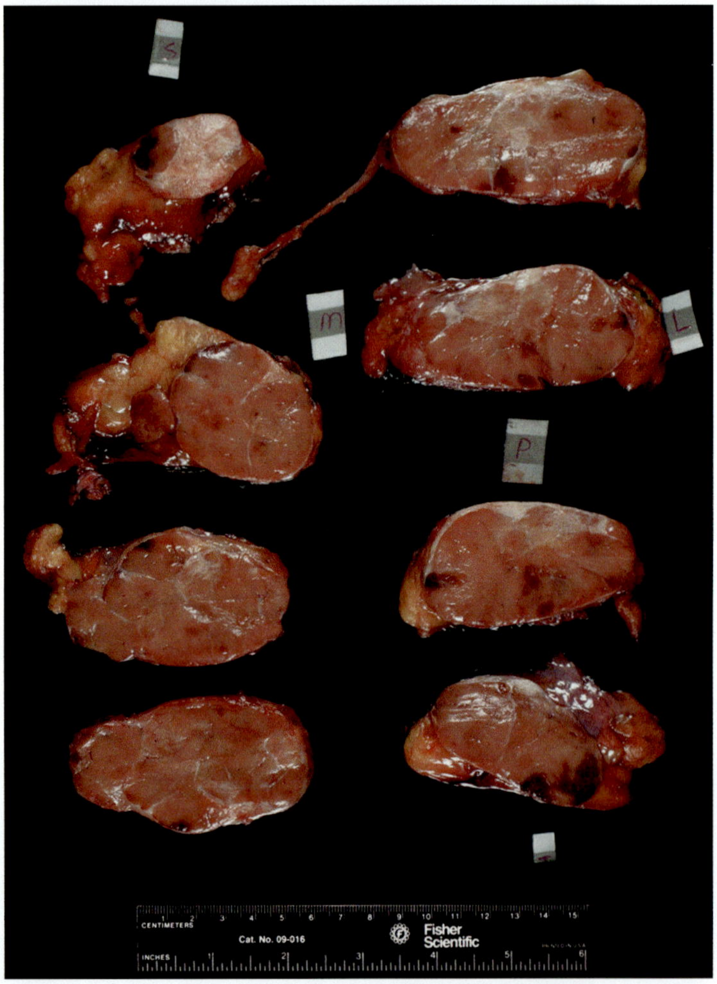

Fig. 7.17 A common practice for us in the gross evaluation of these tumors is not only serially sectioning the tumor to properly evaluate the possibility of invasion but also to provide our own markings (in this case letters) to determine from where the sections were taken, so that in case we need to go back to the specimen, we can find our way back to the area in question

largest dimension, or it can reach over 10 cm in greatest diameter. Therefore, it is important to pay closer attention to the macroscopic features of the tumor and try to correlate those with the histological characteristics of the tumor. Special attention should be given to:

1. Cystic tumor in which the cystic nature of the tumor may obscure the real underlying process. Tumors may show only focal cystic changes or prominent cystic structures similar to those seen in thymic cysts (Figs. 7.18, 7.19 and 7.20).
2. Cystic hemorrhagic and degenerative changes: these tumors are usually large tumors in which the tumor may show solid areas alternating with cystic areas. In some tumors, prominent hemorrhagic changes may be easily identified. Proper sampling of these tumors is essential (Figs. 7.21, 7.22, 7.23 and 7.24).
3. The surface of these tumors may also be smooth and showing streaks of fibrous tissue (Fig. 7.25). On the contrary, other tumors showed marked macroscopic nodularity (Fig. 7.26), while others still may show ill-defined borders and become suspicious for invasion (Fig. 7.27). It is very important to properly sample those areas.
4. Even in cases that appear to be well-circumscribed, we proceed with serially sectioning the tumor and then extensively sample the tumor (Fig. 7.28).
5. Even though in the majority of cases it is difficult to predict the type of histological features that any given tumor can have, in some cases, when the tumor shows solid areas accompanied with focal areas of degeneration, hemorrhage, or necrosis, we have been able to correlate those features with some atypical thymomas (Fig. 7.29a, b).
6. Contrary to primary thymomas, the macroscopic features of recurrent thymomas are different. In general, something that we have observed in our experience with 250 cases and from which we proposed our staging system is that primary thymomas generally involve adjacent structures by continuity. Essentially, the tumor overruns pleural, lung, or pericardium. However, in recurrent tumors, the tumor involves adjacent structures by the presence of several nodules of different sizes, which may be spread in the pleura, lung, and pericardium or in the mediastinal compartment (the so-called pleural dissemination) (Fig. 7.30a, b).

Histopathological Features

Even though great emphasis is placed on histological classification of thymomas, in daily practice, there is one important step that generally takes place before a resection is performed, and that is a mediastinal biopsy. This initial step is essential in the management of patents with mediastinal tumors, as this initial interpretation forms the basis for further treatment and the consideration for surgical resection. Therefore, in this section we will divide the interpretation of thymomas in two different aspects:

- Handling of biopsy material
- Interpretation of surgical resection

Handling of Biopsy Material

Contrary to the issue of sampling to document tumor heterogeneity of thymomas, biopsy material represents exactly the opposite. Even though there has been a review manuscript on the "guidelines" to report small biopsies from mediastinal masses [136], such a review is based essentially on supposition rather than on practice. The authors essentially listed in a table all the different tumors of the mediastinum, but, as the information is presented, it becomes apparent that there is lack of experience in dealing with some of the most pertinent issues. When it comes to the diagnosis of thymoma via mediastinal biopsies, some of the most important aspects that must be known are basic clinical demographics such as age of the patient, gender, and imaging. As we have pointed out

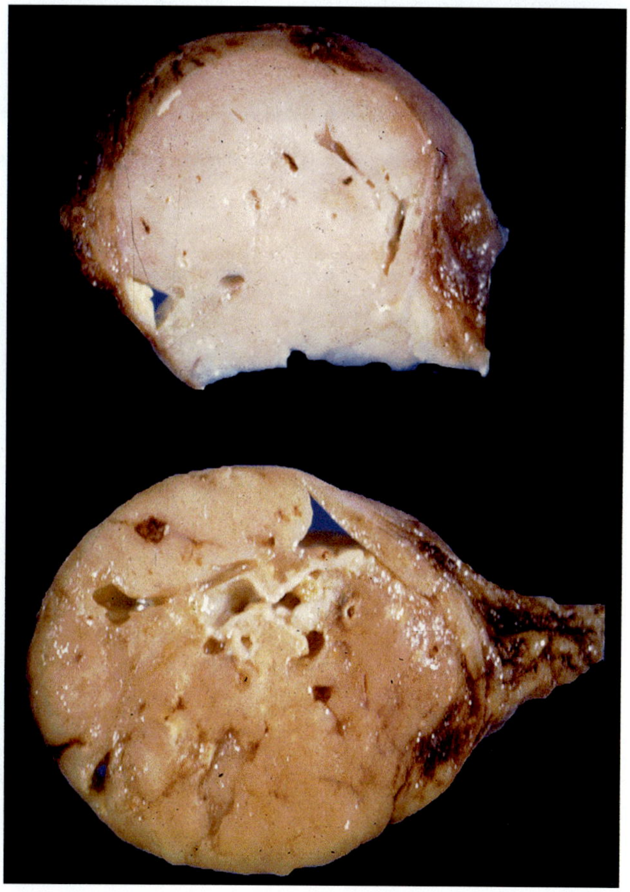

Fig. 7.18 Cystic thymoma in which the majority of the specimen is rather solid with only focal cystic areas

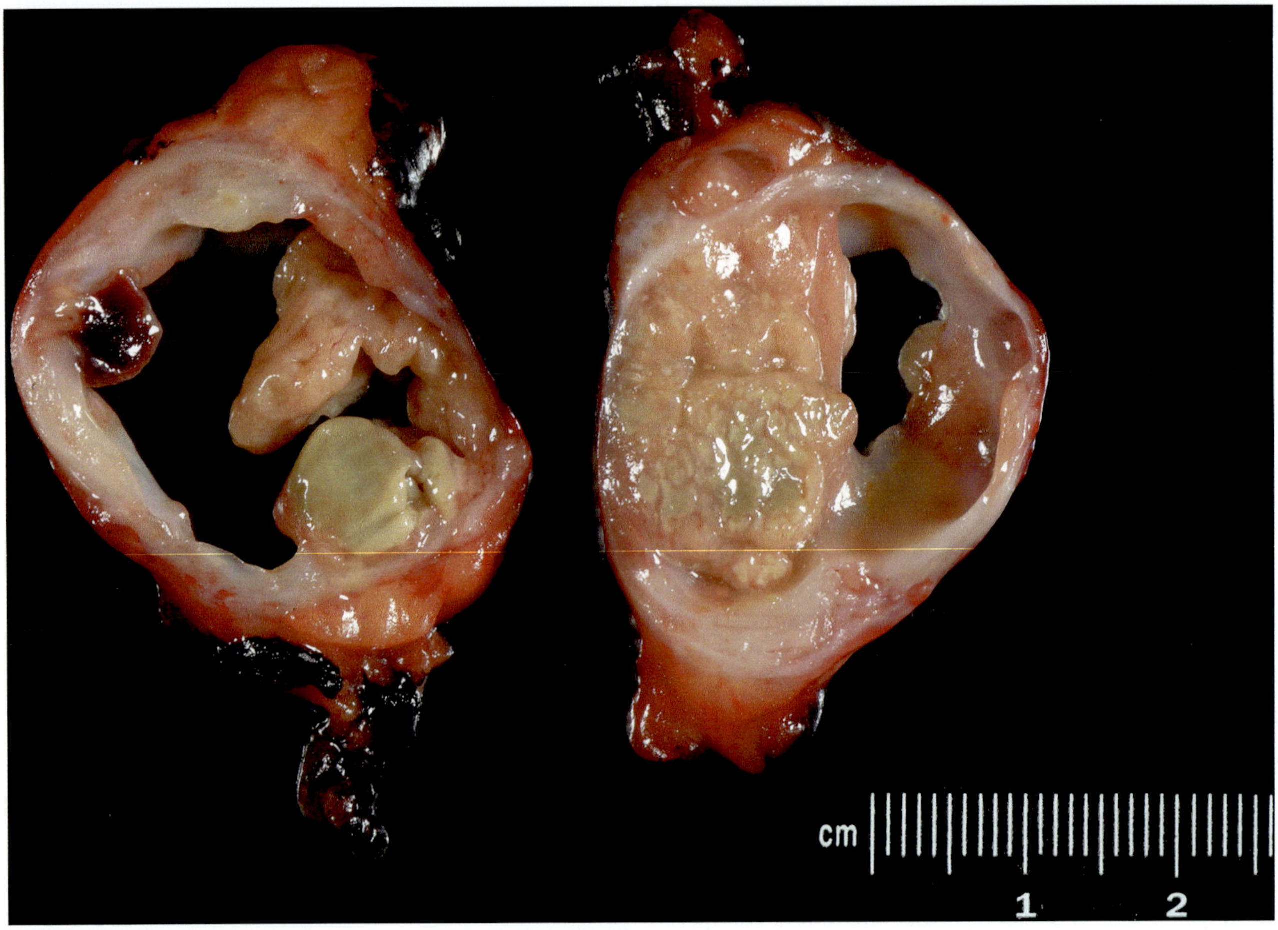

Fig. 7.19 Cystic thymoma in which tumor shows solid and cystic areas

Fig. 7.20 Predominantly cystic thymoma with focal areas of hemorrhage

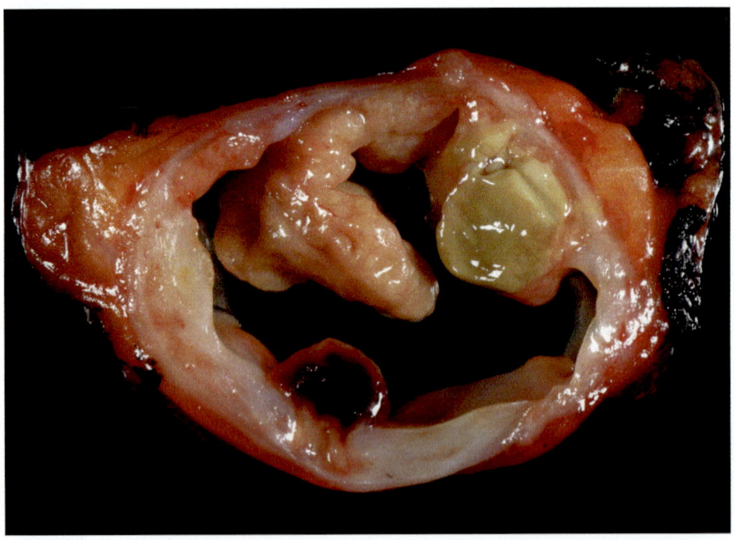

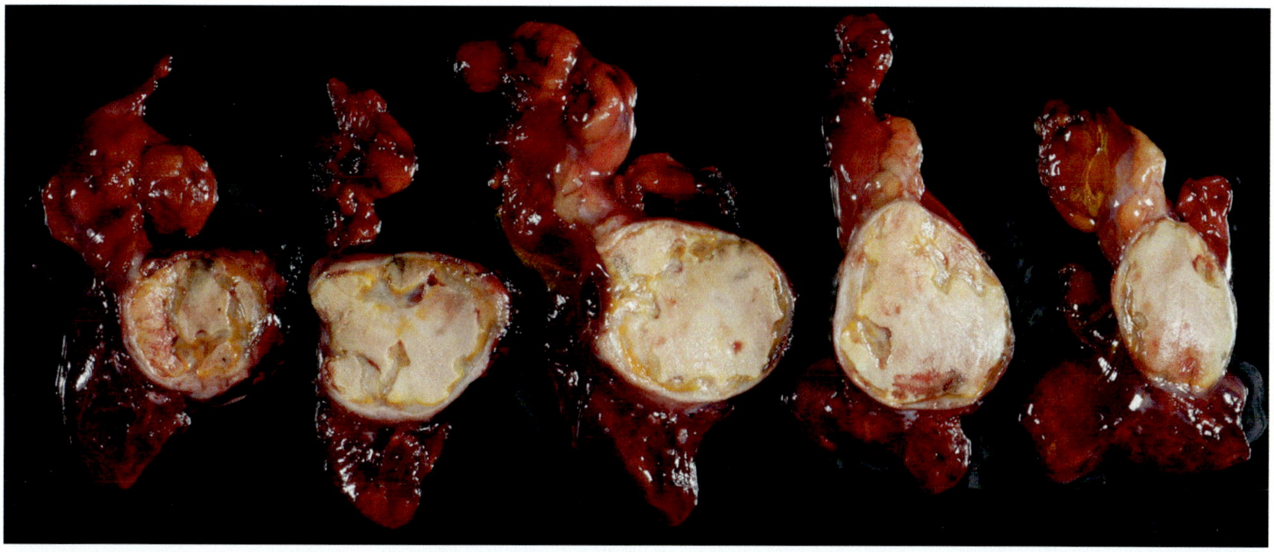

Fig. 7.21 Thymoma showing focal areas of necrosis and degeneration

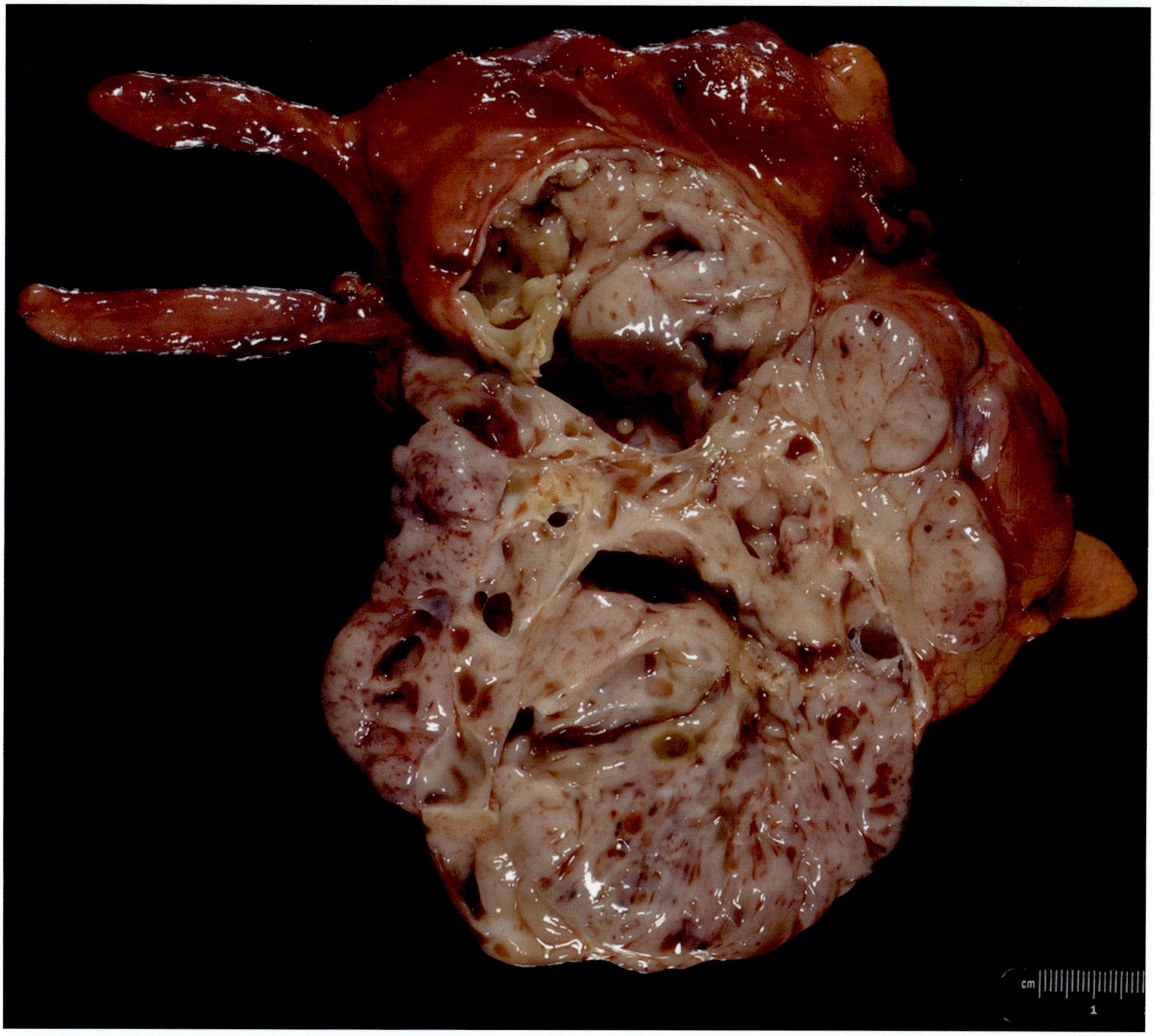

Fig. 7.22 Thymoma showing cystic, solid, and focal areas of degeneration

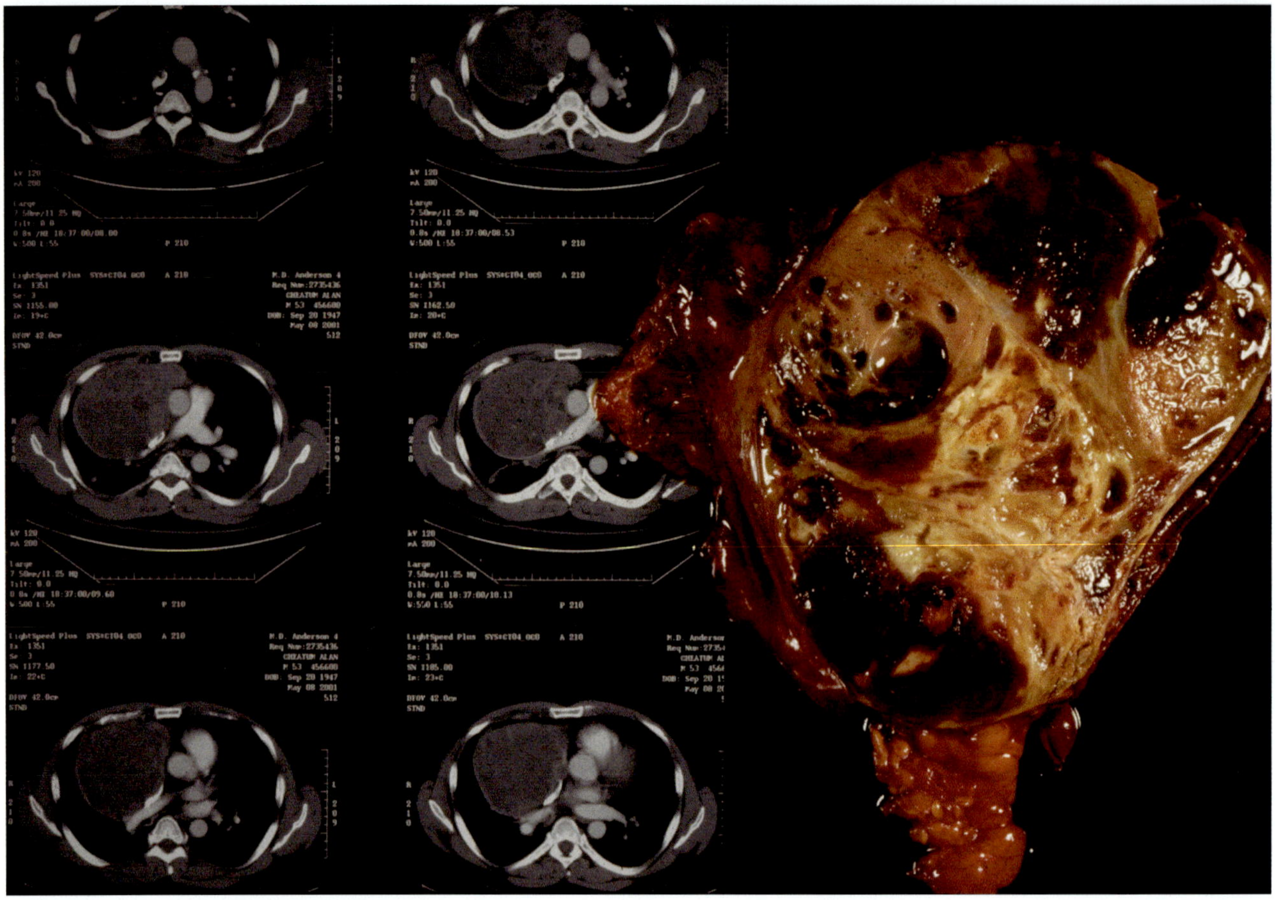

Fig. 7.23 Large thymoma showing areas of cystic and hemorrhagic changes; note the comparison with the thoracic films

previously in this chapter, the diagnosis of thymoma needs to be carefully considered in patients under 30 years of age, as, even though we are fully aware that they occur, they represent a small proportion. Gender becomes important; since the consideration is germ cell tumor (GCT), it is also known that GCT are tumors almost exclusively occurring in males. Therefore, since the authors of that review [136] mentioned every possibility in the mediastinum, they essentially lost perspective of the real interpretation of the biopsy material and the information that needs to be conveyed to the surgeon or oncologists. Any practicing surgical pathologist needs to know the information that the treating physician is looking for and communicate such information in unambiguous terms so that the patient is followed appropriately. The biopsy sample just represents a small snapshot of the tumor present in the mediastinal compartment. In addition, one important purpose for the mediastinal biopsy is to rule out the possibility of tumors that may not require surgical intervention, tumors that need to be treated initially with chemotherapy such as lymphoma or germ cell tumor, or any other tumors that may require different types of medical treatment.

Regarding specifically the issue of the diagnosis of thymoma in small biopsies, we recommend that, because of the limited sample available for interpretation, histological classification of the tumor should be carefully worded as there is more than a 50% possibility that, once a resection is available, the tumor in question will show mixed histologies, which in essence will dilute the use of any histological classification. In addition, we have observed several different scenarios that a pathologist may face during the interpretation of a biopsy specimen in which thymoma is the leading diagnosis:

1. *The sample is composed predominantly of lymphocytes.* Generally, the clinical history of a mediastinal mass is provided, and the biopsy is obtained. In this particular setting, there are some important considerations before a definitive interpretation of thymoma is made (Fig. 7.31a–d):
   (a) Normal thymus and lymphocyte-rich thymomas may look very much alike, and, even though one can perform immunohistochemical stains, the use of the most common stains in the setting of thymoma will also be positive in the normal thymus (see Chap. 1 in

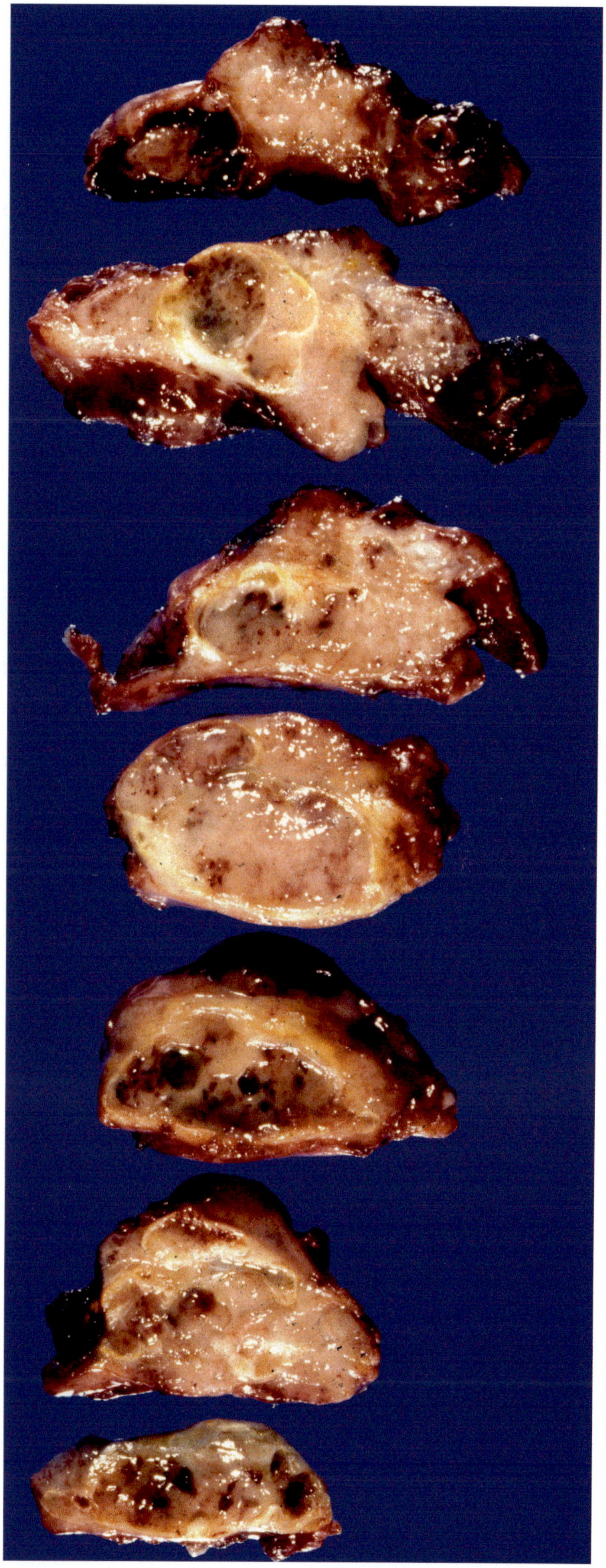

Fig. 7.24 Thymoma with degenerative and hemorrhagic changes serially sectioned

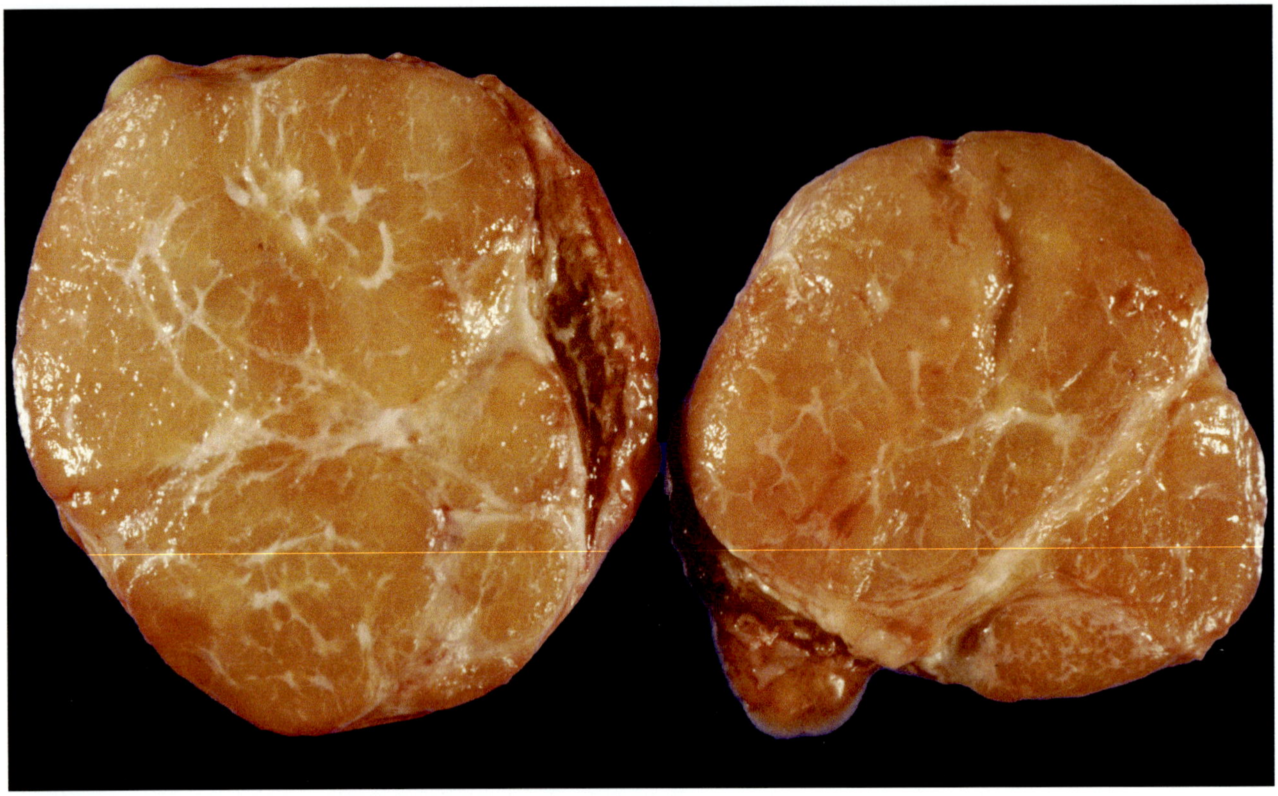

Fig. 7.25 Thymoma showing smooth surface and easily identifiable streaks of fibrous tissue, giving a lobular appearance of the tumor

this text). Therefore, final interpretation of thymoma may need to wait until after another possible biopsy is obtained or a surgical resection takes place due to the presence of an anterior mediastinal mass. However, it is important to keep in mind that in our experience, we have evaluated biopsies from primary mediastinal tumors in which the initial biopsy just shows normal thymic tissue, while the true neoplasm is of different lineage.

(b) *Thymic hyperplasia*: Often, the clinical information obtained in these cases is also of an anterior mediastinal mass. The biopsy will likely show abundance of lymphocytes, which in a limited sample may lead to the incorrect interpretation of thymoma. The same as with normal thymus, the immunohistochemical analysis of these cases will provide limited information. In this setting as well as in the setting of the normal thymus, the most important consideration to exclude will be that of lymphoma. However, ruling out lymphoma does not mean necessarily that the biopsy should be interpreted as thymoma.

(c) *Multilocular thymic cyst (MTC)*: One common feature of MTC is lymphoid hyperplasia, which in turn may be the site from where the biopsy may be obtained, thus, once again leading the possibility of interpreting the biopsy as unequivocal thymoma.

2. *The sample is composed of spindle cells*: This particular setting is also often seen in biopsy material. In this scenario, even though the interpretation may seem easier, the considerations are different:

(a) *Primary mediastinal spindle cell sarcoma:* It is important to be aware that primary sarcoma of the mediastinum, although rare, occurs, namely, as synovial sarcoma, monophasic variant. These tumors may also show positive staining although focal for keratin. However, in this setting, other stains such as keratin 5/6 may help in the final interpretation. In cases in which such concern is strong, then the use of molecular analysis is indicated (Fig. 7.32a, b).

(b) *Reactive spindle cells*: This represents another pitfall in interpretation, and we have seen this particular sce-

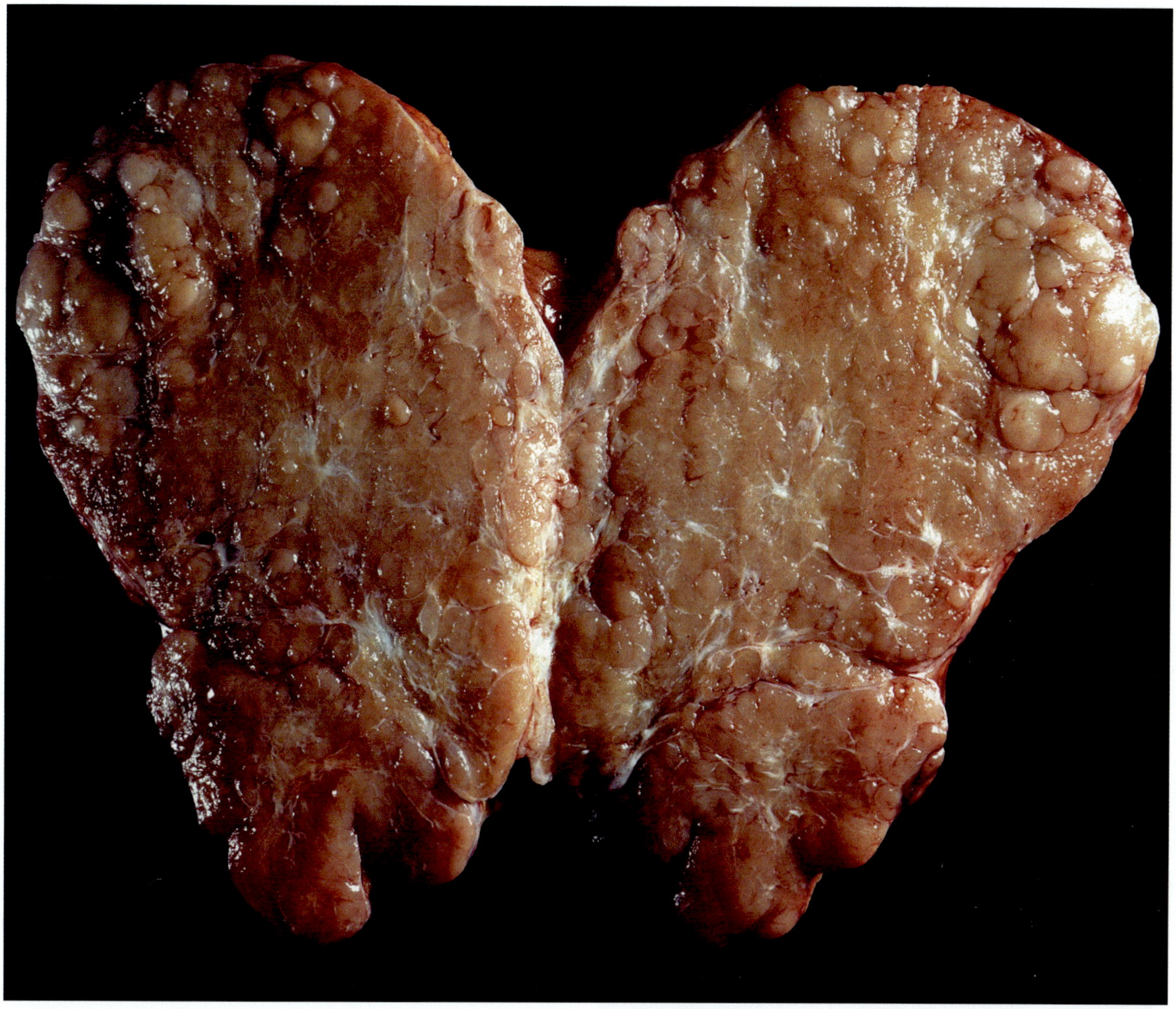

Fig. 7.26 Thymoma showing marked nodularity at the cut surface

nario in infarcted and hemorrhagic thymomas or in benign cystic lesions of the mediastinum, in which the biopsy most likely represents the fibrotic areas with reactive changes. Also in this scenario, the use of immunohistochemical analysis will provide limited value (Fig. 7.33a, b).

3. *The sample clearly shows a thymic epithelial neoplasm*: However, even though the sample is adequate for diagnosis, a clear distinction between an atypical thymoma and thymic carcinoma cannot be clearly determined (Fig. 7.34a, b). In such cases, even the most sophisticated immunohistochemical analysis may not be fool-proof for making such a distinction. In those cases, we advise to define the tumor as thymic epithelial neoplasm, and then to offer a comment about both possibilities, and the difficulty in arriving at a more definitive diagnosis. Such information, even though it may appear to be incomplete, is actually helpful as both entities – thymic carcinoma and atypical thymoma – are surgically treated, and one has essentially excluded the possibility of a germ cell tumor or lymphoma, which may require a different approach. However, in some cases, small biopsies can

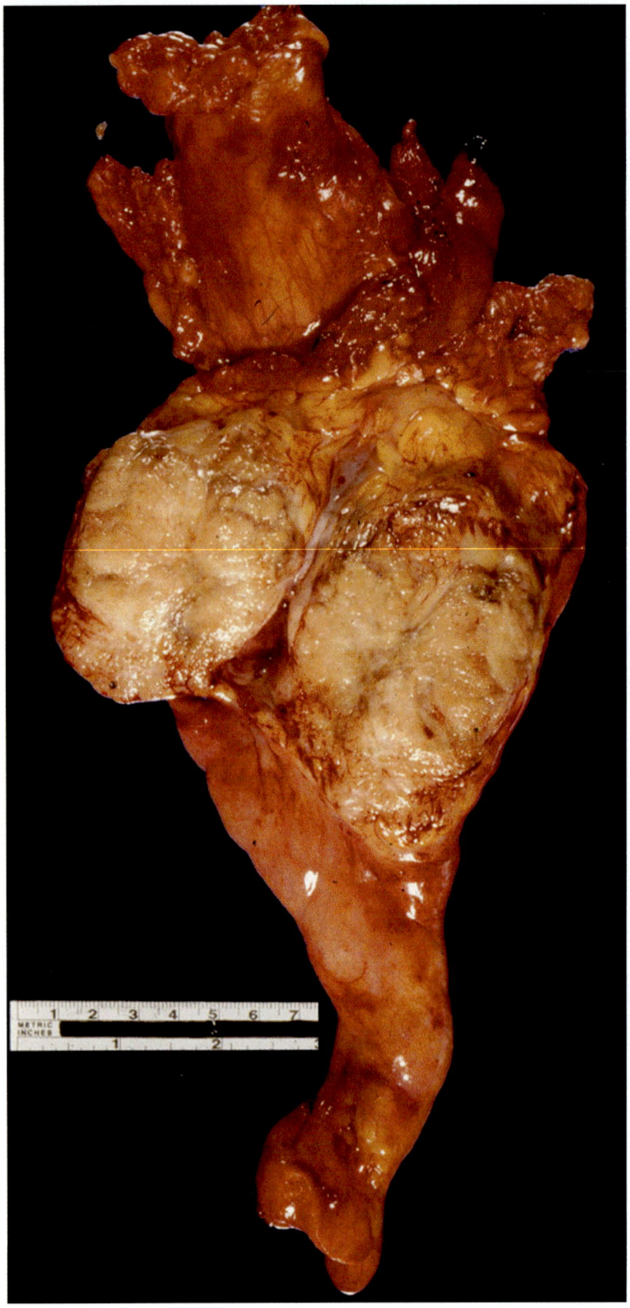

Fig. 7.27 Thymoma showing areas in which the tumor is at least suspicious for invasion

clearly point toward a more appropriate diagnosis of atypical thymoma (Fig. 7.34c–e).

4. *The sample shows thymoma and another malignancy*: This is the most unusual scenario, as to actually have two different tumors in a small sample is quite unusual. However, in this setting, one may overlook the presence of another tumor besides the thymoma, which may again impact the treatment options. We have had the opportunity to see unusual associations of not only spindle cell thymoma with carcinoma but also spindle cell thymoma and germ cell tumors such choriocarcinoma (Fig. 7.35a–e).
5. *The sample shows an unusual histology*: It is very important to keep in mind that thymomas are very heterogeneous tumors, which have no pathognomonic immunophenotype. Therefore, the presence of an unusual histology may prompt a different interpretation for an unusual case of thymoma, which may also impact treatment decisions.

Surgical Resections

As we have stated previously, we take particular interest in making sure that these cases get properly sampled. Once the sampling issue is done, then we analyze every component of these tumors and make a final interpretation for histological classification. In this final interpretation, we follow the nomenclature of thymoma (WHO types A, B1, and B2) and atypical thymoma (WHO type B3). However, it is important to highlight that the conventional histological classification is not always possible, and several specific growth patterns have been reported in the literature. Herein, we will address the conventional growth pattern and all those different specific types. In addition, we have included other growth patterns that over the years, we have been able to observe. Table 7.2 depicts the histological variability in terms of growth patterns that we have observed in thymomas. In addition, Figs. 7.36 and 7.37 depict the age distribution and the histopathological breakdown of thymomas.

Conventional Thymomas

Thymomas with Lymphocytes

As we have previously stated, in this group of tumors, we include those that have been recognized in different nomenclatures as lymphocyte-rich, cortical, WHO type B1, and mixed thymoma – lymphoepithelial, cortical, and WHO type B2. In our recent study of 1470 cases [29], these tumors represented 31% of the total and 51.9% of the invasive tumors in that category. Therefore, one can estimate that from the total number of these types of thymoma, half of these tumors may be invasive at the time of diagnosis.

Histologically, in the tumor in which the characteristic feature is the predominantly lymphocytic, the low power view of these tumors may show three different growth patterns: (1) lobulated growth pattern in which the lobules are separated by bands of fibroconnective tissue or extensive areas of hyalinization (Fig. 7.38a–d); (2) the tumor does not have well-formed lobules, but there is the presence of collagenous material admixed with the biphasic populations of lymphocytes and epithelial cells (Fig. 7.39a–d); and (3) diffuse growth pattern in which the tumor shows sheets of

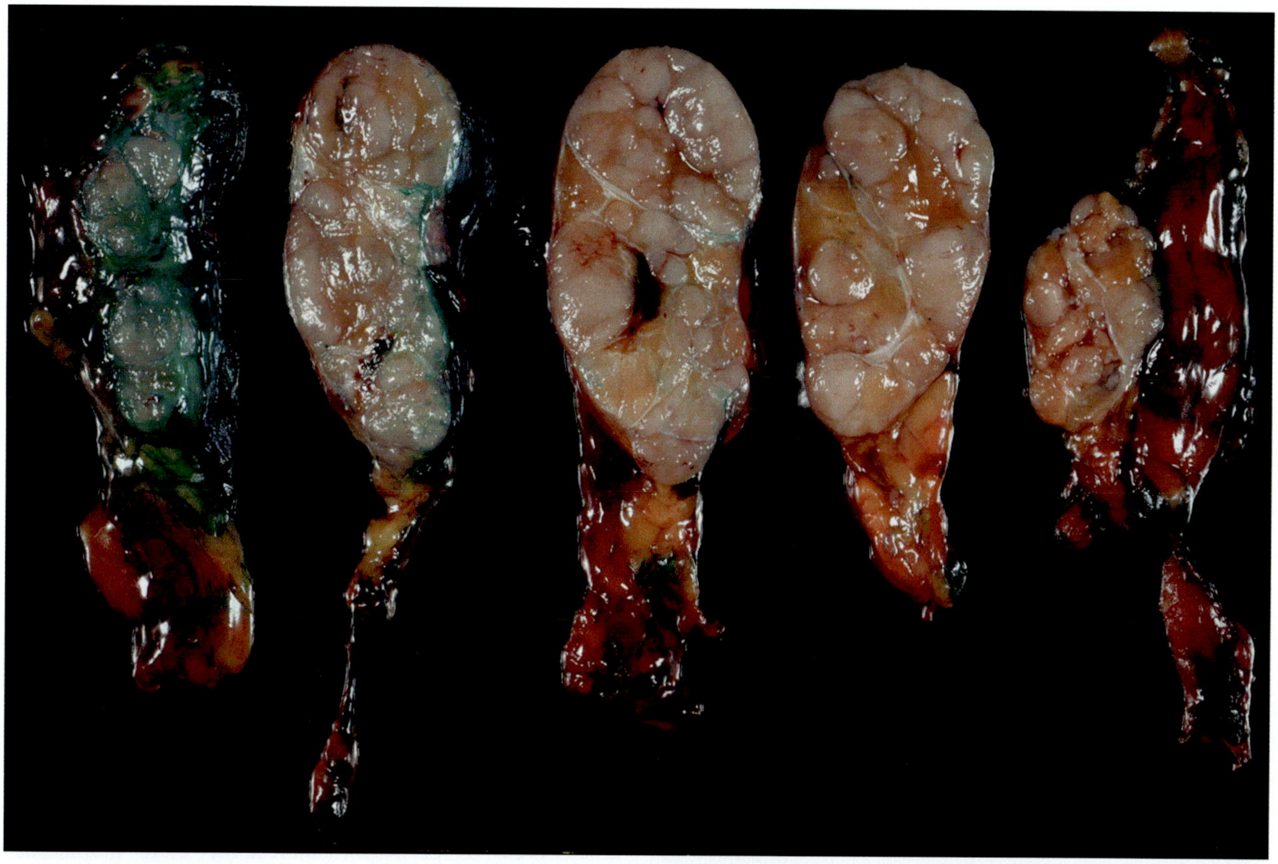

Fig. 7.28 Well-circumscribed thymoma serially sectioned to properly determine not only capsular integrity by microscopic examination but also to determine the areas that required sampling

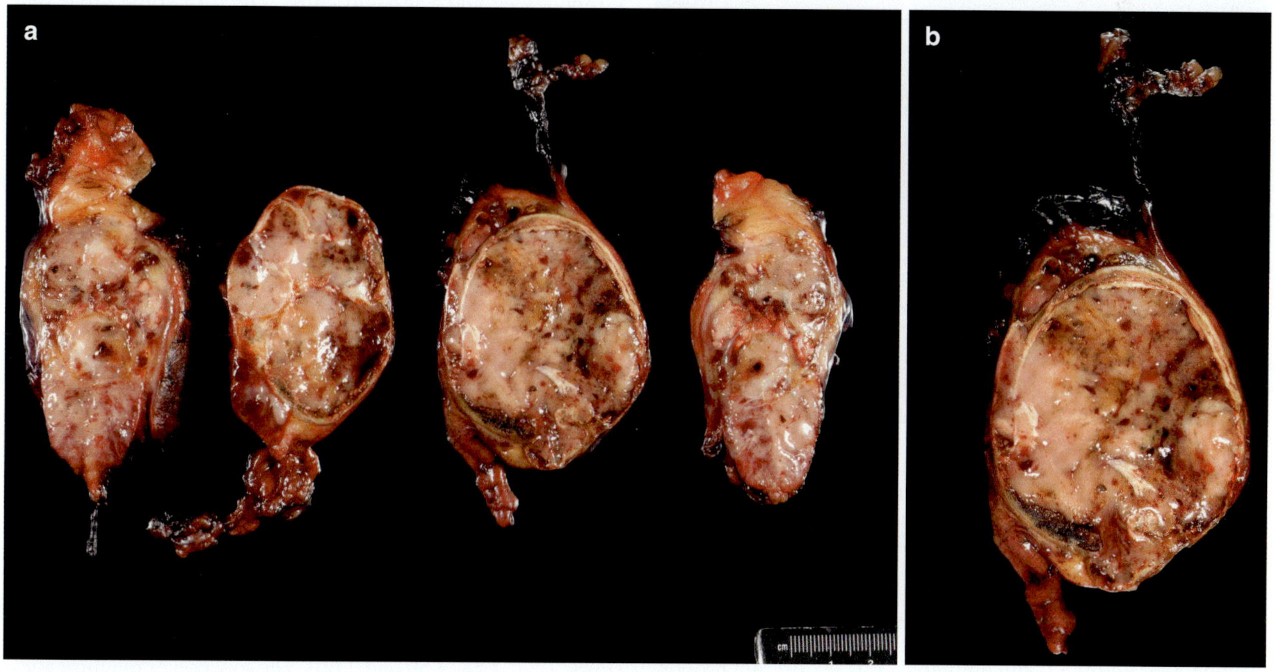

Fig. 7.29 (**a**, **b**)Thymoma showing solid areas admixed with focal areas of degeneration, hemorrhage, and necrosis. In our experience, in some cases these macroscopic changes should alert to the possibility of atypical thymoma

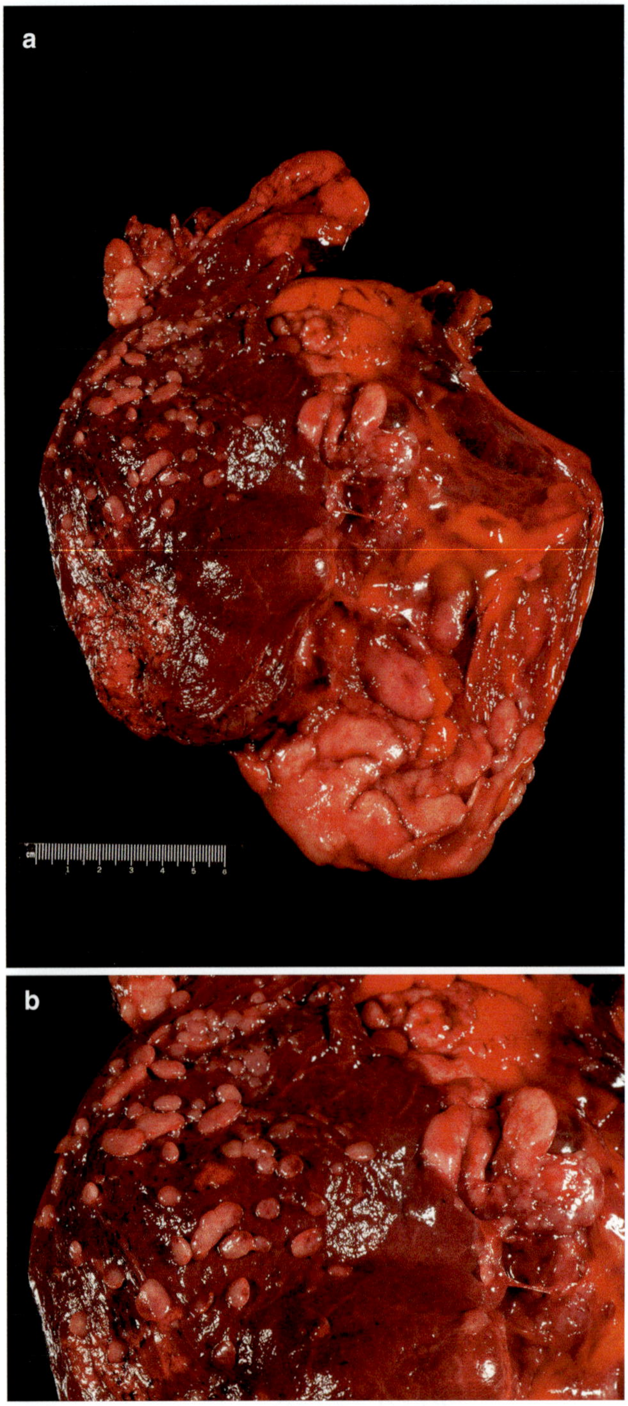

Fig. 7.30 (**a**) Recurrent thymoma showing multiple nodules in the pleura and lung, (**b**) closer view of the multiple nodules in the lung and pleura. This is a feature of recurrent thymomas, which likely has been termed "pleural dissemination." This type of pattern would be highly unusual in primary thymomas

lymphocytes admixed with epithelial cells in different proportions (Fig. 7.40). In some cases, the tumor may have dilated hemorrhagic areas, which may impart a vascular appearance to the tumor (Fig. 7.41). Higher magnification of these tumors characteristically shows predominantly lymphocytes with minimal component of epithelial cells. The lymphocytic component may show atypia and mitotic activity. In other areas, the tumor may show the characteristic perivascular spaces. The epithelial cells are of medium size with indistinct cell borders, round nuclei, and some with prominent nucleoli. Generally, mitotic activity is either minimal or absent within the epithelial component of the tumor (Fig. 7.42a–c). Other features that may be seen in these tumors include the presence of a germinal centers, and Hassall's corpuscles (Fig. 7.43), germinal centers without Hassall's corpuscles (Fig. 7.44), the presence of numerous Hassall's corpuscles (Fig. 7.45), and collections of macrophages (Fig. 7.46). In addition, the presence of perivascular spaces is a feature that helps in the diagnosis of thymoma (Fig. 7.47a, b).

On the other hand, in a tumor in which there appears to be an equal number of lymphocytes and epithelial cells, low power views can be similar to those with predominantly lymphocytes. The low power view may be of an invasive or an encapsulated tumor (Fig. 7.48). The tumor may show extensive lobulation with tumor nodules separated by thick fibroconnective tissue (Fig. 7.49) or extensive fibrocollagenous areas (Fig. 7.50a, b). In other areas, the tumor may show striking presence of vascular spaces (Fig. 7.51a–c). Other uncommon features may be the presence of extensive edematous areas (Fig. 7.52), cholesterol cleft granulomas (Fig. 7.53), areas of fibrinous changes (Fig. 7.54), or a pseudopapillary change (Fig. 7.55). Higher magnification of these tumors shows the presence of fairly equal number of lymphocytes and epithelial cells, which in some areas may have the presence of Hassall's corpuscles (Fig. 7.56a–c).

Spindle Cell Thymoma

Contrary to the conventional lymphocytic thymomas, spindle cell thymomas may show high variability in their growth patterns [137]. Although the basic morphology is that of a spindle cellular proliferation composed of fusiform cells with scant cytoplasm, elongated nuclei, dispersed chromatin, and inconspicuous nucleoli, the tumor cells may be arranged in ways that may mimic other epithelial or mesenchymal neoplasm. The specific growth patterns that have been described for these tumors are presented separately in this chapter. From the statistical point of view, spindle cell thymomas represent approximately 13% of the bulk of thymomas. Herein, we will highlight some other features that we have encountered in our daily practice (Fig. 7.36).

Spindle cell thymomas, just like any other histopathological type, can be either an encapsulated tumor, minimally invasive, or invasive involving adjacent anatomical structures (Figs. 7.57, 7.58, 7.59 and 7.60). The low power magnification of these tumors can show essentially different growth patterns: (1) lobulated, (2) diffuse, and (3) vascular or HPC growth pattern (Figs. 7.61, 7.62, 7.63, 7.64 and 7.65). In the diffuse

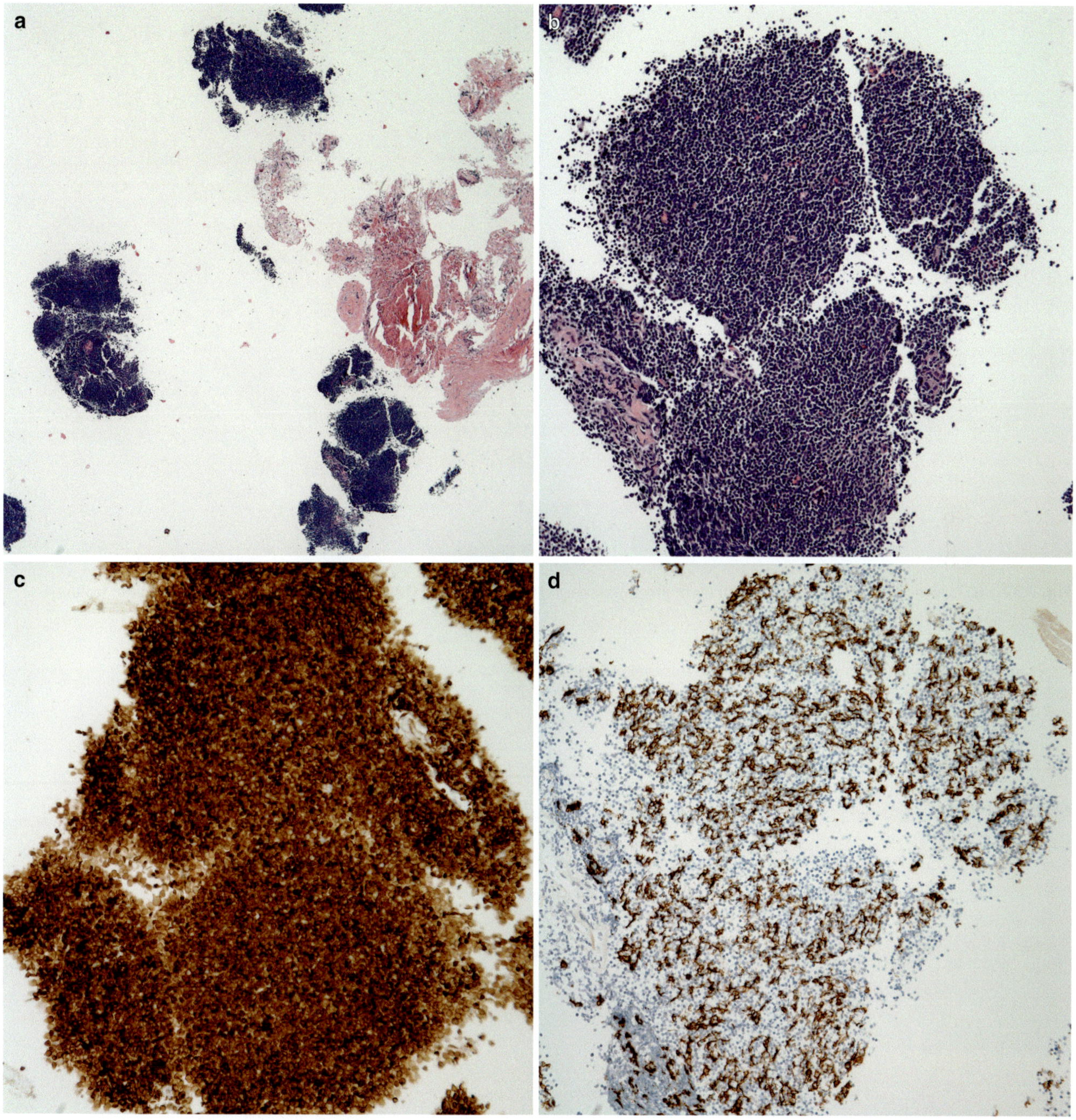

Fig. 7.31 (**a**) Mediastinal biopsy in which the low power is that of predominantly lymphocytic proliferation. (**b**) Higher magnification shows a dual population of lymphocytes and epithelial cells. (**c**) CD3 shows strong positive reaction basically obscuring the presence of epithelial cells. (**d**) Keratin stain showing the presence of epithelial cells. Once again, these features could be seen in thymoma, normal thymus, or thymic lymphoid hyperplasia

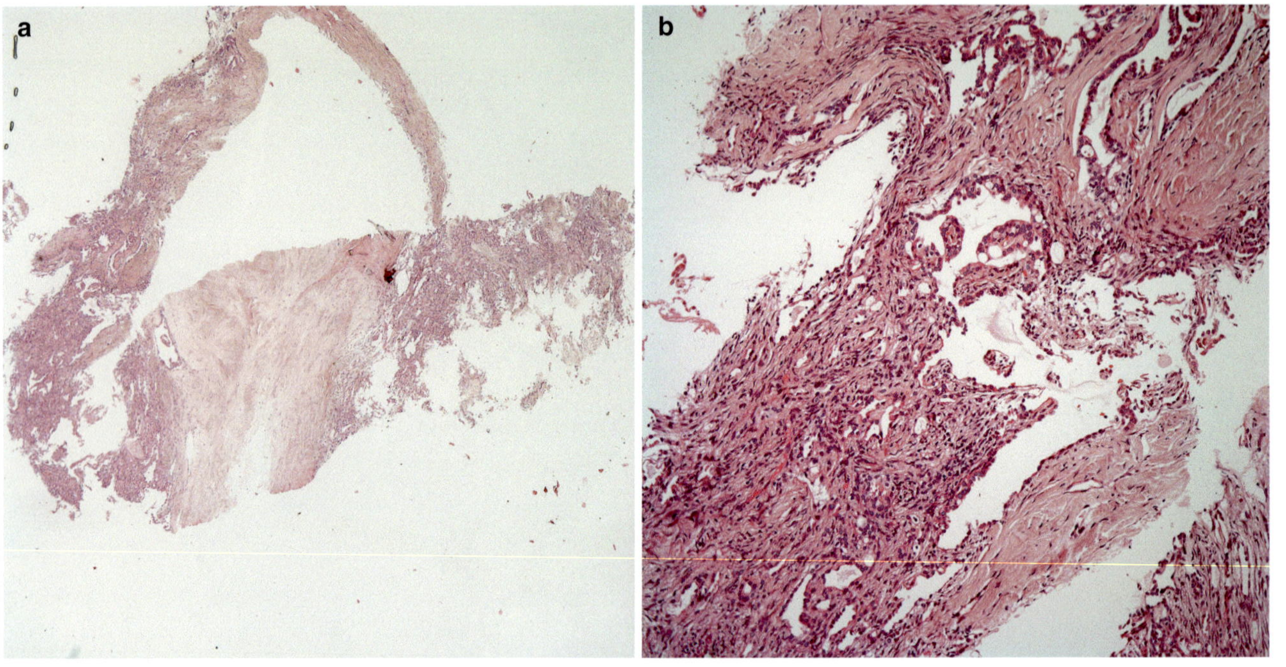

Fig. 7.32 (**a**) Low power view of a spindle cell thymoma mimicking synovial sarcoma. (**b**) It appears as if the tumor has biphasic features

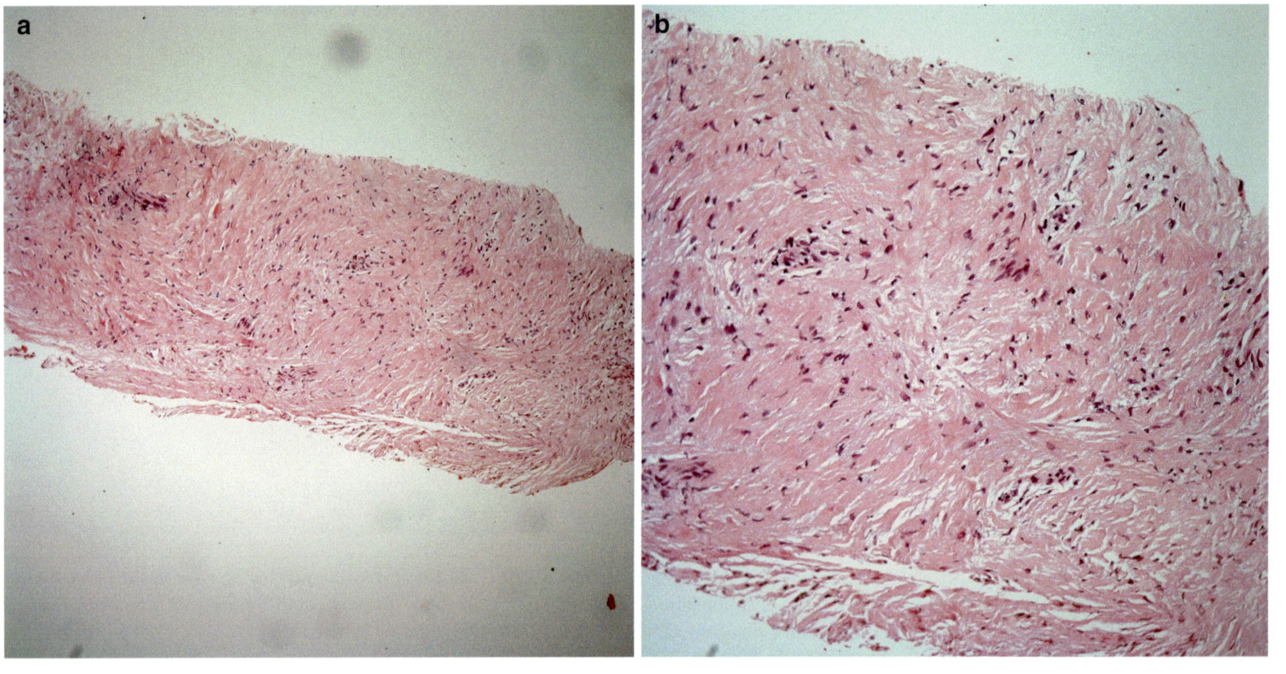

Fig. 7.33 (**a**) Low power view of a mediastinal biopsy showing dense fibrocollagenous tissue, (**b**) higher magnification showing some spindle cells (fibroblasts)

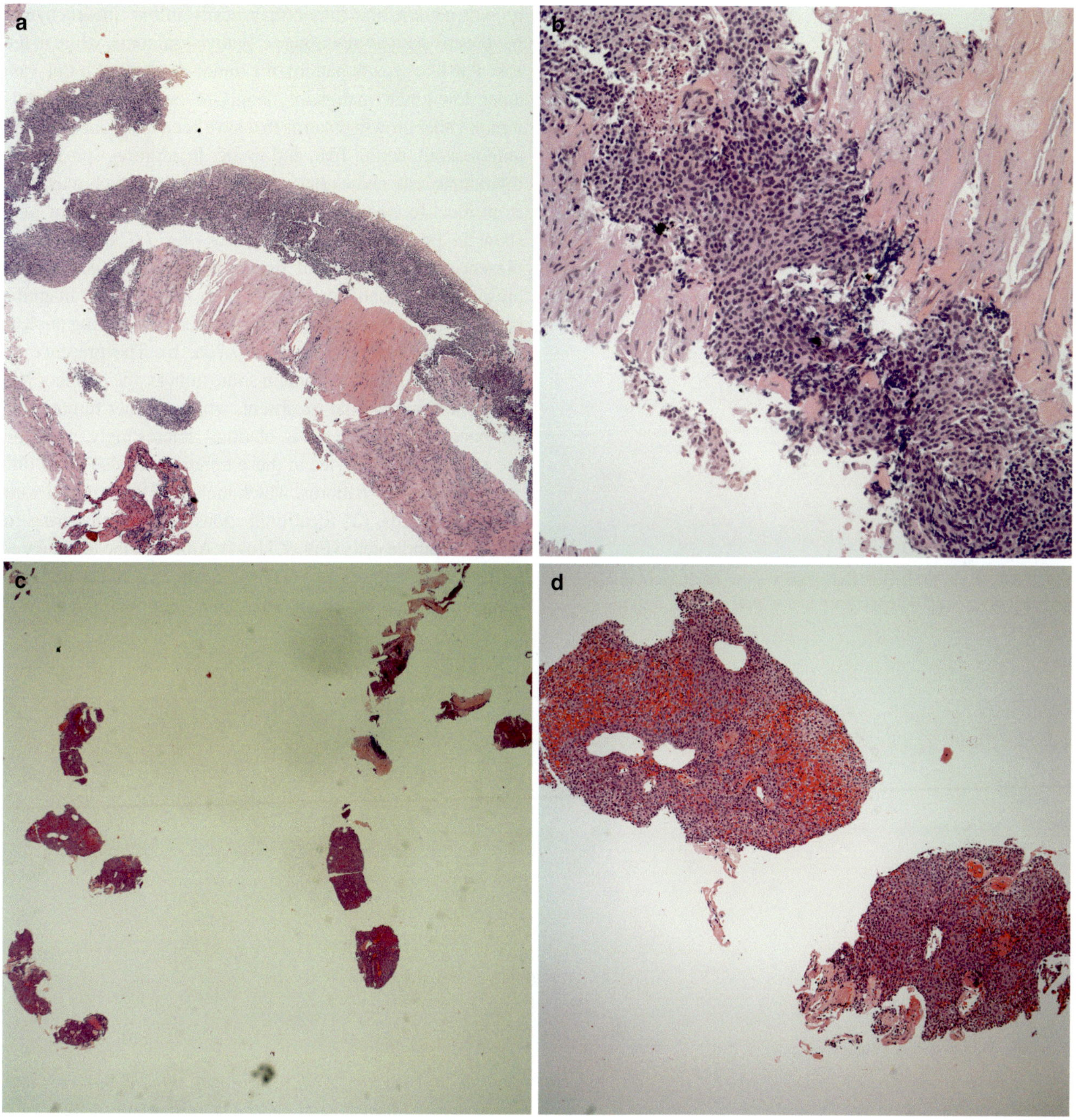

Fig. 7.34 (**a**) Low power view of a mediastinal biopsy which even at this power shows an epithelial neoplasm. (**b**) Higher magnification may create problems in interpretation as to whether it represents atypical thymoma or thymic carcinoma. (**c**) Panoramic view of a mediastinal biopsy. (**d**) The histological features are highly suggestive of an atypical thymoma

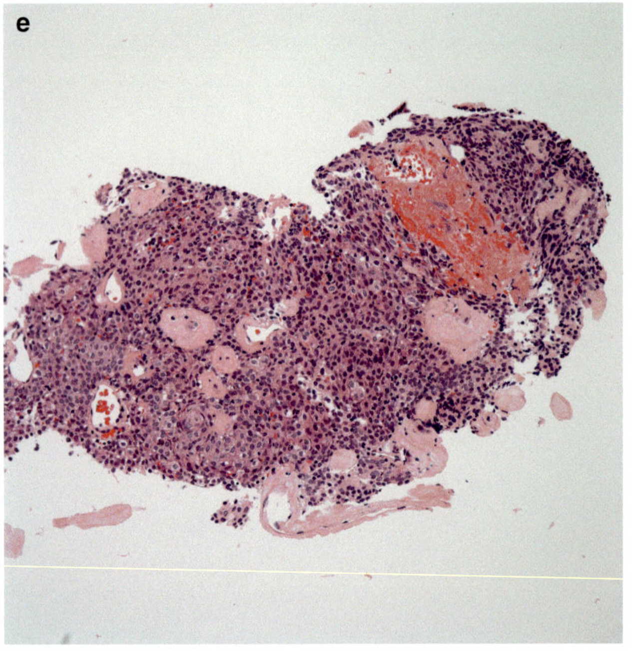

Fig. 7.34 (continued) (**e**) High power view most compatible with atypical thymoma; note the presence of perivascular spaces

growth pattern, the tumor may easily mimic mesenchymal neoplasms such as monophasic synovial sarcoma, while in the vascular-like growth pattern, the tumor may mimic a true vascular low-grade malignant neoplasm or a solitary fibrous tumor. Other growth patterns that have been mentioned include angiomatoid, neural-like, and cystic. In addition, spindle cell thymomas may show areas of hyalinization, which may vary from focal to extensive (Fig. 7.66a–f). Also, the tumor may show the presence of vascular spaces (Fig. 7.67a–d), variable presence of collections of macrophages (Fig 7.68a–d), and presence of Hassall's corpuscles (Fig. 7.69). Higher magnification is that of a spindle cellular proliferation lacking nuclear atypia or mitotic activity (Fig. 7.70a, b). The presence of lymphocytes is variable, and in some tumors, the lymphocytic component is minimal or absent, while in other tumors, the presence of lymphocytes is obvious. Interestingly, even the presence of lymphocytes in these tumors may also show different distribution patterns, which include (1) intermixed with the spindle cells, (2) focal collections, and (3) clustering in between spindle cells (Fig. 7.71a–f). Although the tendency is to label these tumors as WHO type AB, it is likely that this approach is incorrect as they basically represent spindle cell

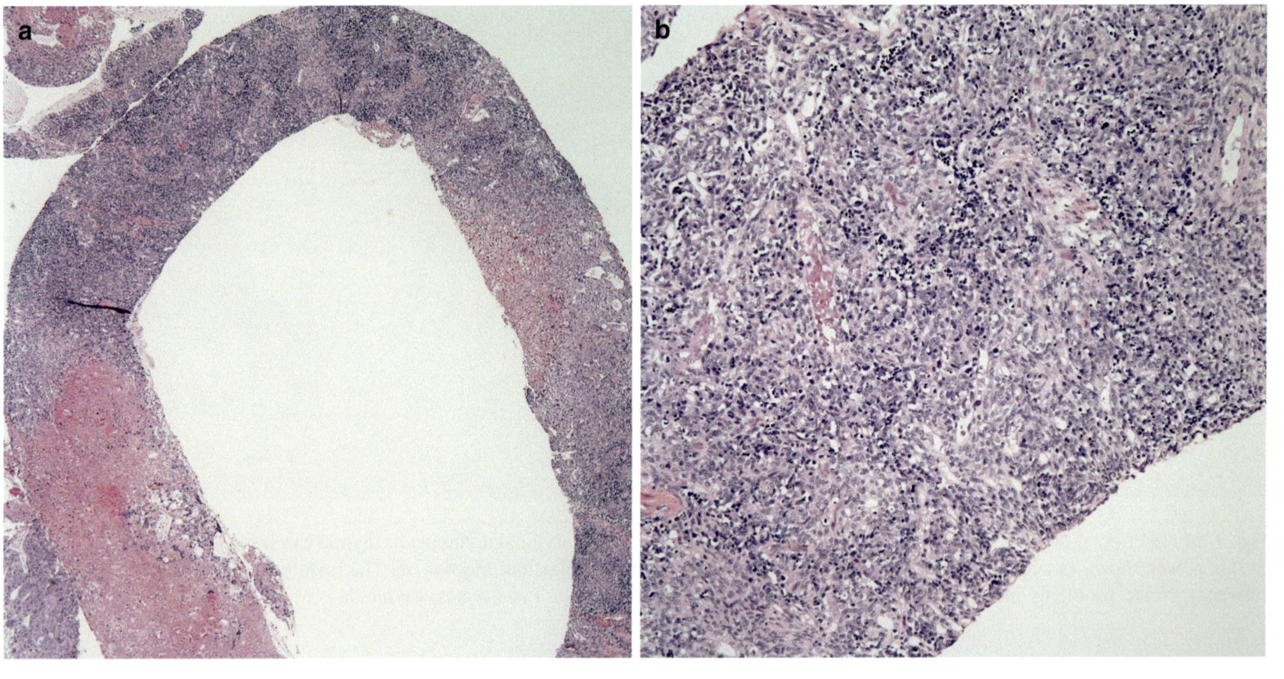

Fig. 7.35 (**a**) Low power view of a mediastinal biopsy showing an unequivocal neoplasm, (**b**) some areas show conventional thymoma

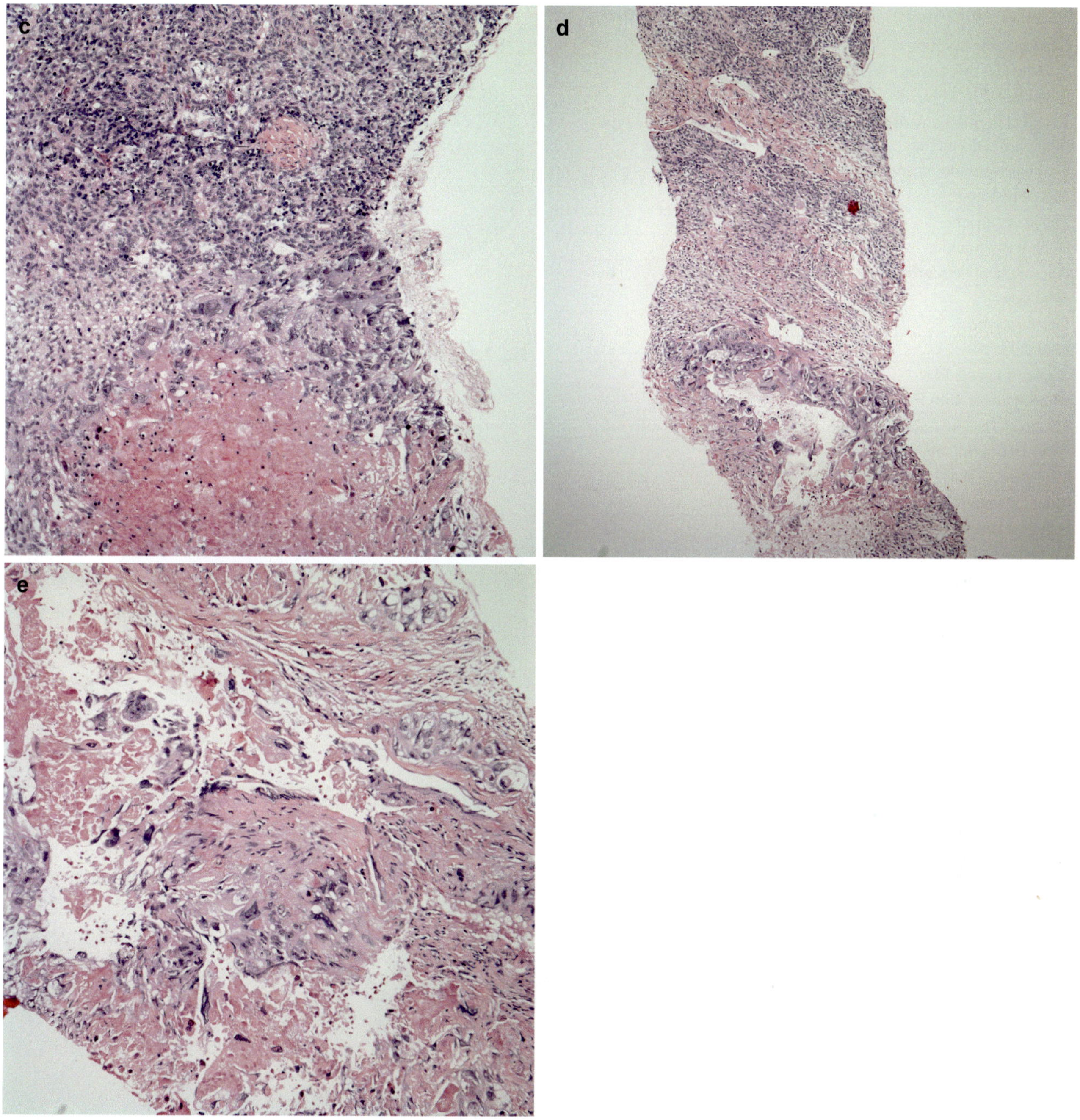

Fig. 7.35 (continued) (**c**) Conventional thymoma mergin with a high-grade malignancy with necrosis (choriocarcinoma), (**d**) different view of a spindle cell thymoma with adjacent choriocarcinoma, (**e**) high power view of choriocarcinoma

Table 7.2 Different growth patterns associated with thymomas

Lymphocytic thymomas (WHO type B1, B2)
Spindle cell thymomas (WHO type A)
Atypical (WHO type B3)
Atypical thymoma with pseudosarcomatous stroma (WHO type metaplastic thymoma)
Combined thymoma and thymic carcinoma
Mixed histologies
Plasma cell rich
Rhabdomyomatous
Necrotic and hemorrhagic
Mucinous
Desmoplastic
Glandular
Signet ring cell-like
Micronodular with B-cell hyperplasia
Cystic and cystic micronodular
Neuroendocrine morphology
Papillary
Ancient changes
Adenomatoid
Giant cells
Other unusual features
Myxoid/edematous
Hydropic-like changes
Alveolar
Angiomatous
Sebaceous
Microvesicular
ameloblastoma-like
Synovial sarcoma-like
Neural-like

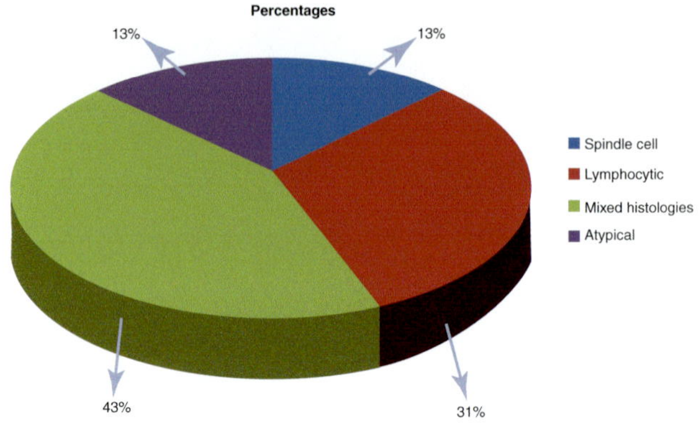

Fig. 7.36 Histological distribution of thymomas based on 1470 cases

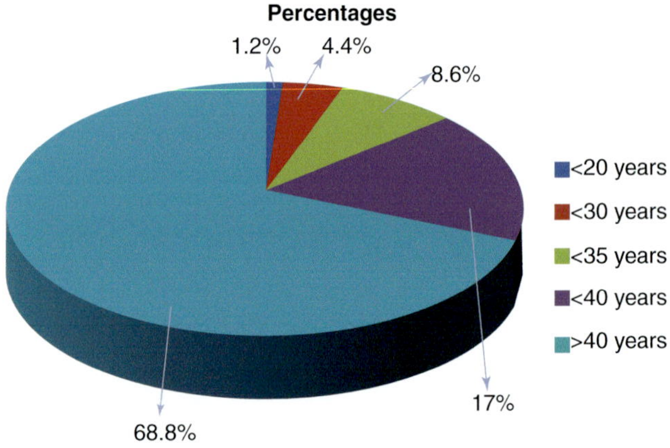

Fig. 7.37 Distribution of thymomas according to age, based on 1470 cases

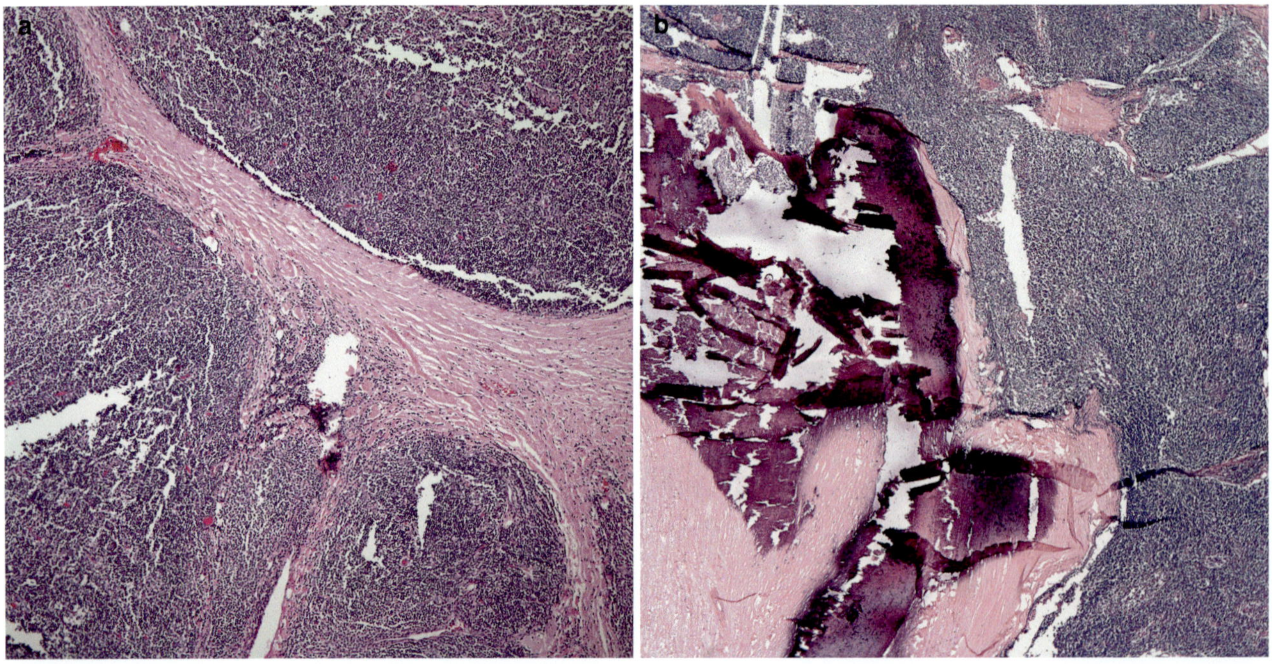

Fig. 7.38 (**a**) Lymphocytic thymoma showing lobulation and thick fibrous bands, (**b**) areas of calcification in fibrous bands

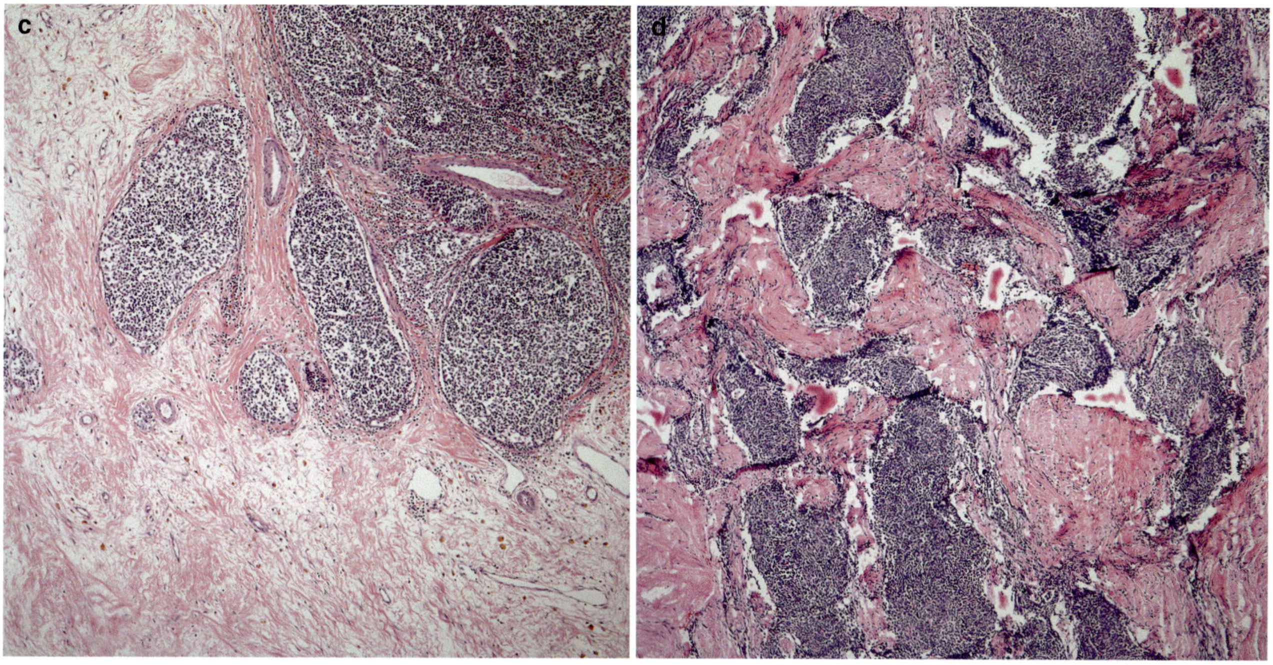

Fig. 7.38 (continued) (**c**) Extensive areas of hyalinization, (**d**) fibrocollagenous bands without forming clear lobulation

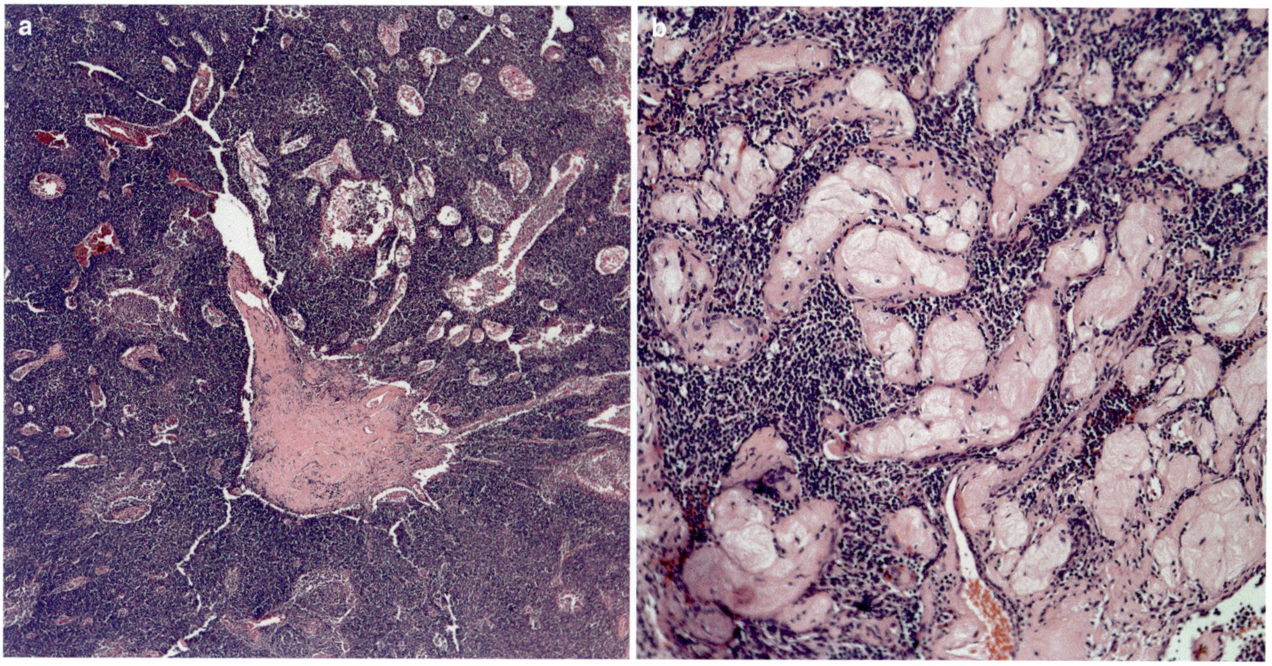

Fig. 7.39 (**a**) Lymphocytic thymoma showing vascular spaces and a central area of hyalinization, (**b**) nodular arrangement of hyalinized areas

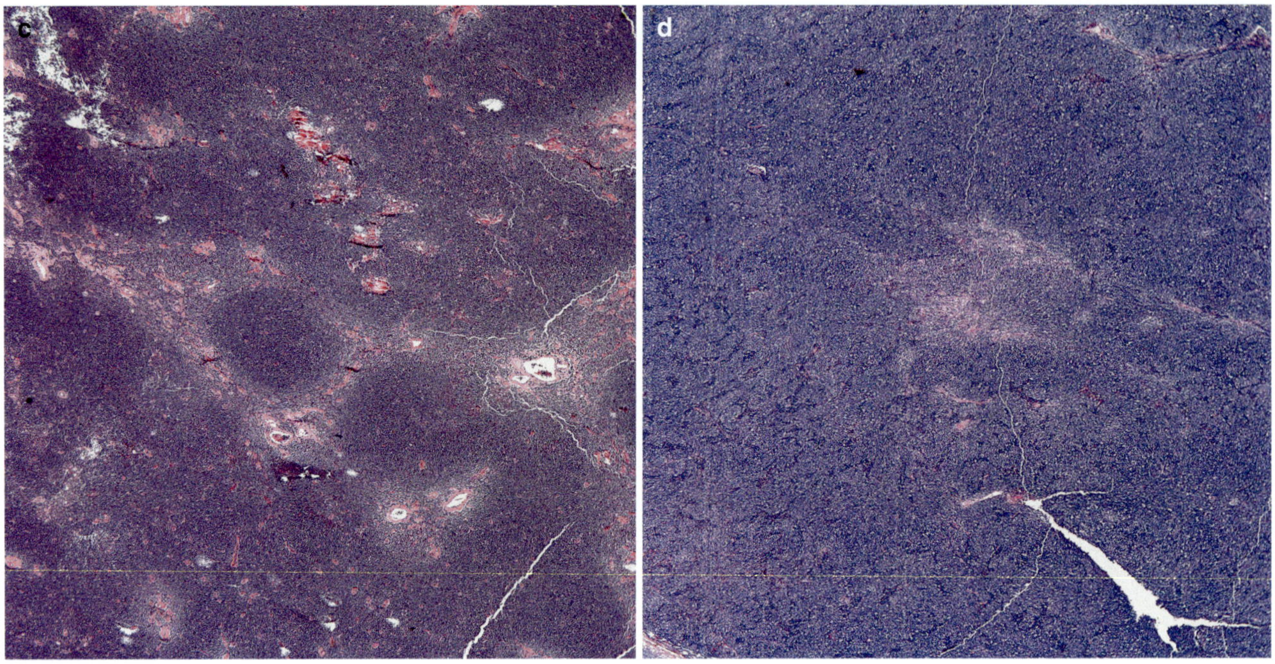

Fig. 7.39 (continued) (**c**) Lymphocytic thymoma with more diffuse pattern and only residual collagenous tissue, (**d**) diffuse pattern of a lymphocytic thymoma

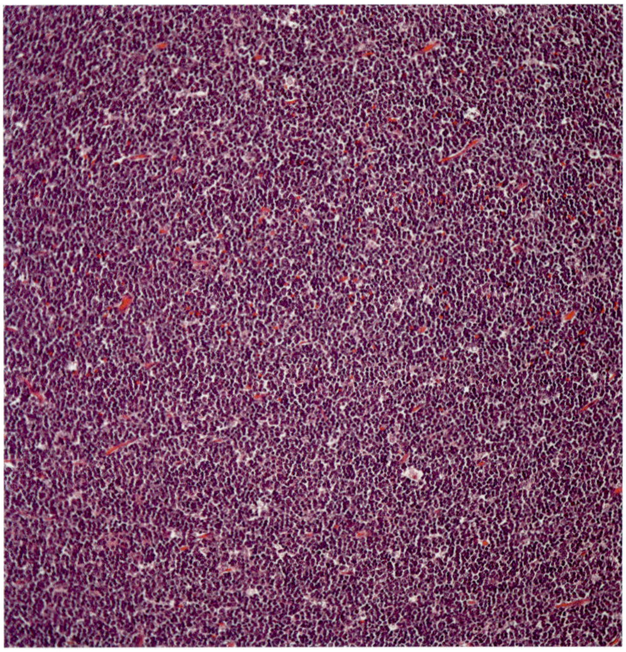

Fig. 7.40 Lymphocytic thymoma with diffuse pattern and absence of fibrocollagen

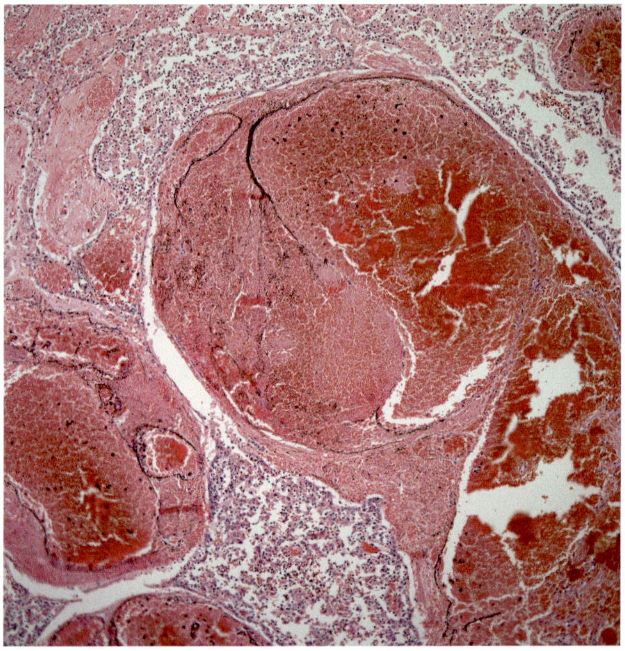

Fig. 7.41 Thymoma with ectatic spaces filled with fresh blood

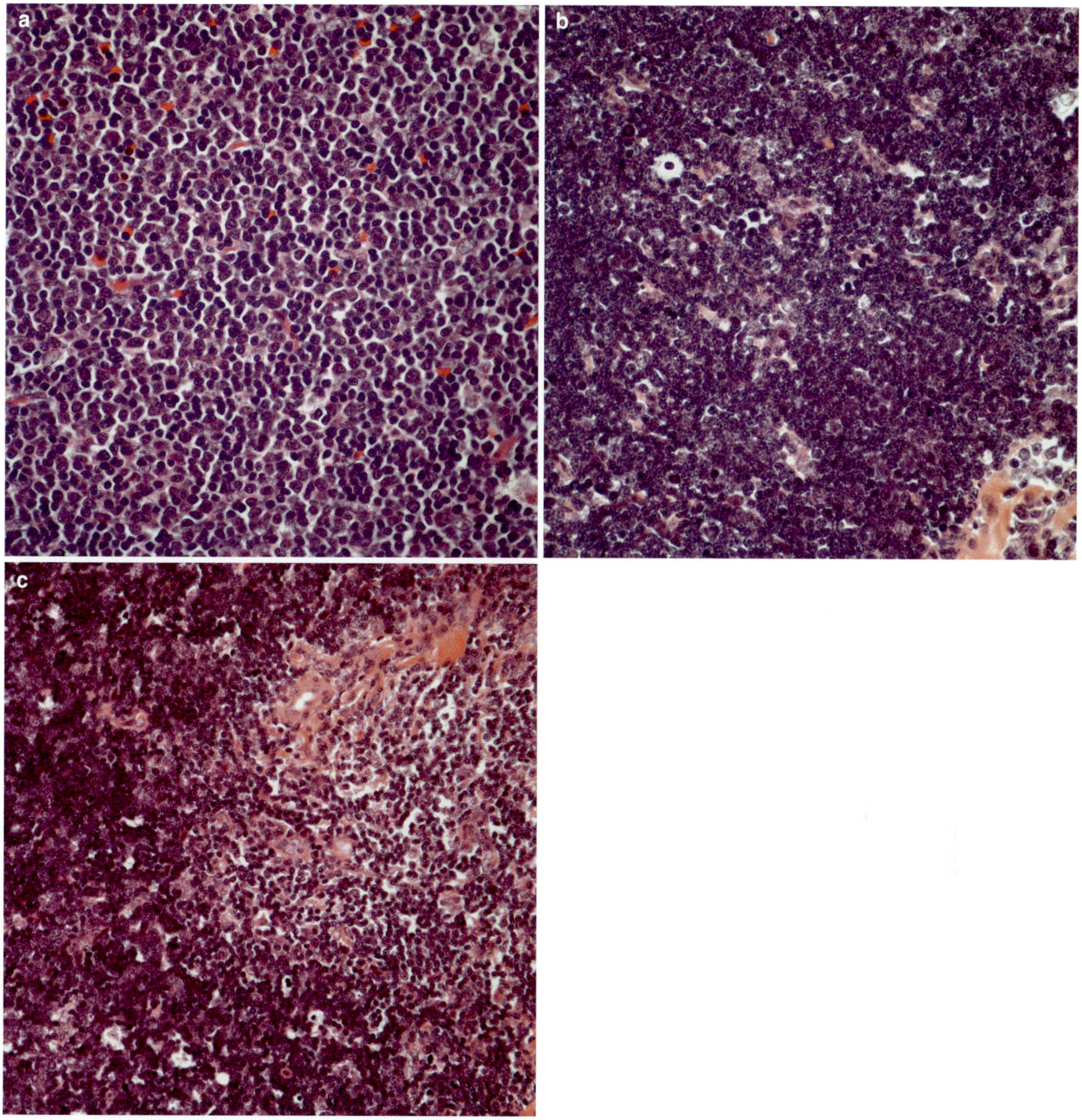

Fig. 7.42 (**a**) Higher magnification of a lymphocytic thymoma showing more lymphocytes than epithelial cells, (**b**) lymphocytic thymoma with more atypia in the lymphocytic component, (**c**) atypical and mature lymphocytes admixed with epithelial cells in a predominant lymphocytic thymoma

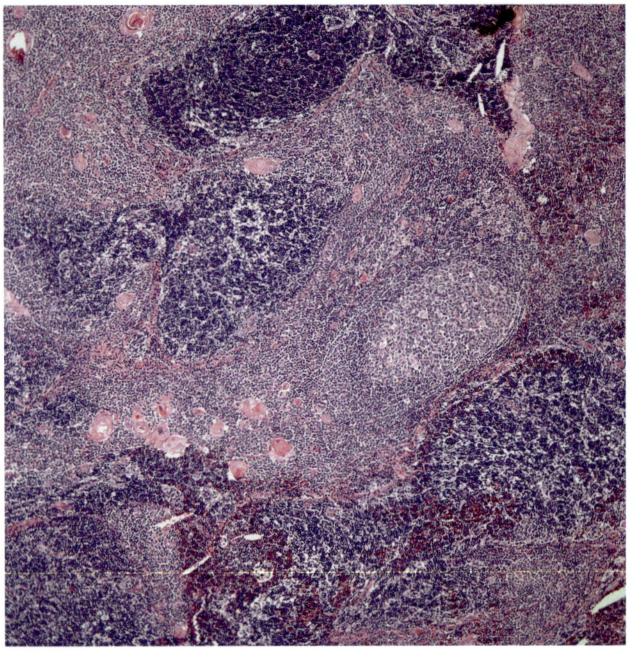

Fig. 7.43 Thymoma with the presence hyperplastic germinal centers and Hassall's corpuscles

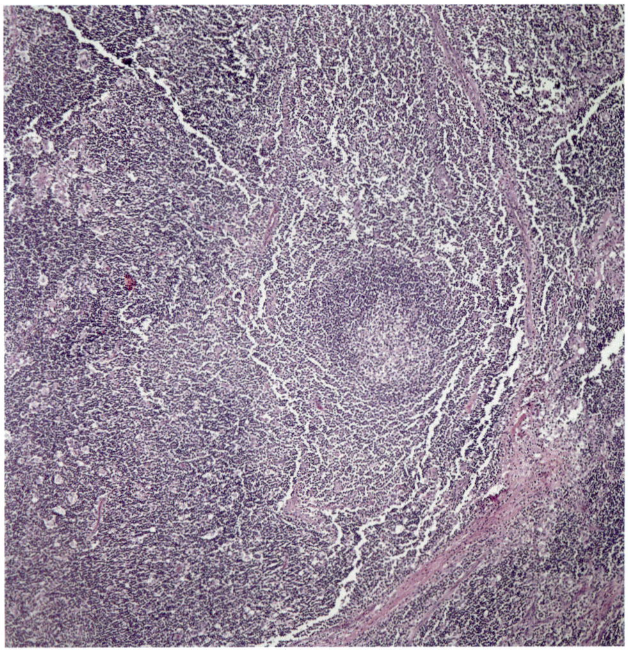

Fig. 7.44 Thymoma with a not so well-formed germinal center

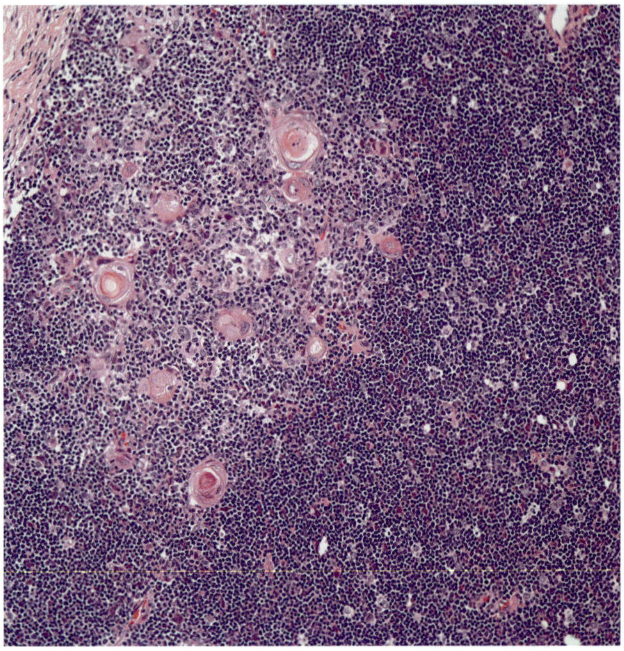

Fig. 7.45 Thymoma with numerous Hassall's corpuscles

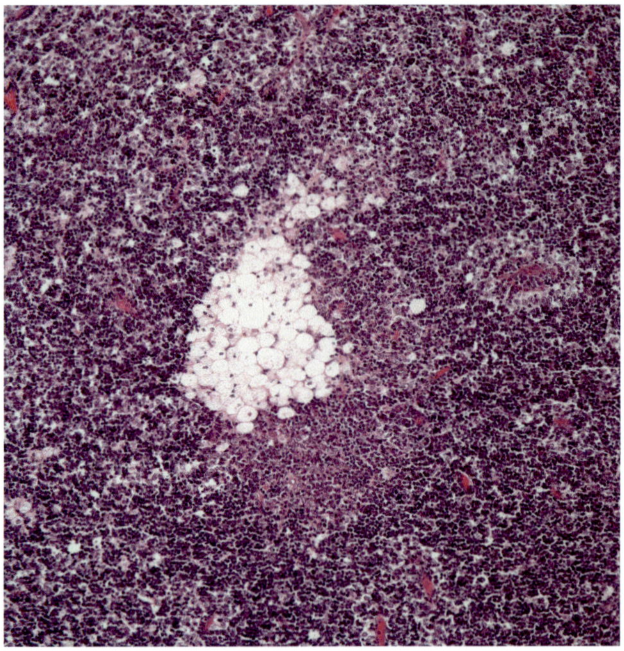

Fig. 7.46 Thymoma with collection of macrophages

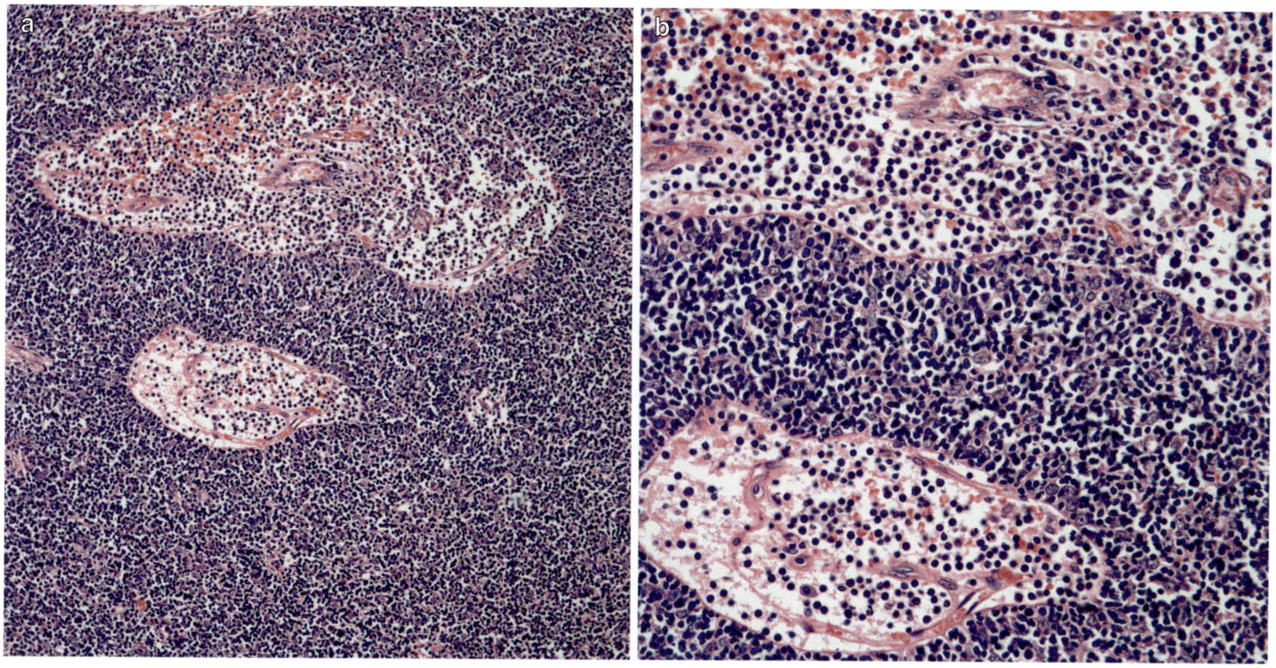

Fig. 7.47 (**a**) Thymoma with easily identifiable vascular spaces, (**b**) vascular spaces with immature lymphocytes

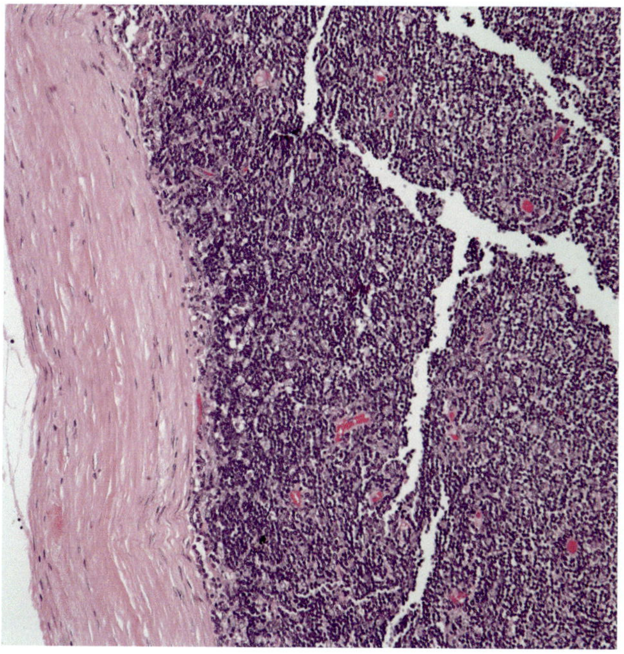

Fig. 7.48 Encapsulate thymoma showing clear circumscription of the tumor

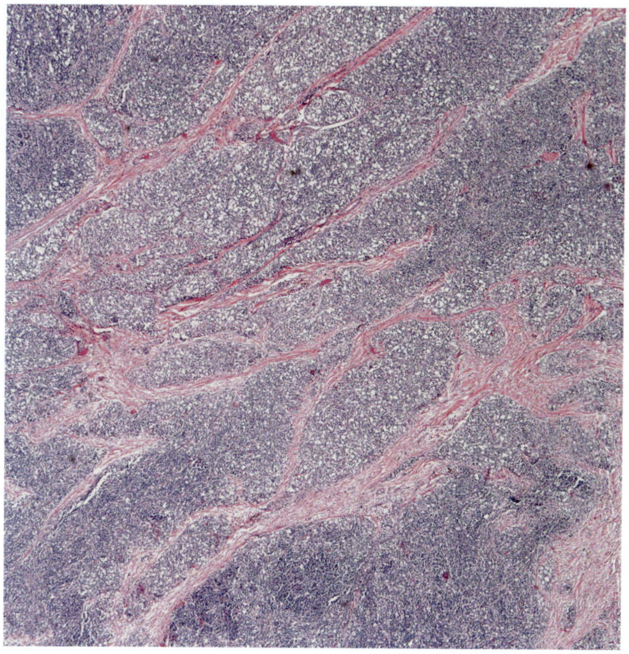

Fig. 7.49 Thymoma showing striking lobulation, and even at this power, the tumor shows approximately equal proportion of lymphocytes and epithelial cells

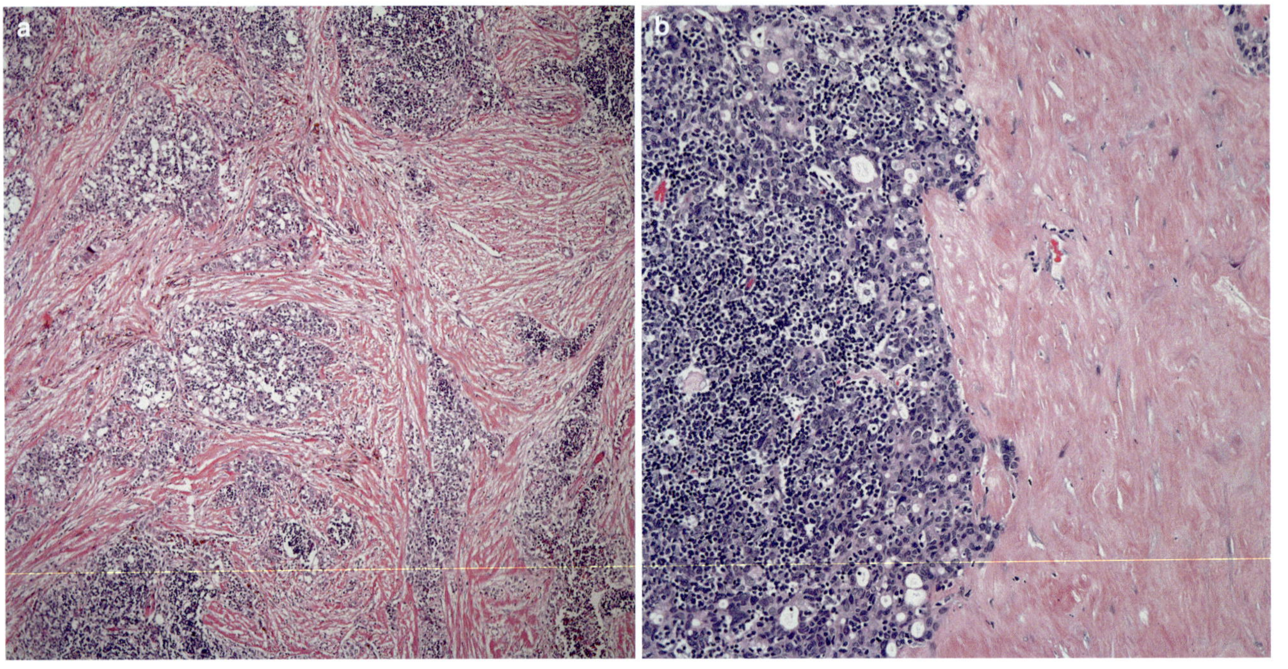

Fig. 7.50 (**a**) Thymoma in areas of fibrocollagen and not well-formed lobulation, (**b**) thymoma with extensive hyalinization

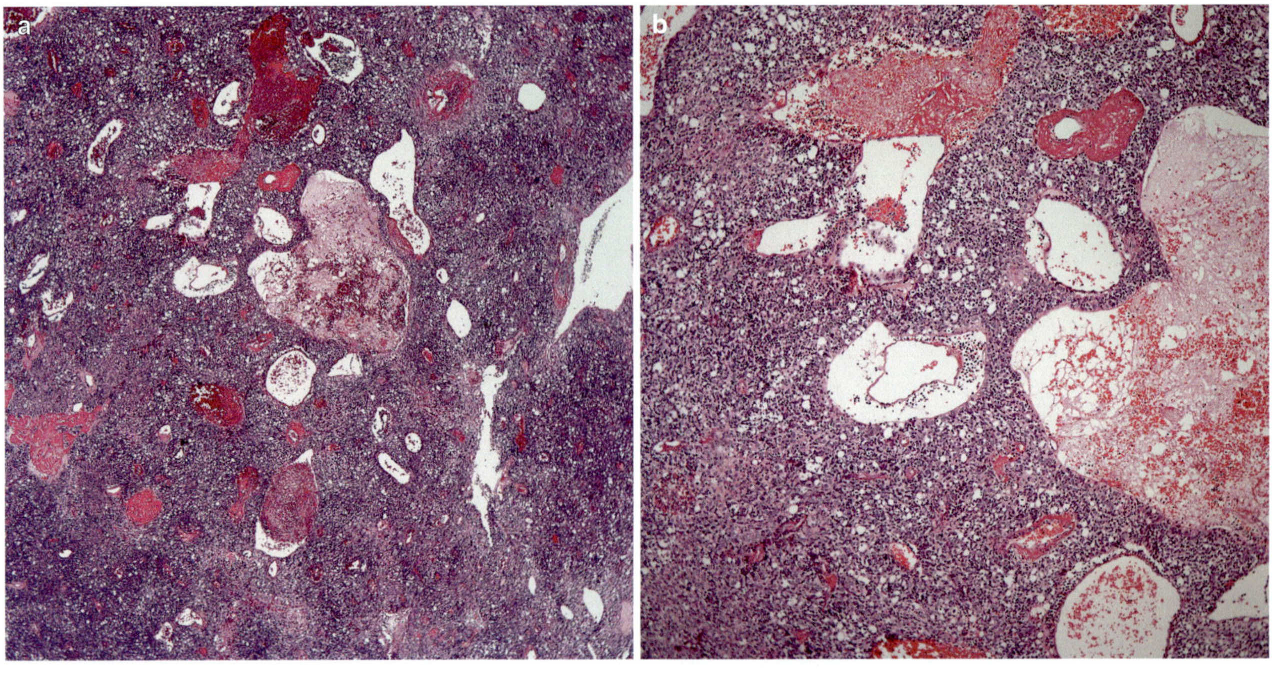

Fig. 7.51 (**a**) Thymoma with prominent vascular spaces, (**b**) closer view at the vascular spaces and the biphasic cellular proliferation

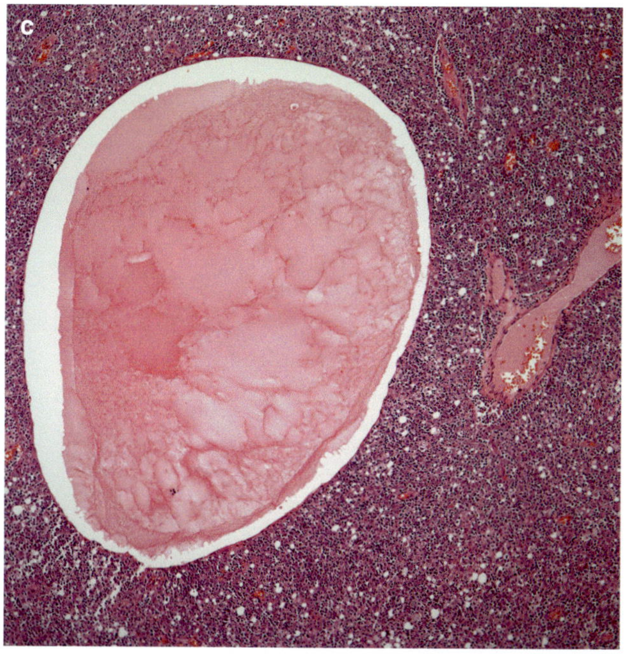

Fig. 7.51 (continued) (**c**) Rare cystic changes in an otherwise solid tumor

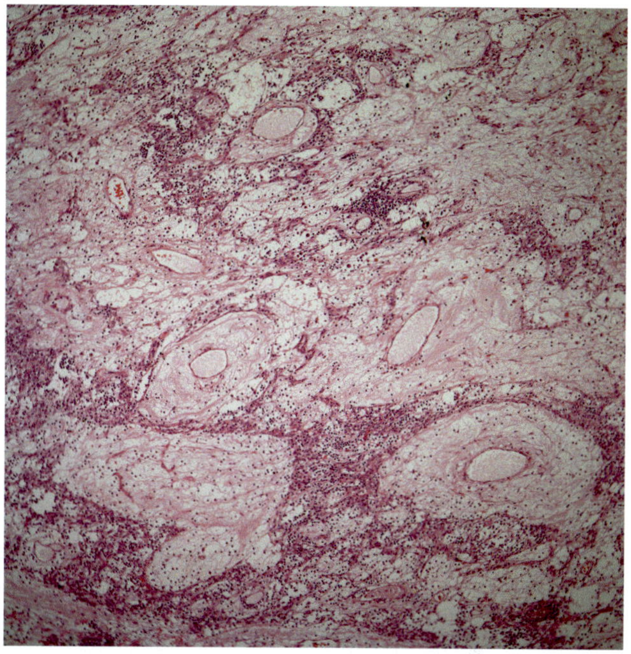

Fig. 7.52 Thymoma with extensive hyalinization around vascular spaces

thymomas with lymphocytes. The equivalent is atypical thymomas in which the tumor is predominantly epithelial, but in areas in which the tumor shows lymphocytes, appending another letter or number to an already unscientific schema will be inappropriate.

Pan and colleagues [138] reported a series of 81 cases of spindle and mixed spindle lymphocytic thymomas which the authors labeled as type A and type AB. Interestingly, 12% of the cases reported by the authors were of the micronodular type, which in essence represents thymomas with B-cell hyperplasia, an entity already well known in the literature. In addition, the authors reported that 90% of the mixed spindle/lymphocytic thymomas were positive for CD20. Regardless of the presence of lymphocytes in the spindle cell thymomas, we have already reported 41 cases of invasive spindle cell thymoma from a cohort of 250 cases [106], while in the most recent cohort of 1470 cases [29], we identify 48.7% of these tumors to be in different pathological stages of invasion. For all practical purposes, the presence or absence of lymphocytes in a spindle cell thymoma does not provide any special distinction regarding invasiveness or encapsulation, which is the most reliable parameter to predict clinical outcome.

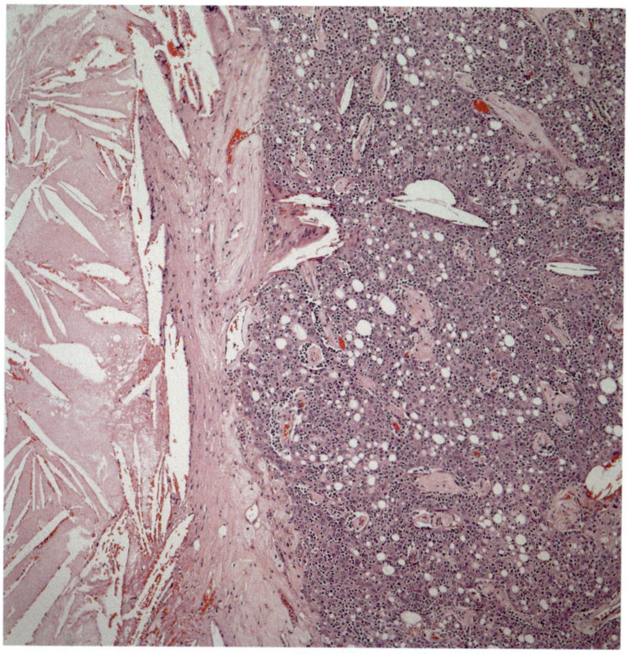

Fig. 7.53 Thymoma with adjacent cholesterol cleft granuloma

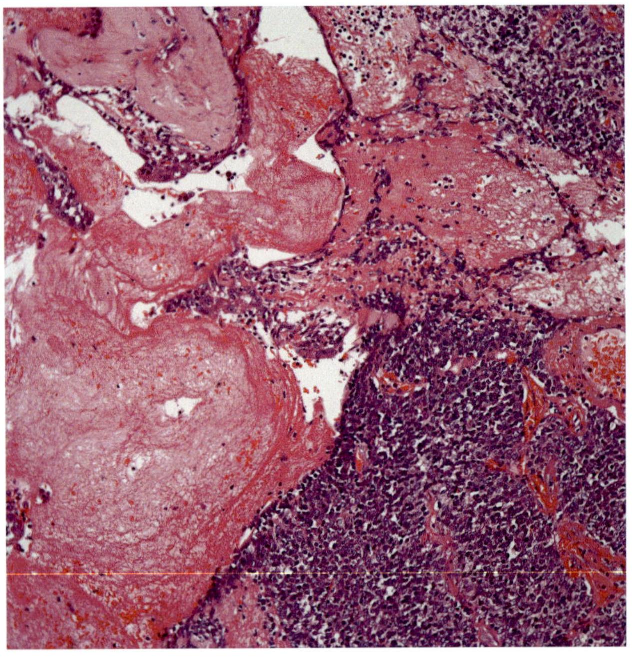

Fig. 7.54 Thymoma with areas of fibrinous exudate

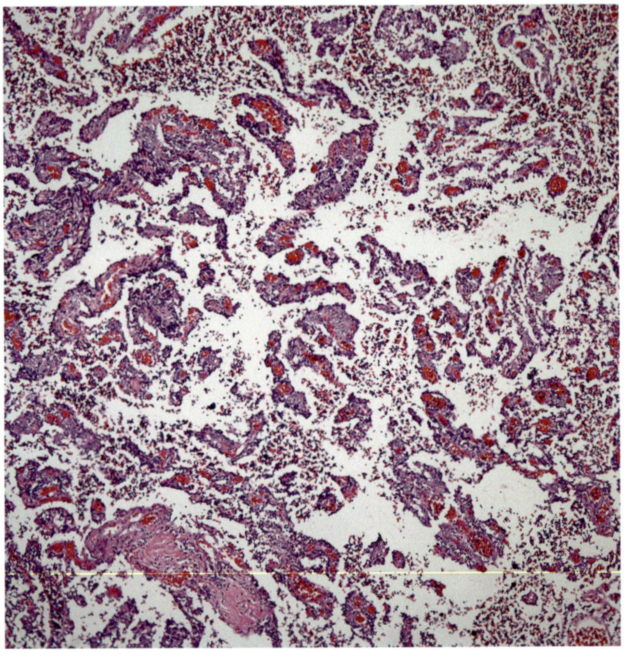

Fig. 7.55 Focal areas of pseudopapillary formation in an otherwise solid tumor

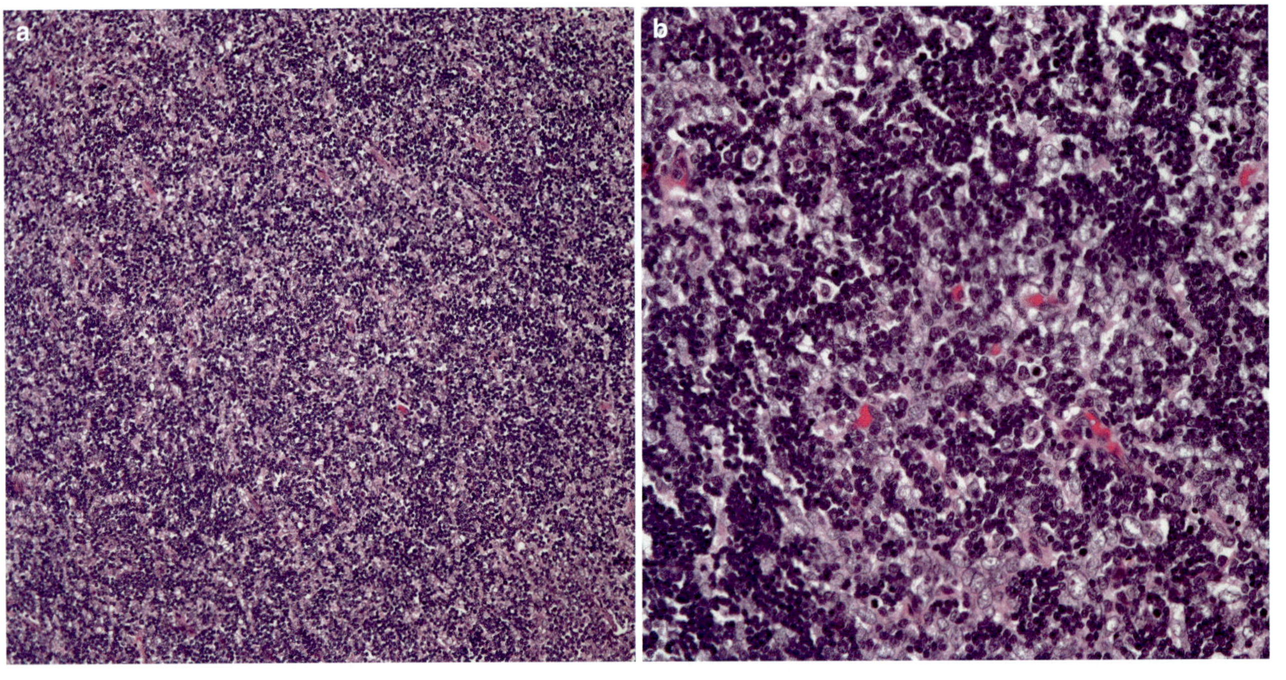

Fig. 7.56 (**a**) Thymoma with equal proportion of lymphocytes and epithelial cells and a diffuse growth pattern, (**b**) higher magnification showing the dual population of lymphocytes and epithelial cells

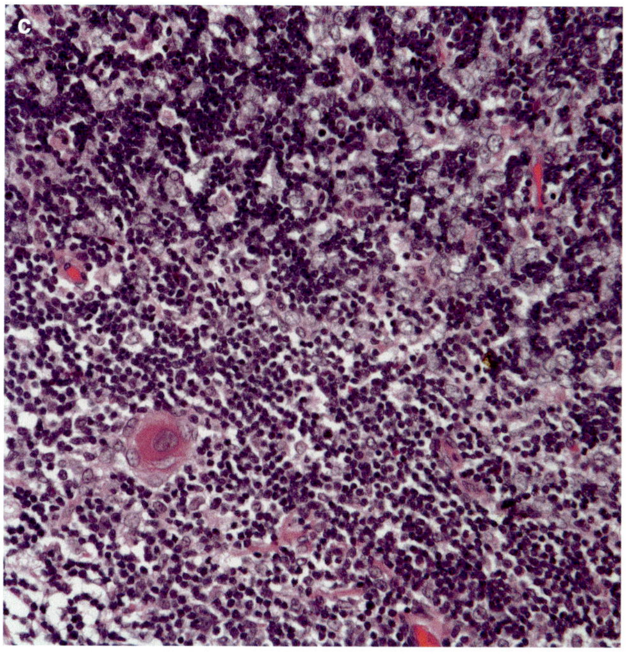

Fig. 7.56 (continued) (**c**) Dual cell population with occasional Hassall's corpuscles

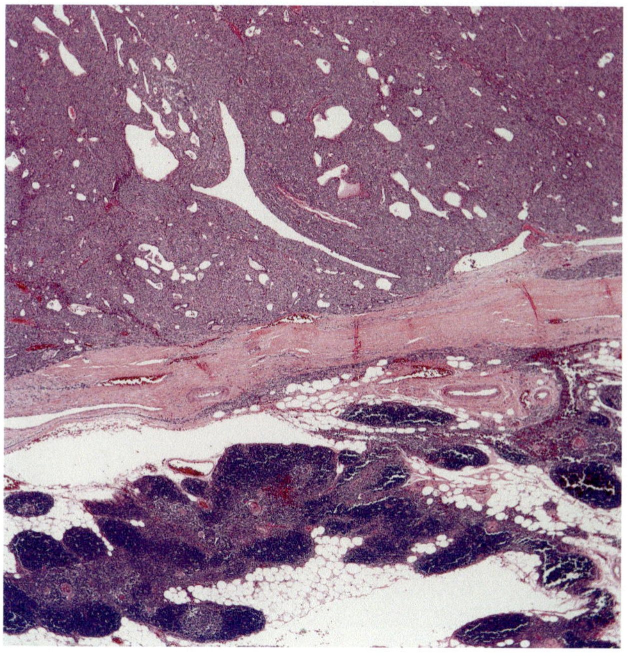

Fig. 7.57 Well-encapsulated thymoma

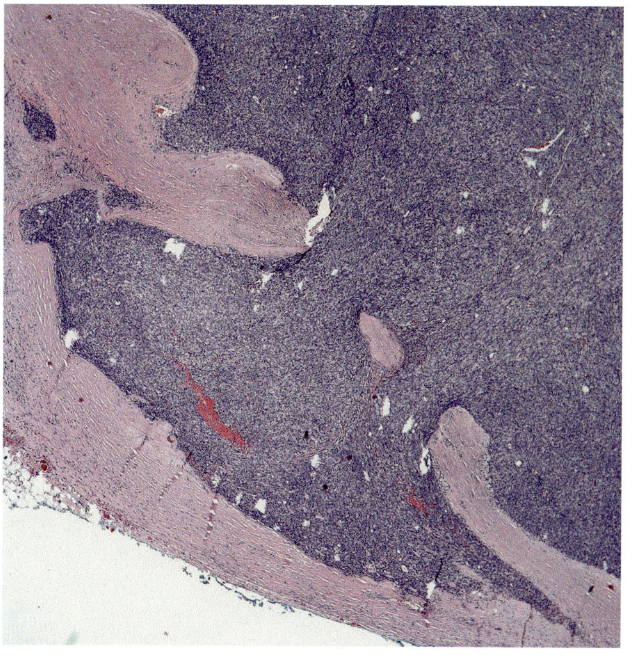

Fig. 7.58 Thymoma with capsular invasion but the tumor does not invade through the capsule

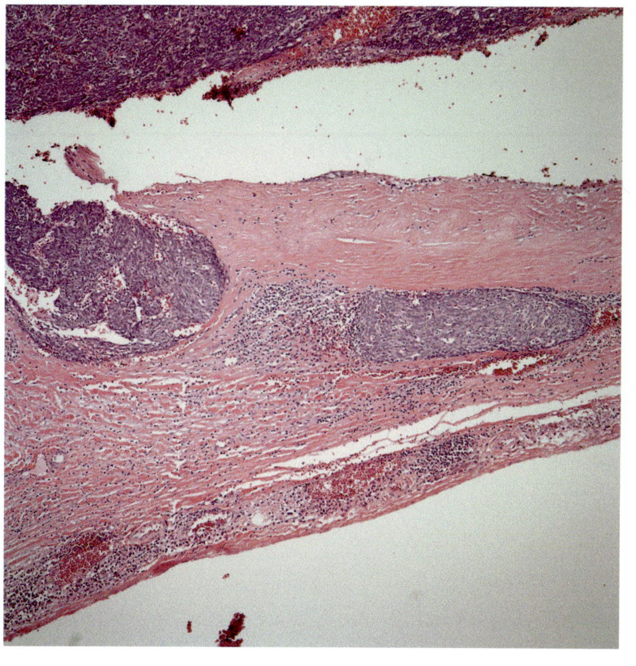

Fig. 7.59 Thymoma with capsular invasion but not breaching the capsule

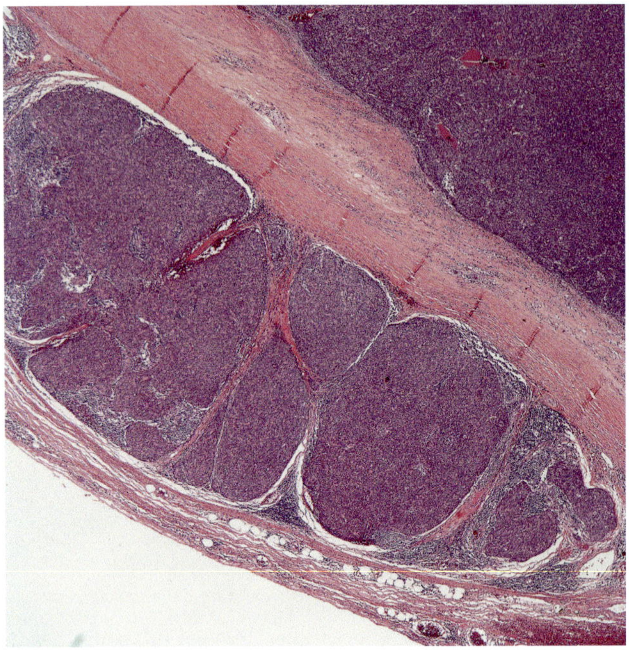

Fig. 7.60 Thymoma with invasion through the capsule: minimally invasive thymoma

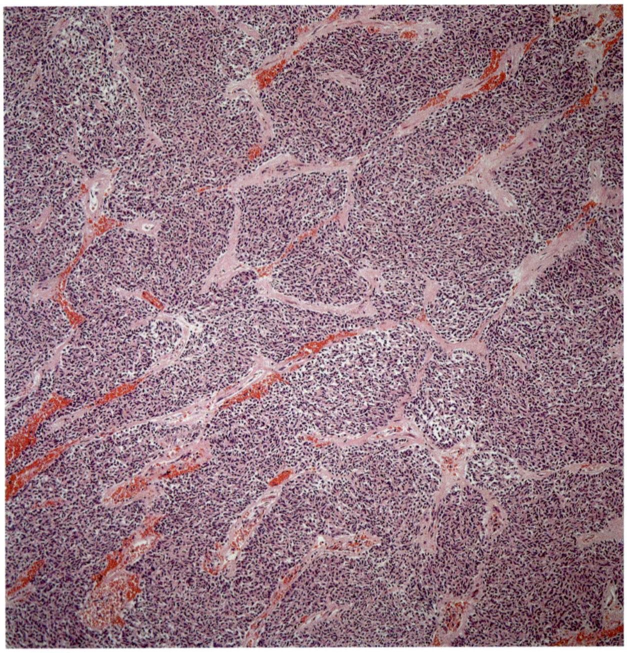

Fig. 7.61 Spindle cell thymoma showing lobulation

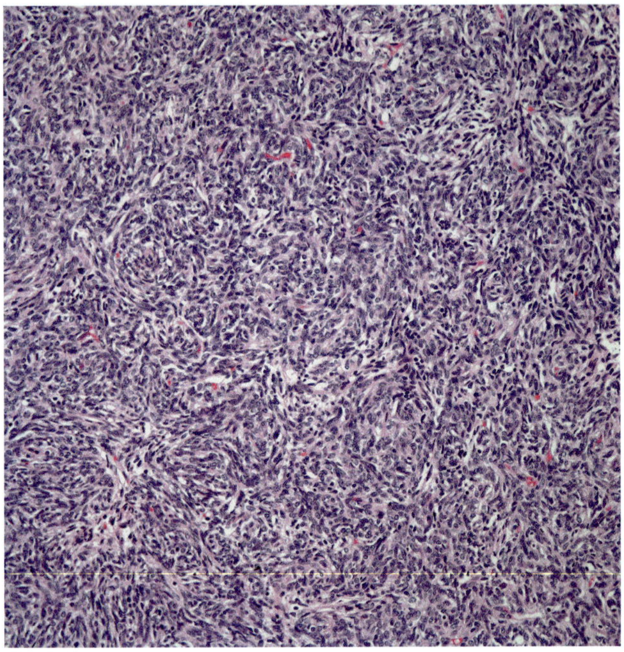

Fig. 7.62 Spindle cell thymoma with more diffuse pattern

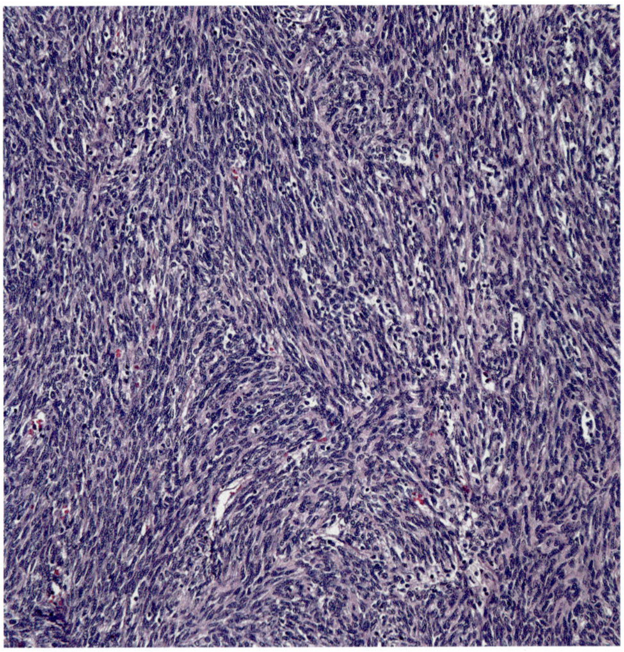

Fig. 7.63 Diffuse pattern of spindle cell thymoma mimicking sarcoma

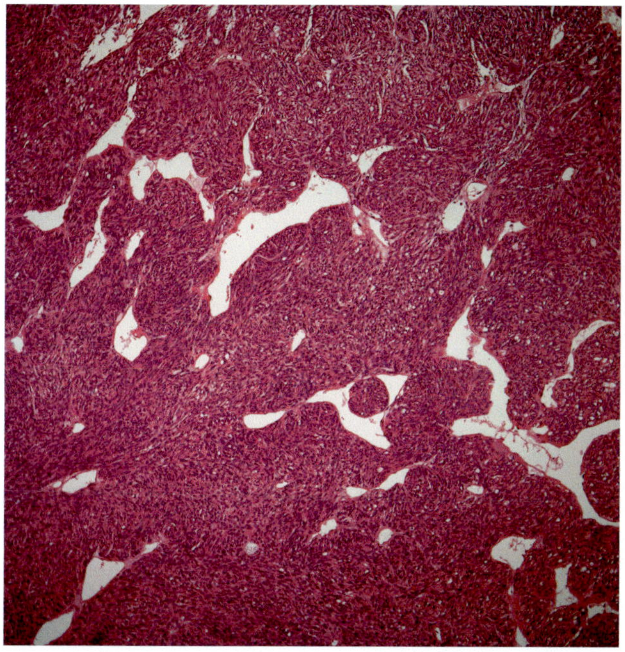

Fig. 7.64 Spindle cell thymoma with hemagiopericytic (HPC) pattern

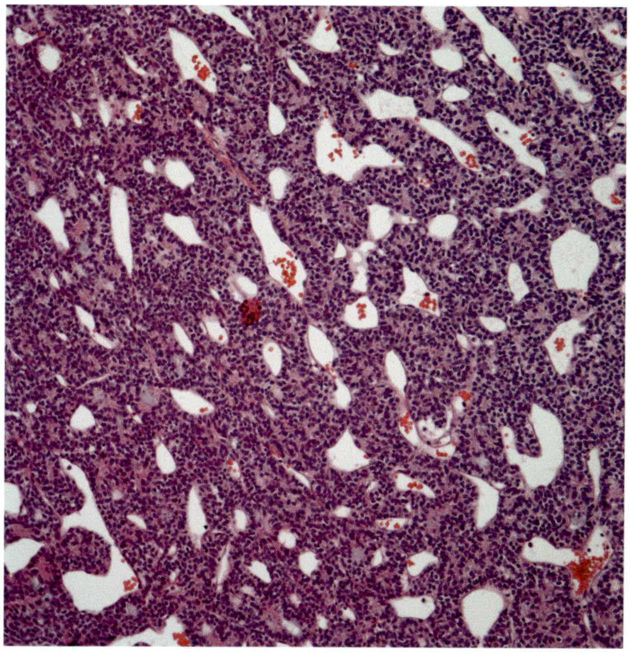

Fig. 7.65 HPC pattern in a thymoma with more oval cells

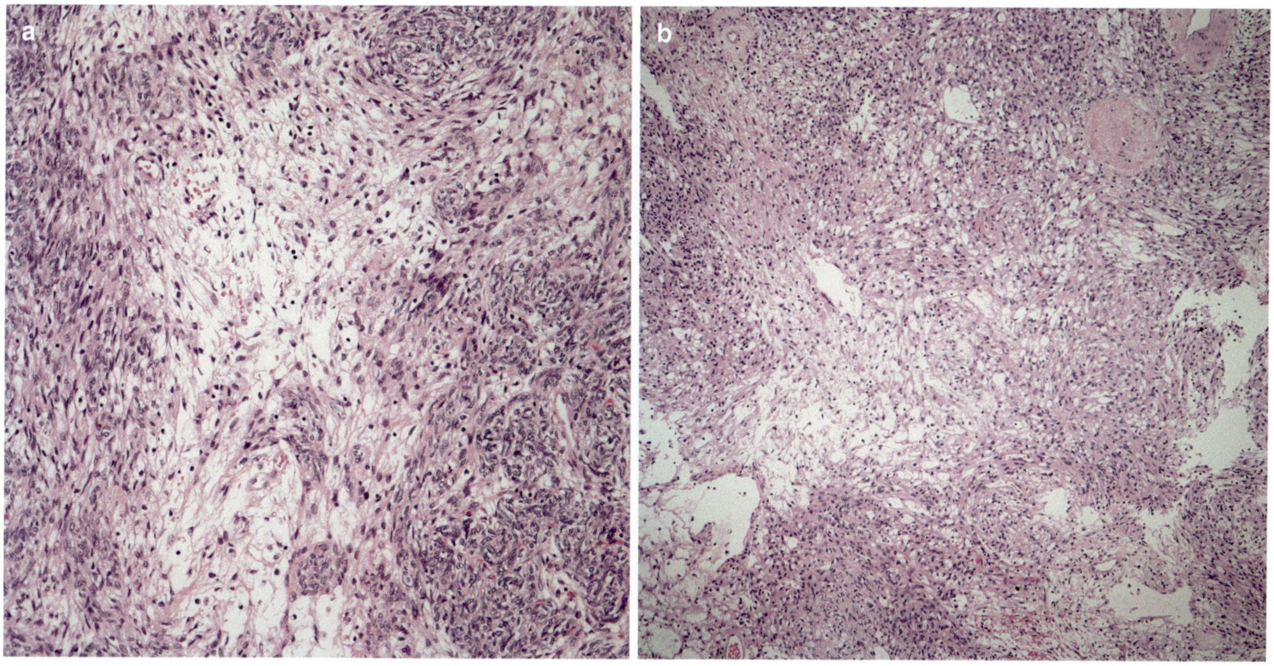

Fig. 7.66 (**a**) Spindle cell thymoma with focal areas of hyalinization, (**b**) hyalinization and edematous changes with focal microcystic changes

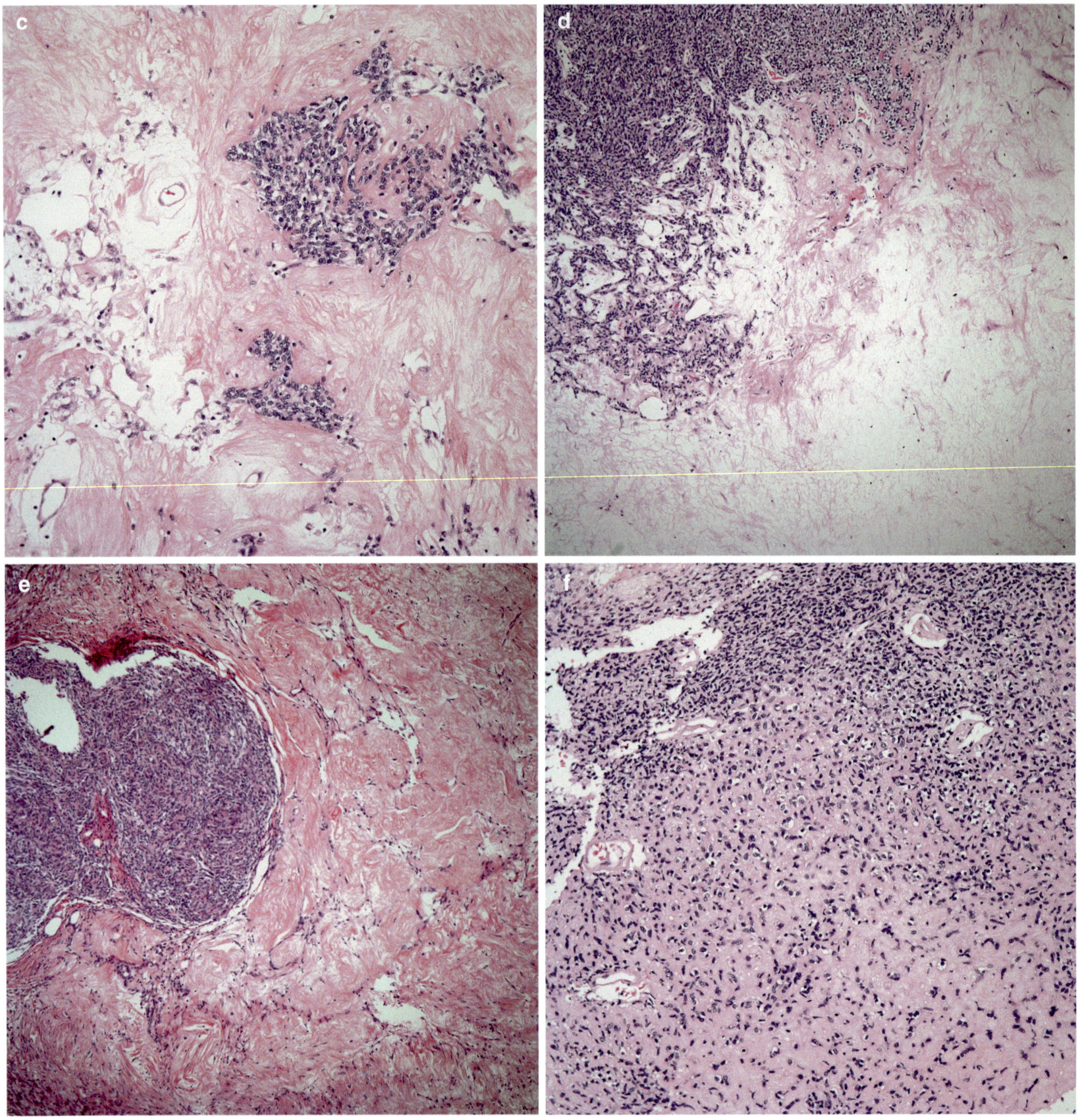

Fig. 7.66 (continued) (**c**) Extensive hyalinization in a spindle cell thymoma, (**d**) extensive edematous changes adjacent to spindle cell thymoma, (**e**) hyalinization with outlines of spindle cells and nodular area of spindle cell thymoma, (**f**) dense hyalinization osteoid-like change in spindle cell thymoma

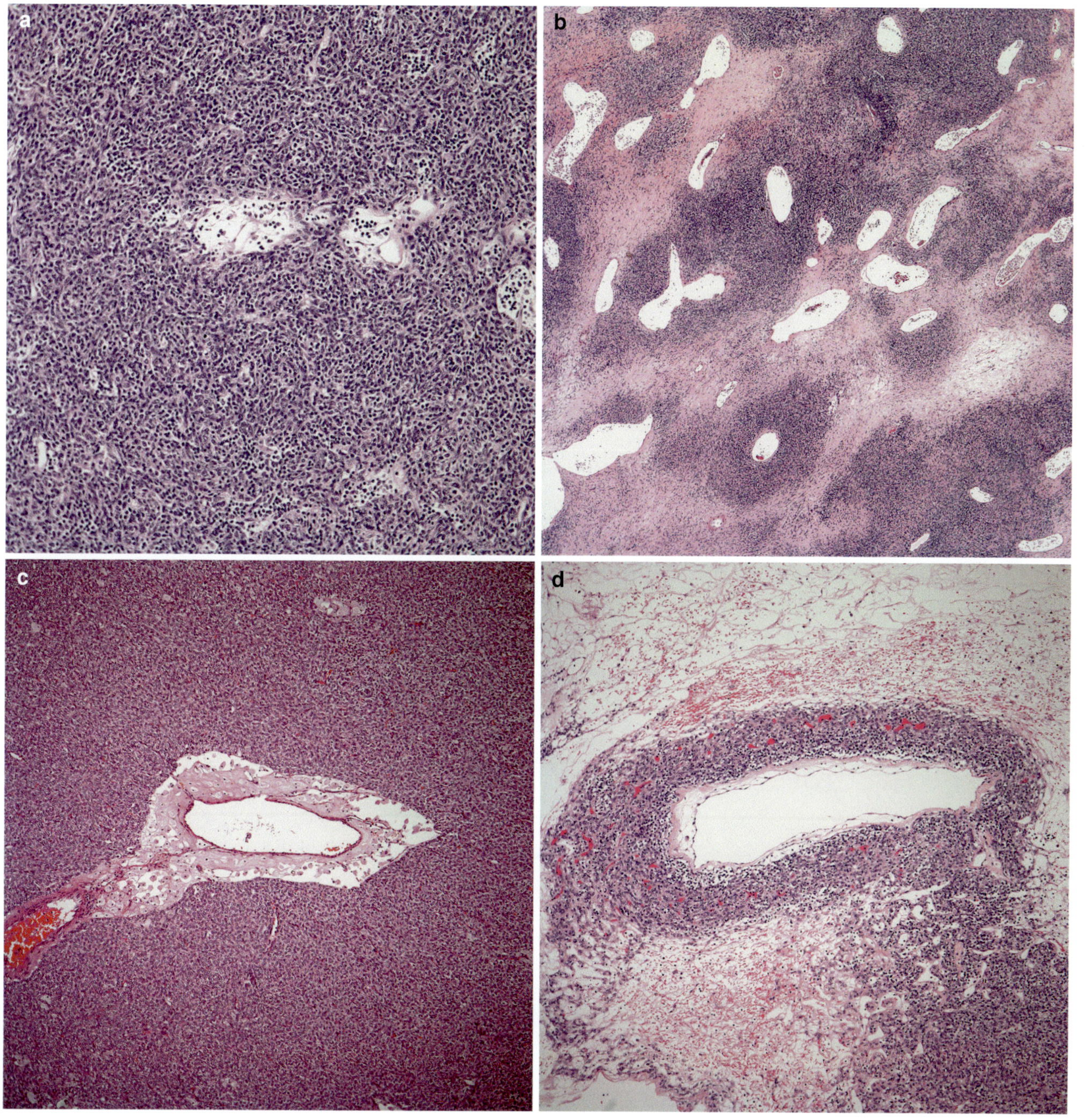

Fig. 7.67 (**a**) Spindle cell thymoma with lymphocytes and focal vascular spaces, (**b**) prominent vascular spaces with hyalinization and tumor spindle cells, (**c**) spindle cell thymoma with prominent vascular space, (**d**) spindle cell thymoma with spindle cells surrounding vascular spaces

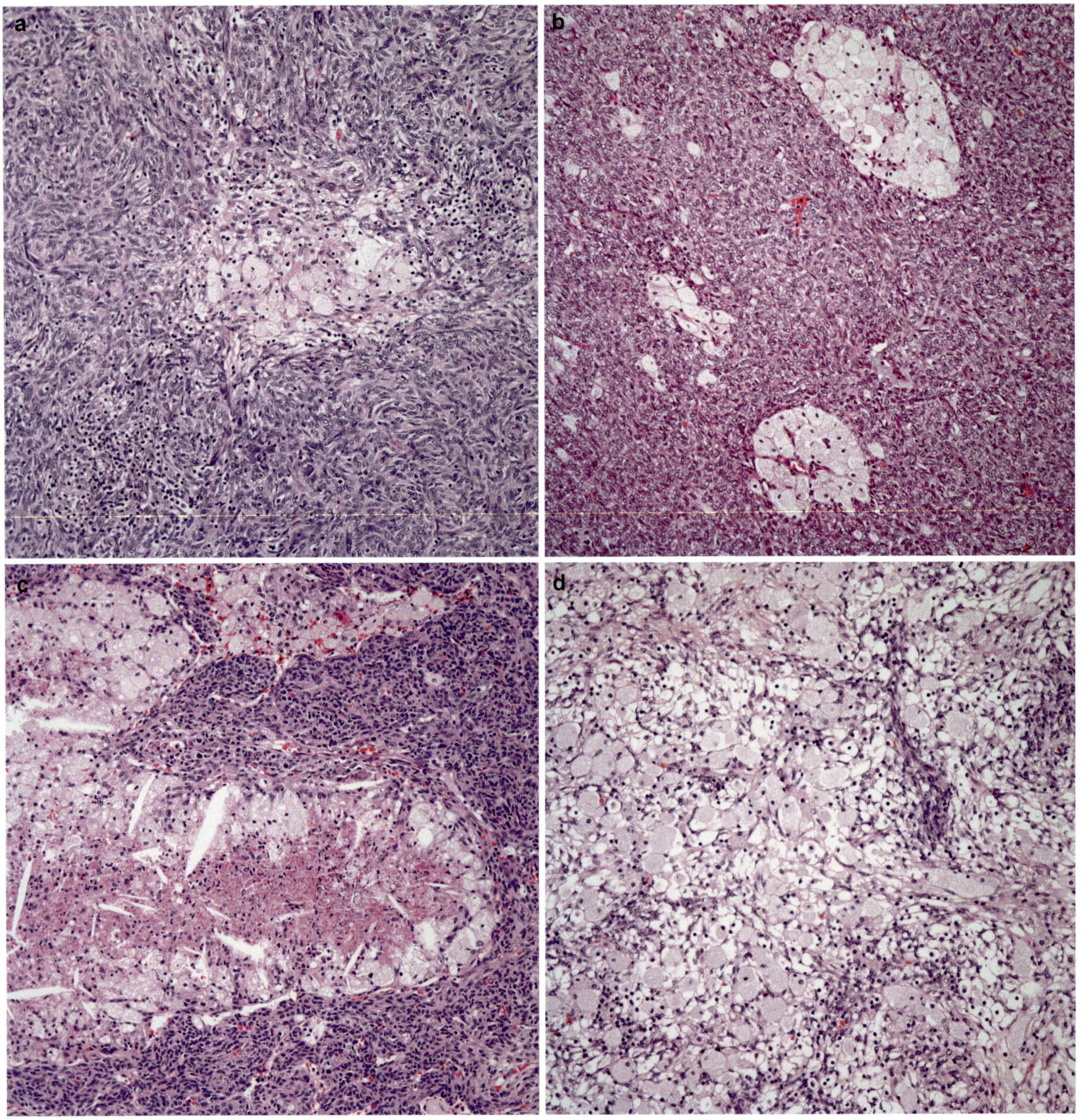

Fig. 7.68 (**a**) Spindle cell thymoma with focal collection of macrophages, (**b**) nodular collections of macrophages in spindle cell thymoma, (**c**) spindle cell thymoma with collections of macrophages and cholesterol cleft granuloma, (**d**) extensive deposition of macrophages in spindle cell thymoma – xanthomatous thymoma

Atypical Thymoma

This term encompasses terms that have been used for similar tumors including epithelial-rich thymoma [42, 52], well-differentiated thymic carcinoma [139, 140], and the WHO translator of B3 thymoma. In the original description by Bernatz and colleagues [42], the authors clearly separated tumors depending on the proportion of lymphocytes present in any given tumor: lymphocyte-rich, mixed or the so-called lymphoepithelioma (equal proportion of lymphocytes and epithelial cells), and epithelial-rich thymoma, which is a tumor in which the proportion of lymphocytes is reduced in comparison to other thymomas. However, in 1992, Kirchner and colleagues [139] described 26 thymic tumors that the authors interpreted as well-differentiated thymic carcinoma, making special reference to the low-grade nature of the tumor and the relationship to cortical thymoma. The age of these patients ranged from 14 to 76 years, and 77% of the patients had a history of MG. Important to highlight is that the majority of the tumors were invasive. Interestingly, the authors stated that the invasiveness of this tumor is higher than the "cortical" thymomas but lower than other thymic carcinomas. In addition, the authors stated that this tumor needed to be separated from the "benign" epithelial-rich thymoma. More interesting is that the follow-up provided of up to 15 years showed that two patients died of recurrence and two additional patients had recurrence. In the same year, Pescarmona and colleagues [140], following the same thinking, reported 15 additional cases of this entity with similar findings and histological features, and added that the designation of well-differentiated carcinoma is justified because of cytological atypia and retention of some organotypical histological features. Here are a few important issues that are important to highlight: (1) judging by the illustrations provided, it appears that what the authors have described is

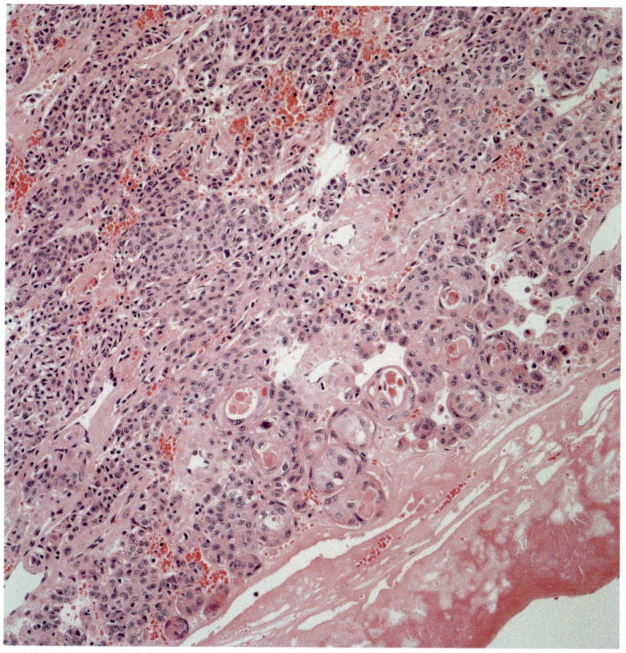

Fig. 7.69 Spindle cell thymoma with Hassall's corpuscles

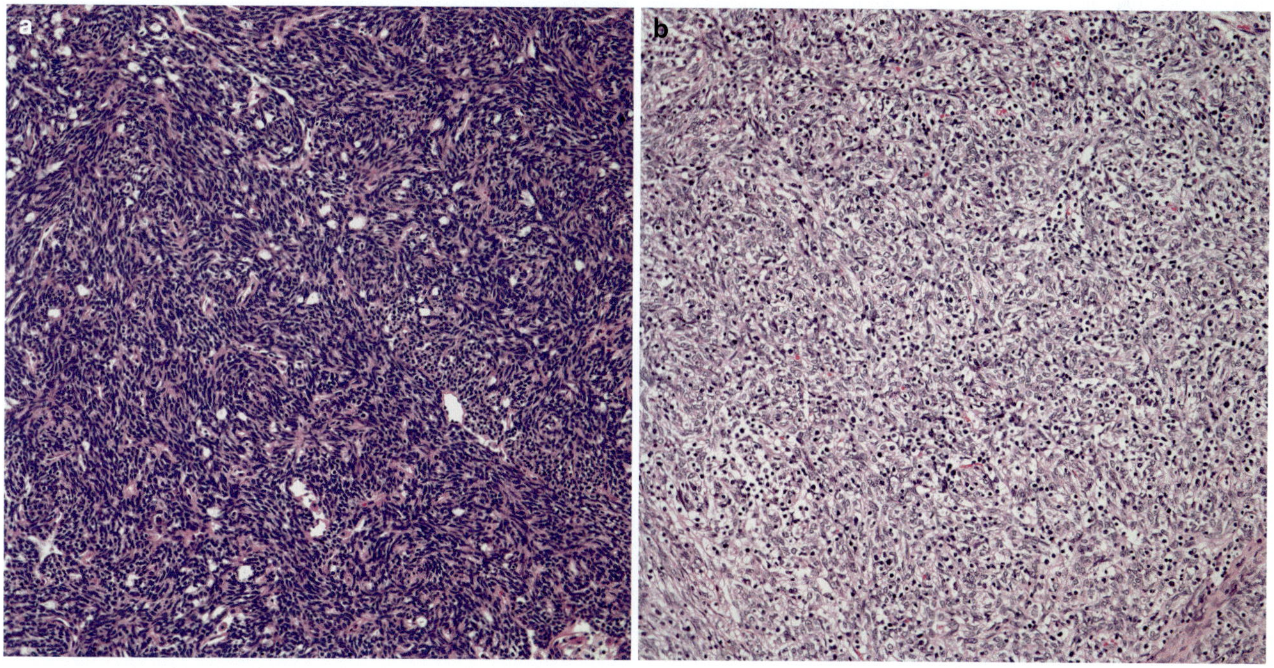

Fig. 7.70 (**a**, **b**) Higher magnification of two different aspects of spindle cell thymoma showing lack of nuclear atypia or mitotic activity

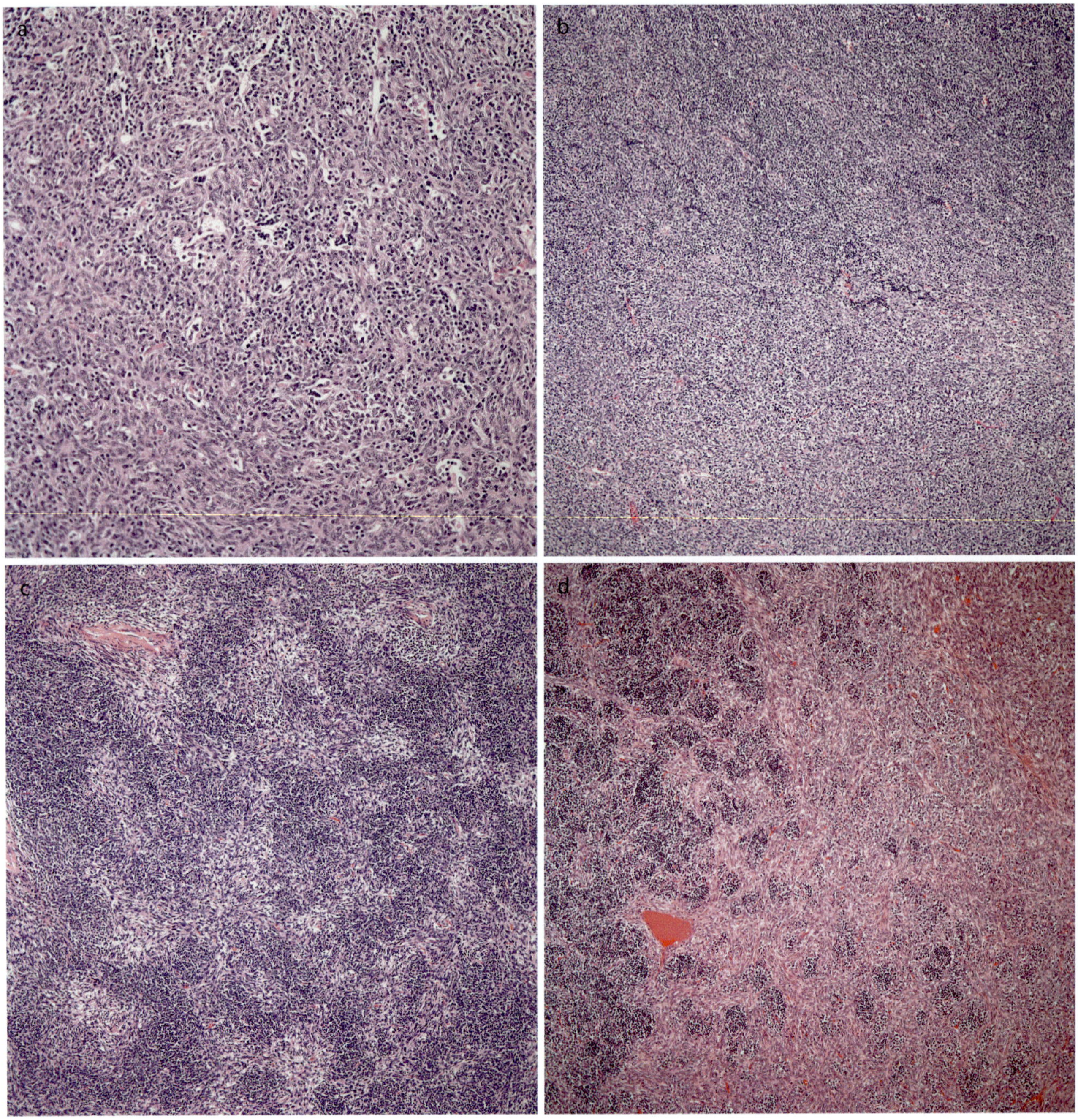

Fig. 7.71 Spindle cell thymomas may also show lymphocytes in different proportions: (**a**) focal clusters of lymphocytes, (**b**) transitional areas with and without lymphocytes, (**c**) spindle cells separated by cluster of lymphocytes, (**d**) clustering of lymphocytes admixed with spindle cells

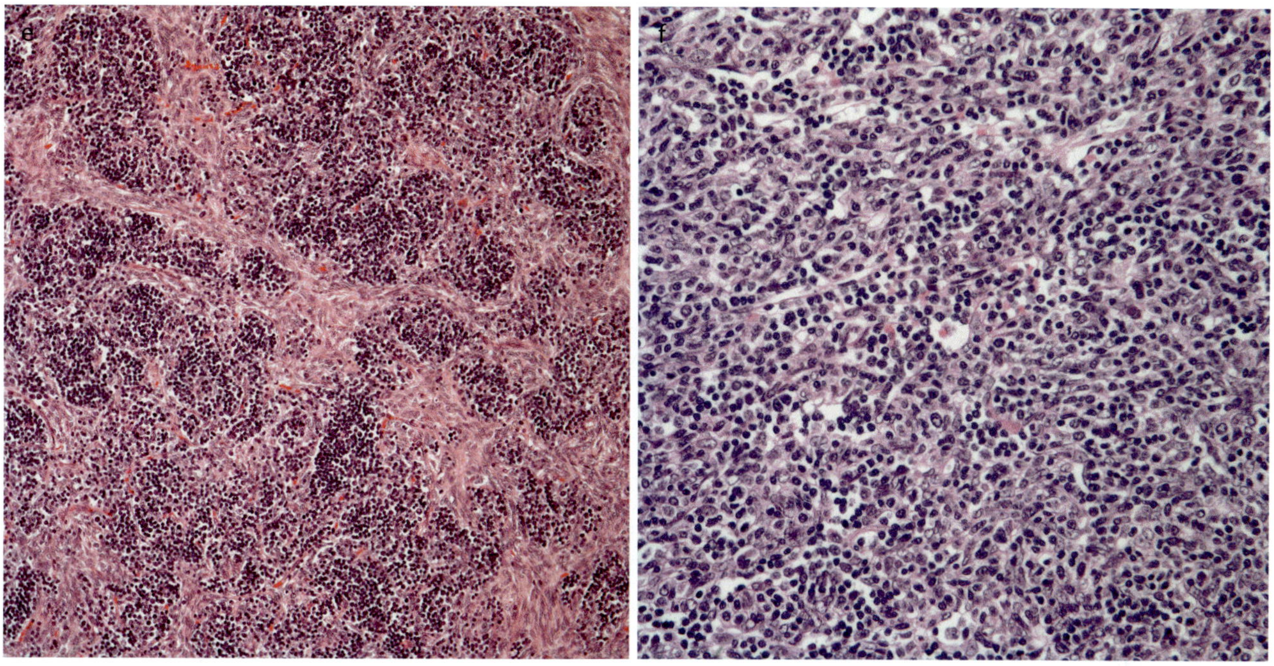

Fig. 7.71 (continued) (**e**) Higher magnification of the lymphocytes and spindle cells, (**f**) in focal areas the proportion of spindle cells and lymphocytes is almost equal

essentially the same tumor already labeled epithelial-rich thymoma by Bernatz [42]; (2) judging by the provided follow-up of up to 15 years, this is also very much in keeping with the behavior of invasive thymomas rather than thymic carcinoma; and (3) the tumors described by the authors had nothing to do with the already described well-differentiated thymic carcinoma already described by Shimosato and colleagues [141]. However, this error in interpretation paved the way later on so that the WHO members of 1999 [102] would introduce a "translator" to account for this tumor in comparison to the epithelial-rich thymoma and decided to use the letters and numbers. At this point, it is important to stress that, based on the available literature and by driving an analogy between the so-called well-differentiated thymic carcinoma and the epithelial-rich thymoma, it is evident that the histological features and clinical behavior of this entity are closer to thymoma than to carcinoma, and, in doing so, the concept of atypical thymoma is best suited for an entity that has intermediate features between thymoma and thymic carcinoma. In addition, morphologically, atypical thymoma still preserves the organotypical features of thymoma—lobulation (Fig. 7.72), fibrous septa (Fig. 7.73a–e), and perivascular spaces (Fig. 7.74a–c). However, the tumor may also show a more diffuse growth pattern without lobulation (Fig. 7.75a–c). In some cases, the tumor may show ectatic areas mimicking a vascular neoplasm (Fig. 7.76a–e), while in some tumors, the pattern may mimic a neuroendocrine neoplasm (Fig. 7.77a–e). Also, collections of macrophages may be seen in different proportions as well as the presence of cholesterol cleft granulomas (Fig. 7.78a–c). The epithelial cellular proliferation is composed of round to polygonal cells with abundant cytoplasm, large vesicular nuclei, some cells with prominent nucleoli, and occasional mitotic figures (Fig. 7.79a–h) [142]. More importantly, the population of lymphocytes in these tumors is scant but remains as T-immature lymphocytes (Fig. 7.80a–c). Small series of cases using the terminology of atypical thymoma have been presented in the literature, reinforcing previously stated issues [143]. It is of interest to note that, despite the fact that the WHO authors have introduced a translator for the different classifications, in a recent publication, Nonaka and colleagues [144] reported 13 spindle cell thymomas under the designation of "atypical type A." Although we are in agreement that atypical thymomas come in different forms and shapes (Fig. 7.81a–e), it is rather ambiguous to mix two different views. In the Suster-Moran classification system, the thymic epithelial neoplasms are viewed as thymoma, atypical thymoma, and thymic carcinoma. On the contrary, the WHO uses letter and numbers, which now – by adding "atypical" to type A – just adds to the confusing views that such a translator has created over the years. More distressing is to see that in the more recent version of the publication of the WHO, when it comes to clinical behavior and prognosis, atypical thymoma is handled with pathological staging while, for the other types of thymoma considered, histological classification is predictable of prognosis. Such inconsistencies represent the degree of misunderstanding and limitations created by the WHO translator.

More recently, the issue of the classification of atypical thymoma in relation to other thymomas and the staging of these tumors was clarified in a large cohort of cases. We evaluated 1470 thymomas of which 186 corresponded to atypical thymomas, representing approximately 12.7% of the entire group. Of this group of 186 atypical thymomas, 139 were invasive tumors in different pathological stages, which is about 75% of the cases. Therefore, when a survival curve was analyzed, the separation of thymomas and atypical thymomas became statistically significant [29], a finding that had already been identified with a smaller cohort of 250 cases in which no statistical significance was observed by separating tumors by specific histologies [105], namely, the proposed translator of the WHO.

Thymomas with Mixed Histologies

Thymomas with mixed histologies represent the bulk of the tumors rendering any histological classification virtually useless if adequate sampling is performed. Not only is the majority of thymomas represented by tumors with mixed histologies, but a significant percentage of these tumors belong to special categories in which any histopathological classification becomes meaningless. In our study with 1470 thymomas, the tumors with mixed histologies were by far more common than any particular histological group. Figure 7.36 depicts the breakdown by histology based on this study.

In terms of histological features, these tumors may exhibit a wide range of histological combinations including spindle, atypical lymphocytic, or unusual growth patterns of thymomas. Essentially, we have seen every possible combination not only with the conventional histologies but also with conventional histologies with unusual histological growth patterns. Some of the possible combinations include predominantly lymphocytic thymomas with spindle cell thymomas in which the spindle cell thymoma may be side by side with the lymphocytic thymoma or have other unusual growth patterns such as cystic changes (Fig. 7.82a, b). Similarly, thymomas with mixed cellularity of equal proportions of lymphocytes and epithelial cells merging with spindle cell thymoma (Fig. 7.83) or with atypical thymoma (Fig. 7.84a–c) are commonly seen. Also, atypical thymoma in association with lymphocytic thymoma is not unusual (Fig. 7.85a, b). Other unusual features that may be seen in some cases are the presence of atypical thymomas with lymphocytes merging with areas lacking lymphocytes (Fig. 7.86a, b) and the presence of spindle cell thymomas with and without lymphocytes (Fig. 7.87).

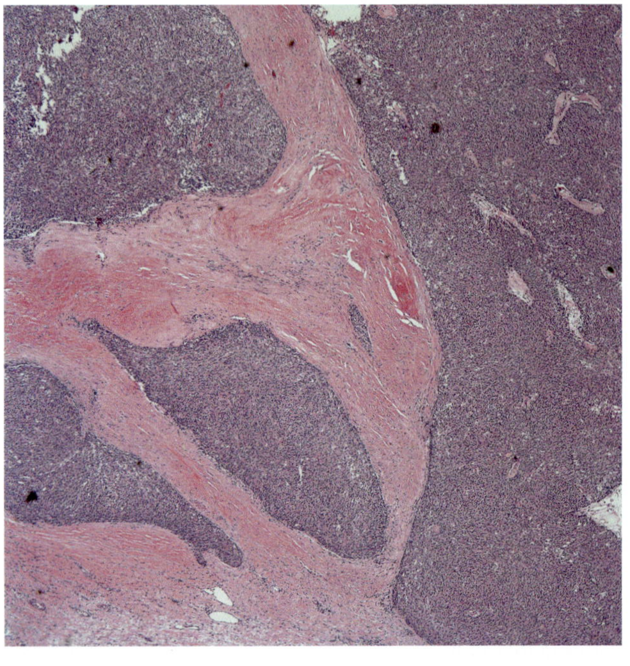

Fig. 7.72 Atypical thymoma showing thick fibrous bands and lobulation

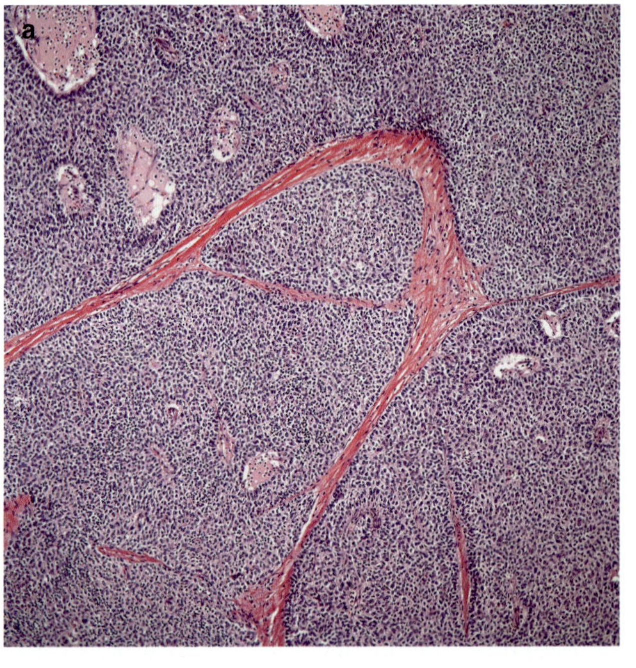

Fig. 7.73 (**a**) Atypical thymoma showing lobules separated by thin fibrocollagenous bands

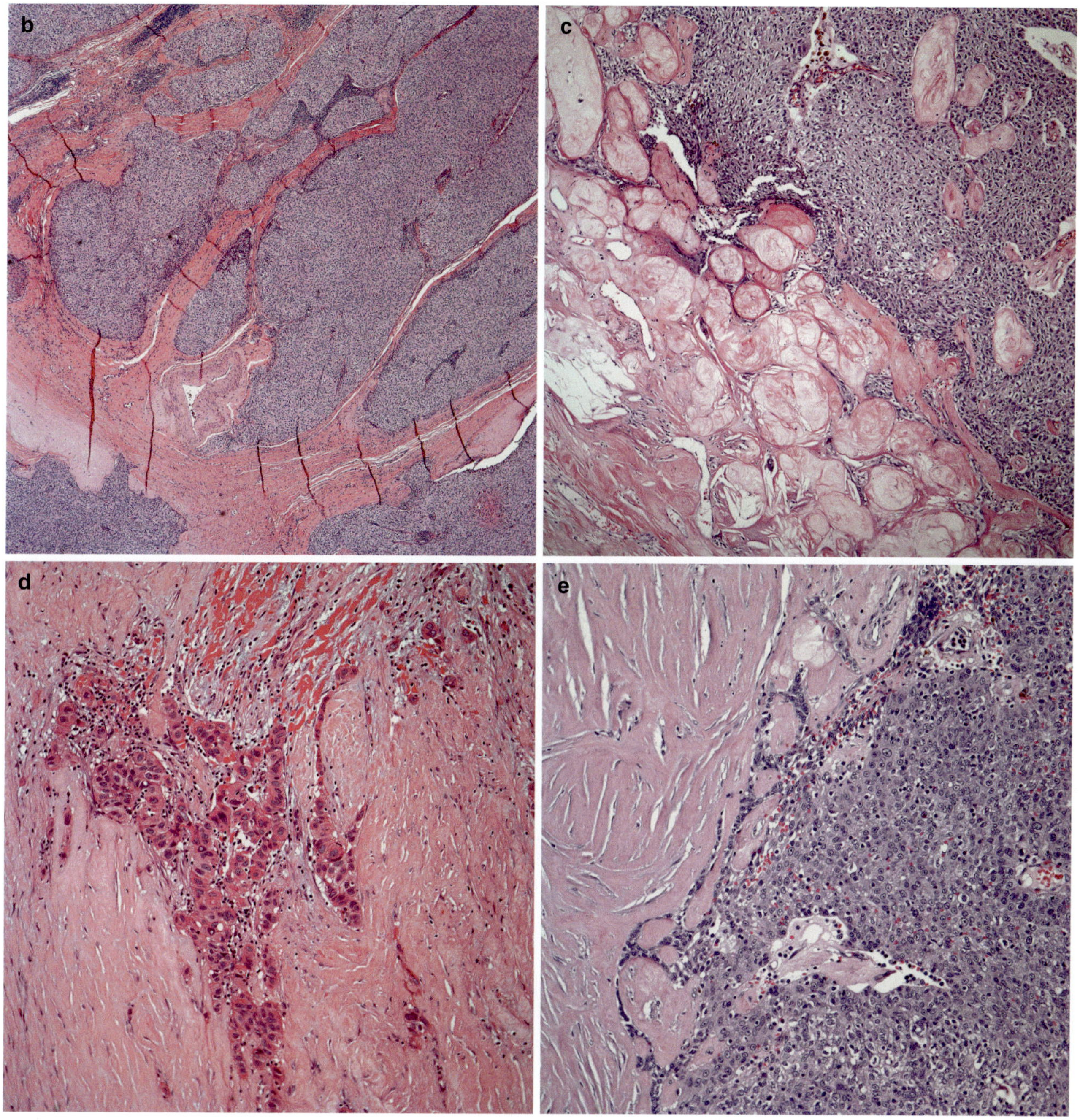

Fig. 7.73 (continued) (**b**) Thick fibrocollagen separates lobules of different sizes, (**c**) nodular hyalinization in an atypical thymoma, (**d**) extensive hyalinization with only focal areas of atypical thymoma, (**e**) thick collagen bands with hyalinization of vascular spaces

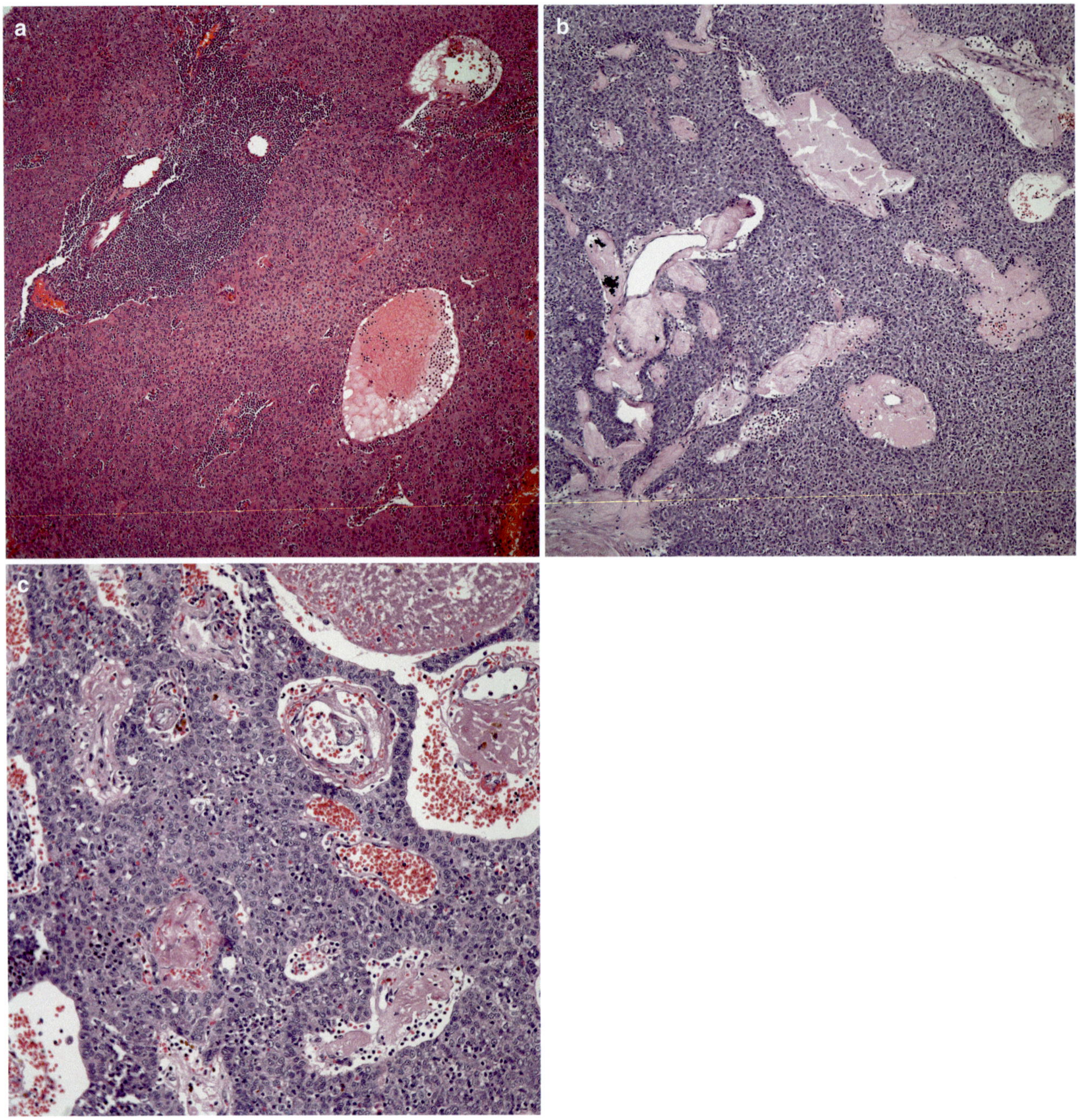

Fig. 7.74 (**a**) Atypical thymoma with prominent vascular spaces and collection of lymphocytes, (**b**) atypical thymoma with hyalinization of vascular spaces, (**c**) atypical thymoma and vascular spaces with fibrinous exudates and hyalinization

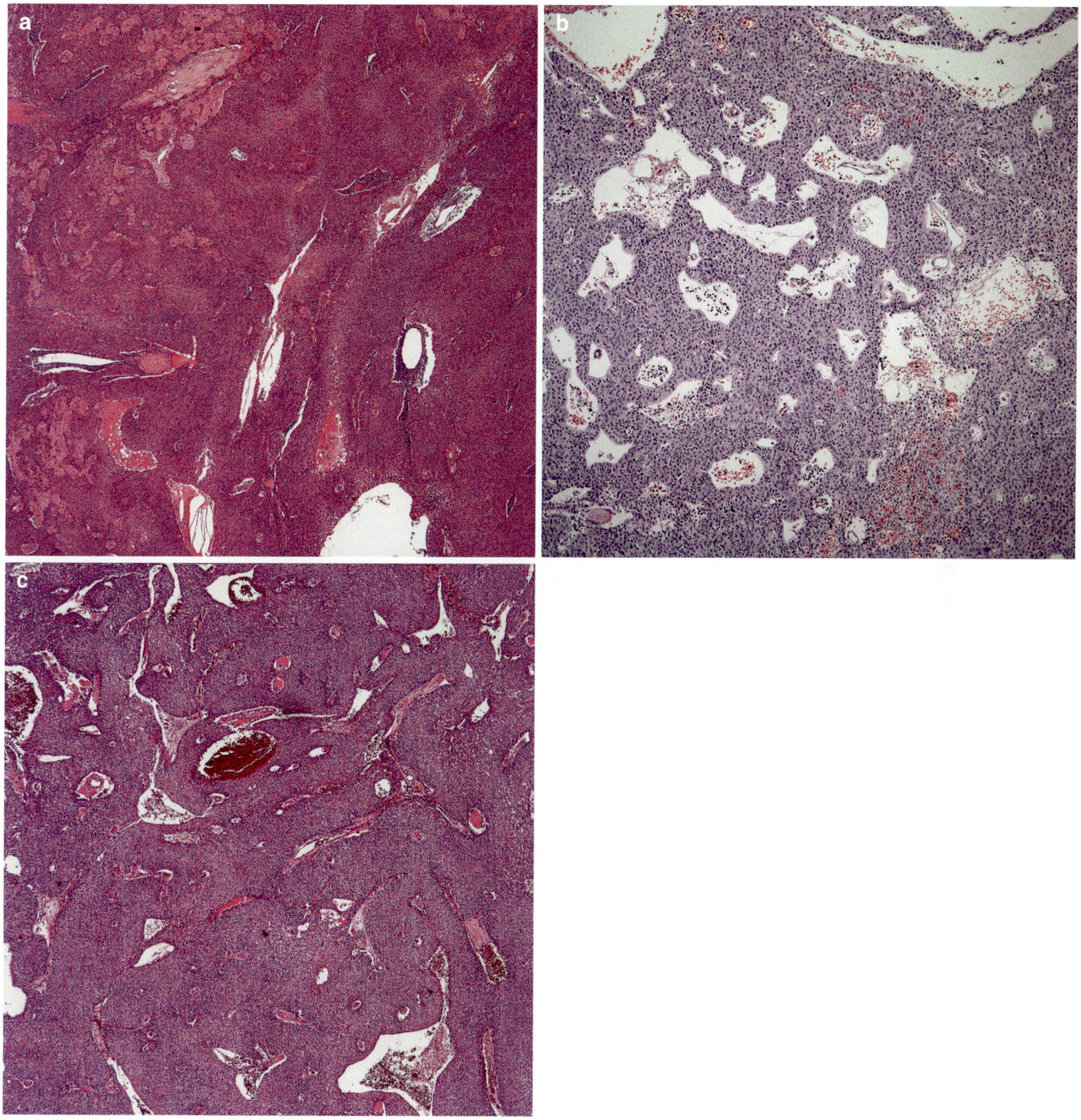

Fig. 7.75 (**a**) Atypical thymoma with diffuse pattern, (**b**) atypical thymoma with numerous vascular spaces, (**c**) atypical thymoma showing ribbons of tumors cells

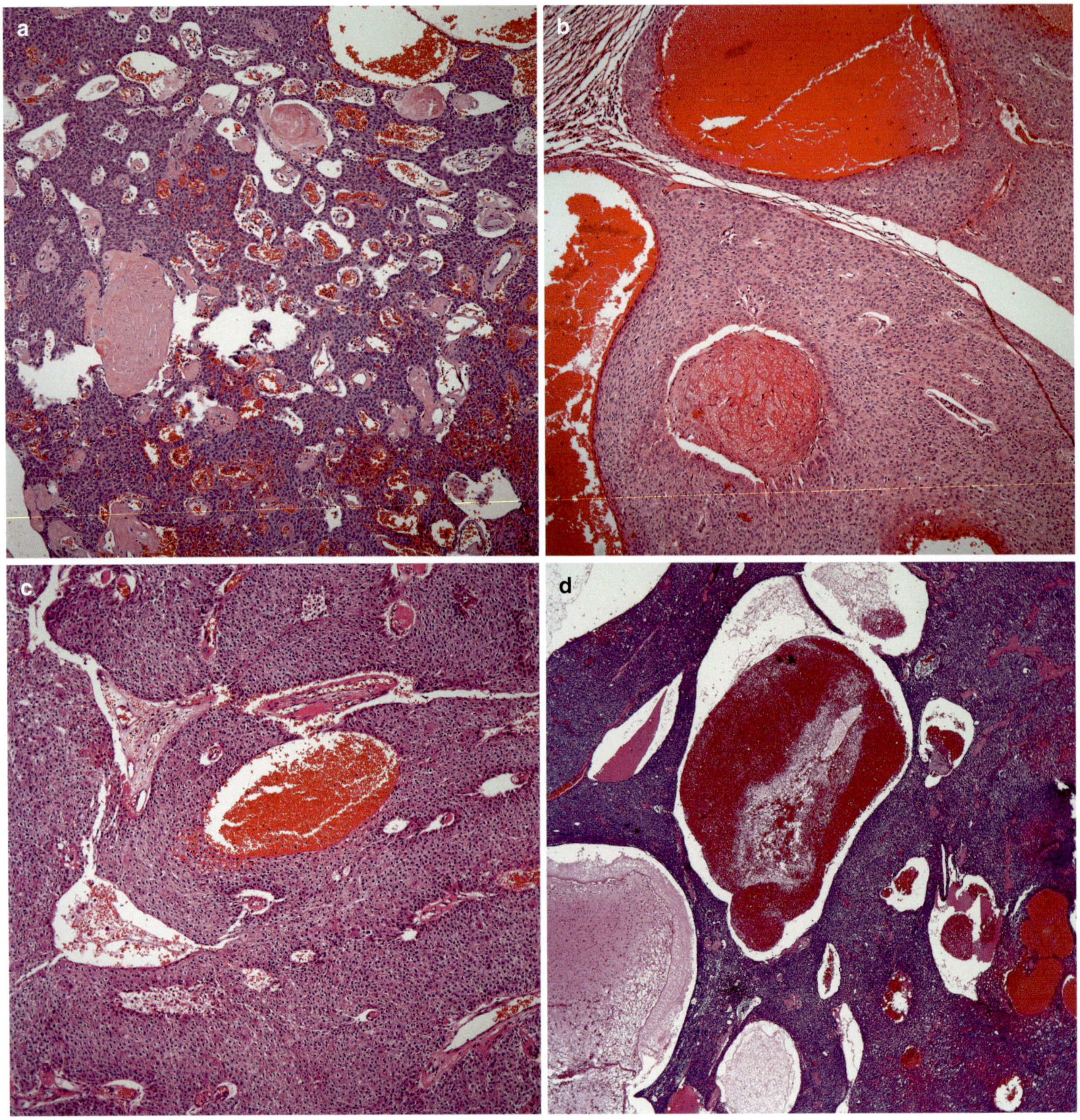

Fig. 7.76 (**a**) Atypical thymoma with numerous ectatic vascular structures mimicking a vascular tumor, (**b**) atypical thymoma with cystic areas with hemorrhage, (**c**) sheets of tumor cells with focal areas of hemorrhage, (**d**) prominent cystically dilated areas containing fresh blood

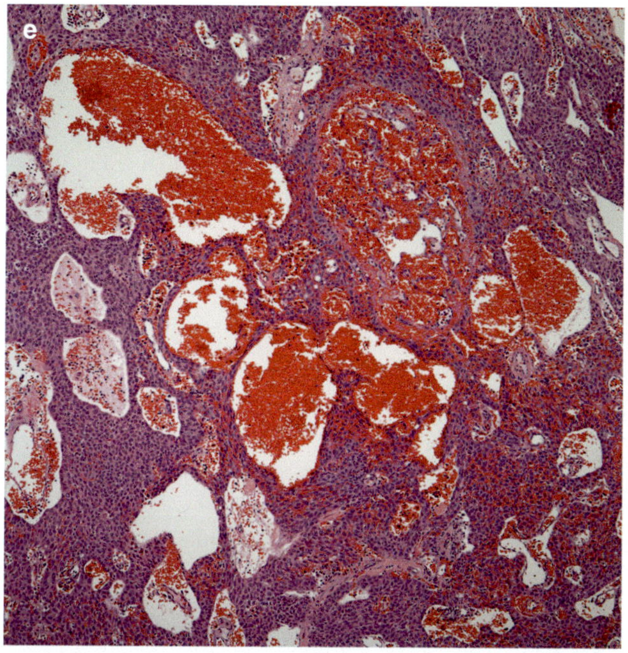

Fig. 7.76 (continued) (**e**) Atypical thymoma with cystic areas containing blood and mimicking a vascular tumor

Specific Growth Patterns

Cystic Thymomas

The occurrence of cystic thymomas is likely underreported and possibly under-recognized as, often once the diagnosis of thymoma is made, other morphological features are not reported. In a review of 93 mediastinal tumors, Dyer [145] described five cases of cystic thymoma in patients between 21 and 53 years of age; two of these patients had a history of MG. Grossly, the tumors were described as cystic, and the histology of the tumors showed different conventional growth patterns. Suster and Rosai [146], in a more direct approach to the issue of cystic thymomas, described ten cases of such variant. The patients ranged in age from 23 to 81 years. Histologically, the features of these tumors are somewhat similar to those observed by Dyer and consist of large cystic spaces separated by thick, fibrous walls, which may show inflammation, cholesterol cleft granulomas, hemorrhage, and focal necrosis. In addition, areas of more conventional thymoma may be present, which may be represented by thymomas with predominant lymphocytic component, mixed epithelial-lymphocytic, or spindle cell thymoma. In

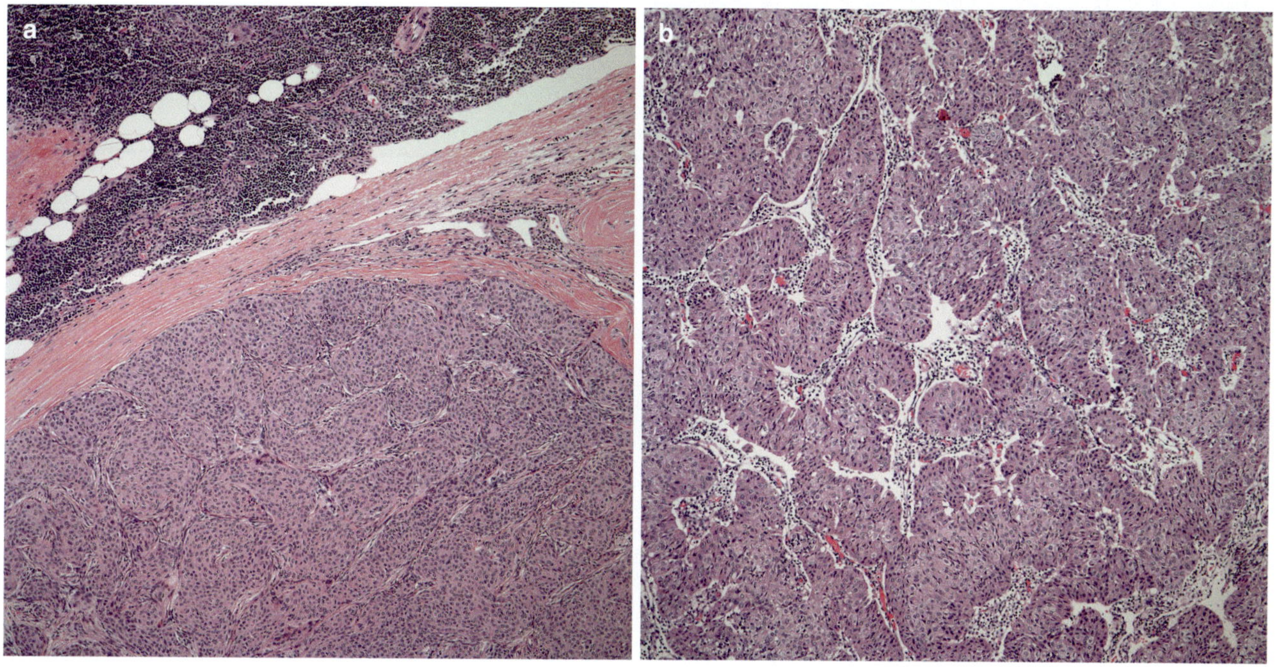

Fig. 7.77 (**a**) Atypical thymoma with a nested pattern, (**b**) ribbons of tumor cells mimicking a paraganglioma

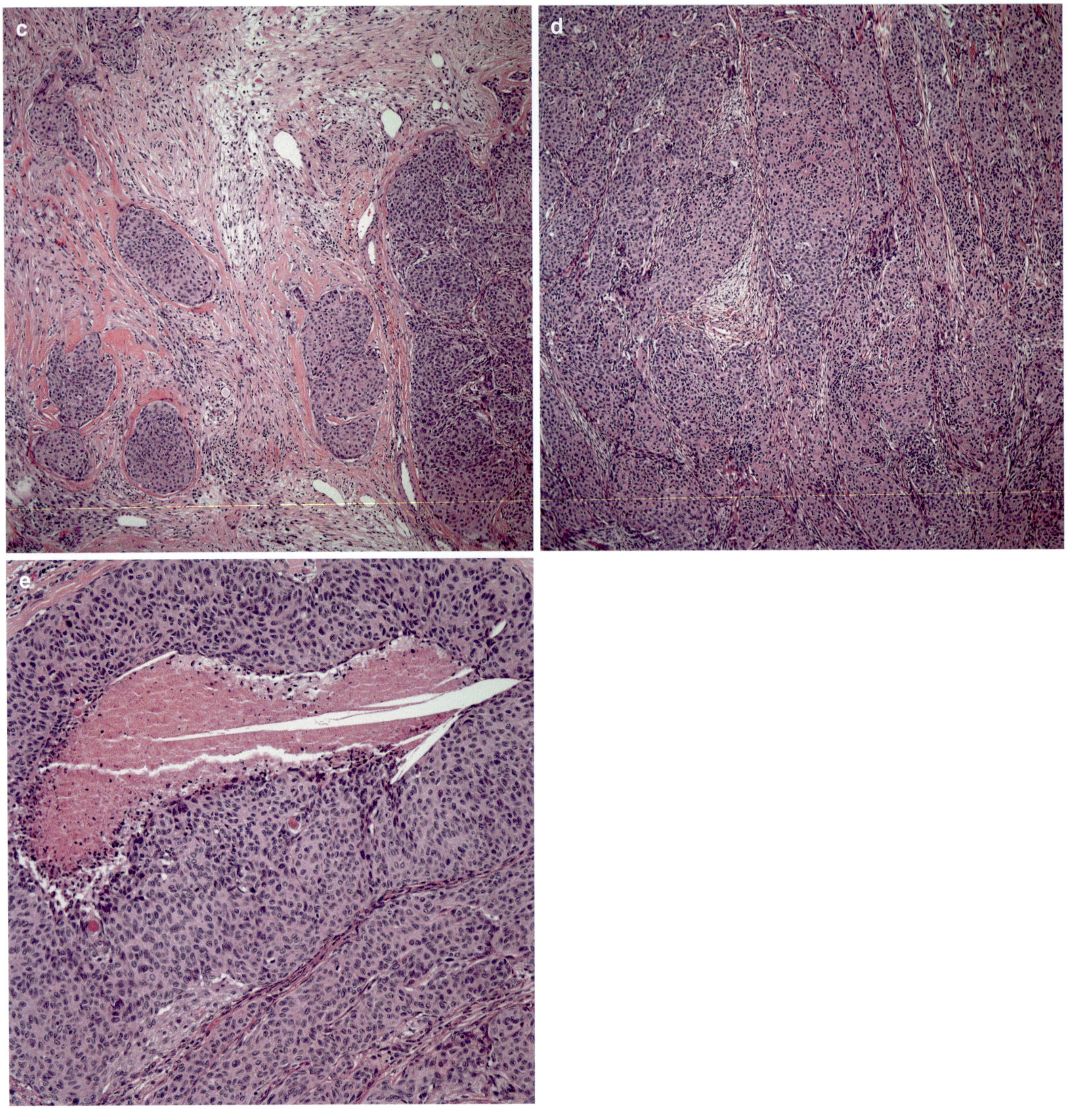

Fig. 7.77 (continued) (**c**) Atypical thymoma with extensive collagenization, (**d**) atypical thymoma with nuclear atypia and rosette-like formation, (**e**) atypical thymoma with focal comedo-like necrosis

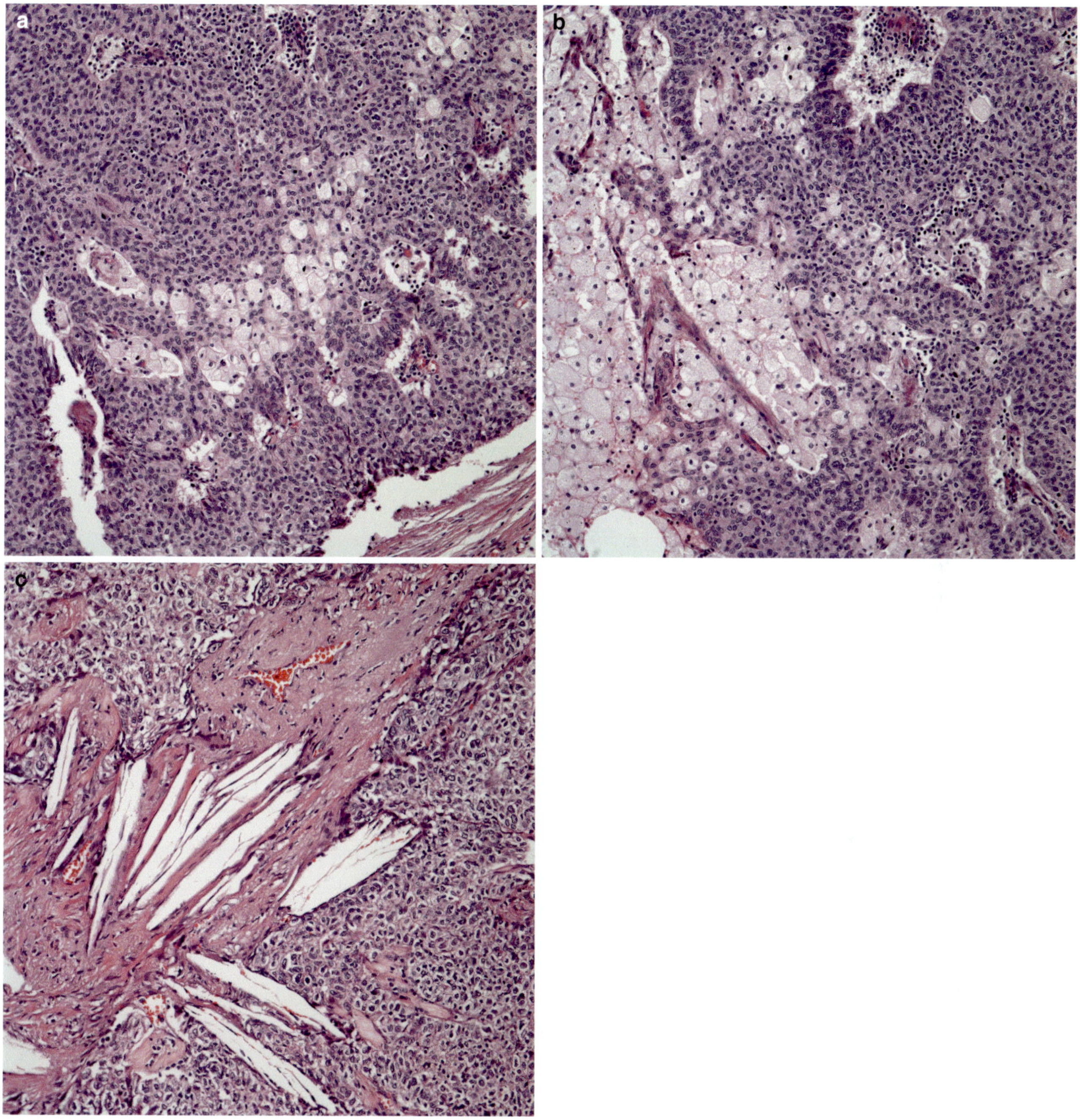

Fig. 7.78 (**a**) Atypical thymoma with focal collection of macrophages, (**b**) more extensive areas of macrophages admixed with atypical thymoma, (**c**) atypical thymoma and cholesterol cleft granuloma

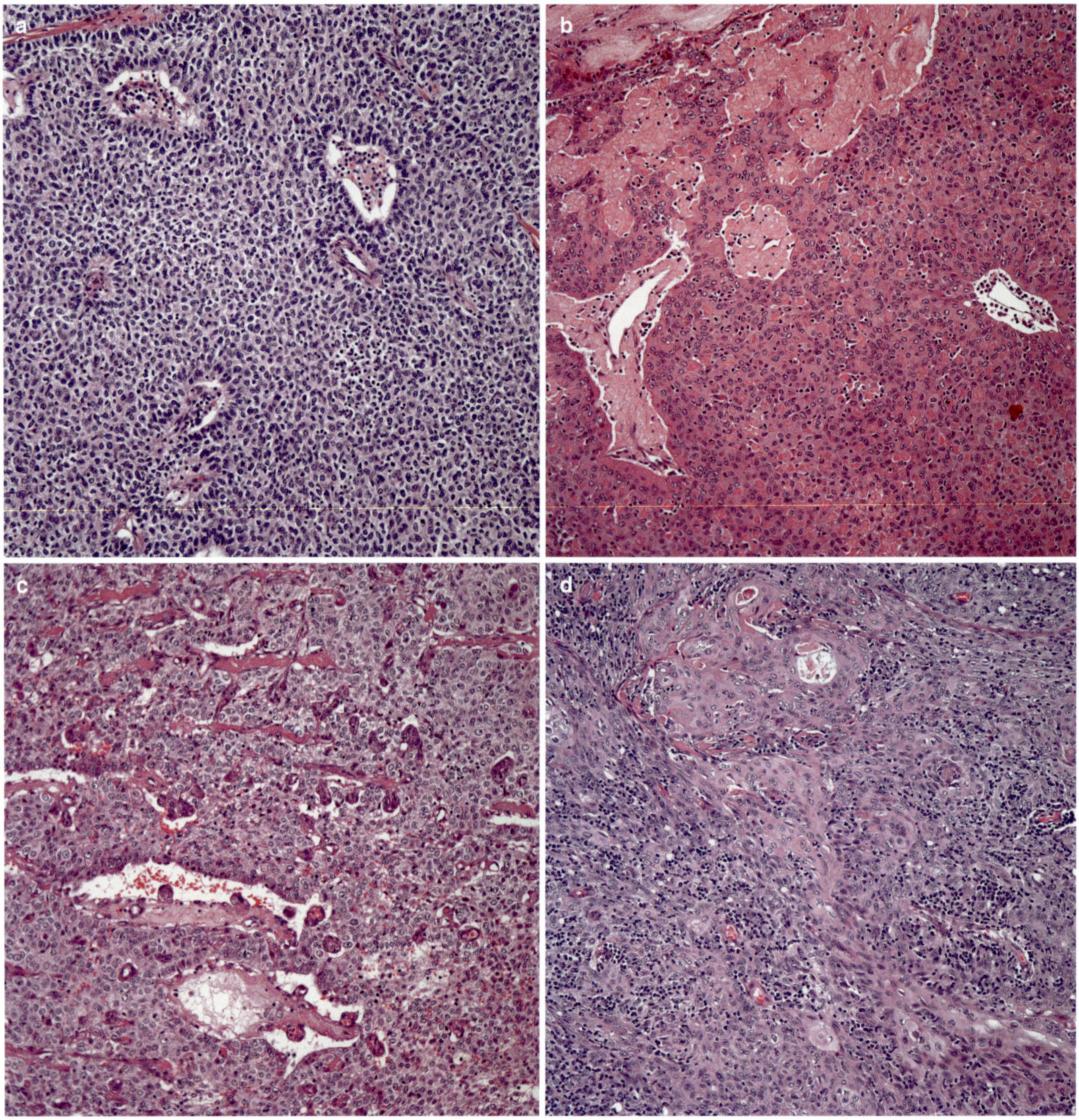

Fig. 7.79 (**a**) Atypical thymoma with palisading of the nuclei around vascular spaces, (**b**) atypical thymoma with hyalinization of vascular spaces, (**c**) atypical thymoma with nuclear atypia, (**d**) atypical thymoma with focal areas of keratinization

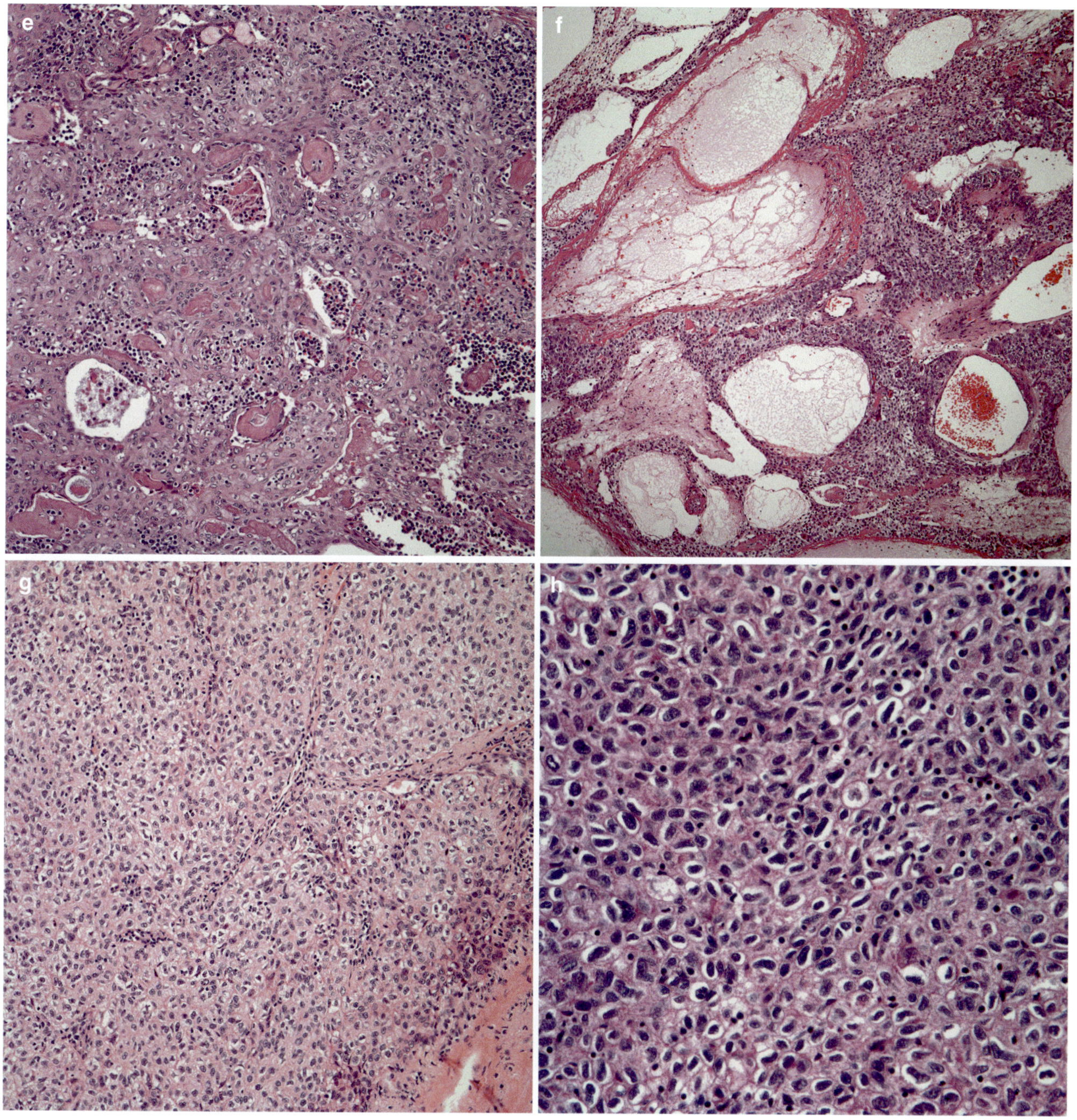

Fig. 7.79 (continued) (**e**) Atypical thymoma with more extensive areas of keratinization, (**f**) atypical thymoma with edematous and fibrinous areas, (**g**) higher magnification shows medium-sized cells with round nuclei and prominent nucleoli, (**h**) atypical thymoma shows mild to moderate nuclear atypia

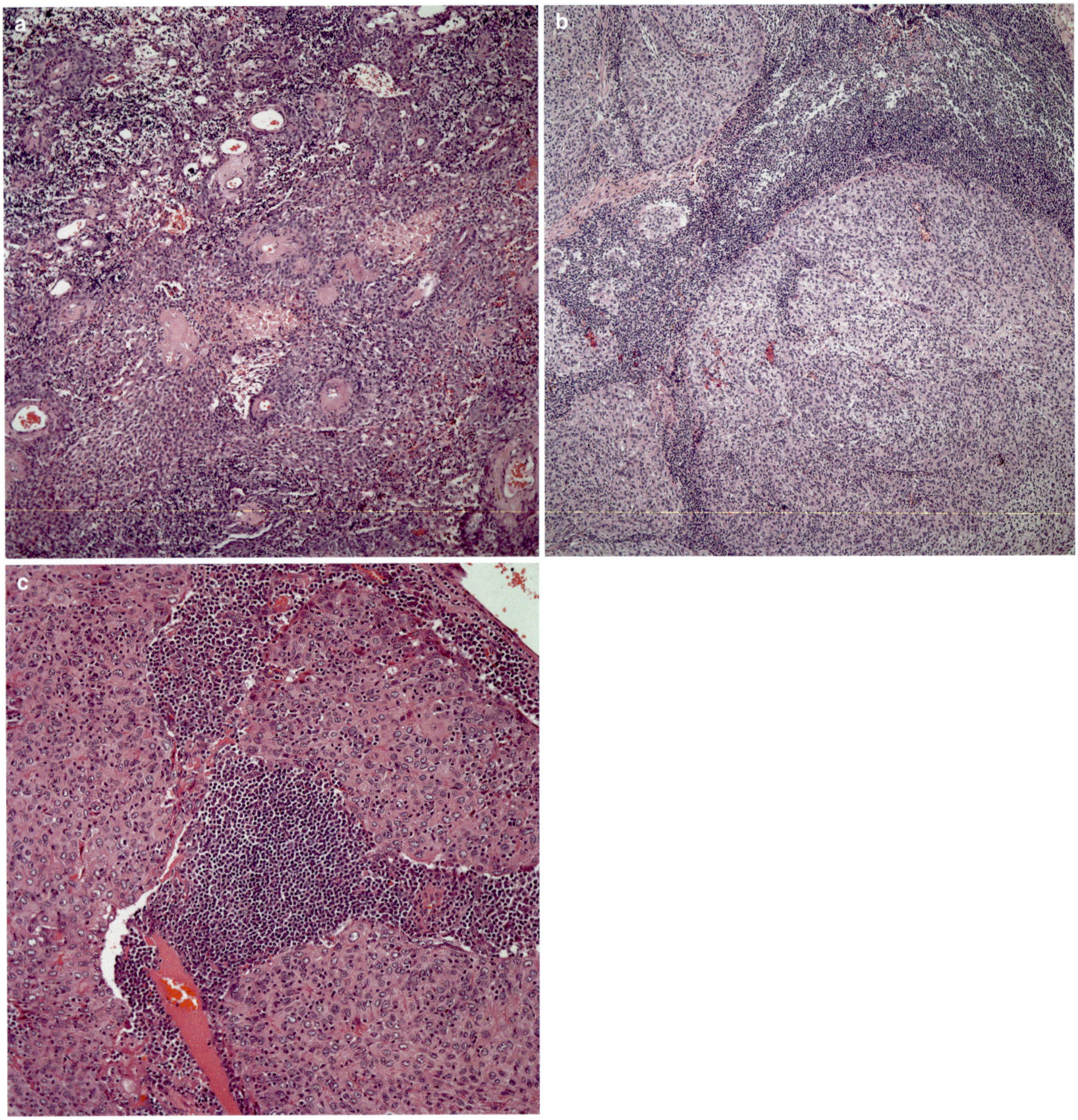

Fig. 7.80 (**a**) Atypical thymoma with focal areas of lymphocytes, (**b**) lobules of atypical thymoma separated by lymphocytes, (**c**) atypical thymoma with focal collections of lymphocytes

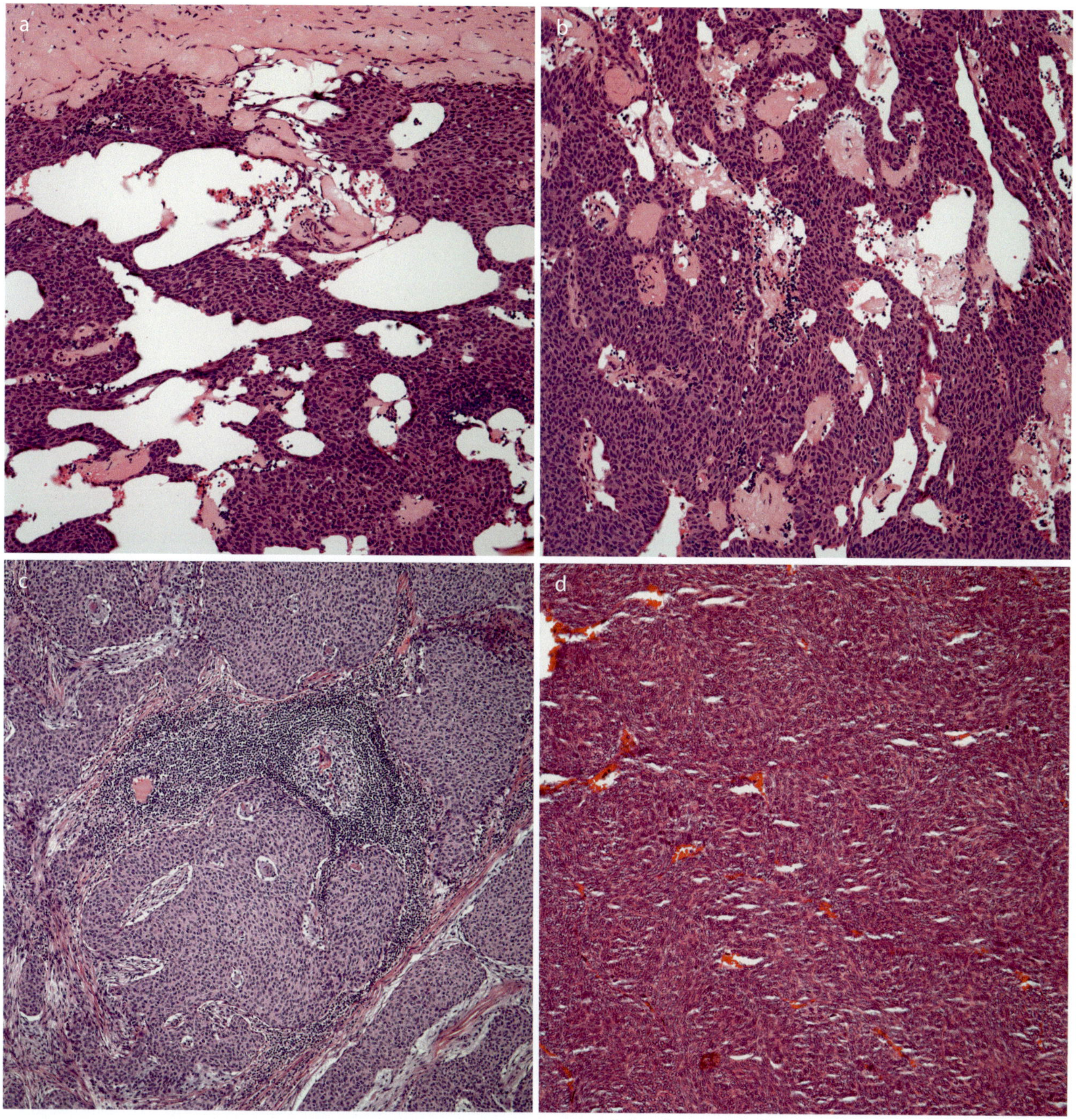

Fig. 7.81 (**a**) Spindle cell atypical thymoma, (**b**) atypical spindle cell thymoma with perivascular spaces and focal hyalinization, (**c**) atypical spindle cell thymoma with focal germinal center formation, (**d**) solid and diffuse pattern of atypical spindle cell thymoma

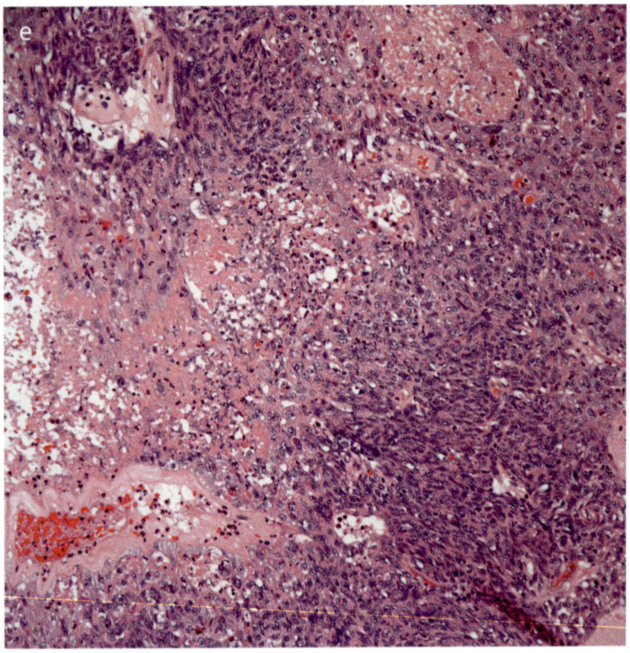

Fig. 7.81 (continued) (**e**) Atypical spindle cell thymoma with focal necrosis

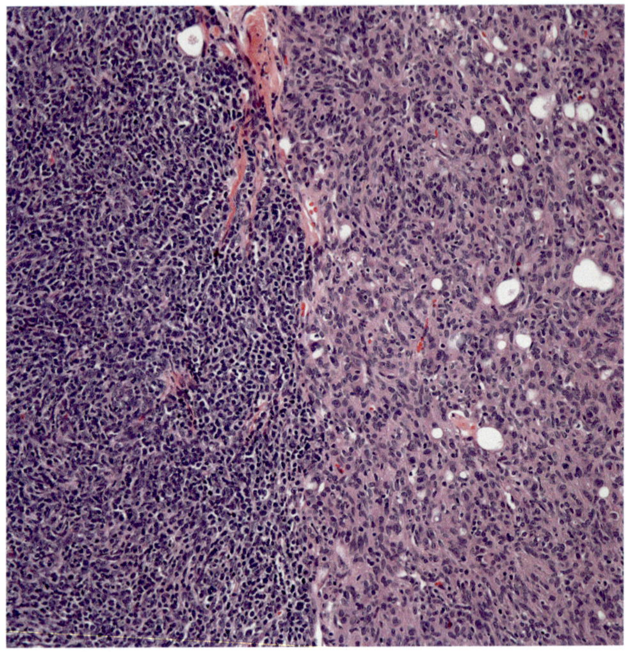

Fig. 7.83 Atypical thymoma mixed with a thymoma with lymphocytes

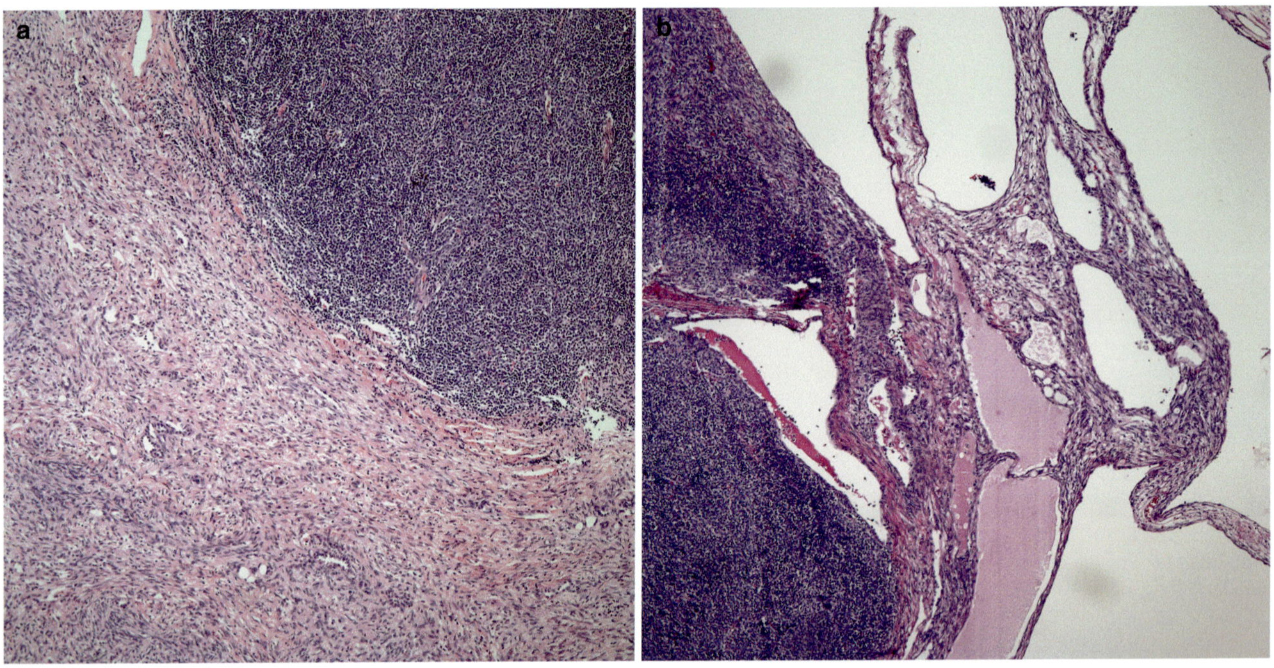

Fig. 7.82 (**a**) Mixed spindle cell thymoma and lymphocytic thymoma almost in equal proportions, (**b**) cystic spindle cell thymoma mixed with lymphocytic thymoma

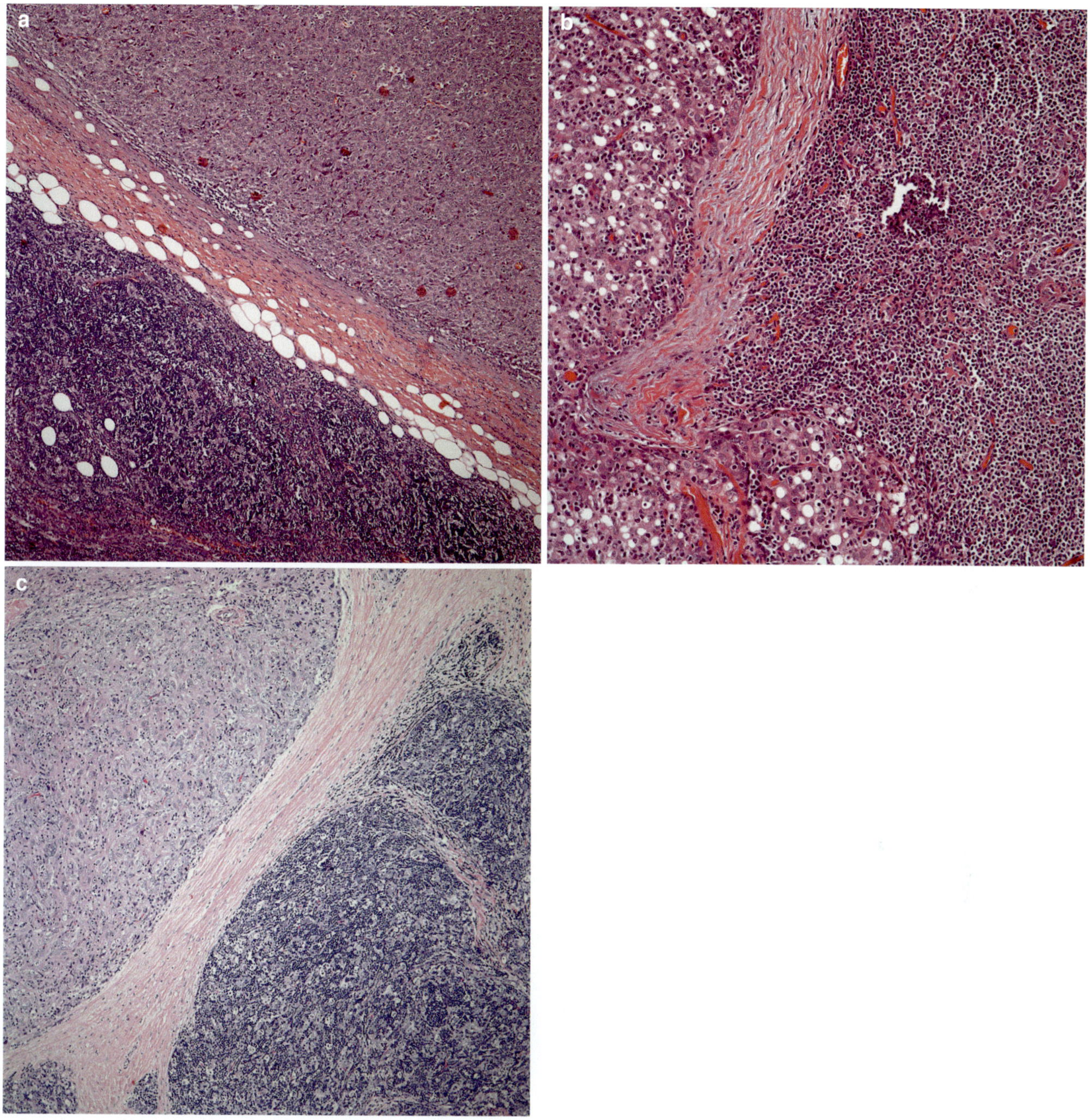

Fig. 7.84 (**a**) Atypical thymoma mixed with a thymoma with approximately equal proportion of lymphocytes and epithelial cells, (**b**, **c**) two different areas: one composed of thymoma with lymphocytes and the other of atypical thymoma, in (**c**) more cellular atypia in the atypical thymoma

some thymomas, the so-called areas of medullary differentiation may be present (presence of Hassall's corpuscles). Other common features associated in the thymoma areas include the presence of perivascular spaces. Important to highlight is that in the cystic spaces of thymoma, the cysts are generally not lined by any specific type of epithelium (Fig. 7.88). However, in some cases, it is difficult to separate cystic thymomas not otherwise specified from thymomas arising in multilocular thymic cysts, in which the cystic wall may be lined by different types of epithelium (Fig. 7.89a–h). It is also important to highlight that the cystic changes are not specific for some histologies, as we have seen cystic changes occur in spindle cell thymomas (Fig. 7.90) and atypical thymomas (Fig. 7.91). More recently, cystic thymomas have been reported as case reports either in adults or children [147, 148]. In general, the gross features of the resected tumor mass are of great importance in order to correlate the microscopic findings with the macroscopic appearance of the tumor. In cases in which the tumor may have areas of multilocular thymic cyst, it is important to properly evaluate whether the tumor is invasive or encapsulated.

Rhabdomyomatous Thymoma

Myoid cells and striated muscle cells are well known to occur in the normal thymus [149]. In pathological conditions, myoid cells have been described in thymuses of patients with myasthenia gravis [150–152]. However, the presence of myoid cells in association with thymomas is rather rare. Henry reported a single case that the author designated as an "unusual thymic tumor with striated muscle" [153]. In 1984, Murakami and colleagues [154] reported a case that the author described as thymic tumor (thymoma) with massive proliferation of myoid cells. The authors performed electron microscopic studies, which clearly separated the epithelial from the myoid cells. The term rhabdomyomatous thymoma was coined in 1993 with the description of a single case in a 21-year-old asymptomatic patient who presented with anterior mediastinal mass which, at resection, showed the presence of an encapsulated tumor with a dual proliferation of epithelial cells and myoid cells [155]. However, it is important to recognize that the epithelial component of these tumors with rhabdomyomatous differentiation may also be varied. We have seen cases of spindle cell thymomas, atypical thymomas, and lymphocytic thymomas with varying proportions of rhabdoid cells (Fig. 7.92a–g). Immunohistochemical stains for keratin decorated the epithelial component, while desmin and myoglobin were positive in the myoid component (Fig. 7.92h, i). More recently, we have had the opportunity to observe other similar cases occurring in thymomas and thymic carcinomas. Interestingly, the cases have been in adult patients without history of MG. In addition, the histological types of the thymomas have been atypical thymoma and lymphocytic type.

Plasma Cell Thymoma

In general, although plasma cells may be a component of the normal thymus, their presence is rare. In some pathological conditions such as autoimmune diseases, however, plasma cells may be present in the thymic gland [156]. However, in 1994, a description of a thymoma with extensive presence of plasma cells was described in what the authors designated as plasma cell-rich thymoma (Fig. 7.93a–c) [157]. The tumor was described in a 49-year-old man without history of auto-

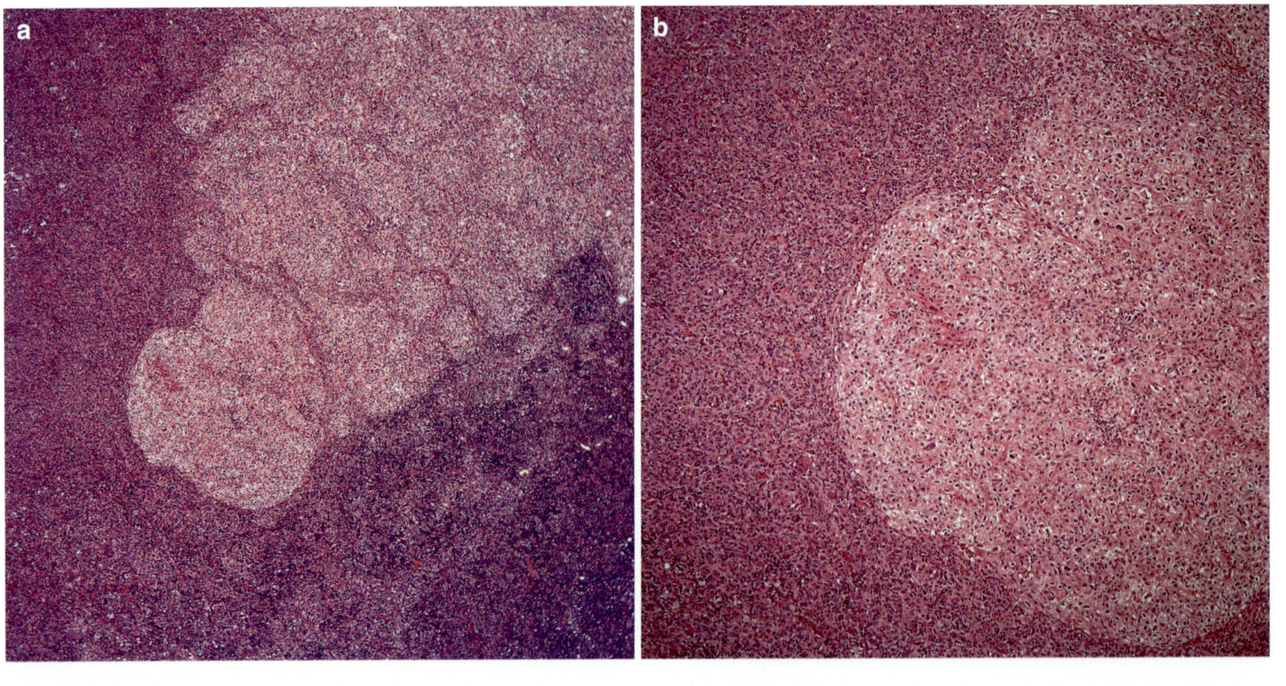

Fig. 7.85 (**a**) Atypical thymoma margin into a lymphocytic thymoma, (**b**) higher magnification shows both components without specific barrier

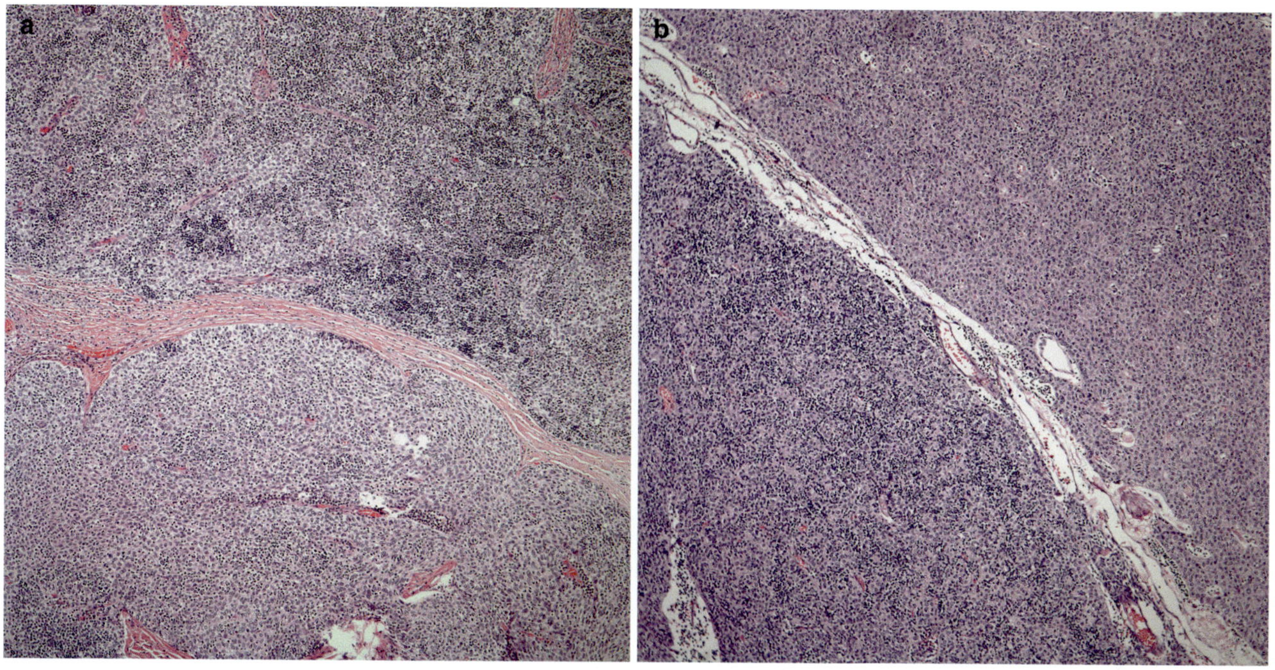

Fig. 7.86 (**a**) Atypical thymoma showing areas with lack of lymphocytes and areas with lymphocytes, (**b**) higher magnification of both components separated by thin strands of collagen

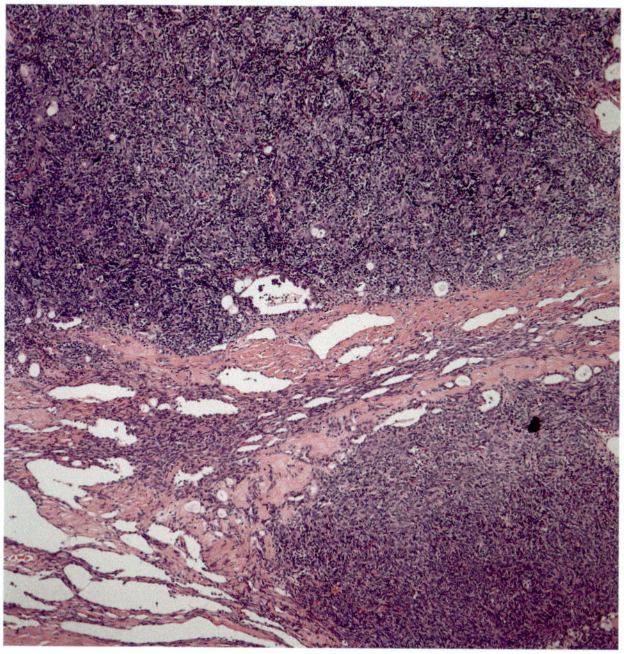

Fig. 7.87 Spindle cell thymoma showing areas with and without lymphocytes

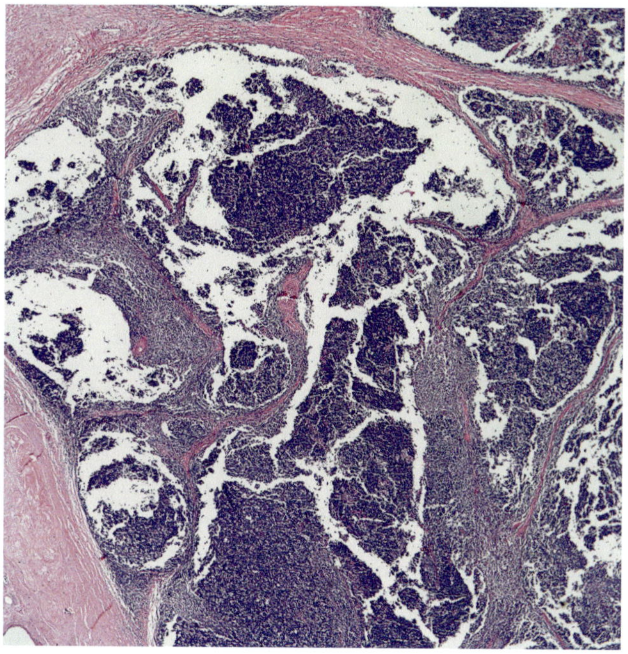

Fig. 7.88 Cystic lymphocytic thymoma

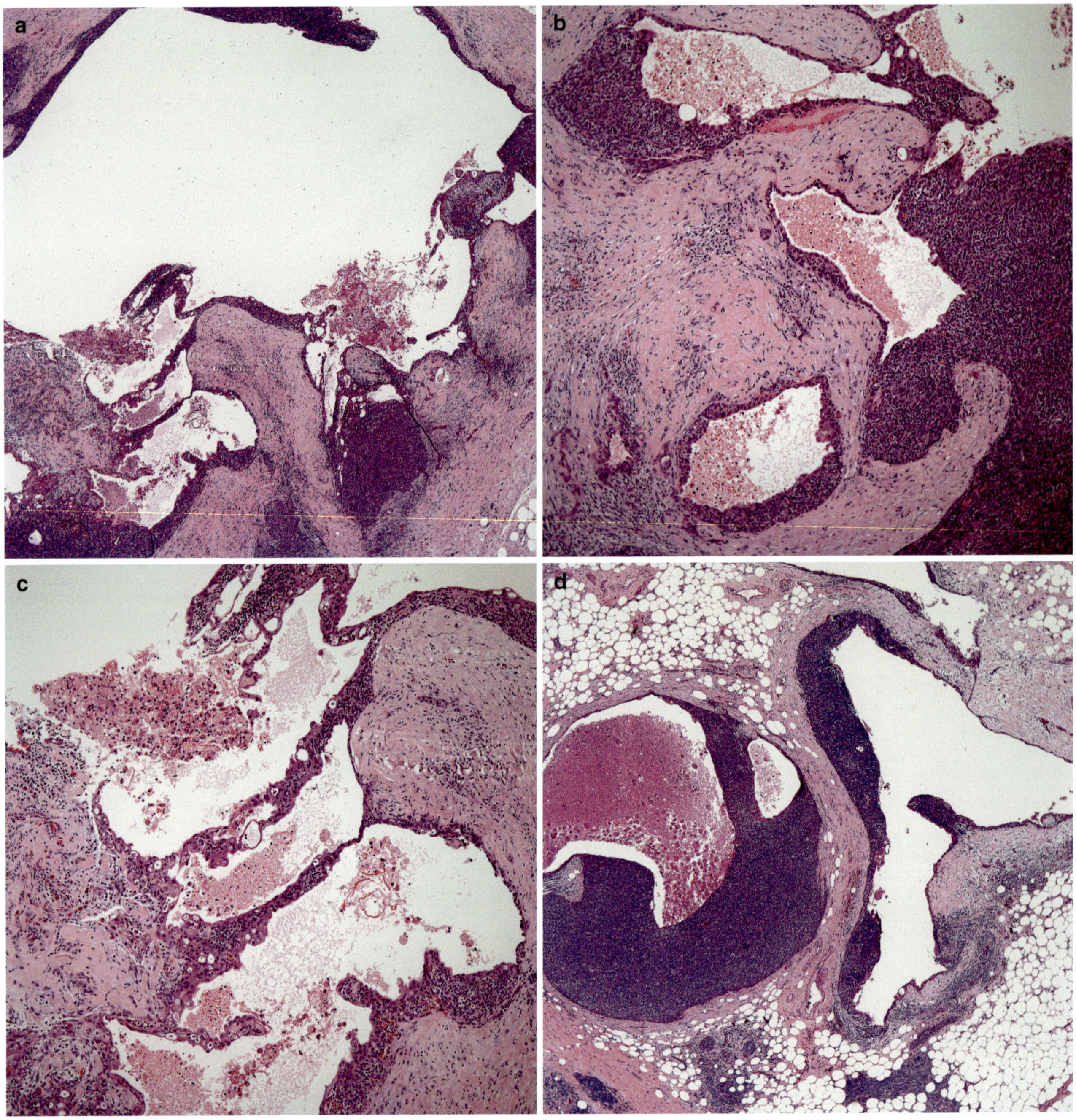

Fig. 7.89 (**a**) Cystic thymoma possibly growing along a MTC, (**b**) higher magnification showing the lymphocytic thymoma and the lining of the cysts, (**c**) closer view of the cystic structures lined by vacuolated and squamous type of epithelium, (**d**) merging areas of cystic thymoma and cystic structures lined by squamous epithelium merging with lymphocytic thymoma

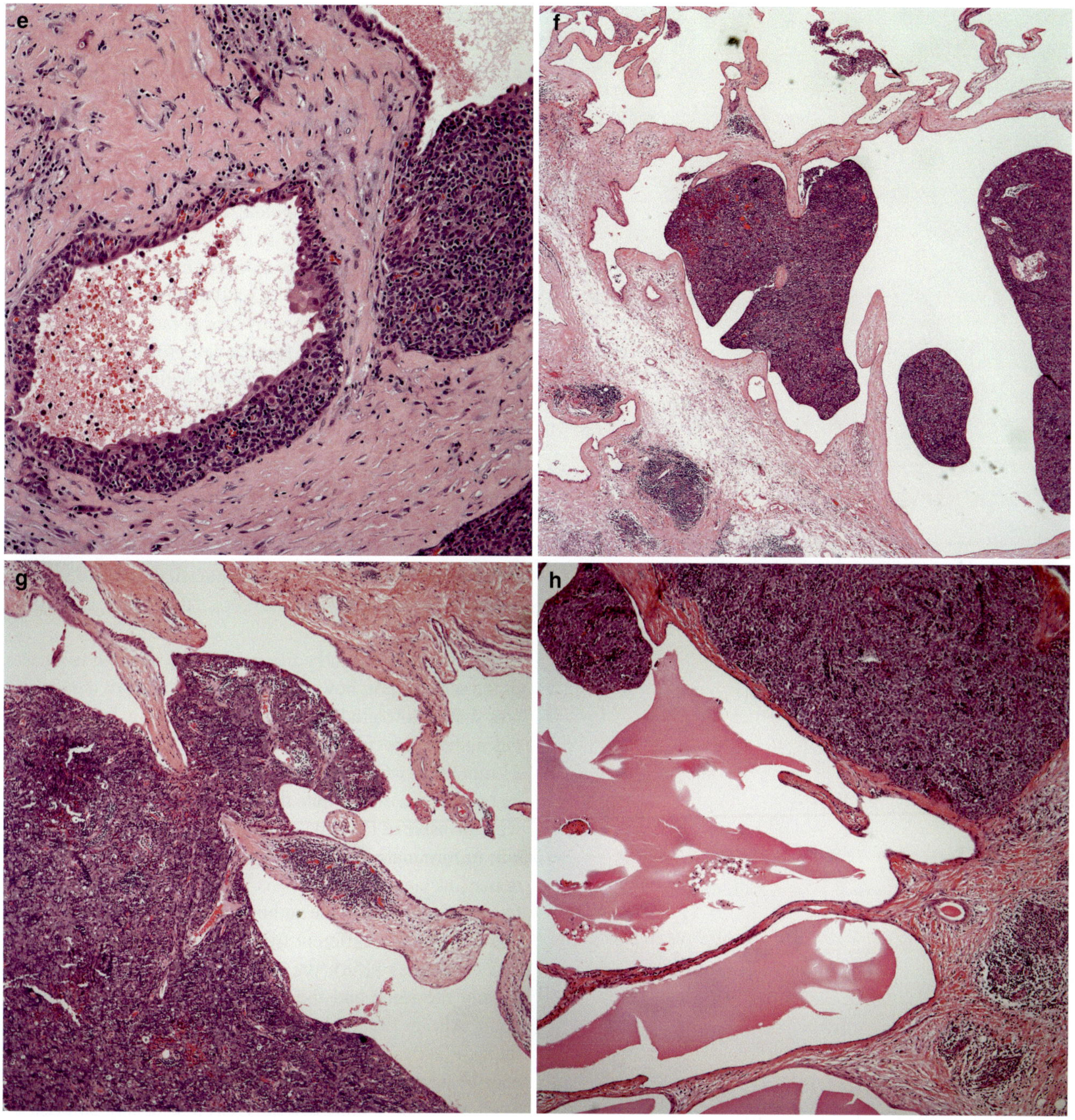

Fig. 7.89 (continued) (**e**) Closer view at the lining of the cyst; at times it is difficult to determine the exact nature of the epithelium, (**f**) prominent cystic areas containing lymphocytic thymoma, (**g**) thymoma with equal proportion of lymphocytes and epithelial cells and cystic structures, (**h**) closer view of the two different components

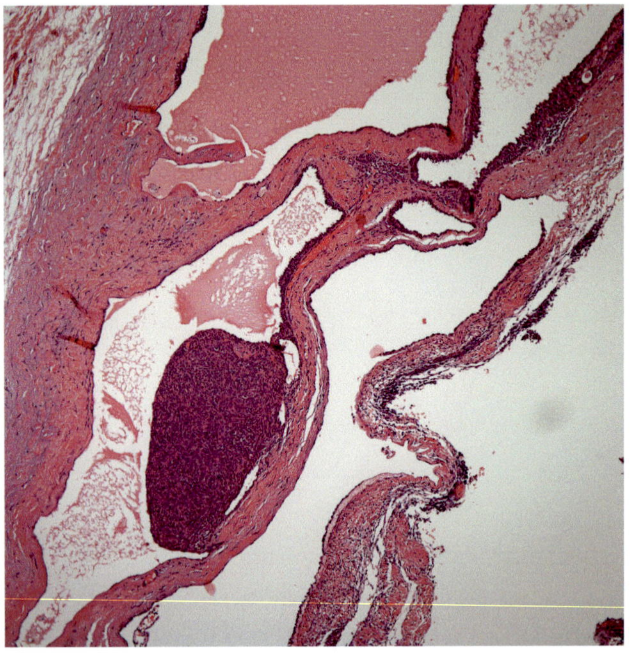

Fig. 7.90 Cystically dilated structures and spindle cell thymoma

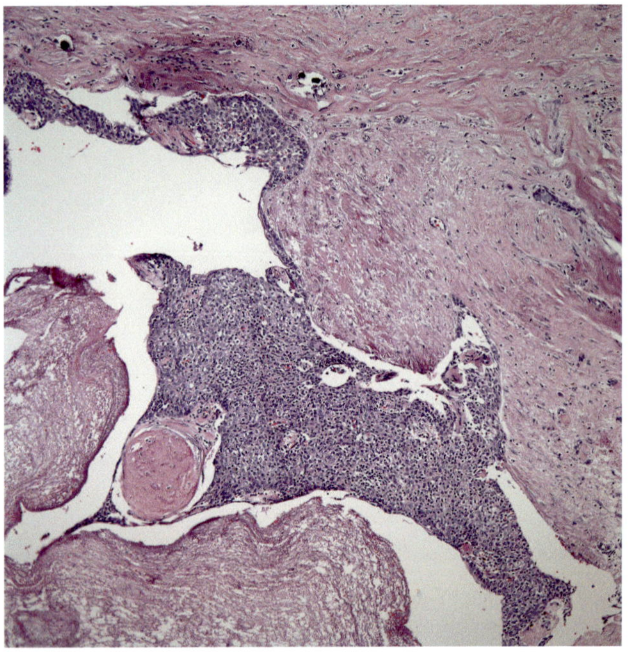

Fig. 7.91 Atypical thymoma with cystic changes

immune disorder including MG. However, subsequently the patient developed polyclonal hypergammaglobulinemia of unknown cause. The plasma cells in this tumor showed polyclonal immunoreactivity for kappa and lambda. The authors concluded that such a case is an extreme case of aberrant immunologic modulation of the thymus to an autoimmune process with massive hyperplasia of the B-cell compartment of the thymus.

Thymoma with Pseudosarcomatous Stroma

This tumor was initially described by Suster [158] in 1997 in a description of six patients with mediastinal tumors that were characterized by the presence of anastomosing islands and cords of oval to polygonal epithelial cells, which in some areas show nuclear atypia and occasional mitotic activity. The epithelial islands are separated by extensive areas composed of a cellular spindle cell proliferation without atypia and/or mitotic activity (Fig. 7.94a–e). In some of these cases, the epithelial component has been of the atypical spindle cell type (Fig. 7.95a, b). By immunohistochemistry, the epithelial islands are positive for keratin (Fig. 7.96) and p40 (Fig. 7.97), while the spindle cell proliferation is negative for keratin and positive for vimentin (Fig. 7.98) and focally for smooth muscle actin. More important to highlight is that, despite some atypical features in these tumors, the follow-up is that of a benign or low-grade neoplasm. In five of the six cases described, the follow-up ranged between 5 and 20 years (mean, 10 years), and no recurrences were observed. Nevertheless, it is also important to highlight that in the original description of the tumor, all the cases described represented encapsulated tumors, thus the uneventful follow-up.

In 1999, Yoneda and colleagues [159] reported five cases of the same tumor; however, the interpretation of the authors was that of low-grade metaplastic carcinoma. Interestingly, the authors provided a follow-up that ranged from 12 to 21 months in which they did not document any recurrence or metastatic disease, despite the fact that some of these tumors were invasive at the time of diagnosis. Therefore, it is difficult to formulate a rationale for the interpretation of "carcinoma," as clearly the tumor is behaving in a more indolent fashion. Even though the authors of this series of cases stated that this tumor is different from the one described by Suster and colleagues [158], the fact is that the two tumors are exactly the same and the behavior is clearly not of carcinoma. Also in 1999, the same group of authors [160] reported the same series of cases in a different journal, the only difference being that in this manuscript one patient had recurrence. Such an event should not be viewed with any surprise as some of the tumors were invasive at the time of diagnosis, and such occurrence commonly happens with garden-variety thymomas. However, in this "new version" by the same group of patients, the authors once again stated incorrectly that "their tumor" is probably different from the one described by Suster and colleagues [158]. In 2001, Noh and colleagues [161] reported a single case of this particular tumor, and the authors stated that in their opinion all the cases described with different names represent the same entity, and the authors of the case report opted for the one proposed by Suster and colleagues [158]. More interesting is that the WHO, without conducting any specific study of their own, decided to change the name of this tumor to what the

WHO authors called "metaplastic thymoma." Of course, with this new terminology, reports of the same entity have been presented, and, needless to say, the results have been the same. Liu and colleagues [162], now using the WHO terminology, reported seven cases of this tumor and found similar follow-up as the one provided in the original report by Suster and colleagues [158]. More recently, this tumor has also been described as a cystic tumor [163]. At this point, it is important to review some concepts regarding this tumor. It is obvious that the authors of the WHO, realizing the error in interpretation by those who interpreted this tumor as "metaplastic carcinoma," decided to play a game of satisfaction by keeping the term "metaplastic" but appending that term to thymoma. However, there is nothing metaplastic about this tumor at all. First of all, the epithelial component without the presence of abundant lymphocytes actually qualifies as an atypical thymoma. The spindle cell component likely originates from the remnants of fibrocollagenous bands that are commonly seen in thymomas. These collagenous bands can have a fibroblastic proliferation, which in thymomas with pseudosarcomatous stroma becomes exuberant forming what the authors of the original interpretation termed "pseudosarcomatous." One can argue that if this is in reality "metaplasia" in which the epithelial cells are transforming into spindle cells, then one would identify it either by immunohistochemistry or electron microscopic evidence of epithelial differentiation in the spindle cell component, which likely is of fibroblastic nature. More worrisome is the fact that names and entities are changed at will without conducting meaningful studies or, worse, without understanding the nature of the entity in question.

Micronodular Thymoma with Lymphoid B-Cell Hyperplasia

This thymoma variant was described originally in 1999 by Suster and Moran [164] in a description of 18 cases which were characterized by the presence of nodules of spindle cells embedded in a lymphoid stroma with prominent germinal centers. The spindle cell nodules are composed of oval cells without nuclear atypia or mitotic activity (Fig. 7.99a–d). Germinal centers are commonly seen, which can be either inconspicuous of showing hyperplastic changes (Fig. 7.99e, f). In some cases, these tumors may show prominent cystic changes (Fig. 7.100a–e). By immunohistochemistry, the epithelial nodules show strong positivity with keratin (Fig. 7.100f), while the lymphoid stroma shows strong positivity with CD45 and CD20 (Fig. 7.100g) and polyclonality with kappa and lambda chains. In addition, other lymphoid markers – including CD3, CD5, CD99, and CD1a – are negative. Clinically, none of the patients originally described had a history of MG or any other autoimmune disease. The clinical follow-up provided in this original manuscript was that observed in conventional thymomas, and in about half of the cases presented,

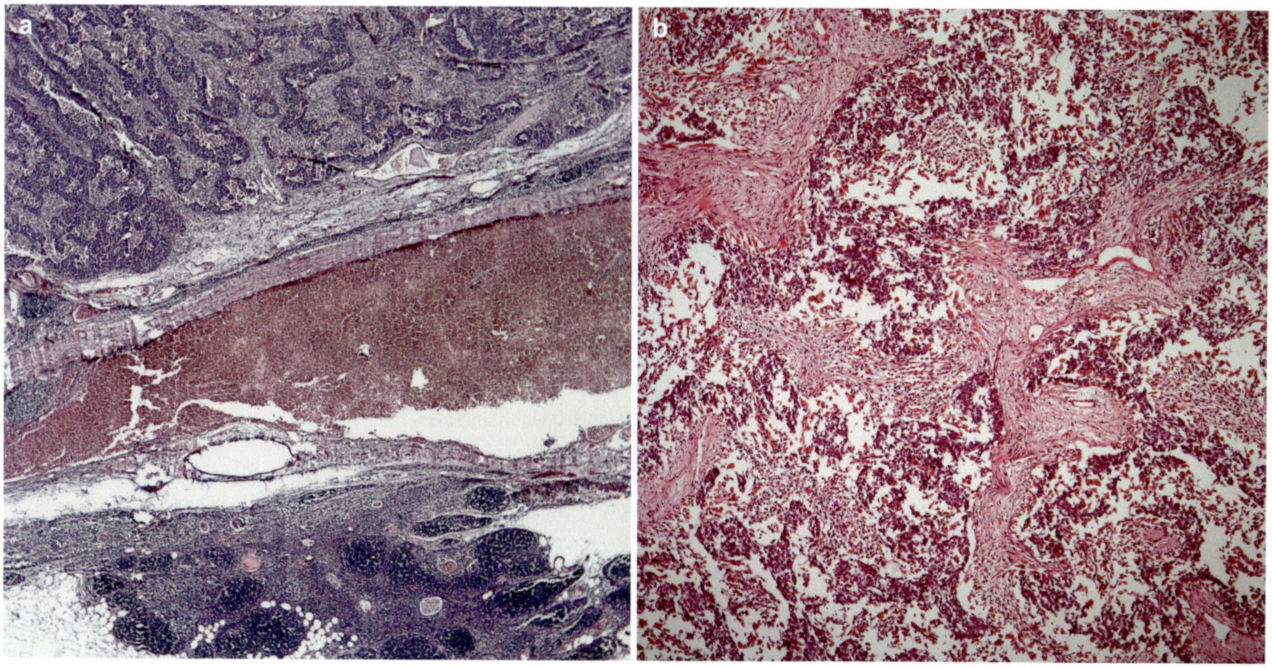

Fig. 7.92 (**a**) Encapsulated rhabdomyomatous thymoma; note the presence of normal thymus in the periphery. (**b**) Rhabdomyomatous thymoma; note the presence of epithelial spindle cells

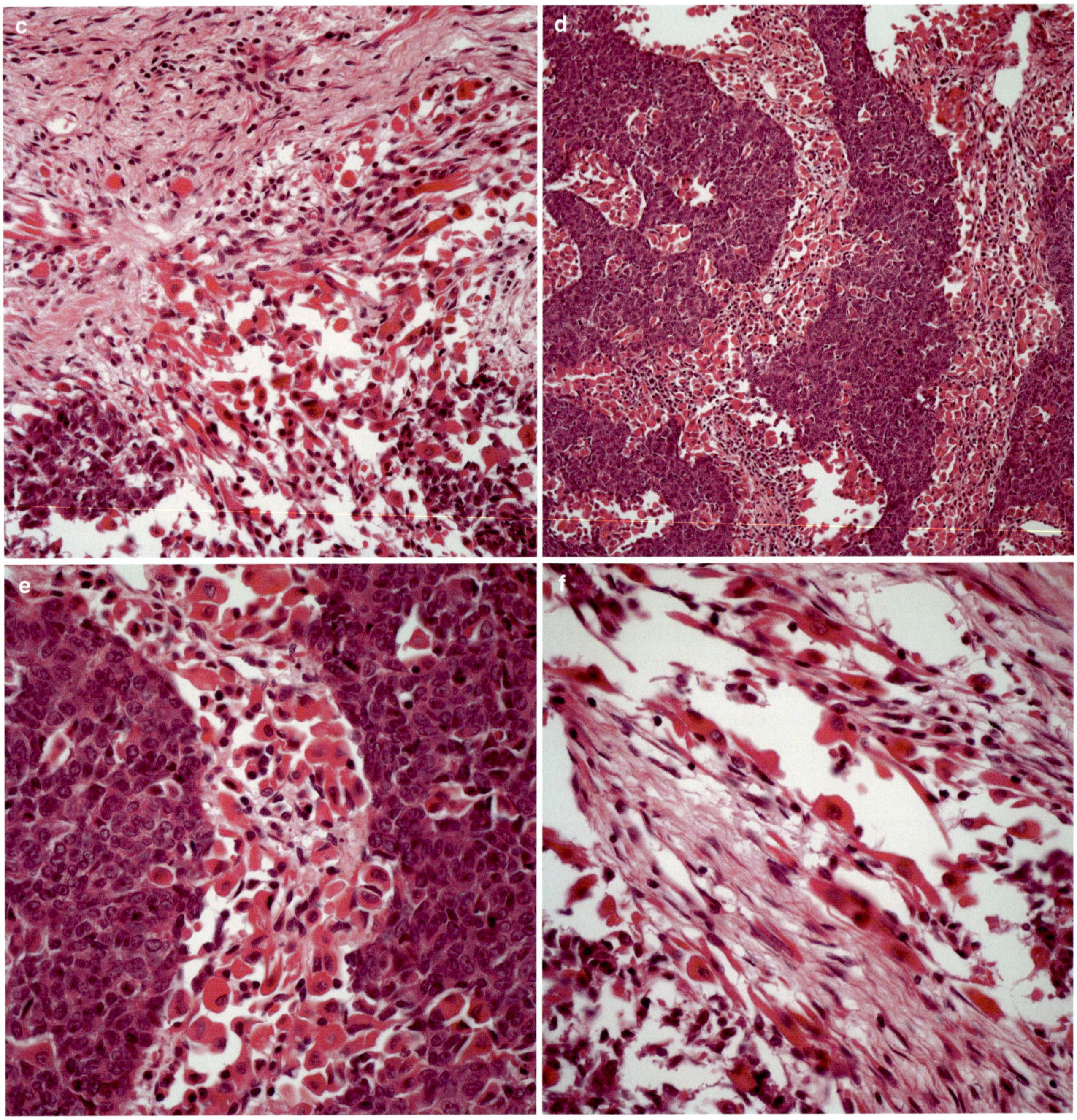

Fig. 7.92 (continued) (**c**) Spindle and oval cells admixed with muscle cells. (**d**) Atypical thymoma and extensive muscle component. (**e**) Closer view of the muscle cells and adjacent epithelial cells. (**f**) Closer view at the muscle cells mixed with spindle cells

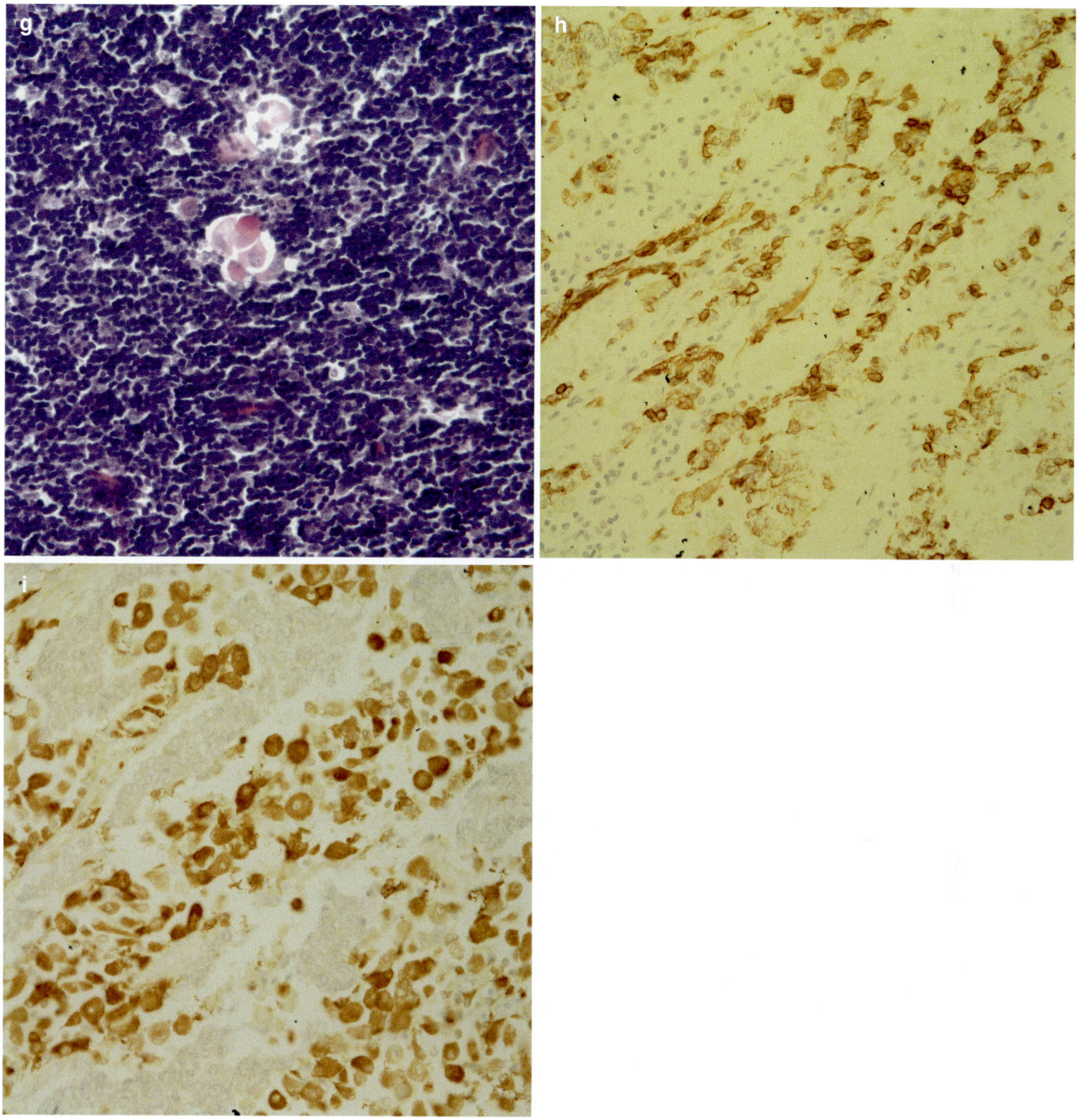

Fig. 7.92 (continued) (**g**) Lymphocytic thymoma with cluster of muscle cells. (**h**) Keratin stain is positive in the epithelial component. (**i**) Myoglobin is positive in the muscle component

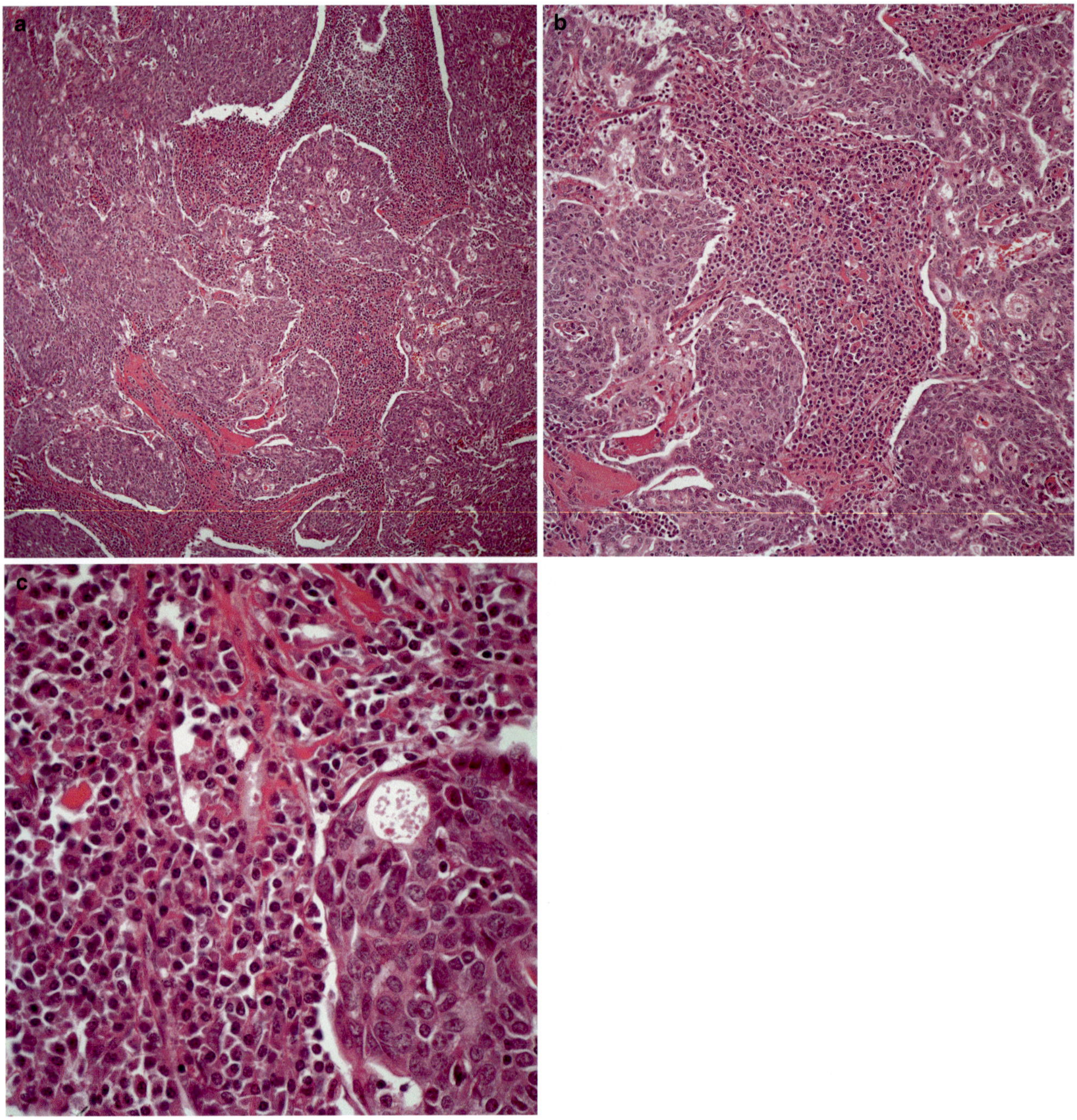

Fig. 7.93 (**a**) Plasma cell-rich thymoma, (**b**) extensive presence of plasma cells admixed with epithelial cells, (**c**) closer view at the mature plasma cells

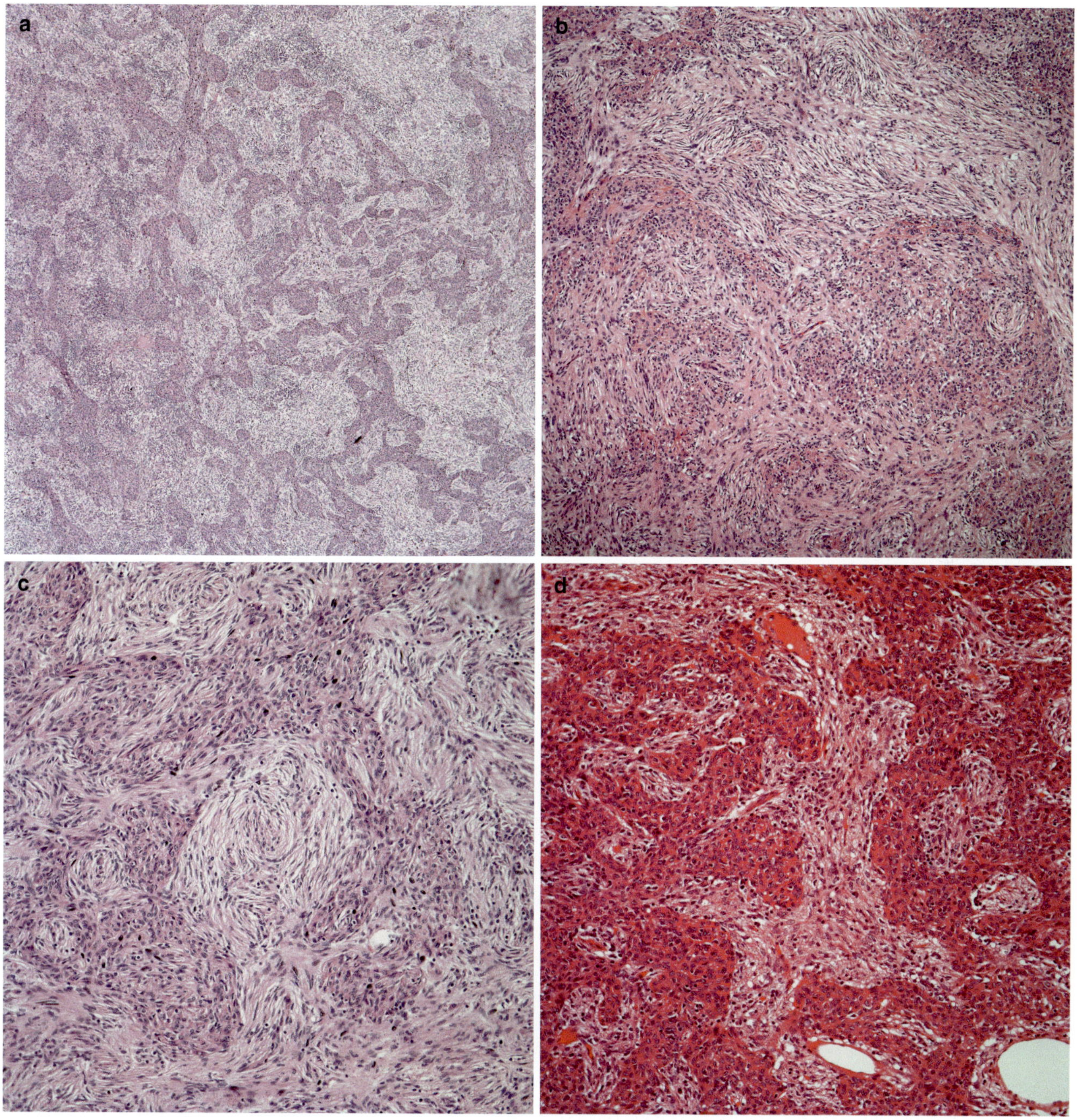

Fig. 7.94 (**a**) Low power view of a thymoma with pseudosarcomatous stroma, (**b**) marked separation of the epithelial component and the spindle component of the tumor, (**c**) closer view does not show nuclear atypia in either component, (**d**) closer view of the spindle cell component with scattered inflammatory cells

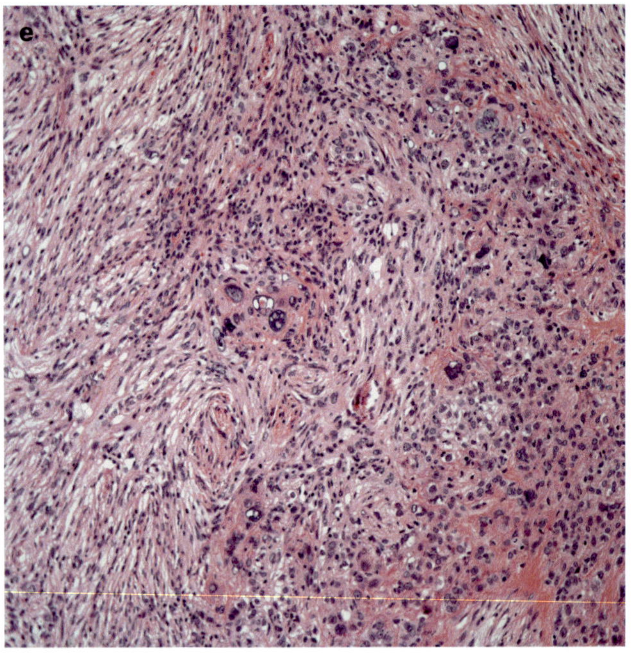

Fig. 7.94 (continued) (**e**) Focal areas with nuclear atypia in the epithelial component of the tumor

the patients were without evidence of recurrence after up to 7 years postsurgical resection. In 2001, Tateyama and colleagues [165] reported 11 additional cases of this variant and separated the tumor into 3 groups depending on the shape of the epithelial, spindle, and polygonal cells. In addition, the authors added a case of lymphoepithelioma-like carcinoma. (for discussion of this latter entity, please refer to the chapter of thymic carcinoma in this text). Interestingly, the author also detected EBV genome in a few lymphocytes of five cases. However, it was concluded that a factual association between EBV and this variant of thymoma could not be established. Strobel and colleagues [166], in a report of this variant of thymoma, stated that abnormal chemokine expression can promote the recruitment of MALT, the emergence of monoclonal B-cells, and subsequent development of lymphoma. In our experience, we have observed such cases in which we have identified the presence of a micronodular thymoma associated with a thymic lymphoma (Fig. 7.101a–d). However, it is impossible to determine whether the first tumor was a lymphoma or a thymoma. Reports of this variant of thymoma associated with thymic lymphoid hyperplasia have also been recorded [167].

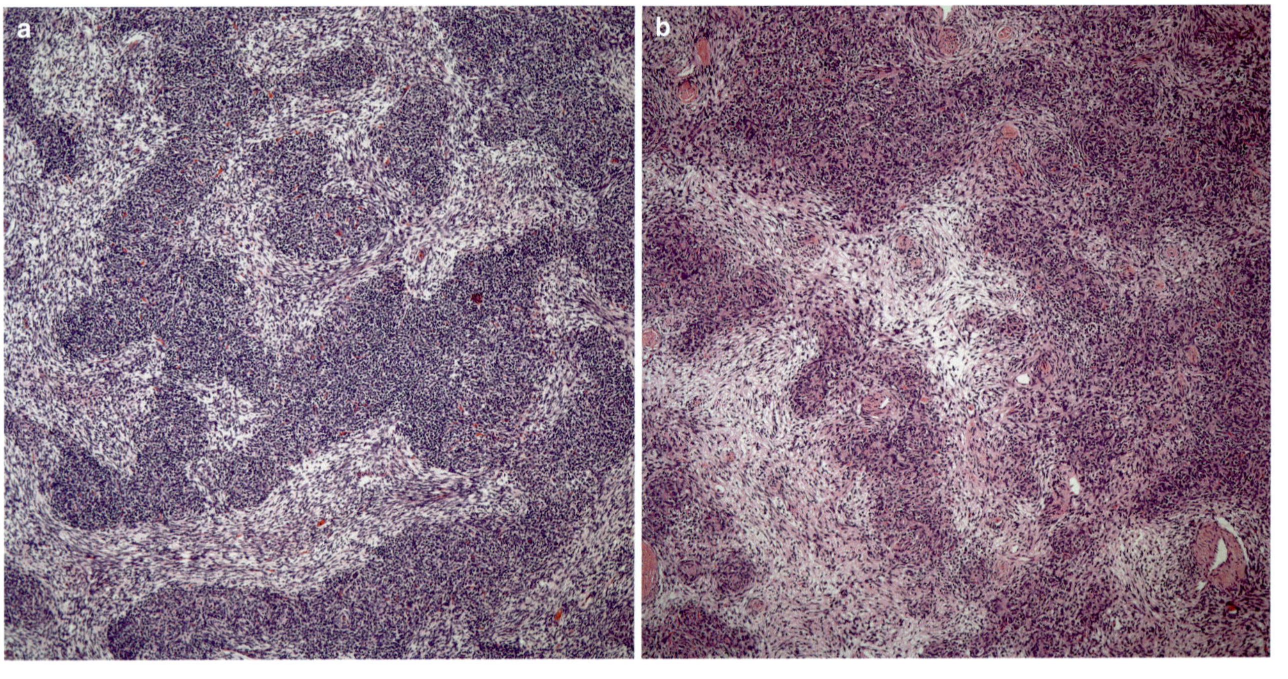

Fig. 7.95 (**a**) Lymphocytic thymoma with similar pattern as that seen in thymoma with pseudosarcomatous stroma, (**b**) closer view shows only focal nuclear atypia

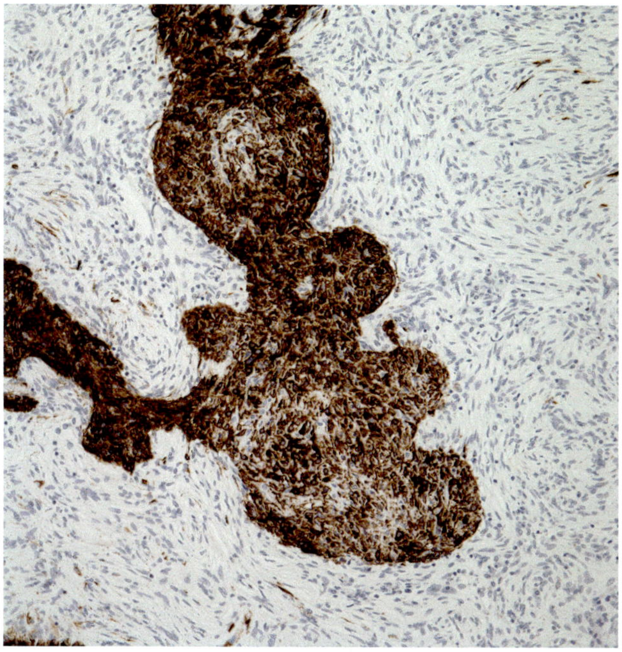

Fig. 7.96 Keratin is positive in the epithelial component of a thymoma with pseudosarcomatous stroma

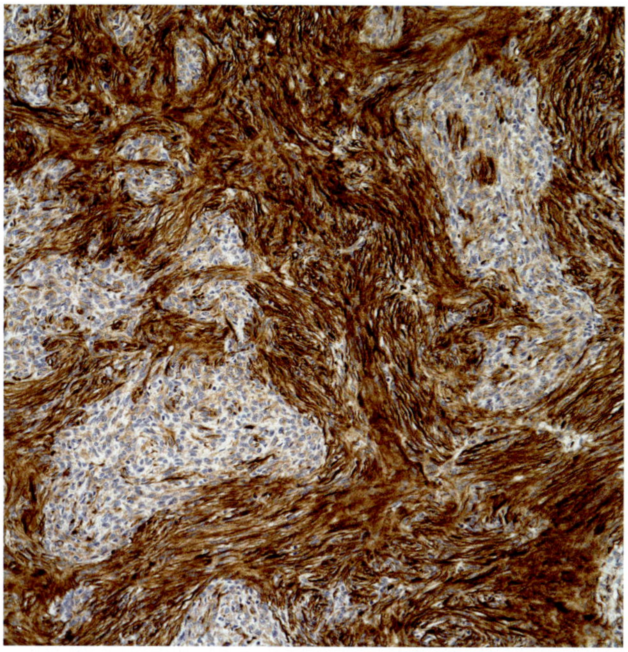

Fig. 7.98 Strong positive with vimentin in the spindle cell component of the thymoma with pseudosarcomatous stroma

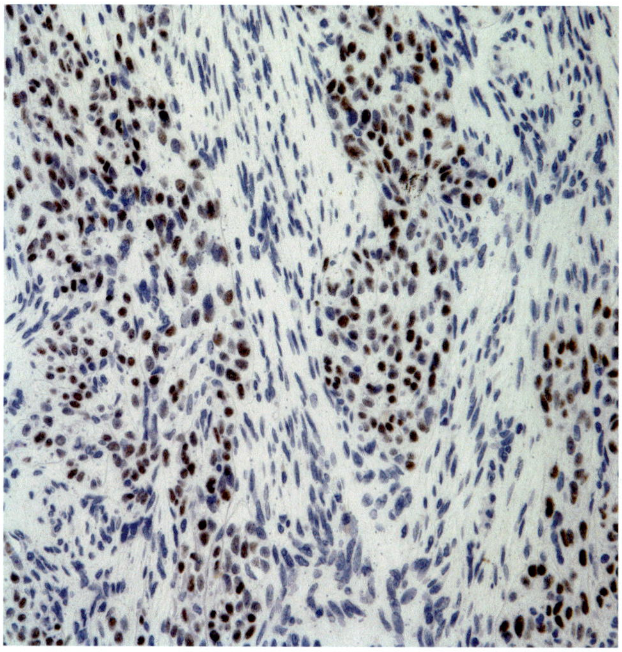

Fig. 7.97 p40 positive in the epithelial component of a thymoma with pseudosarcomatous stroma

Thymoma with Hemorrhage, Necrosis, Infarction, and Cystic Changes

The awareness of all these changes occurring in thymomas was raised in a report of 25 cases demonstrating these changes [168]. The emphasis of this report was to highlight that such changes in an otherwise conventional thymoma do not portent any adverse prognosis. These changes can occur in either encapsulated or invasive thymomas, and the clinical behavior of these tumors will follow the degree of invasiveness at the time of diagnosis. Therefore, pathological staging plays a more significant role than the presence of necrosis or hemorrhage. However, in many cases, the final diagnosis may be more difficult, mainly in cases that have not been sampled properly and in which conventional areas of thymoma are not present. In such cases in which the mediastinal tumor shows cystic, hemorrhagic, and necrotic areas without residual viable tumor, it is highly important to make sure that proper sampling has taken place. Often, in the necrotic areas, it is possible to see the presence of lymphoid component that would suggest the possibility of thymoma (Fig. 7.102a–h). It is also of interest to highlight that, in our experience, we have seen these changes occurring in thymomas with marked lymphocytic component. Also important to highlight is that if proper sampling takes place, at least foci of unequivocal thymoma are encountered, while in other areas, one usually encounters areas of residual thymic epithelium, cholesterol cleft granuloma, and extensive fibrosis with inflammatory reaction.

Ancient (Sclerosing) Thymoma

This is an unusual phenomenon that occurs in a small proportion of thymomas. Kuo [169] reported two cases in 1994 as sclerosing thymoma, suggesting the possibility of regression. In 2004, a series of ten cases with similar features was reported in which the authors' interpretation was that of "ancient changes" occurring in thymomas [170]. The cases described showed extensive areas of hyalinization, which amounted to 85–90% of the tumor. Only focal areas of viable conventional thymoma were present in these cases (Fig. 7.103a–d). In some cases, areas of calcification and cholesterol cleft granulomas may also be seen. We consider that such diagnosis is not difficult to arrive at in resected specimens; however, in small biopsies, due to the presence of extensive hyalinization, the interpretation may be that of sclerosing (fibrosing) mediastinitis. Also important to highlight is the proper sampling of these tumors, which, if not done correctly and extensively, will miss the true nature of the neoplasm.

Adenomatoid Spindle Cell Thymoma

This is an unusual variant of thymoma [171]. The authors reported 20 such cases in which the tumors were characterized by the presence of spindle cell proliferation with an adenomatoid-like appearance and focal areas of signet ring cell-like areas (Fig. 7.104a–c). The majority of the cases reported were encapsulated tumors, while some cases showed transcapsular invasion. Immunohistochemical stains were performed showing tumor cells positive for keratin and scattered cells positive for calretinin and epithelial membrane antigen. Follow-up information in 17 of the 20 cases described showed that all patients were alive and well after a period ranging from 4 to 96 months.

Thymomas with Papillary and Pseudopapillary Features

This variant is rather unusual and was reported in a series of ten spindle cell thymomas [172]. The patients presented with mediastinal tumors that varied in size from 4 to 9 cm in diameter. Histologically, the tumors were characterized by the presence of prominent areas of papillary and pseudopapillary features of variable size, which could be associated with areas of hyalinization. In some cases, the papillary structures showed extensive edematous changes (Fig. 7.105a–g). Seven of the cases described were invasive

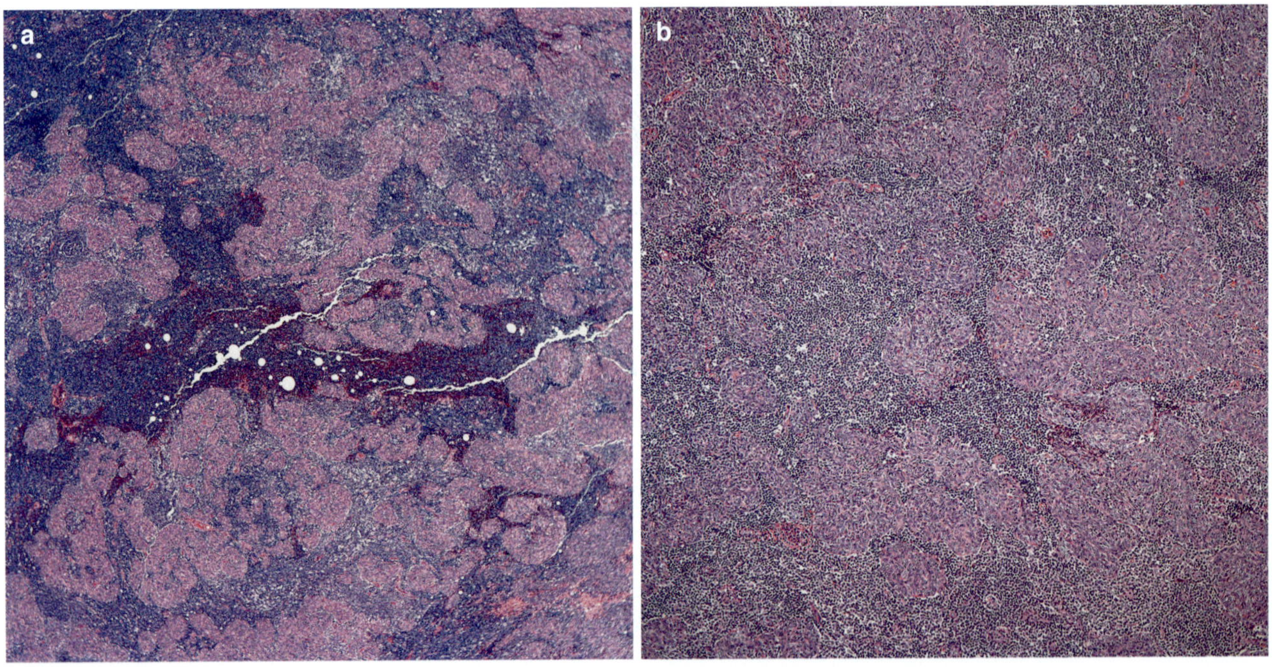

Fig. 7.99 (**a**) Low power view of a micronodular thymoma; (**b**) nodular epithelial islands embedded in a lymphocytic stroma

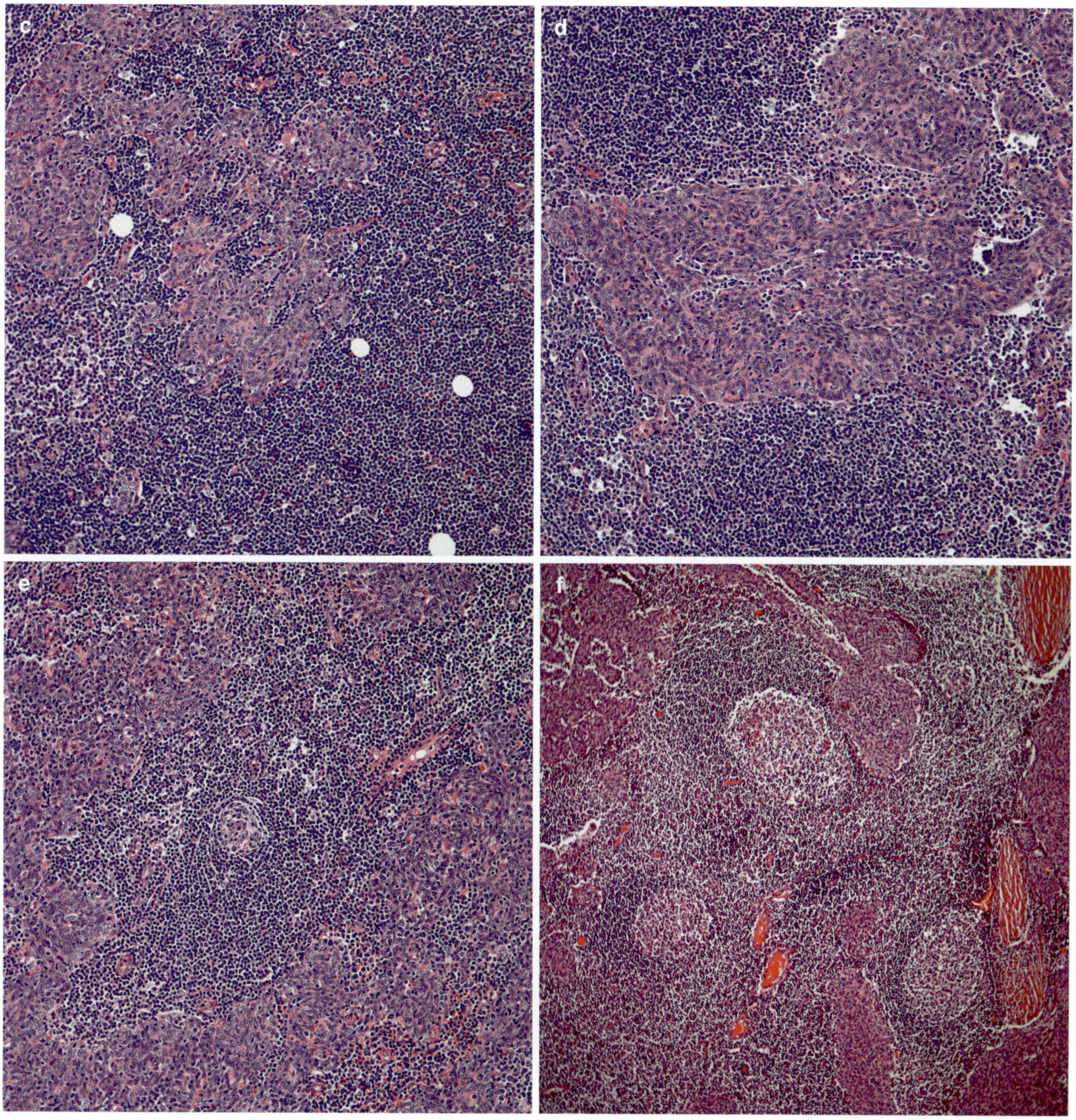

Fig. 7.99 (continued) (**c**) The epithelial component is formed of oval or spindle cells or both, (**d**) nuclear atypia or mitotic activity is commonly absent, (**e**) in some areas germinal centers may be focal, (**f**) in other areas prominent hyperplastic germinal centers are easily identified

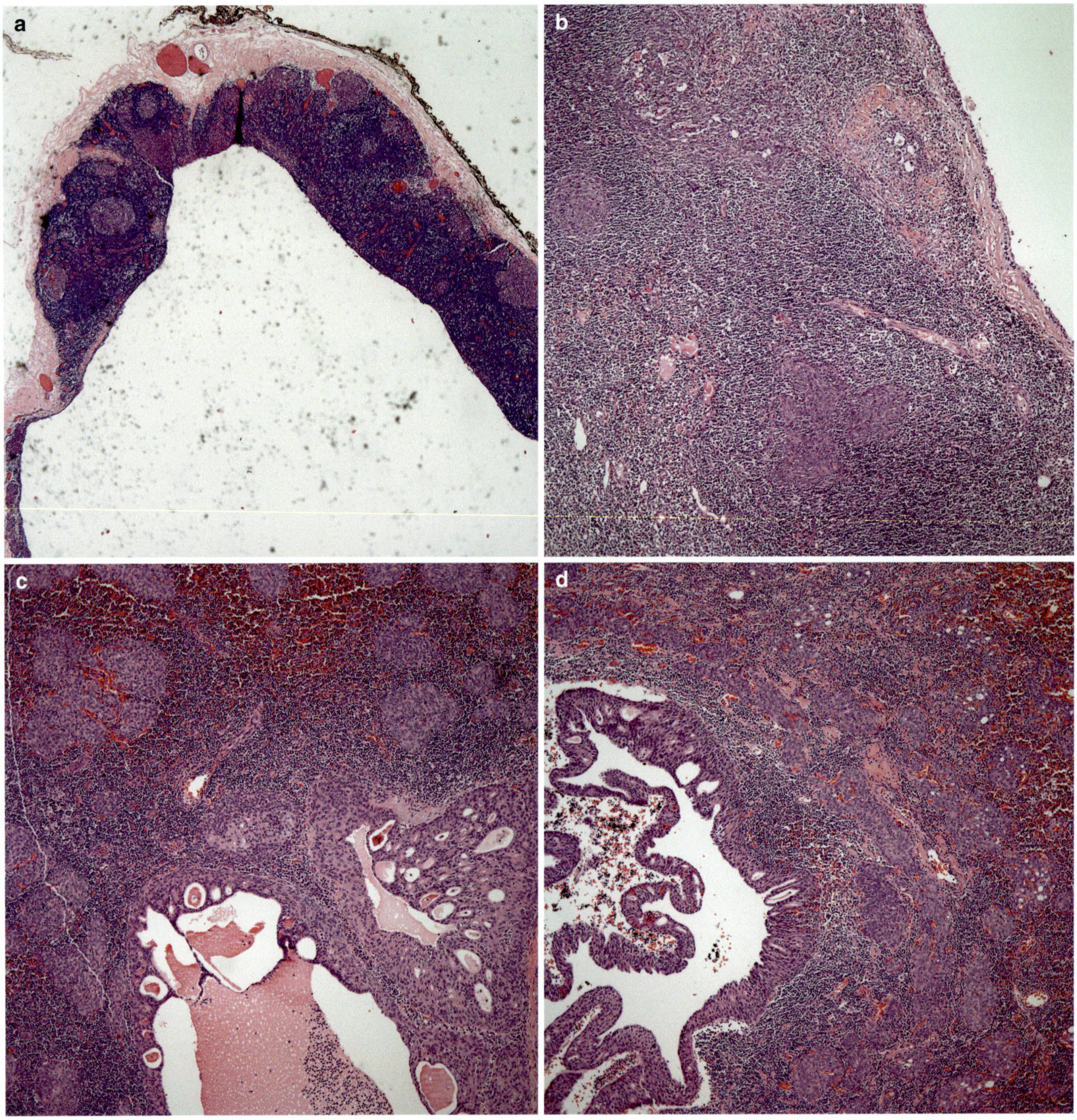

Fig. 7.100 (**a**) Cystic micronodular thymoma, (**b**) the wall of the cyst lined by cuboidal epithelium contains a micronodular thymoma, (**c**) micronodular thymoma with areas of microcystic thymoma, (**d**) micronodular thymoma with focal areas of cystic thymoma

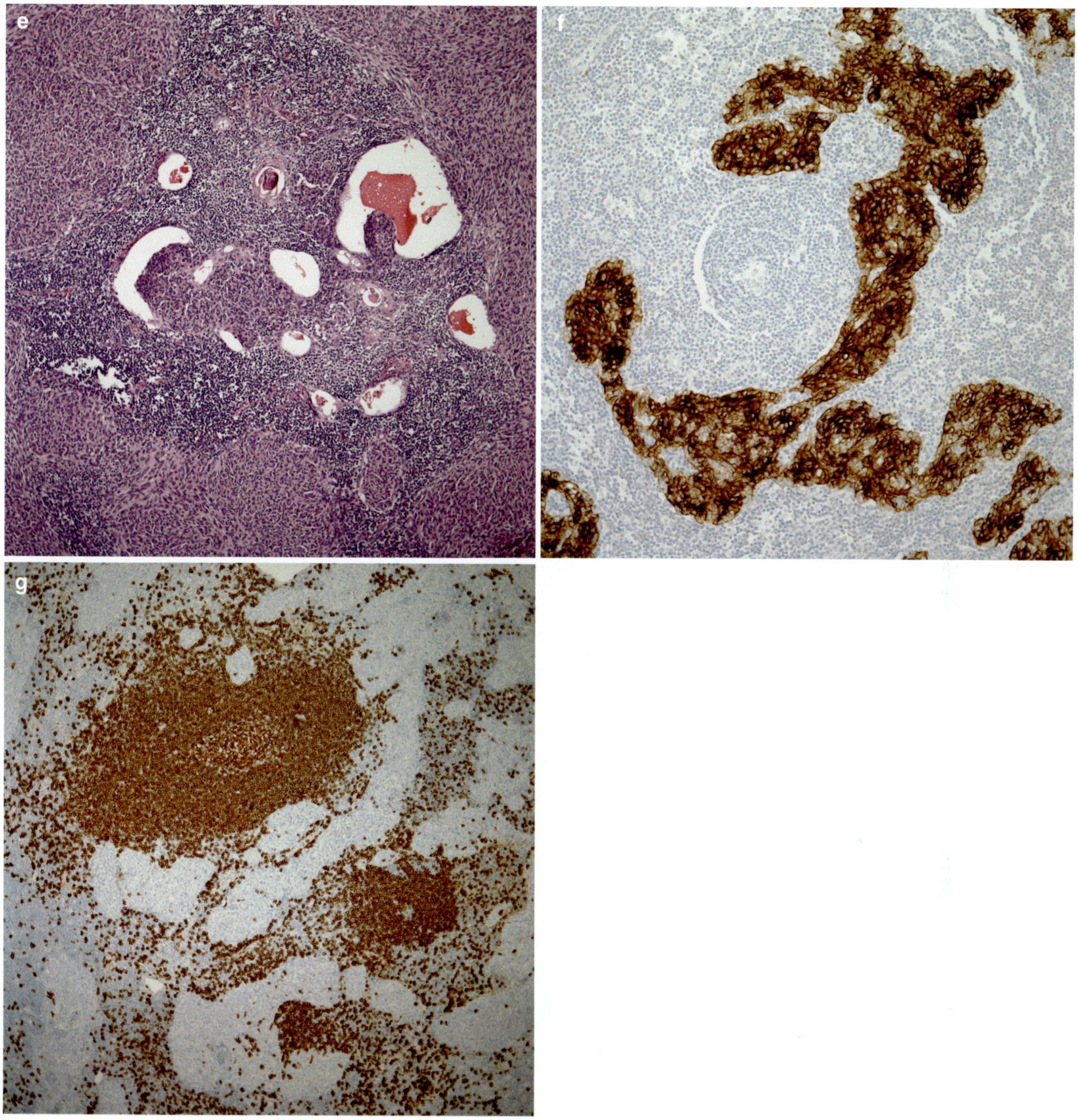

Fig. 7.100 (continued) (**e**) Cystic micronodular thymoma with focal presence of Hassall's corpuscle, (**f**) keratin positive in the epithelial component, (**g**) CD20 positive in the lymphoid component

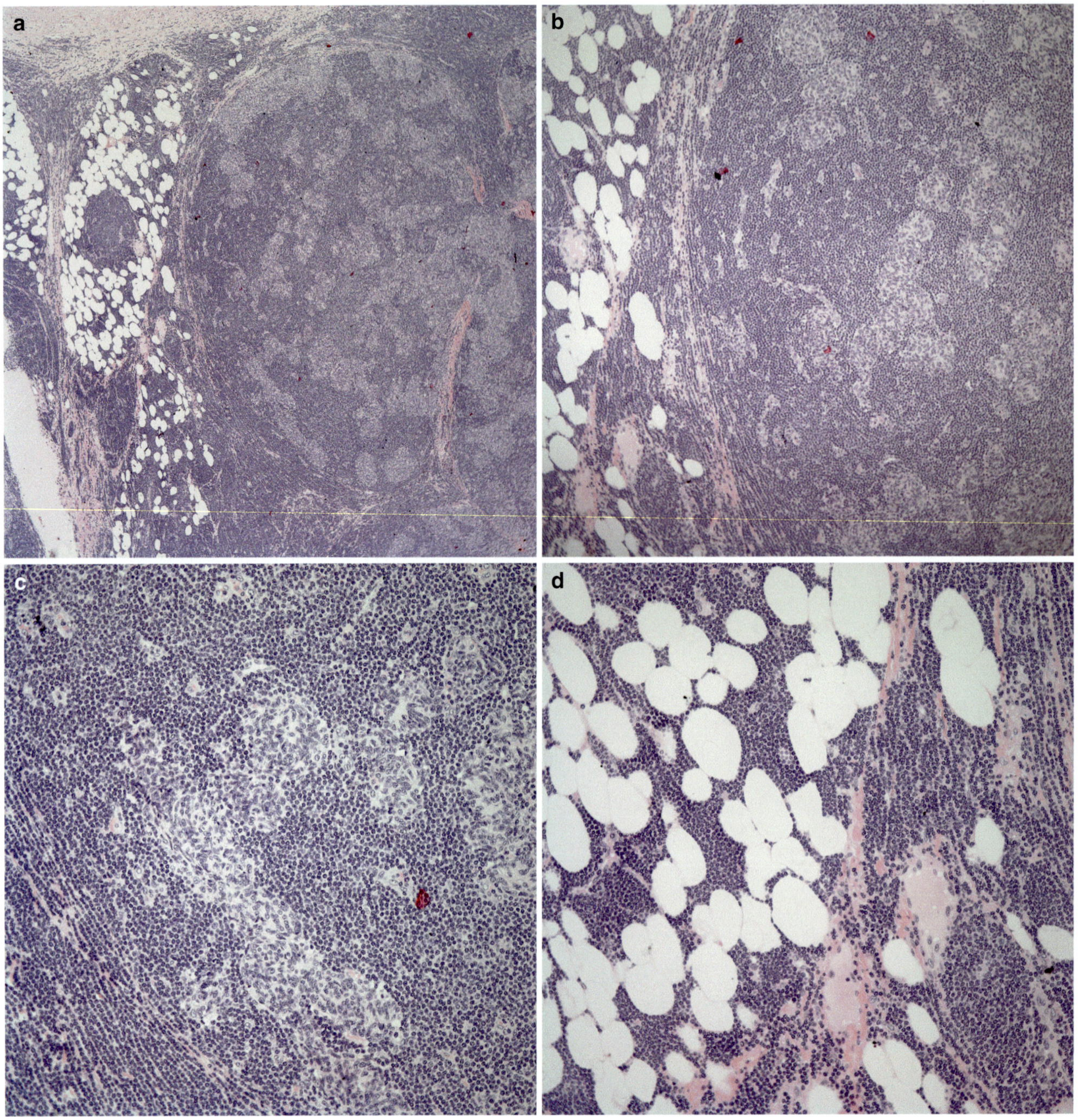

Fig. 7.101 (**a**) Micronodular thymoma growing along a mediastinal lymphoma, (**b**) note the two distinct tumors growing alongside, (**c**) closer view at the micronodular thymoma, (**d**) closer view at the lymphoma infiltrating adipose tissue

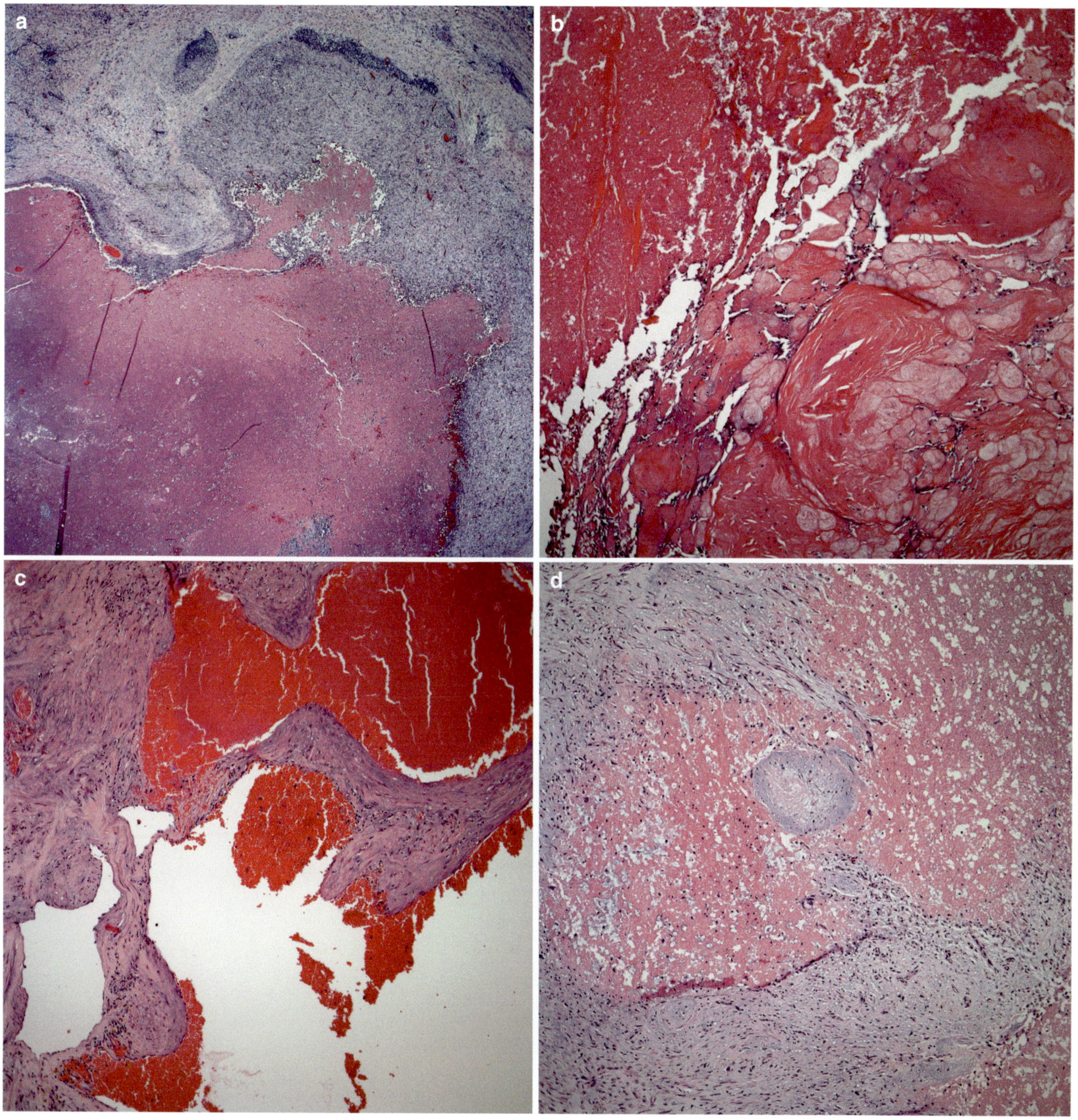

Fig. 7.102 (**a**) Thymoma with extensive areas of hemorrhage and necrosis, (**b**) hemorrhage and extensive hyalinization, (**c**) cystic spaces filled with fresh blood, (**d**) cysts without lining and with fibrosis

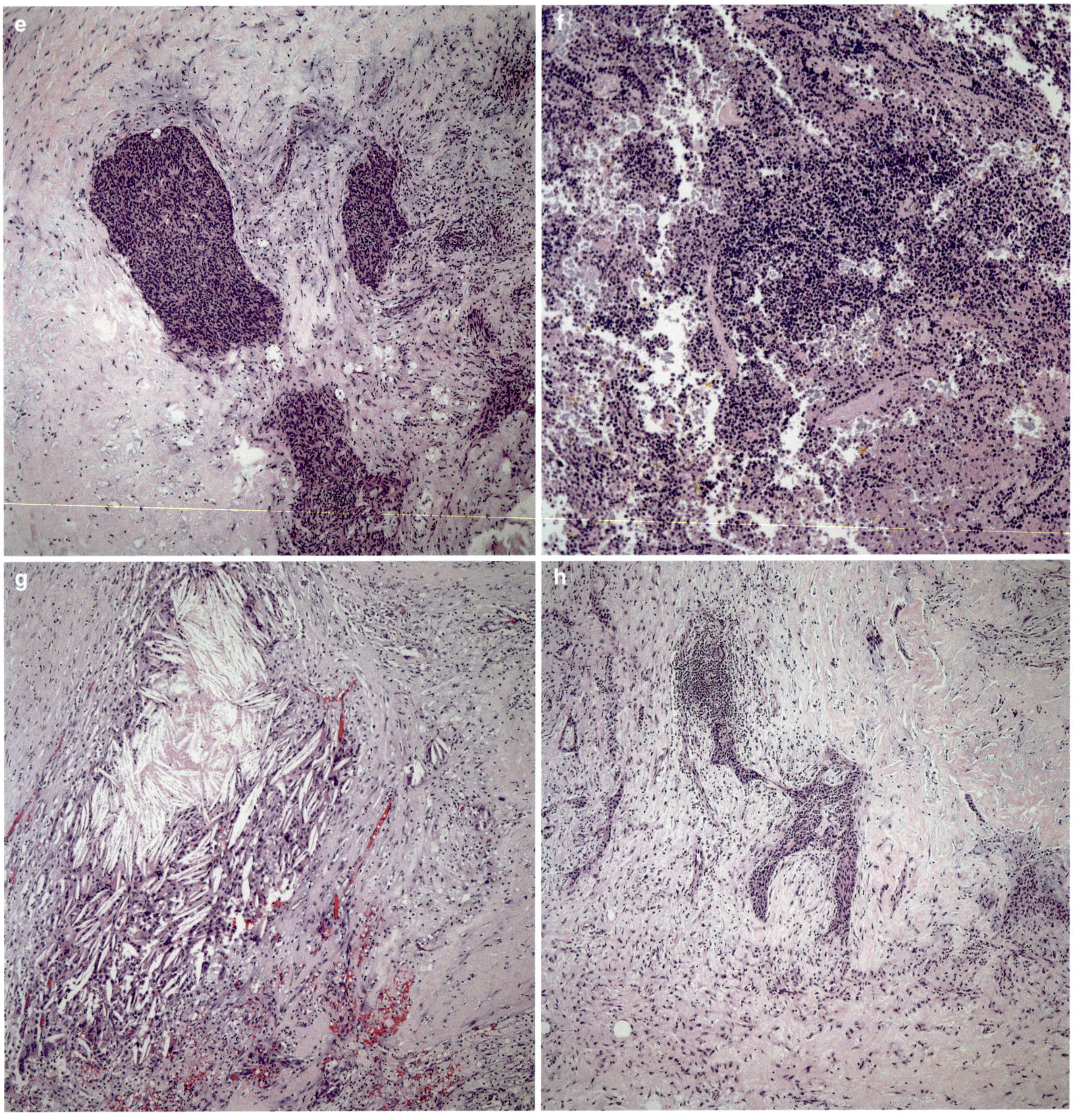

Fig. 7.102 (continued) (**e**) Residual conventional thymoma, (**f**) residual lymphocytic thymoma with extensive necrosis, (**g**) fibrosis and cholesterol cleft granuloma, (**h**) residual thymic epithelium in the walls of the fibrotic cysts

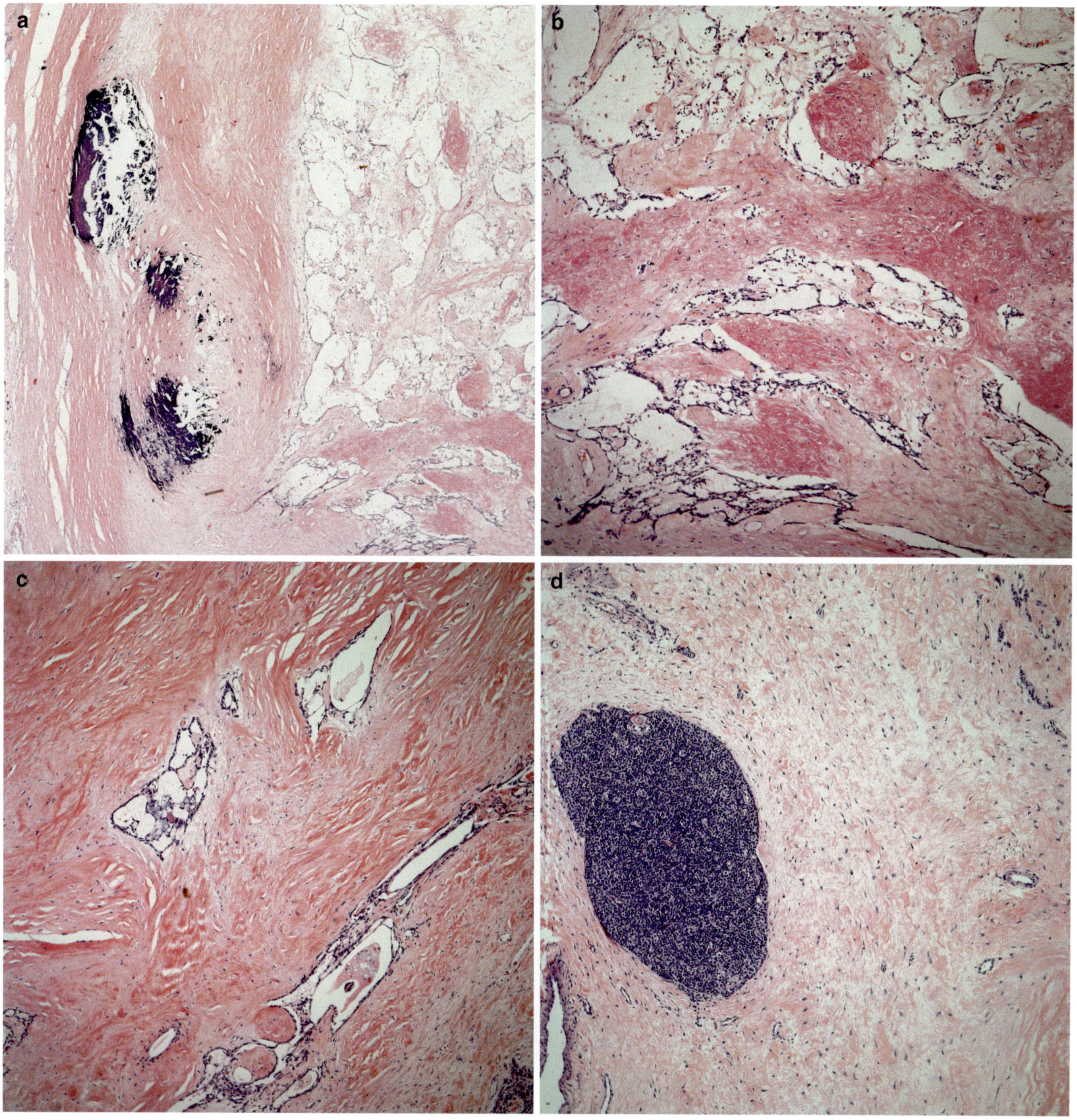

Fig. 7.103 (**a**) Thymoma with ancient changes; note the presence of calcification in the areas of hyalinization. (**b**) Residual outlines of thymoma with extensive hyalinization. (**c**) Focal microcystic thymoma embedded in a hyalinized stroma. (**d**) Focal residual lymphocytic thymoma embedded in a collagenous stroma

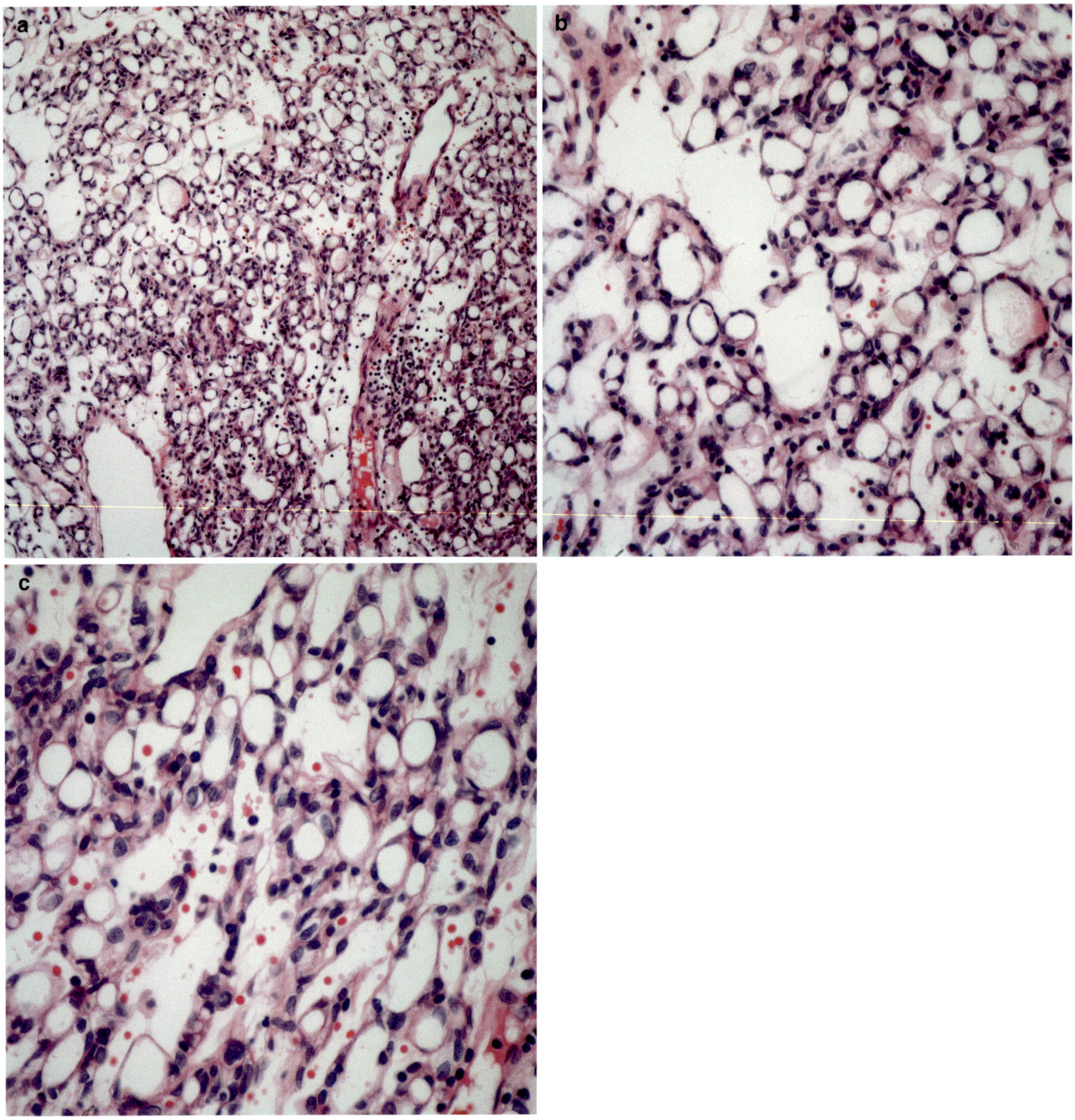

Fig. 7.104 (**a**) Adenomatoid thymoma showing cords of tumor cells, (**b**) closer view shows cells with vacuolated cytoplasm mimicking either signet ring cells or indented mesothelial cells, (**c**) adenomatoid thymoma with oval and spindle cells lacking nuclear atypia and mitotic activity

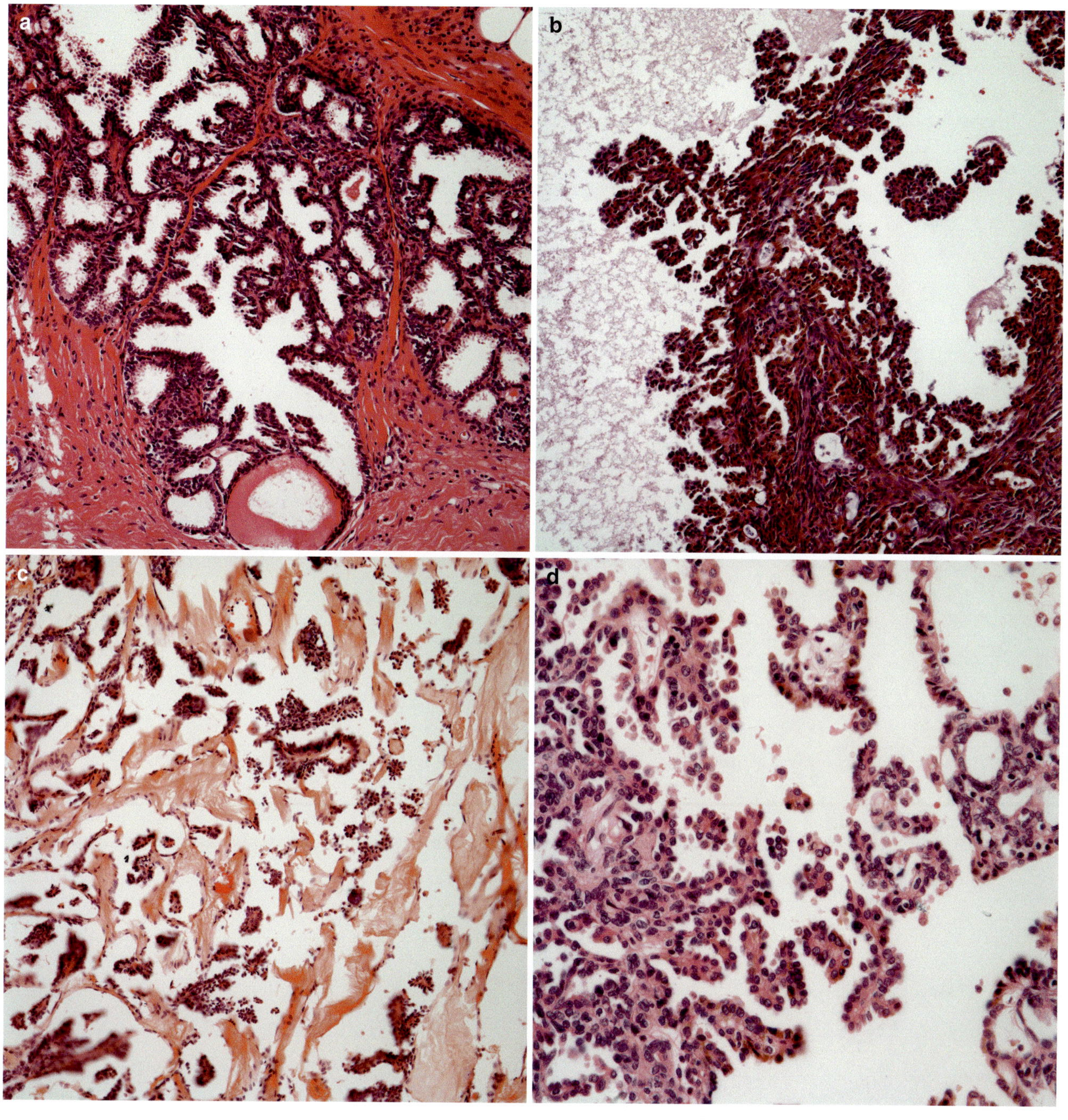

Fig. 7.105 (**a**) Thymoma with prominent papillary features, (**b**) spindle and oval cells with papillary features, (**c**) papillary-like structures and extensive hyalinization, (**d**) pseudopapillary structures lacking nuclear atypia or mitotic activity

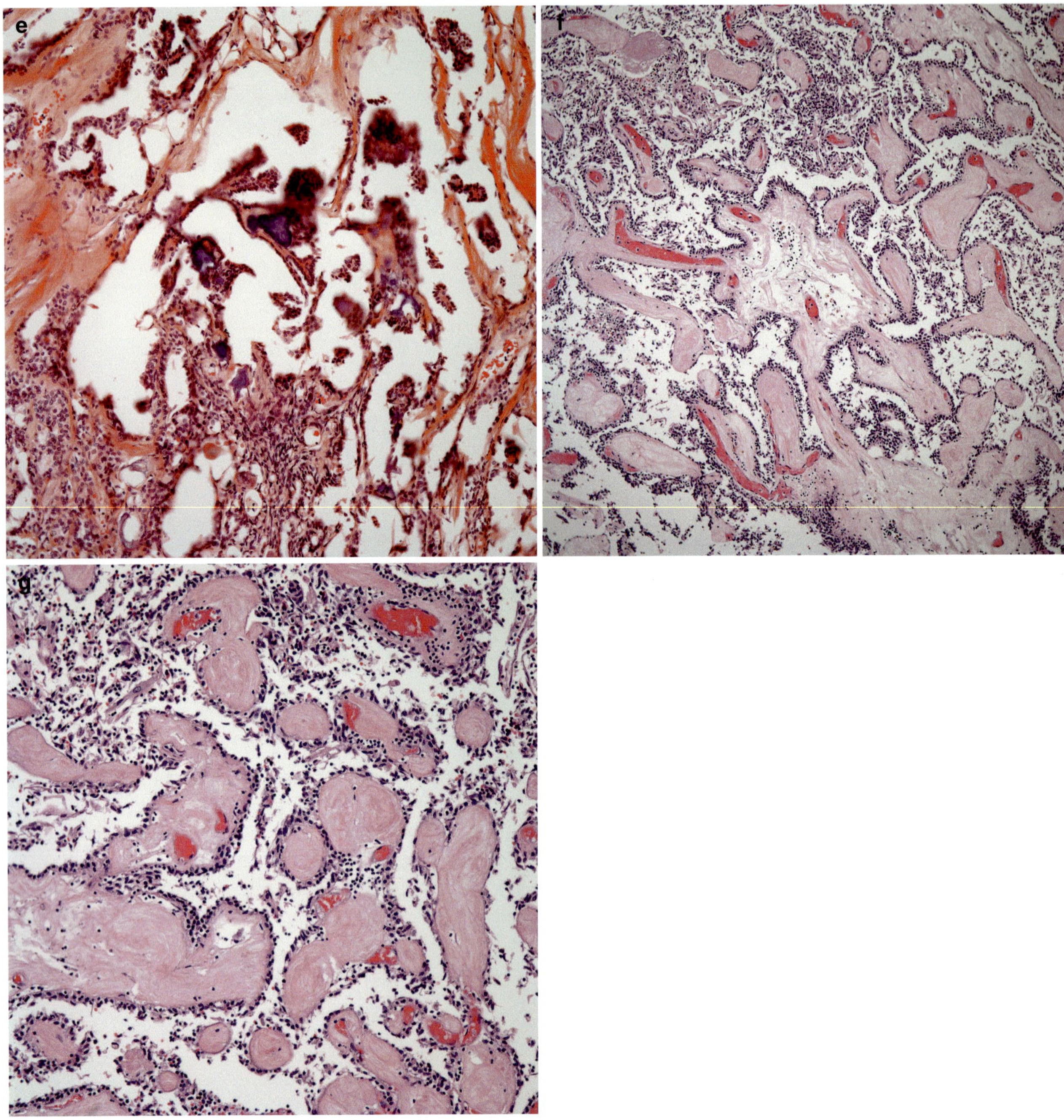

Fig. 7.105 (continued) (**e**) Papillary structures admixed with calcifications, (**f**) papillary-like structures with extensive hyalinization, (**g**) closer view at the hyalinized structures lacking nuclear atypia or mitotic activity

tumors, and three were encapsulated. Immunohistochemical stains showed tumor cells positive for keratin CAM 5.2 and keratin 5/6.

Thymoma with Loss of Keratin Expression and Giant Cells

The presence of giant cells in otherwise conventional cases of thymoma is not unusual. Adam and colleagues [173] reported a series of 14 cases in which the tumor appeared to have reduced expression of keratin, and, in at least three of the cases reported, the tumor did not express keratin at all. However, 13 of the 14 cases reported showed strong nuclear expression for p63. In addition, the authors documented that in 5 of the 14 cases described with keratin-depleted thymomas, giant cells reminiscent of thymic nursing cells were discovered. Some of these giant cells show positive staining for keratin, FOXN1, and p63. As the authors point out in their description, this issue of reduced expression of keratin in thymomas represents a pitfall in the diagnosis, mainly in mediastinoscopic biopsies. However, we consider that the presence of "giant cells" has nothing to do with this reduced expression of keratin as we have had the opportunity to evaluate numerous cases of conventional thymomas with focal presence of giant cells and still the tumors have shown keratin expression (Fig. 7.106a–d). We have observed the presence of these giant cells in different types of thymomas.

Microcystic Thymoma

Although in our experience this pattern is not that uncommon, there are no well-presented clinicopathological correlations highlighting these unusual features in thymomas. Fukuda and colleagues [174] reported two cases of this variant characterized by round cells with ample vacuolated cytoplasm. In our experience, we have seen this pattern admixed with both lymphocytic, spindle, and atypical thymomas (Fig. 7.107a–d). By immunohistochemistry, the tumor cells react in a similar fashion to the garden variety of thymomas. In the cases described by Fukuda and coauthors [174], the authors performed electron microscopic studies and stated that the vacuoles in these cases correspond to excess accumulation of Leu-7-positive material, probably in the cystically dilated endoplasmic reticulum.

Desmoplastic Thymoma

This unusual variant is seen in spindle cell tumors and is characterized by extensive areas of young fibrocollagen and a prominent fibroblastic proliferation associated with scattered areas of conventional spindle cell thymoma (Fig. 7.108a–d) [175]. In the original description of 14 cases, the tumor did not show necrosis, cellular atypia, or mitotic activity. Some of these thymomas may be encapsulated or invasive, and the pathological staging is what will determine biologic behavior. However, in small mediastinoscopic biopsies, the presence of fibroblastic proliferation may be confused with a mesenchymal type of neoplasm.

Thymomas with Glandular Differentiation

This particular variant may be seen in either lymphocytic or spindle cell thymomas. In the original description of 12 cases [176], the authors documented such finding in all the different conventional variants of thymoma. However, in addition to the conventional features, these tumors may also show the presence of glandular structures that may exhibit mucin production. These glandular structures do not show cellular atypia or mitotic activity and are present in a haphazard pattern within the conventional areas of the tumor (Fig. 7.109a–e). Interestingly, some of the glandular structures may show positive staining for EMA and calretinin. The most relevant consideration in a small mediastinoscopic biopsy will be the issue of primary adenocarcinoma of the thymus. However, most adenocarcinomas of the thymus will show more conventional areas of adenocarcinoma with cellular atypia and mitotic activity.

Thymoma with Clear Cell Component

In the past, this particular feature has been associated with thymic carcinomas. However, we documented nine thymoma cases in which the presence of a clear cell component was a significant component of an otherwise conventional thymoma (Fig. 7.110a–d) [177]. These epithelial cells with clear cytoplasm appear to be haphazardly present in different areas of the thymoma; in some cases, these areas can be extensive, taking over about 70–80% of the entire tumor. However, the cells do not show nuclear atypia or mitotic activity. In general, these tumors do not show necrosis or hemorrhage grossly or microscopically. Also important to highlight is that some of these tumors can be invasive or encapsulated. In the report of nine cases with these features, the follow-up presented up to 2 years in some patients showed no recurrence of metastatic disease.

Thymoma with Neuroendocrine Morphology

This unusual growth pattern is seen exclusively in spindle cell thymomas. In a report of 18 cases of thymomas with this particular histology, the tumors were characterized by the presence of spindle cells with rosette-like structures and trabecular, insular, or ribbon-like architecture (Fig. 7.111a–d) [178]. However, in others, the tumor shows more conventional areas of spindle cell thymoma. In the report of 18 cases, 10 of the cases reported were of invasive tumors. Despite the architecture of these tumors, immunohistochemical stains for neuroendocrine markers, chromogranin and synaptophysin, were reported as negative. Because of the occurrence of true neuroendocrine carcinomas of the thy-

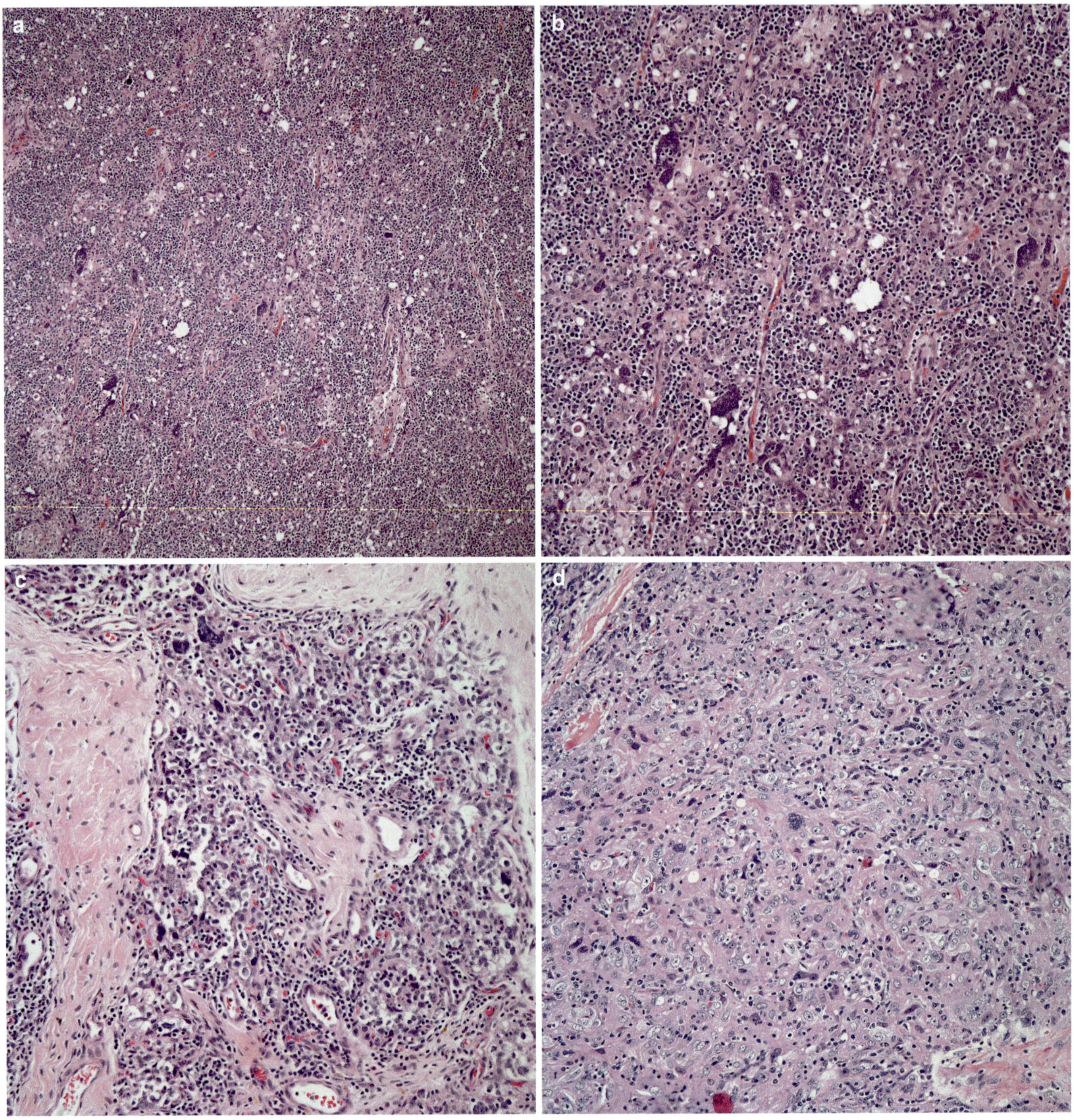

Fig. 7.106 (**a**) Lymphocytic thymoma with numerous giant cells, (**b**) closer view of the multinucleated giant cells in an otherwise garden-variety thymoma, (**c**) the multinucleated giant cells can be seen only focally, (**d**) atypical thymoma with scattered multinucleated giant cells

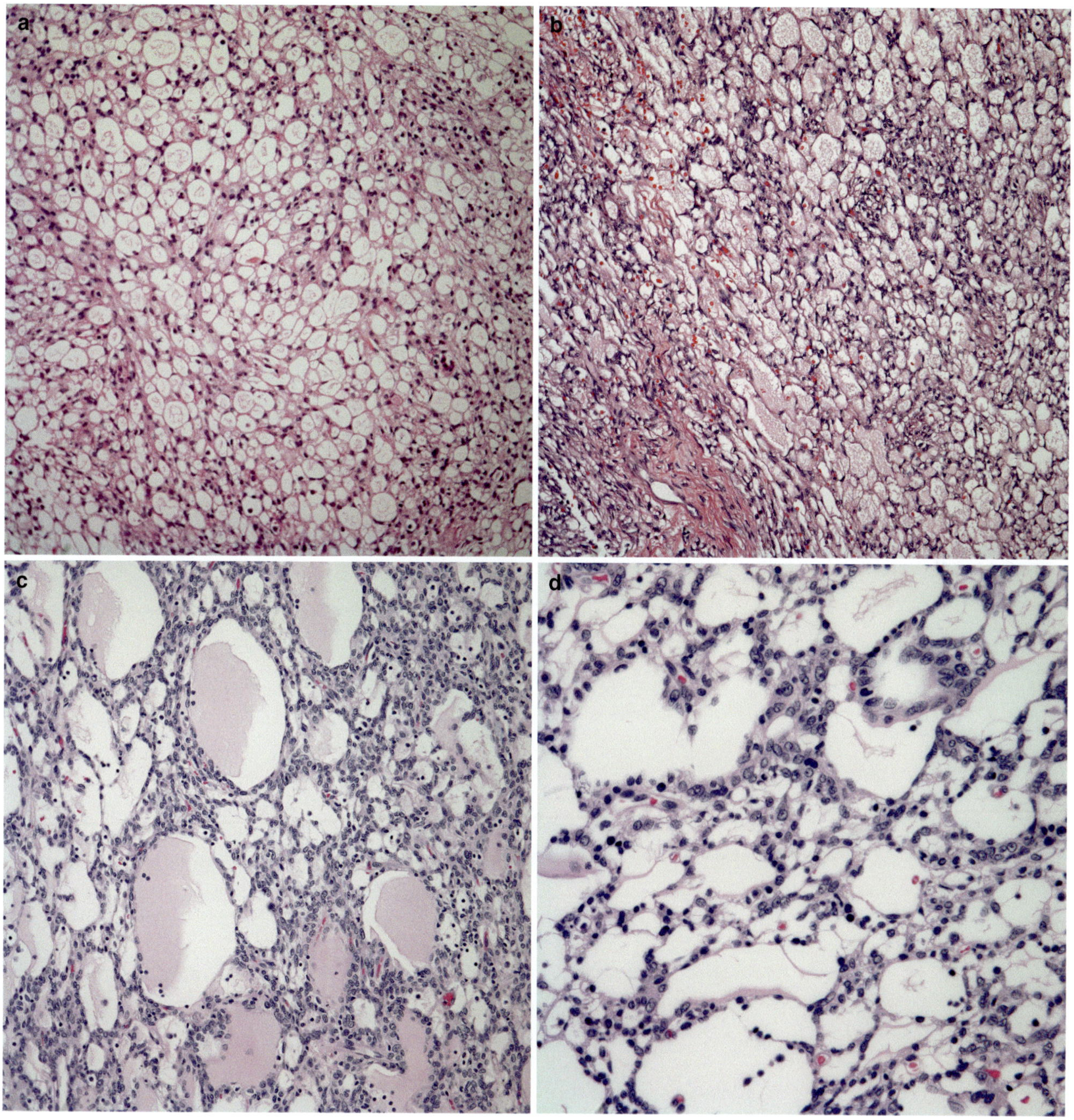

Fig. 7.107 (**a**) Microcystic thymoma showing prominent small cystic structures, (**b**) in some areas the microcysts are filled with fibrinous debris, (**c**) the epithelial cells lack nuclear atypia and mitotic activity. (**d**) Higher magnification showing lack of nuclear atypia or mitotic activity

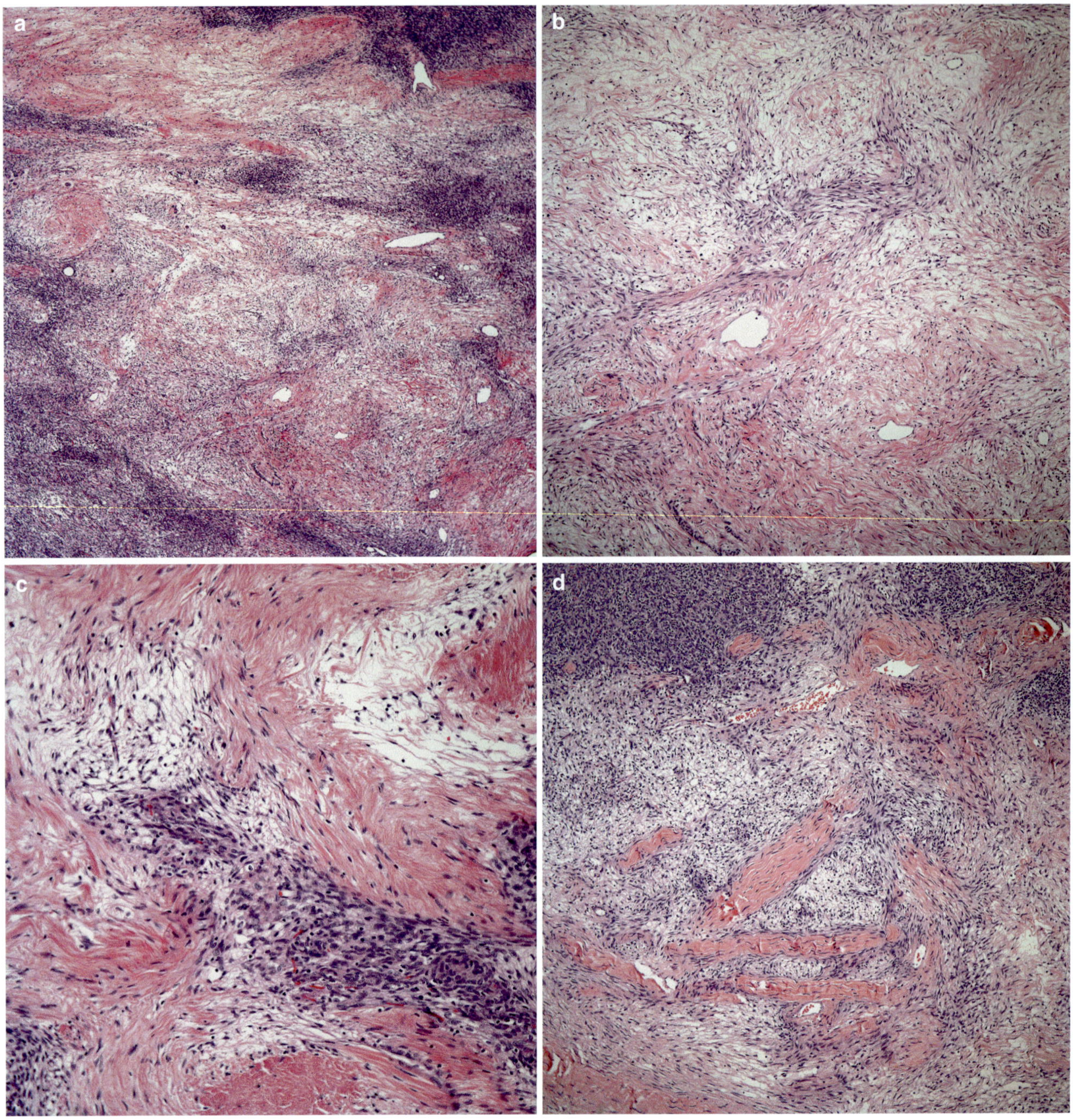

Fig. 7.108 (**a**) Low power view of a desmoplastic thymoma, (**b**) prominent spindle cell proliferation admixed with collagen given the image of a solitary fibrous tumor, (**c**) areas of collagenization admixed with spindle epithelial cells, (**d**) prominent desmoplastic changes with areas of easily identifiable thymoma

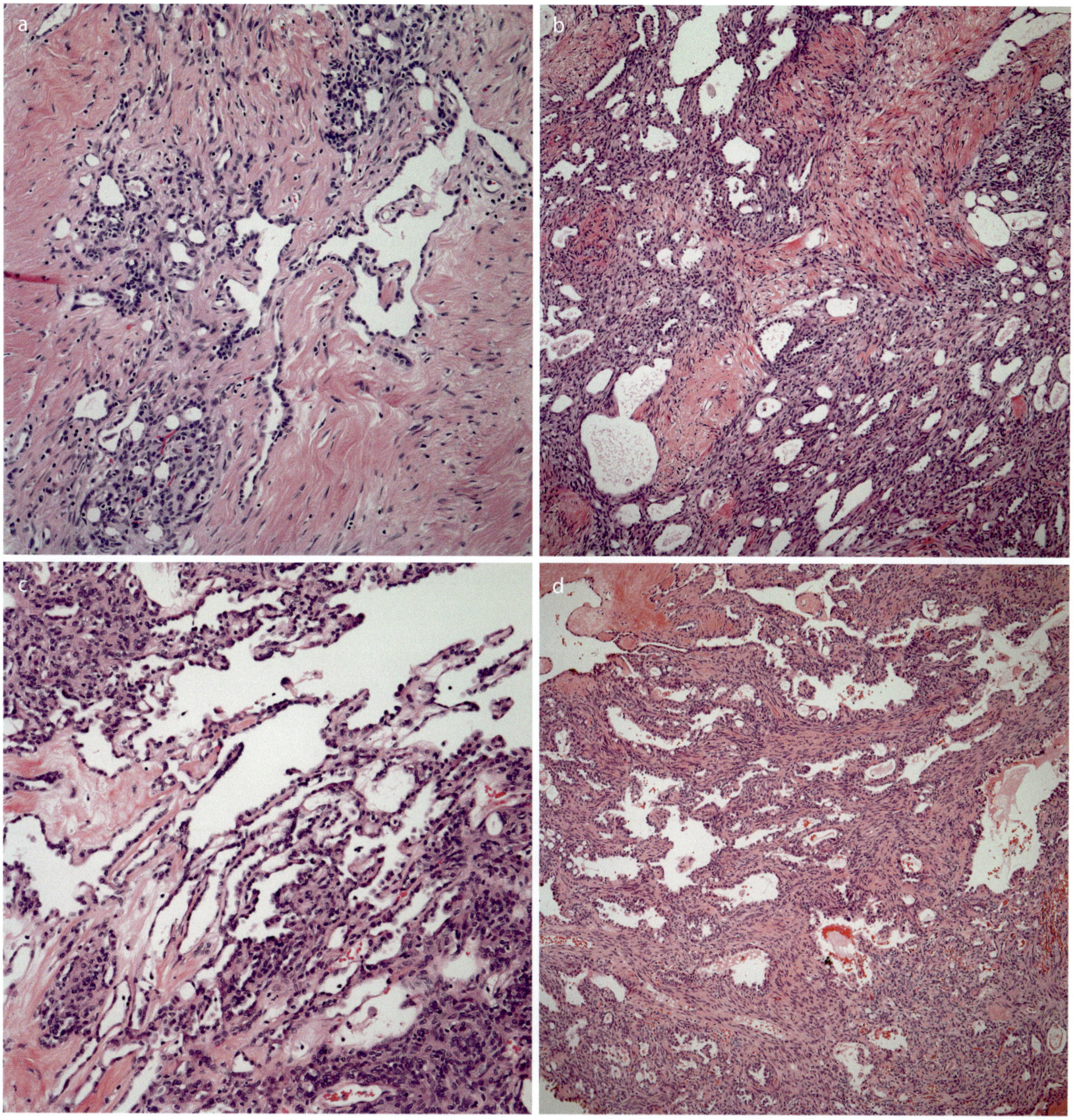

Fig. 7.109 (**a**) Thymoma with prominent glandular-like structures, (**b**) spindle cell thymoma with numerous gland-like structures, (**c**) gland-like structures of different sizes admixed with thymoma, (**d**) better formed glandular-like structures admixed with thymoma given the image of biphasic synovial sarcoma

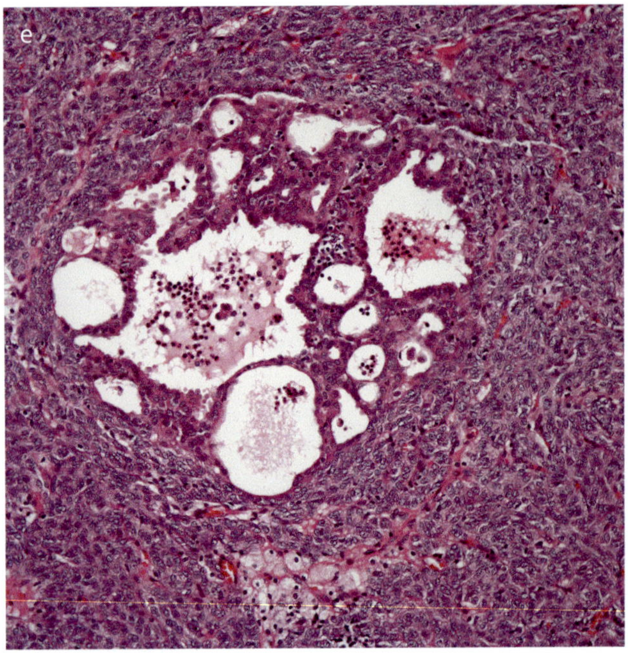

Fig. 7.109 (continued) (**e**) Thymoma with focal collection of macrophages and glandular formation

mus, which may show spindle cell morphology, it is important to separate these two entities in small mediastinoscopic biopsies. In general, thymomas with neuroendocrine morphology are negative for neuroendocrine markers, especially chromogranin.

Thymoma with Signet Ring Cell-Like Features

This unusual pattern may overlap to some extent with other thymomas with adenomatoid and microcystic features. However, in the cases described in a series of ten, the predominant feature of the tumors was that of cords of neoplastic cells embedded in collagenous stroma and composed of cells with vacuolated clear cytoplasm, the nuclei was displaced to the periphery, given the appearance of signet ring cells (Fig. 7.112a–c) [179]. However, the tumor does not show mitotic activity or nuclear atypia, and the presence of lymphocytes is scant. These tumors may be either invasive or encapsulated. The immunohistochemical features of these tumors are essentially the same as the one observed in conventional thymomas.

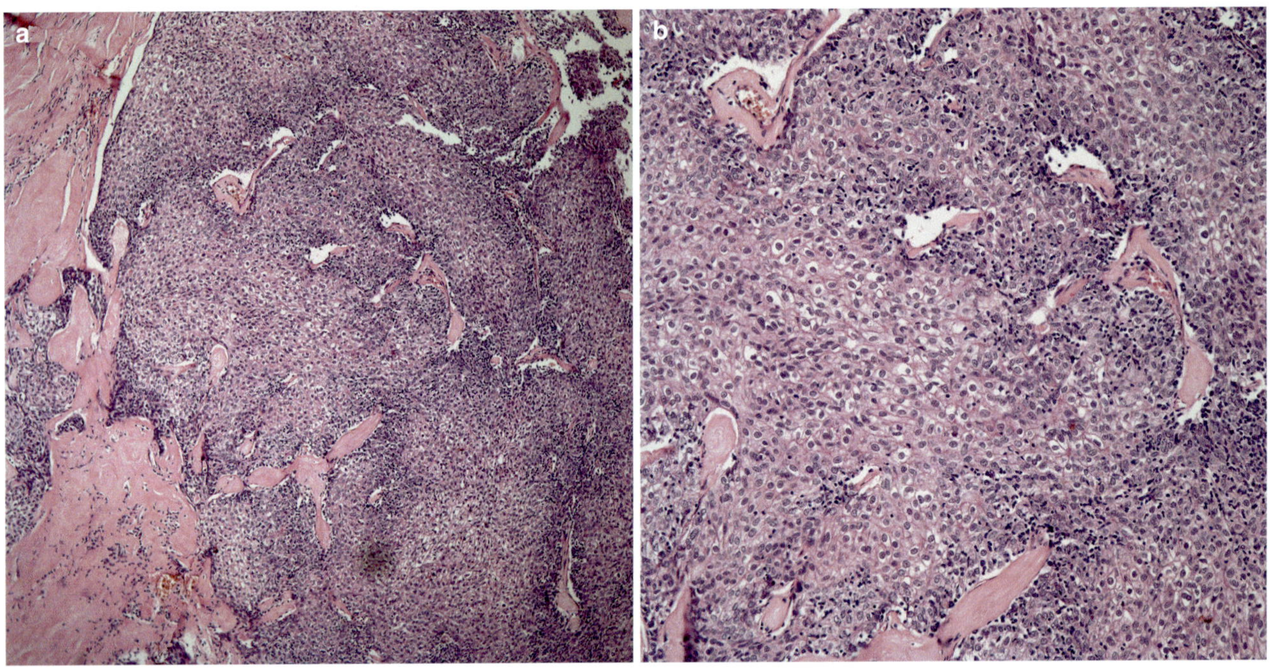

Fig. 7.110 (**a**) Thymoma with prominent clear cell changes, (**b**) higher magnification showing the clear cells with mild atypia

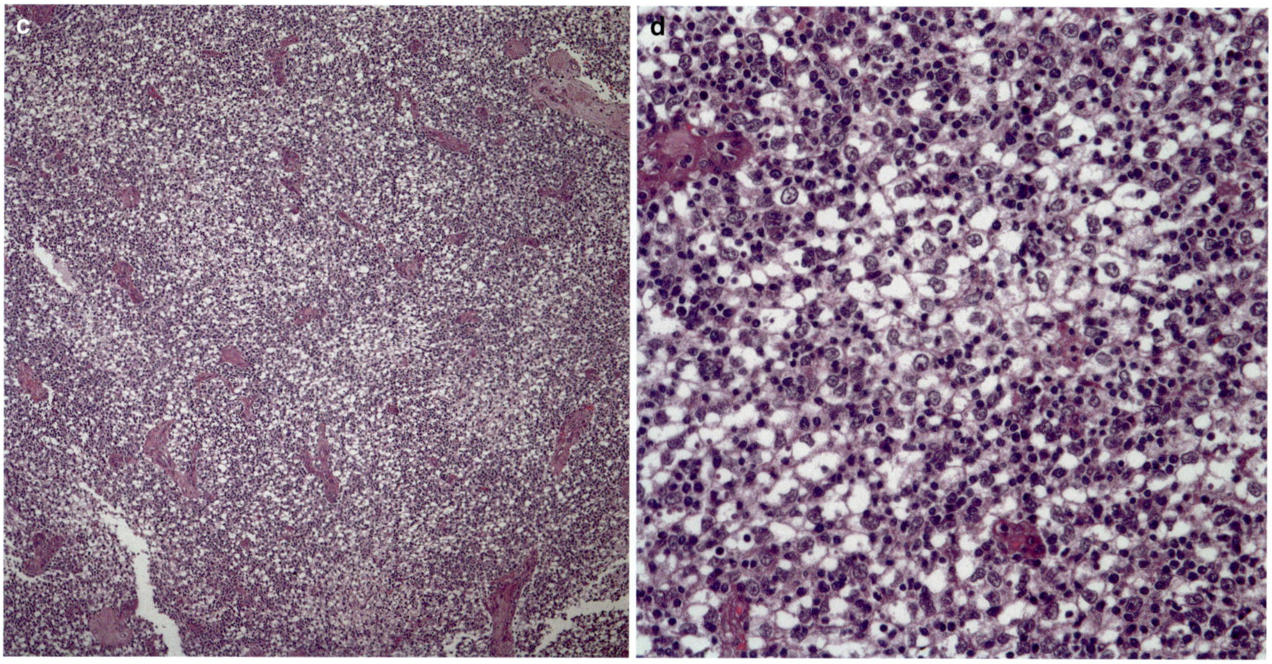

Fig. 7.110 (continued) (**c**) Thymoma with lymphocytes and clear cells, (**d**) higher magnification of the clear cells admixed with lymphocytes

Thymoma/Thymic Carcinoma

The occurrence of this phenomenon of dual tumor is unusual, however not surprising given the heterogeneity of thymomas and the spectrum of differentiation that these tumors may show. One of the largest series of this occurrence reported 22 cases of thymoma/thymic carcinoma [180]. It is important to highlight that such diagnosis is likely not to be rendered on the basis of small biopsies, remembering that it is not advisable to attempt to predict prognosis in cases of thymoma in which there is a limited material for evaluation. In some of the cases described, the histology of these tumors has shown spindle cell thymoma associated with thymic carcinomas or other conventional variants of thymoma associated with thymic carcinoma. However, it is also important to highlight that the association of thymoma with another malignancy is not limited to thymic carcinoma. We have had the opportunity to evaluate thymomas that are associated with thymic adenocarcinomas, neuroendocrine carcinomas, and germ cell tumors [181]. Therefore, we have advised that the final diagnosis of thymoma be performed after evaluation of resected material rather than on small biopsy samples, which will limit the possibility of discovering another associated malignancy. Needless to say, the resected material will provide the necessary information to properly stage the tumor at the time of surgical resection.

Other Unusual Variants of Thymoma

Over the years, we have had the experience to identify other variants of thymoma that are rare and that may pose a significant problem in diagnosis, namely, in mediastinoscopic biopsies. These unusual variants include:

- *Alveolar thymoma*: In this variant, the tumor grows as if forming alveolar spaces, the cells are either spindle or oval and the tumors lack nuclear atypia and mitotic activity (Fig. 7.113a, b).
- *Angiectatic thymoma*: In this growth pattern, the low power view is that of ectatic spaces filled with fresh blood, and the round to oval tumor cells are around the hemorrhagic spaces. However, in other areas, the tumors show a spindle cellular proliferation admixed with reds cells (Fig. 7.114a–c).
- *Thymomas with neural-like pattern*: This tumor is either composed of spindle or oval cells, which may grow in patterns either mimicking schwannoma or meningioma.

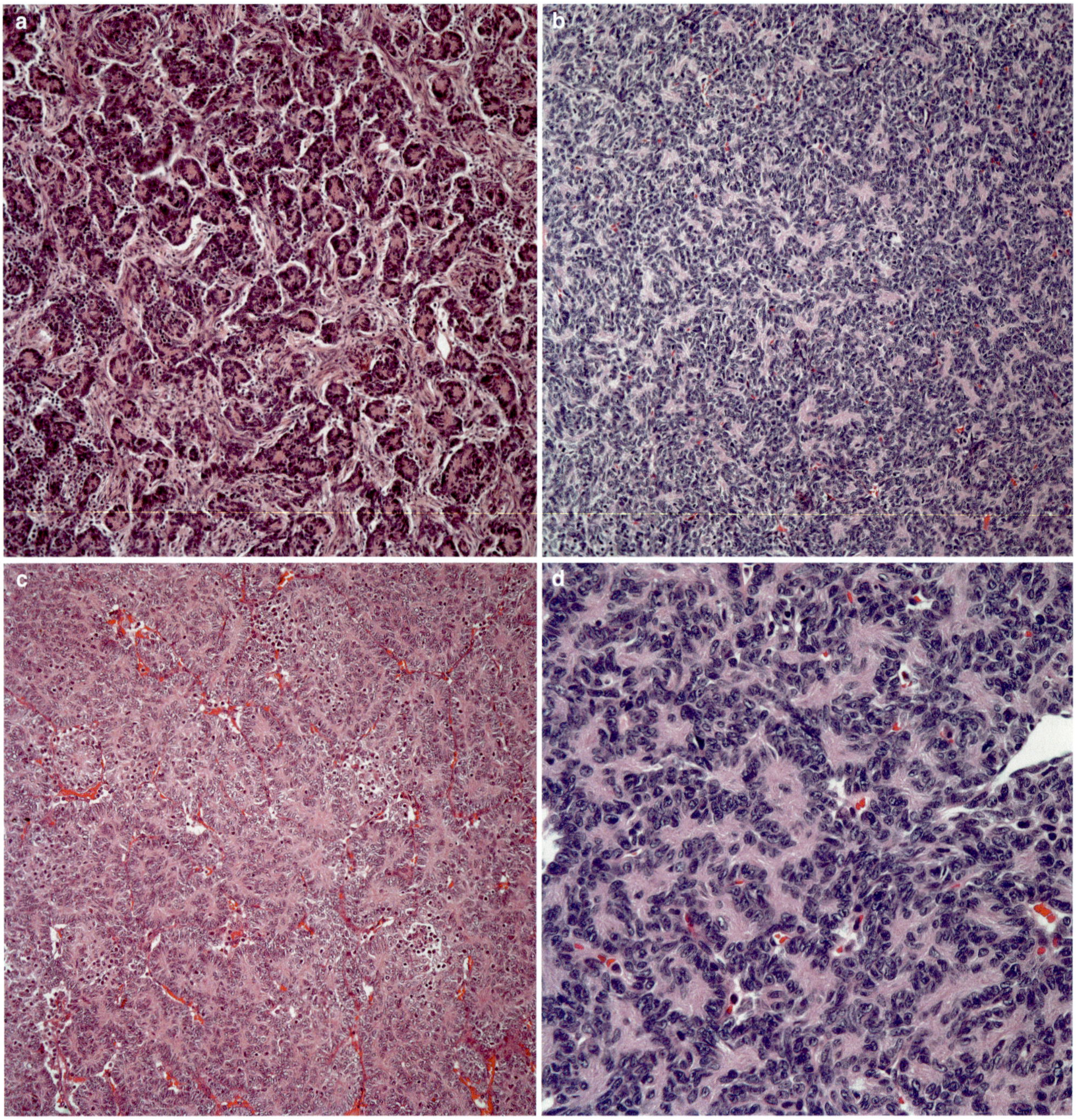

Fig. 7.111 (**a**) Low power view of a spindle cell thymoma with neuroendocrine morphology, (**b**) presence of pseudorosettes, (**c**) higher magnification of the pseudorosettes showing lack of nuclear atypia or mitotic activity, (**d**) oval and spindle cell with fusiform nuclei and prominent nucleoli in some of the cells

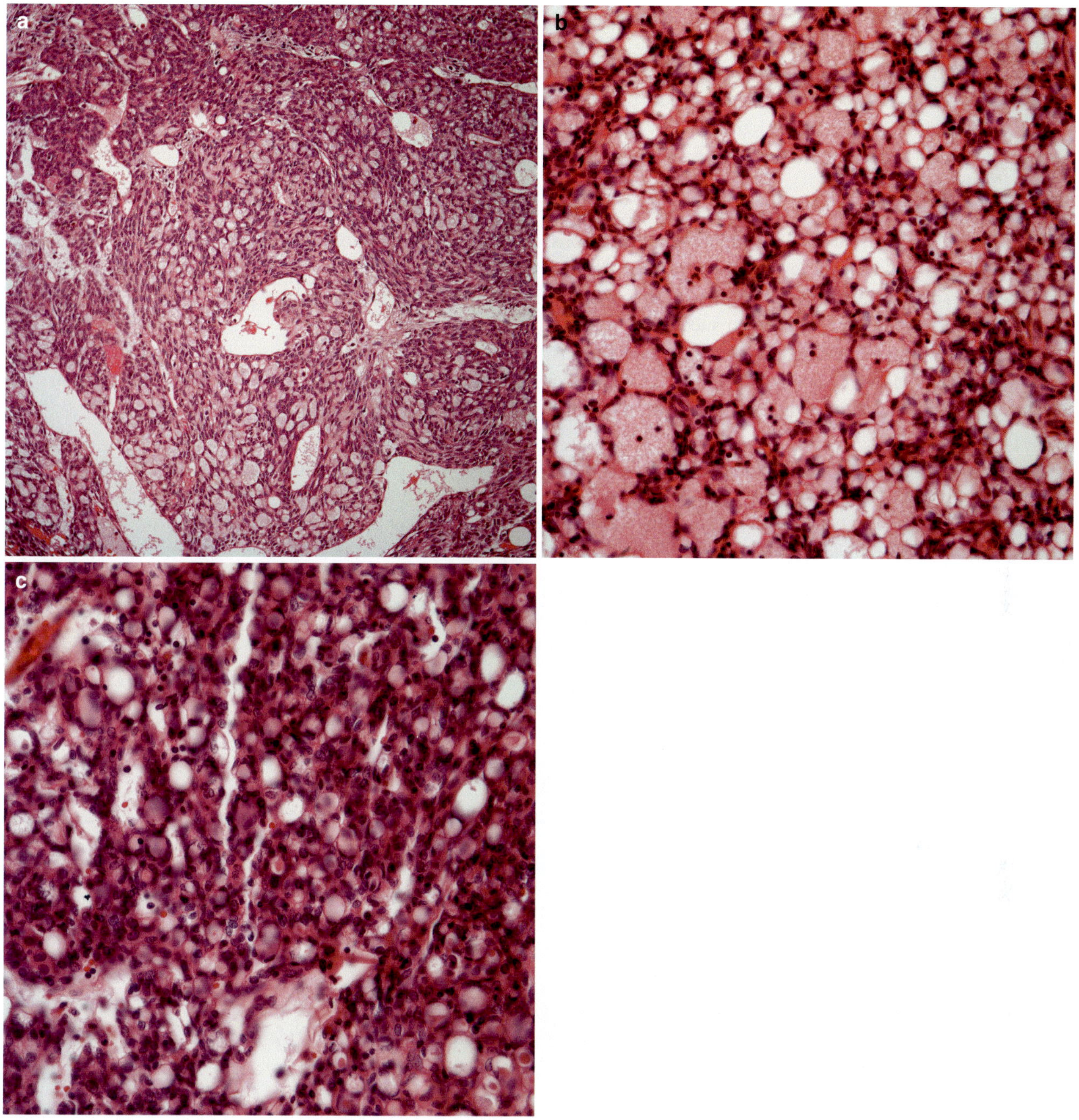

Fig. 7.112 (**a**) Low power view of a thymoma with signet ring cell-like morphology, (**b**) closer view at the signet ring cell-like areas, (**c**) higher magnification lacks nuclear atypia and mitotic activity

In this latter growth pattern, areas of hyalinization are commonly present (Fig. 7.115a, b).

- *Mucinous thymomas*: The production of mucin in otherwise conventional thymoma is also an unusual phenomenon. We have seen mucin production mainly in spindle cell thymomas and in thymomas with papillary features (Fig. 7.116a–d).
- *Thymomas with sebaceous differentiation*: Sebaceous differentiation is an unusual feature in thymomas. Sebaceous differentiation has been observed in the normal thymus and also in some benign salivary gland-type tumors of the thymus. However, we have observed such differentiation in conventional thymomas, mainly those in which there is the presence of Hassall's corpuscles (Fig. 7.117a, b) and also in tumors without the presence of Hassall's corpuscles.
- *Thymomas with extensive presence of Hassall's corpuscles*: Even though such change has been well recorded in the literature and it can occur in any type of thymoma, the presence of extensive areas in which the presence of Hassall's corpuscles is marked is an unusual occurrence (Fig. 7.118a, b).
- *Thymomas with ameloblastic pattern*: This is an unusual growth pattern that can be seen in spindle cell and atypical thymomas. The tumor characteristically shows strands or thymic epithelium with a subtle microcystic growth pattern admixed with more solid areas of an epithelial proliferation (Fig. 7.119a, b). Areas of hyalinization are often encountered, but cellular atypia, necrosis, and mitoses are absent.

Thymomas Without a Well-Formed Capsule or Incomplete Capsule

Even though great emphasis is placed in the assessment of capsular integrity, it is important to highlight that not all thymomas have a well-defined capsule or in some cases the

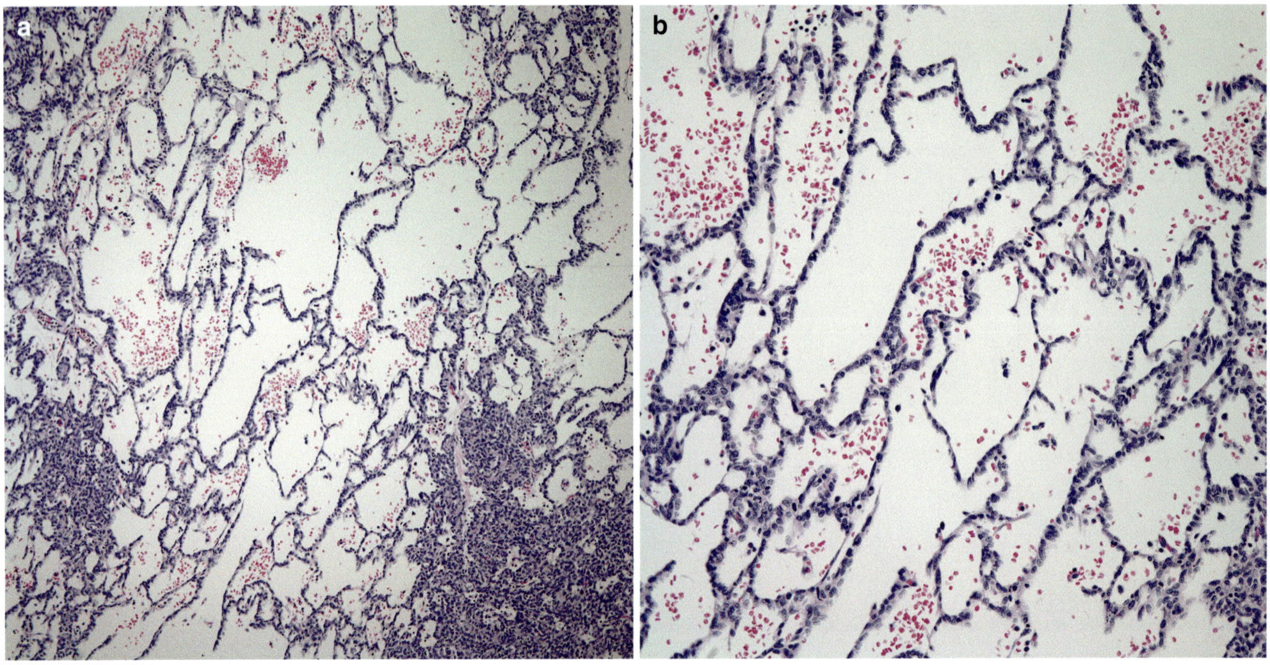

Fig. 7.113 (**a**) Thymoma with prominent alveolar-like pattern, (**b**) closer view is reminiscent of the pulmonary alveoli

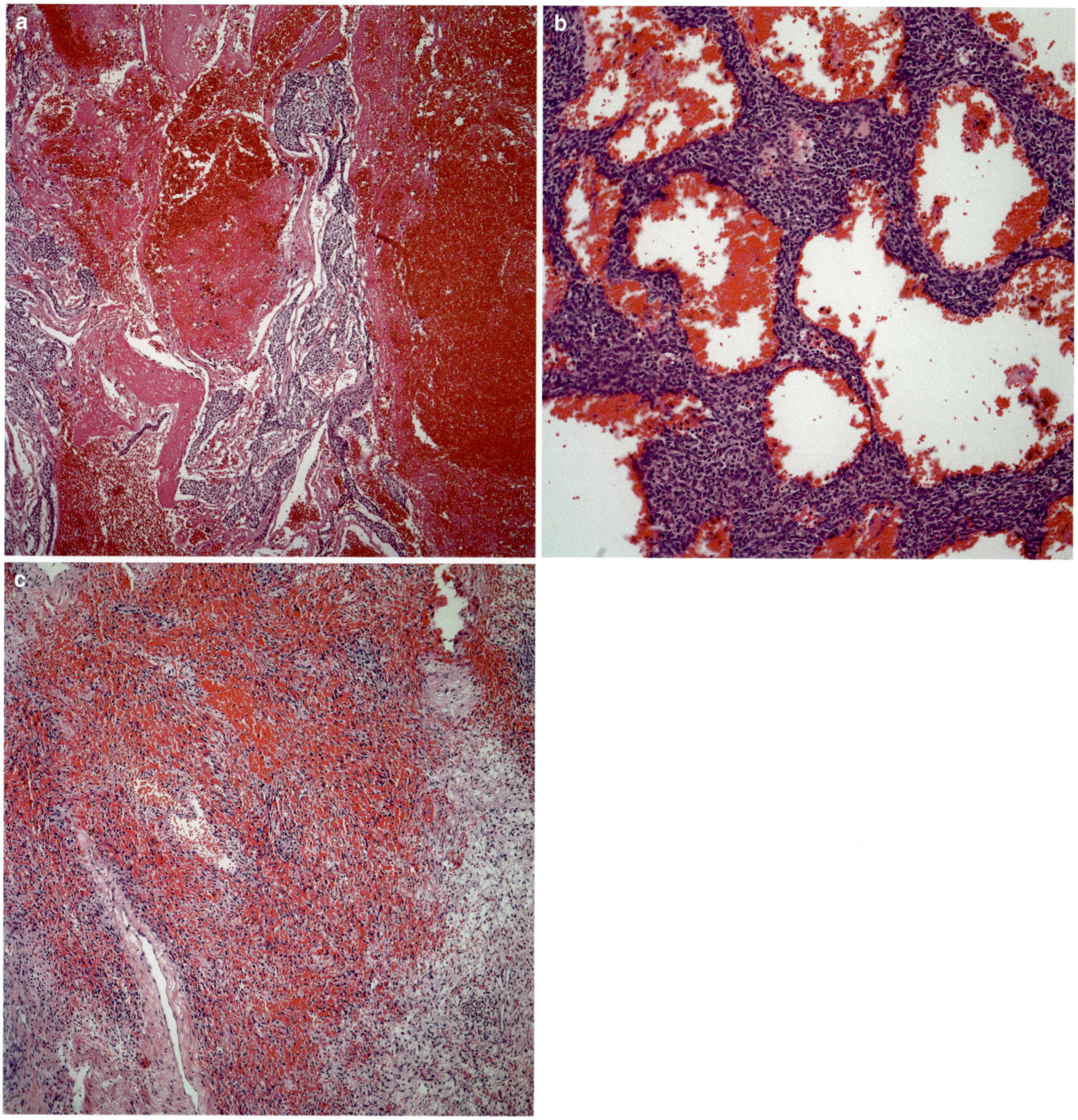

Fig. 7.114 (**a**) Thymoma with prominent angiectatic changes, (**b**) thymoma with dilated vascular-like structures, (**c**) spindle cells admixed with red cells

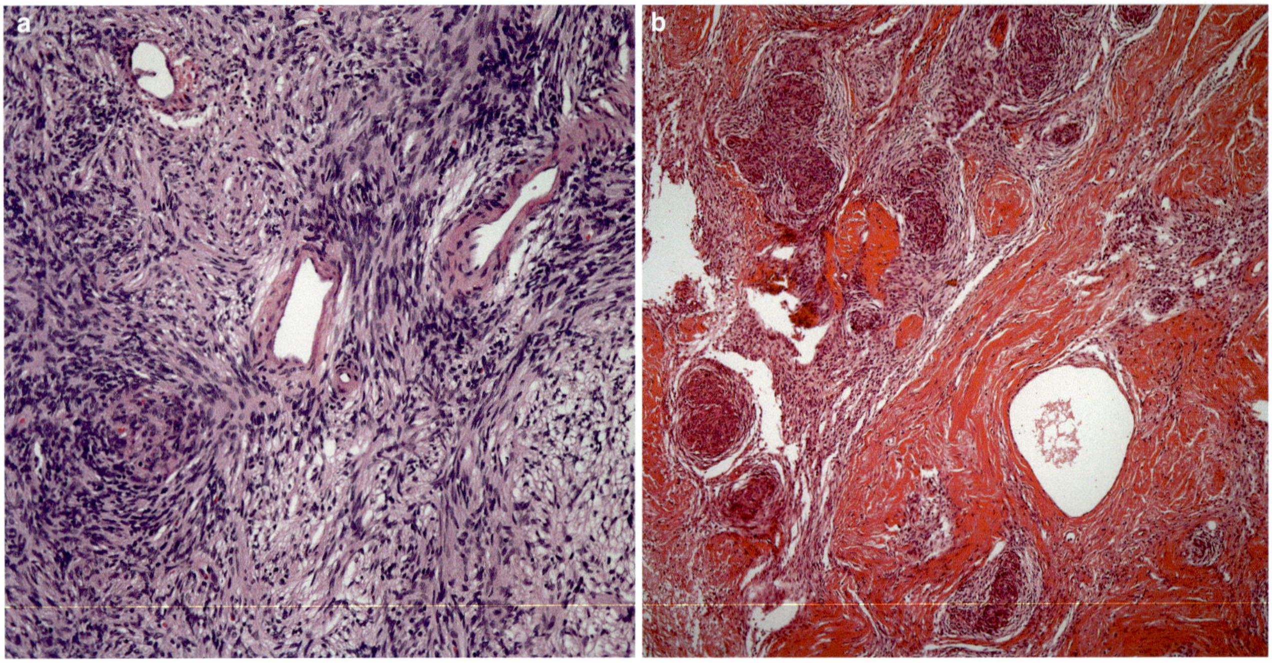

Fig. 7.115 (**a**) Thymoma with neural-like pattern and hyalinized blood vessels, (**b**) spindle and oval cells with extensive hyalinization reminiscent of meningioma

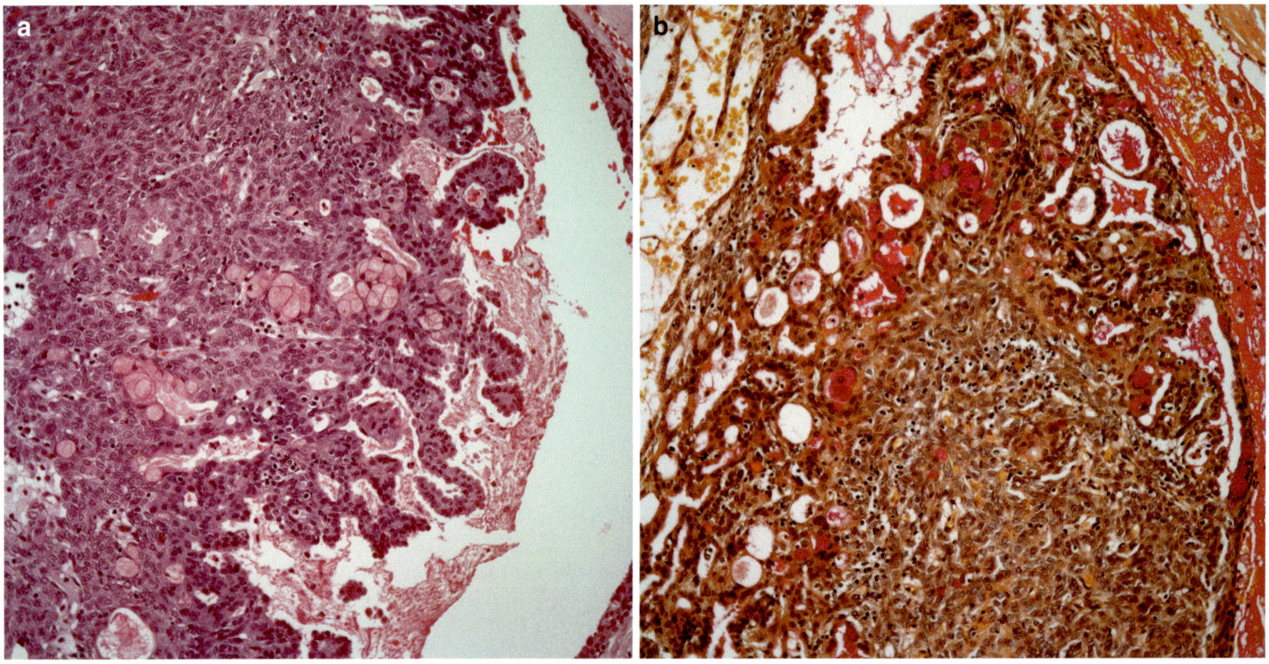

Fig. 7.116 (**a**) Mucinous thymoma; note the presence of mucinophages. (**b**) Histochemical stains for mucicarmine is positive

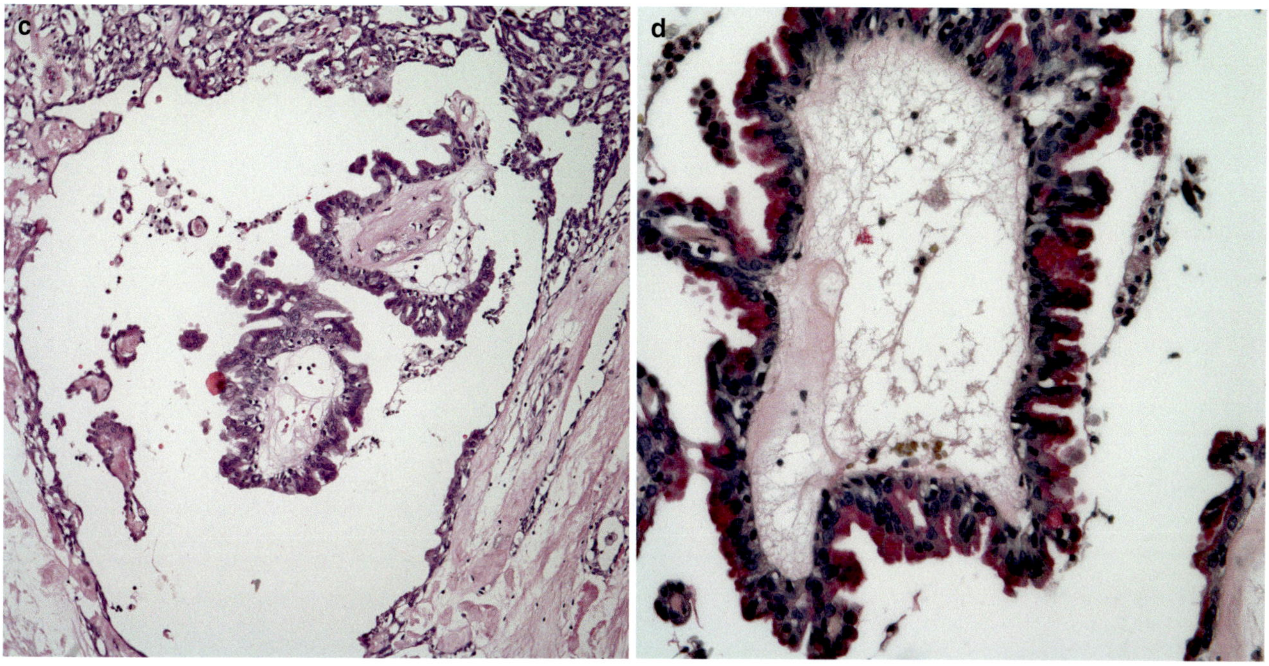

Fig. 7.116 (continued) (**c**) Mucinous papillary thymoma. (**d**) Histochemical stain for mucin is positive

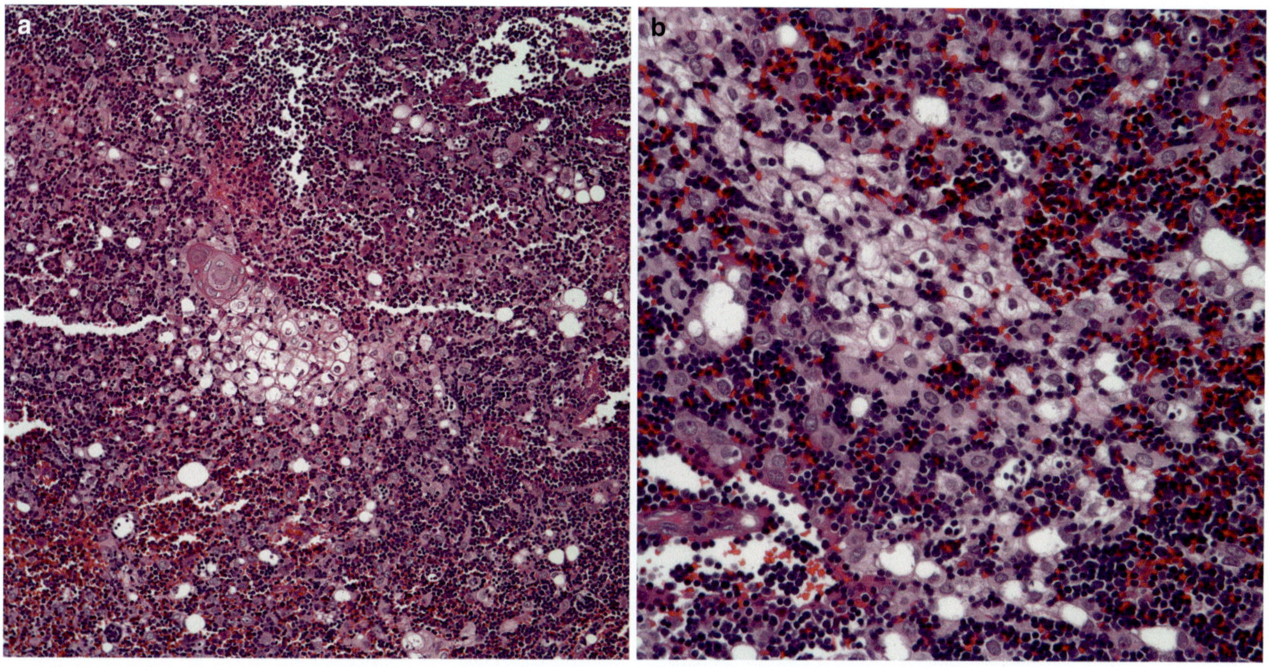

Fig. 7.117 (**a**) Thymoma with sebaceous differentiation; note the presence of the sebaceous component coming off a Hassall's corpuscle. (**b**) Higher magnification of the sebaceous component

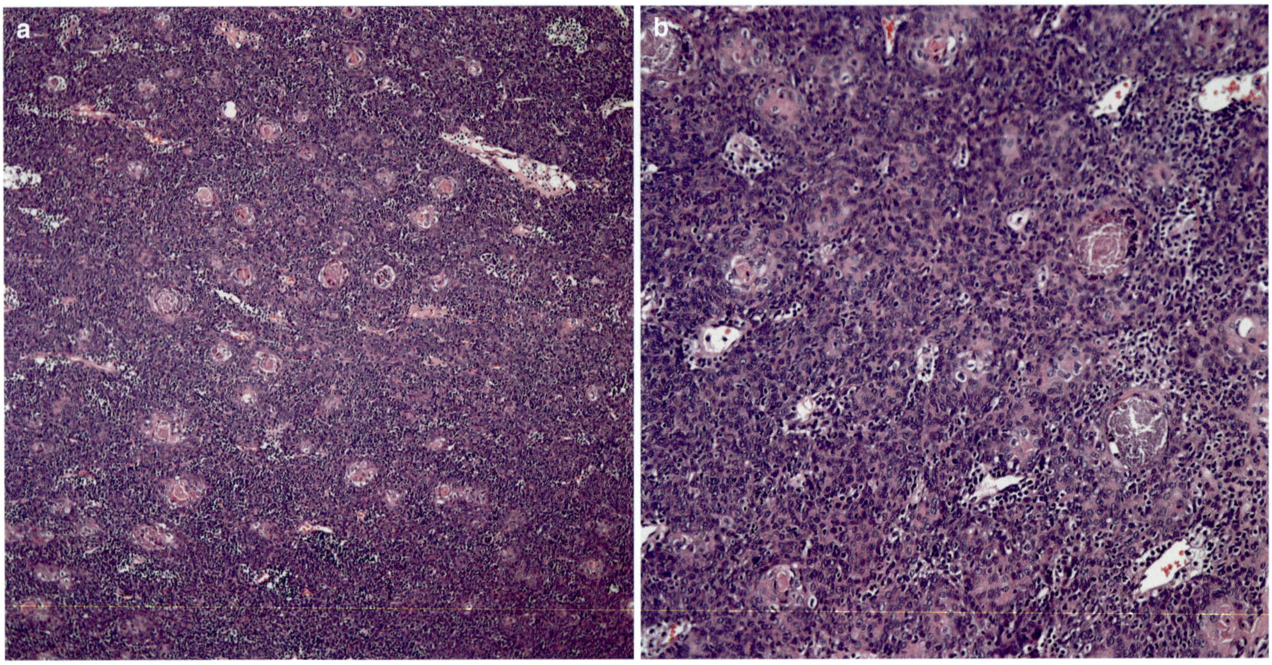

Fig. 7.118 (**a**) Thymoma with extensive presence of Hassall's corpuscles, (**b**) higher magnification shows Hassall's corpuscles with necrotic debris

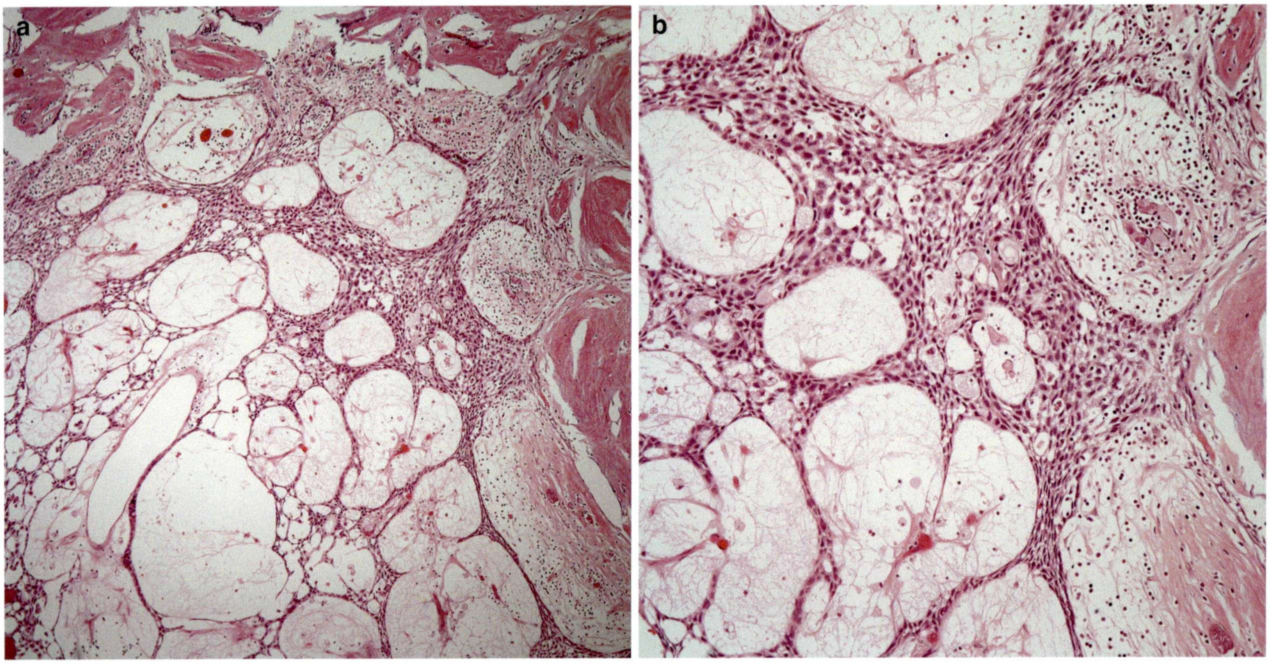

Fig. 7.119 (**a**) Thymoma with ameloblastic-like pattern, (**b**) epithelial cells with lack of nuclear atypia and mitotic activity

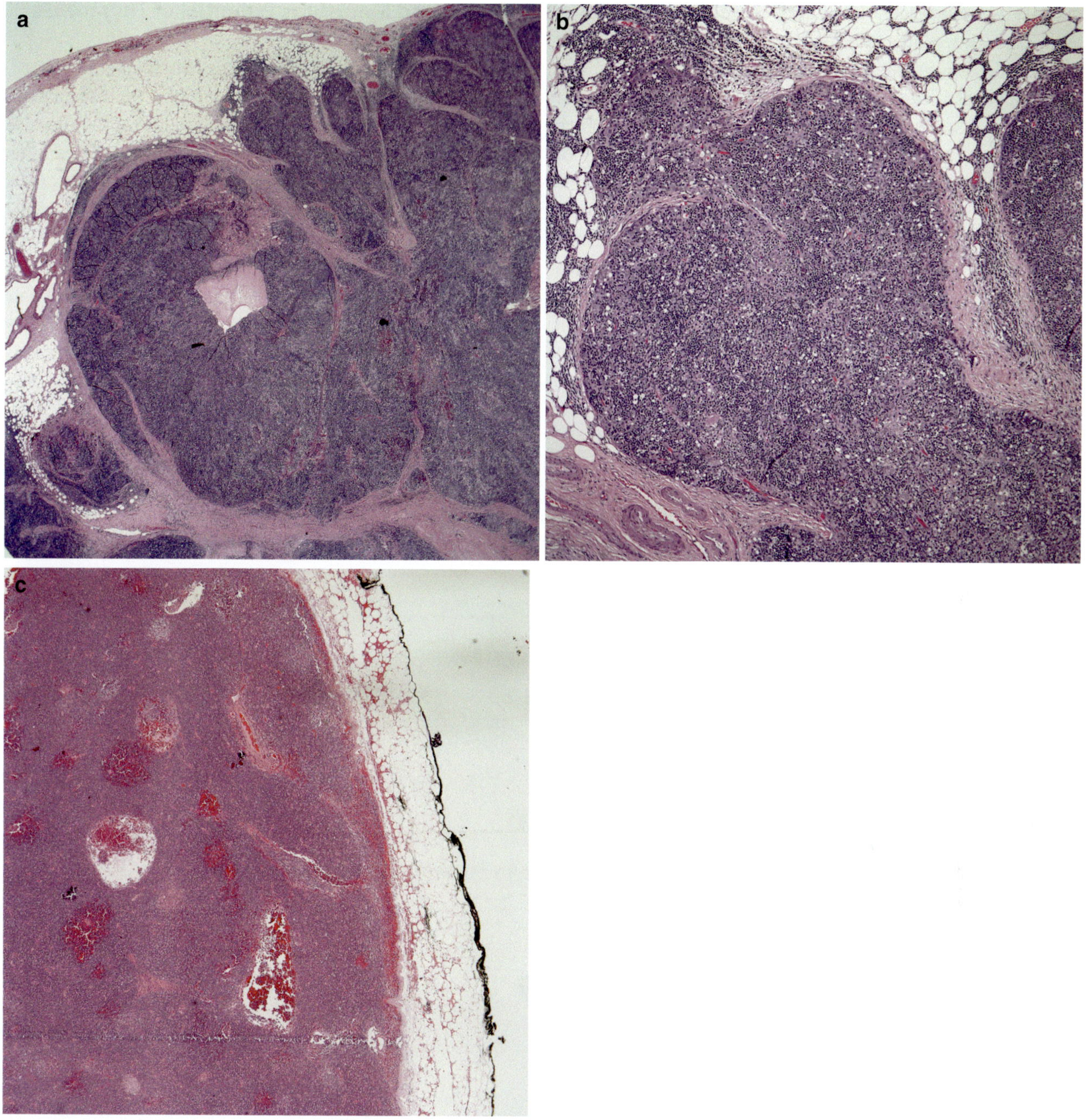

Fig. 7.120 (**a**) Low power view of a thymoma without a capsule; the tumor is in adipose tissue, but the ink border is negative for thymoma. (**b**) Closer view at the infiltration of the tumor into adipose tissue. (**c**) Closer view at the free ink border of resection

capsule is incomplete. Therefore, these cases need to be addressed differently. Current staging systems have not addressed this issue meaningfully.

We have estimated based on our current practice that the percentage of cases in which there is no capsule or in which the capsule is incomplete represents approximately 1–2% of all cases. Since in our daily practice we consistently ink the borders of these tumors, as we have stated previously, according to the manner in which we handle surgical resections, then it is much easier to determine in these tumors without a well-defined capsule, whether the tumor is at the ink border of resection or not (Fig. 7.120a–c). In addition, it is important to highlight that, in our experience with tumors limited to the mediastinum (minimmaly invasive), the survival of those patients is similar to those in whom the tumors are encapsulated. However, once more, it is highly important that the pathologist addresses the issue of whether this particular tumor has a well-defined capsule or an incomplete capsule and whether or not the inked surgical border is free of tumor.

Invasive and Metastatic Potential of Thymomas

As discussed in the section on staging, any thymoma, regardless of its histopathological features, has the potential to invade adjacent organs or to metastasize above the thoracic inlet or below the diaphragm. We have encountered such cases in our daily practice to account for all the histological variants. Invasive disease to the lung and diaphragm as well as metastatic disease to the thyroid, bone marrow, skin, liver, and kidney – although rare – can take place (Fig. 7.121a–i). Therefore, as we have expressed in other chapters of this text, all thymomas should be regarded as potentially malignant tumors capable to invade or metastasize. However, it is very important not to confuse an invasive nodule of a thymoma with metastasis to lymph nodes. Figure 7.122 illustrates such a problem. Even if the tumor nodule is near a lymph node, the lymph node proper is negative in this particular illustration, despite the appearance that the tumor is involving the lymph node.

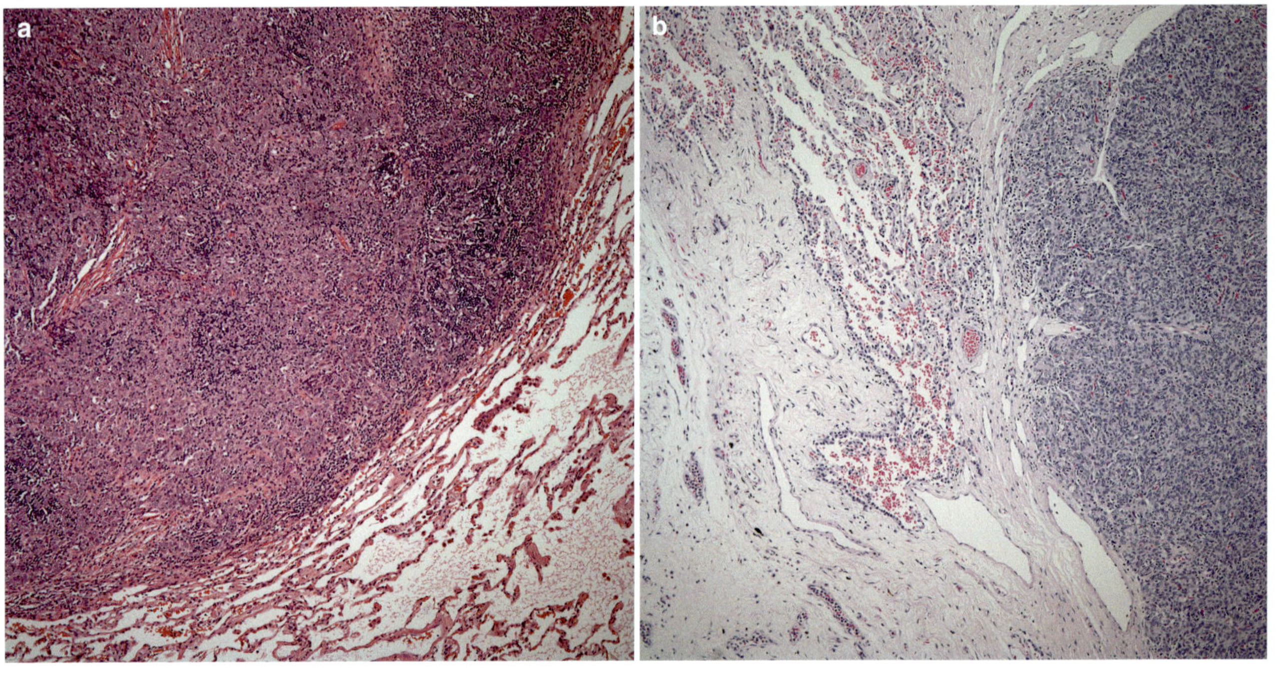

Fig. 7.121 (**a**) Lymphocytic thymoma infiltrating lung parenchyma, (**b**) spindle cell thymoma infiltrating the lung parenchyma,

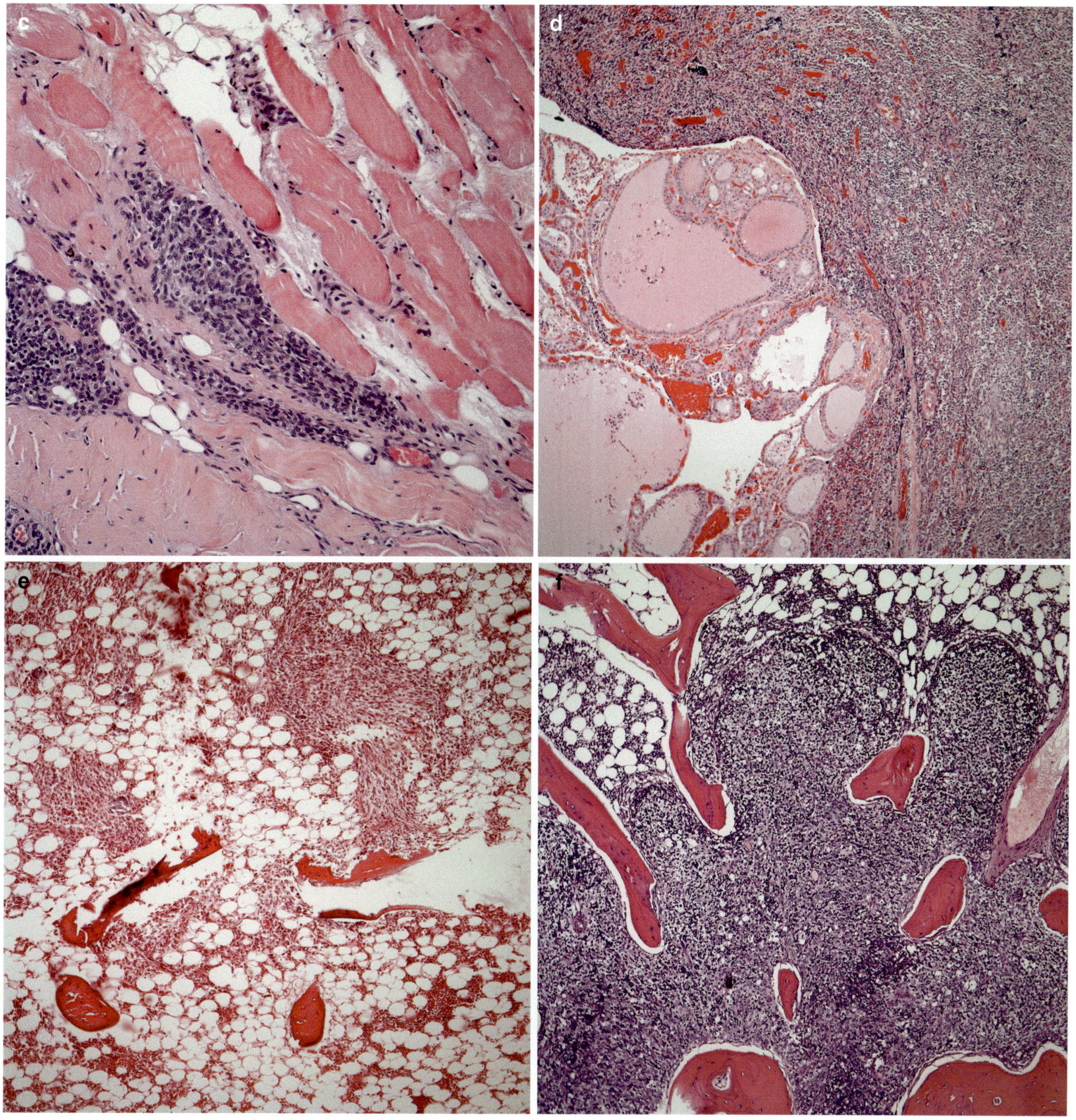

Fig. 7.121 (continued) (**c**) Spindle cell thymoma infiltrating the diaphragm, (**d**) lymphocytic thymoma infiltrating the thyroid gland, (**e**) spindle cell thymoma infiltrating the bone marrow, (**f**) lymphocytic thymoma infiltrating the bone marrow

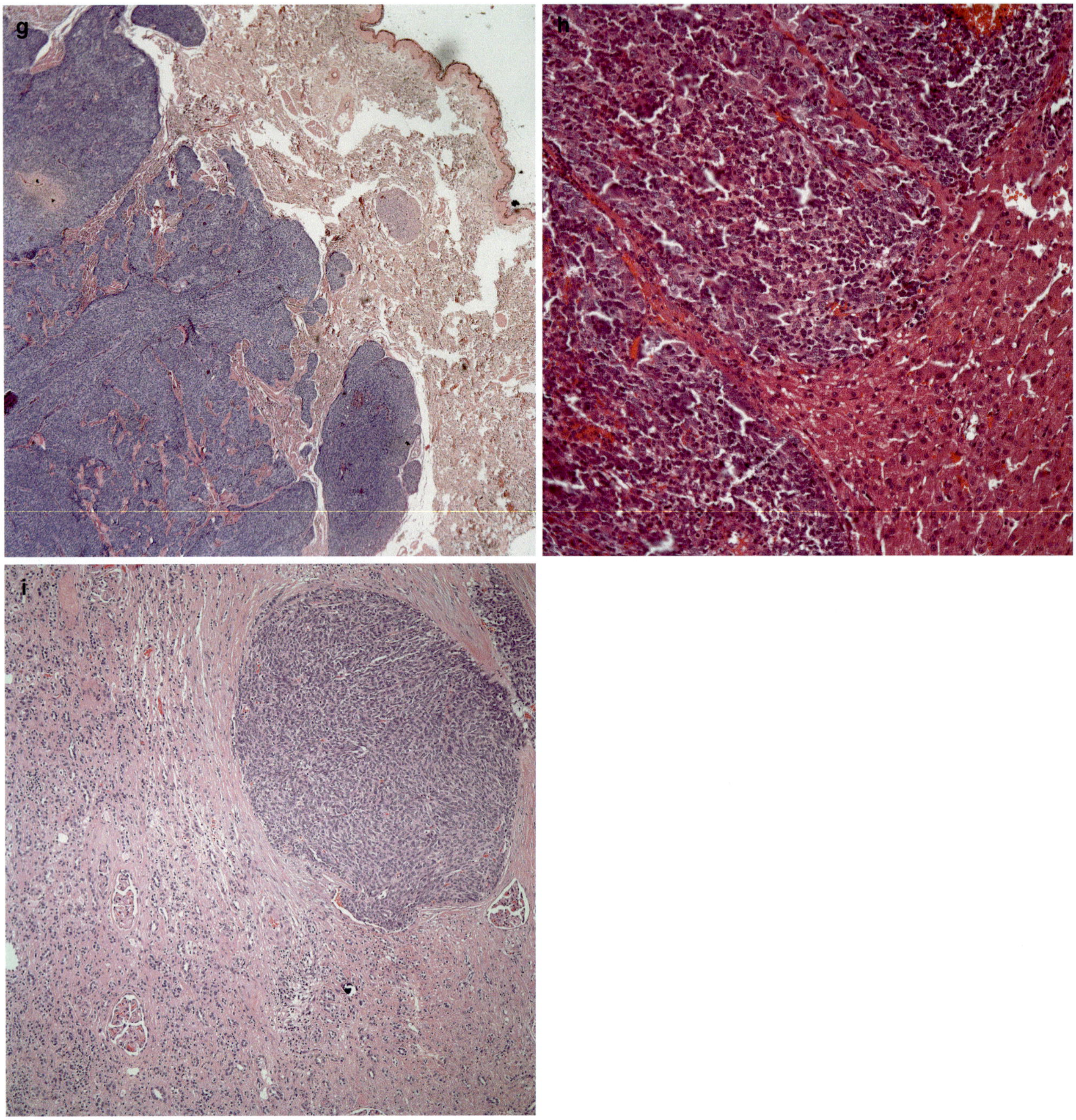

Fig. 7.121 (continued) (**g**) Spindle cell thymoma infiltrating the dermis, (**h**) lymphocytic thymoma infiltrating the liver parenchyma, (**i**) spindle cell thymoma infiltrating the renal parenchyma

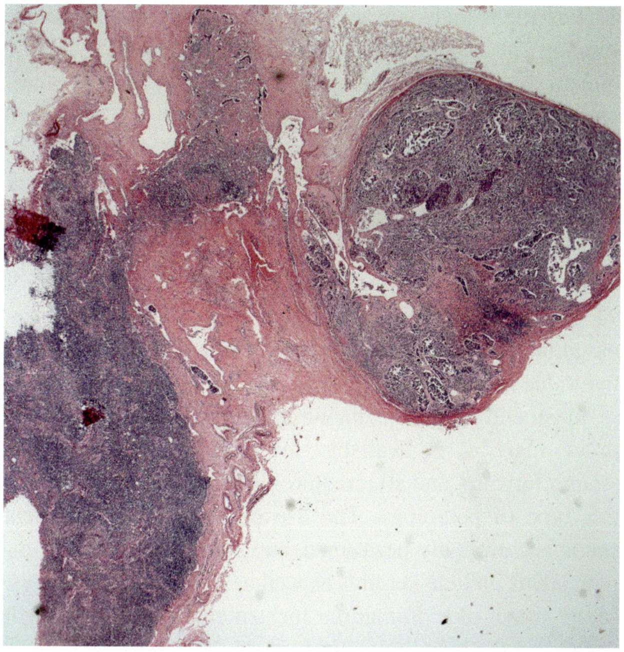

Fig. 7.122 Often a common mistake is to misinterpret a tumor nodule for metastasis to lymph node; note the lymph node is negative, while there is an adjacent tumor nodule

Immunohistochemical and Molecular Features

In the early years of immunohistochemistry, several studies were performed in rather small series of thymomas with the limited immunohistochemistry of the time. Some studies have attempted to identify the origin of the epithelial cells, while other studies have been more general to determine the antigenicity of the epithelial cells with different antibodies. In the decade of the 1980s, efforts were made to categorize the epithelial cells further. Some studies were directed to determine the origin of the epithelial cells, whether from the medulla or the cortex of the thymus. In that regard, the epithelial cells of thymomas have been studied using HLA-DR, anti-HLA-A,B,C, cortical EC,21A6, and keratin 34βE12-IV/82, while the lymphocytes have been evaluated with OK T6, Leu 1, Leu2A, Leu 3a, anti-TdT, and anti S-100 [182–186]. Also, following a similar way of thinking regarding epithelial cells, Ring and Addis [187], Kodama and coauthors [188], and Lee [189] reported small series of thymomas using CAM5.2, Leu 7, HLA-DR, S-100 protein, and CD45 in which the authors observed variable expressions for CAM 5.2 and Leu 7, while the loss of expression for HLA-DR was seen in invasive thymomas in some studies. However, the main driving concepts were to attempt to determine the origin of the epithelial cells. On the other hand, Ruco and coauthors [190] documented the presence of interdigitating reticulum cells in normal thymus and thymomas by staining interdigitating cells for CD45, CD4, HLA-DR, and CD25, while the macrophages were positive for PAM-1/MAC, Leu-M3 (CD14), CD4, and CD11b.

In the 1990s, a few more immunohistochemical studies were presented on thymomas. Mizuno and coauthors [191] reported a study on the distribution of fibronectin and laminin, documenting diffuse or partially intricate network of fibers that contains fibronectin and laminin surrounding tumor cells, especially in spindle cell thymomas, while in other cases their presence was in the septa, blood vessels, and perivascular spaces. Giraud and coauthors [69] reported the presence of thymulin, thymosin α1, and vasopressin in thymomas. Fukai and coauthors [192] reported 81 thymomas (59 encapsulated and 22 invasive) and 14 thymic carcinomas which were evaluated using epithelial membrane antigen (EMA) and encountered that thymic carcinomas express more EMA than thymomas; the authors noted that, when EMA is expressed in thymoma, it is usually in invasive tumors. The same authors, using probably the same material, reported two similar immunohistochemical studies [193, 194]: (1) a study in which the authors used anti-Leu-7, UH-1, and PE-35 monoclonal antibodies, observing positive staining for these antibodies in different compartments, UH-1 reacted with cortical epithelium, Leu-7 was positive in subcapsular-cortical epithelium, and PE-35 reacted with medullary epithelium; and (2) likely the same subset of tumors was evaluated for CK13 and CK18, and the authors arrived at the conclusion that thymic epithelial cells cannot be separated on the basis of keratin expression. Pescarmona and coauthors [195] evaluated the expression of epidermal growth factor (EGF) and nerve growth factor (NGF) receptors in normal thymus and thymomas. The authors encountered that EGF was detected in the subcapsular, cortical, and medullary epithelial cells of the normal thymus, while NGF was detected only in the subcapsular and medullary areas. EGF was expressed by thymomas regardless of their histological features, while NFG was detected in spindle cell thymomas. Wu and coauthors [196] evaluated encapsulated and invasive thymomas for the presence of Epstein-Barr virus by in situ hybridization and reported negative results for the presence of EBV in all thymomas evaluated. Chan and coauthors [197] evaluated O13 (MIC2) in hyperplastic thymus and thymomas and encountered that, in the hyperplastic thymus, MIC2 is expressed in most of the lymphocytes of the cortex while in fewer (about 5%) of the lymphocytes of the medulla. Also, a similar finding was encountered in thymomas. A similar study by Dorfman and Pinkus [198] also identified the expression of CD99 in thymomas. Stefanaki and coauthors [199], in a study of 31 thymomas, identified the expression of p53, mdm2, p21/waf1, and bcl-2 proteins in different proportions depending on the histology of the tumor. In a study by Yang and coauthors [200], the authors evaluated 62 thymomas using

PCNA and Ki67 and identified that PCNA labeling indices were considerably higher than those of Ki-67. Hishima and coauthors [201], in a study of thymomas, thymic carcinomas, and neuroendocrine carcinomas, identified the expression of synaptophysin in atypical thymomas more often than in conventional thymomas. On the other hand, thymomas with expression of B-cells or T-cell lymphocytosis have also been described [202–204].

In more recent years, different aspects of the antigenicity of thymomas have been presented with different goals. Sonobe and coauthors [205] studied the expression of CD44v6 in an attempt to determine possible biologic behavior of thymomas. The authors reported 108 thymomas identifying 70 cases with negative results, 20 weakly positive, and 18 strongly positive. The authors concluded that CD44v6 correlates with tumor staging (Masaoka staging). Lexiev and coauthors [206] evaluated 17 cases of thymoma using lymphoid and neuroendocrine markers and encountered that thymomas associated with autoimmune disease have a significant population of CD20-positive lymphocytes, while CD57's strong positive reaction suggests the possibility of a neuromuscular disorder, namely, MG. Interestingly, the authors concluded that CD5 has limited value, as both thymomas and thymic carcinomas may show positive staining for this antibody. Nonaka and coauthors [207] evaluated 58 thymomas and 17 thymic carcinomas using Foxn1 and CD205, identifying Foxn1 diffuse positive nuclear staining in all thymomas (WHO types A and B) but only focal in thymic carcinoma. CD205 shows positive cytoplasmic staining in most thymomas and variable focal staining in thymic carcinomas. Also, the expression of p63 in thymoma and the normal thymus was evaluated by Dotto and coauthors [208], who identified that all 66 thymomas and 14 thymic carcinomas were positive for p63 staining. Wu and coauthors [209] also evaluated the expression of p63 and X-linked inhibitor of apoptosis protein (XIAP) in thymomas, finding all 12 cases of thymomas positive for p63 and 9 of the 12 positive for XIAP. The authors stated that the level of expression does not correlate with capsular integrity. Kaira and coauthors [210] evaluated the expression of MUC1 in thymic epithelial neoplasms (thymoma and thymic carcinoma) and reported that the overexpression of MUC1 was 94% (16/17) in thymic carcinomas and 0% (0/5) in thymoma (WHO type B3). Cimpean and coauthors [211] looked into the expression of SOX2 in five normal thymuses and ten thymomas, identifying that the expression of SOX2 in thymomas is increased parallel to the pathological stage. In a more specific approach, we recently evaluated 30 spindle cell thymomas for the expression of keratins, TTF1, S-100 protein, CD34, chromogranin, synaptophysin, EMA, calretinin, desmin, smooth muscle actin, and Bcl-2 [212]. We encountered that these tumors express pancytokeratin and keratin 5/6, while all the tumors were negative for S-100, keratin 20, chromogranin, and desmin. However, 83% of the spindle cell thymomas showed variable positive staining for keratin 7 and Bcl-2. In addition, 97% of the tumors showed focal staining for calretinin, 23% for synaptophysin, and 13% for smooth muscle actin. One case showed positive staining for TTF1, while CD34 and EMA were negative. Also, we conducted a study to evaluate the expression of PD-1 and PD-L1 in 74 thymomas and 26 thymic carcinomas [213]. PD-2 was observed positive in 46 of 74 thymomas and 6 of 26 thymic carcinomas, while PD-L1 was positive in 47 of 74 thymomas and 14 of 26 thymic carcinomas. However, based on the results obtained, we considered that the predictive value in terms of prognosis remains uncertain.

In general terms, the diagnosis of thymoma, when appropriate material is available for interpretation, is rather straightforward, and all it requires is to have experience with this type of pathology. The use of immunohistochemical stains is commonly performed, and some of the most common stains include keratins as well as lymphocytic markers. More often, the immunohistochemical stains used will depend on the histological features of the thymoma. In lymphocytic thymomas (Fig. 7.123a), the use of keratin (Fig. 7.123b) and lymphoid markers such as CD5 (Fig. 7.123c) and Tdt (Fig. 7.123d) are commonly performed, while for thymomas with more epithelial component, keratin 5/6 and p40 are commonly used. In cases of spindle cell thymoma, the use of other stains to rule out the possibility of a spindle mesenchymal neoplasm may take place; however, it is important to keep in mind that spindle cell thymomas besides pan-keratin and keratin 5/6 may also show focal positive staining for smooth muscle actin and Bcl-2 (Fig. 7.124a–d), which could be misinterpreted if proper attention is not given to the morphology of the tumor.

Regarding molecular analysis for thymomas, similar to the experience with immunohistochemistry, the field has moved as knowledge is gained. Unfortunately, due to limited knowledge regarding the differences between thymoma and thymic carcinoma, some review articles seem to be rather confusing, as the terminology applied is either not up to date or plainly just incorrect [214].

In 1995, Hayashi and coauthors [215] evaluated the expression of epidermal growth factor (EGF), EGF-receptor, p53, v-erb B, and ras p21 in thymomas in order to evaluate the progression of this tumor. The authors concluded that p53 may be implicated in the initial stages of tumorigenesis, and that increased expression of EGF and EGFR may play a role in thymoma progression. Weirich and coauthors [216] evaluated p53 in thymic epithelial neoplasms by immunohistochemistry and PCR-based single-stranded conformation and DNA sequencing. The authors included thymic carcinoma, "malignant thymomas," and "benign thymomas," which one could assume represented examples of invasive and encapsulated thymomas. In the group of invasive thymomas, the author identified frequent p53 alterations but without p53

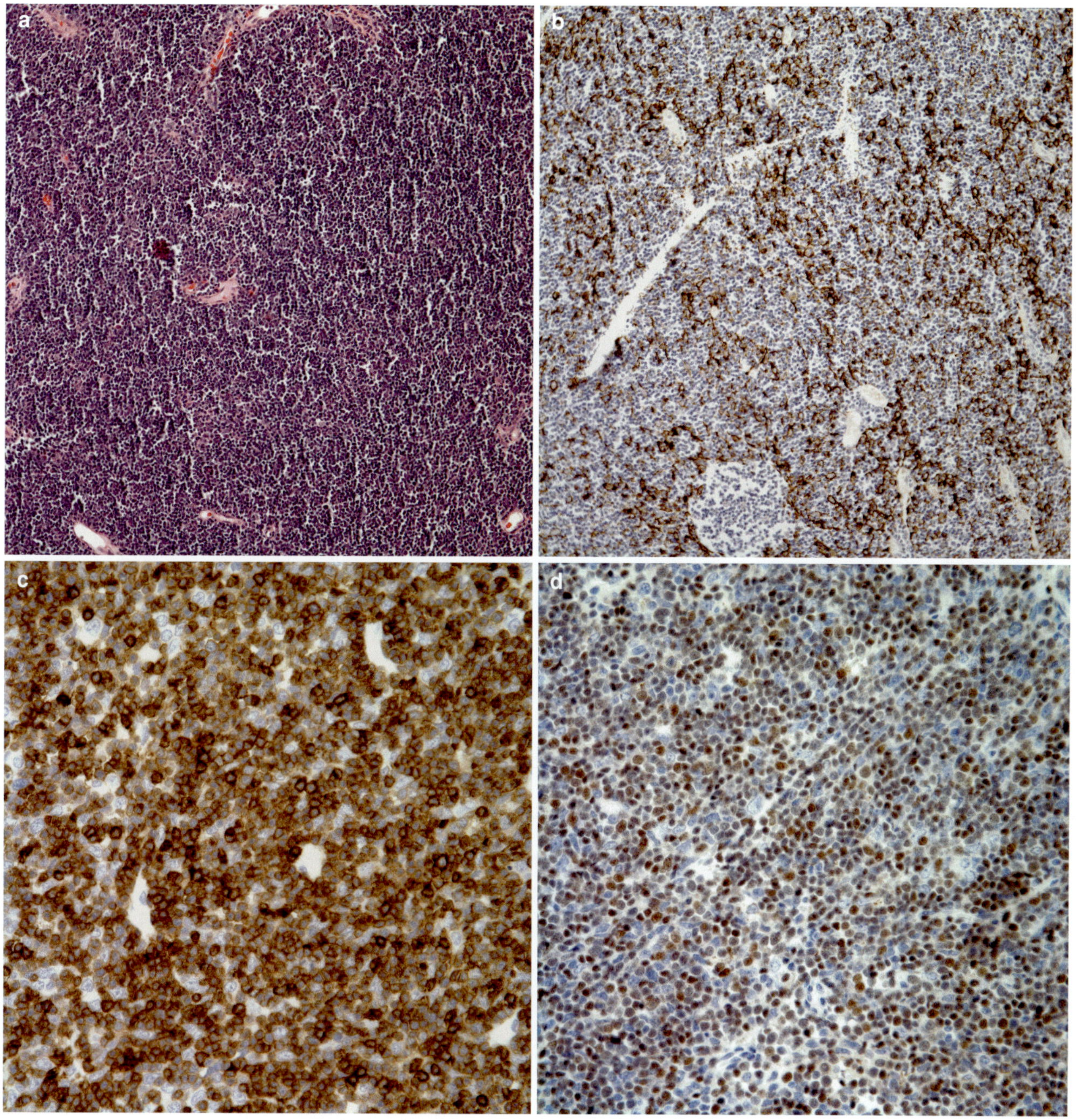

Fig. 7.123 (**a**) Commonly used immunohistochemical stains in a lymphocytic thymoma, (**b**) keratin decorates the epithelial cells, (**c**) CD5 immunostain decorated the lymphocytic component, (**d**) Tdt immunostains decorate the T-lymphocytes

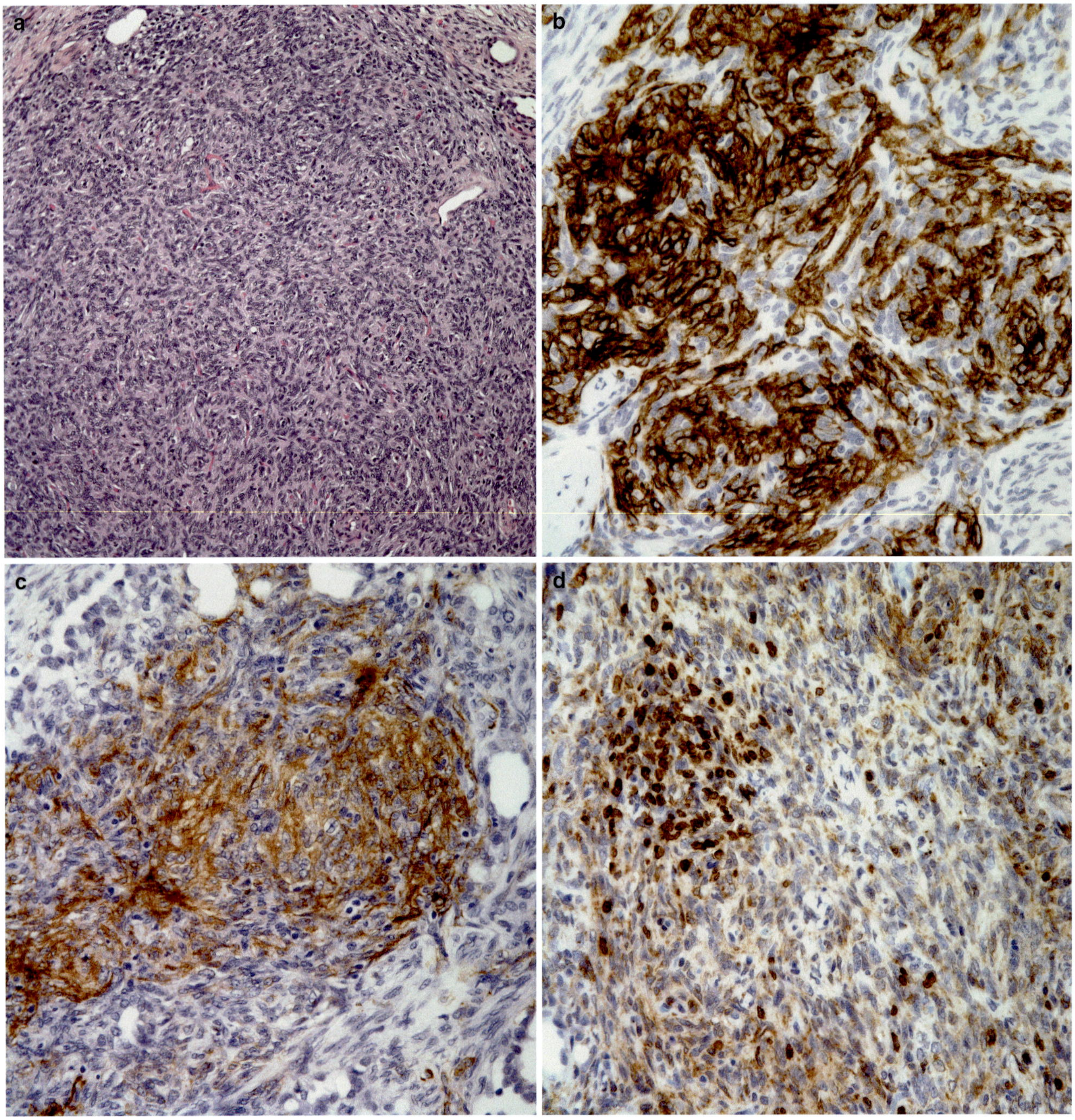

Fig. 7.124 (**a**) Spindle cell thymoma, (**b**) positive staining for keratin 5/6, (**c**) focal positive staining for smooth muscle actin, (**d**) focal positive staining for Bcl-2

gene, while, in encapsulated thymoma, p53 alterations were rare and p53 gene mutations were not identified. Pan and coworkers [217] evaluated the expression of apoptosis-related markers and HER-2/neu in normal thymus, thymomas, and thymic carcinomas. The authors identified that even though thymomas were positive for p53, they were low expressors and negative for Bcl-Xl, p21, and cyclin D1 and inconsistent BAX. Thymomas did not express HER-2/neu, except focally in two cases with lymphocytic component. In 2006, Chang and coworkers [218] evaluated STAT3 (signal transducers and activators of transcription 3) in normal thymuses of different ages, thymomas, and thymic carcinomas by immunohistochemistry. The authors identified that activated STAT3 was noted at a significantly higher frequency in thymomas with lymphocytic component in contrast with those thymomas with less lymphocytic component. In addition, activated STAT3 tended to have higher correlation with MG and to be less aggressive. Suzuki and coworkers [219] also evaluated the expression and mutation of EGFR in thymic epithelial tumors using PCR and did not detect EGFR gene mutation in 38 thymomas studied. However, the authors identified higher EGFR expression in invasive thymomas. Similar experience was also reported by Meister and coworkers [220] in a study of 20 thymomas of different histologies. In a different study, Yoh and coworkers [221] evaluated the prevalence of EGFR and KIT mutations by PCR and direct sequencing in 24 thymomas, encountering EGFR mutation in two thymomas, and the EGFR mutations were missense mutations (L858R and G863D) in exon 21. However, EGFR protein was expressed in 71% of thymomas. KIT mutations were not present in thymomas. Also, Tsuchida and coworkers [222] evaluated gene mutations in KIT-positive in 20 thymomas and 17 thymic carcinomas and showed that KIT- and CD5-positive staining occurred only in thymic carcinoma. Girard and coworkers [223], in what the authors called "comprehensive genomic analysis," profiled for mutations in genes encoding components of the EGFR and KIT signaling pathways and also assessed EGFR and KIT expression by immunohistochemistry in 38 thymomas of different histologies and 7 thymic carcinomas. The authors found that one thymoma harbored KRAS mutations (G12A), while another thymoma had G13A HRAS mutations. The authors concluded that their "comprehensive" genomic analysis suggests that thymic carcinomas are molecularly distinct from thymomas. The Eastern Cooperative Oncology group study evaluated 42 patients entered onto E1C97 with the goal of determining whether EGFR immunoreactivity correlated with outcomes and to identify new biologic markers for potential target therapy [224]. Immunohistochemical analysis for Her2/neu, EGFR, and C-kit was performed and scored on a scale from 0 to 3+. The authors encountered that EGFR immunoreactivity of 2+ or 3+ was associated with more aggressive thymomas. EGFR immunoreactivity was not consistently seen with thymic carcinoma, while Her/2neu immunoreactivity was negative in all tumors. The authors concluded that high EGFR immunoreactivity is seen in more aggressive thymic neoplasms. However, regardless of classification, the presence of EGFR in tumor cells (1+, 2+, and 3+) is associated with improved performance-free survival and a trend for better overall survival.

Based on the available data on molecular studies attempting to identify targets for the treatment of invasive thymomas, there is nothing that can be conclusively stated. However, it is likely that as new discoveries take place, those can be applied to the best treatment and outcome of patients with these tumors.

References

1. Castleman B. Tumors of the thymus gland, Atlas of Tumor Pathology, Section V, Fascicle 19. Washington, DC: Armed Forces Institute of Pathology; 1955.
2. Rosai J, Levine GD. Tumors of the thymus, Atlas of Tumor Pathology, 2nd series, Fascicle 13. Washington, DC: Armed Forces Institute of Pathology; 1975.
3. Shimosato Y, Mukai K. Tumors of the thymus, Atlas of Tumor Pathology, 3rd series, Fascile. Washington, DC: Armed Forces Institute of Pathology; 1999.
4. Engels EA, Pfeiffer RM. Malignant thymoma in the United States: demographic patterns in incidence and associations with subsequent malignancies. Int J Cancer. 2003;105:546–51.
5. Siesling S, van der Zwan JM, Izarzugaza I, Jaal J, Treasure T, Foschi R, et al. Rare thoracic cancers, including peritoneum mesothelioma. Eur J Cancer. 2012;48:949–60.
6. Engels EA. Epidemiology of thymoma and associated malignancies. J Thorac Oncol. 2010;5:S260–5.
7. Shier KJ. The thymus according to Schambacher: medullary ducts and reticular epithelium of thymus and thymomas. Cancer. 1981;48:1183–99.
8. Zhou R, Zettl A, Strobel P, Wagner K, Müller-Hermelink HK, Zhang S, et al. Thymic epithelial tumors can develop along two different pathogenetic pathways. Am J Pathol. 2001;159:1853–60.
9. Manley NR, Blackburn CC. A developmental look at thymus organogenesis: where do the non-hematopoietic cells in the thymus come from? Curr Opin Immunol. 2003;15:225–32.
10. Hale LP. Histologic and molecular assessment of human thymus. Ann Diagn Pathol. 2004;8:50–60.
11. Cheney RT. The biologic spectrum of thymic epithelial neoplasms: current status and future prospects. JNCCN. 2010;8:1322–8.
12. Suster S. Diagnosis of thymoma: my approach. J Clin Pathol. 2006;59:1238–44.
13. Suster S, Moran CA. Histologic classification of thymoma: the World Health Organization and beyond. Hematol Oncol Clin North Am. 2008;22(3):381–92.
14. Pescarmona E, Rendina EA, Venuta F. Recurrent thymoma: evidence for histological progression. Histopathology. 1995;27:445–9.
15. Suster S, Moran CA. Primary thymic epithelial neoplasms with combined features of thymoma and thymic carcinoma. A clinicopathological correlation of 22 cases. Am J Surg Pathol. 1996;20:1469–80.
16. Stoll DB, Lublin F, Brodovsky H, Laucius JF, Patchefsky A, Cooper H. Association of subacute motor neuropathy with thymoma. Cancer. 1984;54:770–2.
17. Guillan RA, Zelman S, Smalley RL, Iglesias PA. Malignant thymoma associated with myasthenia gravis and evidence of extrathoracic metastases. Cancer. 1971;27:823–30.

18. Tandan R, Taylor R, DiCostanzo DP, Sharma K, Fries T, Roberts J. Metastasizing thymoma and myasthenia gravis. Cancer. 1990;65:1286–90.
19. Patten SF, Dijkstra JWE. Associations of pemphigus and autoimmune disease with malignancy or thymoma. Int J Dermatol. 1994;33:836–42.
20. Miura K, Sasaki C, Katsushima I, Ohtomo T, Sat S, Demura H, et al. Pituitary-adrenocortical studies in a patient with Cushing's syndrome induced by thymoma. J Clin Endocrinol. 1967;27:631–7.
21. Korn D, Gelderman A, Cage G, Nathanson D, Strauss AJ. Immune deficiencies aplastic anemia and abnormalities of lymphoid tissue in thymoma. NEJM. 1967;276:1333–9.
22. Anderson ET, Vye MV. Dysproteinemia of the myeloma type associated with a thymoma. Ann Intern Med. 1967;66:141–9.
23. Gilbert EF, Harley JB, Anido V, Mengoli HF, Hughes JT. Thymoma, plasma cell myeloma, red cell aplasia and malabsorption syndrome. Am J Med. 1968;44:820–9.
24. Friedman HD, Inman DA, Hutchinson RE, Poiesz BJ. Concurrent invasive thymoma and T-cell lymphoblastic leukemia and lymphoma: a case report with necropsy findings and literature review of thymoma and associated hematologic neoplasm. Am J Clin Pathol. 1994;101:432–7.
25. Lishner M, Ravid M, Shapira J, Radnay J, Amiel A, Leytin V, et al. Deta-T-lymphocytosis in a patient with thymoma. Cancer. 1994;74:2924–9.
26. Skinnider LF, Alexander S, Horsman D. Concurrent thymoma and lymphoma: a report of two cases. Hum Pathol. 1982;13:163–6.
27. Tormoehlen LM, Pascuzzi RM. Thymoma, myasthenia gravis, and other paraneoplastic syndromes. Hematol Oncol Clin North Am. 2008;22:509–26.
28. Okuma Y, Hosomi Y, Watanabe K, Yamada Y, Horio H, Maeda Y, et al. Clinicopathological analysis of thymic malignancies with a consistent retrospective database in a single institution: from Tokyo metropolitan cancer center. BMC Cancer. 2014;14:349–57.
29. Weissferdt A, Kalhor N, Bishop J, Jang SJ, Ro J, Petersson F, et al. Thymoma: a clinicopathological correlation of 1470 cases. Hum Pathol. 2018;73:7–15.
30. Reid H, Marcus R. Thymoma with a report of 5 cases. Br J Surg. 1937;xxxvi(143):271–9.
31. Andrus W, Foot NC. Report of a large thymic tumor successfully removed by an operation. J Thorac Surg. 1937;6:648.
32. Wilson FN, Pritchard JE. Malignant thymoma. Can Med Assoc J. 1945;53:444–54.
33. Symmers D. Malignant tumors and tumor-like growths of the thymic region. Ann Surg. 1932;95:544–72.
34. Ewing J. Neoplastic diseases: a treatise of tumors. 4th ed. Philadelphia: Saunders; 1940. p. 1160.
35. Hellwig CA. Malignant thymoma: clinical-pathological study of eight cases. Surg Gynecol Obstet. 1941;73:851–63.
36. Lowenhaupt E. Tumors of the thymus in relation to thymic epithelial anlage. Cancer. 1948;1:547–62.
37. Seybold WD, McDonald JR, Clagett OT, Good CA. Tumors of the thymus. J Thorac Surg. 1950;20:195–214.
38. Effler DB, McCormack LJ. Thymic neoplasms. J Thorac Surg. 1956;31:60–77.
39. Thomson AD, Thackray AC. The histology of tumours of the thymus. Br J Cancer. 1957;11:348–57.
40. Lattes R, Jonas S. The pathological and clinical features in eighty cases of thymoma. Bull N Y Acad Med. 1957;33:145–7.
41. Andritsakis GD, Sommers SC. Criteria for thymic cancer and clinical correlations of thymic tumors. J Thorac Surg. 1959;37:273–90.
42. Bernatz PE, Harrison EG, Clagett OT. Thymoma: a clinicopathologic study. J Thorac Cardiovasc Surg. 1961;42:424–44.
43. Lattes R. Thymoma and other tumors of the thymus. Cancer. 1962;15:1224–60.
44. Mottet NK. Malignant thymoma. Am J Clin Pathol. 1964;41:61–71.
45. Rachmaninoff N, Fentress V. Thymoma with metastasis to the brain. Am J Clin Pathol. 1964;41:618–25.
46. Minkowitz S, Solomon L, Nicastri AD. Cytologically malignant thymoma with distant metastasis. Cancer. 1968;21:426–33.
47. Rosen VJ, Christiannen TW, Hughes RK. Metastatic thymoma presenting as solitary pulmonary nodule. Cancer. 1966;19:527–32.
48. Gravanis M. Metastasizing thymoma. Am J Clin Pathol. 1968;49: 690–6.
49. Fechner RE. Recurrence of noninvasive thymomas: report of four cases and review of the literature. Cancer. 1969;23:1423–9.
50. Toker C. Thymoma. An ultrastructural study. Cancer. 1968;21: 1157–63.
51. Levine GD, Bensch KG. Epithelial nature of spindle cell thymoma: an ultrastructural study. Cancer. 1972;30:500–11.
52. Bernatz PE, Khonsari S, Harrison EG, Taylor WF. Thymoma: factors influencing prognosis. Surg Clin N Am. 1973;53:885–92.
53. Jain U, Frable WJ. Thymoma: analysis of benign and malignant criteria. J Thorac Cardiovasc Surg. 1974;67:310–21.
54. Salyer WR, Eggleston JC. Thymoma: a clinical and pathological study of 65 cases. Cancer. 1976;37:229–49.
55. LeGolvan D, Abell MR. Thymomas. Cancer. 1977;39:2142–57.
56. Bergh NP, Gatzinsky P, Larsson S, Lundin P, Ridell B. Tumors of the thymus and thymic region: I. Clinicopathological studies on thymomas. Ann Thorac Surg. 1978;25:91–8.
57. Wilkins EW, Castleman B. Thymoma: a continuing survey at the Massachusetts General Hospital. Ann Thorac Surg. 1979;28: 252–6.
58. Pascoe HR, Miner MS. An ultrastructural study of nine thymomas. Cancer. 1976;37:317–26.
59. Cossman J, Deegan MJ, Schnitzer B. Thymoma: an immunologic and electron microscopic study. Cancer. 1978;41(6):2183–91.
60. Shellito J, Khandekar JD, McKeever WP, Vick NA. Invasive thymoma responsive to oral corticosteroids. Cancer Treat Rep. 1978;62:1397–400.
61. Boston B. Chemotherapy of invasive thymoma. Cancer. 1976;38:49–52.
62. Masaoka A, Monden Y, Nakahara K, Tanioka T. Follow-up study of thymoma with special reference to their clinical stages. Cancer. 1981;48:2485–92.
63. Verley JM, Hollmann KH. Thymoma: a comparative study of clinical stages, histological features, and survival in 200 cases. Cancer. 1985;55:1074–6.
64. Marino M, Muller-Hermelink HK. Thymoma and thymic carcinoma: relation of thymoma epithelial cells to the cortical and medullary differentiation of thymus. Virchows Arch A Pathol Anat Histopathol. 1985;407:119–49.
65. Kirchner T, Schalke B, Buchwald J, Ritter M, Marx A, Müller-Hermelink HK. Well-differentiated carcinoma. An organotypical low-grade carcinoma with relationship to cortical thymoma. Am J Surg Pathol. 1992;16:1153–69.
66. Muller-Hermelink HK, Marino M, Palestro G, Schumacher U, Kirchner T. Immunohistological evidences of cortical and medullary differentiation in thymoma. Virchows Arch A Pathol Anat Histopathol. 1985;408:143–61.
67. Kirchner T, Schalke B, Marx A, Muller-Hermelink HK. Evaluation of prognostic features in thymic epithelial tumors. Thymus. 1989;14:195–203.
68. Kirchner T, Muller-Hermelink HK. New approaches to the diagnosis of thymic epithelial tumors. Prog Surg Pathol. 1989;10: 167–89.
69. Giraud F, Fabien N, Auger C, Girod C, Loire R, Monier JC. Human epithelial thymic tumours: heterogeneity in immunostaining of epithelial cell markers and thymic hormones. Thymus. 1990;15:15–29.
70. Dawson A, Ibrahim NBN, Gibbs AR. Observer variation in the histopathological classification of thymoma: correlation with prognosis. J Clin Pathol. 1994;47:519–23.

71. Pan CC, Wu HP, Yang CF, Chen WY, Chiang H. The clinicopathological correlation of epithelial subtyping in thymoma: a study of 112 consecutive cases. Hum Pathol. 1994;25:893–9.
72. Kornstein MJ, Curran WJ, Turrisi AT, Brooks JJ. Cortical versus medullary thymomas: a useful morphologic distinction? Hum Pathol. 1988;19:1335–9.
73. Pescarmona E, Rosati S, Pisacane A, Rendina EA, Venuta F, Baroni CD. Microscopic thymoma: histological evidence of multifocal cortical and medullary origin. Histopathology. 1992;20:263–6.
74. Pescarmona E, Rendina EA, Venuta F, Ricci C, Ruco LP, Baroni CD. The prognostic implications of thymoma histologic subtyping. A study of 80 consecutive cases. Am J Clin Pathol. 1990;93:190–5.
75. Ricci C, Rendina E, Pescarmona E, Baroni CD. Correlations between histological type, clinical behavior, and prognosis in thymoma. Thorax. 1989;44:455–60.
76. Ho FCS, Fu KH, Lam SY, Chiu SW, Chan AC, Müller-Hermelink HK. Evaluation of a histogenetic classification for thymic epithelial tumours. Histopathology. 1994;25:21–9.
77. Tan PH, Sng ITY. Thymoma – a study of 60 cases in Singapore. Histopathology. 1995;26:509–18.
78. Close PM, Kirchner T, Uys CJ, Muller-Hermelink HK. Reproducibility of a histogenetic classification of thymic epithelial tumours. Histopathology. 1995;26:339–43.
79. Kuo TT, Lo SK. Thymoma: a study of the pathologic classification of 71 cases with evaluation of the Muller-Hermelink system. Hum Pathol. 1993;24:766–71.
80. Quintanilla L, Wilkins EW, Ferry JA, Harris NL. Thymoma – morphologic subclassification correlates with invasiveness and immunohistologic features: a study of 122 cases. Hum Pathol. 1993;24:958–69.
81. Quintanilla L, Wilkins EW, Choi N, Efrid J, Hug E. Thymoma: histologic subclassification is an independent prognostic factor. Cancer. 1994;74:606–17.
82. Hofmann W, Moller P, Manke HG, Otto HF. Thymoma: a clinicopathologic study of 98 cases with special reference to three unusual cases. Pathol Res Pract. 1985;179:337–53.
83. Maggi G, Giaccone G, Donadio M, Ciuffreda L, Dalesio O, Leria G, et al. Thymomas: a review of 169 cases, with particular reference to results of surgical treatment. Cancer. 1986;58: 765–76.
84. Lewis JE, Wick MR, Scheithauer BW, Bernatz PE, Taylor WF. Thymoma: a clinicopathologic review. Cancer. 1987;60:2727–43.
85. Pich A, Chiarle R, Chiusa L, Ponti R, Geuna M, Casadio C, et al. Long-term survival of thymoma patients by histologic pattern and proliferative activity. Am J Surg Pathol. 1995;19:918–26.
86. Nakahara Y, Ohno K, Hashimoto J, Maeda H, Miyoshi S, Sakurai M, et al. Thymoma: results with complete resection and adjuvant postoperative irradiation in 141 consecutive patients. J Thorac Cardiovasc Surg. 1988;95:1041–7.
87. Wick MR, Nichols WC, Ingle JN, Bruckman JE, Okazaki H. Malignant, predominantly lymphocytic thymoma with central and peripheral nervous system metastases. Cancer. 1981;47: 2036–43.
88. Needles B, Kemey N, Urmacher C. Malignant thymoma: renal metastases responding to cis-platinum. Cancer. 1981;48:223–6.
89. Elert O, Buchwald J, Wolf K. Epithelial thymus tumors – therapy and prognosis. Thorac Cardiovasc Surg. 1988;36(2):109–13.
90. Chahinian AP, Bhardwaj S, Meyer R, Jaffrey IS, Kirschner PA, Holland JF. Treatment of invasive or metastatic thymoma: report of eleven cases. Cancer. 1981;47:1752–61.
91. Cocconi G, Boni C, Cuomo A. Long-lasting response to cis-platinum in recurrent malignant thymoma. Case Rep Cancer. 1982;49:1985–7.
92. Kosmidis PA, Iliopoulos E, Pentea S. Combination chemotherapy with cyclophosphamide, Adriamycin, and vincristine in malignant thymoma and myasthenia gravis. Cancer. 1988;61:1736–40.
93. Campbell MG, Pollard R, Al-Sarraf M. Complete response in metastatic malignant thymoma to cis-platinum, doxorubicin, and cyclophosphamide: a case report. Cancer. 1981;48:1315–7.
94. Curran WJ, Kornstein MJ, Brooks JJ, Turrisi AT. Invasive thymoma: the role of mediastinal irradiation following complete or incomplete surgical resection. J Clin Oncol. 1988;6:1722–7.
95. Goldel N, Boning L, Fredrik A, Hölzel D, Hartenstein R, Wilmanns W. Chemotherapy of invasive thymoma: a retrospective study of 22 cases. Cancer. 1989;63:1493–500.
96. Park HS, Shin DM, Lee JS, Komaki R, Pollack A, Putnam JB, et al. Thymoma: a retrospective study of 87 cases. Cancer. 1994;73:2491–8.
97. Wang LS, Huang MH, Lin TS, Huang BS, Chien KY. Malignant thymoma. Cancer. 1992;70:443–50.
98. Monden Y, Tanioka T, Maeda M, Masaoka A, Nakahara K, Kawashima Y, et al. Malignancy and differentiation of neoplastic epithelial cells of thymoma. J Surg Oncol. 1986;31:130–8.
99. Levine GC, Rosai J. Thymic hyperplasia and neoplasia: a review of current concepts. Hum Pathol. 1978;9:495–515.
100. Kuo TT. Cytokeratin profiles of the thymus and thymomas: histogenetic correlations and proposals for a histological classification of thymomas. Histopathology. 2000;36(5):403–14.
101. Moran CA, Suster S. Current status of the histologic classification of thymoma. Int J Surg Pathol. 1995;3:67–72.
102. World Health Organization International Histological Classification of Tumours. Histological typing of tumours of the Thymus. Rosa J. in collaboration with L.H. Sobin and Pathologists in 8 countries. 2nd ed. Berlin Heidelberg: Springer-Verlag; 1999.
103. Suster S, Moran CA. Thymoma, atypical thymoma, and thymic carcinoma: a novel conceptual approach to the classification of thymic epithelial neoplasms. Am J Clin Pathol. 1999;111:826–33.
104. Harris NL, Muller-Hermelink HK. Thymoma classification: a Siren's song of simplicity. Am J Clin Pathol. 1999;112:229–303.
105. Moran CA, Weissferdt A, Kalhor N, Solis LM, Behrens C, Wistuba II, et al. Thymoma I: a clinicopathologic correlation of 250 cases with emphasis on the World Health Organization Schema. Am J Clin Pathol. 2012;137:444–50.
106. Moran CA, Kalhor N, Suster S. Invasive spindle cell thymomas (WHO type A): a clinicopathologic correlation of 41 cases. Am J Clin Pathol. 2010;134:793–8.
107. Kornstein MJ. Thymoma classification: my opinion. Am J Clin Pathol. 1999;112:304–7.
108. Suster S, Moran CA. Thymoma classification: the ride of the Valkyries. Am J Clin Pathol. 1999;112:308–10.
109. Moran CA, Suster S. On the histologic heterogeneity of thymic epithelial neoplasms. Am J Clin Pathol. 2000;114:760–6.
110. Chen G, Marx A, Wen-Hu C, Yong J, Puppe B, Stroebel P, et al. New WHO histologic classification predicts prognosis of thymic epithelial tumors. Cancer. 2002;95:420–9.
111. Nakagawa K, Asamura H, Matsuno Y, Suzuki K, Kondo H, Maeshima A, et al. Thymoma: a clinicopathologic study on the new world health organization classification. J Thorac Cardiovasc Surg. 2003;126:1134–40.
112. Okamura M, Ohta M, Tateyama H, Nakagawa K, Matsumura A, Maeda H, et al. The World Health Organization histologic classification system reflects the oncologic behavior of thymoma. Cancer. 2002;94:624–32.
113. World health Organization Classification of Tumours. In: Travis WD, Brambilla E, Muller-Hermelink HK, Curtis CC, editors. Pathology & genetics – tumorus of the lung, pleura, thymus, and heart. Lyon: IARC Press; 2004.
114. Chalabreysse L, Roy P, Cordier JF, Loire R, Gamondes JP, Thivolet-Bejui F. Correlation of the WHO schema for the classification of thymic epithelial neoplasms with prognosis. A retrospective study of 90 tumors. Am J Surg Pathol. 2002;26:1605–11.

115. Rieker RJ, Hoegel J, Morresei-Hauf A, Hofmann WJ, Blaeker H, Penzel R, et al. Histologic classification of thymic epithelial tumors: comparison of established classifications schemes. Int J Cancer. 2002;98:900–6.
116. Kim DJ, Yang WI, Choi SS, Kim KD, Chung KY. Prognostic and clinical relevance of the world health organization schema for the classification of thymic epithelial tumors. A clinicopathologic study of 108 patients and literature review. Chest. 2005;127:755–61.
117. Kim HK, Choi YS, Kim J, Shim YM, Han J, Kim K. Type B thymoma: is prognosis predicted only by world health organization classification? J Thorac Cardiovasc Surg. 2010;139:1431–15.
118. Rena O, Papalia E, Maggi G, Oliaro A, Ruffini E, Filosso P, et al. World Health Organization histologic classification: an independent prognostic factor in resected thymomas. Lung Cancer. 2005;50:59–66.
119. Su XY, Wu WL, Liu N, Zhang S-F, G-D L. Thymic epithelial tumors: a clinicopathologic study of 249 cases from a single institution. Int J Clin Exp Pathol. 2014;7:7760–7.
120. Moran CA, Walsh G, Suster S, Kaiser L. Thymoma II: a clinicopathologic correlation of 250 cases with a proposed staging system with emphasis on pathologic assessment. Am J Clin Pathol. 2012;137:451–61.
121. Zucalli PA, Di Tommaso L, Petrini I, Battista S, Lee HS, Merino M, et al. Reproducibility of the WHO classification of thymomas: practical implications. Lung Cancer. 2013;79:236–41.
122. Guerra F, Rendina EA, Venuta F, Margaritora S, Ciccone AM, Novellis P, et al. Does the world health organization histological classification predict outcomes after thymomectomy? Results of a multicenter study on 750 patients. Eur J Cardiothorac Surg. 2015;48:48–54.
123. Marx A, Strobel P, Badve S, Chalabreysse L, Chan JK, Chen G, et al. ITMIG consensus statement on the use of the WHO histological classification of thymoma and thymic carcinoma: redefined definitions, histological criteria, and reporting. J Thorac Oncol. 2014;9:596–611.
124. Ströbel P, Kurrer MO, Marx A, Marchevsky AM, Badve S, Marom EM, Travis W, Brambilla E, Burke A, Nicholson A. Tumours of the thymus. In: Travis WD, Brambilla E, Burke AP, Marx A, Nicholson AG, editors. WHO classification of tumours of the lung, pleura, thymus, and heart. Lyon: IARC; 2015.
125. SRY C, Suster S. Primary thymic epithelial neoplasms in children. Am J Surg Pathol. 1991;15:466–74.
126. Pescarmona E, Giardini R, Brisigotti M, Callea F, Pisacane A, Baroni CD. Thymoma in childhood: a clinicopathological study of five cases. Histopathology. 1992;21:65–8.
127. Gamondes JP, Balawi A, Greenland T, Adleine P, Mornex JF, Zhang J, et al. Seventeen years of surgical treatment of thymoma: factor influencing survival. Eur J Cardiothorac Surg. 1991;5:124–31.
128. Macchiarini P, Chella A, Ducci F, Rossi B, Testi C, Bevilacqua G, et al. Neoadjuvant chemotherapy, surgery, and postoperative radiation therapy for invasive thymoma. Cancer. 1991;68:706–13.
129. Fornaseiro A, Daniele O, Ghiotto C, Sartori F, Rea F, Piazza M, et al. Chemotherapy of invasive thymoma. J Clin Oncol. 1990;8:1419–23.
130. Loehrer PJ, Kim KM, Aisner SC, Livingston R, Einhorn LH, Johnson D, et al. Cisplatin plus doxorubicin plus cyclophosphamide in metastatic or recurrent thymoma: final results of an intergroup trial. J Clin Oncol. 1994;12:1164–8.
131. Yokoi K, Matsuguma H, Nakahara R, Kondo T, Kamiyama Y, Mori K, et al. Multidisciplinary treatment for advanced invasive thymoma with cisplatin, doxorubicin, and methylprednisolone. J Thorac Oncol. 2007;2:73–8.
132. Kim ES, Putnam JB, Komaki R, Walsh GL, Ro JY, Shin HJ, et al. Phase II study of a multidisciplinary approach with induction chemotherapy, followed by surgical resection, radiation therapy, and consolidation chemotherapy for unresectable malignant thymoma: final report. Lung Cancer. 2004;44:369–79.
133. Kunitoh H, Tamura T, Shibata T, Takeda K, Katakami N, Nakagawa K, et al. A phase II trial of dose-dense chemotherapy, followed by surgical resection and/or thoracic radiotherapy, in locally advanced thymoma: report of a Japan clinical oncology group trial (JCOG 9606). Br J Cancer. 2010;103:6–11.
134. Kondo K. Therapy for thymic epithelial tumors. Gen Thorac Cardiovasc Surg. 2014;62:468–74.
135. Weissferdt A, Moran CA. The impact of neoadjuvant chemotherapy on the histopathological assessment of thymomas: a clinicopathological correlation of 28 cases treated with a similar regimen. Lung. 2013;191:379–83.
136. Marchevsky A, Marx A, Strobel P, Suster S, Venuta F, Marino M, et al. Policies and reporting guidelines for small biopsy specimens of mediastinal masses. J Thorac Oncol. 2011;6:S1724–9.
137. Weissferdt A, Moran CA. The histomorphologic spectrum of spindle cell thymoma. Hum Pathol. 2014;45:437–45.
138. Pan CC, Chen WYK, Chiang H. Spindle cell and mixed spindle/lymphocytic thymomas: an integrated clinicopathologic and immunohistochemical study of 81 cases. Am J Surg Pathol. 2001;25:111–20.
139. Kirchner T, Schalke B, Buchwald J, Ritter M, Marx A, Müller-Hermelink HK. Well-differentiated thymic carcinoma: an organotypical low-grade carcinoma with relationship to cortical thymoma. Am J Surg Pathol. 1992;16:1153–69.
140. Pescarmona E, Rosati S, Rendina EA, et al. Well-differentiated thymic carcinoma: a clinic-pathological study. Virchows Arch A. 1992;420:179–83.
141. Shimosato Y, Kameya T, Nagai K, Suemasu K. Squamous cell carcinoma of the thymus. Analysis of eight cases. Am J Surg Pathol. 1977;1:109–21.
142. Suster S, Moran CA. Primary thymic epithelial neoplasms: current concepts and controversies. In: Fechner RE, Rosen PP, editors. Anatomic pathology. Chicago: ASCP Press; 1997. p. 1–19. ASCP Reviews in Pathology.
143. Baran JL, Magro CM, King M, Williams TE Jr, Ross P Jr. Atypical thymoma: a report of seven patients. Ann Thorac Surg. 2004;78:411–6.
144. Nonaka D, Rosai J. Is there a spectrum of cytologic atypia in type A thymomas analogous to that seen in type B thymomas? A pilot study of 13 cases. Am J Surg Pathol. 2012;36(6):889–94.
145. Dyer NH. Cystic thymoma and thymic cysts. Thorax. 1967;22:408–21.
146. Suster S, Rosai J. Cystic thymomas: a clinicopathologic study of ten cases. Cancer. 1992;69:92–7.
147. Rieker RJ, Aulmann S, Schnabel P, Sack FU, Otto HF, Mechtersheimer G, et al. Cystic thymoma. Pathol Oncol Res. 2005;11:57–60.
148. Honda S, Morikawa T, Sasaki F, Okada T, Naito S, Itoh T, et al. Cystic thymoma in a child: a rare case and review of the literature. Pediatr Surg Int. 2007;23:1015–7.
149. Hayward AR. Myoid cells in the human foetal thymus. J Pathol. 1972;106:45–8.
150. Van de Velde RL, Friedman NB. Thymic myoid cells and myasthenia gravis. Am J Pathol. 1970;59:347–67.
151. Van de Velde RL, Friedman NB. The thymic "myoidzellen" and myasthenia gravis. JAMA. 1966;198:197–8.
152. Henry K. Mucin secretion and striated muscle in the human thymus. Lancet. 1966;1:183–5.
153. Henry K. An unusual thymic tumor with striated muscle (myoid) component. Br J Dis Chest. 1972;66:291–9.
154. Murakami S, Shamoto M, Miura K, Takeuchi J. A thymic tumor with massive proliferation of myoid cells. Acta Pathol Jpn. 1984;34:1375–83.

155. Moran CA, Koss MN. Rhabdomyomatous thymoma. Am J Surg Pathol. 1993;17:633–6.
156. Goldstein G. Thymic plasma cells. JAMA. 1967;6:220.
157. Moran CA, Suster S, Koss MN. Plasma cell-rich thymoma. Am J Clin Pathol. 1994;102:199–201.
158. Suster S, Moran CA, Chan KC. Thymoma with pseudosarcomatous stroma: report of an unusual histologic variant of thymic epithelial neoplasm that may simulate carcinosarcoma. Am J Surg Pathol. 1997;21:1316–23.
159. Yoneda S, Marx A, Heimann S, Shirakusa T, Kikuchi M, Müller-Hermelink HK. Low-grade metaplastic carcinoma of the thymus. Histopathology. 1999;35:19–30.
160. Yoneda S, Marx A, Muller-Hermelink HK. Low-grade metaplastic carcinomas of the thymus: biphasic thymic epithelial tumors with mesenchymal metaplasia – an update. Pathol Res Pract. 1999;195:555–63.
161. Noh TW, Kim SH, Lim BJ, Yang WI, Chung KY. Thymoma with pseudosarcomatous stroma. Yonsei Med J. 2001;42:571–5.
162. Liu B, Rao Q, Zhu Y, Yu B, Zhu HY, Zhou XJ. Metaplastic thymoma of the mediastinum: a clinicopathologic, immunohistochemical, and genetic analysis. Am J Clin Pathol. 2012;137:261–9.
163. Poorabdollah M, Mehdizadeh E, Mohammadi F, Sabeti S. Metaplastic thymoma: report of an unusual thymic epithelial neoplasm arising in the wall of a thymic cyst. Int J Surg Pathol. 2009;17:51–4.
164. Suster S, Moran CA. Micronodular thymoma with lymphoid B-cell hyperplasia: clinicopathologic and immunohistochemical study of eighteen cases of a distinctive morphologic variant of thymic epithelial neoplasm. Am J Surg Pathol. 1999;23:955–62.
165. Tateyama H, Saito Y, Fujii Y, Okumura M, Nakamura K, Tada H, et al. The spectrum of micronodular thymic epithelial tumours with lymphoid B-cell hyperplasia. Histopathology. 2001;38:519–27.
166. Strobel P, Marino M, Feuchtenberger M, Rouzière AS, Tony HP, Wulbrand U, et al. Micronodular thymoma: an epithelial tumour with abnormal chemokine expression setting the stage for lymphoma development. J Pathol. 2005;207:72–82.
167. Mezni F, Braham E, Ayadi A, Ismail O, Kilani T. Micronodular thymoma with lymphoid stroma: report of two cases and particular association with thymic lymphoid hyperplasia in one case. Pathology. 2006;38:586–8.
168. Moran CA, Suster S. Thymoma with prominent cystic and hemorrhagic changes and areas of necrosis and infarction: a clinicopathologic study of 25 cases. Am J Surg Pathol. 2001;25:1086–90.
169. Kuo T. Sclerosing thymoma – a possible phenomenon of regression. Histopathology. 1994;25:289–91.
170. Moran CA, Suster S. "Ancient" (sclerosing) thymoma: a clinicopathologic study of 10 cases. Am J Clin Pathol. 2004;121:867–71.
171. Weissferdt A, Kalhor N, Suster S, Moran CA. Adenomatoid spindle cell thymomas: a clinicopathological and immunohistochemical study of 20 cases. Am J Surg Pathol. 2010;34:15644–1549.
172. Kalhor N, Suster S, Moran CA. Spindle cell thymoma (WHO type A) with prominent papillary and pseudopapillary features: a clinicopathologic and immunohistochemical study of 10 cases. Am J Surg Pathol. 2011;35:372–7.
173. Adam P, Hakroush S, Hofman I, Reidenbach S, Marx A, Ströbel P. Thymoma with loss of keratin expression (and giant cells): a potential diagnostic pitfall. Virchows Arch. 2014;465:313–20.
174. Fukuda T, Ohnishi Y, Emura I, Tachikawa S. Microcystic variant of thymoma: histological and immunohistochemical findings in two cases. Virchows Arch. 1992;420:185–9.
175. Weissferdt A, Moran CA. Desmoplastic spindle cell thymomas: a clinicopathologic and immunohistochemical study of 14 cases. Hum Pathol. 2013;44:623–7.
176. Weissferdt A, Moran CA. Thymomas with prominent glandular differentiation: a clinicopathologic and immunohistochemical study of 12 cases. Hum Pathol. 2013;44:1612–6.
177. Weissferdt A, Moran CA. Thymomas with extensive clear cell component: a clinicopathologic and immunohistochemical study of nine cases. Am J Clin Pathol. 2016;146:132–6.
178. Weissferdt A, Moran CA. Spindle cell thymomas with neuroendocrine morphology: a clinicopathological and immunohistochemical study of 18 cases. Histopathology. 2014;65:111–8.
179. Weissferdt A, Moran CA. Thymomas with prominent signet ring cell-like features: a clinicopathological and immunohistochemical study of 10 cases. Hum Pathol. 2012;43:1881–6.
180. Suster S, Moran CA. Primary thymic epithelial neoplasms showing combined features of thymoma and thymic carcinoma. Am J Surg Pathol. 1996;20:1469–80.
181. Weissferdt A, Kalhor N, Moran CA. Combined thymoma-thymic seminoma: report of two cases of a heretofore unreported association. Hum Pathol. 2014;45:2168–72.
182. Muller-Hermelink HK, Marino M, Palestro G, Palestro G, Schumacher U, Kirchner T. Immunohistochemical evidences of cortical and medullary differentiation in thymoma. Virchows Arch. 1985;408:143–61.
183. Chilosi M, Iannucci AM, Pizzolo G, Menestrina F, Fiore-Donati L, Janossy G. Immunohistochemical analysis of thymoma. Am J Surg Pathol. 1984;8:309–3318.
184. Van der Kwast TH, van Vliet E, Cristen E, Cristen E, van Ewijk W, van der Heul RO. An immunohistologic study of the epithelial and lymphoid components of six thymomas. Hum Pathol. 1985;16:1001–8.
185. Eimoto T, Teshima K, Shirakusa T, Takeshita M, Okamura H, Naito H, et al. Heterogeneity of epithelial cell and reactive components in thymomas: an ultrastructural and immunohistochemical study. Ultrastruct Pathol. 1986;10:157–73.
186. Sasto Y, Watanabe S, Mukai K, Kodama T, Upton MP, Goto M, et al. An immunohistochemical study of thymic epithelial tumors. Am J Surg Pathol. 1986;10:862–70.
187. Ring NP, Addis BJ. Thymoma: an integrated clinicopathological and immunohistochemical study. J Pathol. 1986;149:327–37.
188. Kodama T, Watanabe S, Sato Y, Shimosato Y, Miyazawa N. An immunohistochemical study of thymic epithelial tumors. I. Epithelial component. Am J Surg Pathol. 1986;10:26–33.
189. Lee D, Wright DH. Immunohistochemical study of 22 cases of thymoma. J Clin Pathol. 1988;41:1297–304.
190. Ruco LP, Rosati S, Monardo F, Pescarmona E, Rendina EA, Baroni CD. Macrophages and interdigitating reticulum cells in normal thymus and in thymoma: and immunohistochemical study. Histopathology. 1989;14:37–45.
191. Mizuno T, Hashimoto T, Masaoka A. Distribution of fibronectin and laminin in human thymoma. Cancer. 1990;65:1367–74.
192. Fukai I, Masaoka A, Hashimoto YY, Mizuno T, Tanamura O. The distribution of epithelial membrane antigen in thymic epithelial tumors. Cancer. 1992;70:2077–81.
193. Fukai I, Masaoka A, Hashimoto YY, Mizuno T, Tanamura O, et al. An immunohistologic study of the epithelial components of 81 cases of thymoma. Cancer. 1992;69:2463–8.
194. Fukai I, Masaoka A, Hashimoto YY, Mizuno T, Tanamura O. Cytokeratin in normal thymus and thymic epithelial tumors. Cancer. 1993;71:99–105.
195. Pescarmona E, Pisacane A, Pignatelli E, Baroni CD. Expression of epidermal and nerve growth factor receptors in human thymus and thymomas. Histopathology. 1993;23:39–44.
196. Wu TC, Kuo TT. Study of Epstein-Barr virus early RNA1 (EBER1) expression by in situ hybridization in thymic epithelial tumors of Chinese patients in Taiwan. Hum Pathol. 1993;24:235–8.
197. Chang JKC, Tsang WYW, Seneviratne S, Pau MY. The MIC2 antibody O13: practical applications for the study of thymic epithelial tumors. Am J Surg Pathol. 1995;19:1115–23.

198. Dorfman DM, Pinkus GS. CD99 (p30/32 –MIC2) immunoreactivity in the diagnosis of thymic neoplasms and mediastinal lymphoproliferative disorders. A study of paraffin sections using monoclonal antibody O13. Am J Surg Pathol. 1996;4:34–42.
199. Stefanaki K, Rontogianni D, Kouvidou CH, Bolioti S, Delides G, Pantelidaki A, et al. Expression of p53, mdm2, p21/waf1, and bcl-2 proteins in thymomas. Histopathology. 1997;30:549–55.
200. Yang W, Efird JT, Quintanilla-Martinez L, Choi N, Harris NL. Cell kinetics study of thymic epithelial tumors using PCNA (PC10) and Ki-67 (MIB-1) antibodies. Hum Pathol. 1996;27:70–6.
201. Hishima T, Fukuyama M, Hayashi Y, Fujii T, Arai K, Shiozawa Y, et al. Neuroendocrine differentiation in thymic epithelial tumors with special reference to thymic carcinoma and atypical thymoma. Hum Pathol. 1998;29:330–8.
202. Kornstein MJ, Kay S. B cells in thymomas. Mod Pathol. 1990;3:61–3.
203. Taubenberger JK, Jaffe ES, Medeiros LJ. Thymoma with abundant L26-positive "asteroid" cells. Arch Pathol Lab Med. 1991;115:1254–7.
204. Medeiros LJ, Bhagat SKM, Naylor P, Fowler D, Jaffe ES, Stetler-Stevenson M. Malignant thymoma associated with T-cell lymphocytosis. Arch Pathol Lab Med. 1993;117:279–83.
205. Sonobe S, Miyamoto H, Nobukawa B, Izumi H, Futagawa T, Ishikawa N, et al. Prognostic value of CD44 isoform expression in thymic epithelial neoplasms. Cancer. 2005;103:2015–22.
206. Alexiev BA, Drachenberg CB, Burke A. Thymomas: a cytological and immunohistochemical study, with emphasis on lymphoid and neuroendocrine markers. Diagn Pathol. 2007;2:13–23.
207. Nonaka D, Henley JD, Chiriboga L, Yee H. Diagnostic utility of thymic epithelial markers CD205 (DEC205) and Foxn1 in thymic epithelial neoplasms. Am J Surg Pathol. 2007;31:1038–44.
208. Dotto J, Pelosi G, Rosai J. Expression of p63 in thymomas and normal thymus. Am J Clin Pathol. 2007;127:415–20.
209. Wu M, Sun K, Gil J, Gan L, Burstein DE. Immunohistochemical detection of p63 and XIAP in thymic hyperplasia and thymomas. Am J Clin Pathol. 2009;131:689–93.
210. Kaira K, Murakami H, Serizawa M, Koh Y, Abe M, Ohde Y, et al. MUC1 expression in thymic epithelial tumors: MUC1 may be useful marker as differential diagnosis between type B3 thymoma and thymic carcinoma. Virchows Arch. 2011;458:615–20.
211. Cimpean A, Encica S, Raica M, Ribatti D. SOX2 gene expression in normal human thymus and thymoma. Clin Exp Med. 2011;11:251–4.
212. Weissferdt A, Hernandez JC, Kalhor N, Moran CA. Spindle cell thymomas: an immunohistochemical sturdy of 30 cases. Appl Immunohistochem Mol Morphol. 2011;19:329–35.
213. Weissferdt A, Fujimoto J, Kalhor N, Rodriguez J, Bassett R, Wistuba II, et al. Expression of PD-1 and PD-L1 in thymic epithelial neoplasms. Mod Pathol. 2017;30(6):826–33.
214. Chau NG, Kim ES, Wistuba I. The multidisciplinary approach to thymoma: combining molecular and clinical approaches. J Thorac Oncol. 2010;5:S313–7.
215. Hayashi Y, Ishii N, Obayashi C, Jinnai K, Hanioka K, Imai Y, et al. Thymoma: tumour type related to expression of epidermal growth factor (EGF), EGF-receptor, p53, v-erb B and ras p21. Virchows Arch. 1995;426:43–50.
216. Weirich G, Schneider P, Fellbaum C, Brauch H, Nathrath W, Scholz M, et al. p53 alterations in thymic epithelial tumours. Virchows Arch. 1997;431:17–23.
217. Pan CC, Chen PCH, Wang LS, Lee J-Y, Chiang H. Expression of apoptosis-related markers and HER-2/new in thymic epithelial tumours. Histopathology. 2003;43:165–72.
218. Chang KC, Wu MH, Jones D, Chen F-F, Tseng Y-L. Activation of STAT3 in thymic epithelial tumours correlates with tumour type and clinical behavior. J Pathol. 2006;210:224–33.
219. Suzuki E, Sasaki H, Kawano O, Endo K, Haneda H, Yukiue H, et al. Expression and mutation statuses of epidermal growth factor receptor in thymic epithelial tumors. Jpn J Clin Oncol. 2006;36:351–6.
220. Meister M, Schirmacher P, Dienemann H, Mechtersheimer G, Schnabel PA, Kern MA, et al. Mutational status of the epidermal growth factor receptor (EGFR) gene in thymomas and thymic carcinomas. Cancer Lett. 2007;248:186–91.
221. Yoh K, Nishiwaki Y, Ishii G, Goto K, Kubota K, Ohmatsu H, et al. Mutational status of EGFR and KIT in thymoma and thymic carcinoma. Lung Cancer. 2008;62:316–20.
222. Tsuchida M, Umezu H, Hashimoto T, Shinohara H, Koike T, Hosaka Y, et al. Absence of gene mutations in KIT-positive thymic epithelial tumors. Lung Cancer. 2008;62:321–5.
223. Girard N, Shen R, Guo T, Zakowski MF, Heguy A, Riely GJ, et al. Comprehensive genomic analysis reveals clinically relevant molecular distinctions between thymic carcinoma and thymoma. Clin Cancer Res. 2009;15:6790–9.
224. Aisner SC, Dahlberg S, Hameed MR, Ettinger DS, Schiller JH, Johnson DH, et al. Epidermal growth factor receptor, C-kit, and Her2/neu immunostaining in advanced or recurrent thymic epithelial neoplasms staged according to the 2004 World Health Organization in patients treated with octreotide and prednisone. An Eastern Cooperative Oncology Group Study. J Thorac Oncol. 2010;5:885–92.

Thymic Carcinoma

8

Introduction

In this chapter, we will discuss the entity known as thymic carcinoma; however, some thymic carcinomas are discussed under tumors of salivary gland origin (mucoepidermoid carcinoma, basaloid carcinoma, and others), while neuroendocrine carcinomas are presented in the chapter on neuroendocrine neoplasms. Therefore, this chapter will contain exclusively non-neuroendocrine and non-salivary gland origin neoplasms. In addition, this chapter will not include the so-called well-differentiated thymic carcinoma [1]. Such a tumor is the equivalent to atypical thymoma (WHO type B3), and it is discussed in the chapter on thymoma in this book. Also, the staging of thymic carcinoma and thymoma is presented in a separate chapter in this text.

The entity known as thymic carcinoma is a clinicopathological condition that until recently has generated more interest, essentially because of its separation from the more common thymic tumor: thymoma. Even though the tumor is likely to have existed long before it became recognized as a different tumor from thymoma, it is also known that thymic carcinoma in general is a rare thymic tumor. In the first series of fascicles of the Armed Forces Institute of Pathology (AFIP) [2] on the tumors of the thymus gland, the author of this important document stated "one should occasionally see a primary squamous cell carcinoma in the anterior mediastinum" and provided one illustration of such an occurrence. The tumor the author described was a well-circumscribed tumor in a patient without evidence of primary tumor elsewhere. In essence, such description and careful evaluation of the possible tumor elsewhere have constituted one of the most important definitions for the entity of thymic carcinoma. In 1975, the second series of fascicles from the AFIP [3] were presented; a few important aspects are worth highlighting: (1) the table of contents of the fascicle does not include any entry on the entity "thymic carcinoma"; (2) in the thymoma section, thymic carcinoma, among other terms, appears as a synonym of thymoma; (3) several of the illustrations are labeled as "malignant thymoma," and it is uncertain whether the authors meant *invasive thymoma* or *thymic carcinoma*; and (4) the illustration presented under the heading of squamous cell carcinoma is exactly the same one published in the earlier first series of fascicles of the AFIP. However, this second series does include thymic carcinoid as a separate entity (now considered a neuroendocrine carcinoma). Thus, based on those two highly important publications, one can gather that the entity known as thymic carcinoma had not been properly recognized and likely lumped in with other cases of thymoma. However, other anecdotal cases of thymic squamous cell carcinoma similar to the one described by Castleman [1] in the AFIP fascicle also were reported by Frank and colleagues [4] in a case with concurrent esophageal leiomyoma and by Watson and colleagues [5].

The first original description of a series of cases of squamous cell carcinomas of the thymus is credited to Shimosato and colleagues [6]. The authors described eight cases of thymic squamous cell carcinomas in seven men and one woman between the ages of 39 and 65 years with no associated paraneoplastic syndrome. Interestingly, in this initial report, one can argue that in six of the cases reported, the tumor extended to the lung, thus raising some concerns about the thymic origin. In one other case, the tumor extended to soft tissue and lymph nodes, while in only one case the tumor was limited to the thymus. Nevertheless, the authors concluded that squamous cell carcinomas of the thymus should be separated from ordinary thymoma and that squamous cell carcinoma involving both the thymus and the lungs should be carefully examined for the primary site.

Since this original description of primary thymic carcinoma, numerous original contributions have been reported, and numerous reviews on the subject have been advanced with different aims but with the goal of advancing the knowledge of thymic epithelial tumors. In 1982, Snover and colleagues [7] described a small series of thymic carcinoma with five different histological variants: mixed small cell undifferentiated/squamous cell carcinoma, basaloid carcinoma, mucoepidermoid carcinoma, clear cell carcinoma,

© Springer Nature Switzerland AG 2019

N. Kalhor, C. Moran, *Mediastinal Pathology*, https://doi.org/10.1007/978-3-319-98980-8_8

and sarcomatoid carcinoma. The authors stated that none of the reported patients had tumors elsewhere, which was used as criteria for inclusion as thymic carcinoma. In addition, the authors stated that "occasional thymomas are unequivocally malignant on cytologic grounds, and those are designated as 'thymic carcinoma.'" Interestingly, when the authors estimated the occurrence of these tumors in the mediastinum, a range of 7–33% is given for the generic term of "malignant thymomas." This report of five cases clearly illustrates the issue that thymic carcinomas are also heterogeneous tumors beyond squamous cell carcinomas. However, this description raises another concern, and that is "cytologic atypia," which oftentimes is difficult to define, and clearly not so well defined in terms of separating thymoma and thymic carcinoma, unless the case is straightforward. In 1998, Suster and Moran [8], in a review manuscript on the spectrum of differentiation and histologic types, stated that, in addition to the previously mentioned features by Snover and colleagues [6] regarding cytologic atypia, it is also important to add the presence of loss of organotypical features of thymic differentiation. Furthermore, the authors stated that there is nothing distinctive or pathognomonic about the histology of thymic carcinoma, making it difficult to determine whether a given tumor represents a primary thymic carcinoma or a metastasis from a different source. In addition, the authors emphasize the spectrum of differentiation that can be seen in these tumors that may range from well-differentiated to poorly differentiated to anaplastic malignancies with different growth patterns. The authors also commented on the overall survival rate of these tumors and stated it to be approximately 33% at 5 years. However, they also noted that the survival is related to the staging of the tumor at the time of diagnosis. In 2005, Suster [9] once again emphasized previously reported concepts on thymic carcinoma, and 10 years later, Moran and Suster [10] stated a similar definition about thymic carcinoma: (1) overt cytologic features of malignancy and (2) absence of organotypical features of differentiation of the thymus. However, the authors added that complete clinical and radiological studies are needed to demonstrate the absence of an occult tumor elsewhere, as there is nothing distinctive or pathognomonic about this histology of thymic carcinoma. The authors also stated that, up to 2008, approximately 200 cases of thymic carcinoma have been reported in the literature. One important fact that needs to be highlighted is that, in many reviews or original presentation of cases, the issue of the incidence of this tumor is rather obscured by the fact that most of those publications also include either invasive thymomas or neuroendocrine carcinomas. Ritter and Wick [11], in 1999 also in a review on primary thymic carcinomas, arrived at a similar conclusion in terms of the definition of the diagnosis. The authors agreed that such diagnosis requires detailed clinical and radiographic information and that the histopathology of these tumors is also varied. Suster and Moran [12], in a conceptual approach to the classification of thymic epithelial tumors, stated that the cytological atypia and the identification organotypical features of differentiation are important clues in separating thymoma from thymic carcinoma. The authors further stated the importance of clinical staging for these tumors. More recently, Weiss [13] reviewed the subject of thymic carcinoma and stated that thymoma and thymic carcinoma have a combined incidence of 0.2–1.5% of all tumors, which may account for 50% of all tumors of the anterior mediastinum. The authors further estimated that thymic carcinoma represents 1% of thymic malignancies, with an estimated incidence of 500 cases per year in the USA.

Based on the different publications on this subject, it is important to highlight that the diagnosis of thymic carcinoma must meet the following criteria:

1. Cytologic atypia
2. Loss of organotypical features
3. Clinical and radiological evidence of absence of tumor elsewhere

Regarding the etiology and pathogenesis of thymic carcinoma, there are two speculative hypotheses to account for their occurrence. The first is that the tumor is a separate entity from thymoma and the tumor arises de novo from cellular precursor either from thymic remnants or from misplaced epithelial elements in the mediastinum. The second hypothesis and the one that we believe more likely explains the occurrence of thymic carcinoma is that thymic carcinoma is part of a spectrum of thymic epithelial neoplasms, having in one end a better differentiated neoplasm with high degree of organotypical differentiation simulating the normal thymus (thymoma) and, at the other end, a tumor that has lost the organotypical features of differentiation and in addition shows cellular atypia (thymic carcinoma). This latter hypothesis is based on the occurrence of thymic epithelial tumors that showed in the same lesion a degree of differentiation that expands from classical thymoma to thymic carcinoma [14, 15]. (See diagrammatic illustrations in the chapter on thymoma.)

Clinical Features

The literature of thymic carcinoma compared to the literature on thymoma is rather limited due to the infrequency of the occurrence of thymic carcinoma. Due to those limitations, large series of thymic carcinomas have been reported, but there are only a few. The majority of reports on thymic carcinoma are small series of cases or isolated case reports.

Wick and colleagues [16], in a retrospective study of 75 years, collected 20 patients that the authors concluded represented thymic carcinomas. The patients were 14 men and 6 women between the ages of 4 and 72 years (average 47.6 years). Clinically, none of the patients reported had any associated condition such as myasthenia gravis (MG), Cushing's syndrome, hypogammaglobulinemia, or aregenerative anemia. The symptoms described for these patients were essentially non-specific and included cough, chest pain, fever, fatigue, night sweats, weight loss, anorexia, and superior vena cava syndrome. Two patients in this study were asymptomatic. In 13 patients, the tumor was totally or subtotally resected by thoracotomy; 18 patients received additional radiation therapy, and 8 patients received chemotherapy. Metastatic disease to the liver, lung, lymph nodes, adrenal glands, and bone was documented in 13 patients. Histologically, 13 tumors corresponded to poorly differentiated carcinomas (lymphoepithelioma-like), two tumors were labeled as spindle cell squamous cell carcinoma, one was labeled as "sarcomatoid" carcinoma, and four tumors were labeled as small cell carcinoma. Fifteen patients died of massive local tumor growth, metastases, or both. The overall average postoperative survival of patients who died of thymic carcinoma was 20 months. In addition, the authors documented two cases in which the patients were alive with recurrence or metastasis 18 and 43 months after surgery. Shimizu and associates [17] reported five thymic carcinomas in four men and one woman between the ages of 50 and 69 years who clinically presented with non-specific symptoms such as chest pain and cough. Interestingly, in three cases, the initial biopsy material was interpreted as thymoma and one as mesothelioma. Complete surgical resection was accomplished only in one patient. Histologically, four cases corresponded to squamous cell carcinomas and one case to small cell carcinoma. The five patients were also treated with radiation and chemotherapy, and metastatic disease to the liver, bone, lymph node, and lung was documented in three patients. Three patients died in a period of 7–38 months, while one was reported to be alive with disease at 9 months, and one additional patient was disease-free at 60 months. Truong and associates [18] also reported 13 cases of thymic carcinoma in 7 men and 6 women between the ages of 30 and 74 years (mean age, 54.2 years) who presented with non-specific symptoms related to mediastinal compression by the tumor. None of the patients described had any paraneoplastic syndrome. Eleven tumors were described as invading adjacent structures, while two tumors were described as "encapsulated." Histologically, seven tumors were labeled as lymphoepithelioma-like, four as small cell carcinomas, one as clear cell, and one additional case as "adenosquamous" carcinoma. Six patients died in a period of 3–36 months due to recurrence or metastasis, and three patients died postoperatively, while four patients were alive without disease at 2–60 months. Similar numbers of cases were also reported by Kuo and associates [19] in nine men and four women between the ages of 19 and 64 years (median age, 40 years), who presented with non-specific symptoms and no history of paraneoplastic syndromes. The authors documented five different histological categories including lymphoepithelioma-like (two cases), clear cell (one case), mixed squamous and small cell carcinoma (two cases), mixed adenosquamous and small cell carcinoma (two cases), and squamous cell carcinoma (six cases). The authors identified that all patients with pure squamous cell carcinoma were alive with a median survival of 27 months and, based on that observation, stated that the prognosis of patients with pure thymic squamous cell carcinoma is better. Hartmann and associates [20], in a review of 20 years, identified 5 cases of thymic carcinoma among 54 mediastinal tumors. The tumors were identified in three women and two men between the ages of 38 and 68 years who presented with non-specific symptoms, and no paraneoplastic syndrome was identified. Histologically, three tumors corresponded to lymphoepithelioma-like, one squamous cell carcinoma, and one "undifferentiated" carcinoma. The five patients died of tumor in a period of no more than 20 months. Hsu and associates [21], in a retrospective review of 10 years (1982–1992), reported 20 cases of thymic carcinoma in 9 men and 11 women between the ages of 34 and 70 years (mean, 51.4 years). The presence of MG was not reported in any patient but no additional clinical symptomatology was provided for this group of patients. Histologically, eight tumors were squamous cell carcinomas, seven "undifferentiated" carcinomas, one lymphoepithelioma-like carcinoma, one clear cell, one mucoepidermoid carcinoma, and two carcinoid tumors. The authors documented an overall cumulative survival of 45.9% at 3 years and 34.4% at 5 years, while the median survival times for patients with complete and incomplete resection were 39 months and 14 months, respectively. Patients who received postoperative radiation therapy had a median survival time of 39 months, while those who did not receive radiation therapy had a median survival time of 15 months. Regarding histological features, the authors estimated a median survival time for squamous cell carcinoma and undifferentiated carcinoma at 25 and 11 months, respectively. The authors concluded that complete surgical resection, postoperative radiation therapy, and squamous cell histology do not offer significant favorable prognosis even though those features are associated with longer median survival times. Chalabreysse and associates [22] also reported 19 primary thymic carcinomas in 13 men and 6 women between the ages of 29 and 75 years who presented with symptoms of chest pain or superior vena cava syndrome. The histological features of the cases studied are similar to those previously reported in other studies, and the authors also included among these 19 carcinomas 6 neuroendocrine carcinomas and 1 mucoepidermoid carcinoma. Surgical resection was performed in 10 patients, and only in 2 patients was the resection complete; 16 patients received radiation therapy, and 11 received chemotherapy. In 12 patients, the authors documented local or metastatic disease, while 10 patients died due to tumor. The overall survival rate was 14.5% at 5 years. Based on their analysis, the authors concluded that thymic carcinoma has an aggressive behavior and had poor overall prognosis. Yano and associates [23], in a collective retrospective study at a single institution, evaluated 30 thymic carcinomas in 16 men and 14 women between 33 and 84 years (mean: 59 years) who presented with varied non-specific symptomatology but with no paraneoplastic syndrome. Thirteen patients were inoperable, and those patients received either radiation therapy or chemotherapy, while seven patients had complete surgical and ten patients had incomplete surgical resection. Seventeen patients died between 2 and 78 months, while 13 patients were alive between 6 and 232 months (average, 64 months). The authors estimated a 5-year survival rate of 47.5% and a median survival time of 49 months. The authors concluded that resectability was the only prognostic factor, as the authors observed significant better prognosis in cases with total resection. Takeda and associates [24] had a similar experience in their report of 15 patients with thymic carcinoma in which the authors concluded that complete resection is the mainstay of therapy when possible. In this report – which included 12 squamous cell carcinomas, 2 undifferentiated carcinomas, and 1 adenocarcinoma – the median survival was 13 months for patients without resection and 57 months for patients with complete surgical resection. The total 3- and 5-year survival rate was estimated at 51.9% and 39%, respectively. Tomita and coworkers [25] arrived at a similar conclusion in a report of eight thymic carcinomas in two men and six women between the ages of 19 and 67 years (mean: 54.8). No paraneoplastic syndromes or MG was associated with any patient. The histologies observed were five squamous cell carcinomas, one adenosquamous carcinoma, one clear cell carcinoma, and one small cell carcinoma. In a review of 20 years, Liu and coworkers [26] evaluated 614 cases of anterior mediastinal tumors and identified 38 cases that the authors coded as thymic carcinomas, representing in their experience approximately 6.2% of all anterior mediastinal tumors. The tumors were identified in 26 men and 12 women between the ages of 28 and 80 years. Of the 38 patients, 15 had surgical procedures performed; complete resection was done in 8 patients (all these patients had low-grade histology – squamous cell carcinoma), while debulking was performed in the other 7 patients. The remaining 23 patients were treated either with partial resection or only biopsy. Interestingly, three patients were also diagnosed with MG. The histologies of the tumors are similar to those reported in other series of cases. The mean survival time in 35 patients was estimated to be 53 months, with a median of 24 months, while the overall cumulative survival rate was 38% at 3 years and 27% at 5 years. The authors concluded that tumor grade, stage, and resectability influence patients' survival. In a different study focused on the treatment of thymic carcinoma, Ogawa and coworkers [27] evaluated 40 patients who have been diagnosed with thymic carcinoma; 27 patients were treated with complete surgical resection followed by radiotherapy with or without chemotherapy, while 13 were treated with radiation therapy with or without chemotherapy. The overall survival rates at 5 and 10 years for all patients were estimated at 38% and 28%, respectively. Twenty-seven patients (68%) died of tumor, and 13 patients were alive during a period ranging from 44 to 193 months (median, 87 months). The authors concluded that multimodal treatment – complete surgical resection and postoperative radiation therapy with or without chemotherapy – is *curative* therapy for thymic carcinoma. In that regard, unusual cases of thymic carcinoma with KIT and VEGF positivity have been described in which the patient has responded to a molecular targeted-based therapy [28].

One of the largest series of primary thymic carcinomas is the one reported by Suster and Rosai [29], who encountered 60 cases in 36 men and 24 women between the ages of 10 and 76 years. The majority of tumors occurred in patients in the fourth decade of life. Clinically, two patients had a history of MG, and no other paraneoplastic syndromes were identified. Histologically, the cases were separated into low- and high-grade malignancies: 20 cases belong to low-grade tumors (mucoepidermoid carcinoma, basaloid carcinoma, and keratinizing squamous cell carcinoma), while 40 cases belong to high-grade tumors (lymphoepithelioma-like carcinoma, small cell carcinoma, undifferentiated/anaplastic carcinoma, sarcomatoid carcinoma, clear cell carcinoma). In addition, correlations were made by the infiltrative nature of the neoplasm, whether well-circumscribed to the mediastinum or infiltrative. Based on this experience, the authors identified overall survival rates at 1, 3, and 5 years of 56%, 40%, and 33%, respectively. Furthermore, 88% of the patients with infiltrative tumors died of their tumor compared to 16% of patients with well-circumscribed tumors; 84% of patients with high-grade tumors died of tumor, while none of the patients with low-grade tumors died. In addition, the authors concluded that the morphological features of the tumor correlate well with clinical behavior, and that histological type constitutes the most reliable and important predictor of prognosis. In a more recent publication [30] in what constitutes up to now the largest series of cases of thymic carcinoma – this series of cases excluded neuroendocrine carcinomas as their behavior is different – the authors analyzed 65 thymic carcinomas: 38 squamous cell carcinomas (including 3 basaloid carcinomas), 12 undifferentiated carcinomas, 4 lymphoepithelioma-like carcinoma, 3 spindle cell carcinoma, 2 mucinous adenocarcinomas, 2 papillary carcinomas, 2 clear cell carcinomas, 1 rhabdoid carcinoma, and 1 anaplastic carcinoma. Based on this experience, the authors concluded not only that the Masaoka staging system does not reliably predict prognosis but also that the most important parameter to predict prognosis is the lymph node status, regardless of the location of the lymph node. (See staging of thymic carcinoma in the respective chapter on staging.) Follow-up information was documented in 62 patients over a period ranging from 3 to 126 months (mean, 51 months); it was found that 36 patients (58%) were alive, while 26 patients (42%) had died over a period of 1–165 months (mean survival, 47.5 months). The overall survival rate at 3 and 5 years was estimated to be at 76.6% and 65.7%, respectively. The findings lead the authors to propose a different staging system from the one adapted from Masaoka, and to argue that such findings suggest that thymic carcinoma may have a better outcome than previously believed. However, it is also important to note that staging and particularly the presence of lymph node involvement plays a very important role in prognosis.

Pathological Features

Macroscopic Features

The tumor size of thymic carcinoma varies from 2 to more than 10 cm in greatest diameter. The tumors may be well circumscribed or have an infiltrative pattern compromising adjacent structures, including the pleura, pericardium, or lung. The tumors are generally described as tan to white with firm consistency, while areas of hemorrhage and necrosis may also vary from case to case (Fig. 8.1a–c). In some cases, cystic changes may also be identified. The presence of extensive necrosis is commonly associated with high-grade histology.

Histopathological Features

The tumors described in this section will not include mucoepidermoid carcinoma and basaloid carcinoma, as they are presented in the chapter on salivary gland-type tumors, while neuroendocrine carcinomas are presented in the chapter on neuroendocrine neoplasms. In addition, the entity described as "low grade metaplastic carcinoma of the thymus" [31] will not be discussed in this chapter as we consider such designation incorrect because it represents a change in name only from the original description of thymoma with pseudosarcomatous stroma [32], and as such it is discussed in the chapter on thymomas. Therefore, the histology of the tumors discussed herein will be that of non-neuroendocrine tumors and non-salivary gland-type neoplasms. Nevertheless, the spectrum of histopathological growth patterns that has been documented in thymic carcinoma is varied and as such will be presented in this section.

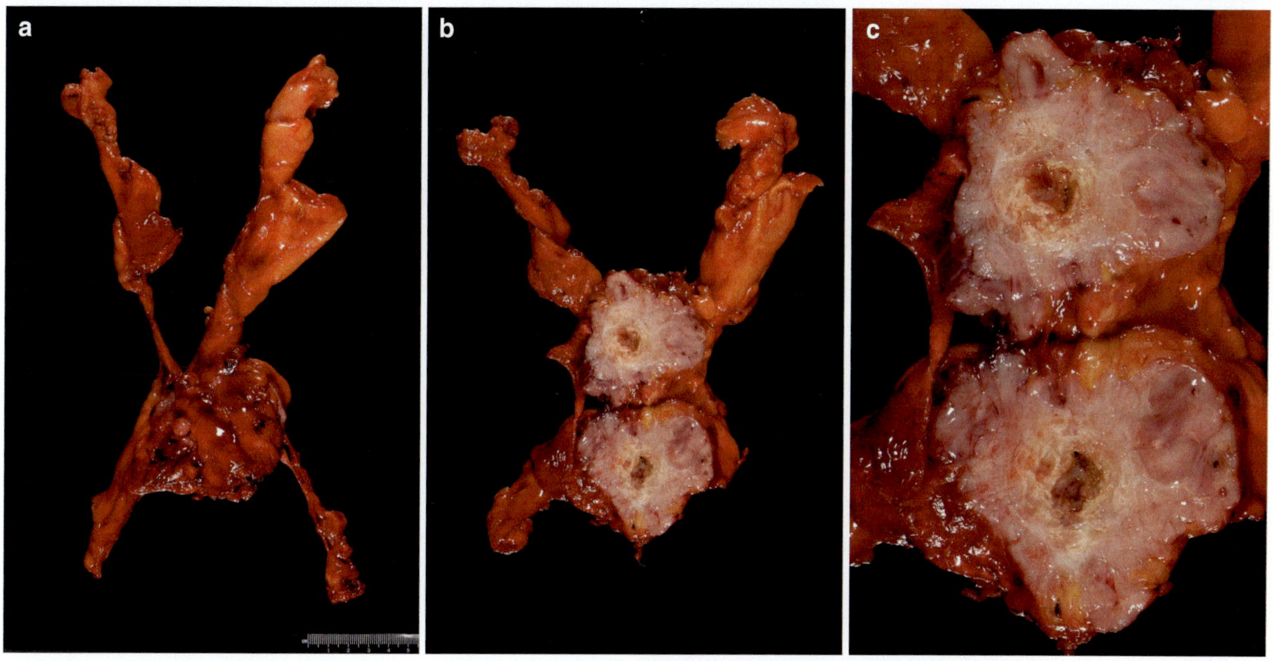

Fig. 8.1 (**a**) Surgical resection of thymic carcinoma; note the presence of a mass within the thymic gland. (**b**) Bisected thymic carcinoma showing infiltrating borders. (**c**) Thymic carcinoma showing focal central necrosis

Squamous Cell Carcinoma

As stated earlier in this chapter, credit for the description of these tumors is given to Shimosato [6], who reported a small series of cases. However, even though the original description emphasizes the well-differentiated nature of these tumors, the fact is that, among squamous cell carcinoma, there is a spectrum that may vary from well to moderately to poorly differentiated squamous cell carcinoma.

In the well-differentiated squamous cell carcinoma, the tumor may show a lobular architecture with varying size islands of tumor cells (Fig. 8.2a–c), which are composed of round or polygonal cells, vesicular nuclei, prominent nucleoli, and abundant eosinophilic cytoplasm (Fig. 8.3a–f). Areas of keratinization with the presence of intercellular bridges are often encountered (Fig. 8.4a–c). The tumor may show cystic changes, and in some cases, the cystic changes are similar to those seen in multilocular thymic cyst (Fig. 8.5a–g). The presence of thymic carcinomas with associated multilocular thymic cyst has been specifically reported in the literature, and this feature is rather unusual. In addition, a variant of cystic well-differentiated squamous cell carcinoma of the thymus has been reported in which the tumors are pre-

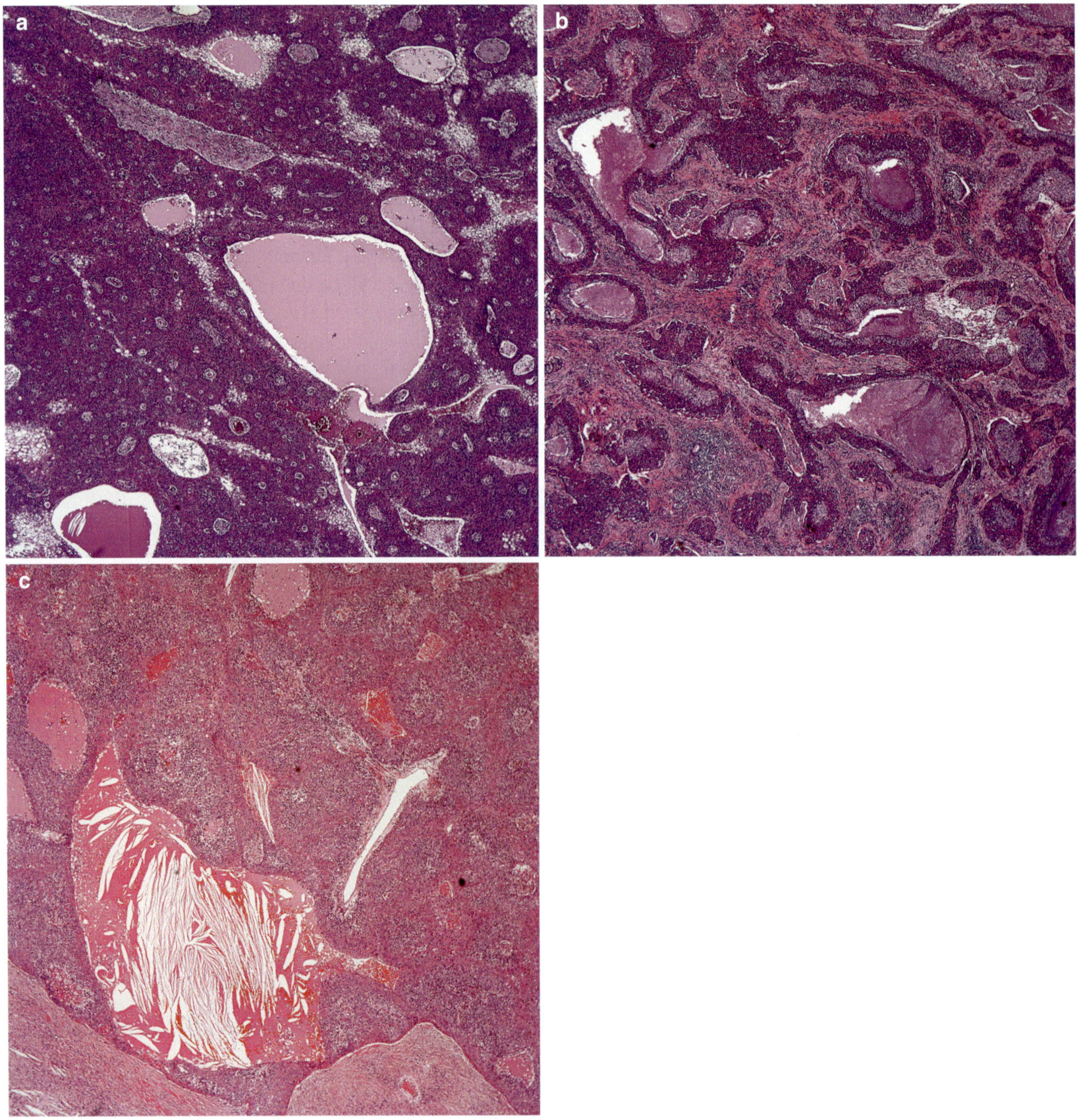

Fig. 8.2 (**a**) Low power view of a thymic carcinoma showing microscopic cystic changes. (**b**) Different growth pattern of a thymic carcinoma with areas of come-like necrosis. (**c**) Sheets of neoplastic cells with focal cholesterol cleft granuloma

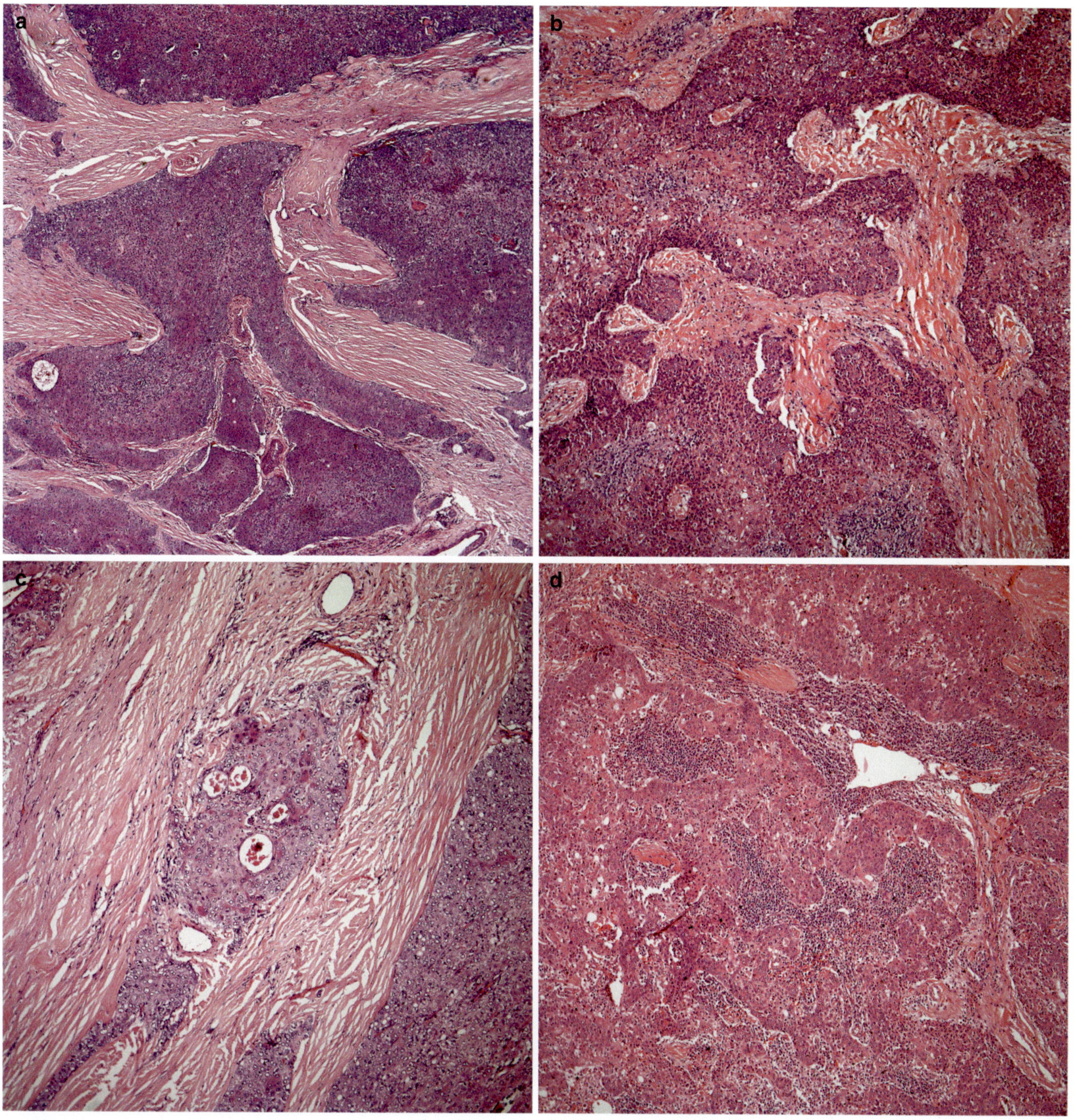

Fig. 8.3 (**a**) Thymic carcinoma showing irregular islands of tumor cells. (**b**) Thymic carcinoma showing sheets of malignant cells without increased mitotic activity. (**c**) Islands of tumor cells embedded in fibro-connective tissue. (**d**) Mixed areas of tumor cells and inflammatory reaction

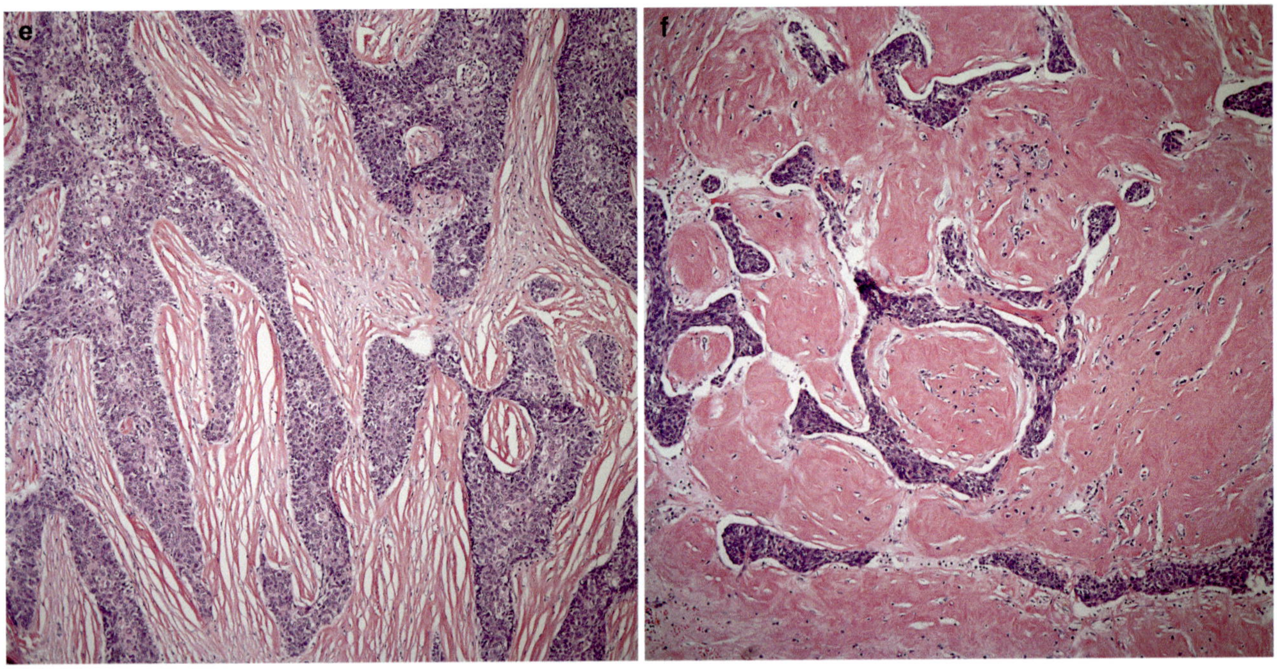

Fig. 8.3 (continued) (**e**) Increased areas of fibroconnective tissue and strips of tumor cells. (**f**) Marked presence of fibroconnective tissue

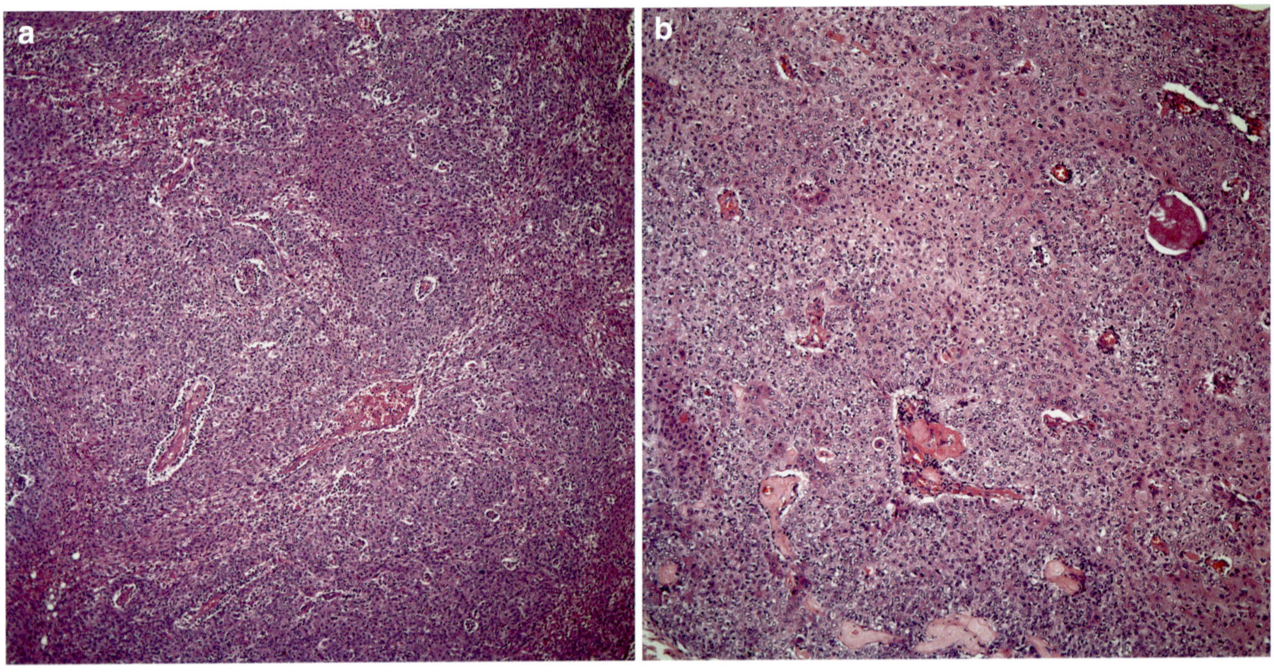

Fig. 8.4 (**a**) Sheets of epidermoid cells in thymic carcinoma. (**b**) Homogeneous cellular proliferation without increased in mitotic activity

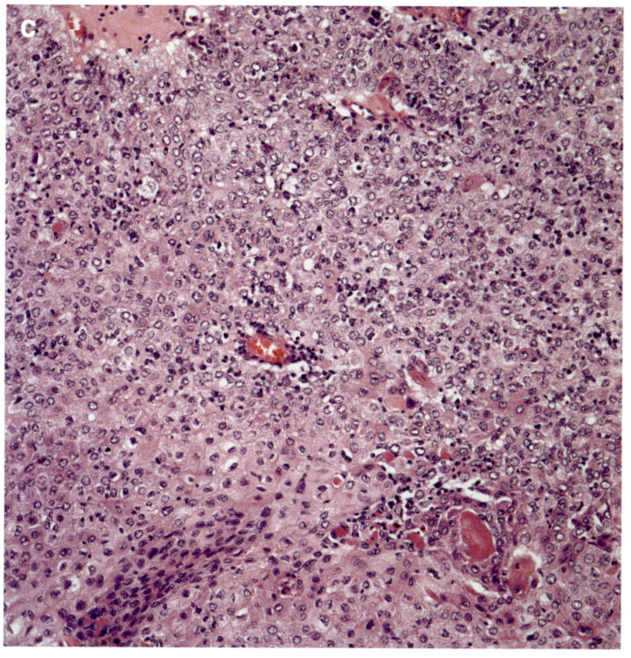

Fig. 8.4 (continued) (**c**) Higher magnification showing mild nuclear atypia and apoptotic nuclei

dominantly cystic with alternating solid areas and evidence of keratinization [33, 34] (Fig. 8.6a–c). Mitotic activity in these tumors (well-differentiated) may be present but usually is not high (Fig. 8.7a–c). Areas of hemorrhage or necrosis are not common (Fig. 8.8a–c).

On the other hand, tumors belonging to the moderately and poorly differentiated categories may be more common in comparison to those of low-grade histology. The low power view of these tumors may also show different growth patterns, which include infiltrating borders (Fig. 8.9), cystic changes, small islands of tumors cells separated by fibroconnective tissue, areas of comedo-like necrosis, tumor necrosis with single cell necrosis, and calcifications (Fig. 8.10a–e). In addition, the tumor may also show irregular lobular architecture, ribbons of tumor cells with abortive germinal centers, extensive hyalinization, and prominent inflammatory changes where the malignant cells can be easily overlooked (Fig. 8.11a–e). Higher magnification of thymic carcinomas shows a neoplastic cellular proliferation composed of medium size cells with round nuclei and prominent nucleoli, mitotic activity is easily identified, areas that can be easily misconstrued as small cell carcinoma may also be present,

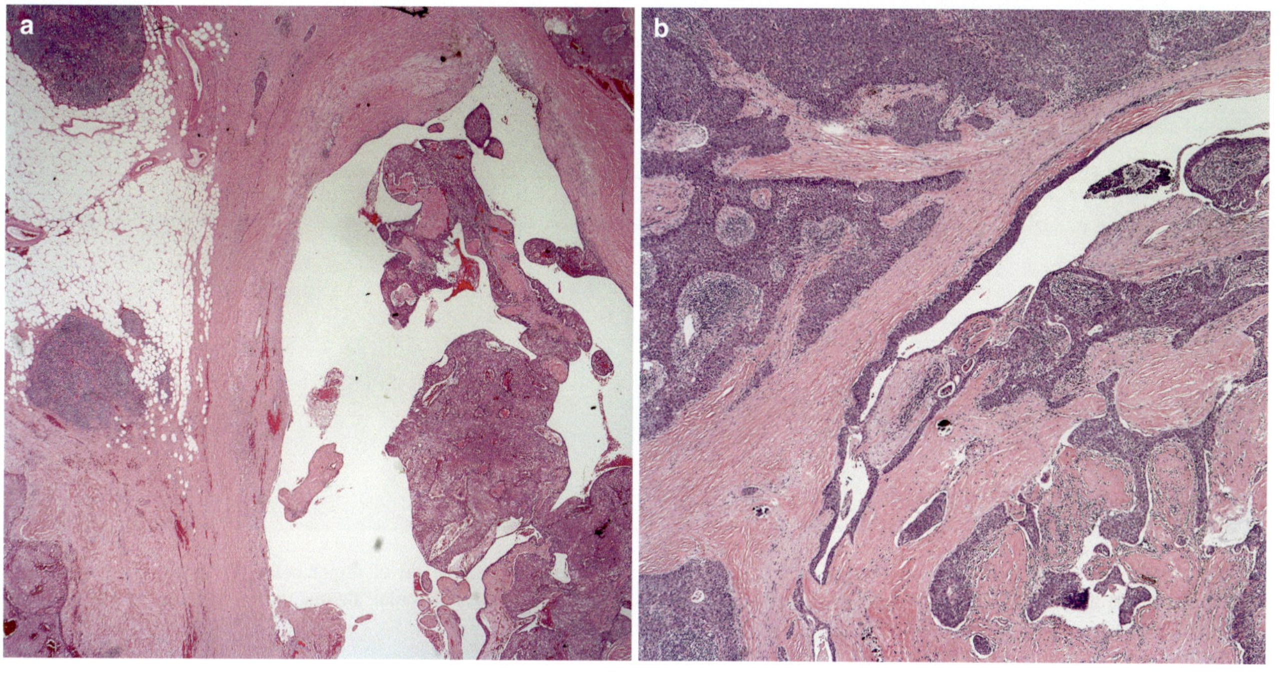

Fig. 8.5 (**a**) Thymic carcinoma with prominent cystic changes. (**b**) Cystic areas showing irregular strips of tumor cells

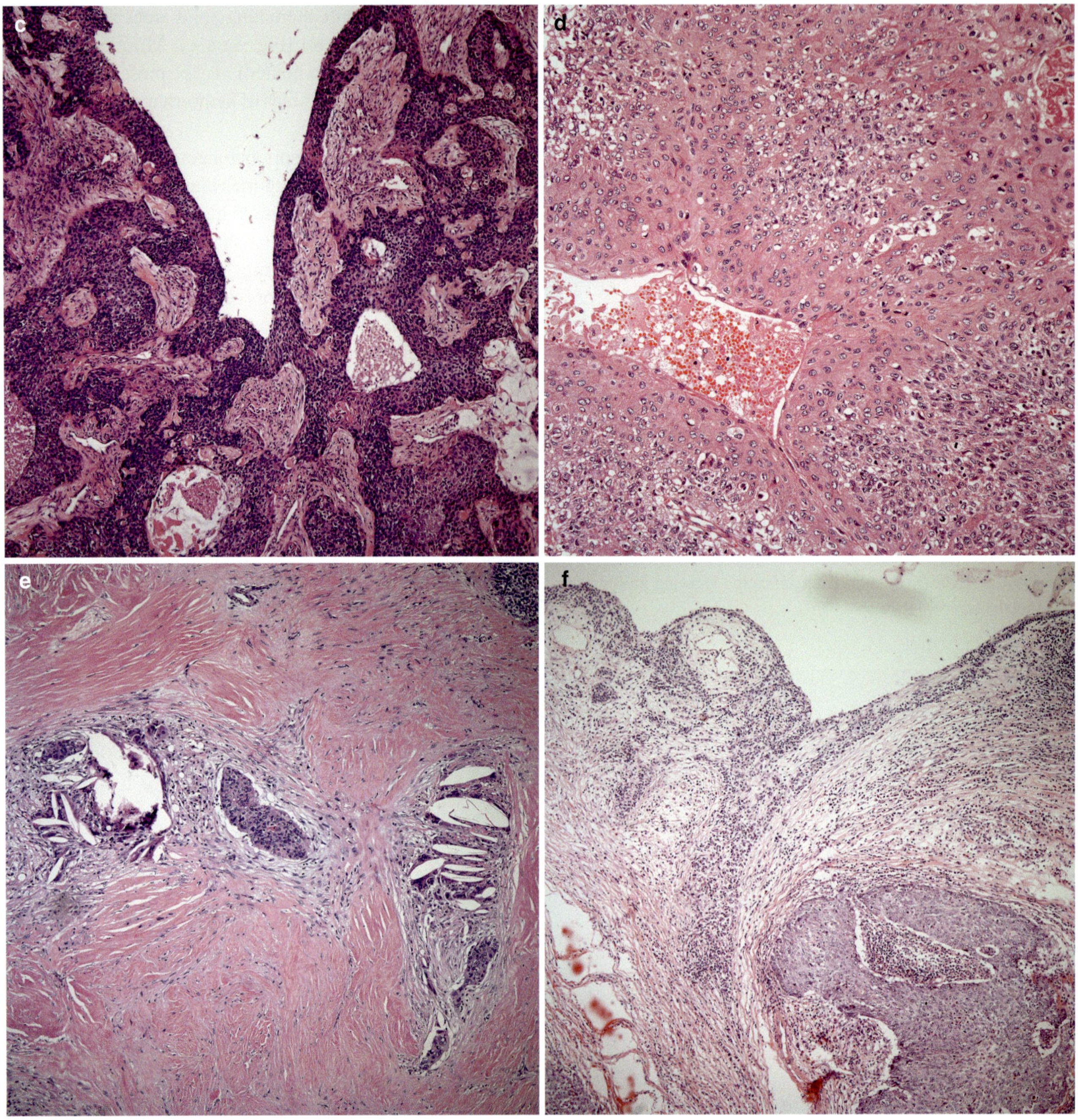

Fig. 8.5 (continued) (**c**) The lining of the cystic area is also involved by carcinoma. (**d**) The wall of a vascular structure is also involved by carcinoma. (**e**) Extensive areas of fibrosis with cholesterol cleft granulomata and small island of tumor cells. (**f**) Cystic areas similar to those seen in multilocular thymic cyst; the wall is involved by carcinoma

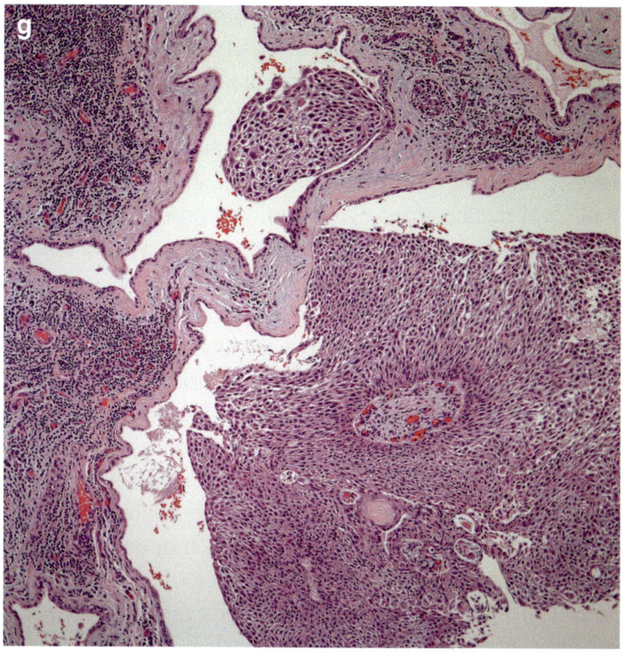

Fig. 8.5 (continued) (**g**) Cystic spaces also involved by carcinoma

and extensive necrosis with only small islands of tumor cells may also be seen (Fig. 8.12a–d). In addition, the presence of keratinization may be seen only focally or may not be present at all. In general terms, the spectrum of thymic squamous cell carcinomas may represent approximately 50–60% of all thymic carcinomas.

Sarcomatoid Carcinoma

Even though this morphological variant of thymic carcinomas has been mentioned in earlier literature, the most comprehensive series of cases is the one presented by Suster and Moran [35] in a description of 16 cases of 7 women and 9 men between the ages of 23 and 82 years. However, the tumor has been documented in other series of cases, and may represent approximately 5% of all thymic carcinomas. The clinical and surgical presentation of these cases is similar to that described in other variants of thymic carcinoma. However, the histopathological features are those of a spindle cell proliferation with varying spectrum of cellular atypia, which in some areas may resemble spindle cell thymoma and in other areas a frank sarcomatoid carcinoma. The tumors show infiltrative pattern, may retain some lobular architec-

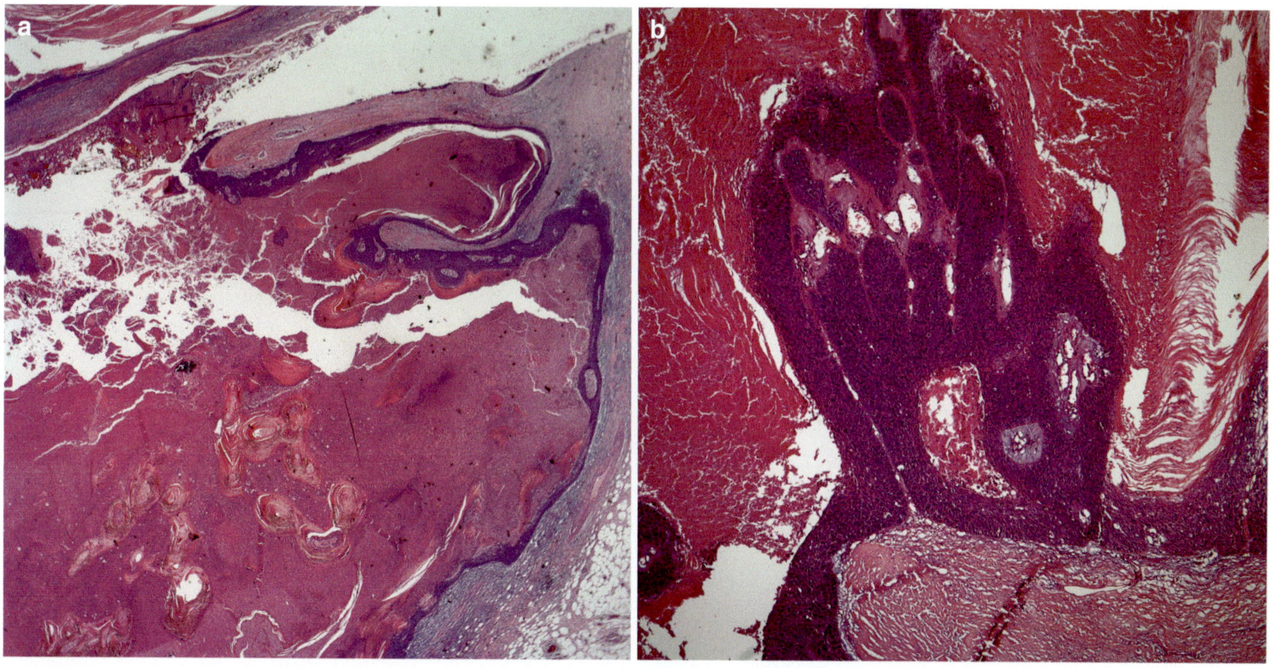

Fig. 8.6 (**a**) Low power view of a cystic keratinizing squamous cell carcinoma. (**b**) Extensive keratinization and verrucous-like proliferation

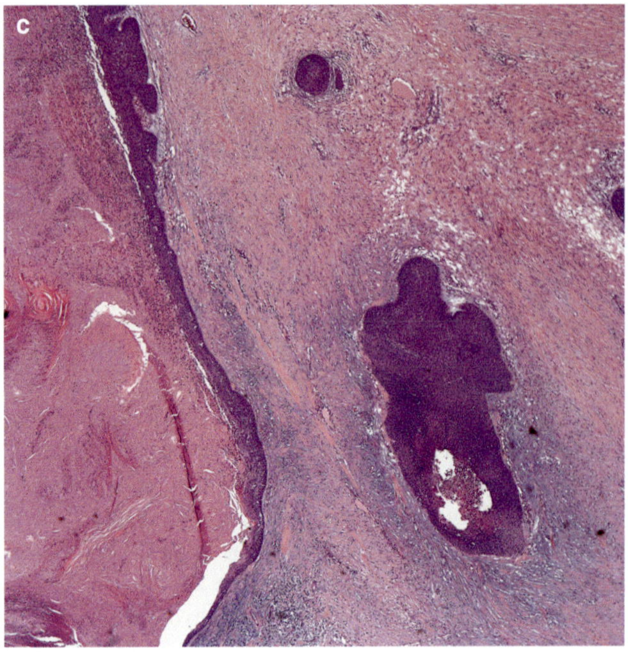

Fig. 8.6 (continued) (**c**) Squamous carcinoma present in the wall of cystic structure

ture, or present with cystic changes similar to those seen in multilocular thymic cyst (Fig. 8.13a–d). The tumor may also show some versatility in the different growth patterns including neural-like, smooth muscle-like, carcinosarcoma-like, and synovial sarcoma-like, among others (Fig. 8.14a–d). Higher magnification of these tumors shows spindle cells with oval nuclei, scant cytoplasm, and prominent nucleoli, while mitotic activity in these tumors may vary from 3 to 10 × 10 hpf (Fig. 8.15a, b). Areas of necrosis and hemorrhage are commonly present. Recently, descriptions of sarcomatoid carcinoma arising in metaplastic thymoma have been reported [36, 37]. However, two issues arise in those cases: (1) the term metaplastic that was coined for these tumors was within thymic carcinoma and not thymoma, as the original description is thymoma with pseudosarcomatous stroma [31, 32], and (2) it appears that this description is a hybrid of two different terms for the same tumor, which in our opinion is thymoma but not metaplastic. However, if we take these reports at face value, then the reported cases belong in the spectrum of thymic epithelial tumors that shares features of thymoma and thymic carcinoma. In that regard, Suster and Moran [14] presented the largest series up to now with 22

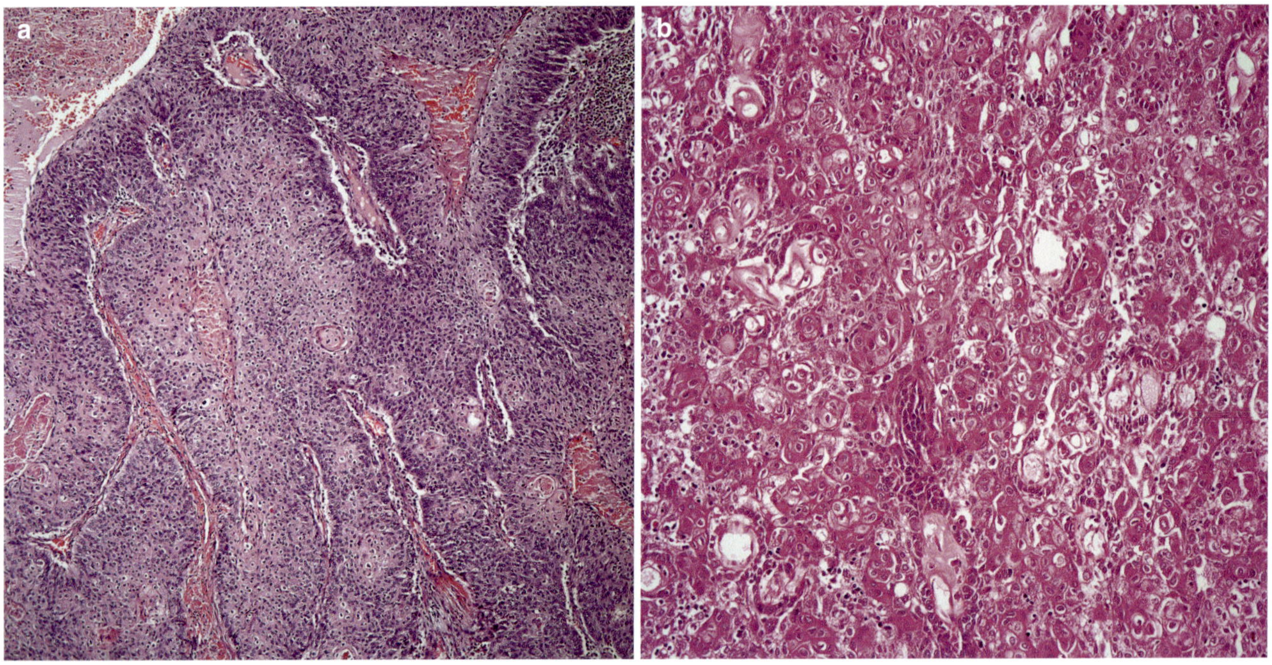

Fig. 8.7 (**a**) Thymic squamous carcinoma with focal areas of keratinization. (**b**) More extensive keratinization

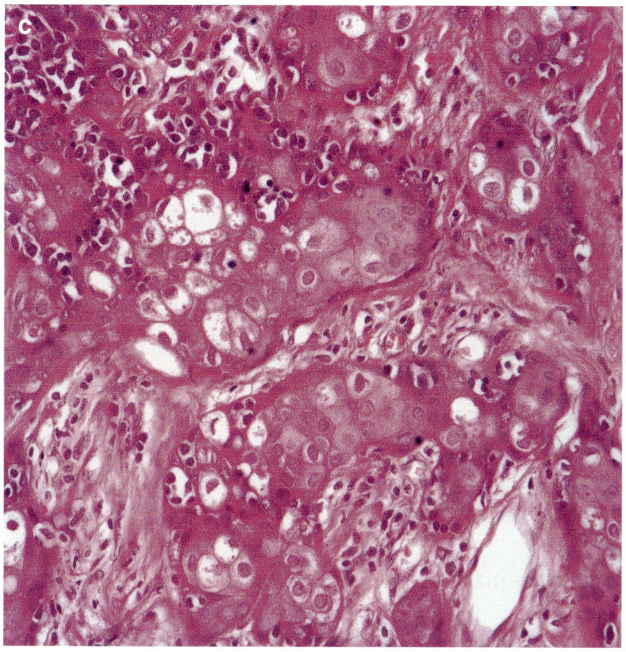

Fig. 8.7 (continued) (**c**) Higher magnification showing keratinizing areas with mild nuclear atypia and absent mitotic activity

patients: 16 men and 6 women between the ages of 23 and 83 years. The cases reported included several different permutations between thymoma and thymic carcinoma in different proportions. Therefore, those cases of sarcomatoid carcinoma arising in metaplastic thymoma only expand the spectrum of such associations.

Undifferentiated Carcinoma

This type of thymic carcinoma represents a minority of the cases; however, it may represent approximately 15% of all thymic carcinomas. Essentially, the tumor is composed of sheets or islands of neoplastic cells without any morphological differentiation toward squamous cell or neuroendocrine carcinomas. The tumors show marked cellular atypia and increased mitotic activity of more than 10 × 10 hpf (Fig. 8.16a–e). In addition, areas of necrosis and hemorrhage are commonly seen. Nonaka and coworkers [38] reported five cases of this type of carcinoma in which the tumor was associated with what the author designated as "Castleman's disease-like reaction." Interestingly, the authors also stated that this type of carcinoma might have an indolent behavior, as their five patients were alive after a period ranging from 1

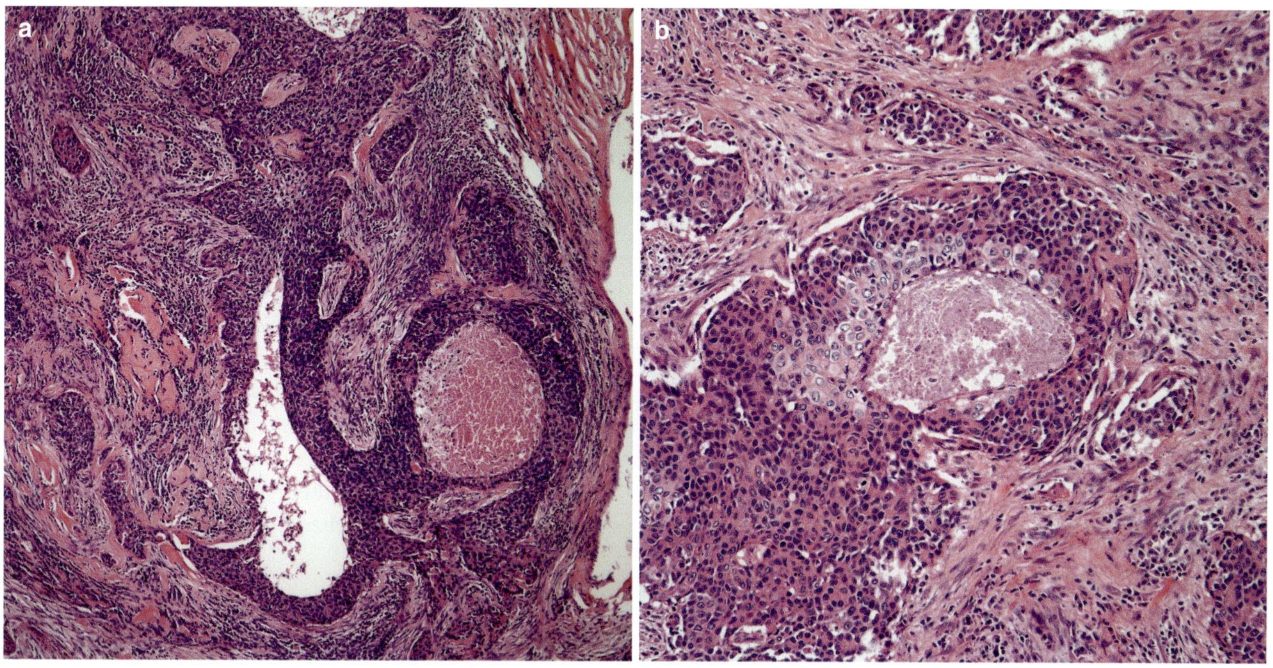

Fig. 8.8 (**a**) Thymic carcinoma with focal areas of necrosis and inflammatory reaction. (**b**) Focal comedo-like necrosis

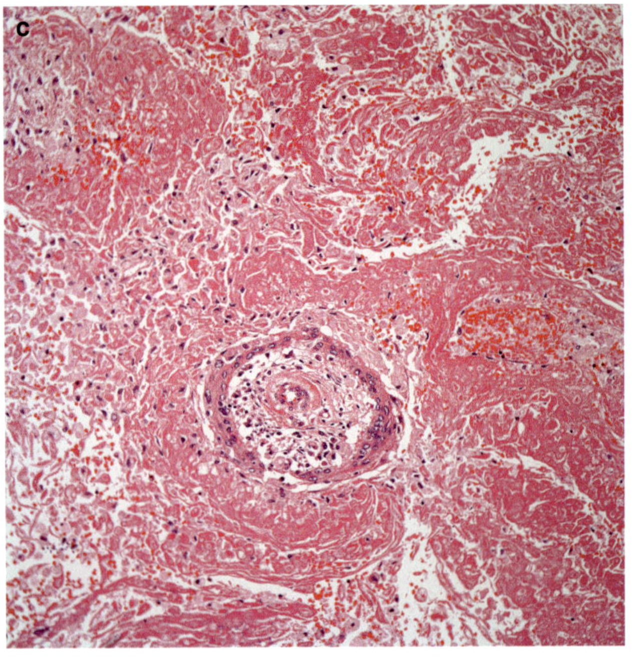

Fig. 8.8 (continued) (**c**) Extensive keratin debris with little viable tumor

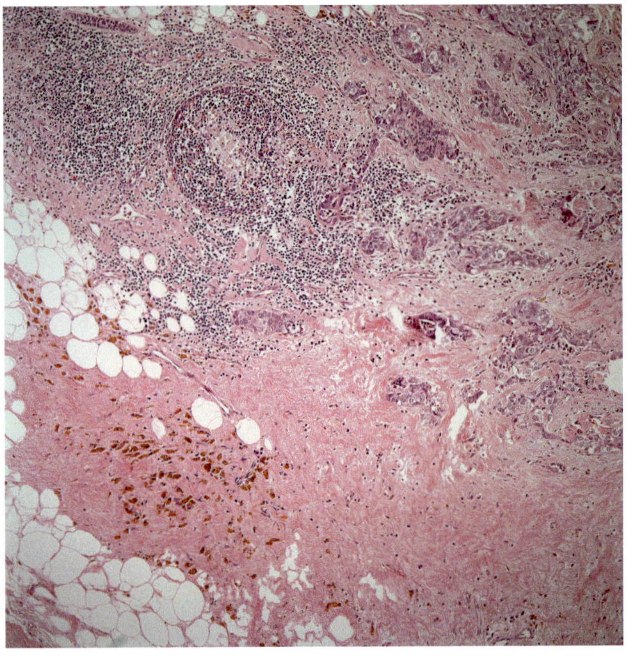

Fig. 8.9 Thymic carcinoma showing infiltrative growth pattern into adipose and perithymic tissue

to 22 years. However, it is important to mention that in four of those patients, the tumor was limited to the anterior mediastinum and complete surgical resection was performed. In one other patient, only biopsy material was done followed by radiation therapy, but no tumor extension outside of the mediastinum was documented. Therefore, it is possible that it is not that this histology follows a good clinical course, but rather the extent of disease, which in these cases appears to be limited to the anterior mediastinum. Thus, this speaks more in favor of staging rather than histology as the driver of the clinical course. We have encountered similar tumors in which the histology is more worrisome, as the tumors may show focal areas of spindle cells admixed with round cells and prominent germinal centers, some of them with a vessel crossing the germinal center in a manner that mimics the hyaline vascular type of Castleman's disease (Fig. 8.17a–c).

Lymphoepithelioma-Like Carcinoma

This particular variant of thymic carcinoma may represent approximately no more than 10% of all thymic carcinomas. The tumors characteristically show a syncytial growth pattern composed of large cells with ill-defined borders, vesicular nuclei, and prominent nucleoli. The tumor cells or islands of tumor cells are embedded in an inflammatory stroma composed predominantly of lymphocytes with scattered plasma cells. Areas of necrosis and hemorrhage are not prominent in these tumors, while the mitotic activity is variable and may range from <10 × 10 hpf to >10 hpf (Fig. 8.18a–g). It is of interest to highlight that reports of this type of thymic carcinoma associated with Epstein-Barr virus (EBV) have been reported in the literature. Dimery and coworkers [39] reported a case of thymic carcinoma in a 30-year-old woman who had serological evidence of infection with EBV, and Southern blot analysis showed the presence of the viral genome in the tissue. Leyvraz and coworkers [40] described a similar occurrence in a 19-year-old young man with thymic carcinoma. The authors concluded that the presence of EBV-associated nuclear antigen (EBNA) in the carcinoma cells and the high level of viral genome detected in the DNA suggest a role of the EBV in the genesis of this type of thymic carcinoma, similar to that seen in nasopharyngeal carcinoma.

Papillary Carcinoma

Even though this tumor is presented here as specific variant of thymic carcinoma, it is very likely that it is part of the spectrum of thymic adenocarcinoma, as we have reported; (see the section on adenocarcinoma in this chapter). However,

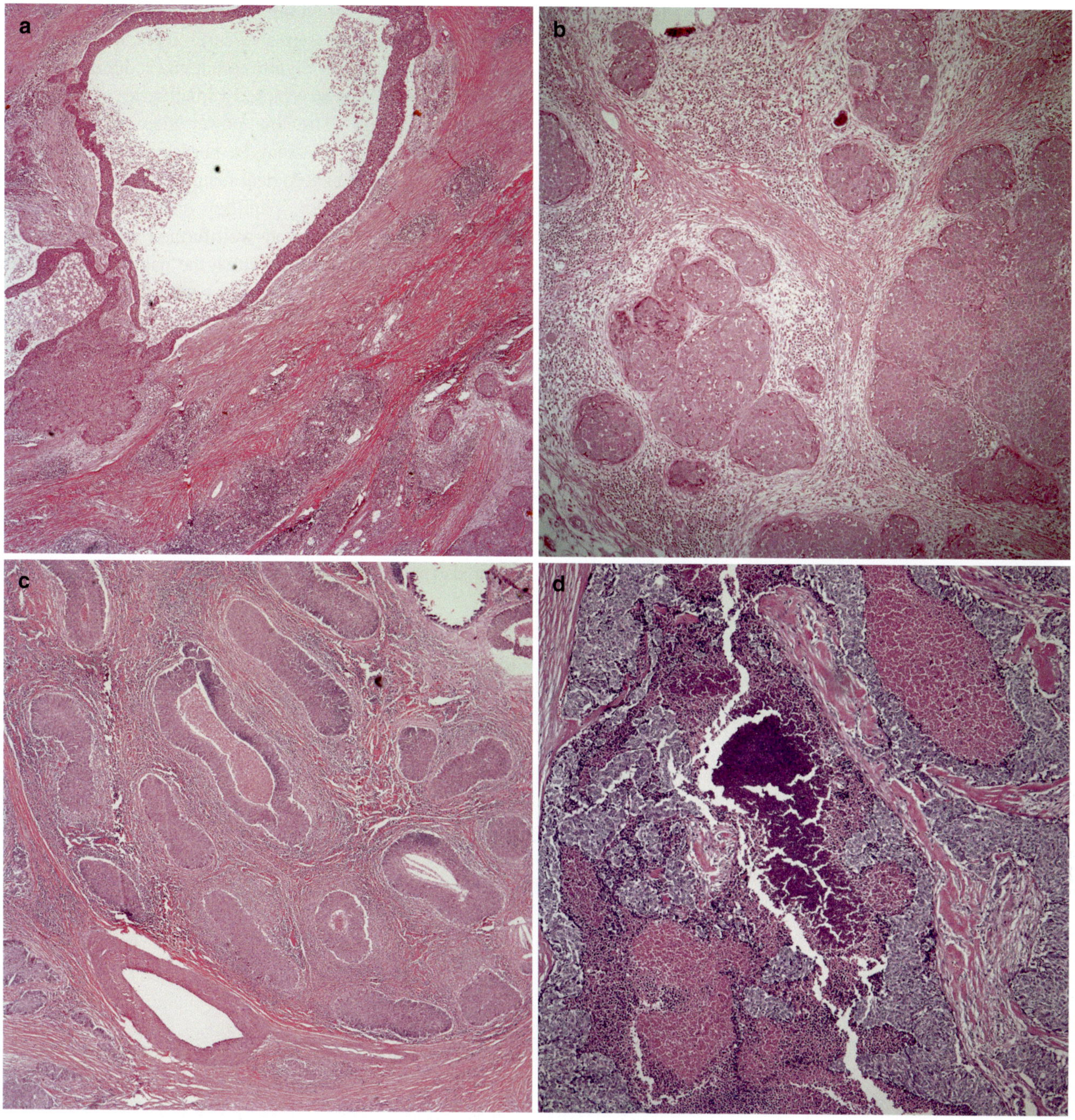

Fig. 8.10 (**a**) Thymic carcinoma with cystic changes. (**b**) Small islands of tumors cells separated by fibroconnective tissue and inflammatory reaction. (**c**) Thymic carcinoma with comedo-like necrosis and inflammatory reaction. (**d**) Thymic carcinoma with extensive necrosis and single cell necrosis

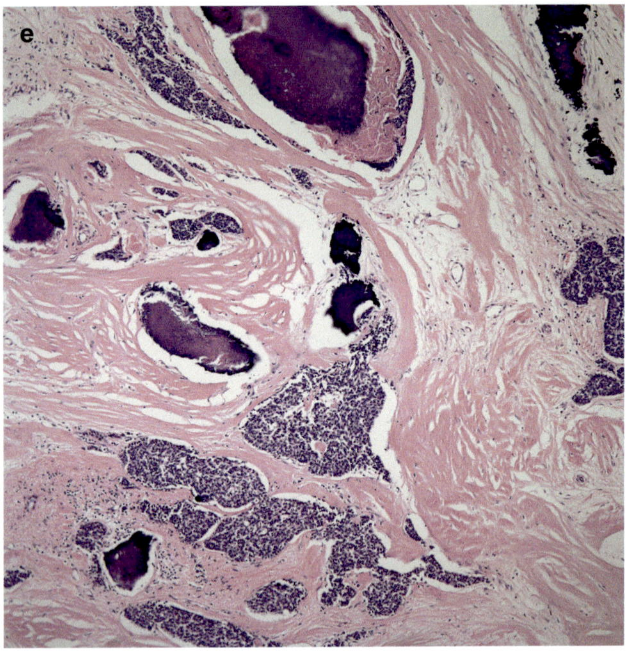

Fig. 8.10 (continued) (**e**) Thymic carcinoma with numerous calcifications

this is another type of carcinoma that – even though it has been reported in some series of cases – credit for a report highlighting this type of thymic carcinoma is due to Matsuno and coworkers [41], who reported a small series of four cases with this histology. The low power view is of a well-circumscribed tumor that may be bordered by remnants of thymic tissue. Other histological features include a complex papillary growth pattern, papillary structures containing foamy histiocytes, loose and well-formed papillary structures, and solid-like areas in which the papillary structures are compressed (Fig. 8.19a–e). The papillary growth pattern may be formed by papillary structures without a fibrovascular core, with a fibrovascular core, with a mixture of these and compressed, and with a complex pattern (Fig. 8.20a–d). At higher magnification, these papillary structures can be lined by low cuboidal epithelium, columnar epithelium, clear cells with nuclear atypia, and/or columnar-like type of epithelium (Fig. 8.21a–d). Nuclear atypia and mitotic activity are variable, but in general the tumor does not show increased mitotic activity. Some cases have been reported in which the tumor also shows combined features of thymoma and thymic

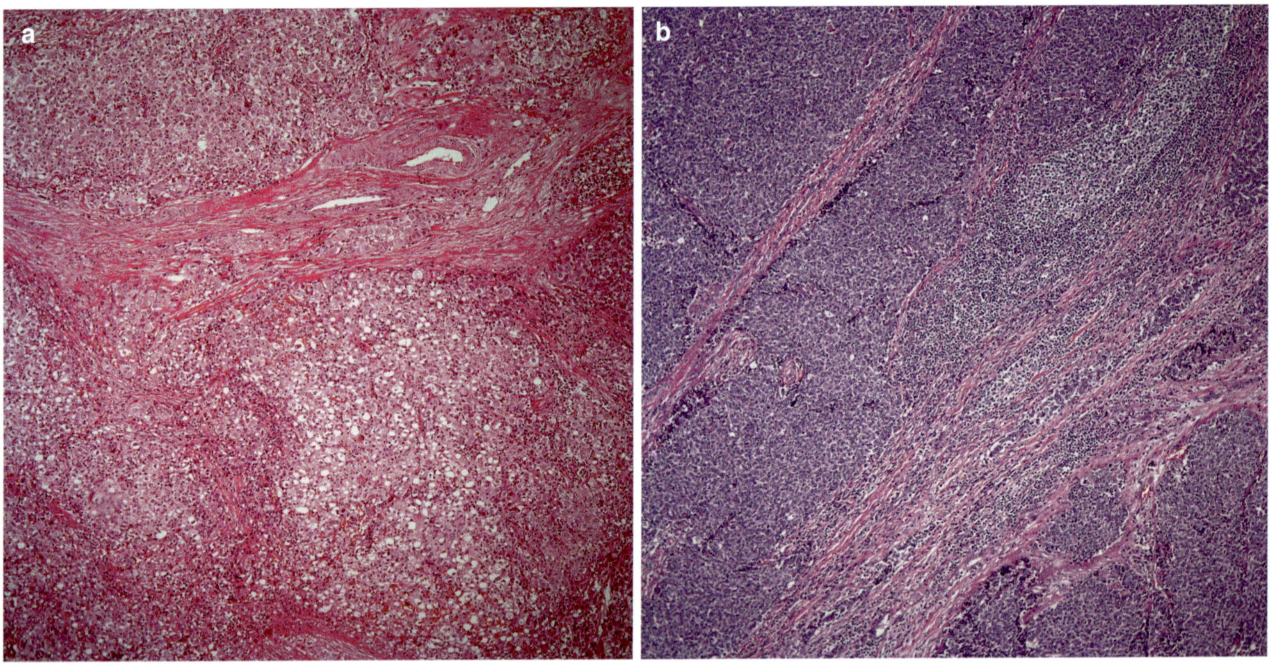

Fig. 8.11 (**a**) Thymic carcinoma with irregular lobules of tumor cells. (**b**) Thymic carcinoma with sheets of tumors cells and presence of abortive germinal center

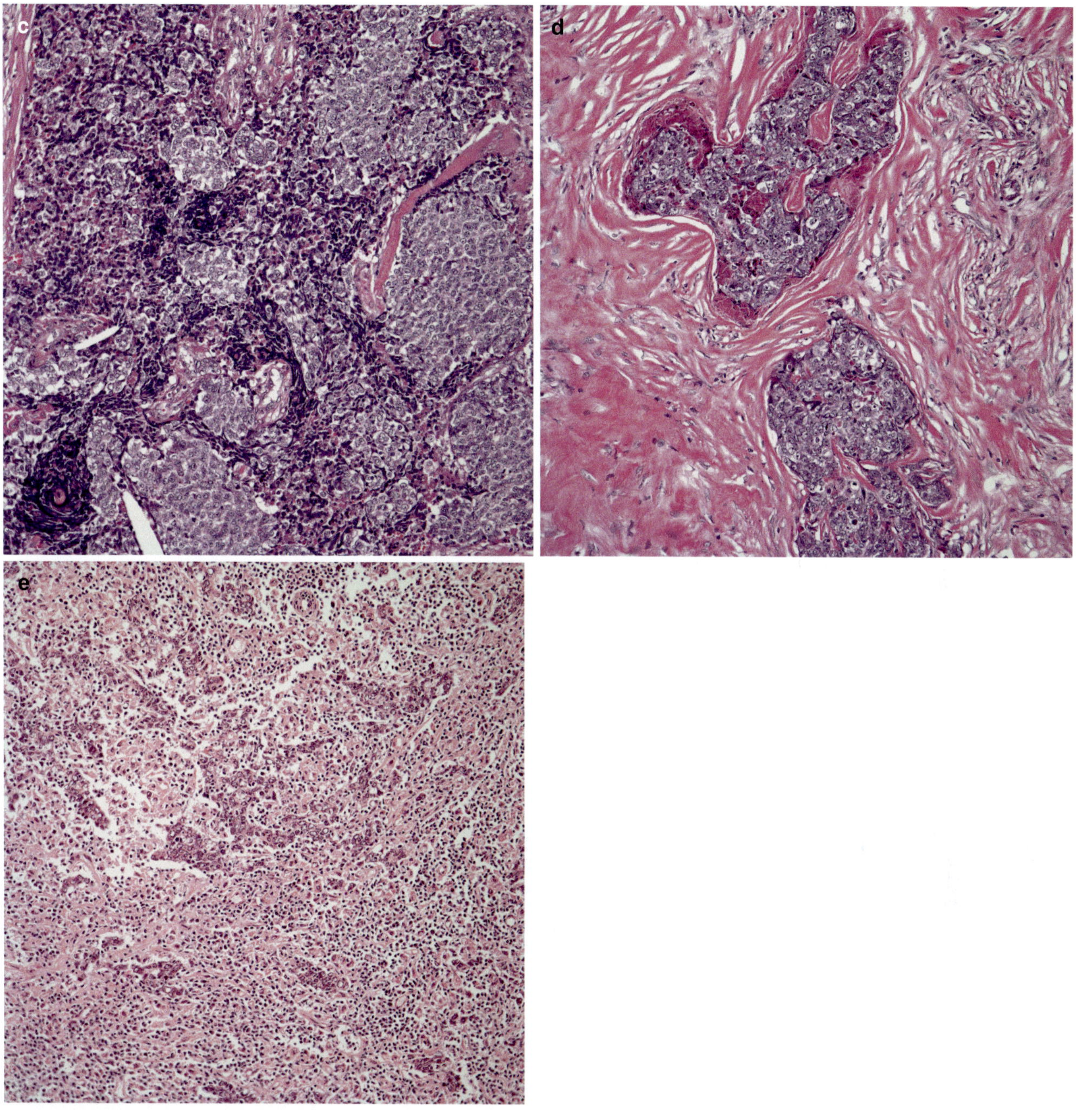

Fig. 8.11 (continued) (**c**) Thymic carcinoma with areas of crush artifact. (**d**) Thymic carcinoma with extensive hyalinization. (**e**) Thymic carcinoma with extensive inflammatory reaction

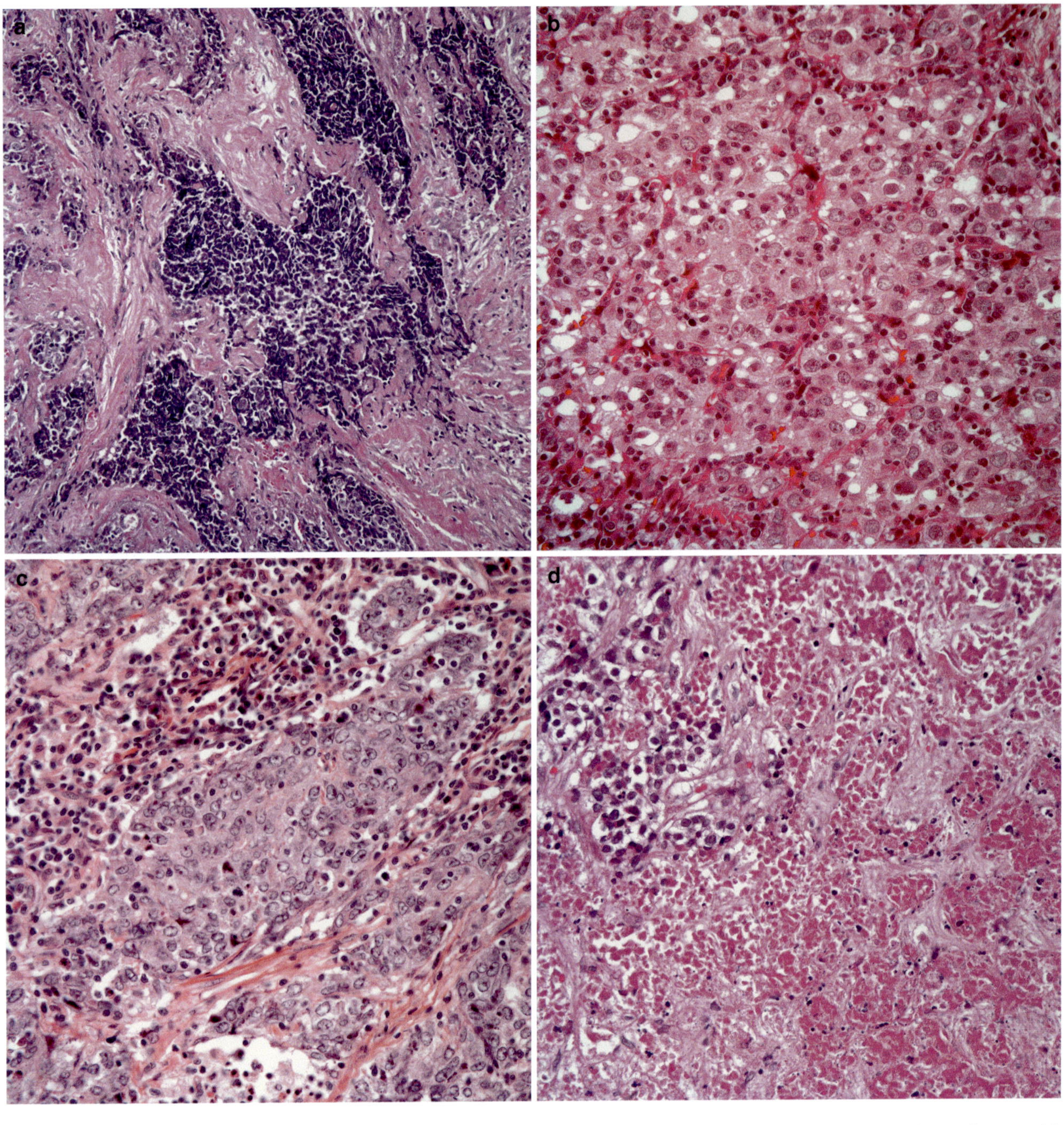

Fig. 8.12 (**a**) Thymic carcinoma with areas mimicking small cell carcinoma. (**b**) Higher magnification of a thymic carcinoma showing medium size cells with round nuclei and prominent nucleoli. (**c**) Thymic carcinoma showing mitotic activity. (**d**) Thymic carcinoma with extensive areas of necrosis

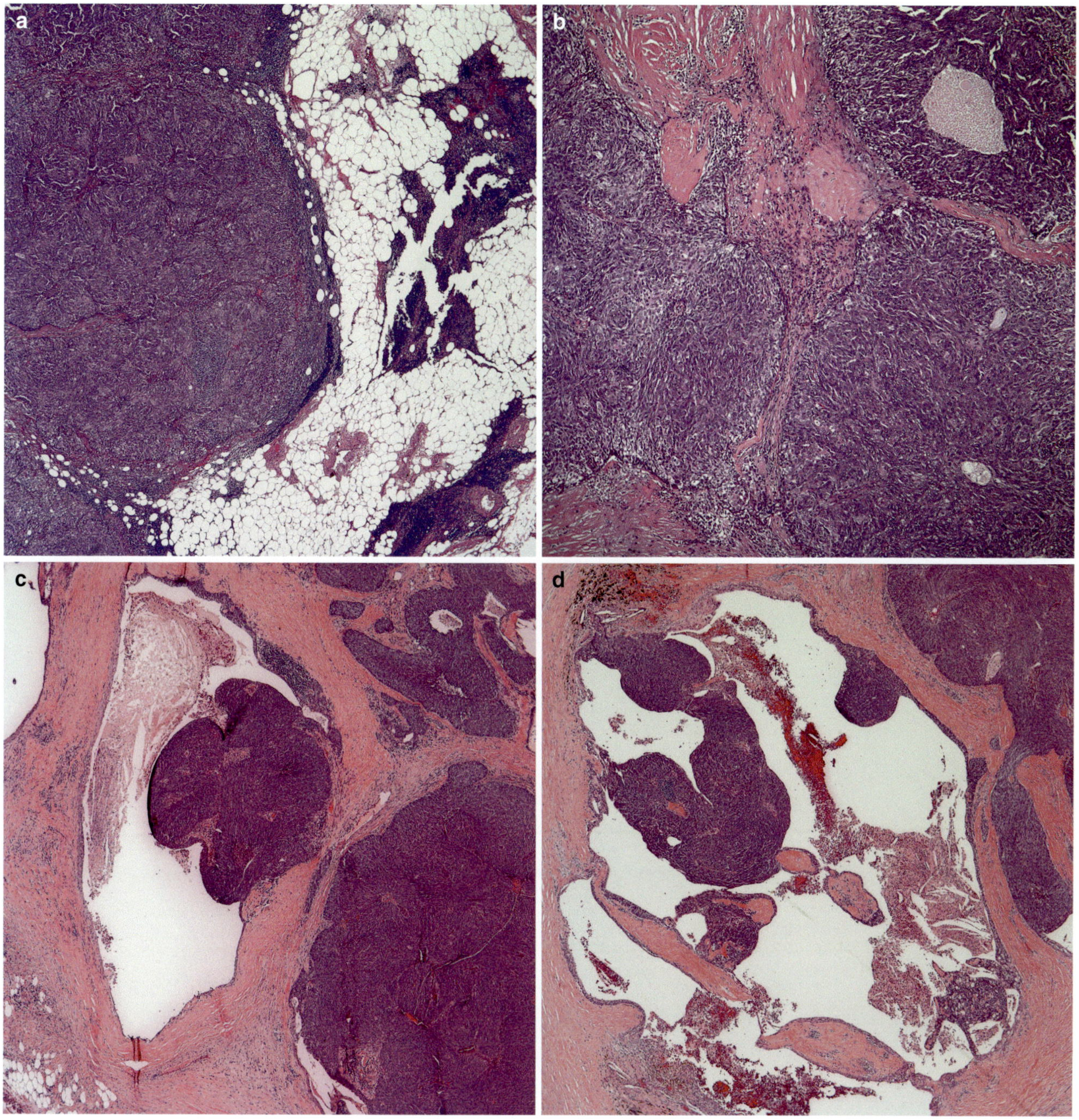

Fig. 8.13 (**a**) Spindle cell thymic carcinoma penetrating perithymic adipose tissue. (**b**) Spindle cell thymic carcinoma preserving some lobular architecture. (**c**) Spindle cell thymic carcinoma with cystic changes. (**d**) Cystic changes similar to those in multilocular thymic cyst

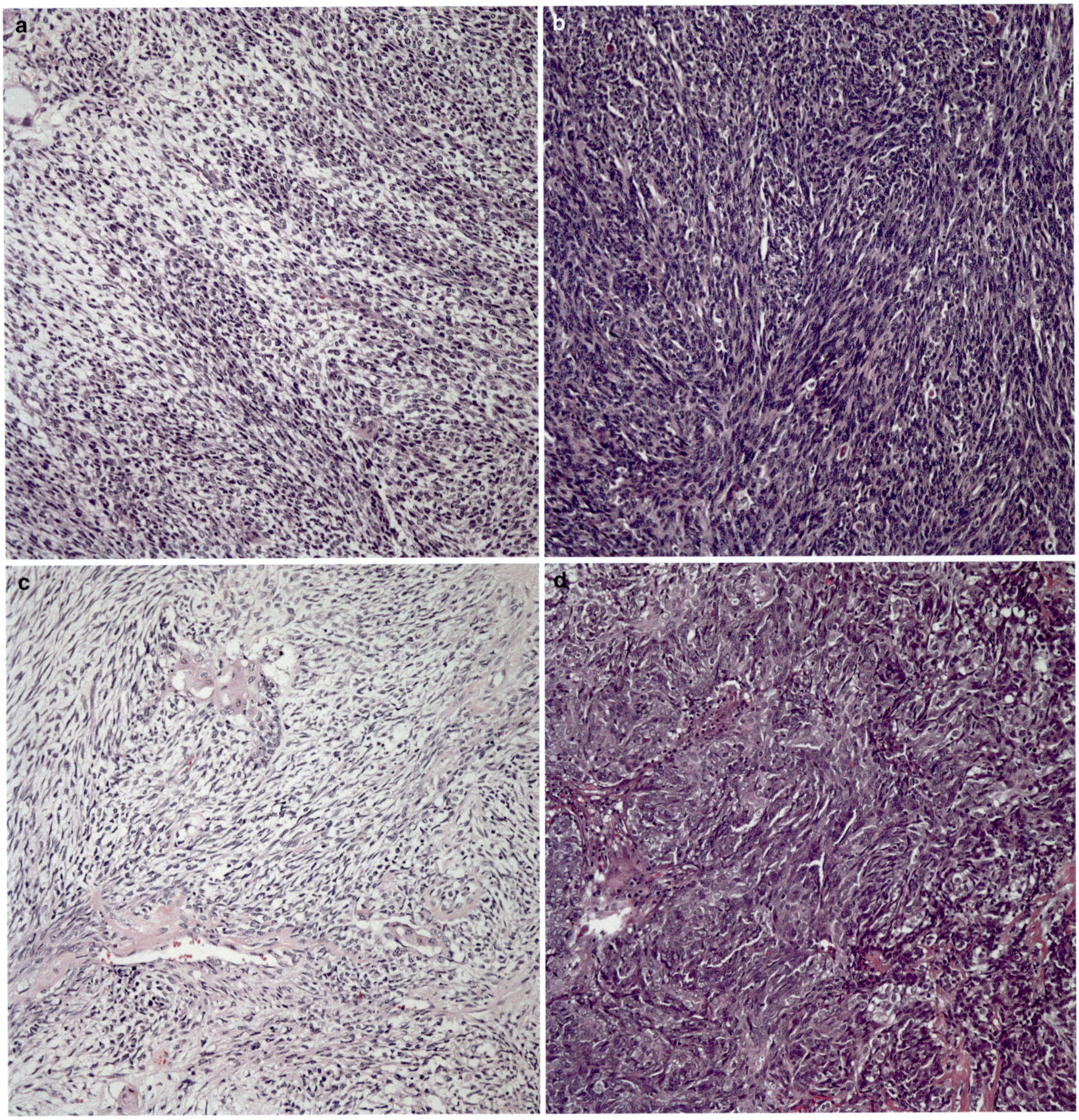

Fig. 8.14 (**a**) Spindle cell thymic carcinoma with a subtle neural-like pattern. (**b**) Spindle cell thymic carcinoma with a smooth muscle-like pattern. (**c**) Spindle cell thymic carcinoma with carcinosarcoma-like pattern; note the presence of an island of classic squamous cell carcinoma. (**d**) Spindle cell thymic carcinoma with synovial sarcoma-like areas

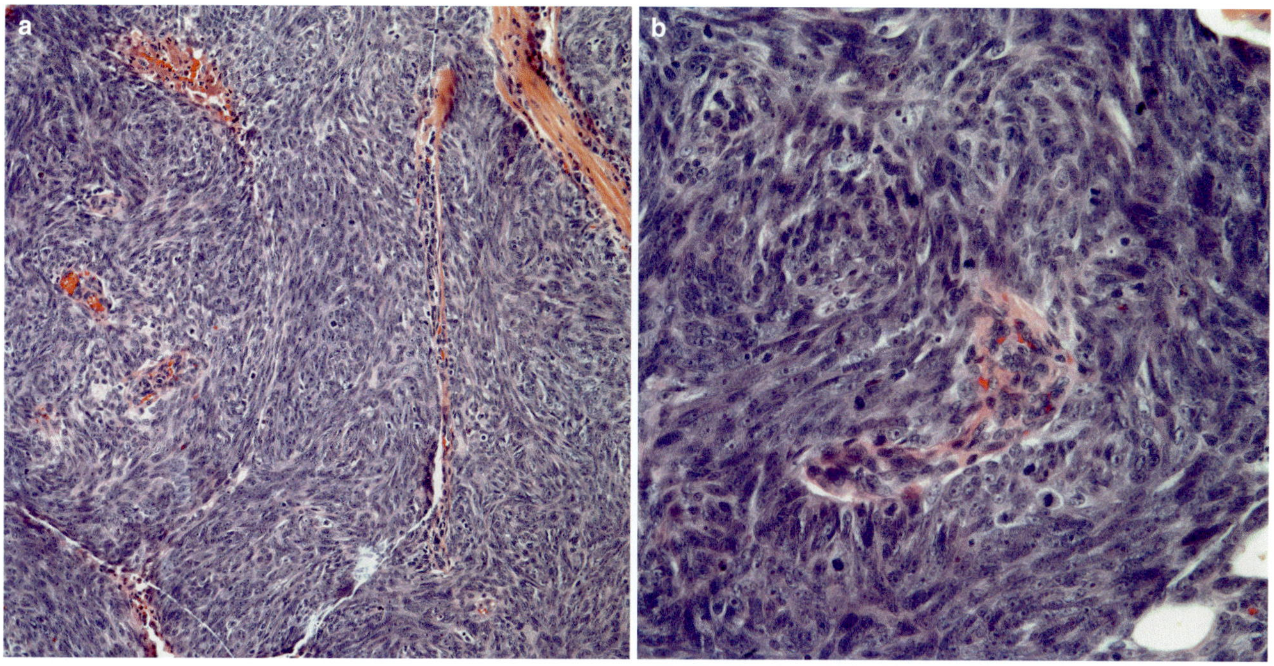

Fig. 8.15 (**a**) Higher magnification of spindle cell thymic carcinoma showing fusiform cells, with scant cytoplasm, oval nuclei, and prominent nucleoli. (**b**) Spindle cell thymic carcinoma with mitotic activity

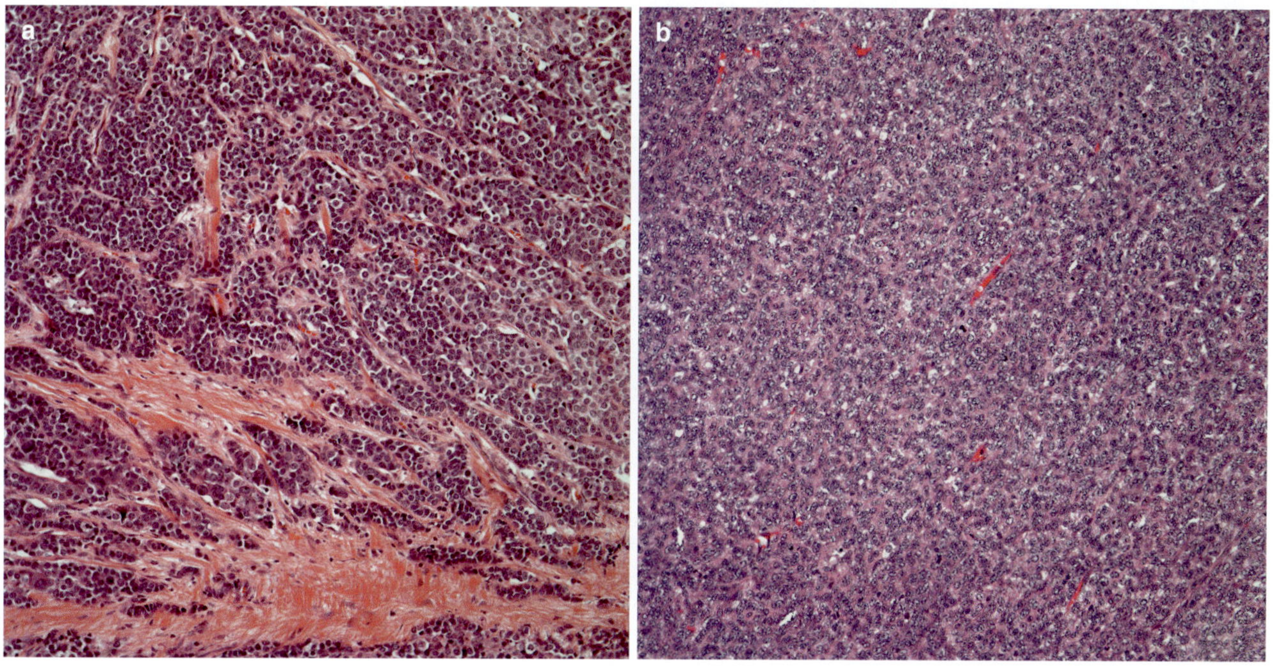

Fig. 8.16 (**a**) Undifferentiated thymic carcinoma showing ribbons of tumor cells. (**b**) undifferentiated thymic carcinoma showing sheets of neoplastic cells

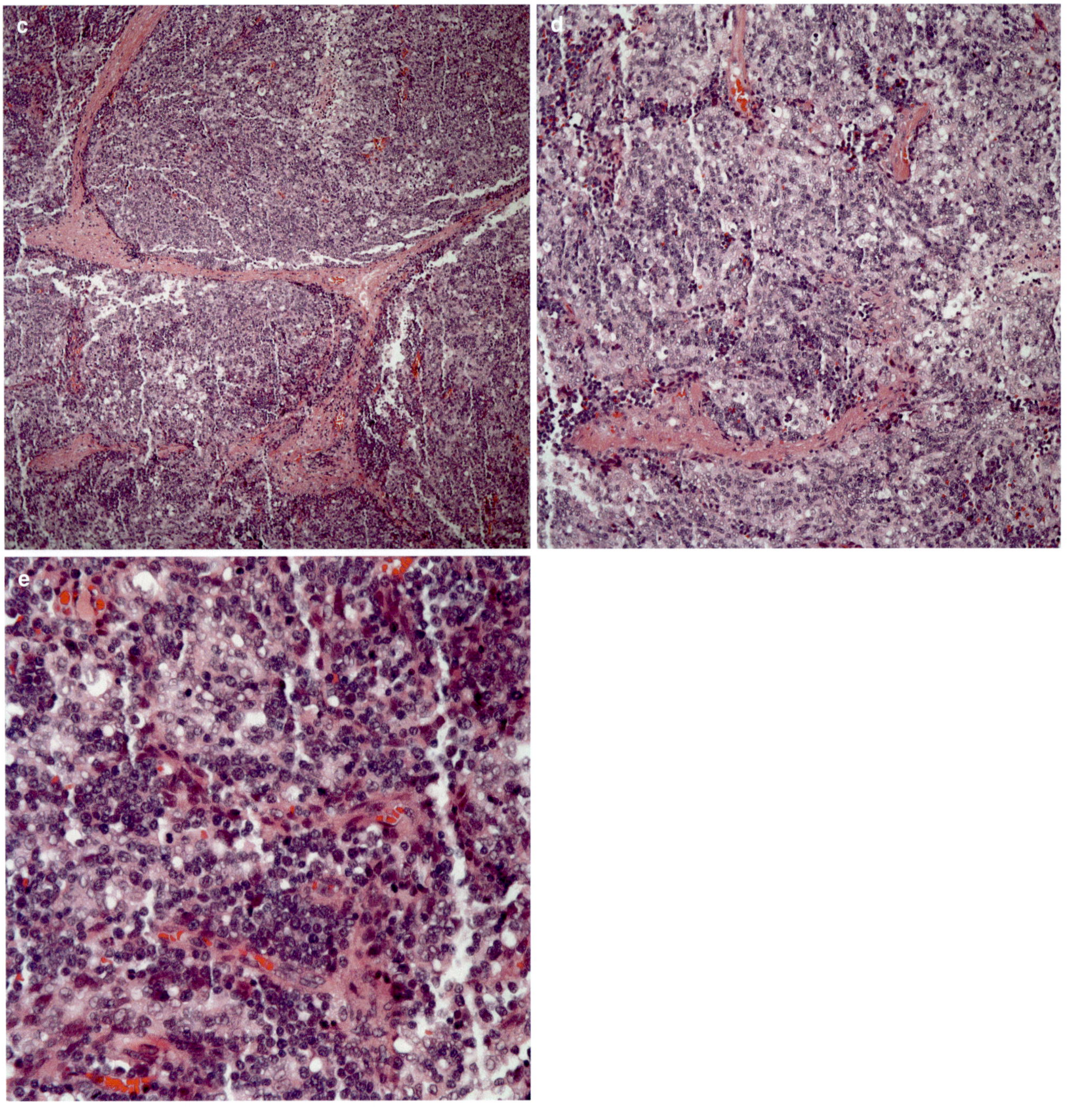

Fig. 8.16 (continued) (**c**) Low power view of an undifferentiated thymic carcinoma showing lobulation. (**d**) Cellular atypia and absence of an inflammatory reaction in undifferentiated thymic carcinoma. (**e**) Mitotic figures are easily encountered

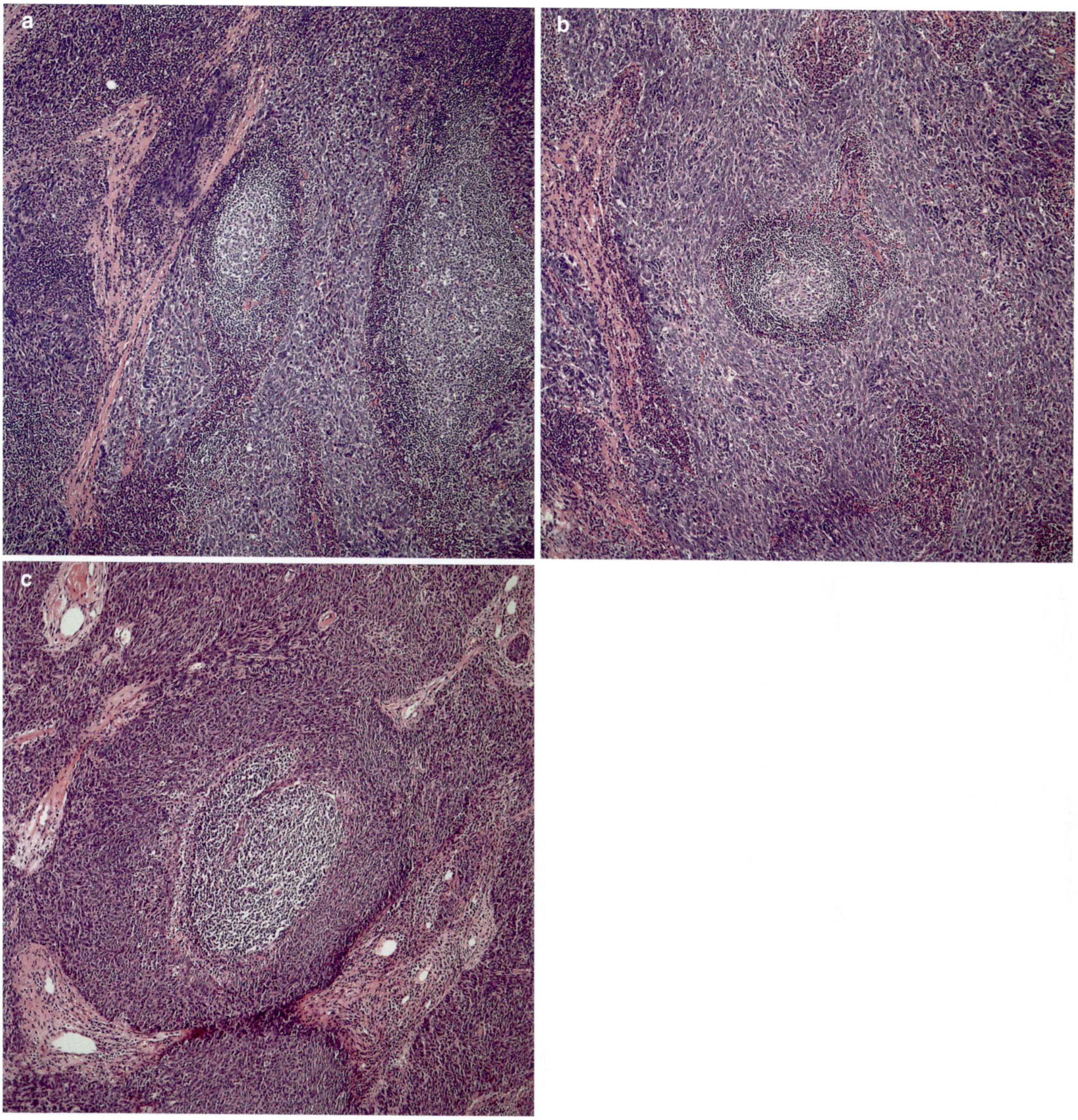

Fig. 8.17 (**a**) Undifferentiated thymic carcinoma with prominent germinal centers. (**b**) Undifferentiated thymic carcinoma with mixture of round and spindle cells circling a germinal center. (**c**) Similar area of prominent germinal center with features mimicking Castleman's disease

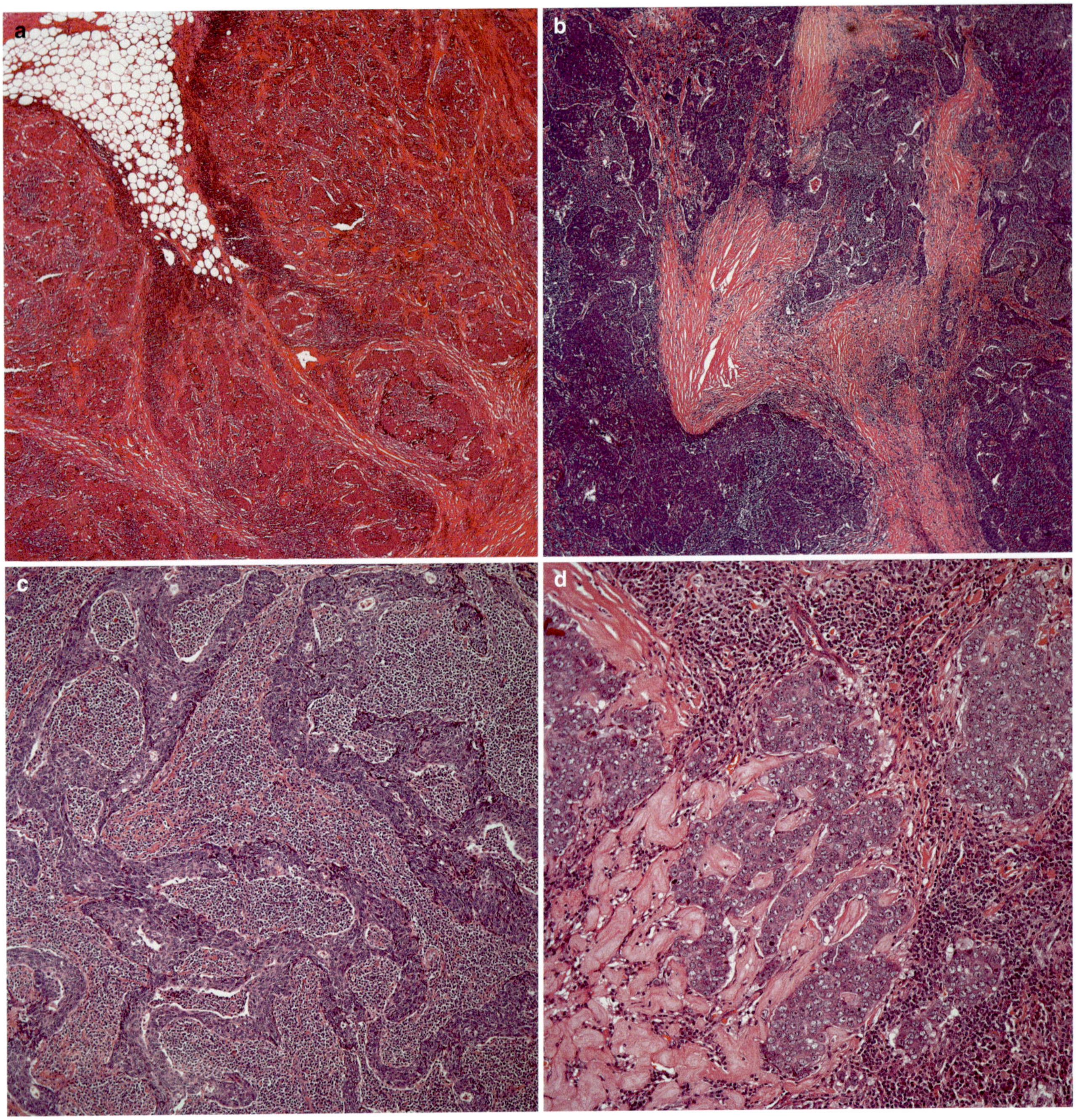

Fig. 8.18 (**a**) Low power of a lymphoepithelioma-like carcinoma of the thymus infiltrating thymic and adipose tissue. (**b**) Lymphoepithelioma-like carcinoma with islands of tumor cells. (**c**) Ribbons of tumor cells embedded in an inflammatory background. (**d**) Tumor cells embedded in amyloid-like reaction admixed with inflammatory cells

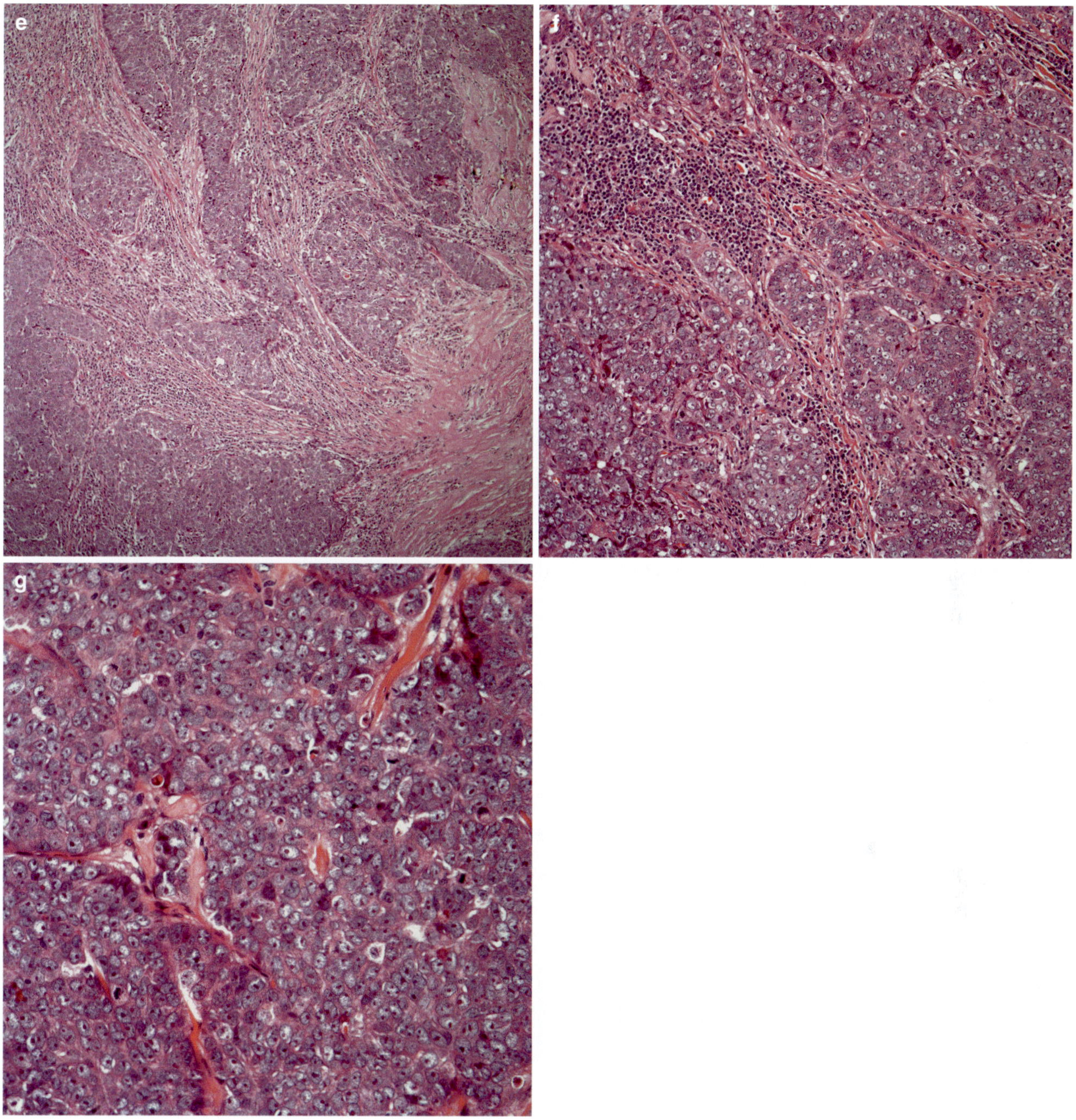

Fig. 8.18 (continued) (**e**) Tumor islands infiltrating fibroconnective tissue in an irregular growth pattern. (**f**) Tumor composed of medium-sized cells with round nuclei and prominent nucleoli. (**g**) Mitotic activity is easily encountered

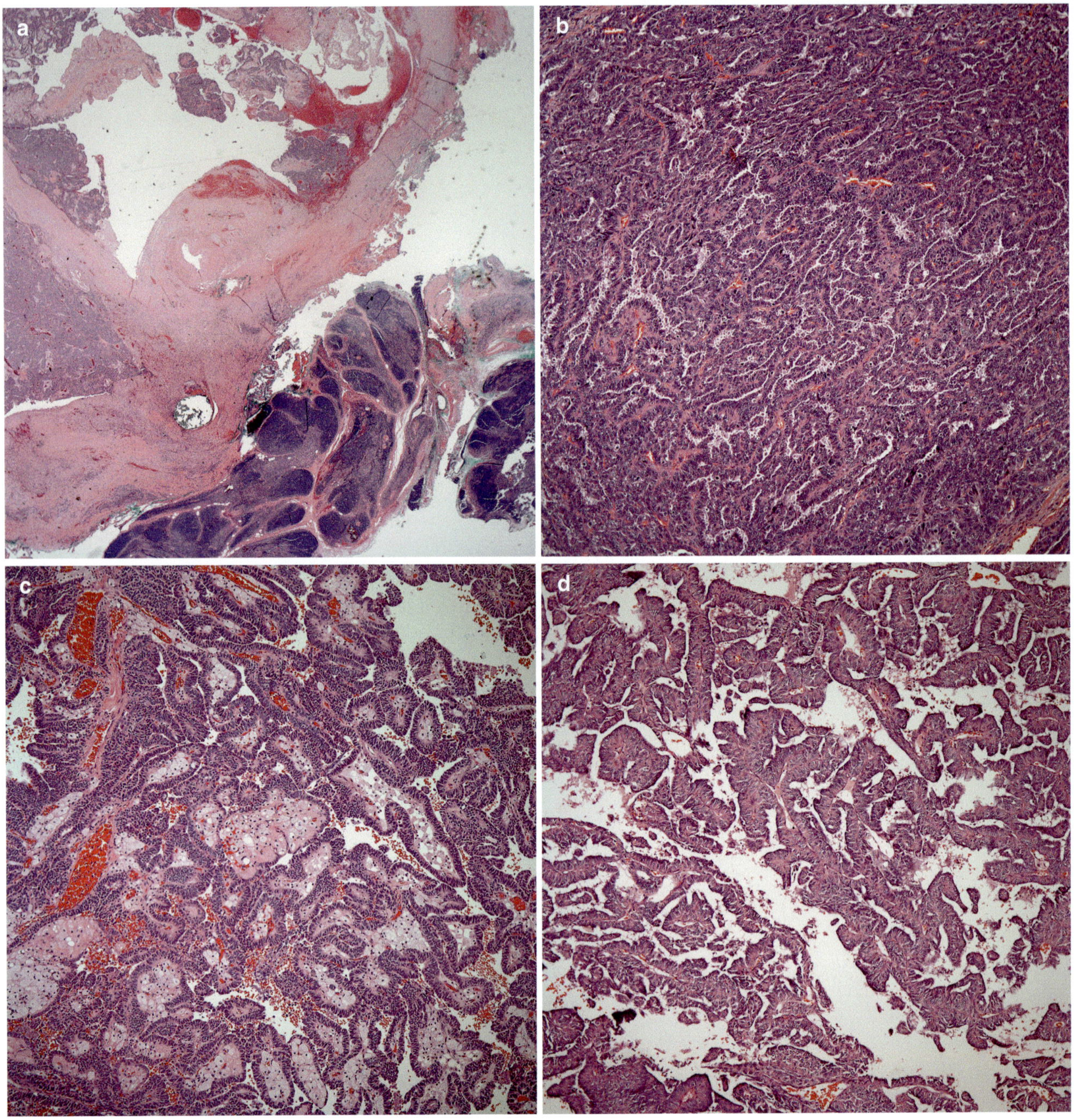

Fig. 8.19 Different growth patterns of papillary thymic adenocarcinoma. (**a**) Cystic tumor with a rim of thymic tissue in the periphery. (**b**) Tightly packed papillary structures arranged in a complex pattern. (**c**) Papillary structures filled with foamy macrophages. (**d**) Slimmed papillae with fibrovascular cores

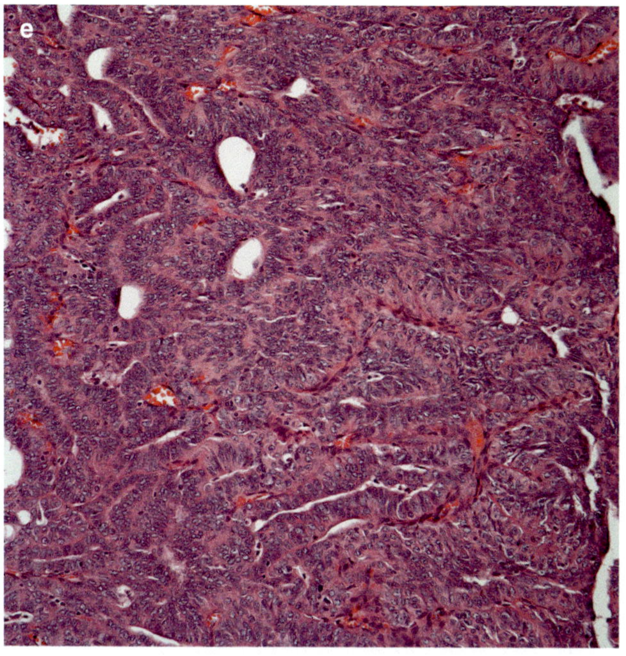

Fig. 8.19 (continued) (**e**) Solid-like areas in which the papillae are compressed

carcinoma. In general terms, thymic papillary carcinomas are rare and account for no more than 2–3% of these tumors. In addition, we have reported another variant in a recent publication on thymic adenocarcinomas in which the tumor shows a micropapillary growth pattern. Characteristically, micropapillary structures are floating in empty spaces separated by thin fibroconnective tissue. Psammoma bodies are common, and the micropapillae are lined by low cuboidal epithelium. Mitotic activity, nuclear atypia, and necrosis are generally absent (Fig. 8.22a–c).

Clear Cell Carcinoma

Snover and Rosai originally mentioned this type of thymic carcinoma in their publication on the "five distinctive histological variants," as the authors reported one case among others [7]. In addition, it has been anecdotally recorded in other series of thymic carcinomas as well as in case reports [42, 43]. The case described by Wolfe and colleagues [42] was in a 33-yer-old man with symptoms of fatigue and weight loss who showed an anterior mediastinal mass upon thoracic imaging. The case reported by Stephens and colleagues [43]

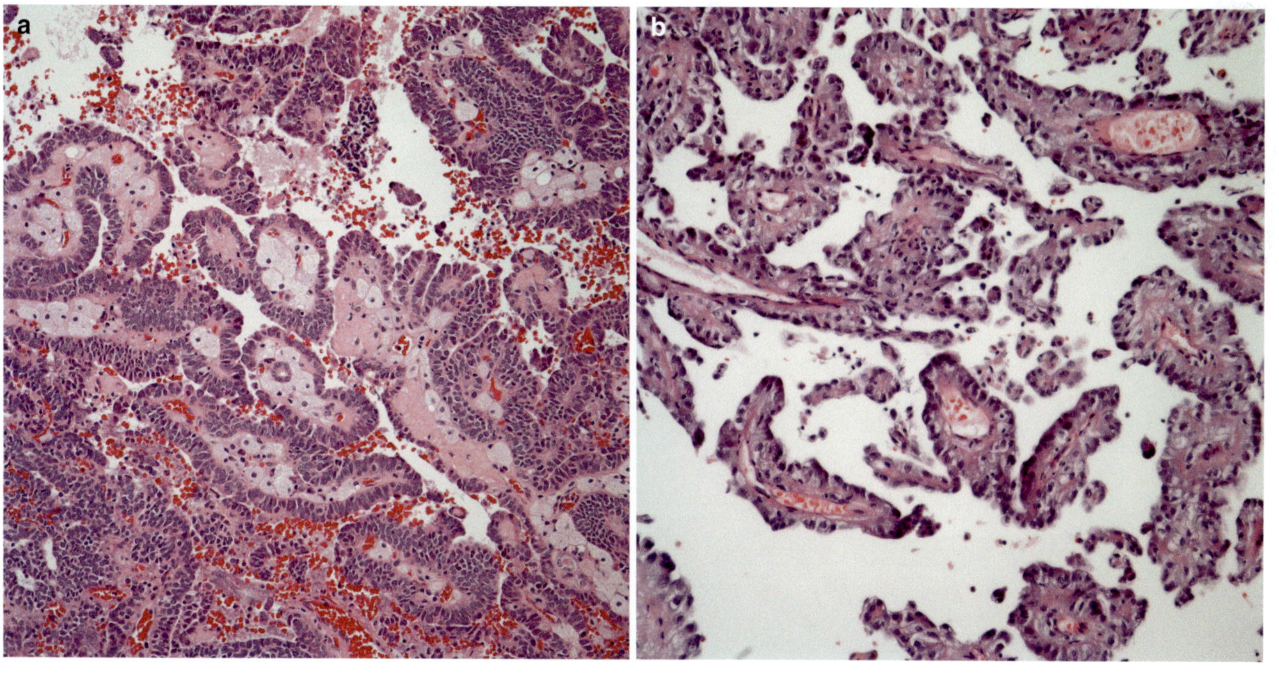

Fig. 8.20 Intermediate view of papillary thymic adenocarcinoma. (**a**) Papillary structures without significant nuclear atypia or mitotic activity. (**b**) Papillary structures of different sizes and shapes with fibrovascular core

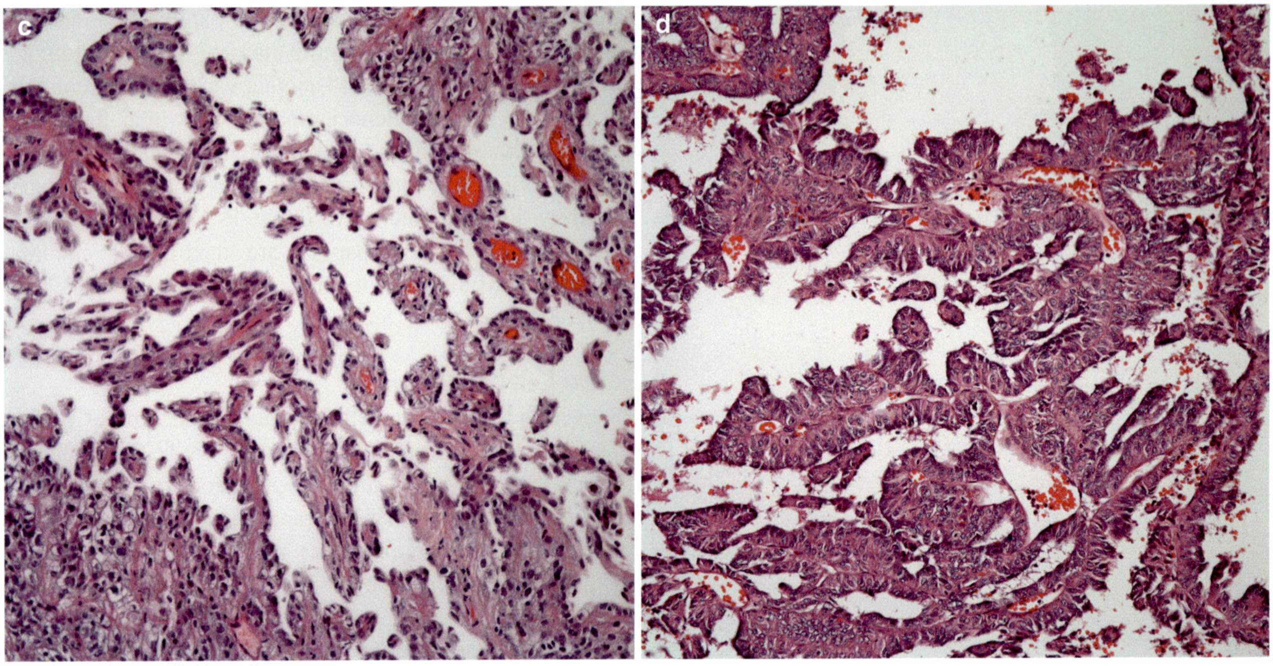

Fig. 8.20 (continued) (**c**) Elongated and compressed papillary structures. (**d**) Well-formed papillary structures with fibrovascular core

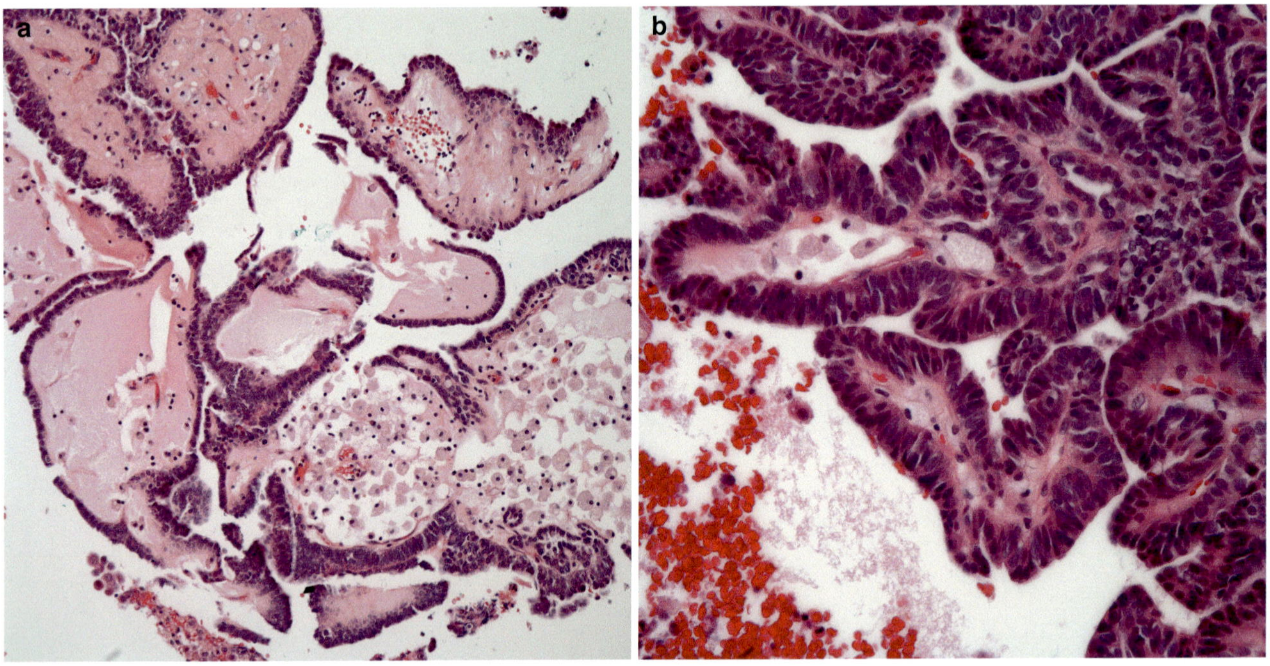

Fig. 8.21 High power view of papillary thymic adenocarcinoma. (**a**) Papillae lined by low cuboidal epithelium with minimal nuclear atypia and absent mitotic activity. (**b**) Papillary structures lined by columnar epithelium

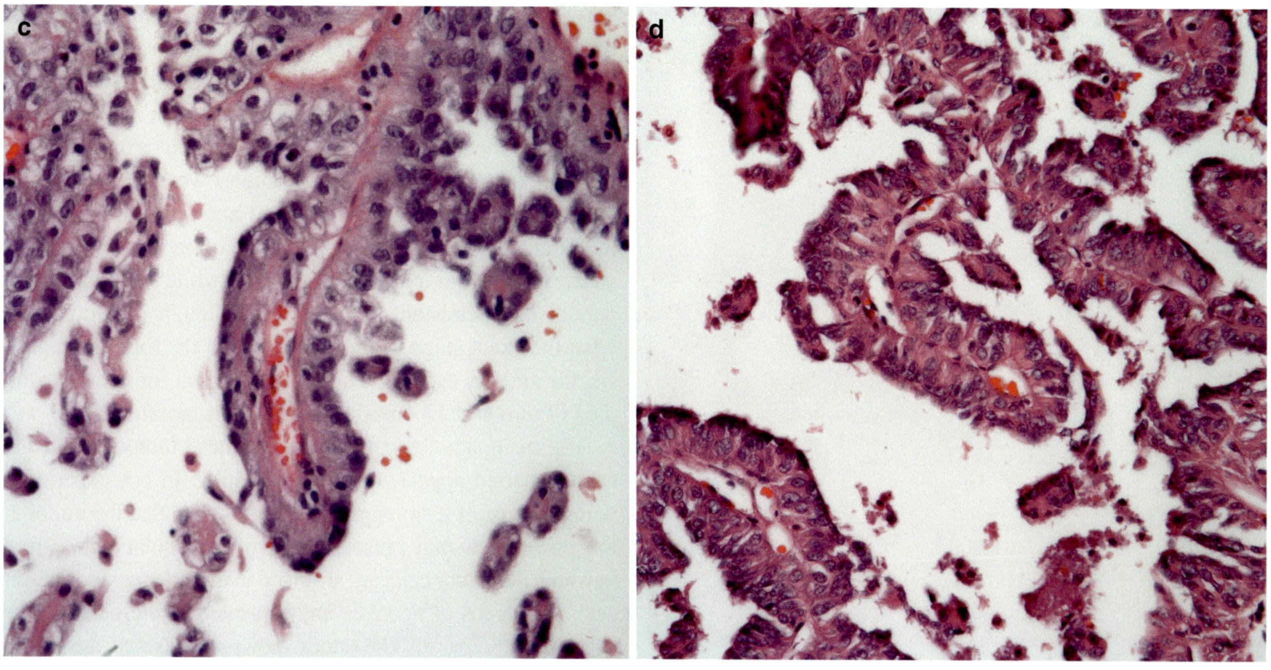

Fig. 8.21 (continued) (**c**) Papillary structures lined by cells with clearing of the cytoplasm and showing nuclear atypia. (**d**) Papillary structures lined with columnar-like type of epithelium

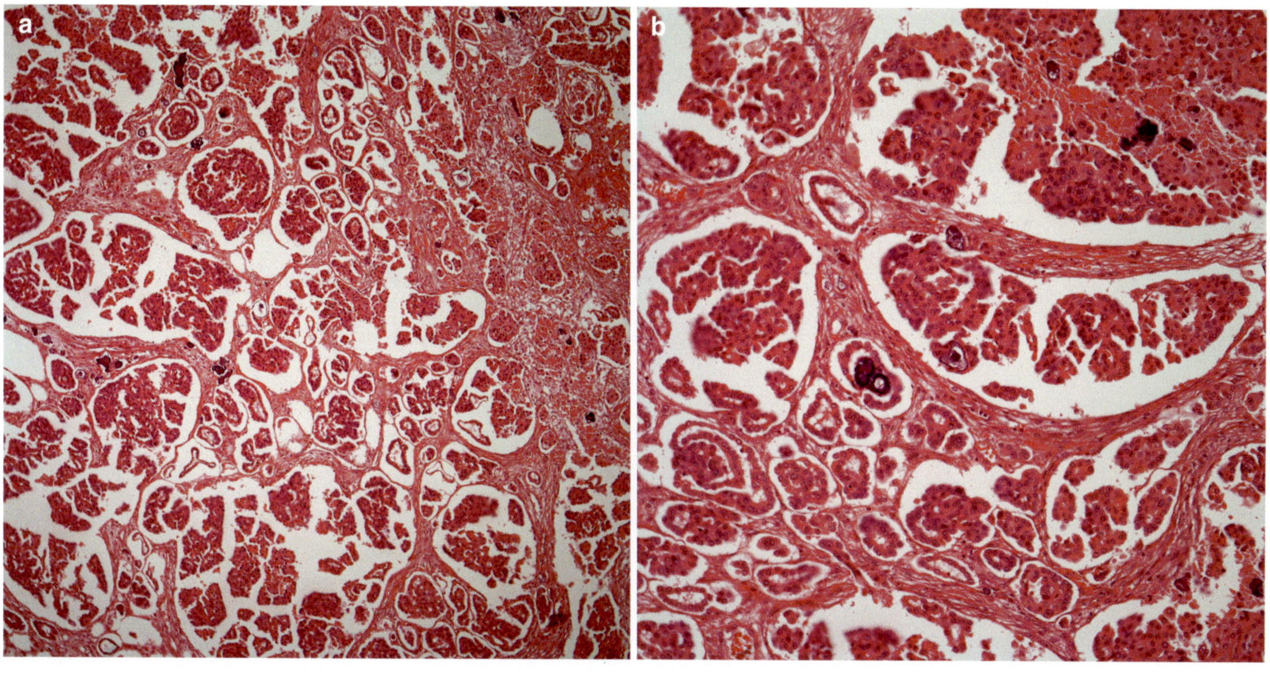

Fig. 8.22 Thymic micropapillary adenocarcinoma. (**a**) Micropapillae floating in empty spaces. (**b**) Micropapillae with scattered psammoma bodies

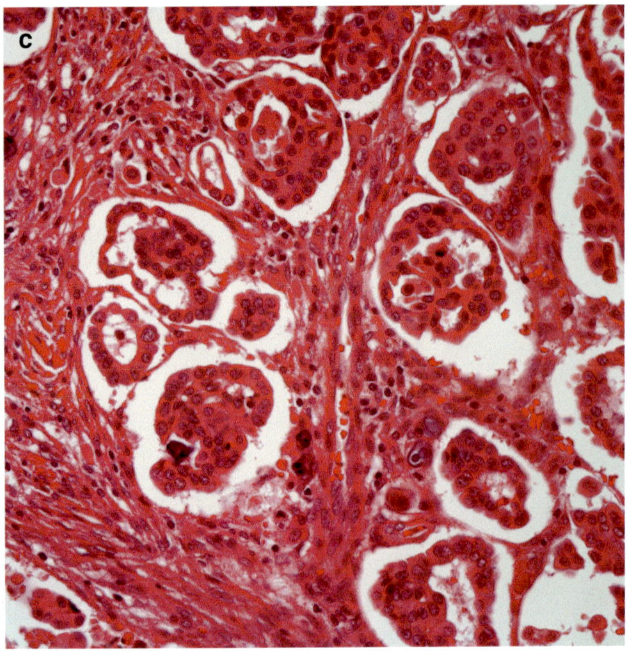

Fig. 8.22 (continued) (**c**) Micropapillae lined by low cuboidal epithelium with absent nuclear atypia or mitotic activity

was in a 72-year-old man who was asymptomatic, and the mediastinal mass was encountered during routine imaging. Hasserjian and colleagues [44] reported the largest series of thymic carcinomas with clear cell features in a report of eight cases: five men and three women between the ages of 36 and 84 years (mean, 52 years). Two patients were asymptomatic, and the remaining patients showed non-specific symptoms including dyspnea and chest pain. Follow-up information showed that four patients had died, while one additional patient had persistent disease. Even though it is not clear what the exact stage of the tumor was at the time of diagnosis, the authors estimated a median survival for patients who died of tumor at 13 months (range, 4–24 months).

The histopathological features of these tumors in all the cases reported appear to be fairly similar. In our experience with this type of histology, we have observed that the tumor at low power view may preserve some of the lobular architecture in which the tumor cells are arranged in irregular nests of tumor cells with areas of necrosis and separated by fibroconnective tissue (Fig. 8.23a, b). The tumor shows sheets or cords of neoplastic cells, composed of round to oval cells with clear cytoplasm, round nuclei, and inconspicuous nucleoli (Fig. 8.24a–c).

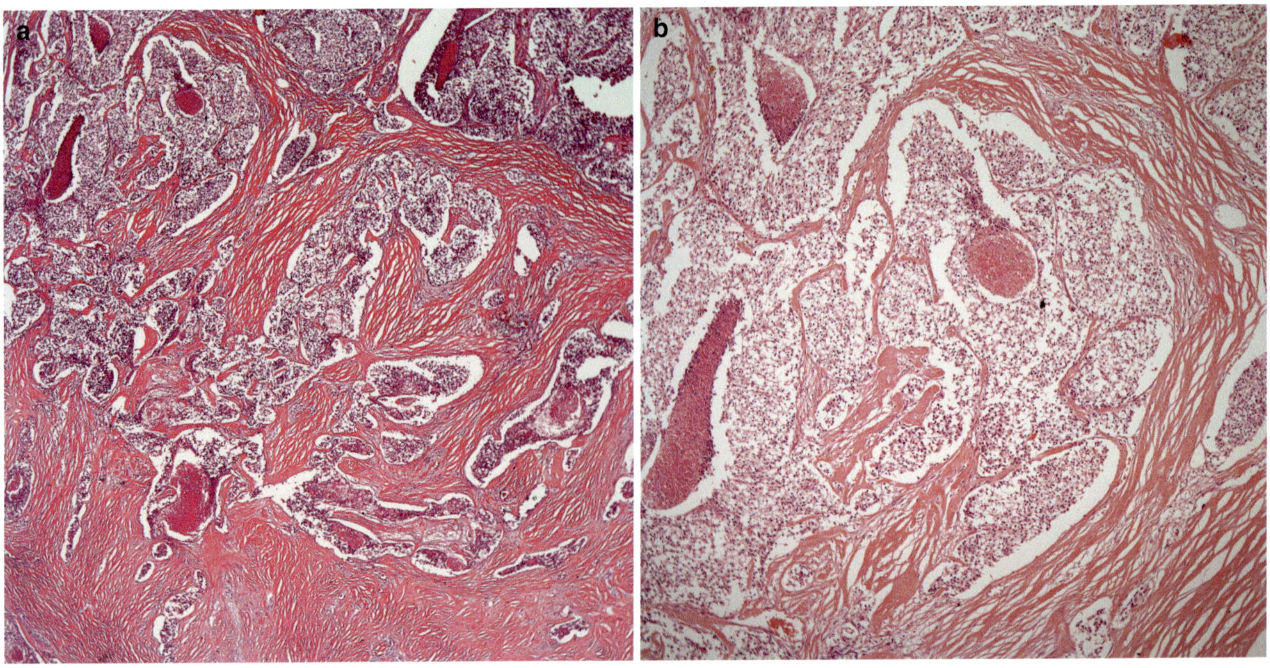

Fig. 8.23 Low power view of thymic carcinoma with clear cells features. (**a**) Tumor still preserves some lobular architecture, form by irregular nests of tumor cells. (**b**) Nests of tumor cells with necrosis, separated by fibroconnective tissue

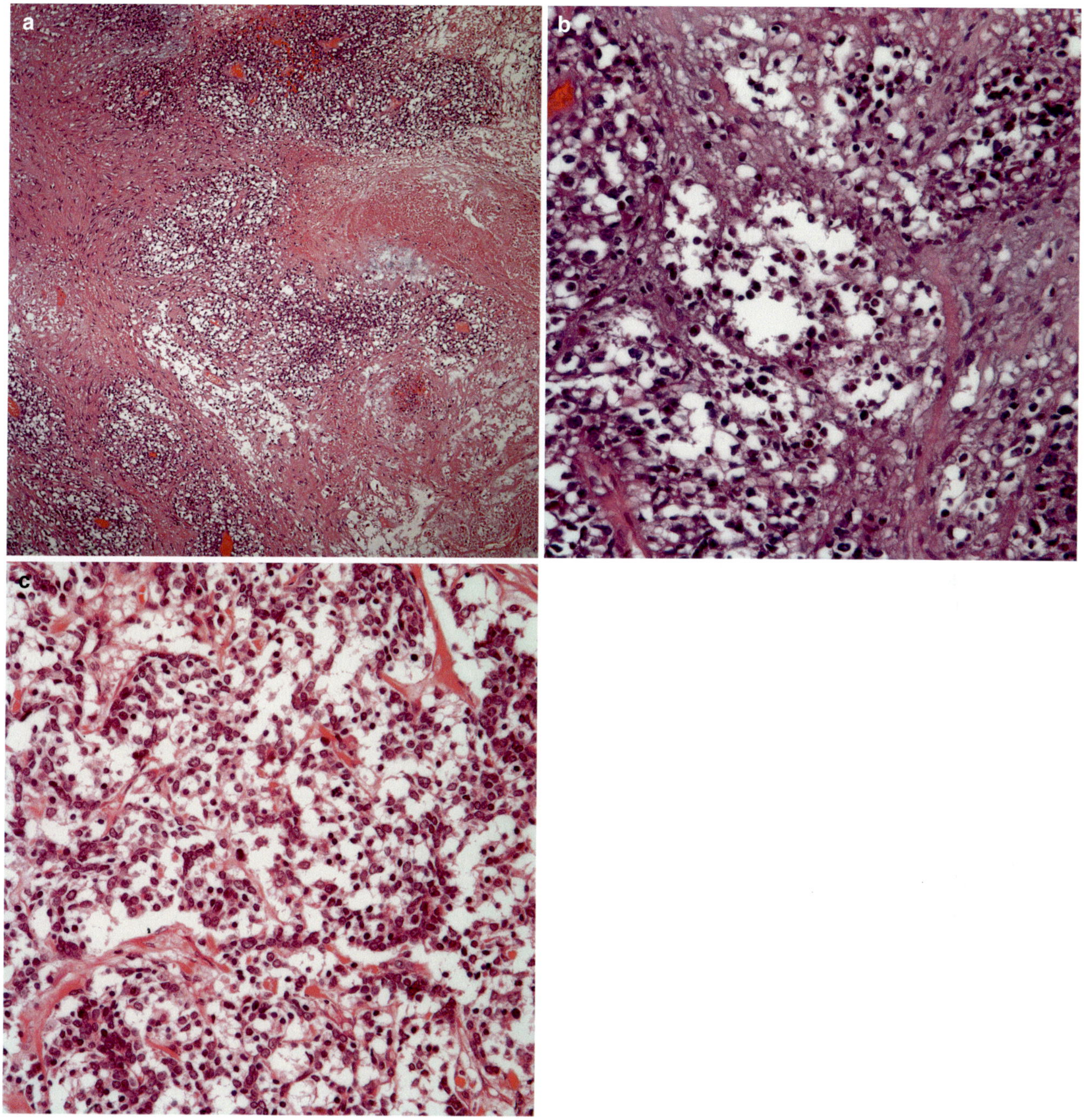

Fig. 8.24 Intermediate power view of thymic carcinoma with clear cell features. (**a**) Sheets of tumor cells admixed with necrotic areas. (**b**) Small nests of tumor cells with apoptotic nuclei. (**c**) Fairly homogeneous cellular population with mild nuclear atypia

Cellular atypia is not marked, and mitotic activity is variable and can be as high as 10 × 10 hpf (Fig. 8.25a–c). The tumor does not show glandular differentiation nor the presence of goblet cells. A focus of squamous cell differentiation has been reported in a single case. Lymphocytes are scant and generally admixed with tumor cells. Histochemical stain for periodic acid-Schiff (PAS) shows the presence of intracellular glycogen, while mucicarmine histochemical stain is generally negative for intracellular mucin. In general, thymic carcinomas with clear cell features account for no more than 3% of all thymic carcinomas.

Rhabdoid Carcinoma

This is a rare variant of thymic carcinoma representing no more than 1% of all these tumors. Tropani and colleagues [45] in 2003 reported what appears to be the first documentation of this unusual variant in a 67-year-old man who presented with chest pain and hemoptysis and who, upon chest imaging, was shown to have an anterior mediastinal mass. A radical thymectomy was performed, obtaining an 8 cm tumor mass, which histologically showed a solid proliferation of neoplastic cells arranged in nests and sheets of large pleomorphic cells with large nuclei and prominent nucleoli. The most salient feature of these tumors is the presence of intracytoplasmic paranuclear inclusions displacing the nuclei to the periphery of the cell. Mitotic activity is variable but easily identifiable. In our experience with these growth patterns, we have seen only a few of these types of cases with similar features as those described by Tropani and colleagues [45] in which the tumor shows a prominent neoplastic cellular proliferation composed of rhabdoid cells arranged in sheets of neoplastic cells (Fig. 8.26a–c).

Hepatoid Carcinoma

This variant of thymic carcinoma was documented by Franke and colleagues [46] in a case report of a 70-year-old woman with symptoms of dyspnea, who was found to have an anterior mediastinal mass. Resection of the mediastinal mass was performed, and the tumor was described as well circumscribed, measuring more than 10 cm in greatest diameter. Histologically, the tumor was described as solid or trabecular sheets of neoplastic cells with a subtle nodular pattern, composed of medium-sized, round cells with round nuclei and prominent nucleoli. Mitotic activity was described as present but not increased. Intraepithelial lymphocytes were not observed. It is possible that this variant of thymic carcinoma may merge with other tumors that in other series of cases have been termed "undifferentiated large cell" carcinoma. In our experience with this type of histology, we have observed a similar growth pattern that is characteristically nodular, and separated by thin fibroconnective tissue with inflammatory cells. These nodules are composed of polygonal cells with ample eosinophilic cytoplasm, round nuclei, and nucleoli. At higher magnification, the tumor cells may have intranuclear inclusion and also show the presence of intracytoplasmic hyaline globules (Fig. 8.27a–d).

Anaplastic Carcinoma

This variant is also rare and may account for approximately 1% of all thymic carcinomas. Once again, this type of carcinoma has been recognized in other series of cases and may be related to tumors that have been coded under different terminology, such as large cell undifferentiated or pleomorphic carcinoma. In 2012, we reported six cases of such a tumor under the designation of "anaplastic carcinoma" [47]. The tumors were described in five women and one man between the ages of 42 and 72 years (mean, 62 years) who presented with non-specific symptoms including cough, dyspnea, and chest pain. Histologically, the tumors are characterized by the presence of islands of tumor cells composed of large polygonal cells with distinct cell borders, basophilic cytoplasm, marked nuclear pleomorphism, and prominent nucleoli. Presence of atypical multinucleated giant cells is often seen haphazardly placed between tumor cells. Mitotic activity is easily identifiable but is not dramatically increased. Follow-up was available in only four of the six cases described and showed that three patients had died between 14 and 63 months after initial diagnosis. It was concluded that thymic anaplastic carcinoma has an aggressive behavior (Fig. 8.28a–c).

Micronodular Carcinoma with Lymphoid Hyperplasia

This variant represents the malignant counterpart of micronodular thymoma with lymphoid hyperplasia described by Suster and Moran in 1999 [48] (see the chapter on thymoma). This thymic carcinoma variant [49] was reported in five patients, three men and two women between the ages of 42 and 78 years (mean: 64 years). Three patients were asymptomatic, while two patients presented with non-specific symptoms of dyspnea and chest pain. Histologically, the tumor characteristically grows in a micronodular fashion with islands of epithelial cells embedded in a lymphoid-rich stroma, which shows florid lymphoid hyperplasia with presence of germinal centers. The epithelial islands, contrary to the thymoma counterpart, show a marked atypical cellular proliferation composed of spindle, round, or oval cells with vesicular nuclei, prominent nucleoli, and moderate eosinophilic cytoplasm. In addition, increased mitotic activity is usually present. Focal keratinization may be seen in some cases. Necrosis may be present, but it is not extensive, when present, it may be in the form of comedo-like type of necrosis (Fig. 8.29a–g).

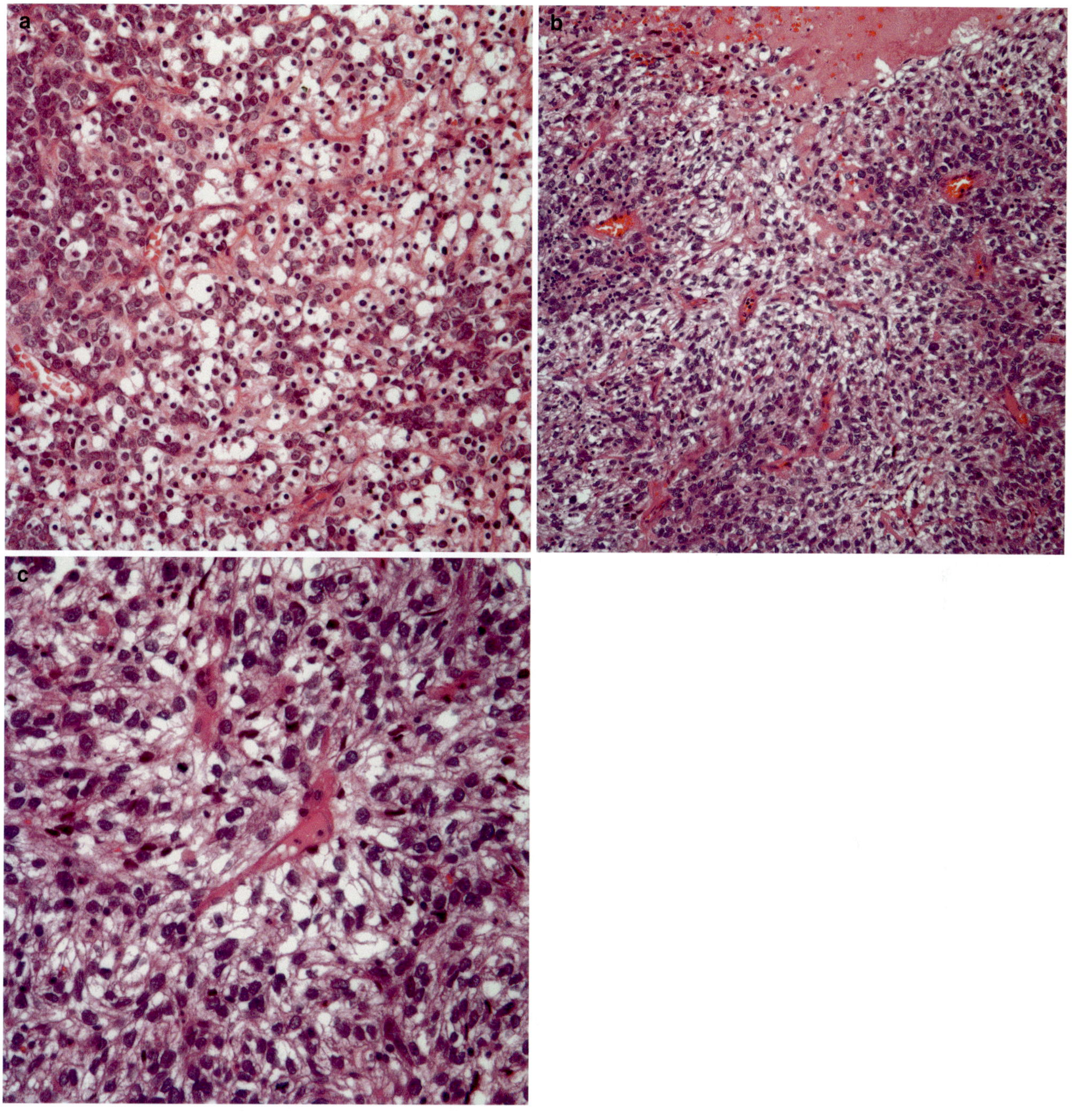

Fig. 8.25 High power view of thymic carcinoma with clear cell features. (**a**) Medium-sized cells with round nuclei, some cells with prominent nucleoli and clear cytoplasm. (**b**) Sheets of tumor cells with clear cytoplasm and a discrete fibrovascular network. (**c**) Moderate nuclear atypia and mitotic activity

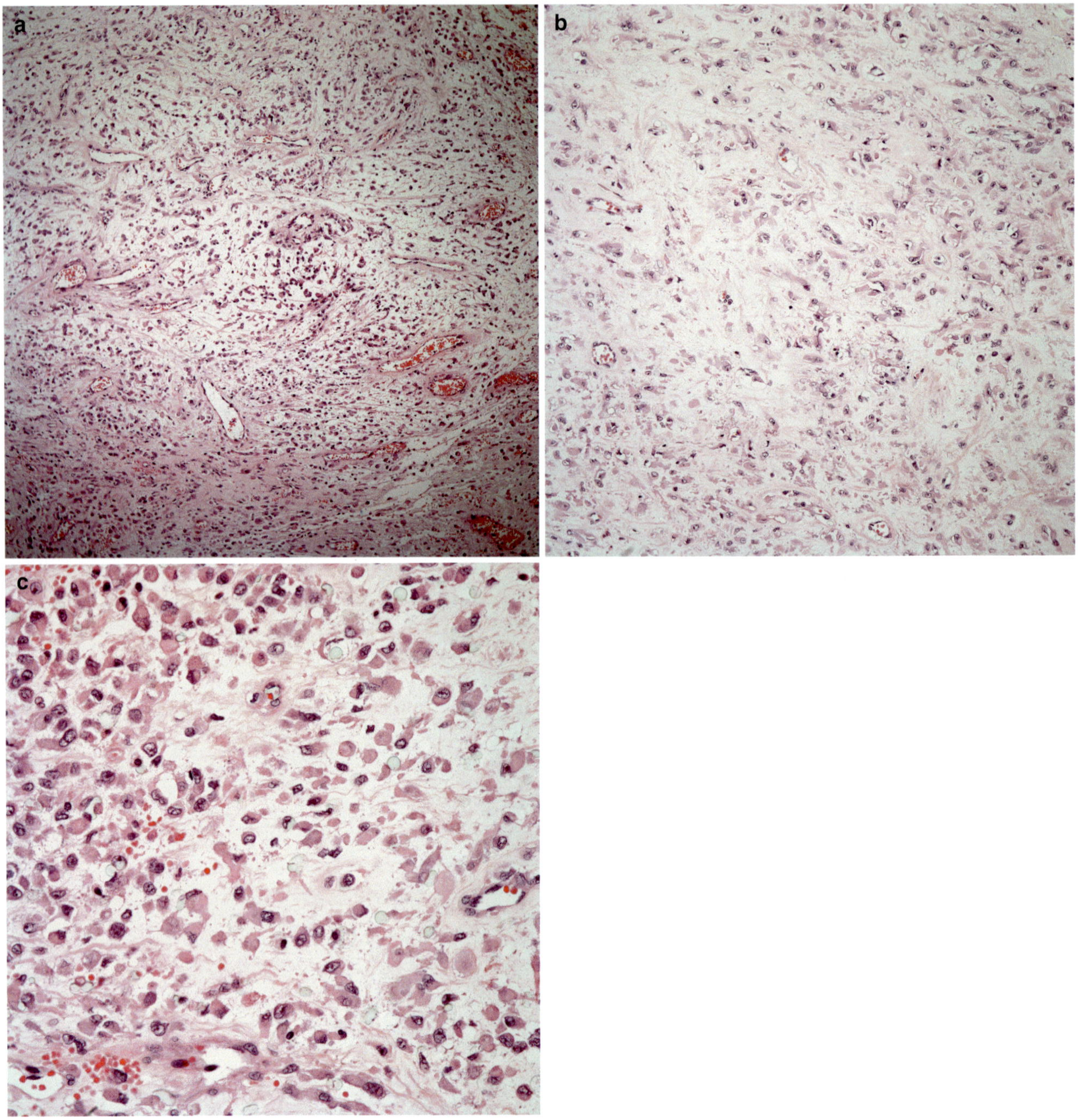

Fig. 8.26 (**a**) Low power view of a primary thymic rhabdoid carcinoma. (**b**) Sheets of tumor cells embedded in a collagenous stroma. (**c**) Tumor cells showing a rhabdoid appearance

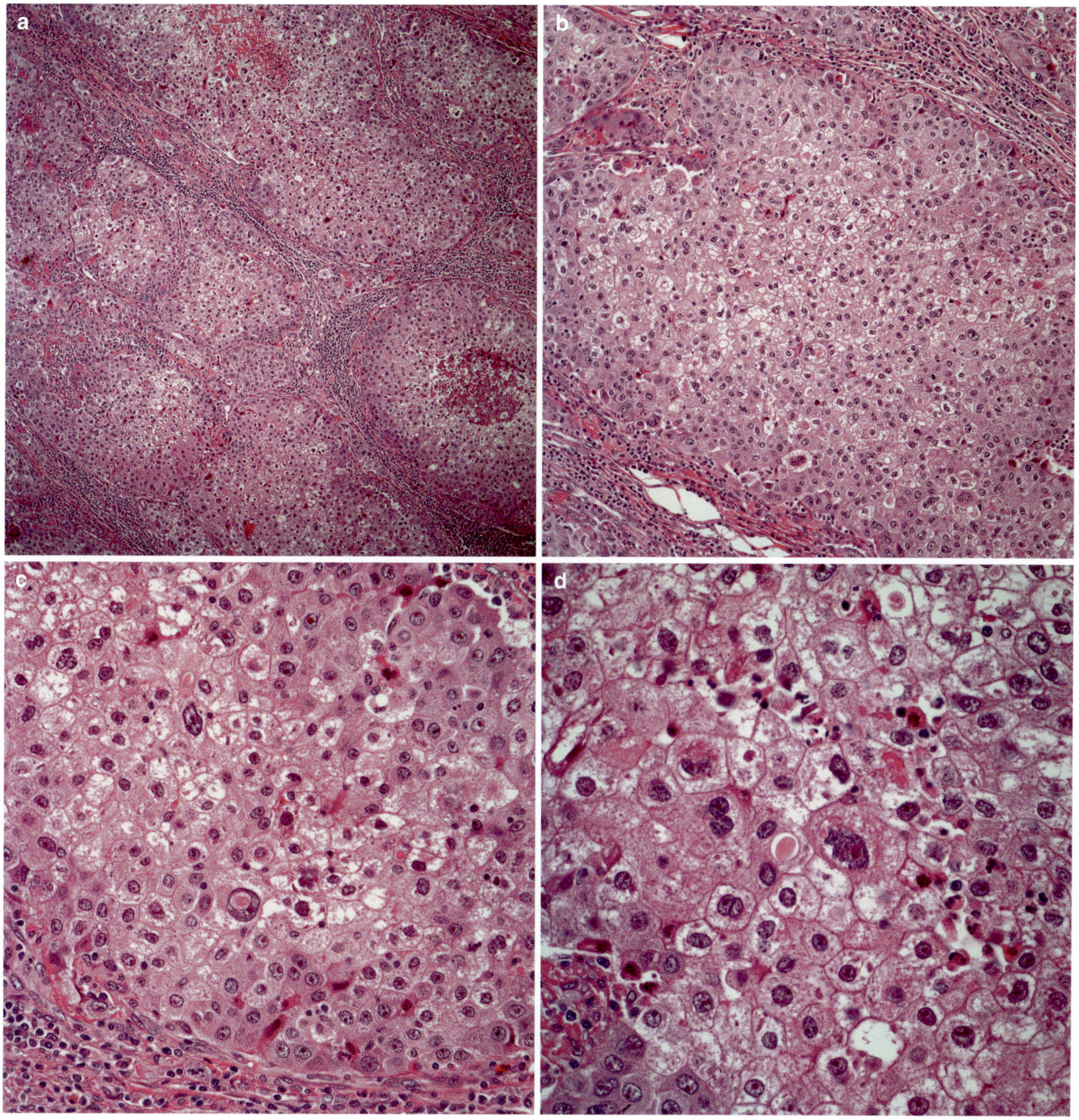

Fig. 8.27 (**a**) Low power view of a hepatoid thymic carcinoma showing a nodular pattern. (**b**) Polygonal cells with ample eosinophilic cytoplasm. (**c**) Presence of intranuclear inclusion. (**d**) Atypical cells with prominent nucleoli and the presence of intracytoplasmic hyaline globules

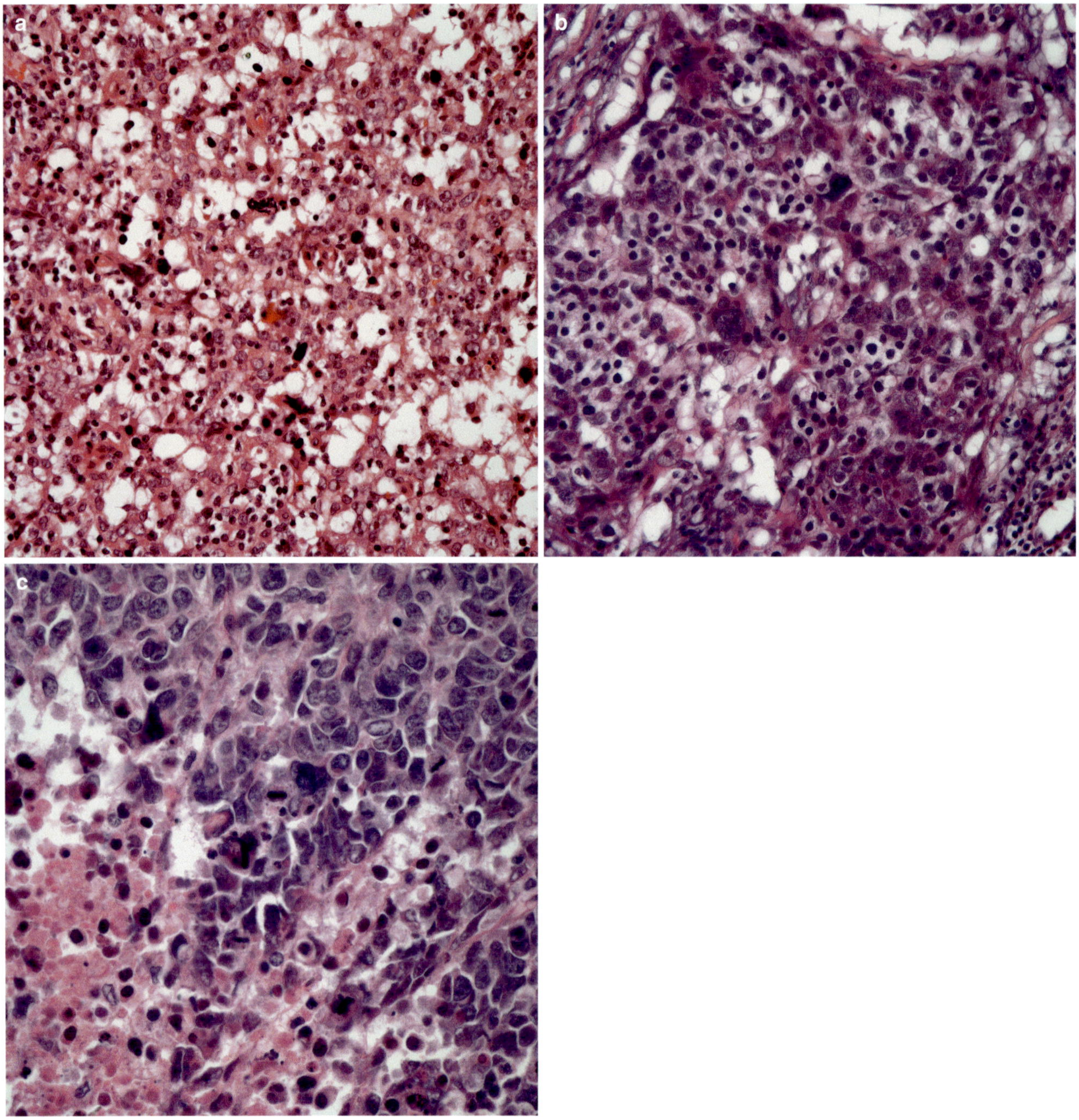

Fig. 8.28 (**a**) Thymic anaplastic carcinoma showing atypical mitotic figures and scattered multinucleated giant cells. (**b**) Multinucleated giant cells with prominent nucleoli. (**c**) Necrosis, multinucleated giant cells, and mitotic activity

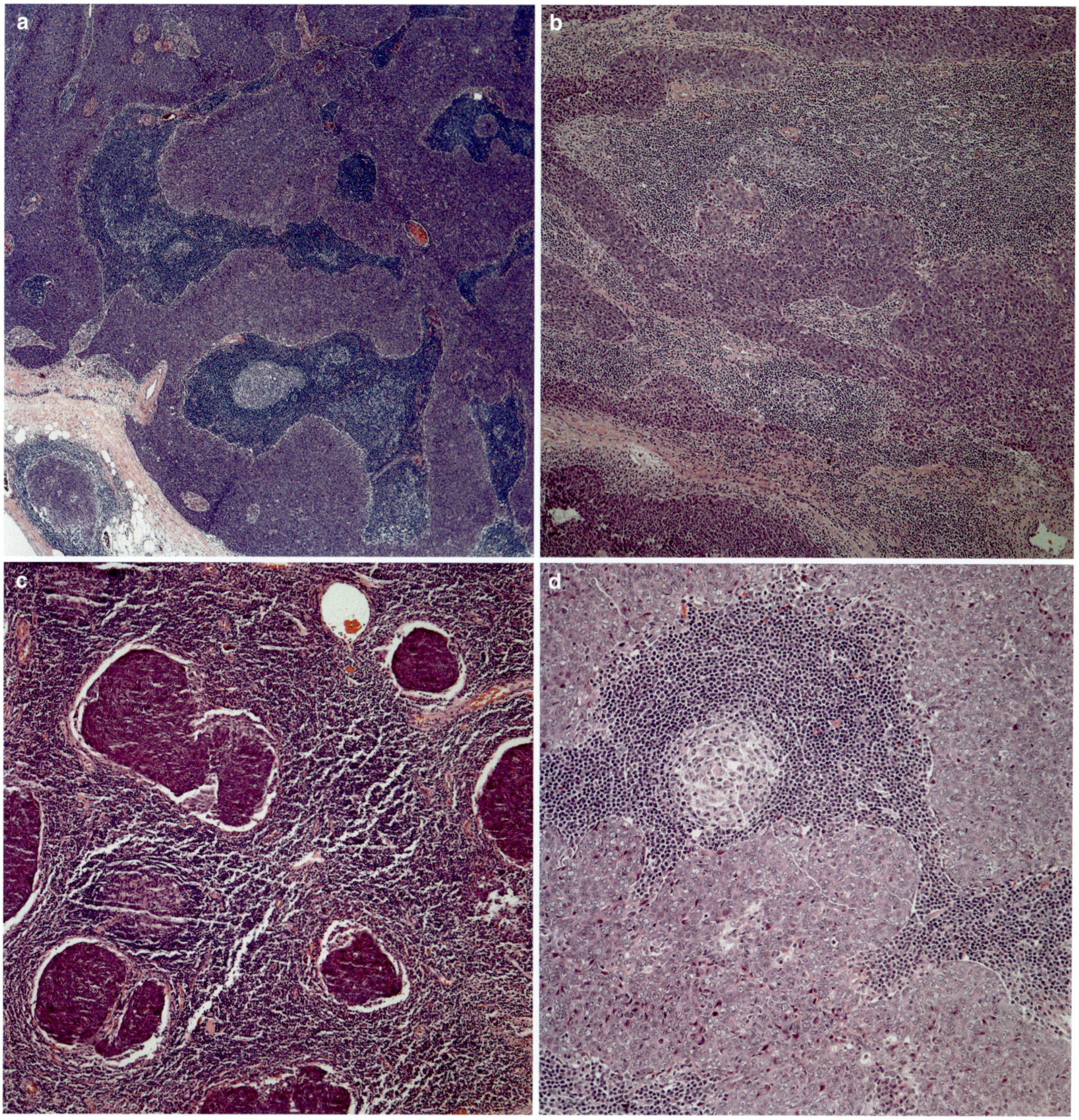

Fig. 8.29 (**a**) Micronodular thymic carcinoma showing nodules of tumor cells with prominent lymphoid hyperplasia. (**b**) Tumor cells growing in ribbons. (**c**) Tumor cells appear to be floating in empty spaces. (**d**) Contrast between the tumor cells and the presence of a germinal center

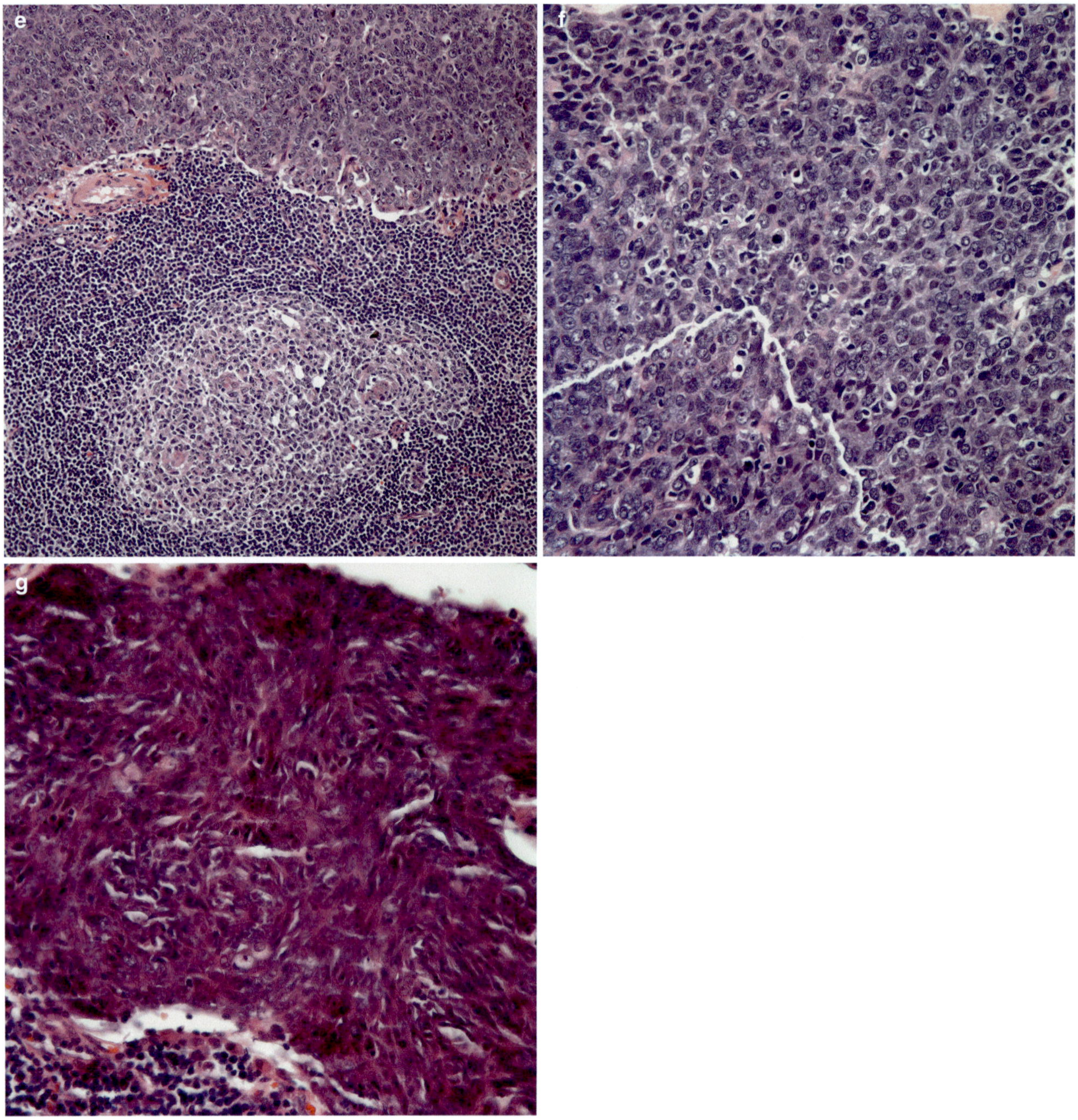

Fig. 8.29 (continued) (**e**) Prominent germinal center and adjacent tumor with cellular atypia and mitotic activity. (**f**) Higher magnification of the tumor cells composed of oval cells with round nuclei, prominent nucleoli, and mitotic activity. (**g**) Tumor cells showing spindle cell features

Other Unusual Variants

Two other additional variants of thymic carcinoma have been described as isolated case reports. However, we have been able to identify additional such cases: thymic carcinoma with rhabdomyomatous component and thymic carcinoma with neuroblastoma. The former unusual variant of thymic carcinoma was described by de Queiroga and colleagues [50] in a description of a 70-year-old woman with a posterior mediastinal mass. Histologically, the tumor showed a high-grade malignancy composed of islands of atypical cells with vesicular nuclei, prominent nucleoli, and increased mitotic activity in association with extensive areas of necrosis. In addition, the malignant epithelial component was associated with a conspicuous cellular proliferation composed of cells with bright eosinophilic cytoplasm and small, round, eccentrically placed nuclei (rhabdomyomatous component) (Fig. 8.30a, b). On the other hand, Alguacil-Garcia and Halliday [51] reported a 60-year-old man who, during a surgical heart procedure, was found to have a small nodule in the left lobe of the thymus. Histologically, the tumor was described as a conventional carcinoma with scattered islands of solid, small round or oval clusters of cells with occasional pseudorosettes embedded in an eosinophilic fibrillary background (neutrophil). Recently, we had the opportunity to see such an occurrence in an adult individual in which the main tumor mass was that of a thymic carcinoma with a separate area of neuroblastoma. In addition, the tumor also showed cystic changes (Fig. 8.31a–d). These two variants of thymic carcinoma are rare and may pose significant problems in interpretation.

Adenocarcinoma

Contrary to the fact that the great majority of thymic carcinomas are represented by squamous cell carcinomas of the different grades of differentiation, the occurrence of thymic adenocarcinoma is unusual, and poses significant problems not only in the diagnosis of the tumor but also in assigning the thymus as the primary site. It is known that in the thoracic cavity, adenocarcinomas are by far more common in the lung, and if to that fact we add that many adenocarcinomas of extrathoracic origin often metastasize to the lung, then the interpretation of primary adenocarcinoma of the thymus requires a more complete clinical and radiological correlation excluding not only a pulmonary adenocarcinoma but also excluding an adenocarcinoma of extrathoracic origin. Nevertheless, primary adenocarcinomas of the thymus have been reported, and rare cases have been included in several series of thymic carcinoma, as other variants of thymic carcinoma. However, in actuality, the reports specifically addressing the issue of thymic adenocarcinoma are limited to a single or three case reports [52–67]. However, it is also important to highlight that many cases that have been coded under the term *papillary carcinoma* may also be grouped under the designation of papillary adenocarcinomas of the thymus, which is a more appropriate terminology. Tumors with that particular histology have already been addressed above. Clinically, thymic adenocarcinomas appear to have a slight predilection for men rather than women in a proportion of 1.5:1 and have been described in young patients as well as in older individuals, ranging in age from 15 to more than 80 years. The symptomatology is varied and non-specific and would include chest pain, shortness of breath, and cough. Even though in several reports the authors have concluded that these tumors with this histology follow an aggressive behavior, there are also reports of patients who have survived 10 years or more without evidence of recurrence or metastasis. In cases in which the tumor has shown an aggressive behavior, the tumor has metastasized to the lung, the liver, or bone.

In general, the frequency of these tumors as primary thymic adenocarcinomas is rare, and up to now there are reports of approximately 50 cases in the literature. However, the histopathological growth patterns described including the papillary growth pattern, have been varied. We recently analyzed 16 primary thymic adenocarcinomas [68] in 9 men and 7 women between the ages of 22 and 68 years. Clinically, the patients presented with non-specific symptoms of cough, chest pain, and dyspnea. Diagnostic imaging in these patients showed an anterior mediastinal mass, and surgical resection of the tumor was performed in those patients. Macroscopically, the tumor size varied between 5 and 14 cm, and some tumors were described as having mucoid changes, while others were described as necrotic or cystic. However, the most important findings of this study were to identify several main growth patterns in these tumors:

- Mucin-rich adenocarcinoma of the so-called colloid carcinoma: in this variant, the tumors show extensive areas of mucinous material in which there may be floating clusters of malignant cells. In some areas, the tumor also shows cystic changes, while in focal areas the tumor may show signet-ring cell appearance (Fig. 8.32a–f).
- Non-mucinous adenocarcinoma: this tumor is characterized by either a proliferation of small to medium size glands or the presence of an intestinal-like growth pattern. In both of these patterns, it is possible to observe well-formed glands with focal areas of necrosis, tumor infiltrating adipose tissue, and cellular atypia with increased mitotic activity. In some cases, one can identify the presence of small glandular proliferation with marked cellular atypia and mitotic activity dissecting fibroconnective and adipose tissue (Fig. 8.33a–h).
- Papillary/micropapillary adenocarcinoma: this tumor is characterized by the presence of well-formed papillary structures with complex arrangement and separated by a delicate network of fibroconnective tissue. Cellular atypia

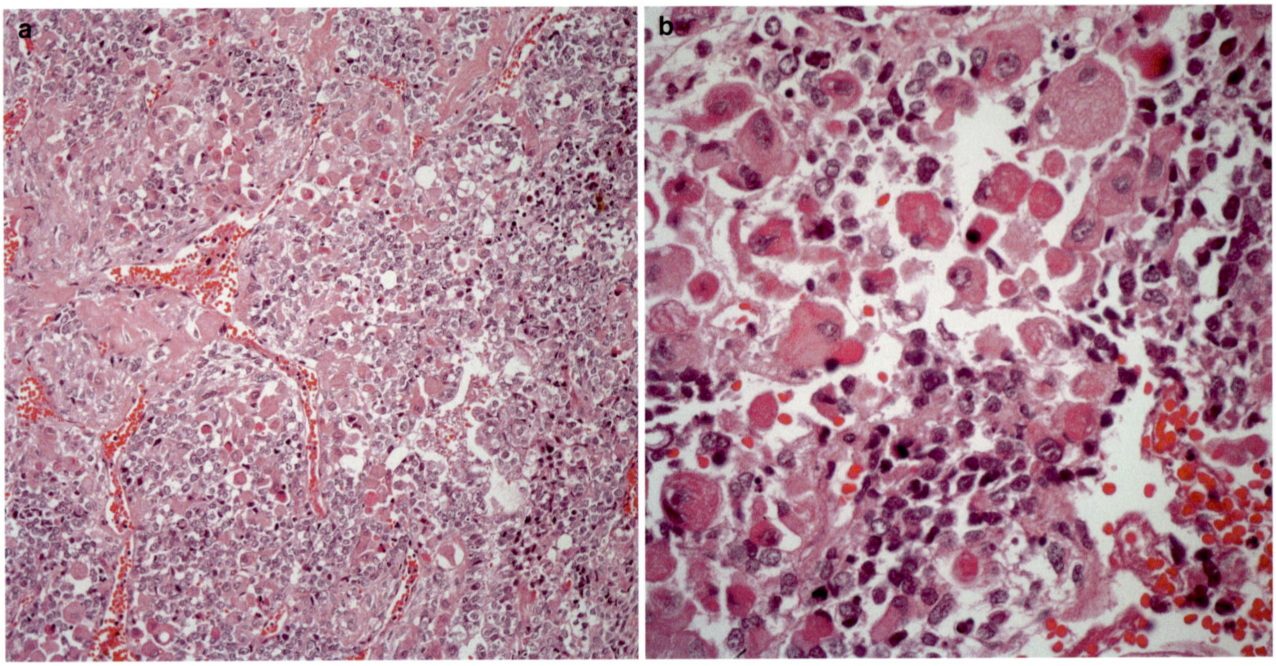

Fig. 8.30 (**a**) Low power view of a rhabdomyomatous thymic carcinoma showing the two different populations of cells. (**b**) Closer view at the rhabdomyomatous component

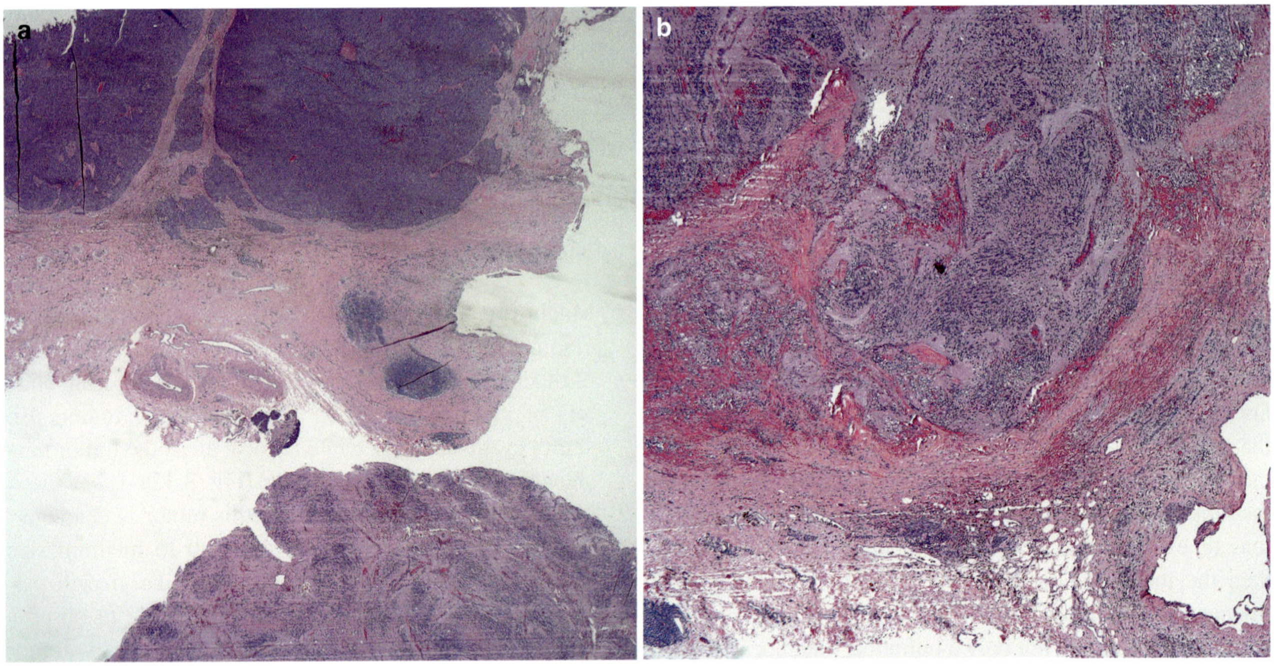

Fig. 8.31 (**a**) Low power view of a mixed thymic carcinoma and neuroblastoma. (**b**) Neuroblastoma with adjacent thymic cystic changes

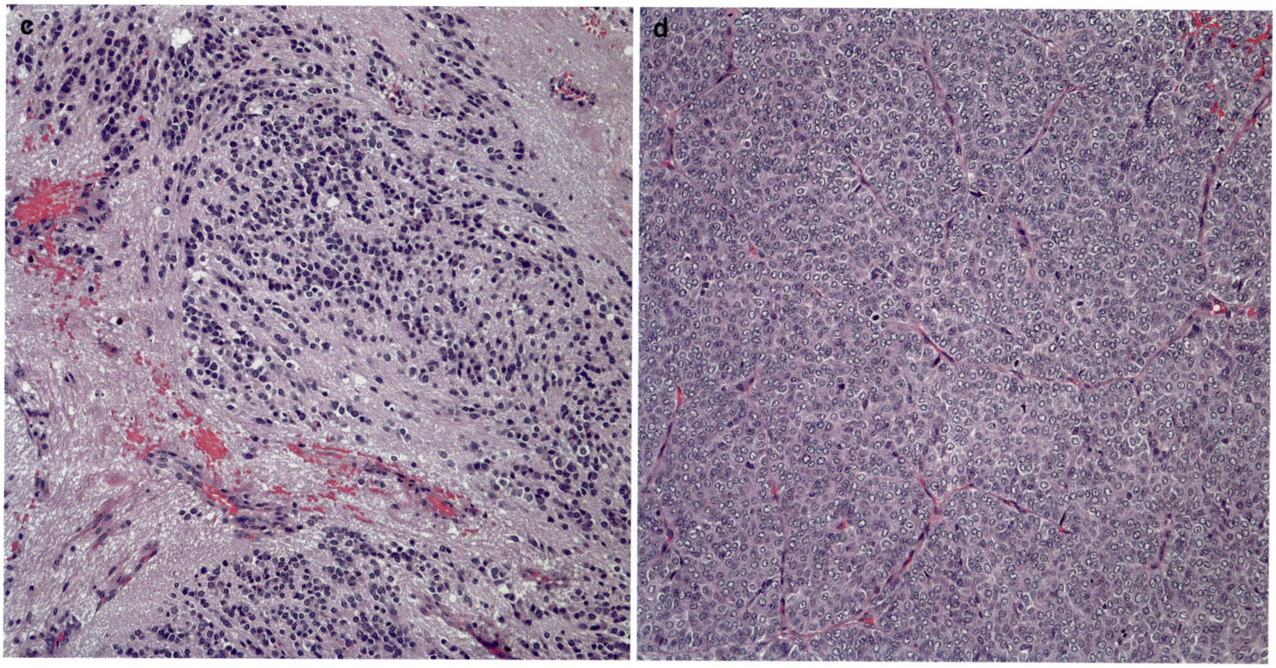

Fig. 8.31 (continued) (**c**) Closer view at the neuroblastomatous component with presence of neurophil. (**d**) Closer view at the thymic carcinoma showing nuclear atypia and mitotic activity

and mitotic activity are easily identifiable. In the micropapillary growth pattern, the tumor appears to be in spaces separated by fibroconnective tissue. The tumor cells are filling those spaces, and psammoma bodies are often present. In this variant, the tumor does not have prominent nuclear atypia or increased mitotic activity; also see papillary carcinoma above.

- In addition, we were able to identify some minor growth patterns that may accompany the main histology of the tumor. These minor patterns include solid areas in which the tumor does not show any glandular differentiation. Also, the minor growth patterns demonstrated the association of thymoma and thymic adenocarcinoma.

Even though we are proponents of the staging of these tumors as the best way to predict prognosis, it is important to highlight that in some cases in which the tumor may show metastatic spread at the time of diagnosis, the clinical follow-up has not been that of a fatal disease. Therefore, it is possible that there may be other mechanisms that may trigger a more rapid course in these cases.

It is also important to highlight the differences that may be observed with the use of immunohistochemical stains in thymic adenocarcinomas. Even though some of these results may correlate with the different histologies present in these tumors, we observed positive staining in tumor cells for keratin 7, keratin 20, CD5 (Fig. 8.34a), CDX2, and CD117 (Fig. 8.34b). Also, important to highlight is that PAX-8 and TTF1 are generally negative in these tumors.

Immunohistochemical and Molecular Features

Due to the rarity of thymic carcinomas, there is somewhat limited information regarding the immunohistochemical profile that those tumors may have. Nevertheless, numerous publications on the subject have been presented, mainly with the idea of attempting to separate thymic carcinomas from others carcinomas of different origin.

Fukai and colleagues [69], in a comparative study of lung carcinoma and thymic carcinoma, analyzed both of these tumors using cytokeratin 7 and 13 and identified that thymic squamous carcinomas were positive for cytokeratin 7 (monoclonal antibody RCK 105) (9/9 cases), while lung carcinomas were negative. Hishima and associates [70], in a study attempting to separate thymic carcinoma from thymoma, studied 23 thymic epithelial tumors, separating them into thymoma, atypical thymoma, and thymic carcinoma. The authors identified CD5 (receptor molecule that signals cell growth in T-cells) as a good marker to separate thymic carcinoma from thymoma; however, the authors also found that CD5 was also expressed in atypical thymomas. Additionally, the authors performed double labeling of tumor cells with CD5 and cytokeratin. In this study, the authors stated that CD5 was not identified in other carcinomas including breast, esophagus, stomach, colon, and uterus. Following this publication, several other studies have documented similar findings. Dorfman and associates [71] evaluated CD5 staining in 24 thymic carcinomas, identifying 16 cases with immunoreactivity to CD5. This staining was seen more often in squamous cell carcinoma (9/16) and less in other types of

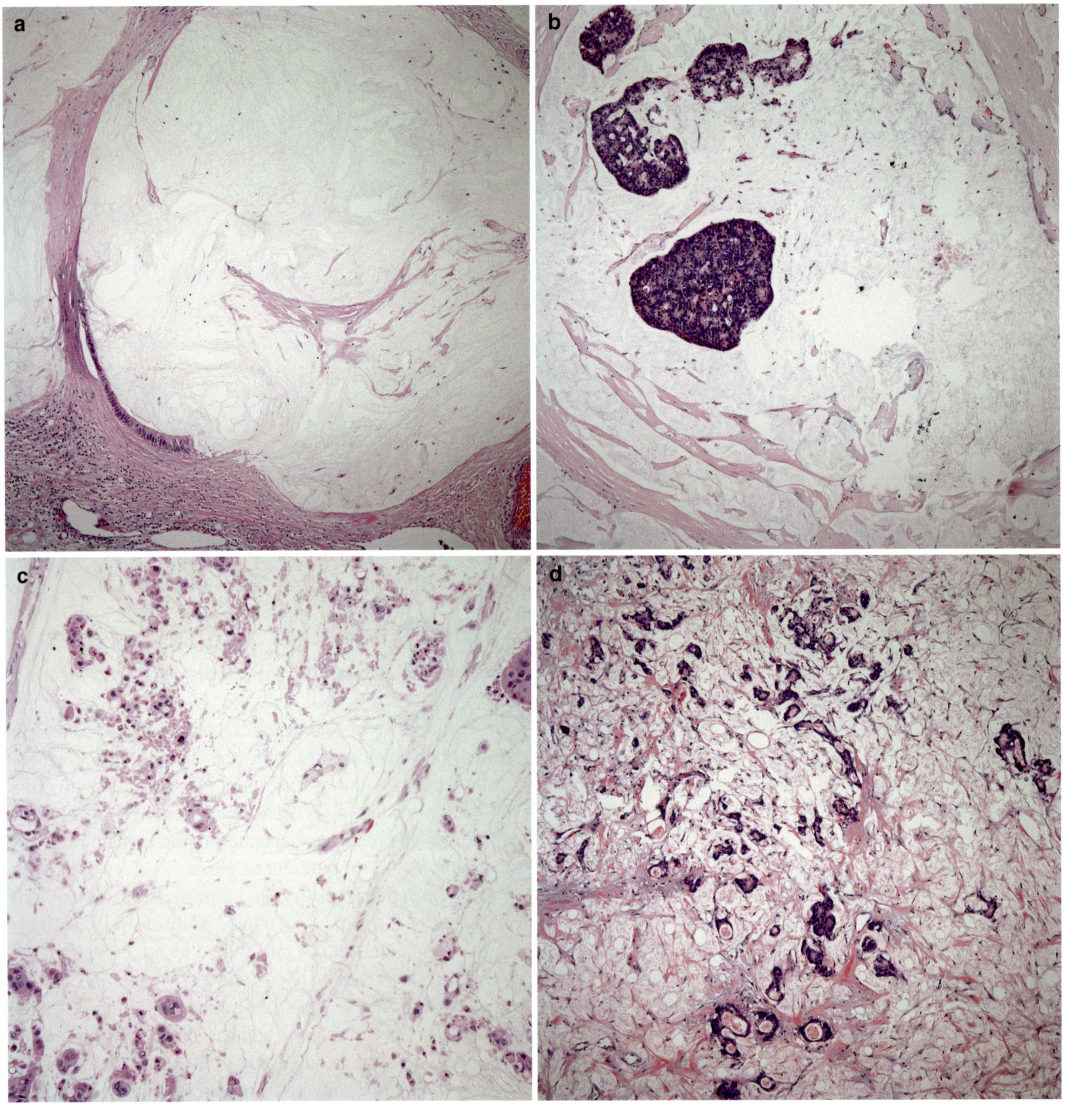

Fig. 8.32 (**a**) Mucinous adenocarcinoma of the thymus showing extensive mucin deposition and only a rim of mucinous epithelium. (**b**) Small islands of malignant cells embedded in mucinous pools. (**c**) Single malignant cells floating in a mucinous pool. (**d**) Well-formed malignant glands embedded in mucinous stroma

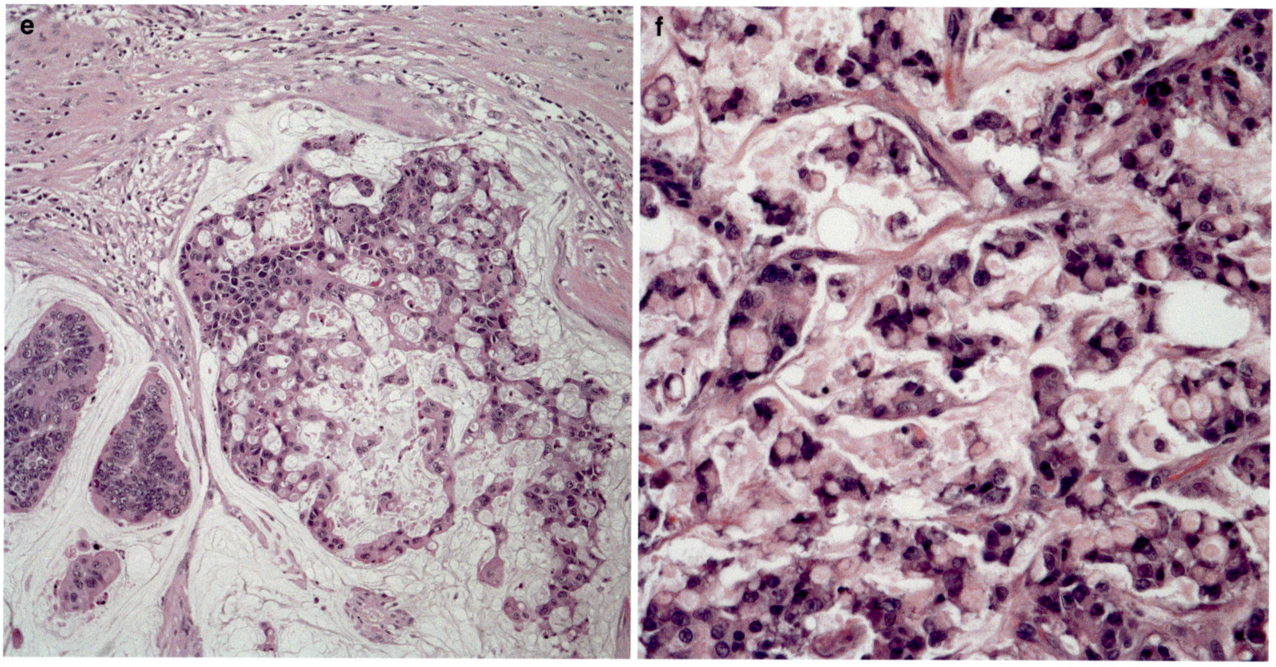

Fig. 8.32 (continued) (**e**) Intra- and extracellular mucinous areas. (**f**) Signet ring-cell areas in a mucinous adenocarcinoma

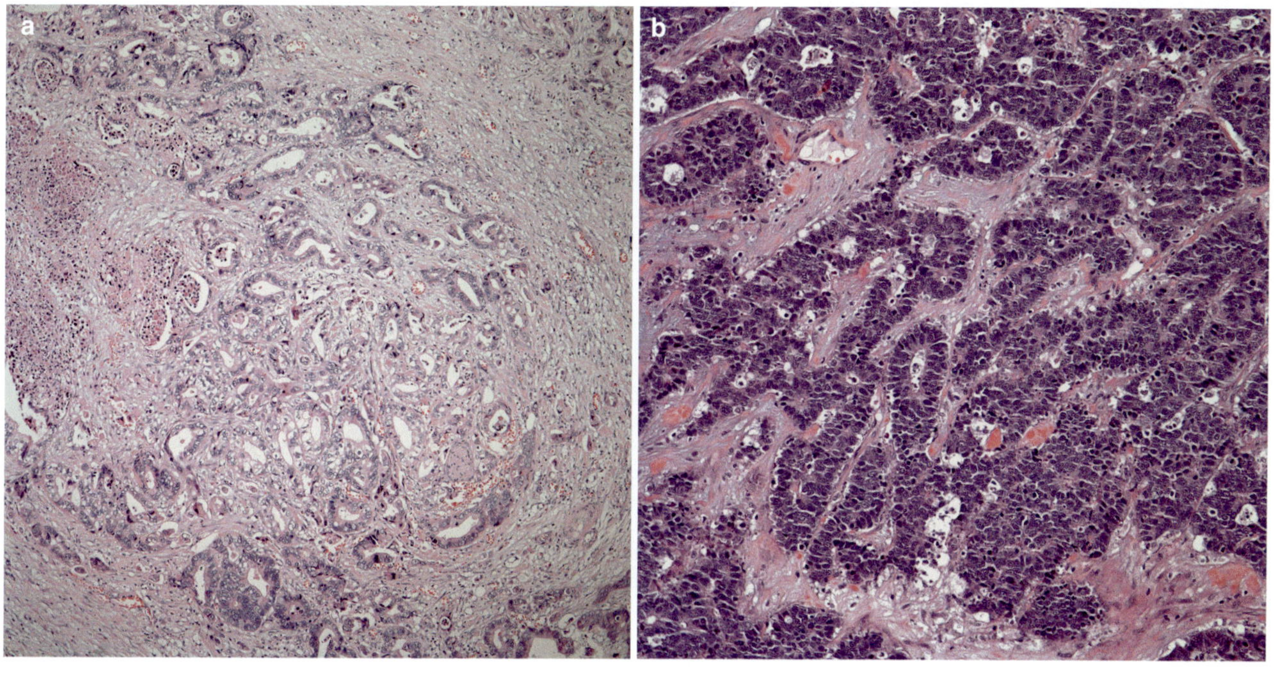

Fig. 8.33 (**a**) Low power view of non-mucinous adenocarcinoma showing a malignant glandular proliferation. (**b**) Small glandular proliferation dissecting fibroconnective tissue

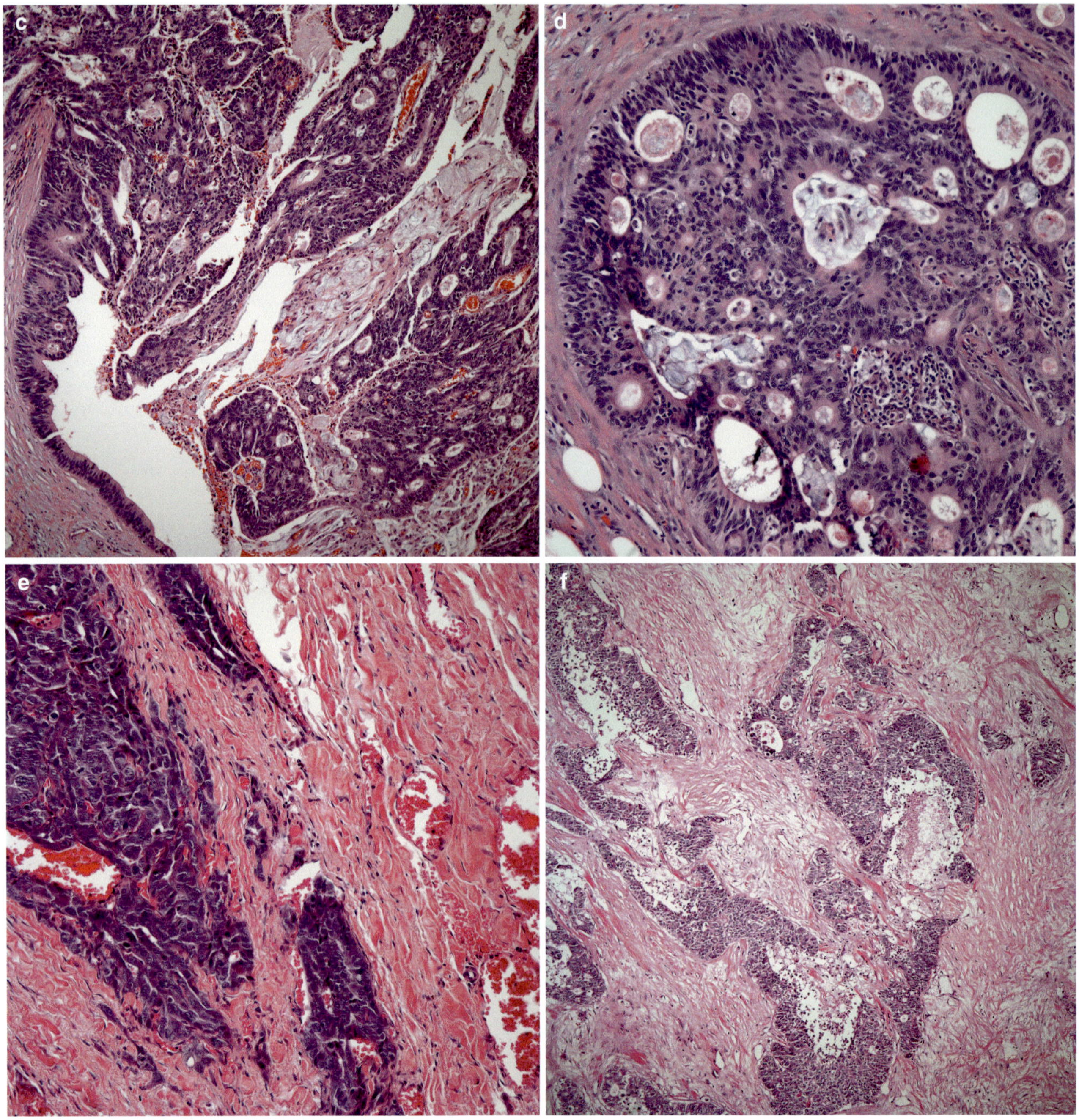

Fig. 8.33 (continued) (**c**) Thymic adenocarcinoma with colonic-like features. (**d**) Malignant gland with luminal mucin. (**e**) Malignant glands with adjacent solid area. (**f**) Irregular islands of malignant cells with glandular formation

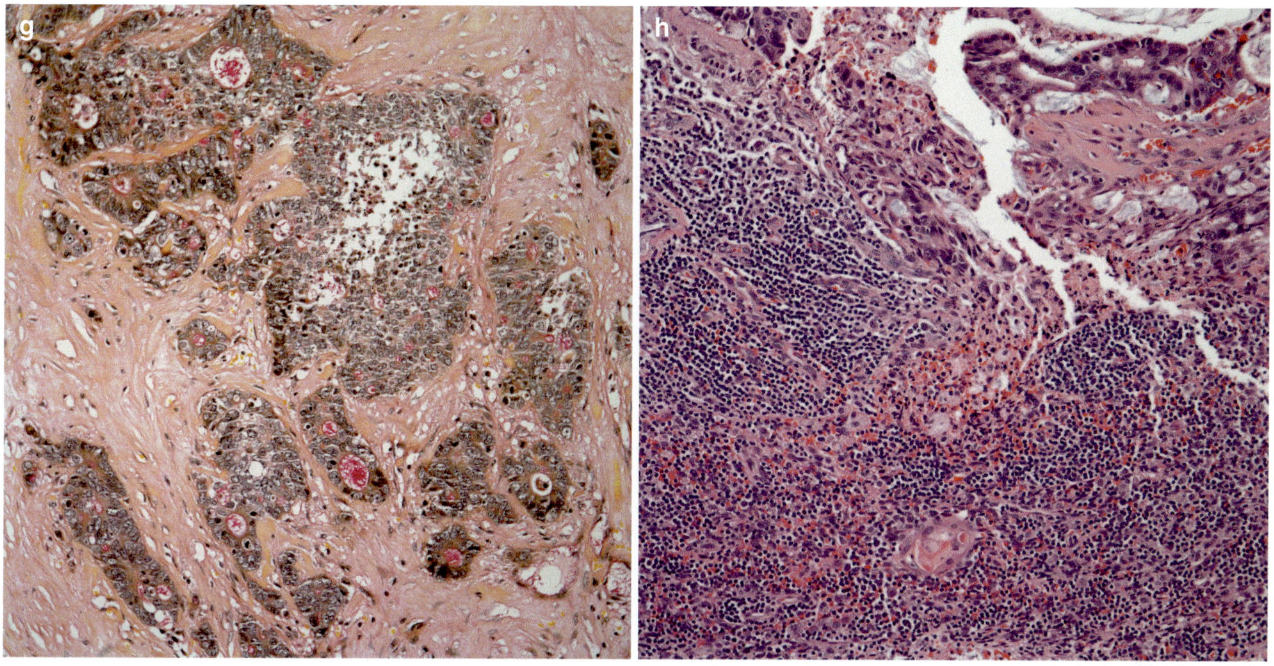

Fig. 8.33 (continued) (**g**) Mucicarmine stain shows intra- and extracellular mucin. (**h**) Adenocarcinoma involving remnant of thymic tissue; note the presence of Hassall's corpuscle

histologies. In addition, the authors stated than none of the 17 thymomas showed any reactivity to CD5 as well as 61 cases of carcinoma of different origin. The authors concluded that CD5 is a useful marker for primary thymic carcinoma. On the other hand, Kornstein and Rosai [72] evaluated 109 thymic tumors and 423 other neoplasms using two different monoclonal antibodies: clone CD5/54/B4 labeled 7/24 thymic carcinomas and none of the other types of tumors, while clone 4C7 labeled 15/24 thymic carcinomas, 2/84 thymomas, and 14/386 other epithelial tumors. In a different study evaluating CD5 (monoclonal antibody CD5-4C7) immunoreactivity, Tateyama and associates [73] stained 73 tumors of different organs including 22 thymomas and 7 thymic carcinomas. All thymic carcinomas showed membranous staining, while four cases of atypical thymoma also showed focal positive staining, and none of the other types of thymoma showed any staining. The authors also documented that positive intracytoplasmic staining was identified in cases of mesothelioma.

Contrary to the emphasis on CD5 as a discriminator of thymoma and thymic carcinoma or thymic carcinoma from other types of carcinomas, more general immunohistochemical panels have been performed in thymic carcinomas. Pomplum and associates [74] evaluated the staining pattern of cytokeratin 7, CD5, CD10, CD1a, and TTF1 in 20 thymic tumors (thymoma, atypical thymoma, and thymic carcinoma) against 10 primary squamous cell carcinomas and 10 large cell carcinomas of the lung. The authors identified 3/10 large cell carcinomas positive for TTF1, while CD5 was positive in 3/6 thymic carcinomas and 1/14 thymomas, with only focal staining in 1/20 lung carcinomas. The staining of CK7 and CD10 did not help in distinguishing thymic or lung origin. In a different study by Pan and associates [75] on thymic carcinoma and thymoma, the authors evaluated 22 thymic carcinoma and 35 thymomas for the staining pattern of calretinin, mesothelin, cytokeratin 5/6, thrombomodulin, HBME-1, Wilms' tumor (WT-1), Ber-Ep4, MOC-31, BG-8, B72.3, CEA, CD15, TTF-1, p63, and CD5. The authors identified that about 33% of thymic carcinomas were positive for calretinin and/or mesothelin, both thymic carcinomas and thymomas were positive for keratin 5/6, HBME-1 was positive in four thymic carcinomas and ten thymomas, and WT-1 was seen positive in one thymic carcinoma. Also, about 70% of thymic carcinomas were positive for Ber-Ep4,

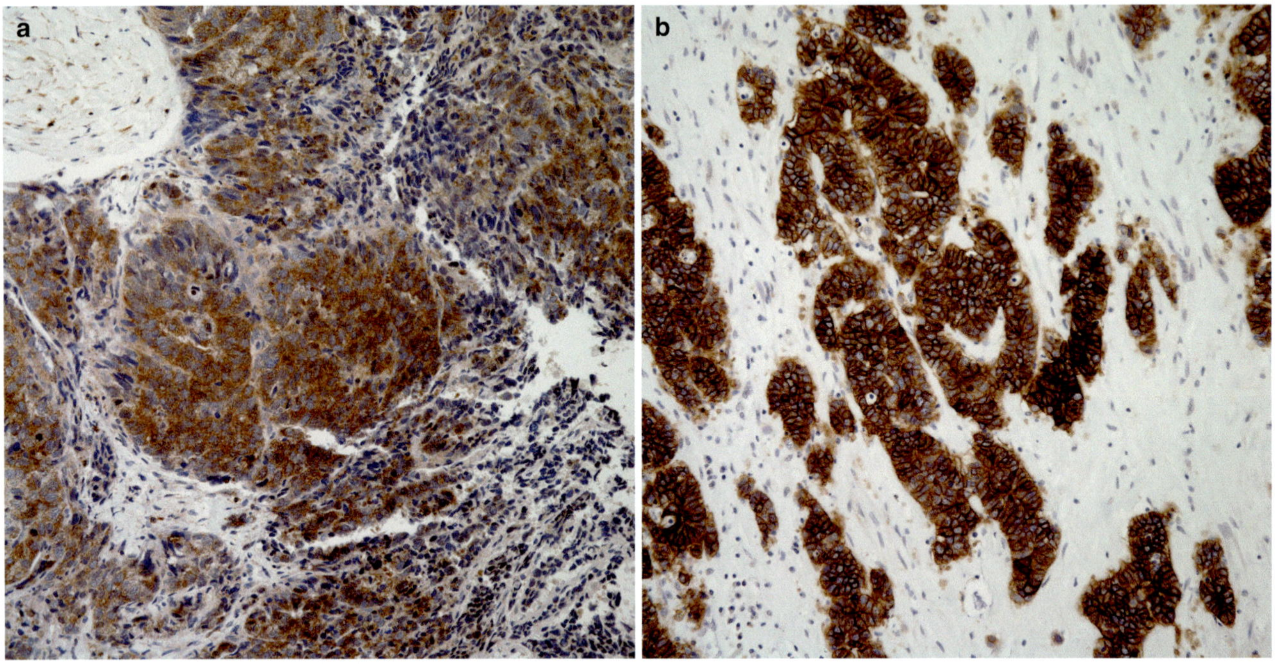

Fig. 8.34 (**a**) Immunohistochemical stain for CD5 showing positive staining in a thymic adenocarcinoma. (**b**) Immunohistochemical staining for CD117 showing positive staining in a thymic adenocarcinoma

BG-8, and CD15. In addition, positive staining in thymic carcinomas was seen for CEA, B72.3, and MOC-31. P63 was positive in all the cases, while CD5 was positive in 9/22 thymic carcinomas. Thrombomodulin and TTF1 were negative in all cases. Nonaka and associates [76] evaluated 58 thymomas and 17 thymic carcinomas using Foxn1 and CD205 (DEC205) and encountered that Foxn1 was diffusely expressed in thymoma, mainly those with lymphocytic component, while it was only focally expressed in thymic carcinoma. Also, CD205 cytoplasmic expression was strong and diffuse in all thymomas, with focal variable intensity in thymic carcinoma. The authors concluded that Foxn1 is a better marker for thymoma and thymic carcinoma than CD5 and CD117. Kojika and associates [77] evaluated the expression of GLUT-1 as a discriminant of atypical thymoma and thymic carcinoma. The authors, using tissue microarray, evaluated 12 thymic carcinomas and 7 atypical thymomas, concluding that GLUT-1 is a good marker to separate atypical thymoma from thymic carcinoma, especially in biopsy specimens.

Also important to highlight is the fact that several authors have identified neuroendocrine differentiation in thymic epithelial tumors [78, 79]. Ishima and associates [78] evaluated nine thymic carcinomas identifying positive staining in seven cases for synaptophysin. Libero and associates [79], in a study of 19 thymic carcinomas, encountered that 10 of the 19 cases (53%) showed immunoreactivity for synaptophysin. In addition, the authors also identified six cases in which there were scattered cells positive for chromogranin. More recently, other markers have been observed to show positive staining in thymic carcinomas, including p63, keratin 5/6, keratin 7, CDX2, FoxN1, CD117, CD205, and calretinin [30]. In addition, thymic carcinomas have shown significant immunohistochemical expression for EGFR, pEGFR, HER2, HER3, TGF alpha, amphiregulin, and epiregulin [80].

Regarding molecular studies on thymic carcinoma, there have been a few attempts to analyze different aspects of this tumor, and a few reviews on this subject have been written [81, 82]. Hirabayashi and associates [83] evaluated thymomas and thymic carcinomas for mutation in p53 and CDKN2 genes using PCR-SSCP and did not identify any mutations of those genes. However, the authors identified one case of thymic carcinoma with hypermethylation in the promoter region of CDKN2. Also, HER gene amplification by FISH and increased EGFR and HER2 gene copy numbers have been reported in thymic carcinomas [80]. Yamaguchi and associates [84] have also reported a single case of thymic carcinoma in which the authors identified deletions in exon 19 of EGFR with PCR method, and also three point mutations, G719A in exon 18, T790M in exon 20, and L858R in exon 21. On this subject, Meister and associates [85] evaluated 20 thymic epithelial tumors (17 thymomas and 3 thymic carcinomas), and even though the authors identified EGFR-positive staining in the majority of cases by immunohistochemistry, none of the cases had sequence alteration in the tyrosine kinase domain of EGFR similar to that seen in lung carcinoma. Yoh and associates [86] evaluated the mutational status of EGFR and KIT in 24 thymomas and 17 thymic carcinomas in which the authors were not able to identify EGFR mutations in thymic carcinoma, while the mutational analysis for KIT showed only missense mutation in exon 11 of a single case of thymic carcinoma. In a similar study of EGFR and KIT in 38 thymomas and 7 thymic carcinomas, Girard and associates [87] identified KIT mutations in thymic carcinomas but no mutations in the EGFR kinase domain. Perhaps more importantly is the fact that in this study squamous cell carcinomas of the thymus and lung were compared, and the findings appear to show a difference, which potentially could be of aid in separating these two tumors. Zettl and coworkers [88], in a study on recurrent genetic aberrations in thymoma and thymic carcinoma, concluded that atypical thymoma (WHO type B3) and thymic squamous cell carcinoma partially share genetic aberrations. Watanabe and coworkers [89] provided their experience with expression of telomerase activity in thymic epithelial neoplasms, namely, thymoma and thymic carcinoma, and identified telomerase activity in these tumors. However, the authors stated that the activity was higher in thymomas than in thymic carcinoma, which could be explained by the presence of immature lymphocytes in thymomas.

NUT Carcinoma

In 1991, Kees and coworkers [90] reported a single case of an intrathoracic poorly differentiated carcinoma in an 11-year-old girl in which the authors performed a chromosomal analysis identifying a translocation t(15;19), which the authors determined had not been previously recorded in the literature. In the same year, Kubonishi and coworkers [91] also described a thymic carcinoma in a 22-year-old female in which the authors also identified a chromosomal translocation t(15;19)(q15;p13) and also arrived at the same conclusion that such translocation had not been previously reported. It is important to highlight that these two publications, although highly important, appear not to have gotten the attention of diagnostic pathologists in general as it took two additional years for another case to be published. In 1993, Lee and coworkers [92] described a disseminated mediastinal carcinoma in a 5-year-old boy who followed a fatal course. In this case, the authors, as in the previous cases, performed a cytogenetic study identifying a chromosomal abnormality t(15;19)(q12;p13.1), concluding that this translocation may be specific for thymic carcinoma and may indicate an aggressive tumor.

In 2001, French and coworkers [93] evaluated 13 carcinomas in patients ranging in age from 3 to 53 years, including 3 thymic, 3 mucoepidermoid, 2 laryngeal, 1 nasopharyngeal, and 4 sinonasal. The goal as explained in the report was to "map" the chromosome 15 and 19 translocation breakpoints by FISH. Interestingly, of the 13 cases studied, the authors detected t(15;19) in only 1 out of the 4 cases of sinonasal carcinoma, while it was not detected in 3 thymic, 3 mucoepidermoid, and 2 laryngeal carcinomas. The authors concluded that their findings reveal a novel oncogenic mechanism in which the chromosome 19 translocation breakpoint interrupts the coding sequence of a bromodomain gene, BRD4, thus implicating BRD4 as a potential partner in a t(15;19)-associated fusion oncogene. Vargas and coworkers [94] also reported similar findings of t(15;19) chromosomal translocation in two young patients, one a 13-year-old with an epiglottic tumor and the other in a 12-year-old with a nasopharyngeal mass. In both of these patients, the tumor followed an aggressive behavior. The authors concluded that these findings are part of a distinct clinicopathological entity characterized by midline carcinoma with rapid fatal course. Sait and coworkers [95] also reported a thymic carcinoma with chromosomal translocation t(1;8)(p13;p11); however, the patient was a 38-year-old man with a tumor characterized by "giant cell features," while Toretsky and coworkers [96] reported another thymic carcinoma in a 15-year-old boy with a complex three-way translocation t(11;15;19). In 2003, French and coworkers [97], following their initial work on BRD4, demonstrated that the chromosome 15 translocation rearranges the novel gene NUT (nuclear protein in testis), resulting in a BRD4-NUT fusion oncogene. The authors added that their finding is the first known fusion oncogene in a highly malignant epithelial neoplasm. In 2008, Stelow and coworkers [98], in a study of 31 cases of undifferentiated carcinomas of the upper aerodigestive tract, introduced the term "NUT midline carcinoma." In this study, 5 of 28 cases showed rearrangements of the NUT and BRD4 genes by FISH, while 3 of the 5 cases also showed diffuse nuclear staining for NUT by immunohistochemistry. In addition, 23 other tumors were also evaluated for NUT immunohistochemistry, which showed mainly focal nuclear staining. The authors concluded that about 20% of these tumors not associated with EBV showed NUT rearrangement by FISH. In addition, the authors were able to document this finding in adult patients and stated that the use of NUT by immunohistochemistry may be a useful method to identify similar tumors. Needless to say, cases outside of the midline have also been encountered to show similar chromosomal translocation. Mertens [99] identified one of these cases in a 10-year-old child with a bone tumor, and den Bakker [100] identified another case in the parotid gland of a 15-year-old male. Based on available literature on this rare type of carcinoma, it is possible that NUT midline carcinoma may account for somewhere between 5% and 20% of poorly differentiated carcinomas, mainly in the midline (Fig. 8.35a, b). However, it is important to highlight that, although most tumors are reported in young patients, adult individuals may also show the chromosomal translocation. Nevertheless, it is difficult to determine which cases need to be tested based on histology alone, and the occurrence of a poorly differentiated carcinoma in the midline in a young patient is the most likely scenario, which triggers the investigation of the translocation. In a recent

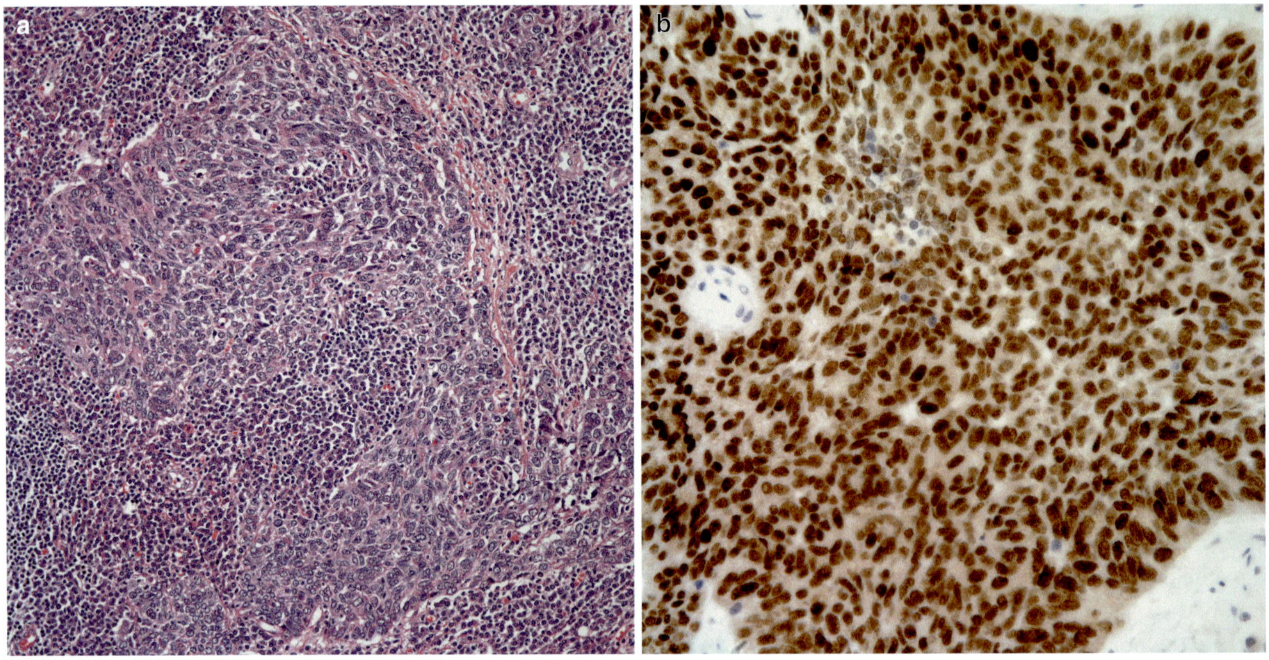

Fig. 8.35 (**a**) Poorly differentiated thymic carcinoma. (**b**) Immunohistochemical staining for NUT showing strong nuclear staining

review on NUT midline carcinomas, French [101] advanced the hypothesis that these tumors may arise from primitive neural crest. However, such a suggestion needs to be properly confirmed.

References

1. Kirchner T, Schlke B, Buchwald J, Ritter M, Marx A, Müller-Hermelink HK. Well-differentiated thymic carcinoma. An organotypical low-grade carcinoma with relationship to cortical thymoma. Am J Surg Pathol. 1992;16:1153–69.
2. Castleman B. Tumors of the thymus gland, Section V, Fascicle 19. Washington, DC: Armed Forces Institute of Pathology; 1955.
3. Rosai J, Levine GD. Tumors of the thymus, 2dn series, Fascicle 13. Washington, DC: Armed Forces Institute of Pathology; 1975.
4. Frank HA, Reiner L, Fleischer FG. Co-occurrence of large leiomyoma of the esophagus and squamous cell carcinoma of the thymus. Report of a case with roentgenologic, pathological, and clinical discussion. NEJM. 1956;255:159–64.
5. Watson RR, Weisel W, O'Conner TM. Thymic neoplasms. A surgical enigma. Arch Surg. 1968;97:230–8.
6. Shimosato Y, Kameya T, Nagai K, Suemasu K. Squamous cell carcinoma of the thymus. Analysis of eight cases. Am J Surg Pathol. 1977;1:109–21.
7. Snover DC, Levine GD, Rosai J. Thymic carcinoma. Five distinctive histological variants. Am J Surg Pathol. 1982;6:451–70.
8. Suster S, Moran CA. Thymic carcinoma: spectrum of differentiation and histologic types. Pathology. 1998;30:111–2.
9. Suster S. Thymic carcinoma: update of current diagnostic criteria and histologic types. Semin Diagn Pathol. 2005;22:198–212.
10. Moran CA, Suster S. Thymic carcinoma: current concepts and histological features. Hematol Oncol Clin N Am. 2008;22:393–407.
11. Ritter JH, Wick MR. Primary carcinomas of the thymus gland. Semin Diagn Pathol. 1999;16:18–31.
12. Suster S, Moran CA. Thymoma, atypical thymoma, and thymic carcinoma: a novel conceptual approach to the classification of thymic epithelial neoplasms. Am J Clin Pathol. 1999;111:826–33.
13. Weiss GJ. Thymic carcinoma: current and future therapeutic interventions. Expert Opin Investig Drugs. 2010;19:1007–16.
14. Suster S, Moran CA. Primary thymic epithelial neoplasms with combined features of thymoma and thymic carcinoma: a clinicopathological study of 22 cases. Am J Surg Pathol. 1996;20:1469–80.
15. Herczeg E, Kahn LB. Primary thymic carcinoma: an unusual case originating in a lymphocytic rich thymoma. Virchows Arch A Pathol Anat Histopathol. 1986;409:163–9.
16. Wick MR, Scheithauer BW, Weiland LH, Bernatz PE. Primary thymic carcinomas. Am J Surg Pathol. 1982;6:613–30.
17. Shimizu J, Hayashi Y, Morita K, Arano Y, Yoshida M, Oda M, et al. Primary thymic carcinoma: a clinicopathological and Immunohistochemical study. J Surg Oncol. 1994;56:159–64.
18. Truong LD, Mody DR, Cagle PT, Jackson-York GL, Schwartz MR, Wheeler TM. Thymic carcinoma: a clinicopathologic study of 13 cases. Am J Surg Pathol. 1990;14:151–66.
19. Kuo TT, Chang JP, Lin FJ, Wu WC, Chang CH. Thymic carcinomas: histological varieties and Immunohistochemical study. Am J Surg Pathol. 1990;14:24–34.
20. Hartmann CA, Roth C, Minck C, Niedobitek G. Thymic carcinoma: report of five cases and review of the literature. J Cancer Res Clin Oncol. 1990;116:69–82.
21. Hsu CP, Chen CY, Chen CL, Lin CT, Hsu NY, Wang JH, et al. Thymic carcinoma. Ten years experience in twenty patients. J Thorac Cardiovasc Surg. 1994;107:615–20.
22. Chalabreysse L, Mastroianni BE, Adeleine P, Cordier JF, Greenland T, Thivolet-Bejui F. Thymic carcinoma: a clinicopathological and immunohistological study of 19 cases. Histopathology. 2004;44:367–74.
23. Yano M, Sasaki H, Yokoyama T, Yukiue H, Kawano O, Suzuki S, et al. Thymic carcinoma: 30 cases at a single institution. J Thorac Oncol. 2008;3:265–9.

24. Takeda S, Sawabata N, Inoue M, Koma M, Maeda H, Hirano H. Thymic carcinoma: clinical institutional experience with 15 patients. Eur J Cardiothorac Surg. 2004;26:401–6.
25. Tomita M, Matsuzaki Y, Edagawa M, Maeda M, Shimizu T, Hara M, et al. Clinical and Immunohistochemical study of eight cases with thymic carcinoma. BMC Surg. 2002;2:3.
26. Liu HC, Hsu WH, Chen YJ, Chan YJ, Wu YC, Huang BS, et al. Primary thymic carcinoma. Ann Thorac Surg. 2002;73:1076–81.
27. Ogawa K, Toita T, Uno T, Fuwa N, Kakinohana Y, Kamata M, et al. Treatment and prognosis of thymic carcinoma: a retrospective analysis of 40 cases. Cancer. 2002;94:3115–9.
28. Li X, Chen Q, Huang W, Ye Y. Response to sorafenib in cisplatin-resistant thymic carcinoma: a case report. Med Oncol. 2009;26:157–60.
29. Suster S, Rosai J. Thymic carcinoma: a clinicopathologic study of 60 cases. Cancer. 1991;67:1025–32.
30. Weissferdt A, Moran CA. Thymic carcinoma, part 1. A clinicopathologic and Immunohistochemical study of 65 cases. Am J Clin Pathol. 2012;138:103–14.
31. Yoneda S, Marx A, Heimann S, Shirakusa T, Kikuchi M, Müller-Hermelink HK. Low-grade metaplastic carcinoma of the thymus. Histopathology. 1999;35:19–30.
32. Suster S, Moran CA. Thymoma with pseudosarcomatous stroma: report of an unusual histologic variant of thymic epithelial neoplasm that may simulate carcinosarcoma. Am J Surg Pathol. 1997;21:1316–23.
33. Weissferdt A, Kalhor N, Moran CA. Cystic well differentiated squamous cell carcinoma of the thymus: a clinicopathological and Immunohistochemical study of six cases. Histopathology. 2016;68:333–8.
34. Weissferdt A, Moran CA. Thymic carcinoma associated with multilocular thymic cyst: a clinicopathologic study of 7 cases. Am J Surg Pathol. 2011;35:1074–9.
35. Suster S, Moran CA. Spindle cell thymic carcinoma: clinicopathologic and Immunohistochemical study of a distinctive variant of primary thymic epithelial neoplasm. Am J Surg Pathol. 1999;23:691–700.
36. Lu H, Gan M, Zhou T, Wang S. Sarcomatoid thymic carcinoma arising in metaplastic thymoma: a case report. Int J Surg Pathol. 2011;19:677–80.
37. Moritani S, Ichihara S, Mukai SY, Inoue S, Yasuda A, et al. Sarcomatoid carcinoma of the thymus arising in metaplastic thymoma. Histopathology. 2008;52:387–411.
38. Nonaka D, Rodriguez J, Rollo JL, Rosai J. Undifferentiated large cell carcinoma of the thymus associated with Castleman disease-like reaction: a distinctive type of thymic neoplasm characterized by an indolent behavior. Am J Surg Pathol. 2005;29:490–5.
39. Dimery IW, Lee JS, Blick M, Pearson G, Spitzer G, Hong WK. Association of the Epstein-Barr virus with lymphoepithelioma of the thymus. Cancer. 1988;61:2475–80.
40. Leyvraz S, Henle W, Chahinian AP, Perlmann C, Klein G, Gordon RE, et al. Association of Epstein-Barr virus with thymic carcinoma. NEJM. 1985;312:1296–9.
41. Matsuno Y, Morozumi N, Hirohashi S, Shimosato Y, Rosai J. Papillary carcinoma of the thymus: report of four cases of a new microscopic type of thymic carcinoma. Am J Surg Pathol. 1998;22:873–80.
42. Wolfe JT, Wick MR, Banks PM, Scheithauer BW. Clear cell carcinoma of the thymus. Mayo Clin Proc. 1983;58:365–70.
43. Stephens M, Khalil J, Gibbs AR. Primary clear cell carcinoma of the thymus gland. Histopathology. 1987;11:763–5.
44. Hasserjian RP, Klimstra DS, Rosai J. Carcinoma of the thymus with clear cell features: report of eight cases and review of the literature. Am J Surg Pathol. 1995;19:835–41.
45. Tropani TH, Tamboli P, Amin MB, Ordoñez NG, Ayala AG, Ro JY. Thymic carcinoma with rhabdoid features. Ann Diagn Pathol. 2003;7:106–11.
46. Franke A, Strobel P, Fackeldey V, Schäfer R, Göller T, Becker HP, et al. Hepatoid thymic carcinoma: report of a case. Am J Surg Pathol. 2004;28:250–6.
47. Weissferdt A, Moran CA. Anaplastic thymic carcinoma: a clinicopathologic and Immunohistochemical study of 6 cases. Hum Pathol. 2012;43:874–7.
48. Suster S, Moran CA. Micronodular thymoma with lymphoid B-cell hyperplasia: clinicopathologic and Immunohistochemical study of eighteen cases of a distinctive morphological variant of thymic epithelial neoplasm. Am J Surg Pathol. 1999;23:955–62.
49. Weissferdt A, Moran CA. Micronodular thymic carcinoma with lymphoid hyperplasia: a clinicopathological and Immunohistochemical study of five cases. Mod Pathol. 2012;25:993–9.
50. De Queiroga EM, Chikota H, Bacchi CE, Moran CA, Suster S. Rhabdomyomatous carcinoma of the thymus. Am J Surg Pathol. 2004;28:1245–50.
51. Alguacil-Garcia A, Halliday WC. Thymic carcinoma with focal neuroblastoma differentiation. Am J Surg Pathol. 1987;11:474–9.
52. Choi WW, Liu YH, Lau WH, Crowley P, Khan A, Chan JK. Adenocarcinoma of the thymus: report of two cases including a previously undescribed mucinous type. Am J Surg Pathol. 2003;27:124–30.
53. Takahashi F, Tsuta K, Matsuno Y, Takahashi K, Toba M, Sato K, et al. Adenocarcinoma of the thymus: mucinous subtype. Hum Pathol. 2005;36:19–223.
54. Sawai T, Inoue Y, Doi S, Ikuta Y, Kimino K, Nakashima M, et al. Tubular adenocarcinoma of the thymus: case report and review of the literature. Int J Surg Pathol. 2006;14:243–6.
55. Kapur P, Rakheja D, Bastasch M, Molberg KH, Sarode VR. Primary mucinous adenocarcinoma of the thymus: a case report and review of the literature. Arch Pathol Lab Med. 2006;130:201–14.
56. Ra SH, Fishbein MC, Baruch-Oren T, Shintaku P, Apple SK, Cameron RB, et al. Mucinous adenocarcinoma of the thymus: report of 2 cases and review of the literature. Am J Surg Pathol. 2007;31:1330–6.
57. Maeda D, Ota S, Ikeda KR, Hata E, Nakajima J, et al. Mucinous adenocarcinoma of the thymus: a distinct variant of thymic carcinoma. Lung Cancer. 2009;64:22–7.
58. Kinoshita F, Shoji F, Takada K, Toyokawa G, Okamoto T, Yano T, et al. Mucinous adenocarcinoma of the thymus: report of a case. Gen Thorac Cardiovasc Surg. 2018;66(2):111–5.
59. Lee Y, Park S, Lee SH, Lee H. Characterization of genetic aberrations in a single case of metastatic thymic adenocarcinoma. BMC Cancer. 2017;17:330.
60. Akiba J, Harada H, Yokoyama S, Hashiguchi T, Kawahara A, Mitsuoka M, et al. Mucinous cystic tumor with CK20 and CDX2 expression of the thymus: is this a benign counterpart of adenocarcinoma of the thymus, enteric type. Pathol Int. 2016;66:29–33.
61. Wang L, Wang D, Quian K, Dehong L, Chen L, Zhao L, et al. Thymic adenocarcinoma associated with thymic cyst: a case report and review of the literature. Int J Clin Exp Pathol. 2015;8:5890–5.
62. Moser B, Schiefer AL, Janik S, Marx A, Prosch H, Pohl W, et al. Adenocarcinoma of the thymus, enteric type: report of 2 cases and proposal for a novel subtype of thymic carcinoma. Am J Surg Pathol. 2015;39:541–8.
63. Maghbool M, Ramzi M, Nagel I, Bejarano P, Siebert R, Saeedzadeh A, et al. Primary adenocarcinoma of the thymus: an immunohistochemical and molecular study with review of the literature. BMC Clin Pathol. 2013;13:17.
64. Abdul-Ghafar J, Yong SJ, Kwon W, Park IH, Jung S-H. Primary thymic mucinous adenocarcinoma: a case report. Korean J Pathol. 2012;46:377–81.
65. Hosaka Y, Tsuchida M, Umezu H, Eimoto T, Hashimoto T, Shinohara H, et al. Primary thymic adenocarcinoma coexisting with type AB thymoma: a rare case with long-term survival. Gen Thorac Cardiovasc Surg. 2010;58:488–91.

66. Morikawa H, Tanaka T, Hamaji M, Ueno Y, Hara A. Papillary adenocarcinoma developed in a thymic cyst. Gen Thorac Cardiovasc Surg. 2010;58:295–7.
67. Kwon AY, Han J, Chu J, Choi YS, Jeong B-H, Ahn M-H, et al. Histologic characteristics of thymic adenocarcinomas: clinicopathologic study of a nine-case series and a review of the literature. Pathol Res Pract. 2017;213:106–12.
68. Kalhor N, Moran CA. Primary thymic adenocarcinomas: a clinicopathological and immunohistochemical study of 16 cases with emphasis on the morphological spectrum of differentiation. Hum Pathol. 2018;74:73–82.
69. Fukai I, Masaoka A, Hashimoto T, Yamakawa Y, Niwa H, Kiriyama M, et al. Differential diagnosis of thymic carcinoma and lung carcinoma with the use of antibodies to cytokeratins. J Thorac Cardiovasc Surg. 1995;110:1670–5.
70. Hishima T, Fukuyama M, Fujisawa M, Hayashi Y, Arai K, Funata N, et al. CD5 expression in thymic carcinoma. Am J Pathol. 1994;145:268–75.
71. Dorfman D, Shahsafaei A, Chan JKC. Thymic carcinoma, but not thymomas and carcinomas of other sites show CD5 immunoreactivity. Am J Surg Pathol. 1997;21:936–40.
72. Kornstein MJ, Rosai J. CD5 labeling of thymic carcinomas and other nonlymphoid neoplasms. Am J Clin Pathol. 1998;109:722–6.
73. Tateyama H, Eimoto T, Tada T, Hattori H, Murase T, Takino H. Immunoreactivity of a new CD5 antibody with normal epithelium and malignant tumors including thymic carcinoma. Am J Clin Pathol. 1999;111:235–40.
74. Pomplun S, Wotherspoon AC, Shah G, Goldstraw P, Ladas G, Nicholson AG. Immunohistochemical markers in the differentiation of thymic and pulmonary neoplasms. Histopathology. 2002;40:152–8.
75. Pan CC, Chen PC, Chou TY, Chiang H. Expression of calretinin and other mesothelioma-related markers in thymic carcinoma and thymoma. Hum Pathol. 2003;34:1155–62.
76. Nonaka D, Henley JD, Chiriboga L, Yee H. Diagnostic utility of thymic epithelial markers CD205 (DEC205) and Foxn1 in thymic epithelial neoplasms. Am J Surg Pathol. 2007;31:1038–44.
77. Kojika M, Ishii G, Yoshida J, Nishimura M, Hishida T, Ota SJ, et al. Immunohistochemical differential diagnosis between thymic carcinoma and type B3 thymoma: diagnostic utility of hypoxic marker, GLUT-1, in thymic epithelial neoplasms. Mod Pathol. 2009;22:1341–50.
78. Hishima T, Fukayama M, Hayashi Y, Fujii T, Arai K, Shiozawa Y, et al. Neuroendocrine differentiation in thymic epithelial tumors with special reference to thymic carcinoma and atypical thymoma. Hum Pathol. 1998;29:330–8.
79. Libero L, Erlandson RA, Rosai J. Neuroendocrine differentiation is a common feature of thymic carcinoma. Am J Surg Pathol. 1998;22:1059–66.
80. Weissferdt A, Lin H, Woods D, Tang X, Fujimoto J, Wistuba II, et al. HER family receptor and ligand status in thymic carcinoma. Lung Cancer. 2012;77:515–21.
81. Strobel P, Hohenberger P, Marx A. Thymoma and thymic carcinoma: molecular pathology and targeted therapy. J Thorac Oncol. 2010;5:S286–90.
82. Weissferdt A, Wistuba II, Moran CA. Molecular aspectrs of thymic carcinoma. Lung Cancer. 2012;78:127–32.
83. Hirabayashi H, Fuji Y, Sakaguchi M, Tanaka H, Yoon HE, Komoto Y, et al. p16^{INKe}, pRB, p53 and cyclin D1 expression and hypermethylation of CDKN2 gene in thymoma and thymic carcinoma. Int J Cancer. 1997;73:639–44.
84. Yamaguchi H, Soda H, Kitazaki T, Tsukamoto K, Hayashi T, Kohno S. Thymic carcinoma with epidermal growth factor receptor gene mutations. Lung Cancer. 2006;52:261–2.
85. Meister M, Schirmacher P, Dienemann H, Mechtersheimer G, Schnabel PA, Kern MA, et al. Mutational status of the epidermal growth factor receptor (EGFR) gene in thymoma and thymic carcinomas. Cancer Lett. 2007;248:181–91.
86. Yoh K, Nishiwaki Y, Ishii G, Goto K, Kubota K, Ohmatsu H, et al. Mutational status of EGFR and KIT in thymoma and thymic carcinoma. Lung Cancer. 2008;62:316–20.
87. Girard N, Shen R, Guo T, Zakowski MF, Heguy A, Riely GJ, et al. Comprehensive genomic analysis reveals clinically relevant molecular distinctions between thymic carcinoma and thymomas. Clin Cancer Res. 2009;15:6790–9.
88. Zettl A, Strobel P, Wagner K, Katzenberger T, Ott G, Rosenwald A, et al. Recurrent genetic aberrations in thymoma and thymic carcinoma. Am J Pathol. 2000;157:257–66.
89. Watanabe M, Shan-kan Y, Sawafuji M, Kawamura M, Horinouchi H, Mukai M, et al. Enhanced expression of telomerase activity in thymoma and thymic carcinoma tissues. A clinicopathologic study. Cancer. 2002;94:240–4.
90. Kees UR, Mulcahy MT, Willoughby MLN. Intrathoracic carcinoma in an 11-year-old girl showing a translocation t(15;19). AM J Pediatr Hematol Oncol. 1991;13:459–64.
91. Kubonishi I, Takehara N, Iwata J, Sonobe H, Ohtsuki Y, Abe T, et al. Novel t(15;19)(q15;p13) chromosome abnormality in a thymic carcinoma. Cancer Res. 1991;51:3327–8.
92. Lee ACW, Kwong YI, Fu KH, Chan GC, Ma L, Lau YL. Disseminated mediastinal carcinoma with chromosomal translocation (15;19). A distinctive clinicopathologic syndrome. Cancer. 1993;72:2273–6.
93. French CA, Miyoshi I, Aster JC, Kubonishi I, Kroll TG, Dal Cin P, et al. BRD4 bromodomain gene rearrangement in aggressive carcinoma with translocation t(15;19). Am J Pathol. 2001;159:1987–92.
94. Vargas SO, French CA, Faul PN, Fletcher JA, Davis IJ, Dal Cin P, et al. Upper respiratory tract carcinoma with chromosomal translocation 15;19. Evidence for a distinct disease entity of young patients with a rapidly fatal course. Cancer. 2001;92:1195–203.
95. Sait SN, Brooks JJ, Ashraf M, Zhang PJ. A novel t(1;8)(p13;p11) in a thymic carcinoma with unusual giant cell features and renal metastasis. Cancer Genet Cytogenet. 2001;124:140–3.
96. Toretsky JA, Jenson J, Sun CC, Eskenazi AE, Campbell A, Hunger SP, et al. Translocation (11;15;19): a highly specific chromosome rearrangement associated with poorly differentiated thymic carcinoma in young patients. Am J Clin Oncol. 2003;26:300–6.
97. French CA, Miyoshi I, Kubonishi I, Grier HE, Perez-Atayde AR, Fletcher JA. BRD4-NUT fusion oncogene: a novel mechanism in aggressive carcinoma. Cancer Res. 2003;63:304–7.
98. Stelow EB, Bellizzi AM, Taneja K, Mills SE, Legallo RD, Kutok JL, et al. NUT rearrangement in undifferentiated carcinomas of the upper aerodigestive tract. Am J Surg Pathol. 2008;32:828–34.
99. Mertens F, Wiebe T, Adlercreutz C, Mandahl N, French CA. Succesful treatment of a child with t(15;19)-positive tumor. Pediatr Blood Cancer. 2007;49:1015–7.
100. Den Bakker MA, Beverloo BH, van den Heuvel-Eibrink MM, Meeuwis CA, Tan LM, Johnson LA, et al. NUT midline carcinoma of the parotid gland with mesenchymal differentiation. Am J Surg Pathol. 2009;33:1253–8.
101. French CA. Demystified molecular pathology of NUT midline carcinomas. J Clin Pathol. 2010;63:492–6.

Neuroendocrine Neoplasms

9

Introduction

Primary mediastinal neuroendocrine neoplasms as they are referred to in this chapter encompass several tumors that do not necessarily share the same histogenesis, biologic behavior, or treatment modalities. In addition, some of these tumors may in turn occur as ectopically placed tissues that may be deposited in the mediastinal compartment. In some of these cases, the embryologic development may be the clue to their occurrence. Nevertheless, this group of tumors ranges from benign tumors to the overtly high-grade malignant tumors. Basically, the group of tumors that more often present as mediastinal tumors are:

- Neuroendocrine carcinomas:
  - Well-differentiated neuroendocrine carcinoma (carcinoid tumor)
  - Moderately differentiated neuroendocrine carcinoma (atypical carcinoid)
  - Poorly differentiated neuroendocrine carcinoma (small cell carcinoma and large cell neuroendocrine carcinoma)
- Paragangliomas
- Parathyroid tumors:
  - Parathyroid adenoma
  - Parathyroid carcinoma
- Thyroid tumors:
  - Intrathoracic goiter
  - Thyroid carcinoma

In practice, these tumors represent only a small percentage of the mediastinal tumors and may account for no more than 10% of primary mediastinal neoplasms. Mediastinal neuroendocrine carcinomas are by far the most common tumors in this family of neoplasms and the ones that deserve special attention as these tumors may follow a more aggressive course.

In general, previously published series of mediastinal tumors do not account for much of the occurrence of neuroendocrine tumors. In 1968, Oldham and colleagues [1] reported 164 cases of mediastinal tumors and cysts without documenting any neuroendocrine carcinoma (carcinoid tumor) and thyroid or parathyroid tumors. In 1971, Wychulis and colleagues [2] documented a 40-year experience by describing 1029 mediastinal tumors, which encompassed the years 1929–1968. The authors documented 56 cases of intrathoracic goiter but no parathyroid tumors or neuroendocrine carcinomas (carcinoid tumor). Interestingly, more recent reports of mediastinal tumors in general have not been able to document a considerable number of cases of neuroendocrine tumors. Blegvad and colleagues [3], in a report of 129 mediastinal tumors, were able to document only 2 cases of neuroendocrine carcinomas, 1 paraganglioma, and 31 intrathoracic goiters. Important to mention is the fact that cases of carcinoma arising in intrathoracic goiters have been described [4]. Adkins and colleagues [5] also presented similar experience documenting 38 cases of mediastinal tumors, encountering only 2 patients with "carcinoid" tumors of thymic origin. However, in general terms, these reports clearly point out that, in general practice, the presence of neuroendocrine tumors, whether they are carcinomas, paragangliomas, or parathyroid tumors, is rare.

Neuroendocrine Carcinomas

Although there is general agreement that the credit for the recognition of neuroendocrine carcinomas (carcinoid tumors) in the mediastinum should be given to Rosai and Higa [6], who in 1972 described eight of these tumors in the mediastinum, it is also important to highlight that in 1963, Pachter and Lattes [7], in a description of uncommon mediastinal tumors, also described four cases, one of which was what the authors called "mediastinal bronchial-type" adenoma, clearly alluding to similar tumors that have already been described in the bronchus, and which at that time were coded as "adenomas," currently regarded as well-differentiated neuroendocrine carcinomas (carcinoid tumor).

© Springer Nature Switzerland AG 2019
N. Kalhor, C. Moran, *Mediastinal Pathology*, https://doi.org/10.1007/978-3-319-98980-8_9

Since Rosai and Higa's [6] description, several reviews and reports on the subject have been presented [8–12]. Some of these reports have been on the histopathologic spectrum, while others have been on the classification of these tumors. However, in most of the series presented, it appears that when these tumors are in the mediastinal compartment, they may show a more aggressive course.

Needless to say, mediastinal neuroendocrine neoplasms, namely, neuroendocrine carcinomas, just like their counterparts in other anatomic areas continue to be the subject of study, controversy, and further analysis.

Clinical Features

The spectrum of clinical syndromes or conditions that have been associated with neuroendocrine carcinomas (carcinoid tumors) is extensive. Conditions such as Cushing's syndrome, polyarthropathy, proximal myopathy, peripheral neuropathy, hyperparathyroidism, Eaton-Lambert syndrome, hypertrophic osteoarthropathy, parathyroid adenoma, cutaneous hyperpigmentation, pericarditis, secretion of ACTH, ADH, parathormone, calcitonin, beta-lipoprotein, serotonin, and multiple endocrine neoplasia (MEN) type I and II [13–34] are among the most commonly reported associations. It has been estimated that about half of all neuroendocrine carcinomas of the thymus are functionally active or associated with MEN syndrome. It is important to highlight that there is not a strong association between thymic neuroendocrine carcinomas and myasthenia gravis or carcinoid syndrome. However, of all previous associations between neuroendocrine carcinomas and other syndromes, it appears that the most important one or at least the most consistent one is the association with MEN syndrome, which in turn may also play a role in the outcome of these patients.

Multiple endocrine neoplasia, type I, or Wermer's syndrome is an autosomal dominant disease that is characterized by the presence of neoplasms that commonly involve parathyroid, pancreas, and pituitary. However, other anatomic structures such as thyroid and adrenal gland may also be involved. In these patients, common manifestations would include hyperparathyroidism or the presence of Zollinger-Ellison syndrome. Rosai and colleagues [13] are also credited for highlighting the association of thymic neuroendocrine carcinomas with multiple endocrine adenomatosis (MEA) after describing three adult patients with such association. The three patients followed a fatal course. In one patient, surgical exploration of the neck revealed the presence of chief cell hyperplasia in three parathyroid glands. At autopsy, adenomatous changes involving pancreas, thyroid, and adrenal were identified. In a second patient, pituitary and parathyroid adenomas were the anatomic structures involved, while in the third patient, symptoms of hyperparathyroidism were identified. Based on the illustrations provided in that report, it is possible that all three mediastinal tumors correspond to what is today considered a moderately differentiated neuroendocrine carcinoma (atypical carcinoid). Interestingly, Rosai and colleagues [13] alluded to the presence of MEN in several cases prior to their report. However, the pathology of the mediastinal lesions is unclear in those cases as they were coded by different names. Nevertheless, it is possible that, using today's nomenclature, some of those lesions may fall into what is known now as neuroendocrine carcinoma, well or moderately differentiated (carcinoid and atypical carcinoid). Important to note is the possible familial occurrence of multiple endocrine adenomatosis or MEN. Manes and Taylor [14] documented a familial case in which parathyroid hyperplasia was the salient feature and in which one member of the family had simultaneous occurrence of parathyroid hyperplasia and thymic neuroendocrine carcinoma. The histology of the thymic tumor appears to have been of the well-differentiated type, with spindle cell morphology. Although MEN type I appears to be more commonly associated with thymic neuroendocrine carcinomas, Marchevsky and Dikman [16] documented a case of a 60-year-old woman with thymic neuroendocrine carcinoma associated with parathyroid hyperplasia, medullary carcinoma of the thyroid, and adrenal neuroma, which the authors interpreted as an incomplete Sipple's syndrome or MEN type II. Based on the illustrations provided of the thymic tumor, it appears to have been of the well-differentiated type (carcinoid tumor). In a separate study analyzing patients diagnosed with MEN type I, Teh and colleagues [35] found 204 patients from 9 Australian and Malaysian MEN type I families. Of those, ten patients had an anterior mediastinal lesion from six unrelated kindreds. Interestingly, in all kindreds, linkage analysis was performed confirming linkage to the MEN type I locus in chromosome 11q13.

Unfortunately, there are not enough series of cases of thymic neuroendocrine carcinomas from where to draw extensive experience. In 1984, Wick and Scheithauer [36] reported a series of 12 patients with thymic neuroendocrine carcinomas in which the patients' ages ranged from 28 to 78 years; 11 patients were men, and 5 of these patients had an associated endocrinopathy. In a previous report, Wick and colleagues [37] had reported seven patients with thymic neuroendocrine carcinomas occurring in five men and two women between the ages of 27 and 67 years. In this group of patients, one patient had an islet cell carcinoma of the pancreas and one other patient had parathyroid hyperplasia. Also in 1996, de Montpreville and colleagues [38] reported patients with thymic neuroendocrine carcinomas occurring in 11 men and 3 women between the ages of 35 and 71 years. Interestingly, in this group of patients, one patient had an associated endocrinopathy, one patient had von Reckinghausen disease, and one other patient had severe psychosis. Similarly, Economopoulos and colleagues [39] reported seven patients with thymic neuroendocrine carcinoma in which none of the patients had an associated endocrinopathy, and the majority of the patients were men (six patients) with ages ranging between 36 and 70 years. In a more exhausting review of mediastinal tumors, Wang and coworkers [40] encountered eight cases of thymic neuroendocrine carcinomas out of 162 patients. In this group, six patients were men and two were women between the ages of 32 and 68 years. Interestingly, only two patients had an associated Cushing's syndrome. More recently, Cardillo and coworkers [41] collected 19 patients with primary neuroendocrine tumors of the thymus over a period of 24 years, with similar demographic features as those previously described in terms of gender and age distribution. Nine of the 19 patients had an associated paraneoplastic syndrome, which was not further specified. Furthermore, Cardillo and coworkers [42] reported their experience with 35 cases accumulated from 5 different institutions. In this particular group of patients, 14 patients had an associated paraneoplastic syndrome. Neary and coworkers [43], in a more direct approach to the association of paraneoplastic syndromes associated with neuroendocrine thymic tumors, reported 12 patients with ACTH-producing thymic tumors. The patients' ages varied from 7 to 51 years (4 patients were children), and 11 of these patients presented with classic Cushing's syndrome at a median age of 21 years. The authors concluded that thymic ACTH-producing neuroendocrine tumor is an aggressive disease, particularly in young patients.

In our experience with 80 cases [44] that we had the opportunity to evaluate, we encountered that the tumor appears to be more common in men in a proportion of approximately 2:1; the age in these patients can be wide, ranging from as young as 16 years to older patients over 90 years of age, with a mean age of 58 years. Most of the tumors, however, appear to be more common in the sixth decade of life among men and in the fourth decade of life for women. Even though in about 28% of the patients the mediastinal mass was found during a routine chest radiograph, about 22% of these patients had an associated endocrinopathy, which included 6% of patients in whom Cushing's syndrome was determined to be associated with the tumor at the time of diagnosis. In addition, another 26% of patients presented with various symptoms, which include chest pain, weight loss, shortness of breath, and superior vena cava syndrome. Interestingly, when compared the age distribution between men and women, there appears to be a slight difference in the appearance of the tumor at certain age. For instance, the tumor appears to be more common in younger women in their 30s, while the tumor in men appears to be more common in their 50s. These demographic and clinical findings are depicted in Figs. 9.1, 9.2, 9.3, and 9.4.

One important issue that needs highlighting is the importance of assessing these neoplasms for what they represent, which essentially is a low- or intermediate-grade carcinoma. For instance, in the report of eight "atypical carcinoid tumors of the thymus" by Valli and coworkers [45], the authors encountered that in four cases in which

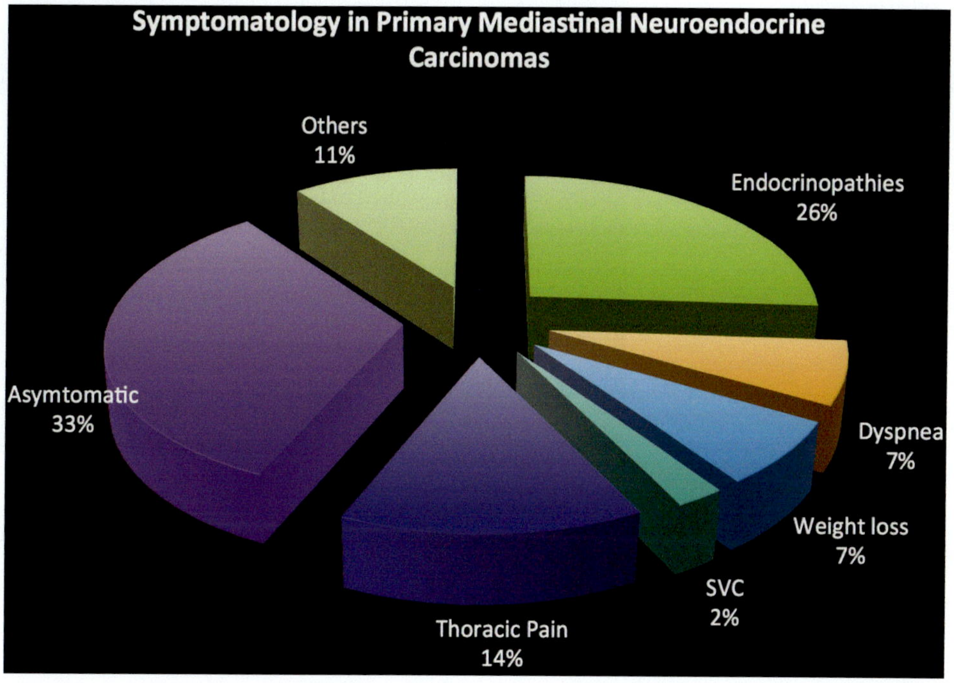

Fig. 9.1 Clinical symptomatology of patients with thymic neuroendocrine carcinomas

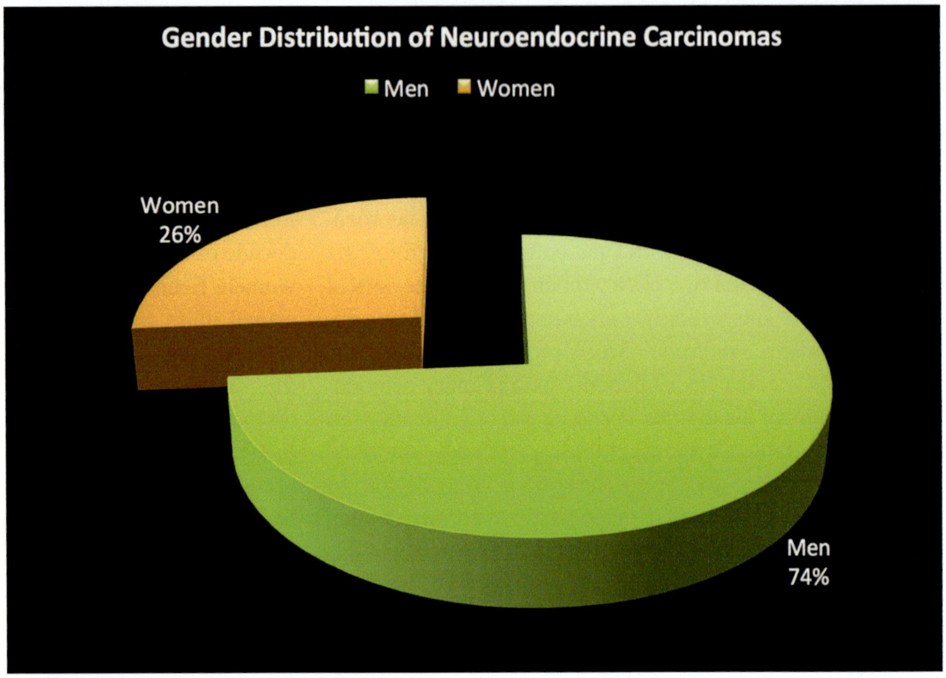

Fig. 9.2 Gender distribution of thymic neuroendocrine carcinomas

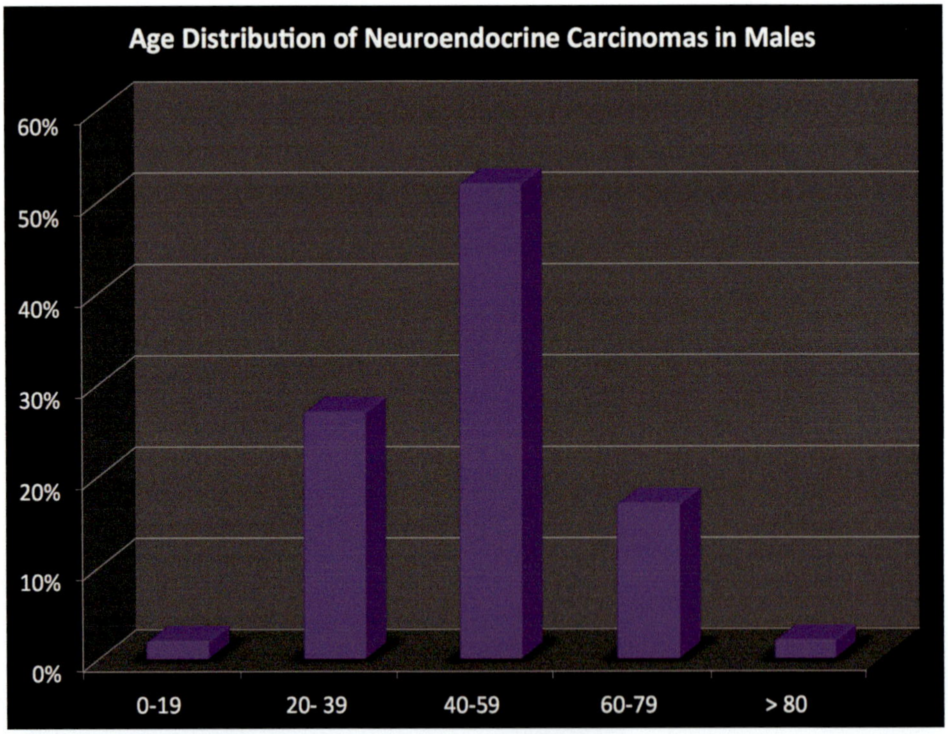

Fig. 9.3 Age distribution of thymic neuroendocrine carcinomas in men

they have follow-up information, even though the authors used the Masaoka staging schema of thymoma, which is clearly inappropriate for these tumors, recurrence and metastatic disease were documented, and three of these four patients died with widespread metastatic disease. In the 19 cases reported by Cardillo and coworkers [41], even though, once again, using an inappropriate schema for staging, the authors stated that the prognosis of these

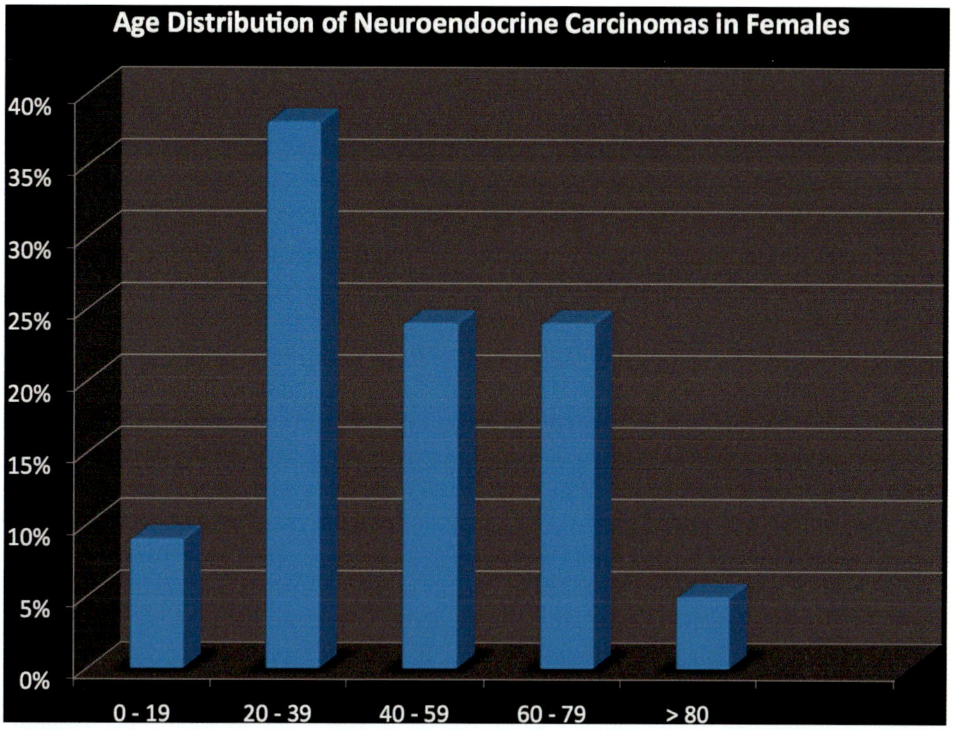

Fig. 9.4 Age distribution of thymic neuroendocrine carcinomas in women

tumors is related to grading, presence of paraneoplastic syndromes, and staging. The same authors [42] in a multicenter experience with 35 cases concluded that size (>7 cm) and proliferation index (ki-67 > 10%) are statistically significant and added a similar statement as in their manuscript with 19 cases that histology, paraneoplastic syndrome, staging, evidence of metastatic disease, and postoperative radiotherapy also impact prognosis. De Montpreville and coworkers [38], in their report of 14 cases, concluded that these tumors should be considered thymic neuroendocrine carcinomas because of their malignant behavior and added that complete surgical resection offers the best hope for a long-term survival. In our experience with 80 cases, we observed after a mean follow-up of 8.6 years that the overall survival for these patients was 28% at 5 years and 10% at 10 years. When further analyzed by histologic grading of the tumor, 32% of patients with low-grade carcinomas (carcinoid tumor) died of tumor, while 48% of patients with intermediate-grade carcinoma (atypical carcinoid) died of tumor in a period of time up to 11 years. In addition, 90% of patients with high-grade carcinoma died of tumor in a period of time up to 7 years. Recurrences were documented in 18 of the 80 patients studied as was metastatic disease to lymph nodes, lungs, bone, chest wall, and liver. Based on the above experience and with the perspective offered by others, it is difficult to argue against the preferred and more accurate terminology of thymic neuroendocrine carcinoma, rather than the ambiguous terminology of neuroendocrine tumor.

Classification

Although the classification of neuroendocrine carcinomas of the thymus appears to be similar to that of lung in terms of names or designations to the different categories of these tumors, there are important subtleties that are important to keep in mind as the criteria for diagnosis of each one of the specific categories of these tumors in the thymus are somewhat different from those in the lung. Interestingly, in the WHO publication of 1999 on the histological typing of tumors of the thymus [46], despite the fact that in a more forward vision of these tumors in the thymus the authors incorporated in parenthesis the term "carcinoma," the definition regarding mitotic activity in the "carcinoid tumor" or well-differentiated neuroendocrine carcinoma was that "mitotic activity is low and necrosis is scanty or absent." However, when the definition of "atypical carcinoid" was presented, not only was the definition regarding the mitotic count stated as "2 × 10/2mm^2," but the designation of carcinoma was also missing, therefore, leading to argue the following: what is the meaning of "mitotic activity low"? In reality, there is only one digit smaller than 2 and that is 1 (of course the absence of value will be 0), but even riskier is the fact that the author left the interpretation of well-differentiated neuroendocrine carcinoma for both low-grade and intermediate-grade tumors. In addition, it is stated that the proportion of "atypical carcinoids" is higher than that of pulmonary carcinoids. That may also be another inaccuracy, as when seen in larger numbers as in the series presented with 80 cases [44], the proportion of low-grade tumors against intermediate-grade tumors (carcinoid versus atypical carcinoid) were not even in a proportion of 2:1. Those numbers are depicted in Fig. 9.5. Such an assessment clearly underrepresents the true nature of these neoplasms and leads to erroneous interpretations and possible treatment options. Unfortunately, such assessment without further analysis was also repeated in the 2004 WHO publication [47] in which these tumors (low and intermediate) were under the designation of "well-differentiated neuroendocrine carcinomas." One would argue that, after such a misrepresentation, the new version of the WHO 2015 [48] would shed more light into the spectrum of two important and yet prognostically different neoplasms. However, in the new version of the WHO 2015 [48], these neoplasms are presented under the heading of thymic neuroendocrine tumors (carcinoid and atypical carcinoid), and it is stated that terms such as well-differentiated neuroendocrine carcinoma are not recommended. Here, it is important to highlight key issues regarding that warning. Indeed, the use of the term well-differentiated neuroendocrine carcinoma should be abandoned when it implies that it represents two different neoplasms, carcinoid and atypical carcinoid; however, it is unclear whether the authors of the WHO meant not to use the term "carcinoma" at all, which would be very much a contradiction to almost everything that has been recorded in more recent literature. Needless to say, such preferential organization was made without conducting a specific clinicopathological study of their own nor citing a specific publication dealing with that specific categorization of tumors. Furthermore, the WHO authors state that the mitotic activity for the low-grade tumor (carcinoid tumor) should be of <2 per 2 mm^2, basically promoting the same criteria that have been put forward with similar tumors in the lung. Regarding that particular topic, the mitotic count issue of low-grade carcinomas (carcinoid tumor) of the lung has been questioned more recently. Tsuta and coworkers [49], in a study of low- and intermediate-grade neuroendocrine carcinomas of the lung (carcinoid and atypical carcinoid) specifically on the issue of mitotic count, analyzed 80 patients and counted mitotic figures using different modalities, which included random count, hot spot count, and the evaluation of the whole section; however, more important was the demonstration that the mitotic count of fewer than 2 mitotic figures per 10 high-power fields is likely incorrect, as it does not provide any meaningful or statistically significant survival prognosis for patients with these tumors. As a matter of fact, when each case was individualized to correlate mitotic count with the 5-year RFS (recurrence-free survival), the results were 0 mitosis, 95.1%; 1 mitosis, 87.5%; 2 mitosis, 75%; and 3 mitosis, 100%. Therefore, the authors had to reset to 3 mitotic figures per 10 high-power fields for the low-grade tumors while 4 to 10 mitotic figures for the intermediate-grade carcinomas. Once these cutoffs were reset, the results clearly show a difference for the 5-year RFS of 93.1% and 0%, respectively ($p = 0.002$). In addition, when the count was on hot spots, the 5-year RFS for tumors with 0–1 mitosis × 10 hpf, 2–10 mitosis × 10 hpf, and more than 11 mitosis × 10 hpf were 95.5%, 94.6%, and 75.2%, respectively. Furthermore, when each case was individualized and correlated with mitotic counts, the 5-year RFS showed 0 mito-

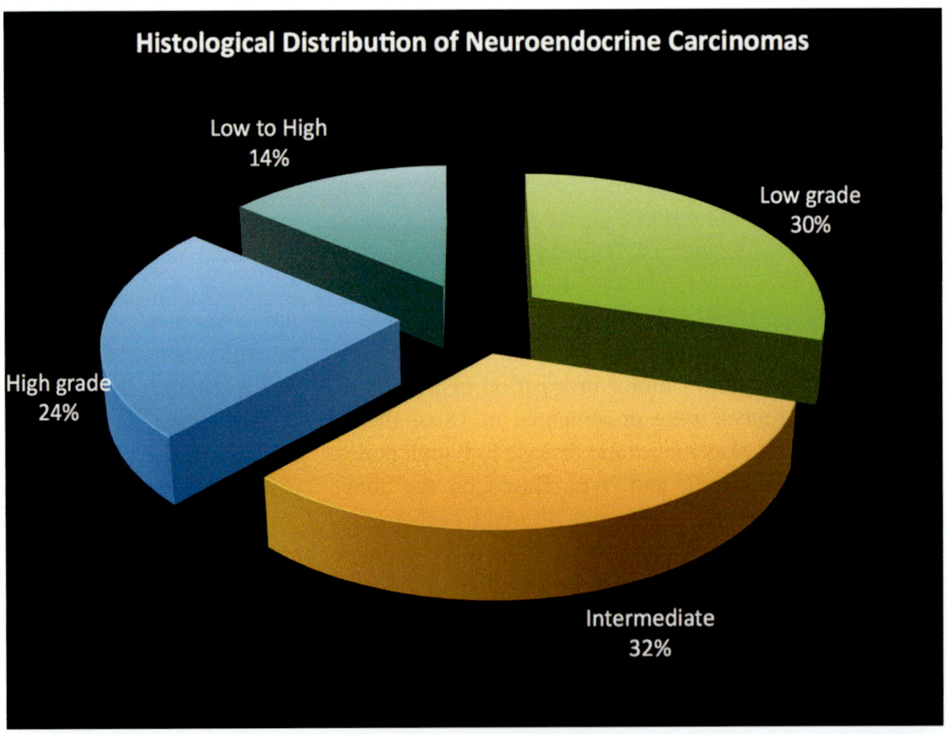

Fig. 9.5 Histological distribution of neuroendocrine carcinomas

sis, 100%; 1 mitosis, 90%; 2 mitosis, 100%; and 3 mitosis, 100%. Thus, the cutoff had to be resetted? to low-grade tumor 0–3 mitosis and intermediate-grade tumor to 4 or more mitotic figure × 10 hpf. Then the 5-year RFS showed 97.4% and 83.4%, respectively. This is similar to our reported experience with 80 thymic neuroendocrine carcinomas in which the mitotic count of 0–3 was assigned to low-grade neuroendocrine carcinoma and 4–10 mitosis × 10 hpf for intermediate-grade neuroendocrine carcinomas. Based on these data, it is likely that not only the WHO is incorrect in their assumption of the number of mitotic figures for the pulmonary low-grade neuroendocrine carcinomas, but also most definitely it is incorrect for the thymic low-grade neuroendocrine carcinomas. Tables 9.1 and 9.2 depict the subtle differences not only in specific nomenclature but also in diagnostic criteria.

In our experience, which up to now remains the largest series of these tumors presented in the literature, a novel classification system with specific histopathological definitions was presented [44]. The study was composed of an analysis of 80 patients with primary thymic neuroendocrine carcinomas ranging from low to intermediate to poorly differentiated carcinomas. In this study, all the different tumor differentiations were observed. Of the 80 cases studied, 29 corresponded to the low-grade tumors, 36 to the intermediate-grade tumors, and 15 to the high-grade tumors. The criteria for diagnosis and inclusion into any of these specific categories as well as its specific nomenclature are as follows:

- Low-grade neuroendocrine carcinoma (well-differentiated neuroendocrine carcinoma, grade I neuroendocrine carcinoma, carcinoid tumor).
  - Predominantly organoid pattern.
  - Small focus of necrosis (punctuate necrosis) may be seen.
  - Mild cytologic atypia.
  - Up to 3 mitotic figures × 10 high-power fields.
  - Vascular invasion may be seen.
- Intermediate-grade neuroendocrine carcinoma (moderately differentiated neuroendocrine carcinoma, grade II neuroendocrine carcinoma, atypical carcinoid).
  - Organoid and diffuse growth pattern.
  - Extensive comedonecrosis or frank necrosis.
  - Moderate cytologic atypia.
  - 4 to 10 mitotic figures × 10 high-power fields.
  - Vascular invasion may be seen.
- High-grade neuroendocrine carcinoma (poorly differentiated neuroendocrine carcinoma, grade III neuroendocrine carcinoma, small cell carcinoma, or large cell neuroendocrine carcinoma).
  - Diffuse growth pattern (loss of organoid pattern).
  - Extensive necrosis.
  - Marked cytologic atypia.
  - >10 mitotic figures per 10 high-power fields.
  - Vascular invasion may be seen.

Table 9.1 Classification schemas for thymic neuroendocrine carcinomas

Moran-Suster[a]	WHO 1999φ	WHO 2004λ	WHO 2015π
Low-grade NE Ca	Classic carcinoid	Well-diff. NE Ca	Typical carcinoid
Intermediate-grade NE Ca	Atypical carcinoid	Well-diff. NE Ca	Atypical carcinoid
High-grade NE Ca	Poorly diff. NE Ca	Poorly diff. NE Ca	Large cell NE carcinoma Small cell carcinoma

φ not based on any clinicopathological study
λ not based on any clinicopathological study
π not based on any clinicopathological study
NE neuroendocrine, *Ca* carcinoma, *Diff* differentiated
[a]Based on a clinicopathological correlation of 80 cases

Table 9.2 Histopathological criteria for the diagnosis of thymic neuroendocrine carcinomas

Feature	Moran-Suster	WHO 1999	WHO 2004	WHO 2015
	Low grade	*Classic carcinoid*	*Well-diff. NE Ca*	*Typical carcinoid*
Mitosis	Up to 3 × 10 hpf	Low	<2 × 10 hpf	<2 × 10 hpf
Necrosis	Small foci	Scanty	No necrosis	No necrosis
Growth pattern	Organoid	Not mentioned	Not mentioned	Not mentioned
	Intermediate grade	*Atypical carcinoid*	*Well-diff. NE Ca*	*Atypical carcinoid*
Mitosis	4–10 × 10 hpf	2–10 × 10 hpf	2–10 × 10 hpf	2–10 hpf
Necrosis	Extensive	Foci of necrosis	Present	Present
Growth pattern	Organoid and diffuse	Not mentioned	Not mentioned	Not mentioned
	High grade	*Poorly diff. Ca*	*Poorly diff. NE Ca*	*Large cell* *Small cell*
Mitosis	>10 × 10 hpf	Not mentioned	>10 × 10 hpf	>10 × 10 hpf
Necrosis	Extensive	Not mentioned	Not mentioned	Frequent
Growth pattern	Diffuse	Not mentioned	Not mentioned	Not mentioned

It is also important to highlight that this stratification and classification of neuroendocrine tumors is based on tumor resections and not on biopsy material. In daily practice, it is more common to have only a mediastinoscopic biopsy available for review. Thus, one is confronted with obvious limitations to provide a specific subclassification of these tumors. In such a situation, as we often do with similar tumors in the lung, the most important separation is with the high-grade tumors such as small cell carcinoma or large cell neuroendocrine carcinoma, which may be followed and treated differently than the lower-grade tumors. Also important to highlight is the possibility of encountering tumors that may show features ranging from low-grade to high-grade histology. In these cases, it is important to assess such histology, which in turn illustrates the limitations that one may encounter with small mediastinoscopic biopsies.

Staging

Due to the rarity of these tumors as primary thymic neoplasms, a more specific staging system has not been officially promoted. Thus, this leaves the staging of these tumors to various schemas that in the majority of the cases have been presented for other more common thymic tumors. However, it is important to highlight that neuroendocrine neoplasms, namely, thymic neuroendocrine carcinomas, are most likely to behave as conventional non-neuroendocrine carcinomas than as thymomas; therefore, the use of schemas proposed for thymomas is likely to show inconsistencies regarding staging and clinical behavior for these tumors. Even though there have been some attempts to use staging for neuroendocrine carcinomas of the thymus, these schemas have lacked universal agreement, and, in some of them, the usefulness has been hampered due to its lack of clarity. For instance, Fukai and coworkers [50] presented a tentative TNM schema and concluded that distant metastasis is the most important prognostic factor, leaving T and N as associated features without any specific clinical impact. Due to these shortcomings, the Masaoka or the Koga-modified Masaoka staging proposal has been used in many cases. However, it is highly important to note that those staging systems were proposed for thymomas and not for thymic carcinoma or neuroendocrine carcinoma, which represent different clinicopathological entities. The fact that these tumors have the potential to spread to lymph nodes, lung, bone, or organs below the diaphragm or above the thoracic inlet [44] should provide a sense of the need to use a more appropriate staging system than the one proposed for thymomas. Therefore, in view of the similar biological behavior of conventional thymic carcinoma to neuroendocrine carcinoma in terms of metastatic spread, we consider that the application of the Weissferdt-Moran [51] proposed staging should be applied not only to conventional thymic carcinoma but also to thymic neuroendocrine carcinoma. A recent review on the topic of staging for thymic tumors addressing these specific issues has been presented in which a comparison of the different schemas is analyzed, with the main emphasis that those schemas presented for thymomas are inadequate for thymic carcinomas or neuroendocrine carcinomas [52]. A comparison of the different schemas for the staging of thymic carcinomas is presented in the chapter on Staging of thymic epithelial neoplasms [Chap. 6].

An illustrative view of the different stages for thymic neuroendocrine carcinoma is presented in Figs. 9.6a–c, 9.7a–c, and 9.8a, b.

a

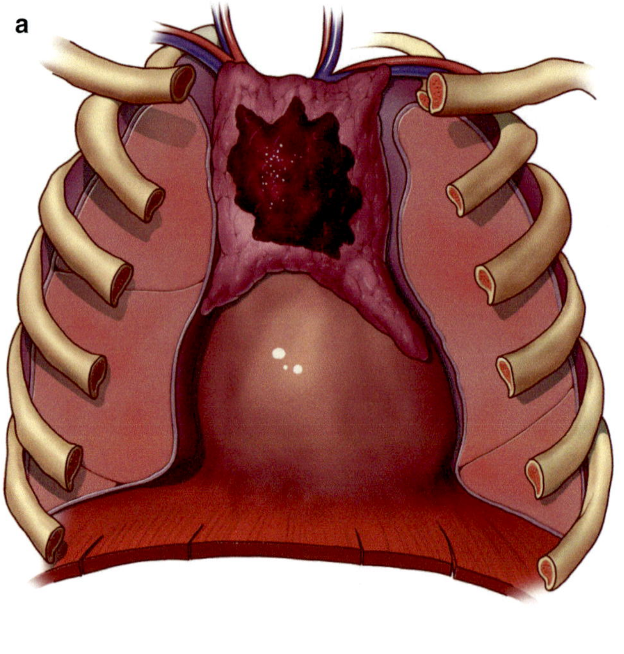

Fig. 9.6 (**a**) Thymic neuroendocrine carcinoma stage I – tumor is confined to the mediastinal compartment (**a**: Copyright © 2016 with permission from Dr. Kalhor and Moran)

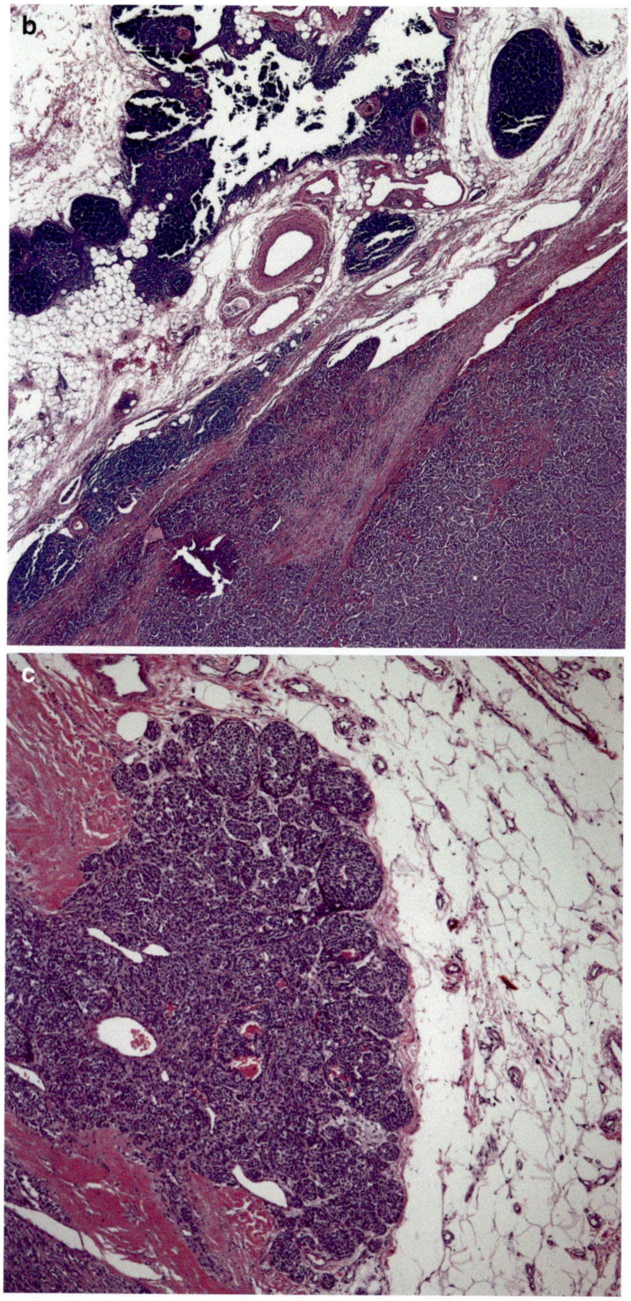

Fig. 9.6 (continued) (**b**) Tumor involves the thymic gland; (**c**) tumor infiltrates into adipose tissue

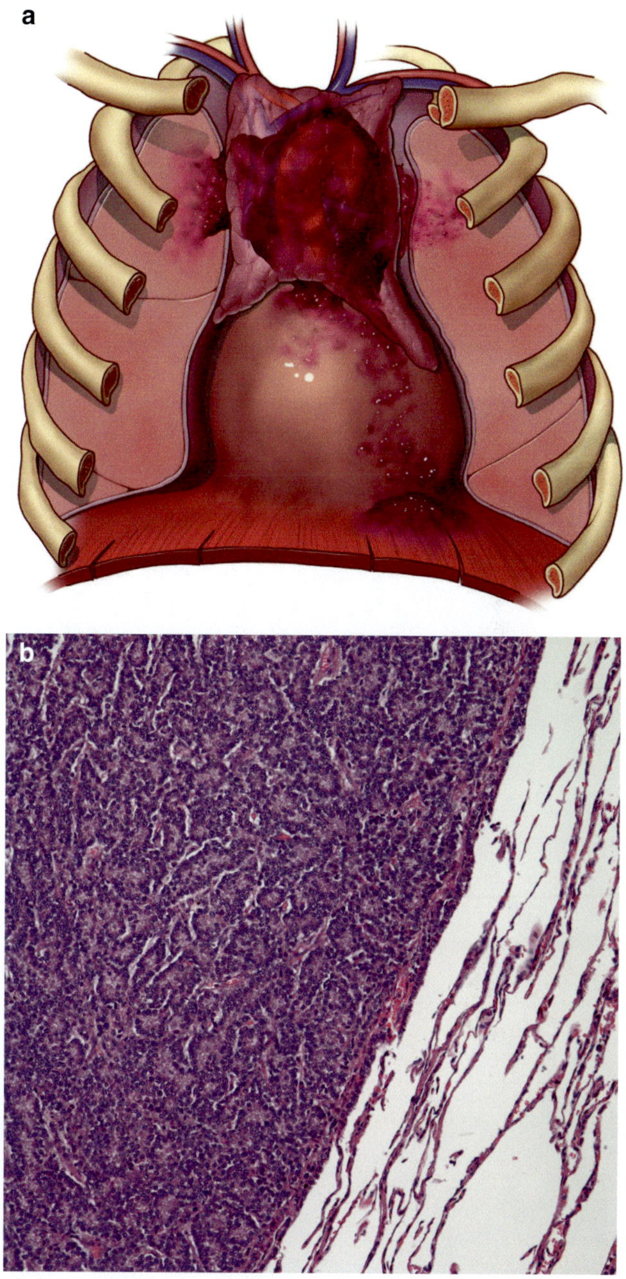

Fig. 9.7 (**a**) Neuroendocrine carcinoma stage II – tumor extends outside of the mediastinal compartment but remains within the thoracic cavity; (**b**) tumors involves lung parenchyma (**a**: Copyright © 2016 with permission from Dr. Kalhor and Moran)

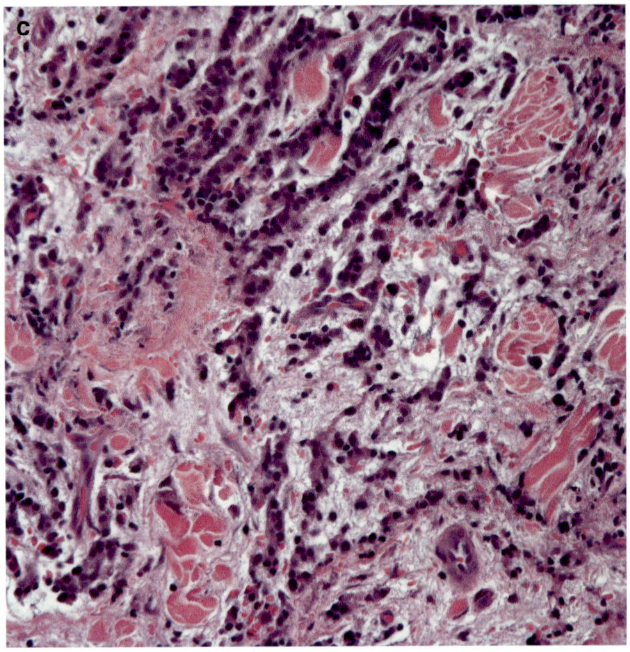

Fig. 9.7 (continued) (c) Tumor involves diaphragm

Pathological Features

Gross Features

The macroscopic features of thymic neuroendocrine carcinomas, either low or intermediate grade, are rather non-specific. These tumors are commonly described as large, soft, and light brown in color. The tumor may measure from a couple of centimeters in greatest diameter to tumors over 15 cm in greatest dimension (Fig. 9.9). The cut surface of these tumors may show a homogeneous rubbery surface, while the presence of areas of hemorrhage and necrosis should alert of the possibility of an intermediate-grade neoplasm. These areas not only need to be documented but also carefully sampled, as the presence of necrosis is part of the criteria for upgrading a neoplasm.

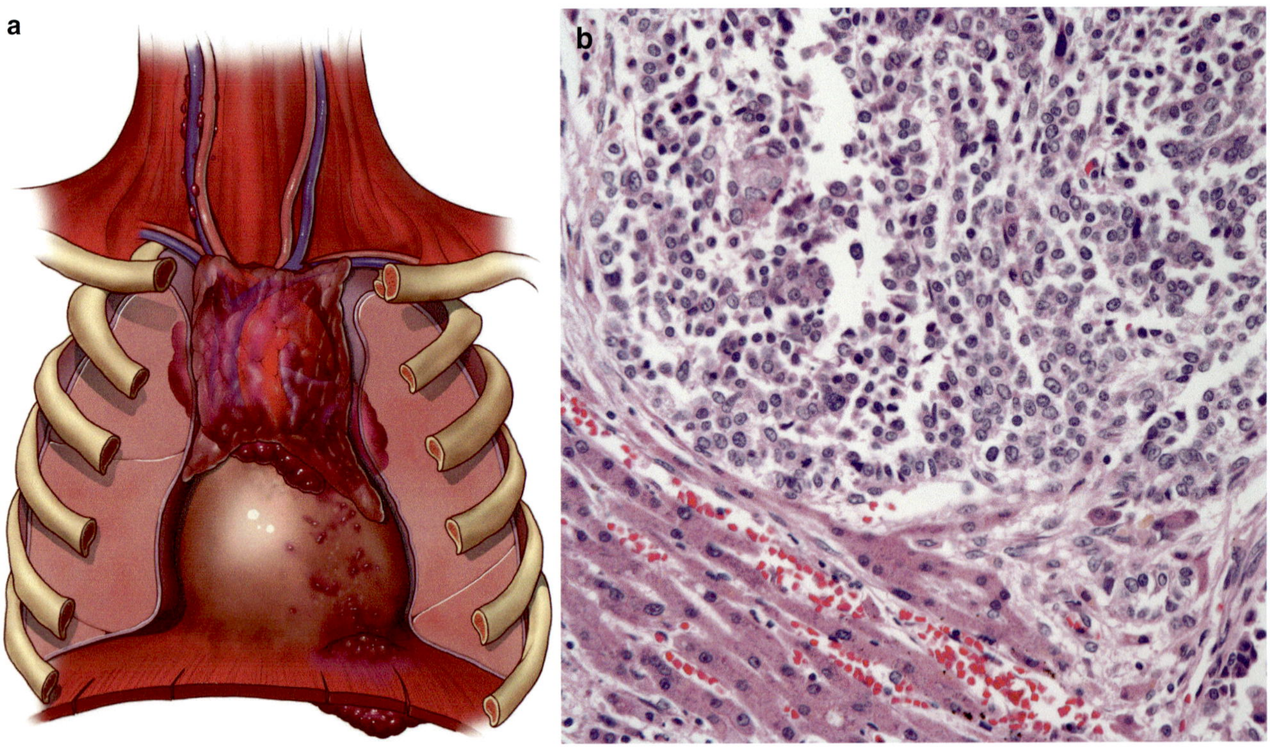

Fig. 9.8 (a) Neuroendocrine carcinoma stage III – the tumor extends above the thoracic inlet or below the diaphragm; (b) metastatic NE carcinoma in the liver. (a: Copyright © 2016 with permission from Dr. Kalhor and Moran)

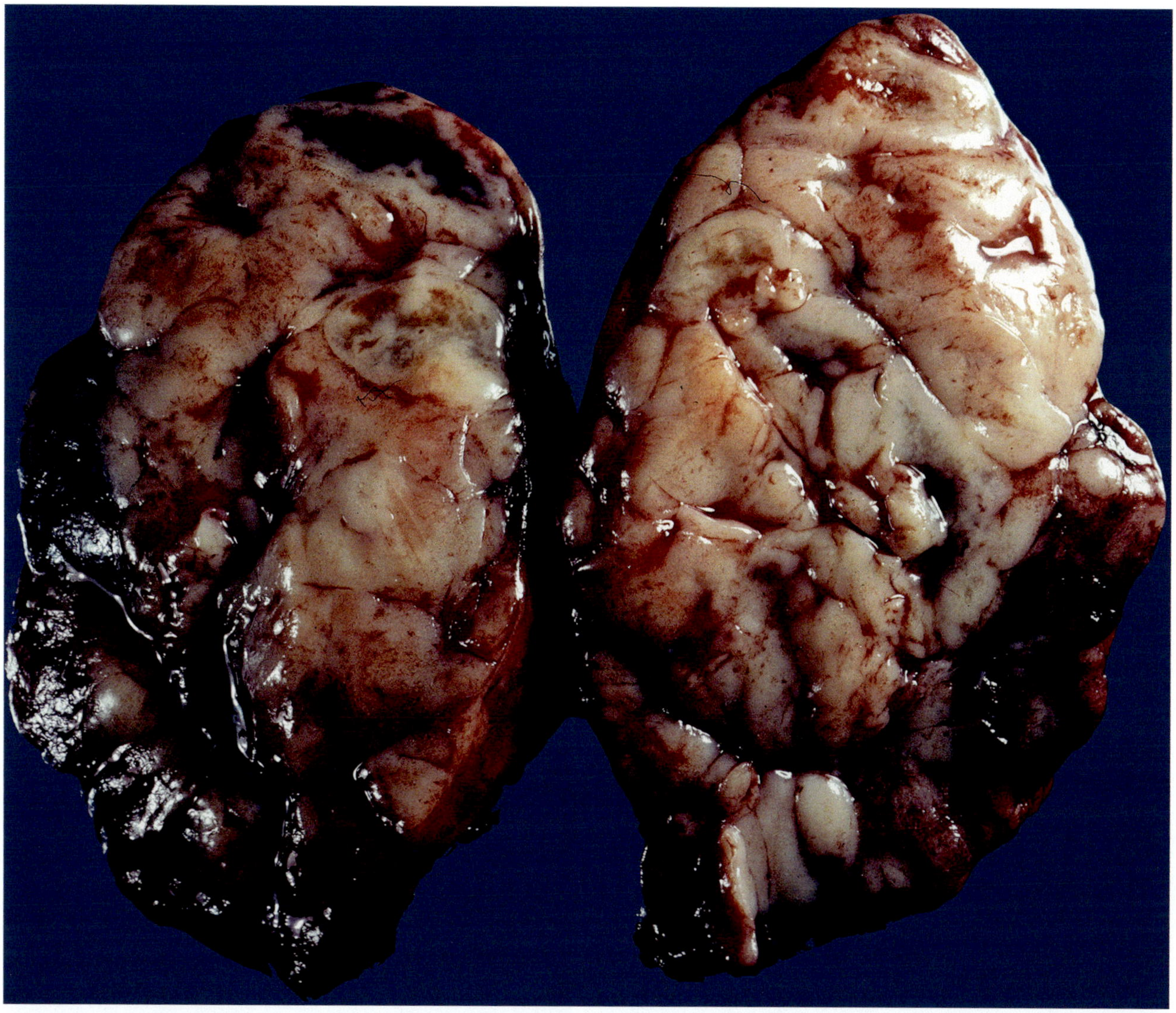

Fig. 9.9 Thymic neuroendocrine carcinoma showing a fleshy homogeneous light brown cut surface

Histopathological Features

The histopathological features ascribed to these tumors have been well presented in the literature, and the basic histopathological features are similar to those tumors in other organ systems such as lung and gastrointestinal tract. Therefore, due to this similarity, it is important to keep in mind the possibility of metastatic disease, as in reality there is not a single histopathological hallmark to separate thymic neuroendocrine carcinomas from those of other anatomic areas. This separation is often performed on clinical and radiological grounds after a good clinical evaluation of these patients.

Low- and Intermediate-Grade Neuroendocrine Carcinomas

Thymic neuroendocrine carcinomas have been the subject of numerous publications either as case reports or small series of cases in which emphasis has been given not only to the morphological aspects of the tumors but also to specific associations of the neuroendocrine neoplasm with other types of histology, or emphasizing a specific clinical feature with the histology of the tumor [53–62]. For instance, Paties and coworkers and Kuo [63, 64] both documented a case in a 62- and 56-year-old men with a mediastinal neoplasm. The authors coded these cases as "multidirectional carcinoma of the thymus with neuroendocrine and sarcomatoid components and carcinoid syndrome." Also, Mizuno and coworkers [65] documented a 60-year-old man with the coexistence of what the authors called "thymic carcinoid and thymoma."

In general, the histopathological features of these tumors include the presence of prominent "organoid" or nested growth pattern in which these nests are surrounded by a delicate fibrovascular septa. In some tumors, the tumor cells may be arranged in cords or ribbons with little intervening stroma. The presence of rosettes may be a common finding in some cases, while in other cases this feature may be subtler and not so easily identified. At higher magnification, the tumor cells are round to oval with moderate amount of cytoplasm and round nuclei with coarse chromatin (Figs. 9.10, 9.11, 9.12, 9.13, 9.14, 9.15, 9.16, 9.17, 9.18, 9.19, 9.20, 9.21, and 9.22). The degree of cellular atypia in the low-grade tumors is rather mild, even though cells with more prominent nucleoli, sporadic mitotic figures, and focal punctuate necrosis may be seen in these tumors (Figs. 9.23 and 9.24). Even though

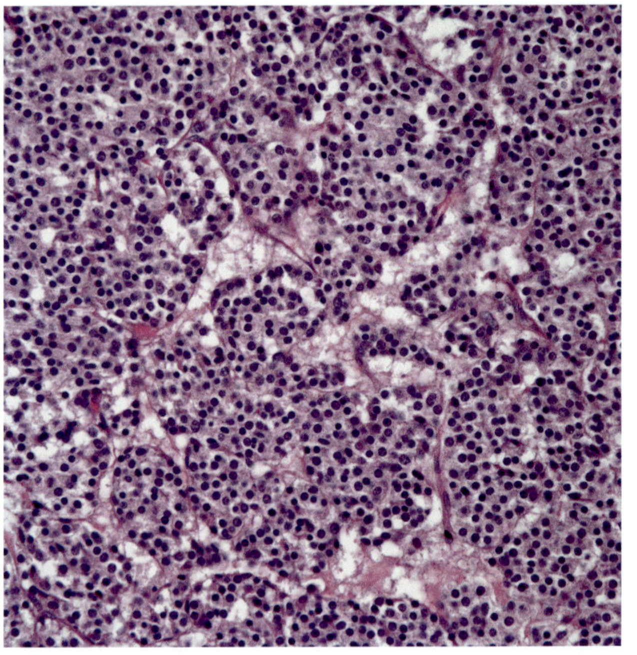

Fig. 9.11 Low-grade neuroendocrine carcinoma showing a fairly homogeneous cellular proliferation with only mild nuclear atypia and absent mitotic activity

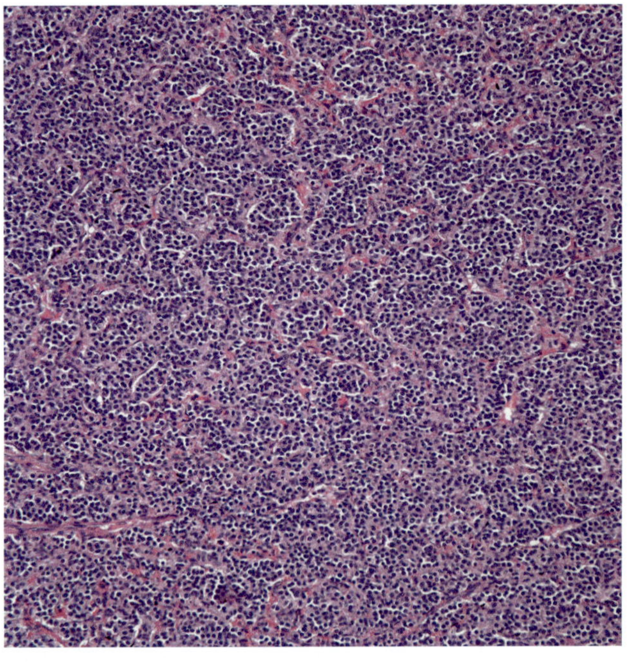

Fig. 9.10 Low-grade neuroendocrine carcinoma showing a well-organized "organoid" growth pattern

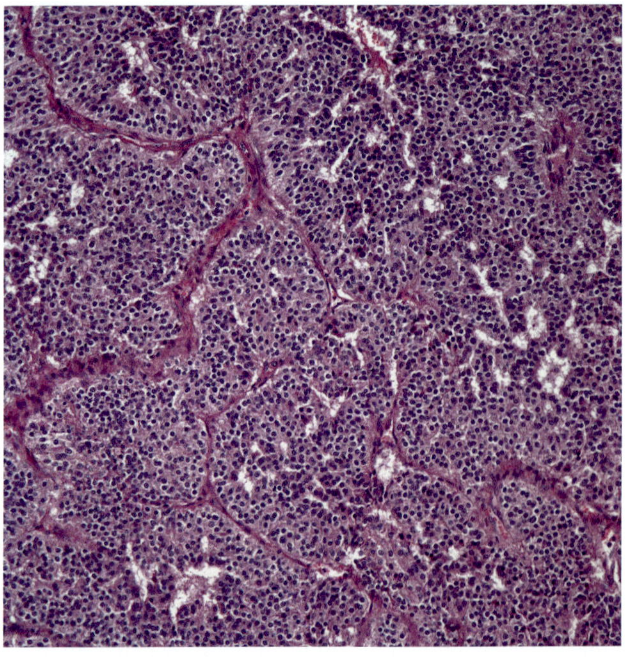

Fig. 9.12 Low-grade neuroendocrine carcinoma showing a nested pattern with a fairly discrete fibroconnective tissue separating tumor nests

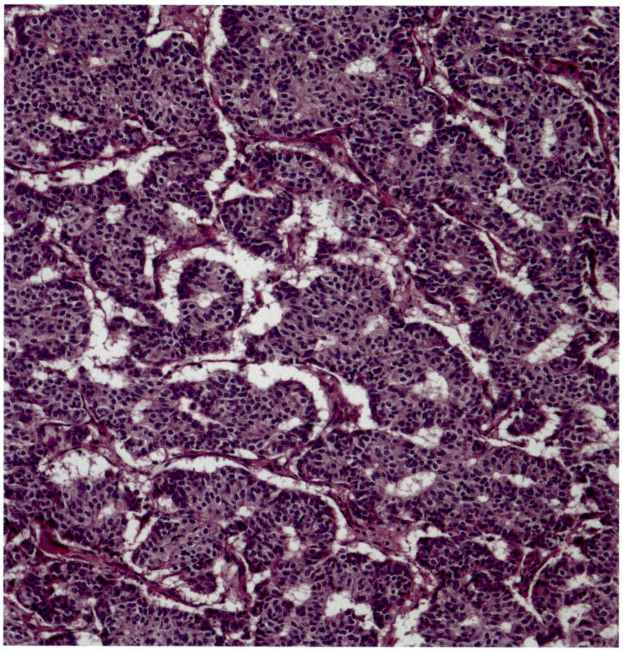

Fig. 9.13 Low-grade neuroendocrine carcinoma showing an organoid pattern with pseudoglandular areas

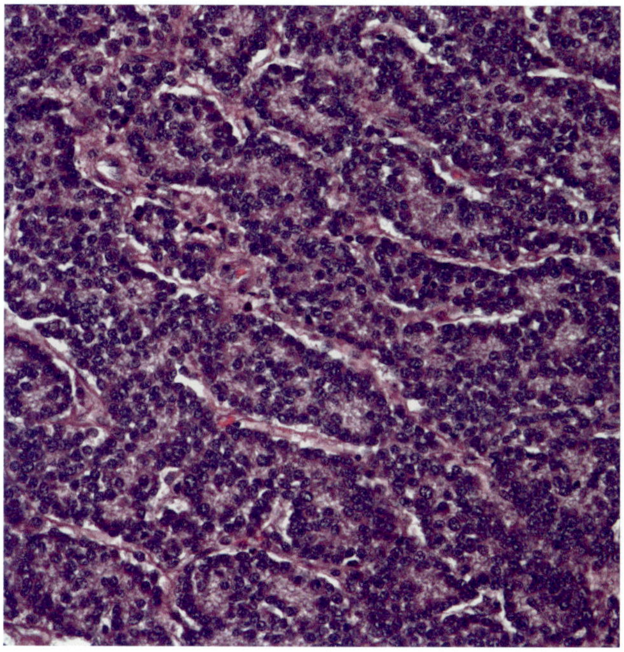

Fig. 9.14 Low-grade neuroendocrine carcinoma showing ribbons of tumor cells

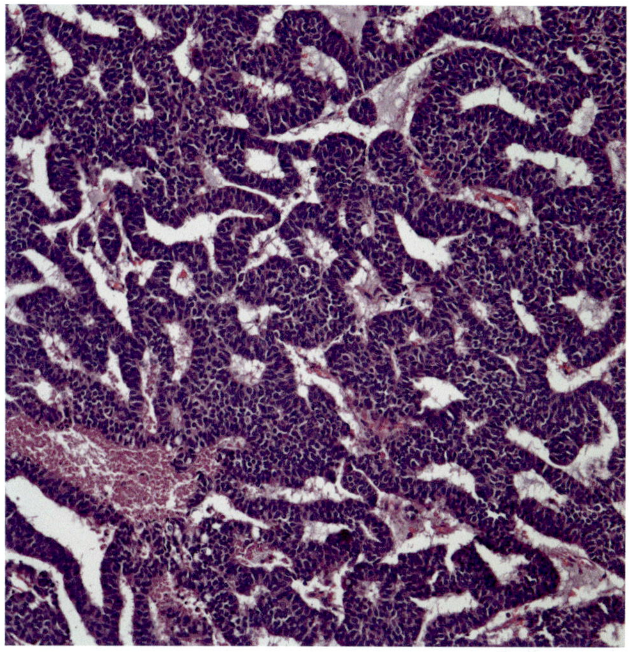

Fig. 9.15 Low-grade neuroendocrine carcinoma showing a more glandular appearance

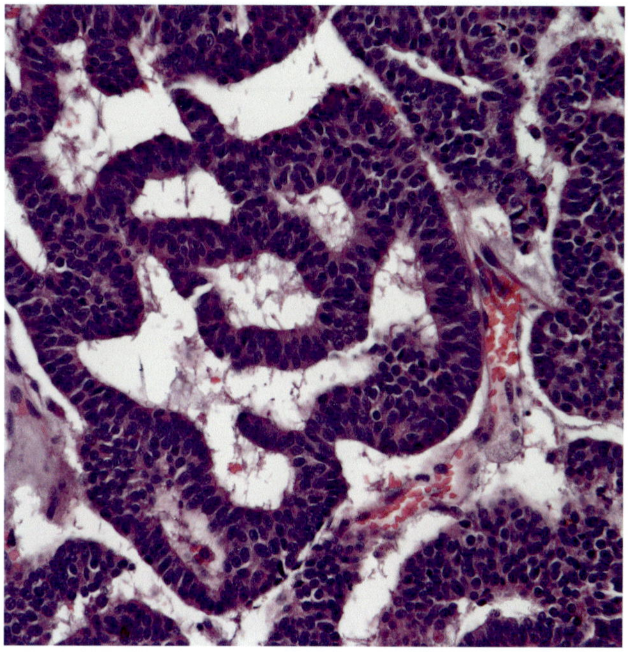

Fig. 9.16 Higher magnification of a low-grade neuroendocrine carcinoma with a glandular appearance

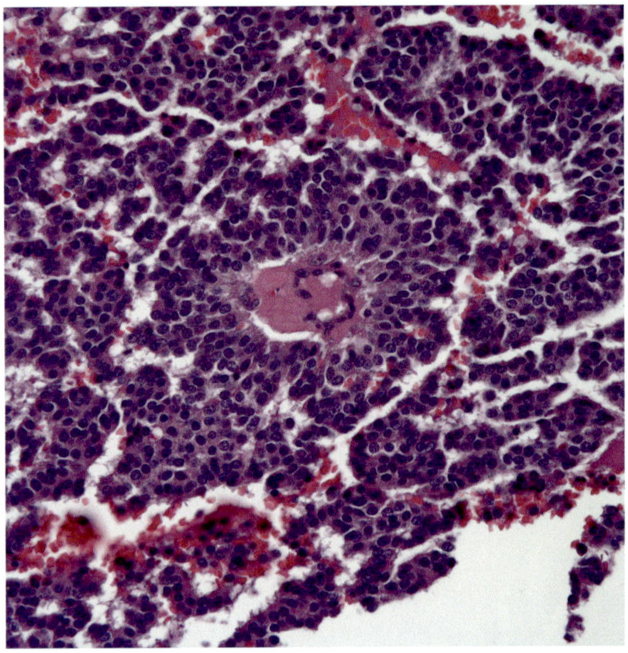

Fig. 9.17 Low-grade neuroendocrine carcinoma showing rosettes

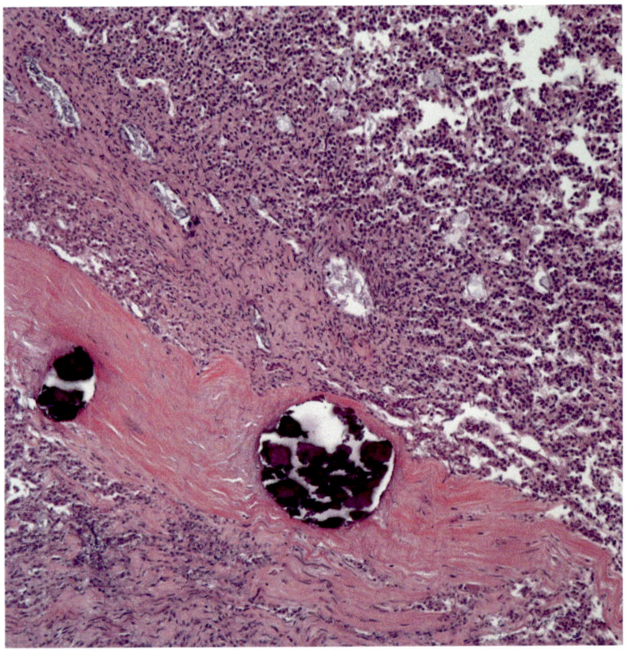

Fig. 9.18 Calcifications present in a low-grade neuroendocrine carcinoma

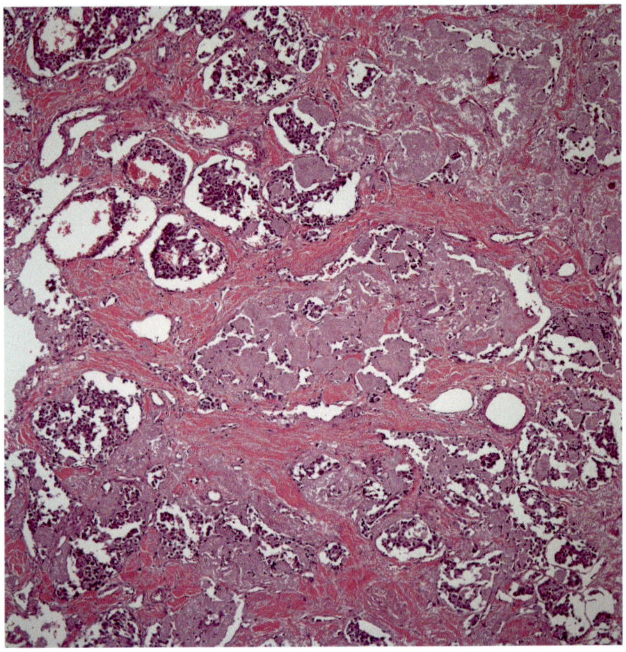

Fig. 9.19 Low-grade neuroendocrine carcinoma with amyloid-like areas

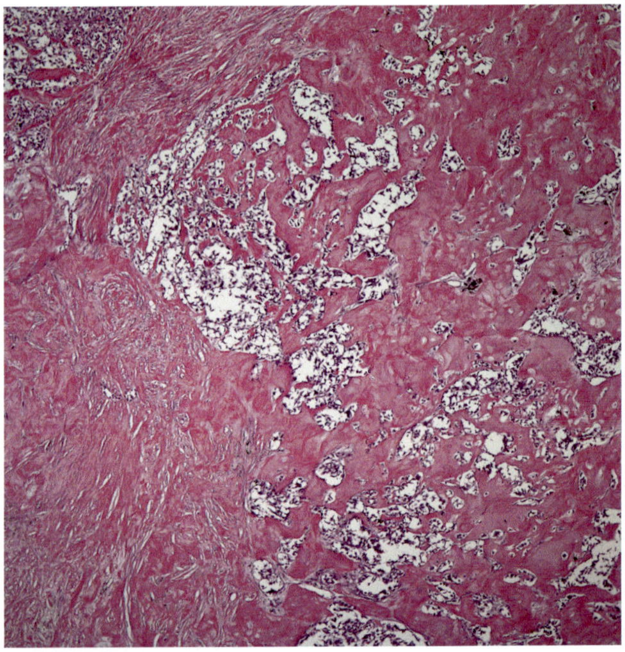

Fig. 9.20 Amyloid-like areas in a low-grade neuroendocrine carcinoma, which is not more than hyalinized fibroconnective tissue

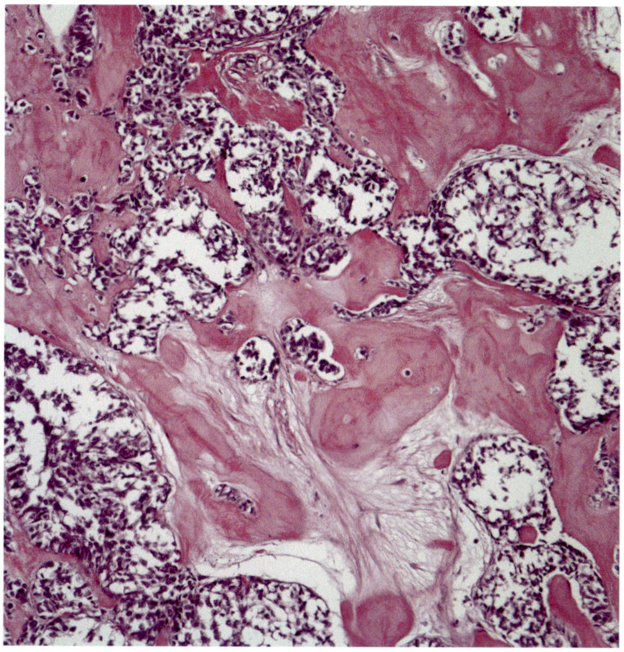

Fig. 9.21 Extensive hyalinization in neuroendocrine carcinoma can pose a challenge in diagnosis

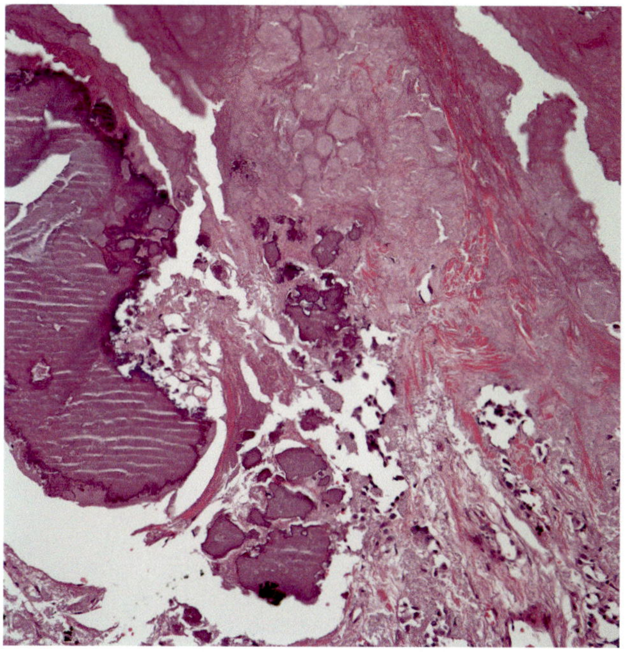

Fig. 9.22 Extensive hyalinization and calcification in a neuroendocrine carcinoma

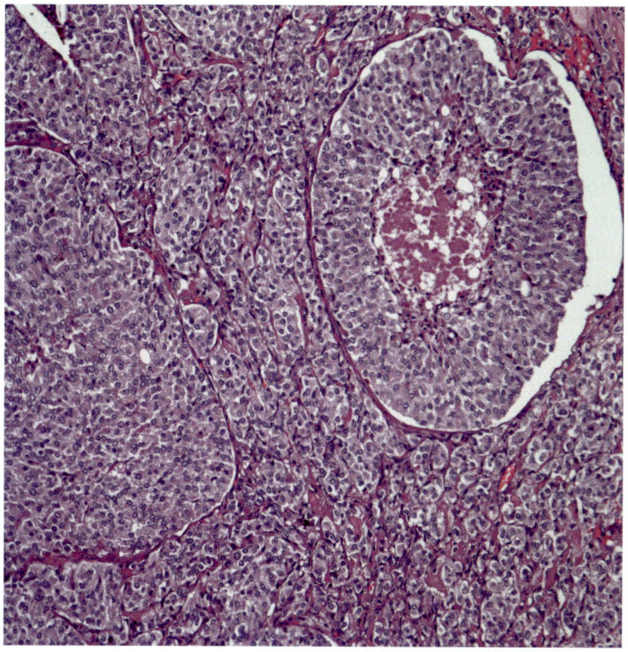

Fig. 9.23 Low-grade neuroendocrine carcinoma with a microscopic focus of necrosis

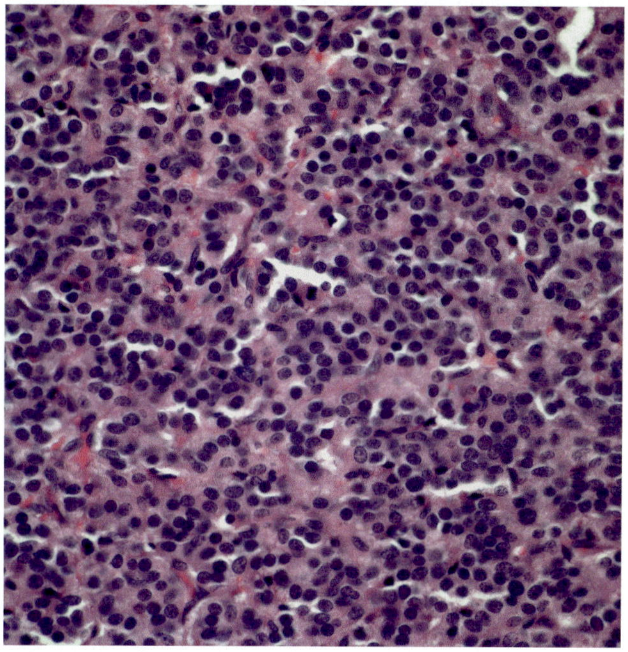

Fig. 9.24 Low-grade neuroendocrine carcinoma showing scattered mitotic figures

similar features may be seen in intermediate-grade tumors, the pattern of growth may be a mixed type in which one can observe the presence of a well-defined nested growth pattern admixed with extensive areas of diffuse, sheetlike growth pattern. The cytological features of these tumors show more pronounced nuclear atypia, and the presence of nucleoli is easier to identify than in the low-grade tumors. However, one important clue to the diagnosis is in the low power view of these tumors, as the presence of areas of comedo-like necrosis is apparent in most of these tumors. As stated in the section on classification of these tumors, the presence of necrosis and mitotic activity in the ranged of 4–10 ×10 hpf should make the classification of these tumors easier (Figs. 9.25, 9.26, 9.27, 9.28, 9.29, 9.30, 9.31, 9.32, 9.33, and 9.34).

In addition, series of different histopathological growth pattern have been described or amplified regarding neuroendocrine carcinoma of the thymus [66–74]. Some of these growth patterns may pose a challenge in the diagnosis and are discussed below.

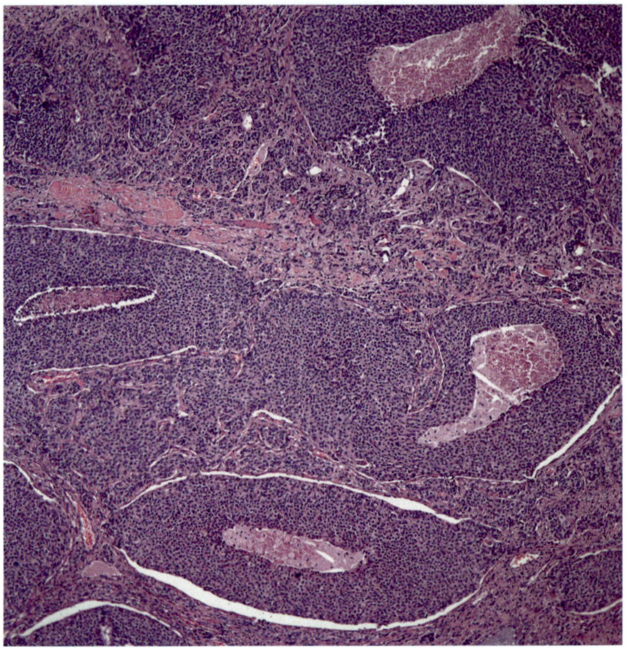

Fig. 9.25 Intermediate-grade neuroendocrine carcinoma showing obvious areas of comedonecrosis

Mucinous

This specific variant is rather unusual as the tumors are characterized by the presence of extensive pools of mucin in which the neoplastic cells are floating within this stroma (Figs. 9.35, 9.36, and 9.37). The neoplastic cells may be arranged in clusters with similar cytologic features as those that have been described in garden-variety cases. In some areas, the tumor may show more solid cellular proliferation in which the tumor may appear as forming glands with a cribriform appearance. Mitotic activity is possible in these cases and may help in properly classifying these tumors.

Angiomatoid

The hallmark of this particular variant is the presence of multiple cystically dilated spaces filled with blood, which at low power magnification resembled a vascular neoplasm. However, upon closer inspection, the cystically dilated spaces are not lined by endothelial cells but rather by neoplastic neuroendocrine cells (Figs. 9.38, 9.39, 9.40, and 9.41).

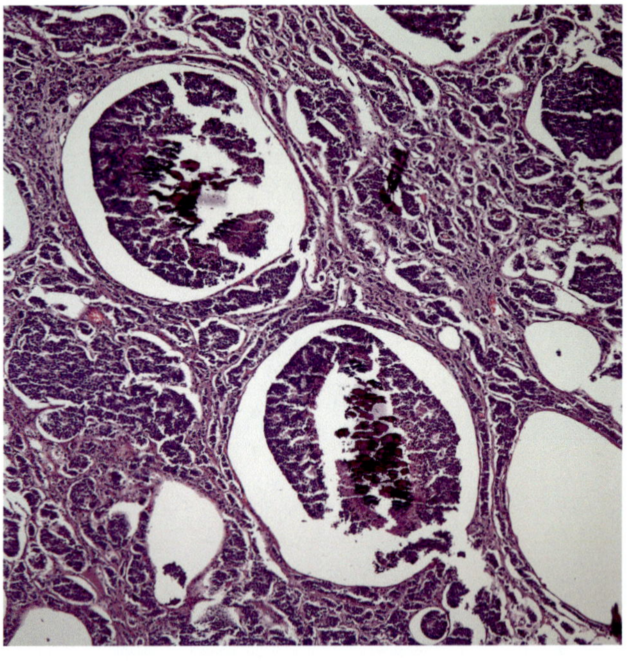

Fig. 9.26 Intermediate-grade neuroendocrine carcinoma showing comedonecrosis and calcifications

Pigmented (Melanocytic)

The presence of melanin pigment associated with neuroendocrine carcinomas may be focal or extensive and may also be seen in any type of growth pattern. When the pigment is

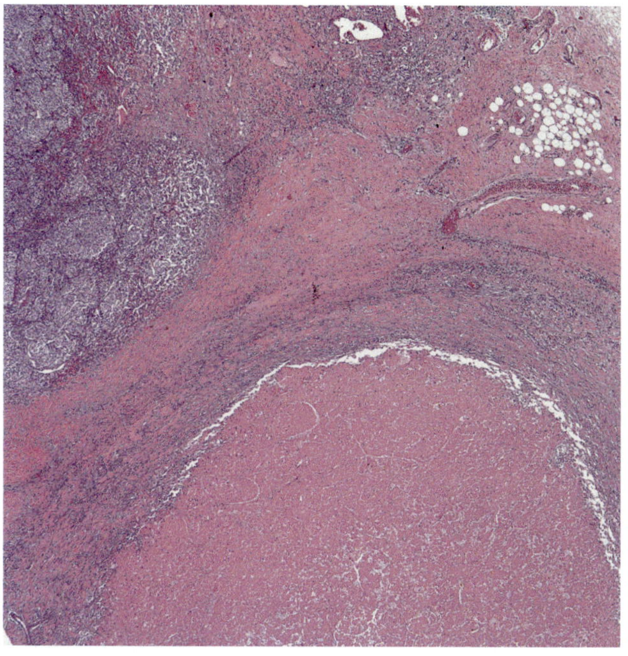

Fig. 9.27 Intermediate-grade neuroendocrine carcinoma showing more extensive areas of necrosis

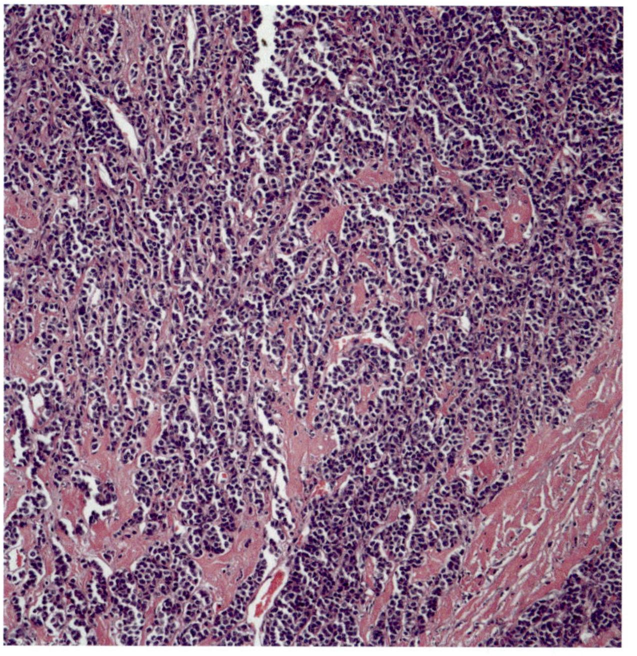

Fig. 9.29 Intermediate-grade neuroendocrine carcinoma showing cords of neoplastic cells

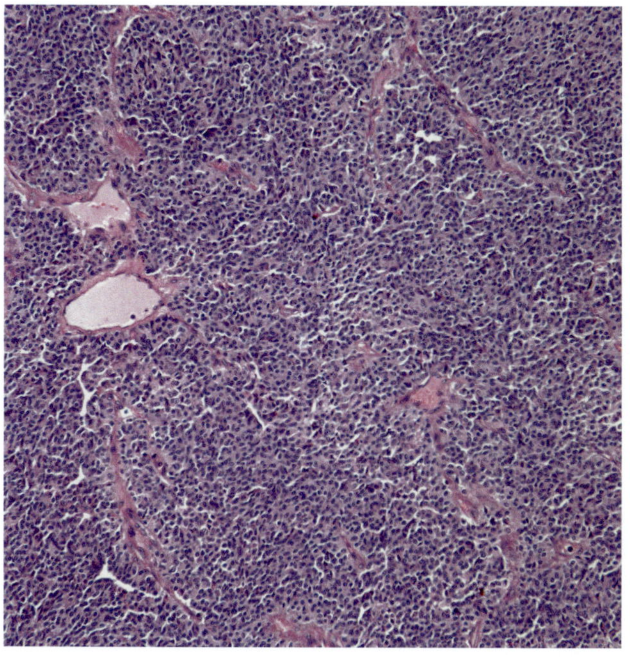

Fig. 9.28 Intermediate-grade neuroendocrine carcinoma showing a more diffuse growth pattern

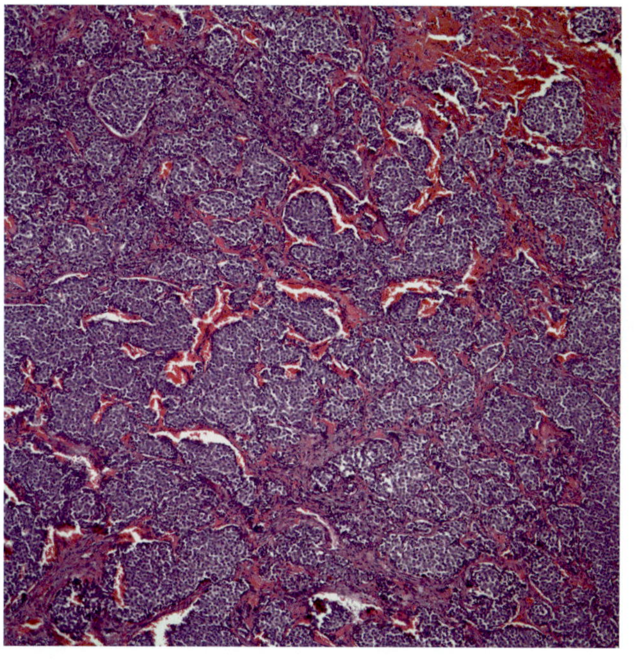

Fig. 9.30 In some areas a more subtle nested pattern may be seen in intermediate-grade neuroendocrine carcinomas

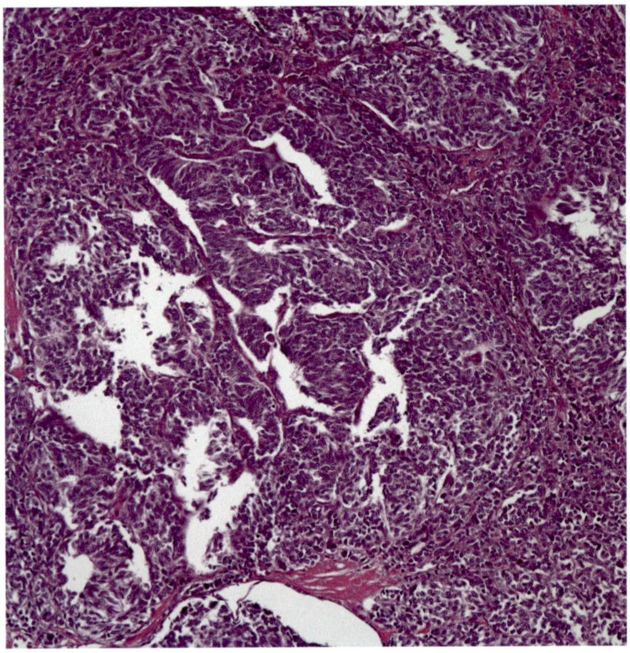

Fig. 9.31 Intermediate-grade neuroendocrine carcinoma showing a more solid growth pattern

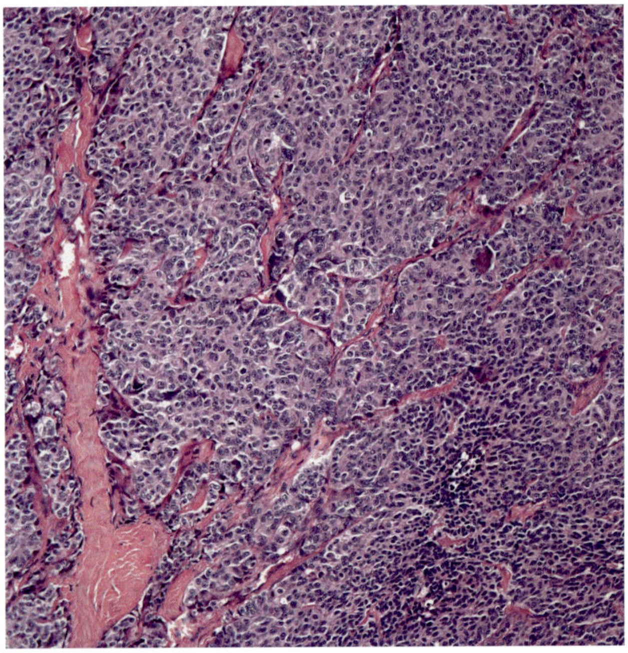

Fig. 9.32 Intermediate-grade neuroendocrine carcinoma showing moderate cellular atypia and mitotic activity

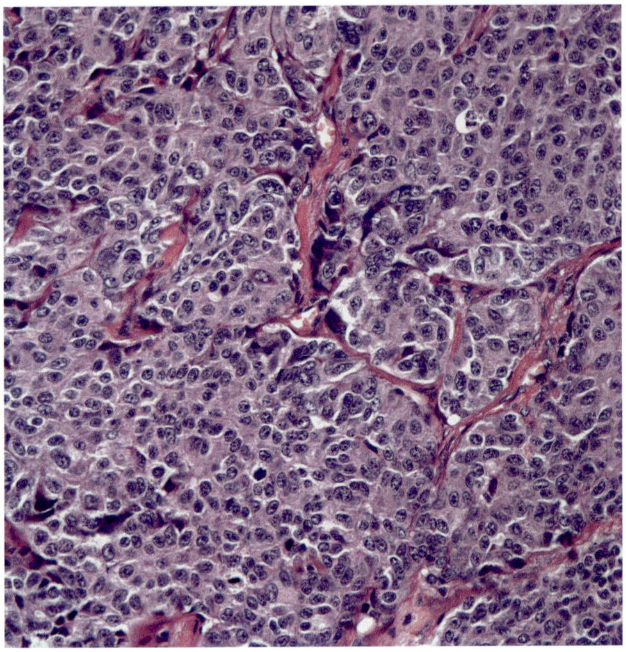

Fig. 9.33 Intermediate-grade neuroendocrine carcinoma showing nuclear atypia and easily identifiable mitotic figures

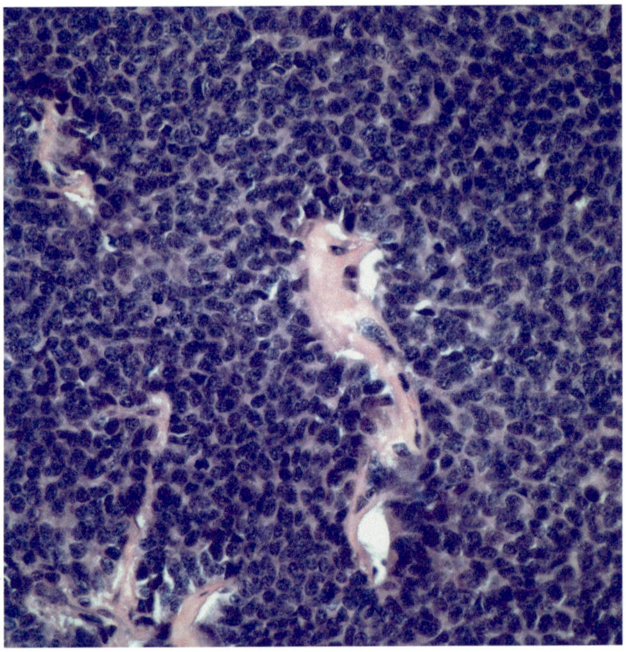

Fig. 9.34 Intermediate-grade neuroendocrine carcinoma showing a solid growth pattern with nuclear atypia and mitotic activity

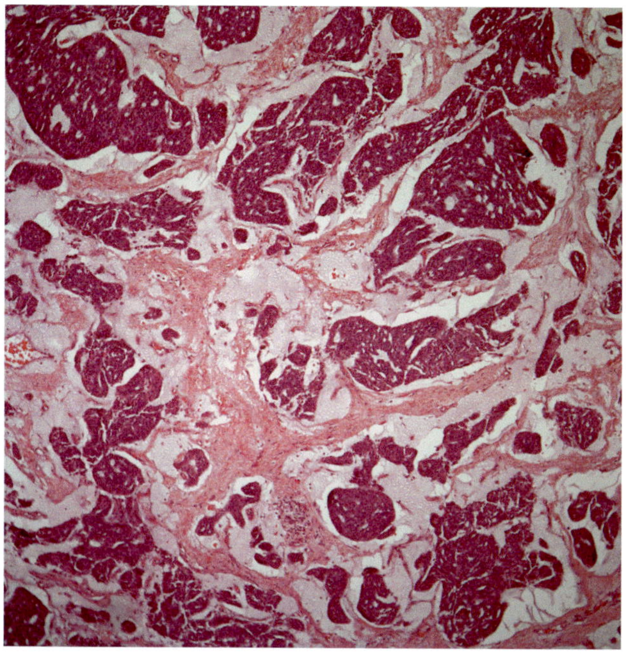

Fig. 9.35 Low power view of a mucinous neuroendocrine carcinoma

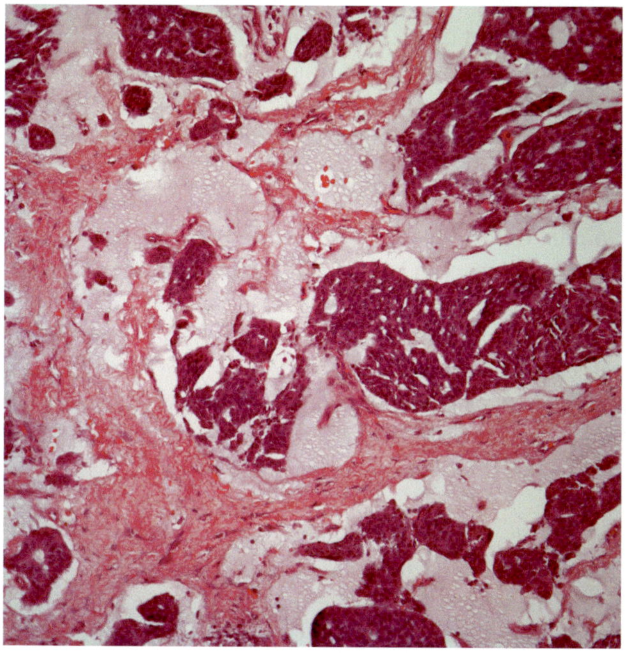

Fig. 9.36 Mucinous neuroendocrine carcinoma showing pools of mucoid material

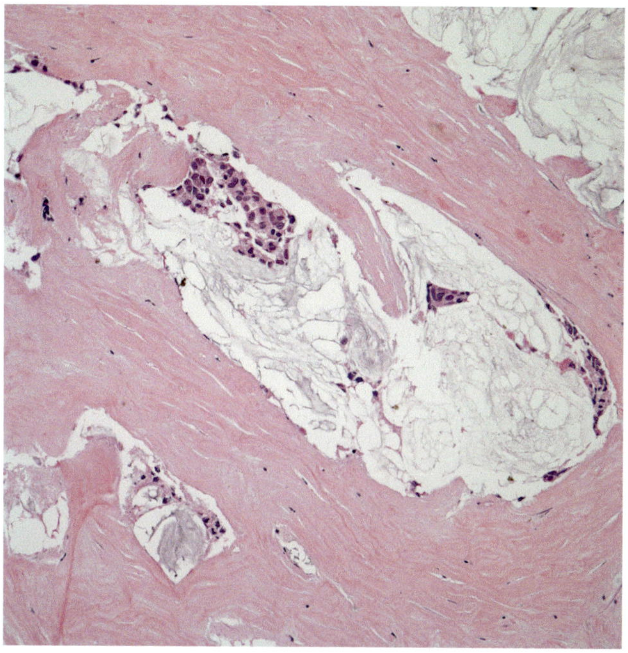

Fig. 9.37 Extensive pools of mucin in neuroendocrine carcinoma

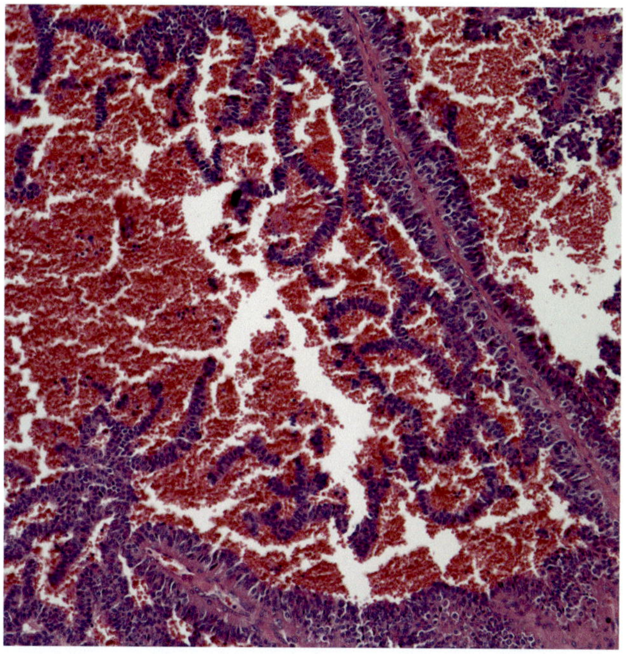

Fig. 9.38 Low power view of an angiectatic neuroendocrine carcinoma

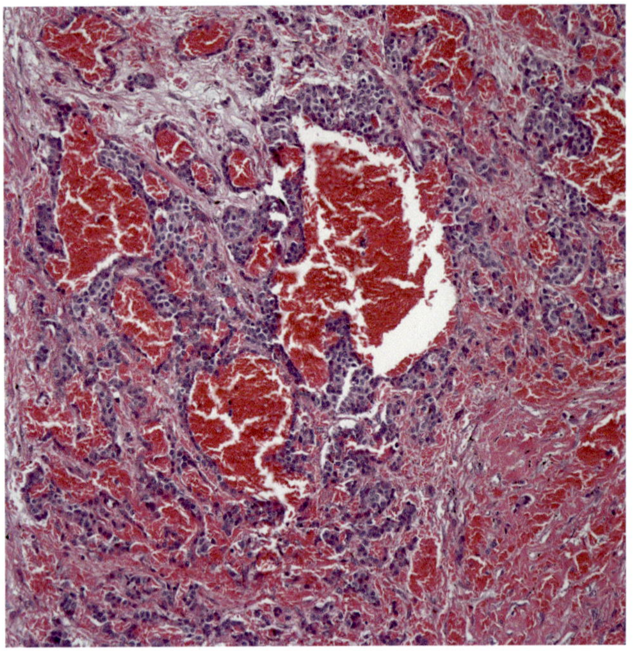

Fig. 9.39 Angiectatic neuroendocrine carcinoma showing areas mimicking a vascular neoplasm

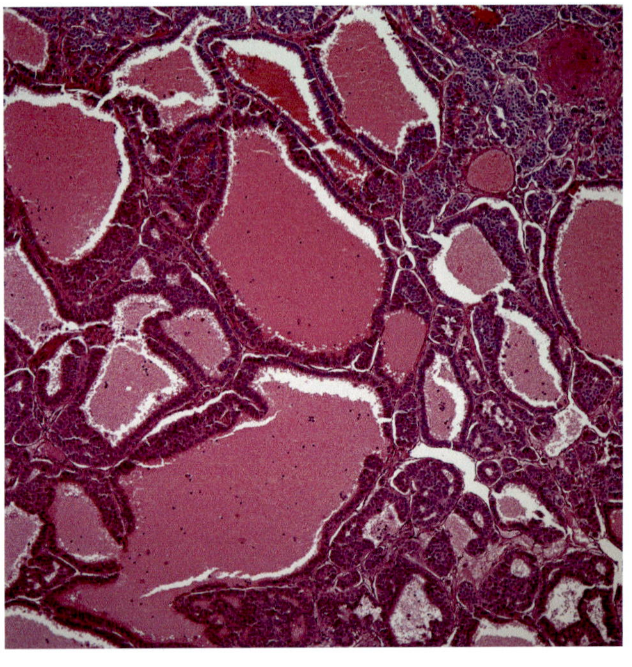

Fig. 9.40 Angiectatic neuroendocrine carcinoma showing dilated spaces occupied by acellular material

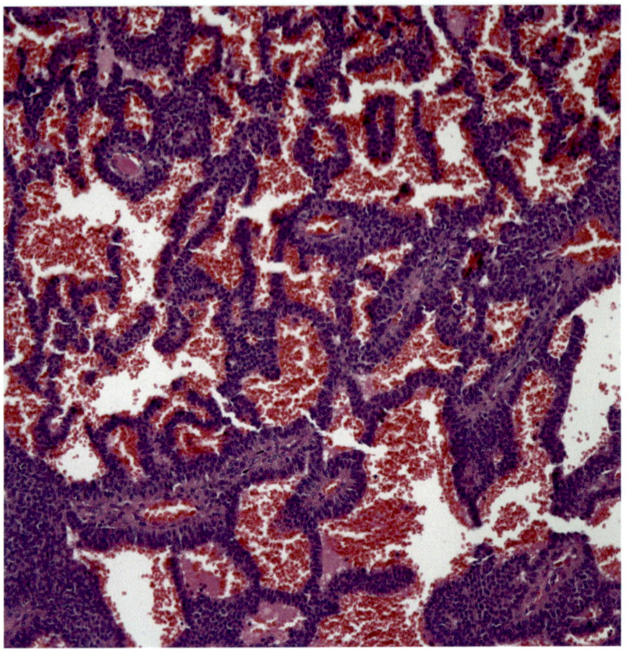

Fig. 9.41 Vascular-like spaces in an angiectatic neuroendocrine carcinoma

extensive, the tumor may resemble other neoplasms, namely, melanoma, in which the presence of pigment is much more common. However, in that setting, the use of immunohistochemistry may be of aid in identifying the true nature of the neoplasm (Fig. 9.42).

Spindle Cell

Neuroendocrine carcinomas may show a distinct growth pattern composed predominantly or exclusively of fusiform cells with elongated nuclei and scant to moderate amounts of cytoplasm. The tumor may also show a subtle hemangiopericytic growth pattern or in some areas a nested growth pattern composed of small nests populated by spindle cells (Figs. 9.43, 9.44, 9.45, 9.46, 9.47, and 9.48).

Oncocytic

The presence of oncocytic changes in neuroendocrine carcinomas may vary from focal change to tumors composed almost exclusively of an oncocytic neoplastic cellular proliferation. The basic growth pattern may show ribbons of neoplastic cells with presence of rosettes, or the tumor may show a nested growth pattern. However, the cell composition is that

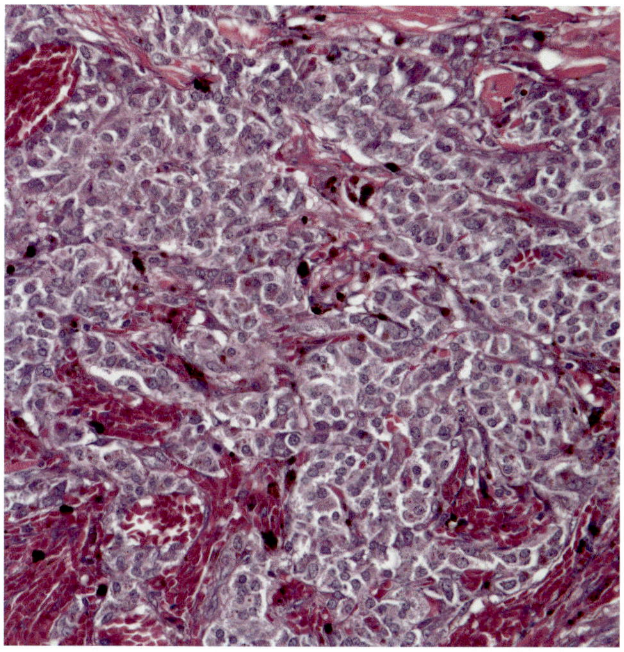

Fig. 9.42 Neuroendocrine carcinoma showing areas of melanin pigment

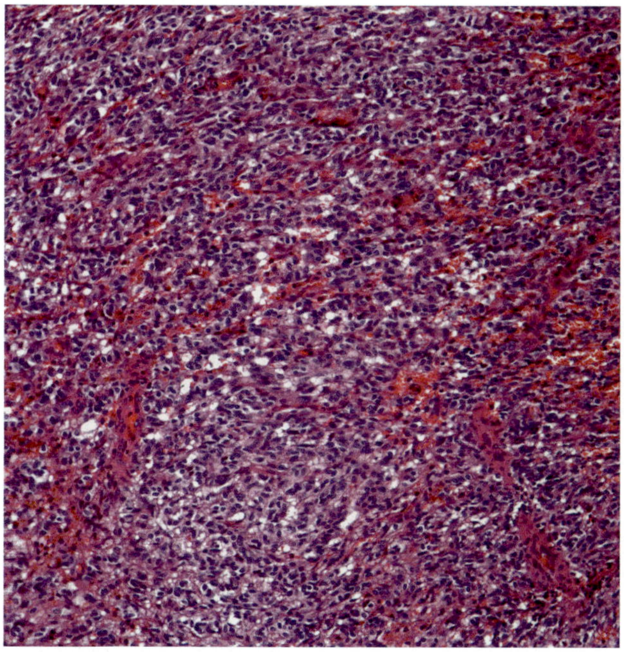

Fig. 9.43 Low power view of a neuroendocrine carcinoma with a spindle cell growth pattern

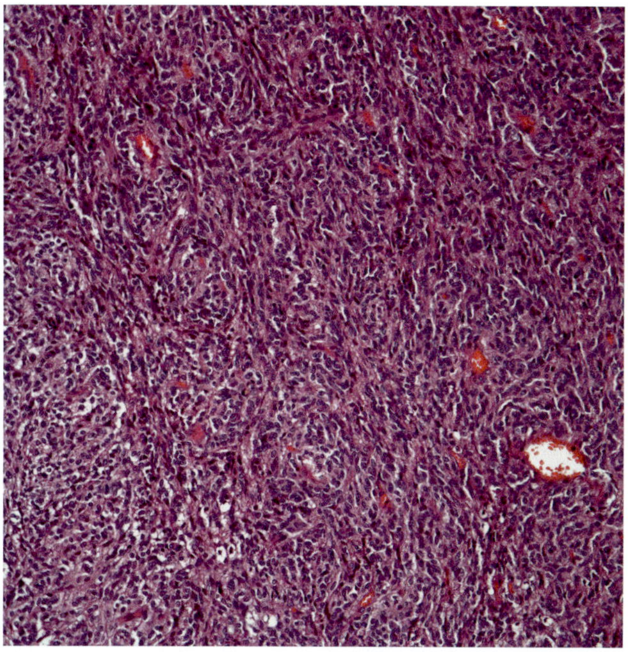

Fig. 9.44 Solid spindle cell growth pattern in a neuroendocrine carcinoma

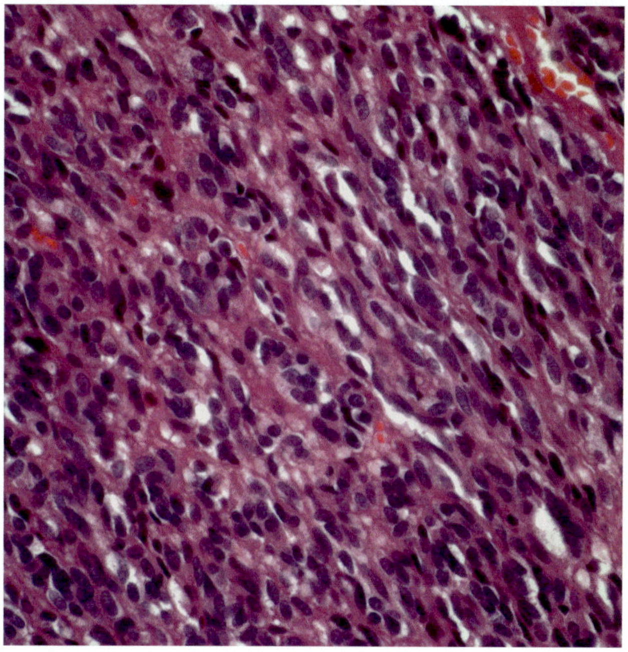

Fig. 9.45 Higher magnification of the spindle cells showing mild nuclear atypia and no mitotic activity

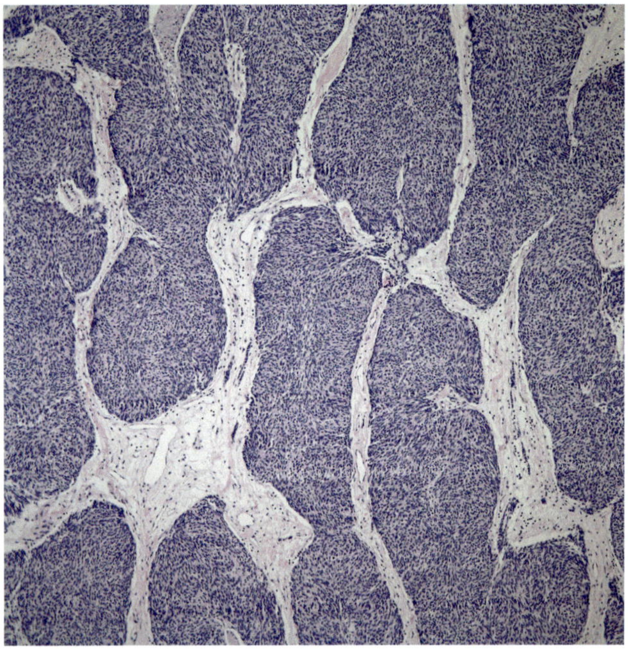

Fig. 9.46 Intermediate-grade neuroendocrine carcinoma with a spindle cell growth pattern

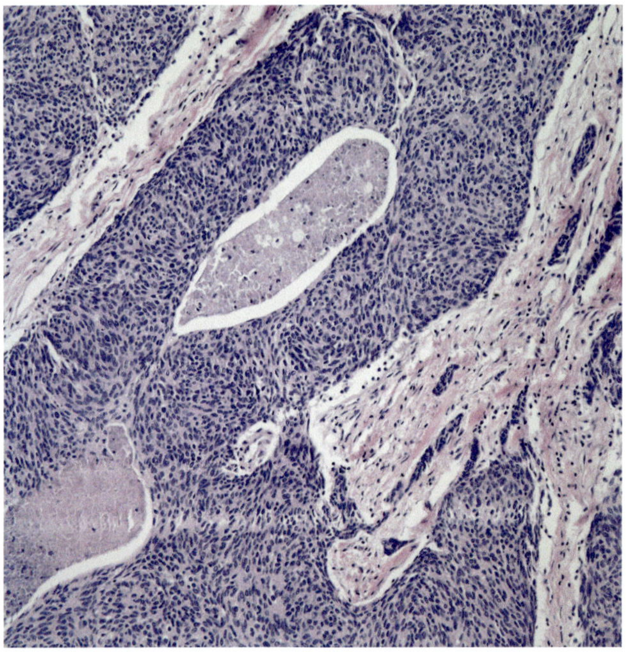

Fig. 9.47 Focal area of comedonecrosis in an intermediate-grade neuroendocrine carcinoma with spindle cell morphology

of relatively larger cells with ample eosinophilic cytoplasm, round to oval nuclei, and in some cells prominent nucleoli may be seen. In this type of neuroendocrine carcinoma, one may be able to identify more nuclear atypia than in the non-oncocytic tumors (Figs. 9.49, 9.50, 9.51, and 9.52).

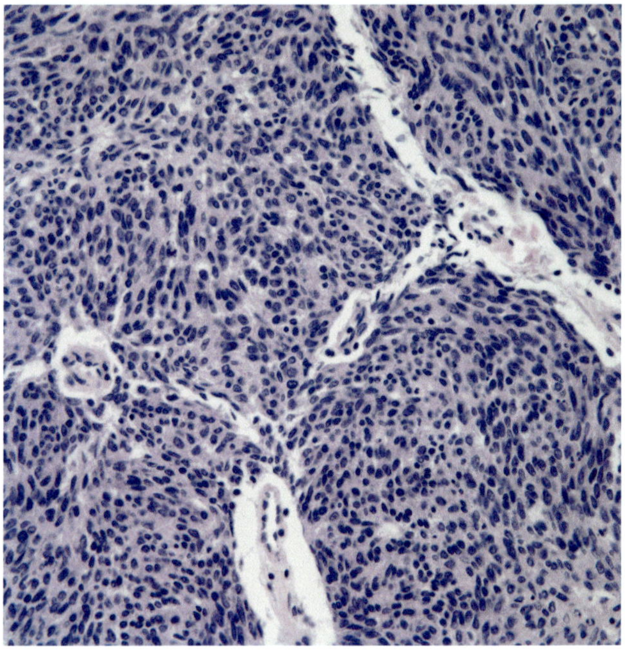

Fig. 9.48 Intermediate-grade spindle cell neuroendocrine carcinoma showing mitotic activity

Cystic

This represents a rather unusual occurrence as the tumor may show predominantly cystic changes similar to those described in multilocular thymic cyst. However, in the walls of the cyst, one can identify the presence of a neuroendocrine neoplastic cellular proliferation, which focally can extend to the surface epithelium lining the cystic structures. These tumoral areas may be focal in some cystic areas, while in others areas the tumor may be more obvious (Figs. 9.53, 9.54, 9.55, and 9.56).

Combined (Low, Intermediate, and High Grade)

Tumors showing transitions between low- and high-grade neuroendocrine carcinomas are unusual but represent a distinct type of malignancy, which may become apparent only after complete resection of the mediastinal tumor. In these cases, low- and intermediate-grade neuroendocrine carcinomas (carcinoid or atypical tumor) are clearly identifiable, while in other areas the tumor is more compatible with a small cell carcinoma. Areas of transition between those two tumors may be observed (Figs. 9.57, 9.58, 9.59, and 9.60)

High-Grade Neuroendocrine Carcinomas

Essentially, there are two types of mediastinal high-grade neuroendocrine carcinomas: small cell carcinoma and large cell neuroendocrine carcinoma [75–77]. In the former, the diagnosis is essentially done on morphological grounds, as the criteria used for these tumors in the thymus are the same as that in the pulmonary small cell carcinomas. However, great care must be taken when

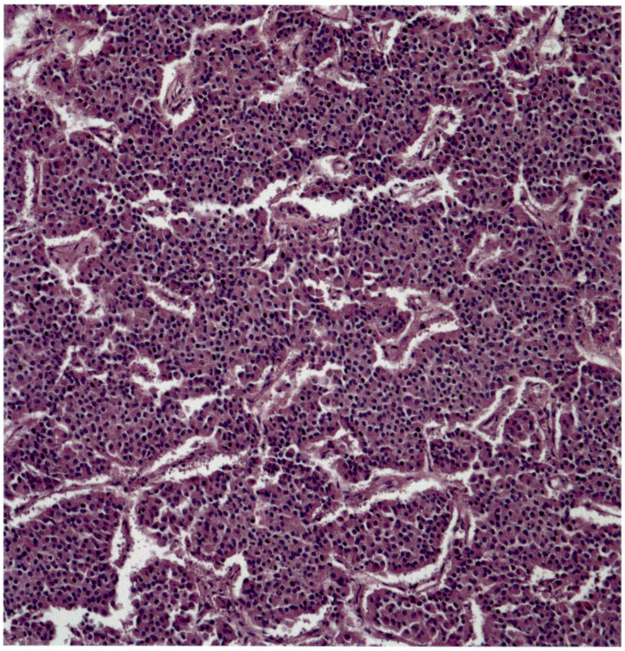

Fig. 9.49 Low power view of an oncocytic neuroendocrine carcinoma

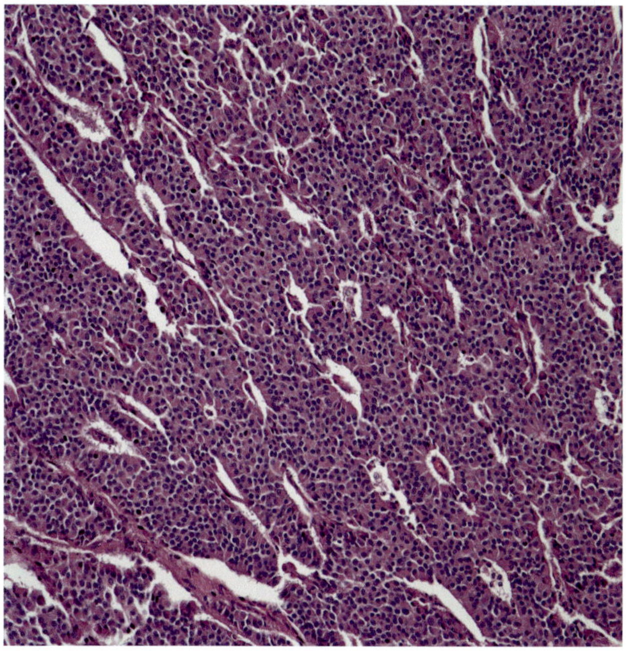

Fig. 9.50 Diffuse and focal glandular areas in an oncocytic neuroendocrine carcinoma

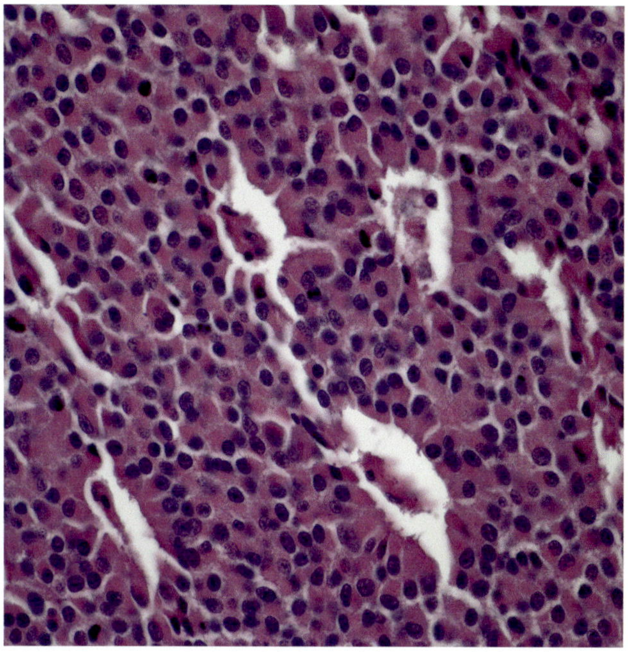

Fig. 9.51 Mitotic activity and nuclear atypia may be seen also in oncocytic neuroendocrine carcinomas

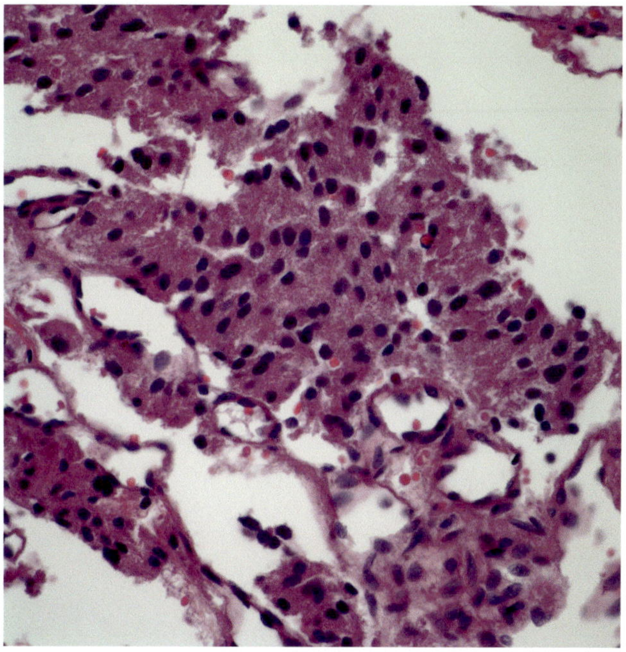

Fig. 9.52 Higher magnification of an oncocytic neuroendocrine carcinoma; note the granular cytoplasm

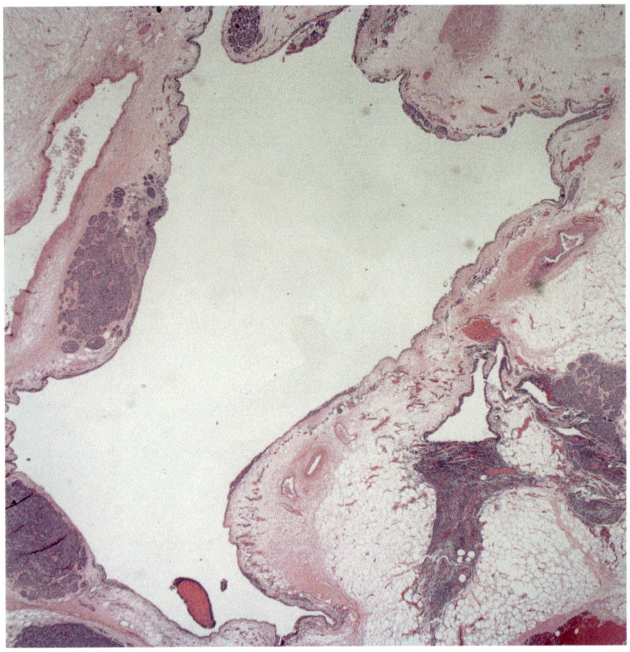

Fig. 9.53 Low power view of a cystic neuroendocrine carcinoma mimicking multilocular thymic cyst

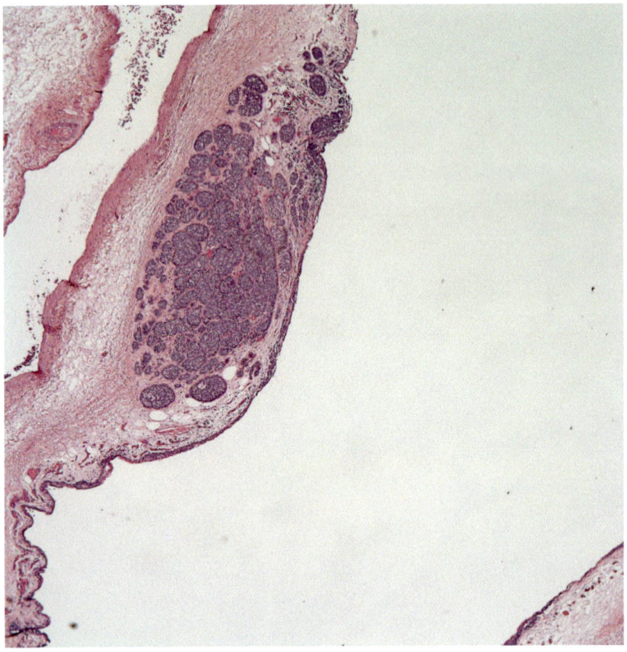

Fig. 9.54 Cystic neuroendocrine carcinoma showing the neoplastic cellular proliferation in the walls of the cyst

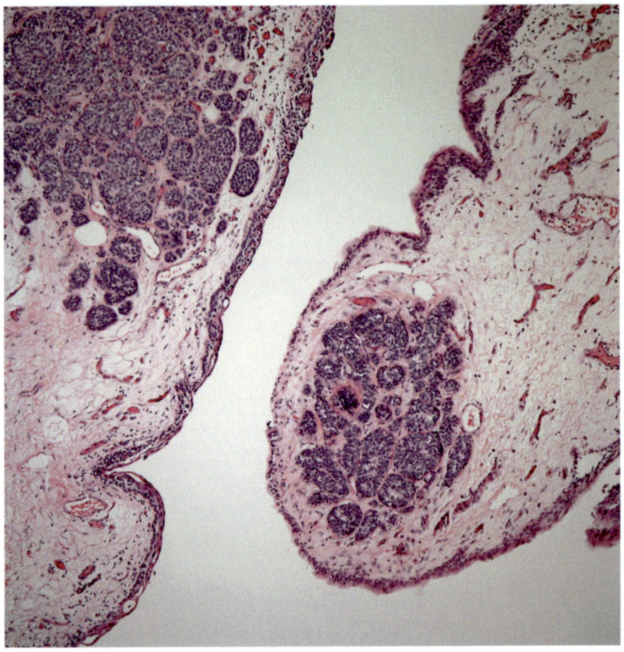

Fig. 9.55 Closer view of the cystic walls containing neoplastic cells

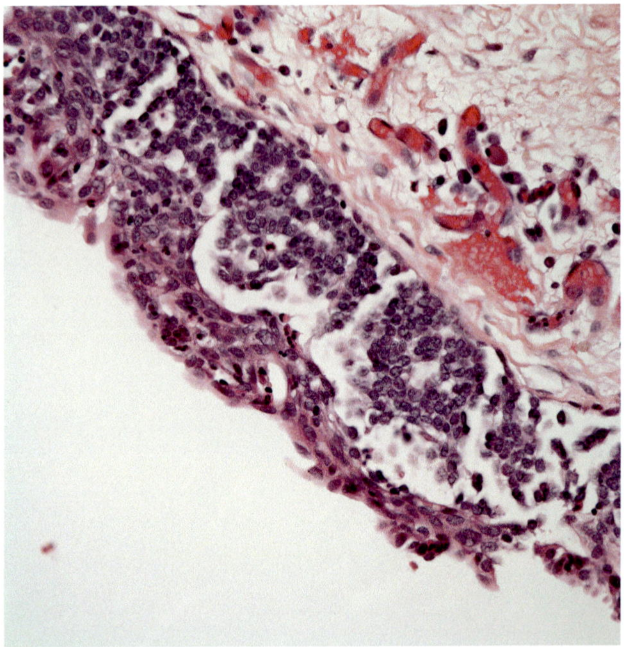

Fig. 9.56 Cystic neuroendocrine carcinoma; note the subtle neoplastic cellular proliferation just underneath the cyst lining

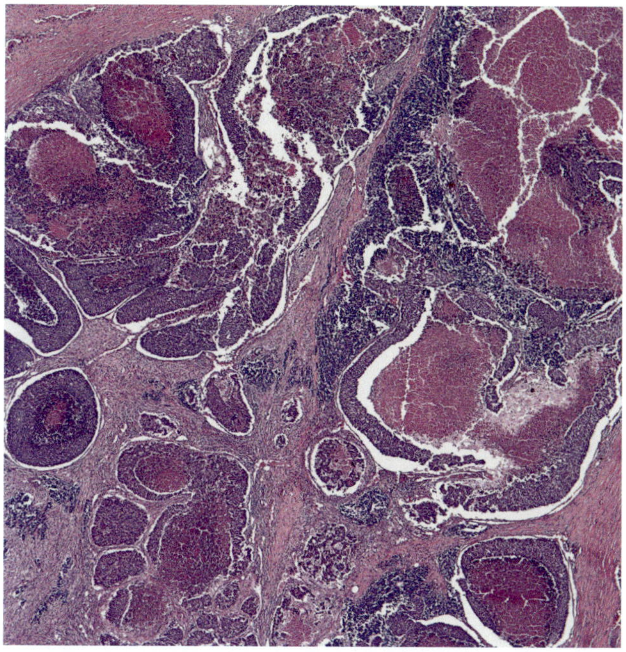

Fig. 9.57 Low power view of a high-grade neuroendocrine carcinoma. The necrosis is obvious

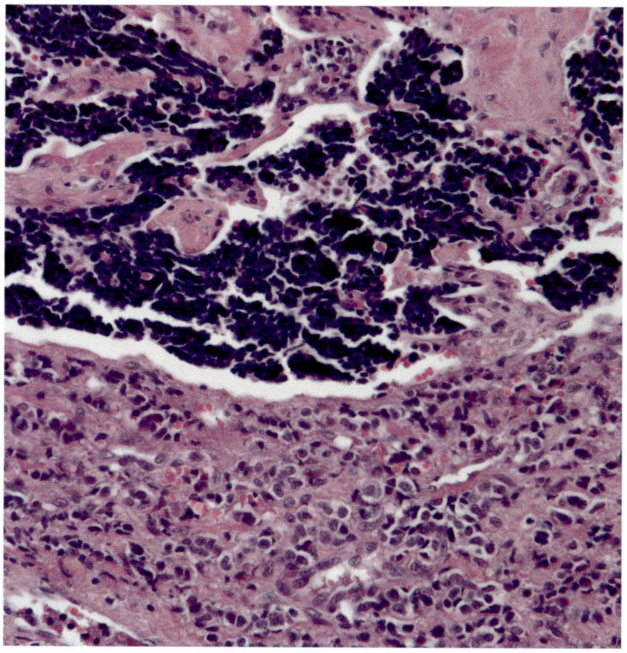

Fig. 9.58 Transitional areas of low- to high-grade neuroendocrine carcinoma (small cell carcinoma)

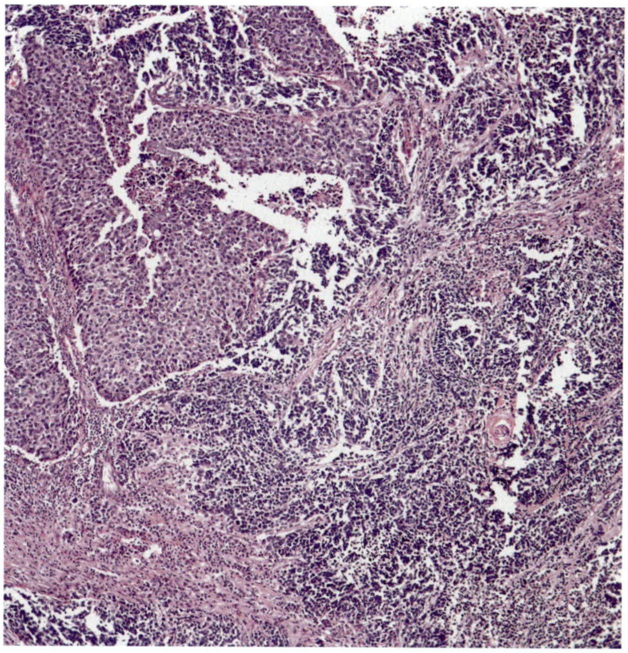

Fig. 9.59 Easily identifiable components of an intermediate-grade and a high-grade neuroendocrine carcinoma

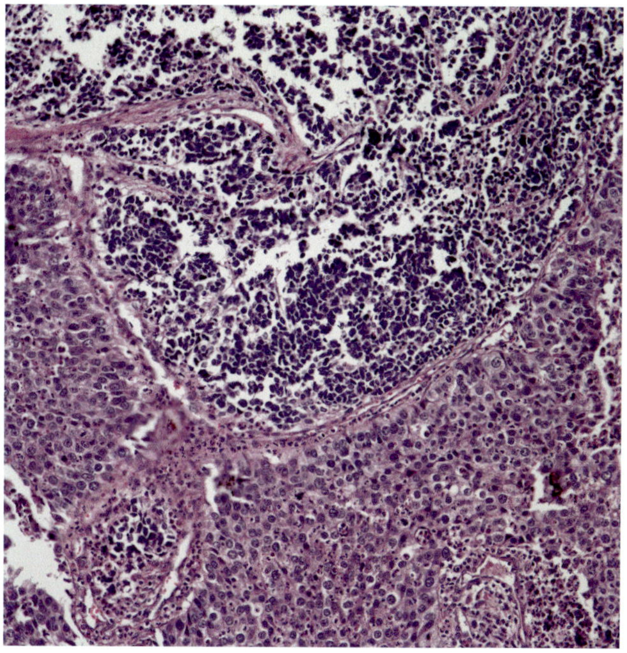

Fig. 9.60 High-grade neuroendocrine carcinoma, small cell type admixed with an intermediate-grade neuroendocrine carcinoma

diagnosing primary thymic small cell carcinoma, as it is not uncommon for a primary lung carcinoma to present with mediastinal involvement. Even though similar warning can be applied to large cell neuroendocrine carcinoma of the thymus, in this particular tumor two different aspects must be carefully analyzed. One is the fact that these tumors must have a neuroendocrine pattern that also shows neuroendocrine differentiation using neuroendocrine markers or electron microscopy. The second aspect may be more complicated as thymic non-neuroendocrine carcinomas may also show areas of positive staining using neuroendocrine markers. However, in these tumors, the growth pattern is not a neuroendocrine growth pattern. Thus, such positive staining should not be construed as specific for the diagnosis of large cell neuroendocrine carcinoma. It is important to highlight that high-grade neuroendocrine carcinomas within the thoracic cavity are much more common in the lung than in the mediastinum, so that every attempt should be made to clinically rule out that possibility. Ultimately, the diagnosis of either one of these tumors lies on the radiological evidence of the absence of tumor in the lung.

Histologically, small cell carcinoma may show extensive areas of necrosis with a rather small neoplastic cellular proliferation composed of cells with round nuclei and finely dispersed chromatin and absence of nucleoli. High mitotic count and apoptotic cells are easily identified. Molding of the nuclei is commonly seen, while the so-called Azzopardi phenomenon may be seen in some cases (Figs. 9.61 and 9.62). On the contrary, large cell neuroendocrine carcinoma by definition is a non-small cell carcinoma with a neuroendocrine growth pattern (ribbon, rosettes, etc.) composed of a neoplastic cellular proliferation of larger cells with round to oval nuclei and prominent nucleoli. Extensive areas of necrosis may be present, and the mitotic activity in these tumors is high. However, the current diagnostic criteria require the presence of positive staining using neuroendocrine markers (chromogranin, synaptophysin, CD56).

Immunohistochemical Features

Table 9.3 depicts some of the most commonly used immunohistochemical stains in the diagnosis of mediastinal neuroendocrine neoplasms. Specific studies on thymic neuroendocrine carcinomas with large series of cases are lacking. However,

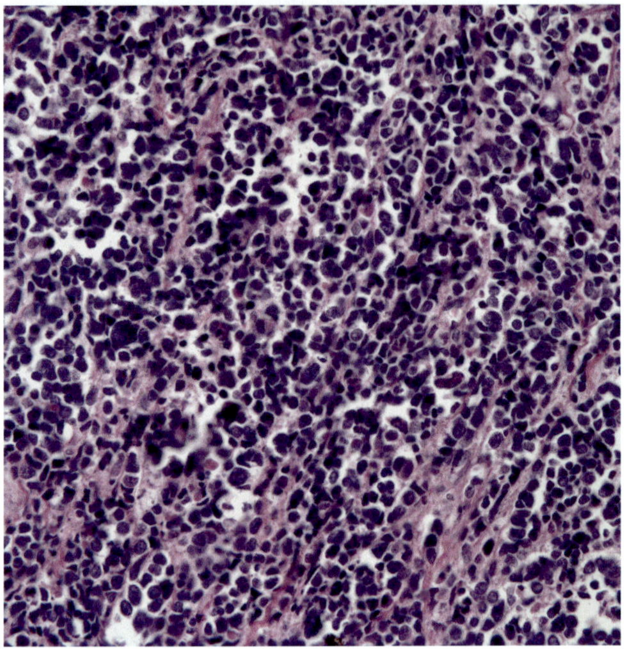

Fig. 9.61 High-grade neuroendocrine carcinoma, small cell type

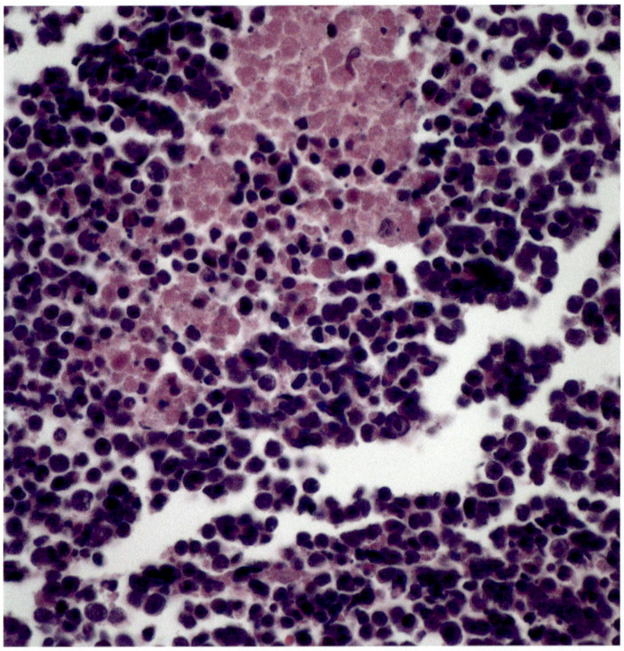

Fig. 9.62 Closer view of a high-grade neuroendocrine carcinoma (small cell carcinoma); note the presence of necrosis and molding

Table 9.3 Commonly used immunohistochemical stains in the diagnosis of mediastinal neuroendocrine neoplasm

Antibody	NE carcinoma	Paraganglioma	Parathyroid adenoma
Chromogranin	Positive	Positive	Positive
Synaptophysin	Positive	Positive	Positive
CD-56	Positive	Positive	Positive
S-100 protein	Positive	Positive	*Negative*
Keratin	Positive	*Negative*	Positive
GATA3	*Negative*	Positive	*Negative*
TTF-1	Positive	*Negative*	*Negative*
Parathyroid hormone	*Negative*	*Negative*	Positive
Histochemical studies			
PAS	*Negative*	*Negative*	Positive
D-PAS	*Negative*	*Negative*	*Negative*
Mucicarmine	Positive in some cases extracellular	*Negative*	*Negative*

the use of immunohistochemistry to aid in the diagnosis of these tumors is well recognized in the literature, and there are several series of cases on this particular topic [44, 78–83]. Essentially, the use of conventional neuroendocrine markers such as chromogranin, synaptophysin, and CD-56 has been shown to aid in the diagnosis. Also important to highlight is that, in unusual cases, calcitonin may also show positive staining in these tumors [80]. In our experience with 40 cases of low- and intermediate-grade neuroendocrine carcinomas of the thymus, we were able to observe that low molecular weight keratin (CAM5.2) stained 100% of the tumors while broad-spectrum keratin stained 88% of them. In addition, chromogranin stained 75%, synaptophysin 72%, and Leu-7 68%. It is important to highlight that only 60% of the cases showed positive staining for both chromogranin and synaptophysin, thus arguing for performing a complete panel rather than just selected immunostains. More recently, in an attempt to separate thymic neuroendocrine tumors, namely, carcinoid and paraganglioma [83], a study of 46 cases was performed which not only used the conventional neuroendocrine markers but also other relatively new markers such as thyroid transcription factor (TTF-1); napsin A, and GATA-3 were added for evaluation. We reported that neuroendocrine carcinoma (carcinoid tumor) showed 100% staining for pan-cytokeratin, while chromogranin A and synaptophysin showed positive staining in 92 and 88%, respectively (Fig. 9.63a–c). Interestingly, TTF-1 was seen positive in 17% of thymic neuroendocrine carcinoma (Fig. 9.63d), while GATA-3 and napsin A were negative in all the cases. In a different study [81], we also attempted to determine the use of polyclonal PAX-8 and TTF-1 to separate thymic from pulmonary neuroendocrine carcinomas. We observed that pulmonary neuroendocrine carcinomas showed polyclonal PAX-8 expression in 8% of the tumors, while TTF-1 was seen positive in 76% of these tumors. On the contrary, thymic neuroendocrine carcinomas showed 32% positive staining for polyclonal PAX-8 and 8% positive staining for TTF-1.

Based on the collected experience with these tumors and their immunohistochemical profile, the use of neuroendocrine markers such as chromogranin and synaptophysin offers a good yield of positivity. The use of other stains such as TTF-1 and polyclonal PAX-8 offers a limited value in the diagnostic aid for these neoplasms. Important to highlight is the use of keratin, either pan-cytokeratin or low molecular weight keratin CAM5.2, which can help in separating these tumors from other neuroendocrine neoplasms that have a different biological behavior, namely, paragangliomas.

One important stain that has generated popularity is the use of Ki67 proliferative marker as an aid in the grading of neuroendocrine carcinomas. Even though it is an important stain, the use of that immunostain to properly grade these tumors may have some limitations. For instance, if the use of the marker is to determine grading of the tumor before resection, then it may prove complicated, as the marker would have to be used in a biopsy specimen, which may not necessarily be representative of the entire tumor. That is especially problematic for mediastinal tumors, which may be larger tumors. Thus, in this setting, the use of the marker may have limitations. On the other hand, if the use of the marker is left for resections, then once again their use may have limitations as the histological evaluation of these tumors in terms of mitotic count, and the presence of necrosis should be easily performed by light microscopy, delegating the use of Ki67 to a lesser importance. More important is the fact that there is not a single study addressing such a feature in thymic neuroendocrine carcinomas. Therefore, any conclusion on that topic would have to be extrapolated from tumors either of lung or gastrointestinal origin, and that may prove not necessarily correct. One other important issue is where to draw the lower and upper limit of the nuclear labeling. It is perhaps safe to assume that low-grade tumors should have <5% of nuclear labeling while high-grade tumors will have easily a nuclear labeling of 90–100%. However, determining the proper labeling range for intermediate-grade tumors may prove more complicated, thus the importance of an accurate histopathological assessment. Important to mention is the fact that even though the use of Ki-67 in the assessment of neuroendocrine carcinomas is

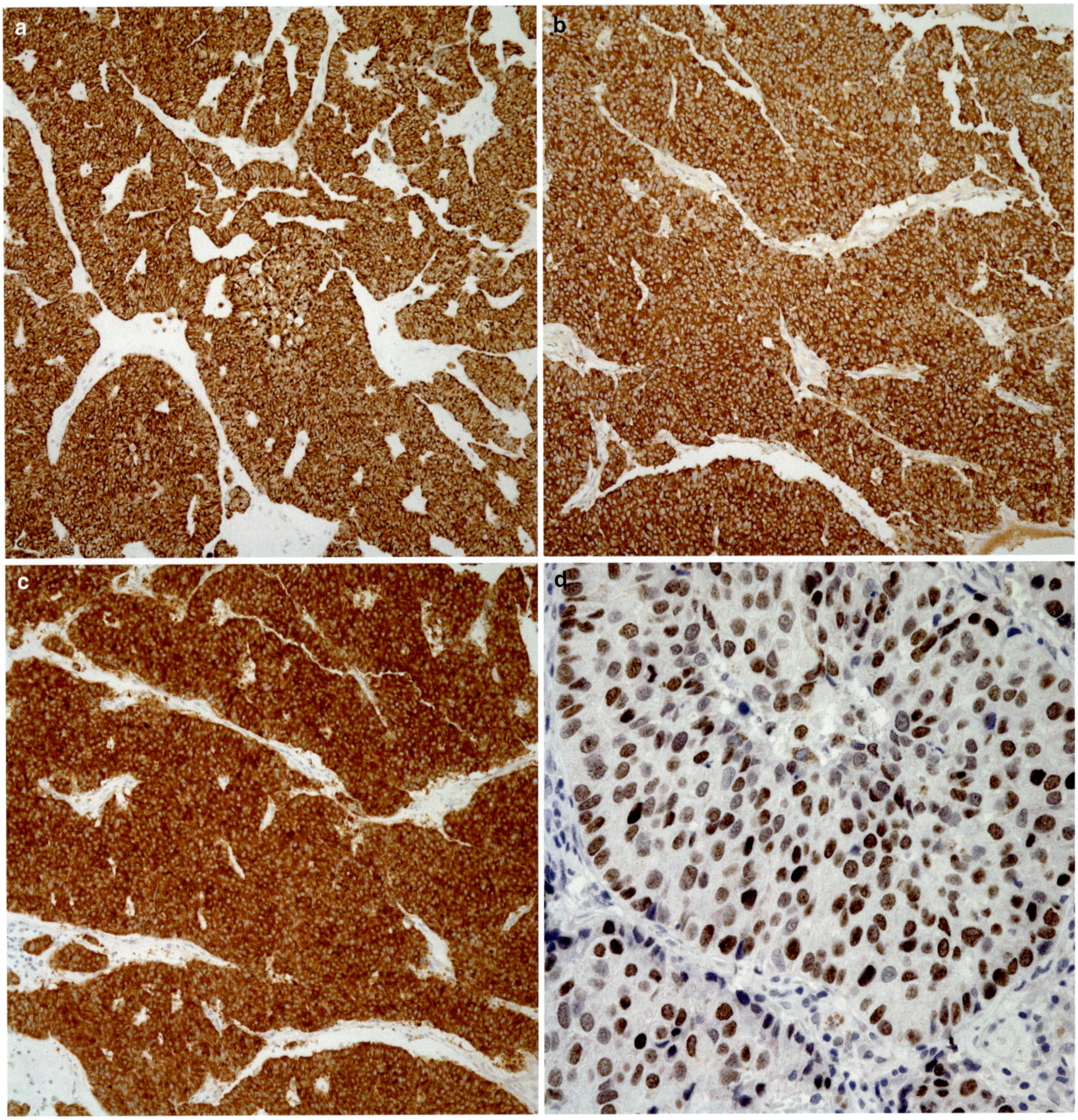

Fig. 9.63 (**a**) positive staining for keratin in a low-grade neuroendocrine carcinoma; (**b**) positive chromogranin stain; (**c**) positive staining for synaptophysin; (**d**) positive nuclear staining for TTF-1

important, the morphological appraisal of the presence of necrosis in these tumors cannot be underestimated, and this assessment can be easily performed by light microscopy. The presence of necrosis plays an important role in the grading of these neoplasms.

It is important to highlight that the use of neuroendocrine markers, such as those that have been mentioned for low- and intermediate-grade tumors, is not needed for the diagnosis of high-grade neuroendocrine carcinomas, except in the setting of the diagnosis of large cell neuroendocrine carcinoma, which requires such positive staining for final diagnosis. For the diagnosis of small cell carcinoma, the presence or absence of positive or negative staining for neuroendocrine markers should not be used as a discriminatory feature. However, if the consideration is another neoplasm, then their use may be appropriate. Table 9.3 depicts some of the most common antibodies used in daily practice for the diagnosis of neuroendocrine neoplasms.

Other Ancillary Studies

In today's practice, the use of immunohistochemistry is widespread in diagnostic surgical pathology in general. Nevertheless, there are other modalities that have been employed with some success and which potentially can be used as either diagnostic tools, or for pure academic curiosity. For instance, Kujari and coworkers [84] evaluated 23 carcinoid tumors by flow cytometry; they concluded that DNA aneuploidy is common in human carcinoid tumors, and may occur in tumors secreting biogenic amines. Fetissof and coworkers [85] evaluated the presence of probable intermediate filaments, which were accompanied by neurosecretory granules, and correlated these findings with a Grimelius histochemical stain. Similarly, Levine and Rosai [72] reported the use of electron microscopy in spindle cell "carcinoid" as a way to aid in the separation of these tumors from spindle cell thymomas. Kay and Wilson [86] reported a thymic ACTH-secreting tumor in which the authors performed electron microscopy, concluding that neurosecretory granules were easily identified in the tumor cells, and added that these granules were similar to those present in similar tumors in the lung. Essentially, the use of histochemical stains like Grimelius or the use of ultrastructural studies can also aid in the diagnosis of neuroendocrine carcinomas, as the presence of neurosecretory granules is rather characteristic in those tumors. However, in current practice the use of those ancillary studies is not as common as it used to be.

Differential Diagnosis

The differential diagnosis of thymic neuroendocrine carcinomas may include a diversity of conditions based on the type and growth pattern of the neuroendocrine carcinoma. However, more important in the assessment of neuroendocrine carcinomas is defining the primary site, as these tumors share similar histopathological features with those tumors arising in the gastrointestinal or pulmonary region. Often, establishing a good clinical and radiological correlation will lead to a more accurate interpretation regarding origin of the neoplasm. Therefore, whether it is a low-, intermediate-, or high-grade neuroendocrine carcinoma, establishing a good clinical and radiological correlation is highly recommended in order to determine a primary site, as such features not only determine prognosis but also lead to possible different treatment options.

From the histopathological point of view, the most important and difficult differential diagnosis is with paraganglioma and ectopic parathyroid adenoma. Both of these tumors may pose a significant problem in a small mediastinoscopic biopsy, and both of these tumors may also show positive staining for neuroendocrine markers. In this setting, if the suspicion is high, then the use of additional immunohistochemical stains such as keratins and parathyroid hormone immunostains may provide important information regarding the true nature of the neoplasm. Paragangliomas are likely to show negative staining for keratin, while parathyroid adenomas are likely to show positive staining for parathyroid hormone. In addition, the clinical information on disturbances in the metabolism of calcium and phosphorous will be relevant information that is generally correlated with parathyroid adenomas. In cases in which the histology of the neuroendocrine carcinoma is that of spindle cells, then spindle cell thymoma becomes an important tumor to exclude. In this setting, the use of neuroendocrine markers should lead to the correct interpretation. In cases in which the tumor shows mucinous component, a metastatic neoplasm from gastrointestinal origin should be carefully considered and properly excluded on clinical and radiological grounds. The use of other immunohistochemical markers such as CDX2 may also provide some additional aid in defining the site of origin of the tumor. When the tumors show prominent oncocytic features, important consideration would include an ectopic or metastatic thyroid carcinoma. Once again, the use of appropriate immunostains such as thyroglobulin, calcitonin, or monoclonal PAX-8 should lead to the correct interpretation.

In short, the differential diagnosis of thymic neuroendocrine carcinomas can be separated into (a) tumors that shared similar immunohistochemical profile and are primary thymic neoplasms, (b) primary thymic tumors that may show similar histopathological features but with different immunohistochemical phenotype, and (c) tumors that may share histological and immunohistochemical features but their primary site is outside of the mediastinal compartment. In all these settings, establishing a close clinical and radiological correlation coupled with proper assessment of the histopathological features of the tumor supported by a proper immunohistochemical profile should lead more often to a more appropriate interpretation.

Paraganglioma

Extra-adrenal paragangliomas are tumors of ubiquitous distribution that have been described in many unusual anatomic areas such as the cauda equine and bladder. In the mediastinum, paragangliomas have been described in either anterior or posterior mediastinal locations [87–108].

Clinical Features

In one of the earlier reports of "intrathoracic pheochromocytoma," Phillips [90] described a single case of a 39-year-old man who presented with cardiac palpitation, throbbing in the head, polyuria, nocturia, and high blood pressure, and stated that a review of the literature had disclosed only 11 other cases in which the adrenal gland was not involved. He also alluded to the finding of chromaffin cells along the entire length of the autonomic nervous system in nests in the autonomic ganglions (paraganglions) or independently as chromaffin bodies (adrenal gland and Zuckerkandl's organ). In 1950, Lattes [91] described four cases of what the author called nonchromaffin paraganglioma of ganglion nodosum, carotid body, and aortic arch bodies, and asserted previous views that these tumors are not part of chromaffin paraganglionic system, and that they belong to an entirely different system. Marshall and Horn [92] studied 19 carotid and jugular body tumors and alluded to prior cases as far back as 1762. Green and Bassett [93] described what the authors called "intrathoracic pheochromocytoma" and accounted for 12 previous cases, of which 9 occurred in men and 3 in women between the ages of 8 and 64 years, with the average age being 30 years. Tama and coworkers [94] described a similar case in a 66-year-old man who presented with superior vena cava obstruction; however, the authors designated this neoplasm as a "chemodectoma of the mediastinum." Pachter in 1963 [95] described eight additional cases under the designation "mediastinal nonchromaffin paraganglioma." The tumors occurred in six women and two men between the ages of 27 and 68 years (average 46.5 years). Six of these patients were asymptomatic, and two others had non-specific symptoms; three of the cases described were incidental findings at autopsy. None of the tumors had clinical or laboratory evidence of hormonal activity, and all the tumors were in the anterior mediastinum. One important issue that is worth mentioning in the cases described by Pacther is that, in one of these cases, the patient had three separate tumors, similar to the case with multiple localizations also described by Lacquet and coworkers [99] in a 31-year-old woman. These cases highlight the issue of the care that must be exercised in rendering these cases as synchronous or metachronous tumors rather than metastatic disease. Olson and Salyer described four cases of their own in three men and one woman between the ages of 16 and 35 years. The authors stated that local recurrence or metastasis could not be predicted on histologic grounds and in their review of the literature concluded that the incidence of metastasis varies and depends on the length of the follow-up. In the cases reviewed by the authors, seven patients were known to have died of disease, with an average survival time of 6 years; four patients lived 8 years or longer. In addition to previous reports on thoracic paragangliomas, there have been cases in which the tumors from the outset have been described as "malignant." Enquist, Victor, and Odze, respectively [96, 97, 105], described three different male patients between the ages of 20 and 59 years, who presented with metastatic disease to the humerus, rib, and chest wall and whose main tumor was either in the anterior or posterior mediastinum. It is also important to recognize that, clinically, extra-adrenal paragangliomas may be associated with other neoplasms including pulmonary chondromas and gastric smooth muscle tumors, which is also known as Carney triad [103, 107]. In our experience with 16 mediastinal paragangliomas [89], the patients were ten men and six women between the ages of 16 and 69 years (mean: 42.5 years); 12 tumors were located in the posterior mediastinum, while 3 tumors were in the anterior mediastinum. In one case, a definitive location was not defined. Follow-up information obtained in 12 patients ranged from 1 to 168 months (mean: 84.5 months). Nine patients (75%) remained alive and well; however, metastatic disease to the bone marrow, lymph node, lung, and pelvis was documented as far as 14 years after initial diagnosis. It was concluded that the only parameter that correlates with aggressive behavior for these tumors is the extent of circumscription and/or local infiltration of the tumor at initial resection. No clinical or histological features were possible to associate with the behavior of these neoplasms; thus, close follow-up is highly recommended for patients with these tumors.

More recently, succinate dehydrogenase (SDH) has been studied in the evaluation of hereditary paragangliomas. Essentially, four subunits are evaluated in this setting, A, B, C, and D, which are the subunits that encode the mitochondrial enzyme succinate dehydrogenase (SDH) [109]. For mediastinal paragangliomas, Sato and coworkers [110] described a 69-year-old Japanese woman with a posterior mediastinal paraganglioma and a novel mutation (P236S) in the SDH subunit B gene (SDHB). The authors stated the relevance of such mutation, as it may be associated with an aggressive behavior. Also, Garibaldi and coworkers [111] reported on a 55-year-old man with hereditary paraganglioma syndrome associated with SDHD gene mutations. The patient is described as having multiple extra-adrenal paragangliomas, including one in the mediastinal para-aortic area. Prodanov and associates [112] also reported on an 8-year-old girl with history of catecholamine excess-related symptoms with a malignant mediastinal paraganglioma associated with SDHB mutations. The authors stated that SDHB mutations in paragangliomas have a higher risk of malignancy.

Pathological Features

Gross Features

These tumors are either well-localized or ill-defined with local invasion into adjacent structures. They are soft, irregular, and tan to brown in color, which at cut surface may show focal areas of hemorrhage; otherwise, the surface is smooth (Fig. 9.64). The tumor also varies in size from a couple of centimeters to tumors over 10 cm in greatest dimension.

Histological Features

These tumors are characterized by a nesting pattern (so-called Zellballen), which is composed of islands of large cells with eosinophilic cytoplasm with round to oval nuclei; some cells may also have prominent nucleoli (Figs. 9.65, 9.66, 9.67, 9.68, 9.69, 9.70, and 9.71). Closer view of these tumors shows areas of prominent cellular pleomorphism, which are characterized by the presence of larger "bizarre" cells with macronuclei and prominent nucleoli (Figs. 9.72, 9.73, and 9.74). Even though mitotic figures may be present, they are scattered despite the prominent cellular pleomorphism that some tumors may have. The tumor also shows the presence of prominent ectatic vessels separating the islands of tumor cells. Even though these tumors show essentially a fairly similar growth pattern, some cases may show some unusual features that may pose a challenge in the evaluation of these

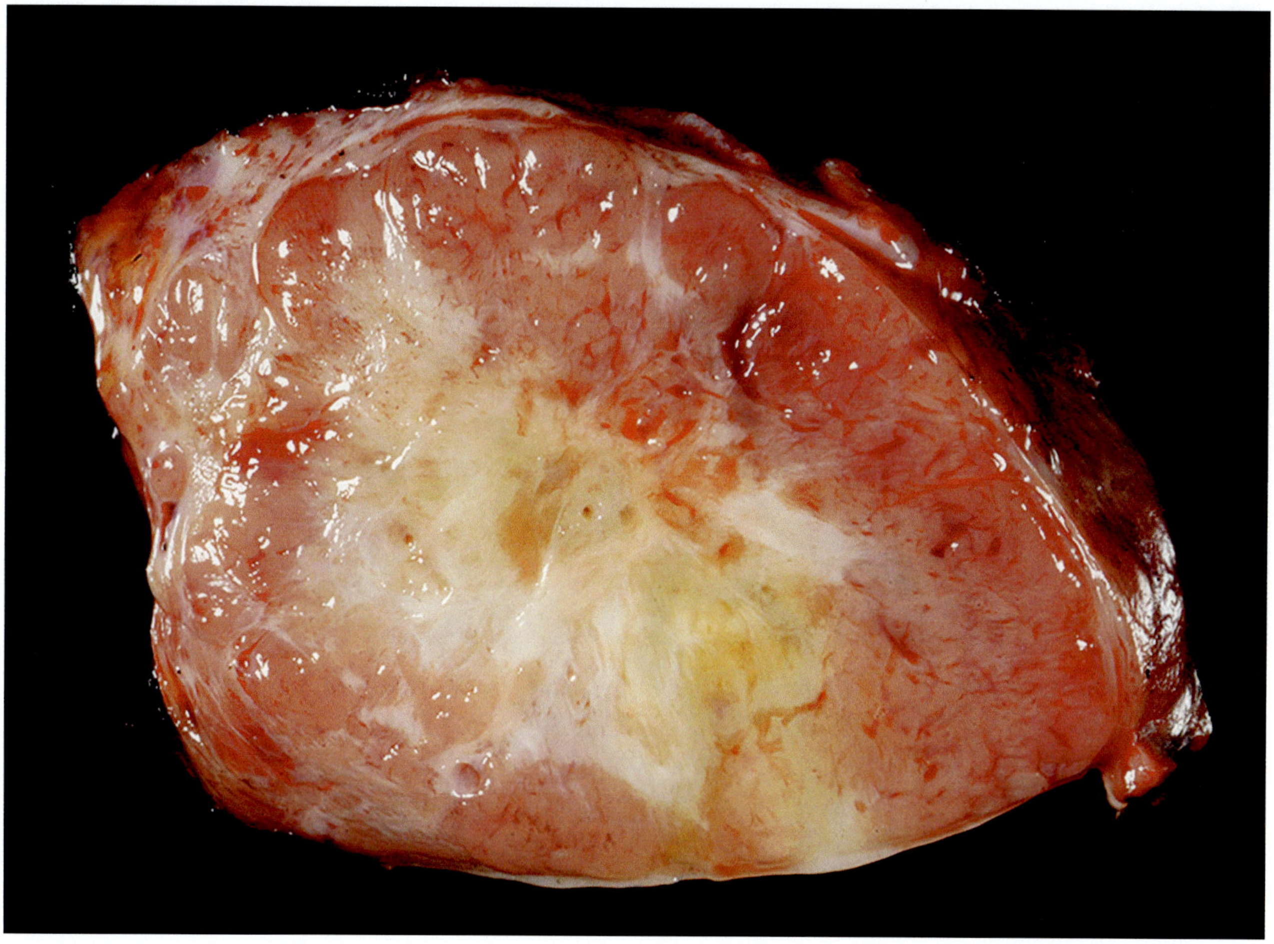

Fig. 9.64 Mediastinal paraganglioma showing a fleshy homogeneous cut surface. The tumor does not show areas of necrosis

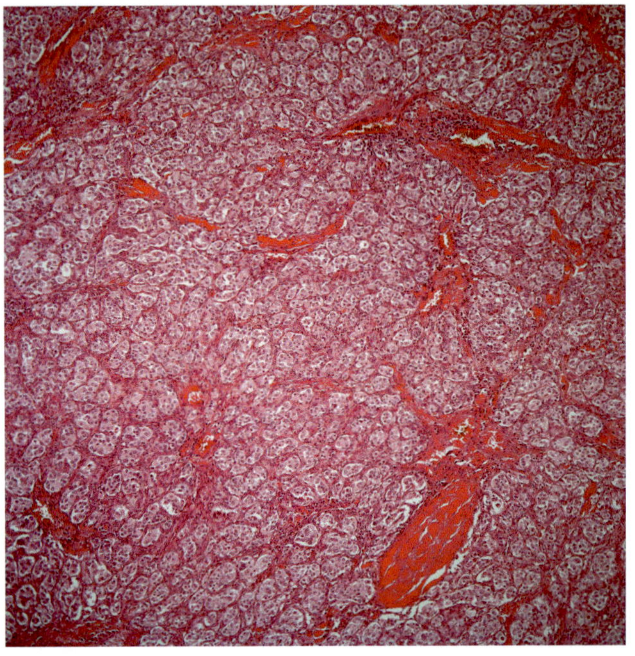

Fig. 9.65 Low power view of a paraganglioma showing the classic so-called zellballen

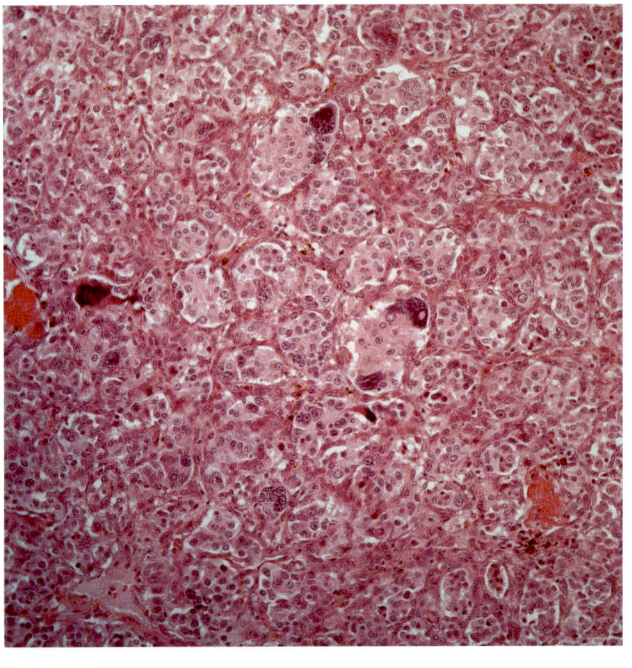

Fig. 9.66 Intermediate magnification of a paraganglioma showing the classic nested growth pattern and easily identifiable nuclear atypia

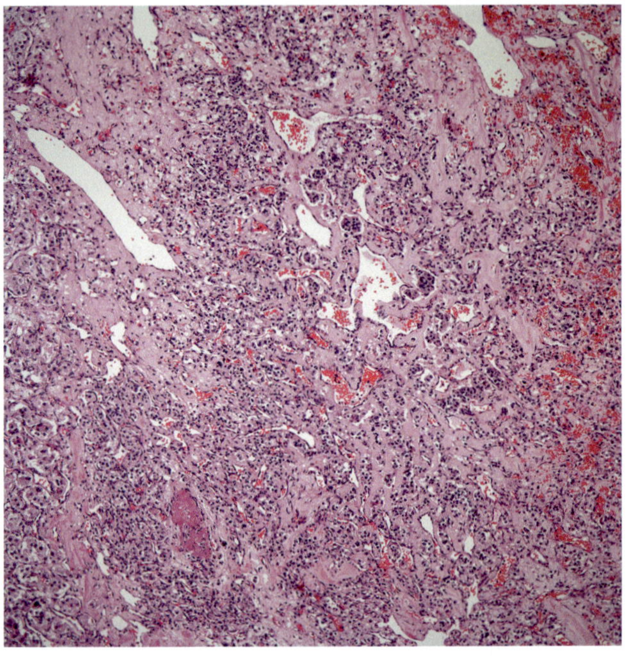

Fig. 9.67 Paraganglioma showing prominent ectatic vessels

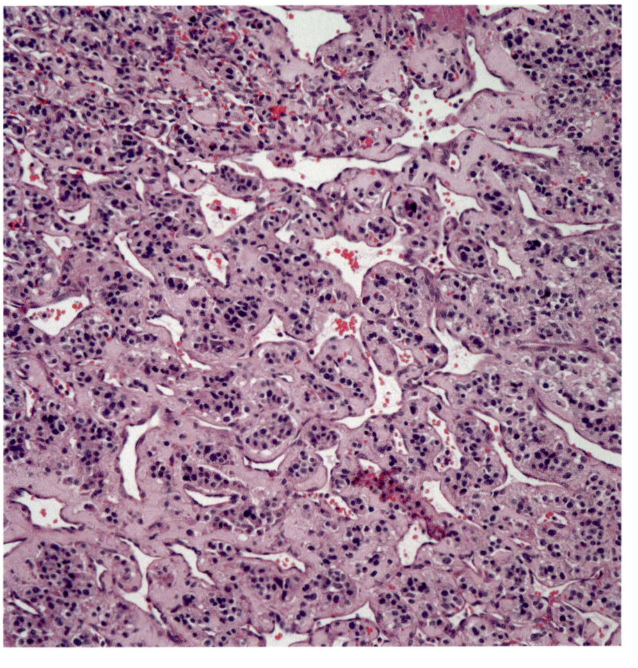

Fig. 9.68 Paraganglioma with an HPC-like growth vascular proliferation

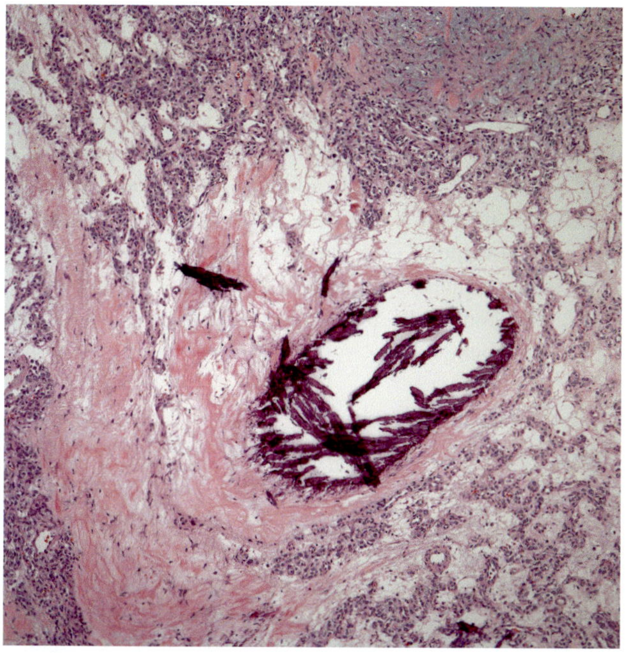

Fig. 9.69 Paraganglioma with extensive calcification

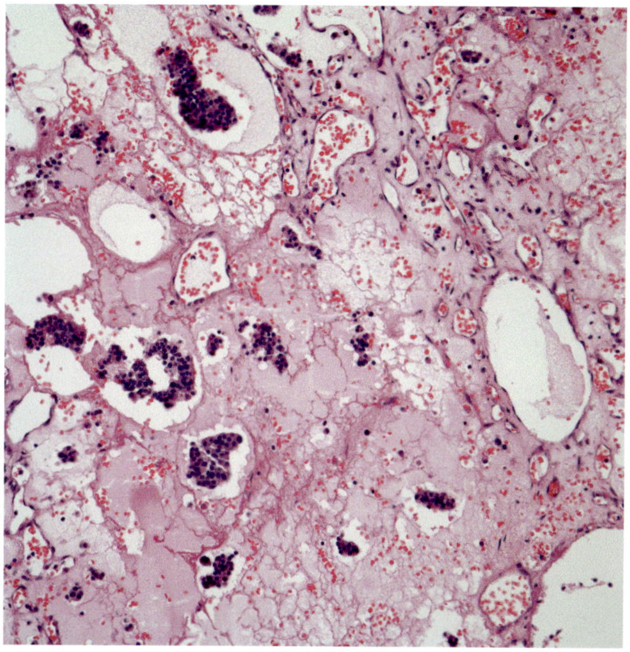

Fig. 9.71 Paraganglioma with extensive hyalinization and only clusters of neuroendocrine cells

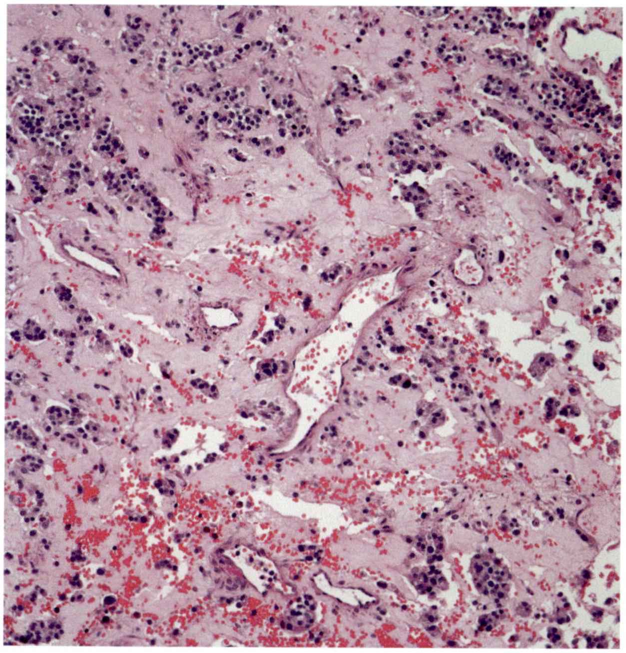

Fig. 9.70 Paraganglioma with more extensive areas of hyalinization

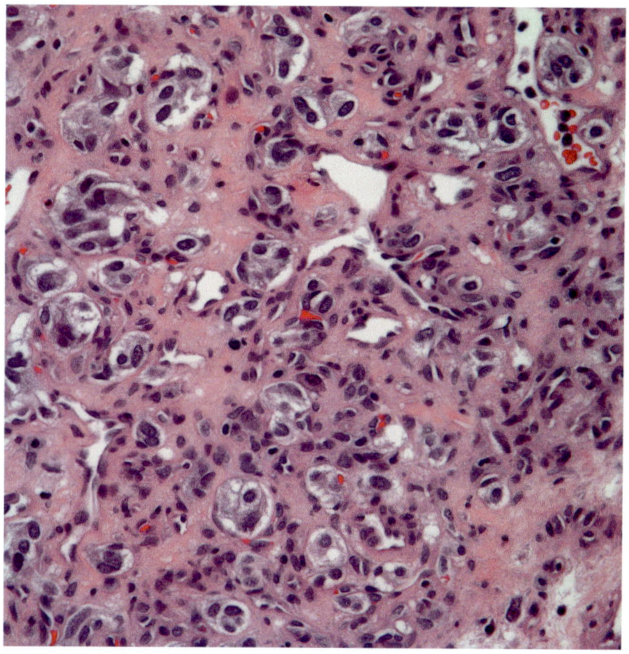

Fig. 9.72 Closer view of a paraganglioma showing nests of neuroendocrine cells with absent of nuclear atypia or mitotic activity

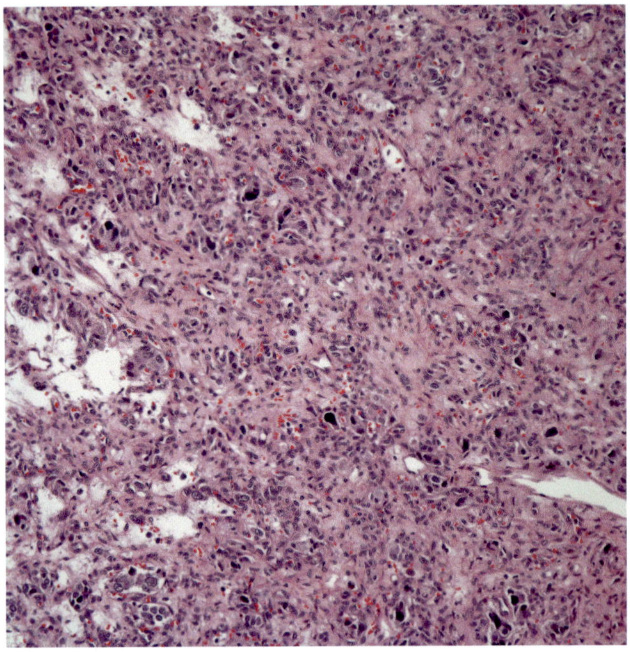

Fig. 9.73 Paraganglioma with easily identifiable cells with macronuclei

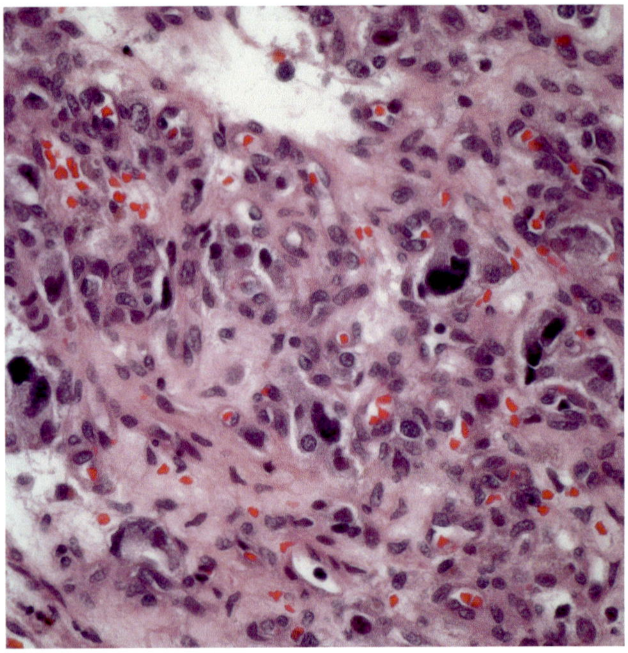

Fig. 9.74 Closer view of a paraganglioma showing bizarre cells with macronuclei

tumors. The presence of spindle cells (Figs. 9.75, 9.76, and 9.77) in which the tumor cells are arranged in a subtle storiform growth pattern may pose a challenge in the definitive diagnosis of these tumors. Also, tumors showing extensive areas of sclerosis (hyalinization) (Figs. 9.78, 9.79, and 9.80) have been described [108]. In addition, an unusual cystic variant of paraganglioma has been described [113]. From the cytologic standpoint, the tumor cells may show a striking granular appearance (Figs. 9.81 and 9.82), oncocytic changes (Figs. 9.83 and 9.84), clear cell cytoplasm (Fig. 9.85), and melanin pigment.

Immunohistochemical Features

By definition, paragangliomas are neuroendocrine neoplasms that may show positive staining for the conventional purported neuroendocrine markers, which include chromogranin, synaptophysin, and CD-56. In addition, S-100 protein may show positive staining in the sustentacular cells, which may be more prominent in those surrounding the epithelioid round cell areas rather than in the spindle cell component that may be present in these tumors. Also, other stains that have shown to be positive in these tumors, even though in a small number of cases, include Leu-enkephalin and neurofilament protein. One important feature with paragangliomas is the negative staining for these tumors with keratin. In a more recent study [83], we identified that paragangliomas may also show positive staining for GATA-3 in approximately 50% of the cases, while the tumors are also negative for TTF-1 and Napsyn, which may also aid in differentiating these tumors from neuroendocrine carcinomas (carcinoid tumors) (Fig. 9.86a–d).

Other Ancillary Studies

The use of ultrastructural studies may also help in the diagnosis of these tumors as the fine ultrastructural features of paragangliomas may show the presence of neurosecretory granules. However, the separation of neuroendocrine carcinomas and paragangliomas solely on ultrastructural grounds may prove to be very difficult as both tumors may show the presence of neurosecretory granules. Grimellius histochemical stain in paragangliomas may also show positive staining in tumor cells. The tumor is negative for PAS with and without diastase.

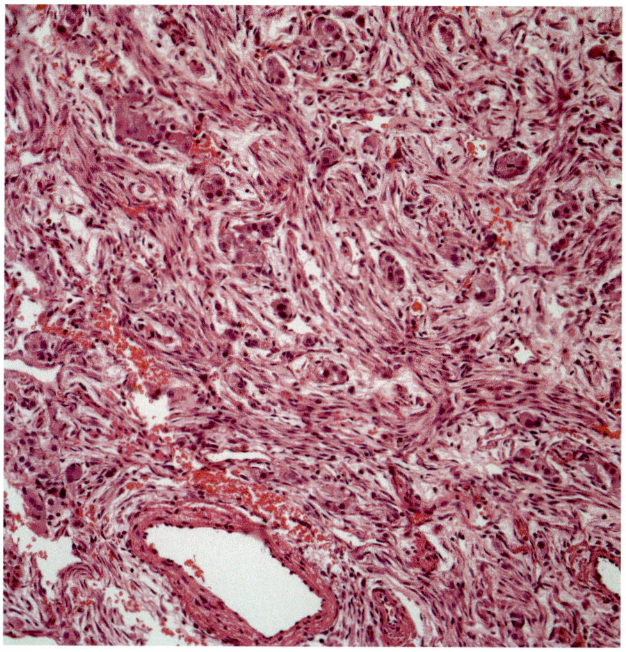

Fig. 9.75 Paraganglioma showing a mixture of round and spindle cells

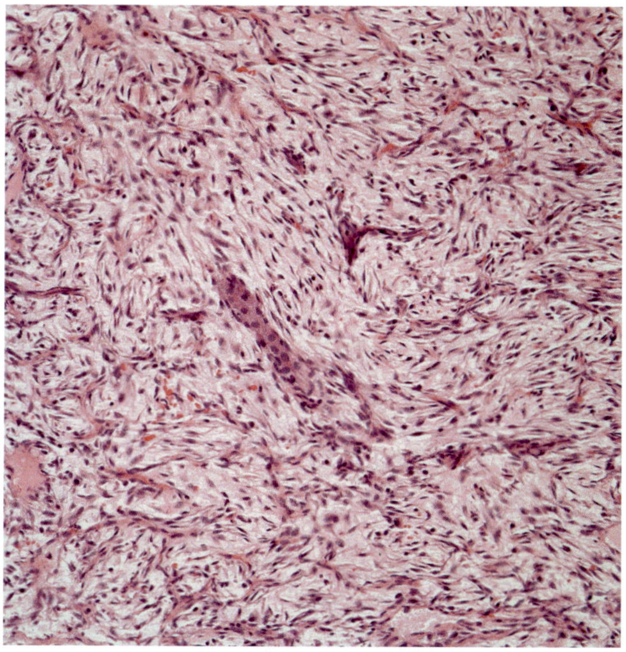

Fig. 9.76 Predominantly spindle cell paraganglioma with only focal round cell component

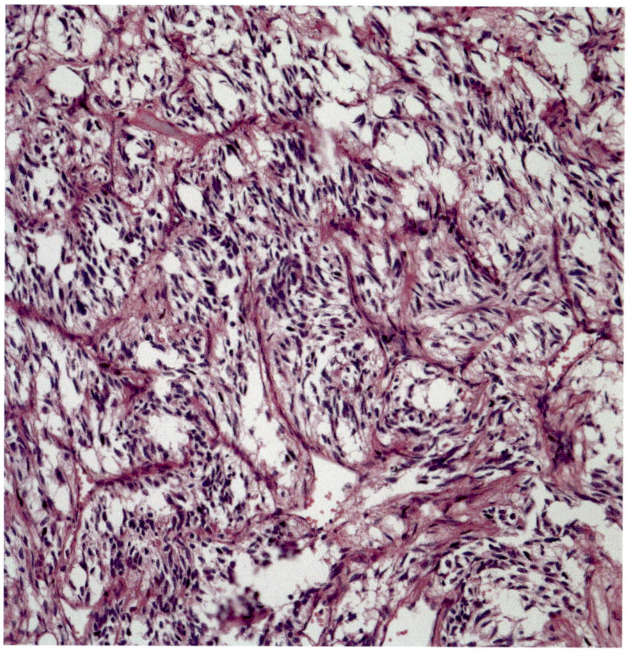

Fig. 9.77 Spindle cell paraganglioma

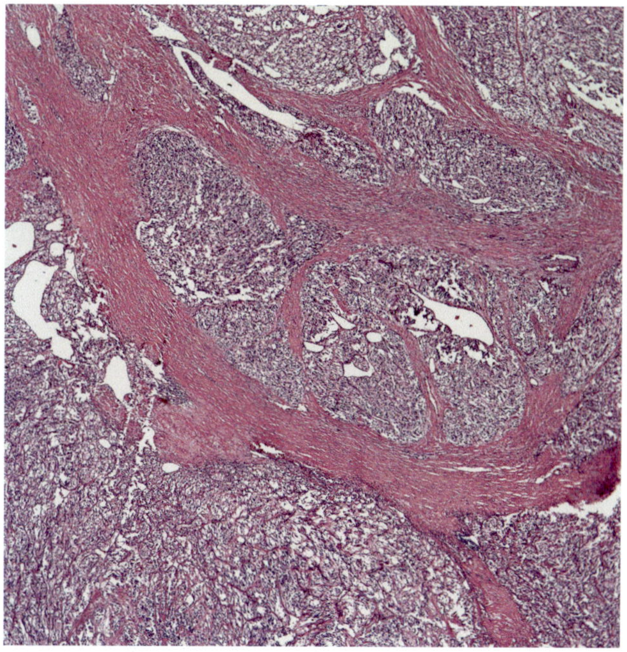

Fig. 9.78 Paraganglioma with extensive areas of thick fibrous bands

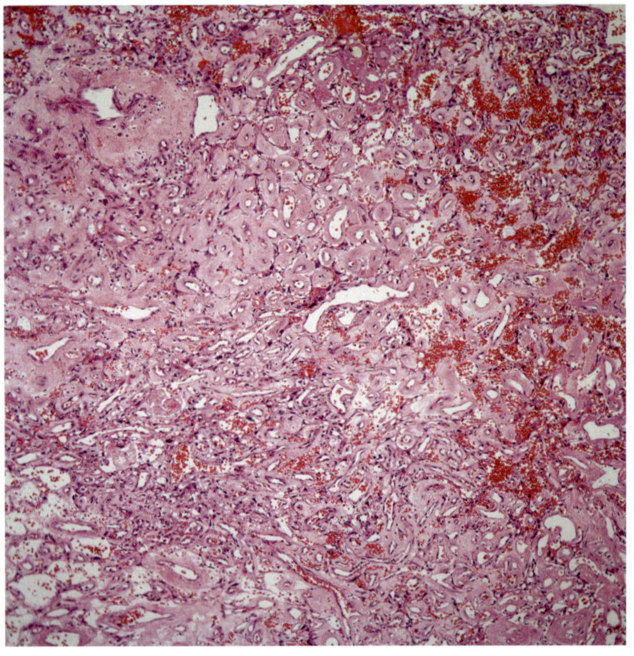

Fig. 9.79 Paraganglioma with extensive vascularity and hyalinization

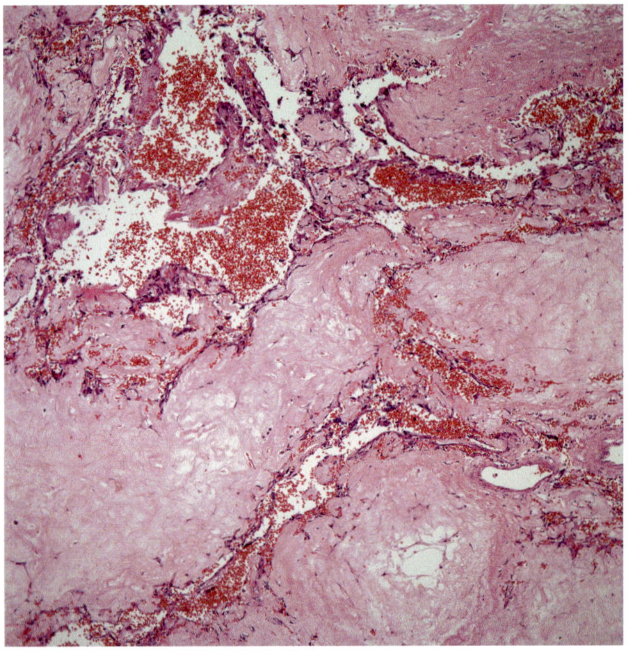

Fig. 9.80 Paraganglioma with extensive hyalinization

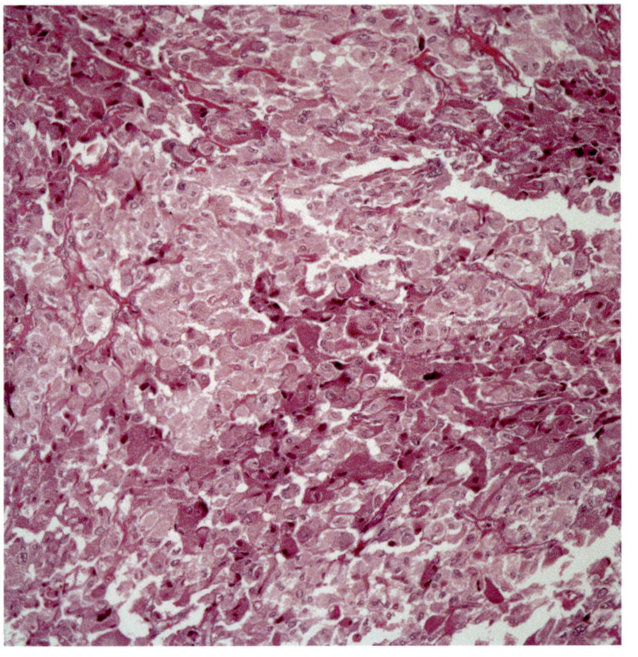

Fig. 9.81 Low power view of a paraganglioma with prominent granular cells

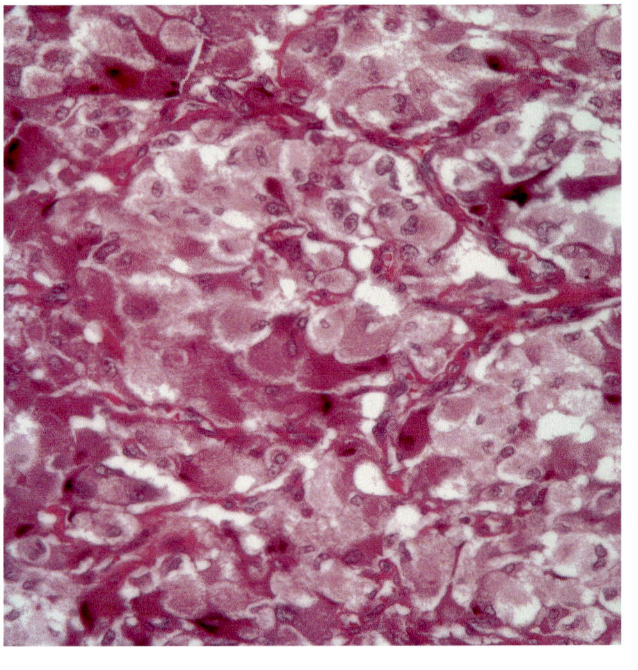

Fig. 9.82 Higher magnification of a granular cell paraganglioma; note the presence of ample granular cytoplasm of the cells

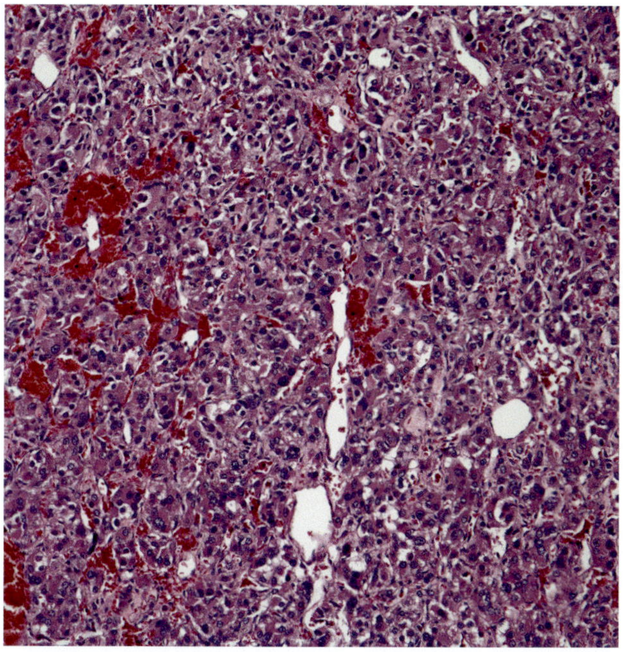

Fig. 9.83 Low power view of an oncocytic paraganglioma

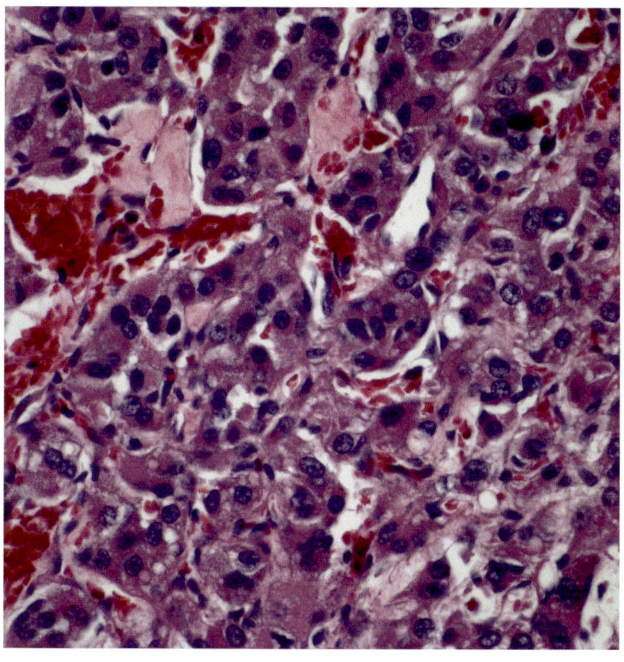

Fig. 9.84 Higher magnification of an oncocytic paraganglioma

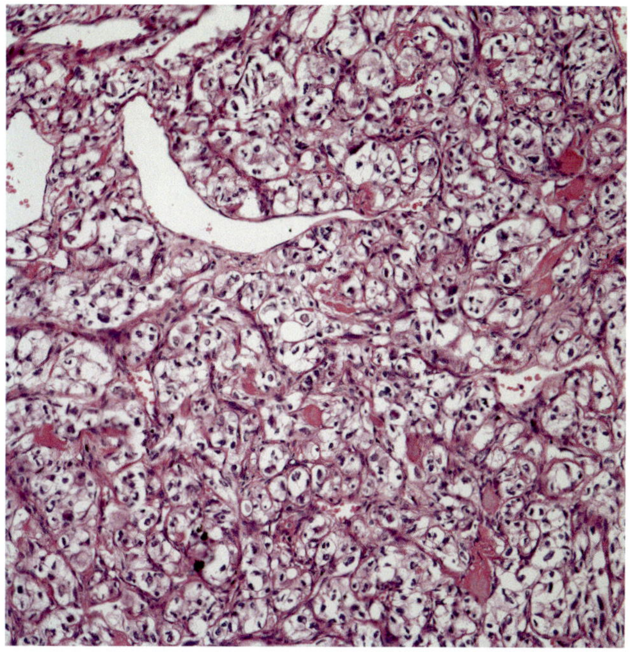

Fig. 9.85 Paraganglioma with prominent clear cell change

Differential Diagnosis

By far, the most important differential diagnosis is separating paragangliomas from neuroendocrine carcinomas and ectopic parathyroid adenomas or carcinoma. In this setting, the use of immunohistochemical stains – mainly the use of keratin coupled with neuroendocrine markers (chromogranin, synaptophysin, and CD-56) – may lead to the correct interpretation, as paragangliomas may show positive staining for neuroendocrine markers but negative staining for keratin and parathyroid hormone.

One other important consideration in the differential diagnosis of these tumors is the evaluation of multicentricity, as these tumors may be present in different locations from where normal paraganglia may exist, and yet the tumor should not be interpreted as metastatic in nature but rather synchronous or metachronous tumors.

On morphological grounds, the tumor that may mimic some of the growth pattern seen in paragangliomas is alveolar soft part sarcoma [114]. Alveolar soft part sarcoma has been described in the mediastinum; however, the tumor will

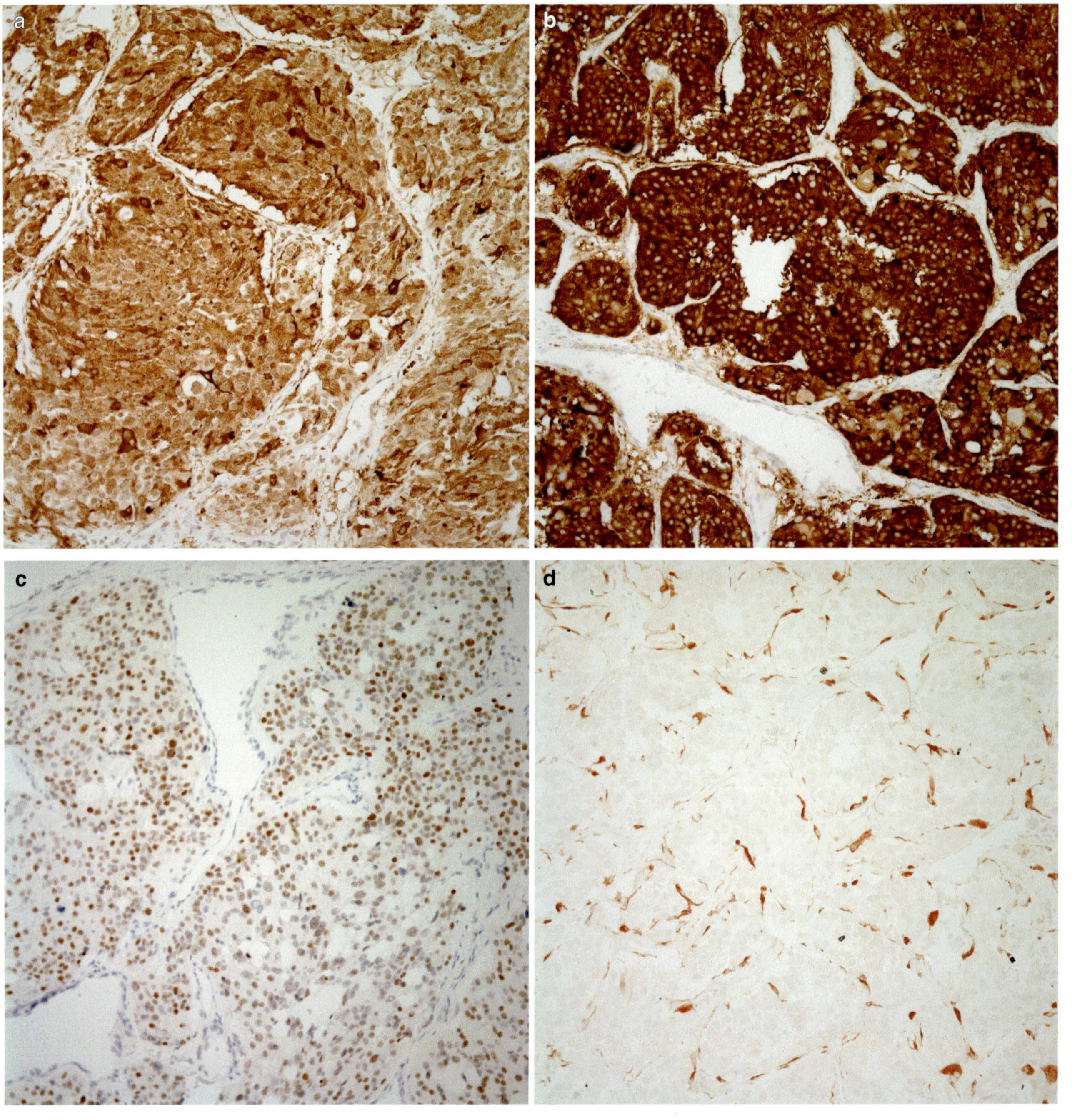

Fig. 9.86 (**a**) paraganglioma showing positive staining for chromogranin; (**b**) positive staining for synaptophysin; (**c**) positive nuclear staining for GATA3; (**d**) positive staining in sustentacular cells for S-100 protein

show negative staining for neuroendocrine markers. Other possible neoplasms that may enter in the differential diagnosis include metastatic renal cell carcinoma and other carcinomas that may have an organoid growth pattern. However, in this context, the use of keratin stain will lead to the correct interpretation.

Parathyroid Tumors

The presence of primary parathyroid tumors in the mediastinal compartment is a rare occurrence and represents a small percentage of these tumors when compared to other mediastinal neuroendocrine neoplasms such as carcinomas (carcinoid tumors) and paragangliomas. Even though parathyroid tumors were described in the mediastinum for more than a century, still these tumors are rare in daily practice and when present may pose a real problem in interpretation.

A possible explanation to account for these tumors may be the embryological development of the parathyroid glands and thymus. Parathyroid glands are formed from the dorsal diverticula of the endothelial cells of the third and fourth pharyngeal pouches. The pair from the fourth pouch is located on each side of the tunica propria of the medial surface of the lateral thyroid lobes at the level of the cricoid cartilage. On the other hand, the pair from the third pouch migrates caudally to the lower border of the thyroid gland. Regarding the primitive thymus, it arises as ventral and medial prolongations on either side from the third pharyngeal pouch. Some additional portions are derived from smaller invaginations of the fourth branchial pouch. The atrophy of the connecting ducts is followed by caudal migration of these cells to form the thoracic thymus [115]. Interestingly, the presence of parathyroid tissue in the thymus appears to be much more common in inferior animals such as rats, rabbits, and hedgehogs. Brewer [115] reported what appears to be one of the earliest observations of this phenomenon in humans in the USA, accounting for four autopsy cases in which the author was able to find two cases of heterotopia of parathyroid in thoracic thymus and two cases of parathyroid nodules in cervical thymus. On the other hand, some authors have actually questioned the name "parathyroid" as it suggests that the glands exist only in a limited area near the thyroid gland [116].

Clinical Features

The hallmark of patients with either parathyroid adenomas or carcinomas in the mediastinum is that of hyperparathyroidism. In 1941, Cope [116] documented his experience with 60 patients with hyperparathyroidism in whom 11 cases of parathyroid adenomas were found in the anterior mediastinum and 5 in the posterior mediastinum. The author estimated that hyperparathyroidism may be secondary to enlarged parathyroid glands in the mediastinum in more than 10% of the cases. Bauer and Federman [117] provide a detailed account of a particular patient who appears to have been one of the earliest cases diagnosed in the USA with hyperparathyroidism secondary to an anterior mediastinal parathyroid adenoma. In 1963, Pachter and Lattes [7] reported their experience with three mediastinal parathyroid tumors. Of the three cases reported, one was a functional parathyroid adenoma in which the patient had symptoms of nephrolithiasis and osteitis cystica. The parathyroid carcinoma was a nonfunctional tumor in which the patient presented with chest pain and no hormonal symptoms, while the additional parathyroid adenoma was an incidental finding during an autopsy procedure. Hardy and associates [118] documented a case in which the patient had four normal cervical parathyroids with an additional large functioning "fifth parathyroid" intrathoracic adenoma. In 1970, Nathaniels and associates [119] reviewed once again the subject of intrathoracic parathyroid tumors and documented that, out of 400 patients treated for hyperparathyroidism, 84 of the parathyroid tumors were located in the mediastinum, 67 in the anterior, and 17 in the posterior mediastinum. Interestingly, the authors also documented that, of the 94 normal parathyroid glands identified in the right neck, 19–20% were located within the thymic capsule in the lower neck or in the substance of the thymus in the anterior mediastinum. Important to mention is the fact that parathyroid cysts similar to those described in the neck have also been described in the mediastinum. Thacker and associates [120] documented a single case of a 46-year-old man with no symptoms of hyperparathyroidism and also provided an account of nine previous cases reported in the literature dating back to 1925. However, Margolis and associates [121] documented a similar case of a mediastinal parathyroid cyst in a 40-year-old man who had metabolic abnormalities, while Simkin [122] documented a 52-year-old man with hyperparathyroidism in association with a mediastinal parathyroid cyst. Eventually, numerous publications on the topic of mediastinal parathyroid cyst have been published in the literature on patients presenting with a diversity of symptoms, while others do not show any symptoms of functioning parathyroid tumor [123–128]. Scholz and associates [129] also documented a 43-year period of time with approximately 1000 patients with hyperparathyroidism. The authors documented 14 cases of mediastinal parathyroid tumors, which were found after one or more cervical explorations. Of the 14 mediastinal tumors, 13 were adenomas and 1 carcinoma; two of the cases were findings at autopsy. Interestingly, the authors also documented five patients in whom abnormalities (hyperplasia or adenoma) in one or more parathyroid glands in the neck were identified. In addition, five patients had a total of five parathyroids including one in the mediastinum. In 1979, Wang and associates [130], in what appears to be the third review from the same institution, presented six additional cases of what the authors called hyperfunctioning supernumerary parathyroid glands, of which four of the patients have mediastinal tumors. Russell and associates [131] described their experience, also in what appears to be the second review from the same institution, with 38 mediastinal tumors requiring mediastinotomy for removal. Except for one of these patients, all had previous parathyroid exploration, while the authors described that "almost all" had significant complications of primary parathyroidism.

In general, regarding the occurrence of parathyroid tumors in the mediastinum, in a review of 285 patients treated surgically for hyperparathyroidism, 22% of the tumors were present in the mediastinum, and 38% of the patients required reoperation for persistent or recurrent hyperparathyroidism. The location of these tumors was more common in the anterior mediastinum at a ratio of approximately 4:1 [132]. Similar findings were also documented by Conn and associates [133], who reviewed 573 patients who had been explored for primary hyperparathyroidism and in whom parathyroid tissue was found in the mediastinum in approximately 11%. In a report more focused toward parathyroid adenomas, Roslyn and Mulder [134] encountered 26 out of 262 patients with persistent primary hyperparathyroidism. Six of these 26 patients had mediastinal parathyroid adenomas. Similar cases of fifth parathyroid adenoma after surgical exploration of the neck have also been documented [135].

Contrary to cases of mediastinal parathyroid adenomas, reports on mediastinal parathyroid carcinomas have been also presented in the literature; almost all of them reported as single case reports [136–140]. Just the same as with the cases reported as adenomas, patients with mediastinal parathyroid carcinomas may also present with functional and nonfunctional tumors. However, it is important to highlight that some metabolic abnormalities have also been associated with other tumors that are not of parathyroid origin. Yoshiike and associates [141] documented a 54-year-old man with a thymic squamous cell carcinoma producing parathyroid hormone-related protein and CYFRA 21-1. Also, Hsiao and associates [142] documented a patient with primary mediastinal B-cell lymphoma secreting parathyroid hormone-related protein who presented with superior vena cava syndrome and hypercalcemia. More recently, we have documented our experience with 17 patients with primary parathyroid tumors [143]. The tumors were equally distributed in both genders as nine tumors were in women and eight in men. All the tumors were located in the anterior mediastinum, and all patients had disturbances in the metabolism. One patient had previous history of neck exploration and secondary hyperparathyroidism due to polycystic kidney disease. One case was encountered at autopsy.

From the radiological point of view, patients with either parathyroid adenoma or parathyroid carcinoma may present with large mediastinal masses, which in turn may be either solid or cystic [144, 145]. However, the definitive diagnosis lies on the histopathological evaluation of the tumor.

Regarding the treatment and prognosis of parathyroid mediastinal tumors, it is linked to the histological type. For those tumors with the histological characteristics of adenoma, complete surgical resection may be the only therapy needed, while for parathyroid carcinoma, not only may the resection be more extensive due to the infiltrative manner of these tumors in the mediastinum, but, in addition, the patients may also be candidates for additional medical treatment with close follow-up.

Pathological Features

Gross Features

The description of most parathyroid adenomas is that of a well-circumscribed tumor mass, which at cut surface shows a homogeneous light brown color. The tumors do not show areas of hemorrhage or necrosis. However, in the macroscopic description of cases in which the histology is that of carcinoma, the tumors may show a more infiltrative nature by compromising more extensive areas within the mediastinum or involve adjacent structures such as the pericardium or mediastinal pleura. In these tumors, areas of hemorrhage or necrosis may be apparent. The size of these tumors varies, and small tumors of about 2 cm as well as large tumor of over 15 cm with large weight have been described (Fig. 9.87).

Histopathological Features

The histopathological features of parathyroid tumors can be subdivided in those seen in (A) parathyroid cyst, (B) parathyroid adenomas, and (C) parathyroid carcinomas. The different morphological patterns would show distinctive characteristics that make them amenable for appropriate interpretation.

Mediastinal parathyroid cyst would show a unilocular cystic structure lined by flatten epithelium and thick wall, which may show inflammatory reaction and underlying adipose tissue. Higher magnification of the walls of the cyst will disclose the presence of a cellular proliferation that may be

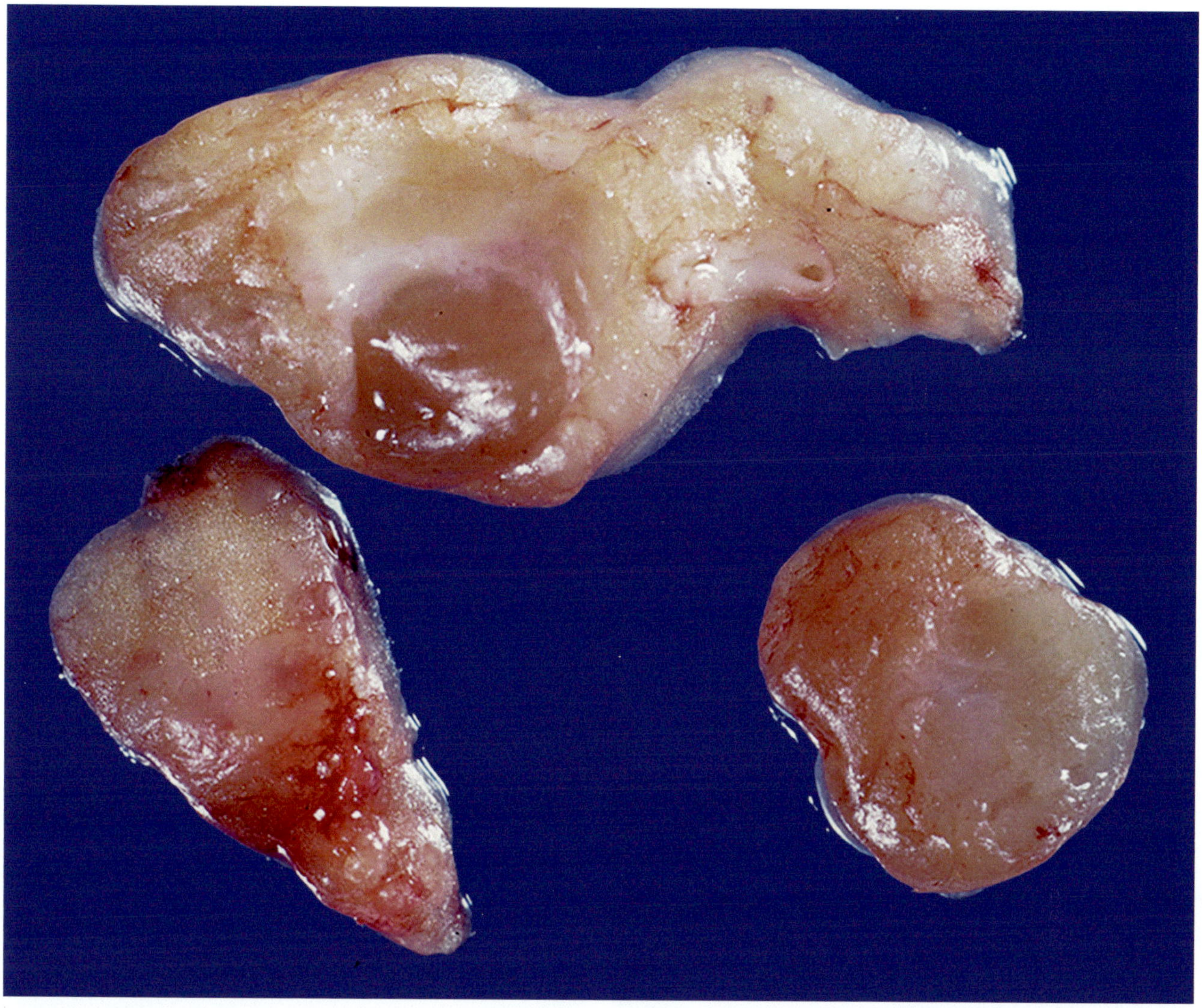

Fig. 9.87 Mediastinal parathyroid adenoma showing a light brown color with the absence of necrosis or hemorrhage

present in sheets of cells or in a subtle nested growth pattern (Fig. 9.88a, b). The cells may show a mixture of oncocytic cells with clear cells (chief cells). This cellular proliferation may extend in varying proportions in the walls of the cystic structures. Areas of necrosis and hemorrhage are generally not present nor are cellular atypia or mitotic activity.

Mediastinal parathyroid adenomas may be further separated in tumors with predominant oncocytic proliferation, chief cells, or a mixture of both. In predominantly oncocytic tumor, the cellular proliferation may be arranged in two forms. One is a more solid cellular proliferation with an organoid growth pattern composed of medium size, oval to polygonal cells with moderate amounts of eosinophilic cytoplasm, round to oval centrally placed nuclei, and in many cells with prominent nucleoli. The other unusual growth pattern is that of a pseudoglandular appearance with similar cytological features as those seen in the solid growth pattern. The presence of areas with numerous pyknotic cells is common. On the other hand, the tumors may be composed predominantly of chief cells in which the tumor cells are arranged in sheets of round to polygonal cells with clear cytoplasm, round to oval nuclei, and inconspicuous nucleoli (Figs. 9.89, 9.90, 9.91, 9.92, 9.93, 9.94, 9.95, 9.96, 9.97, 9.98, and 9.99). Microscopic cystic changes may be seen in both of these growth patterns. Even though the presence of mitotic activity is generally absent, in some cases,

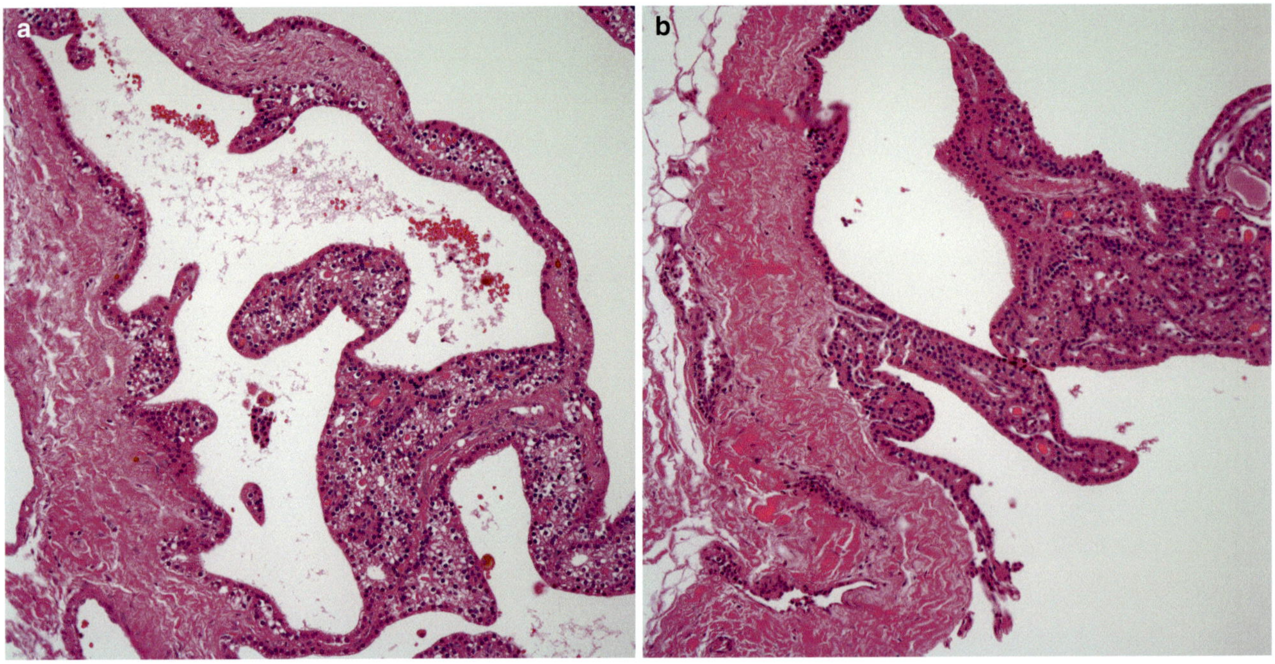

Fig. 9.88 (**a**) Mediastinal parathyroid cyst; note the cystic nature of the tumor; (**b**) mediastinal parathyroid cyst showing a proliferation of neuroendocrine cells

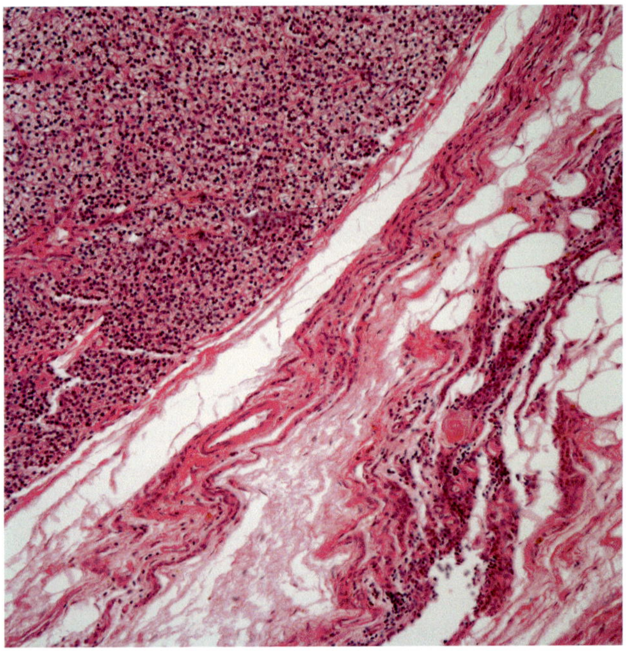

Fig. 9.89 Mediastinal parathyroid adenoma; note the presence of residual thymus in the periphery (Hassall's corpuscle)

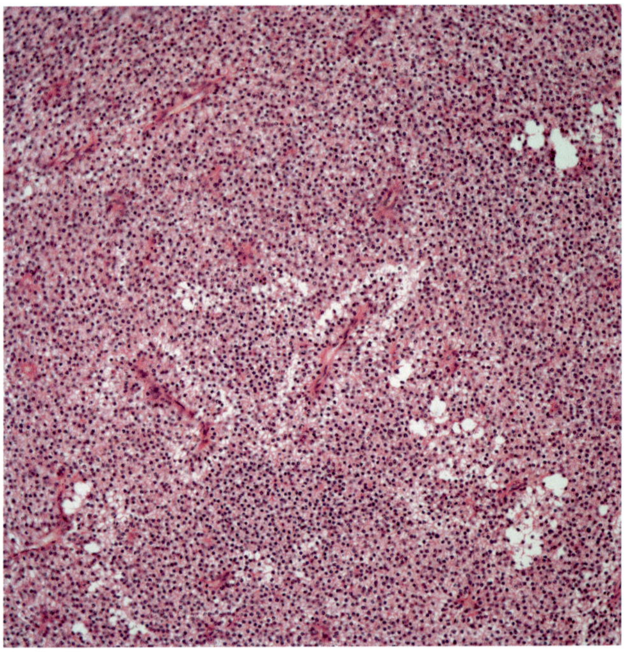

Fig. 9.90 Mediastinal parathyroid adenoma composed predominantly of chief cells

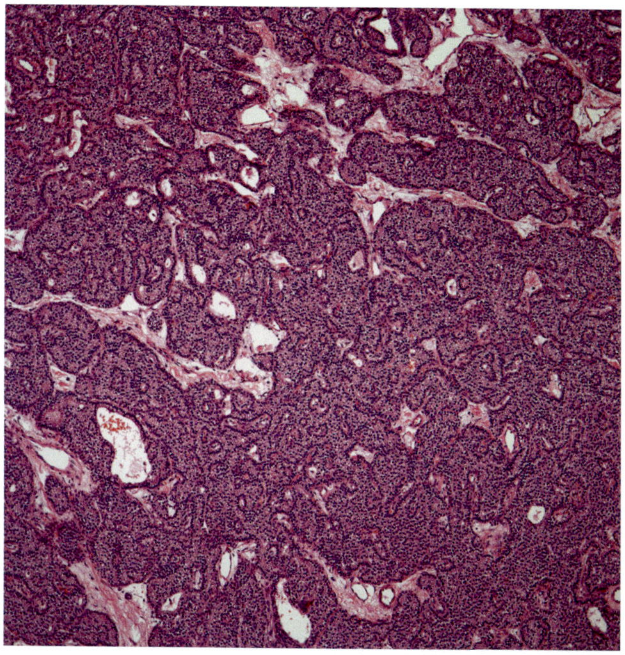

Fig. 9.91 Mediastinal parathyroid adenoma composed predominantly of chief cells in a pseudoglandular growth pattern

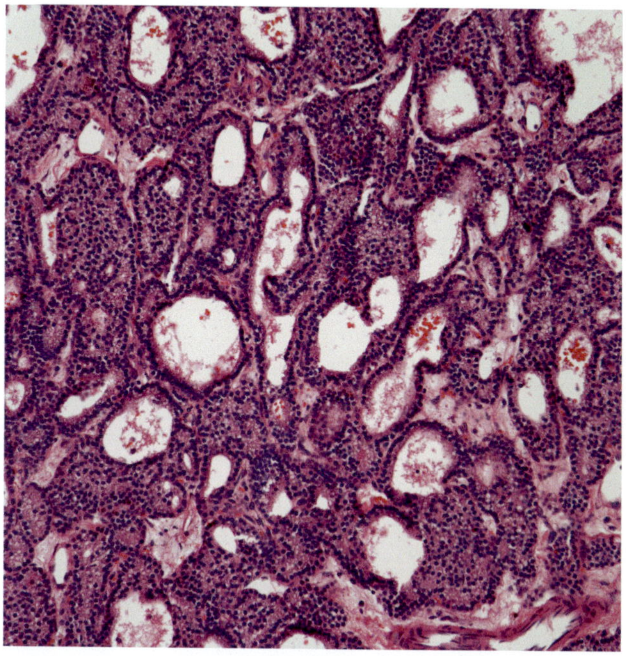

Fig. 9.92 Higher magnification showing a homogeneous cellular proliferation with absence of nuclear atypia or mitotic activity

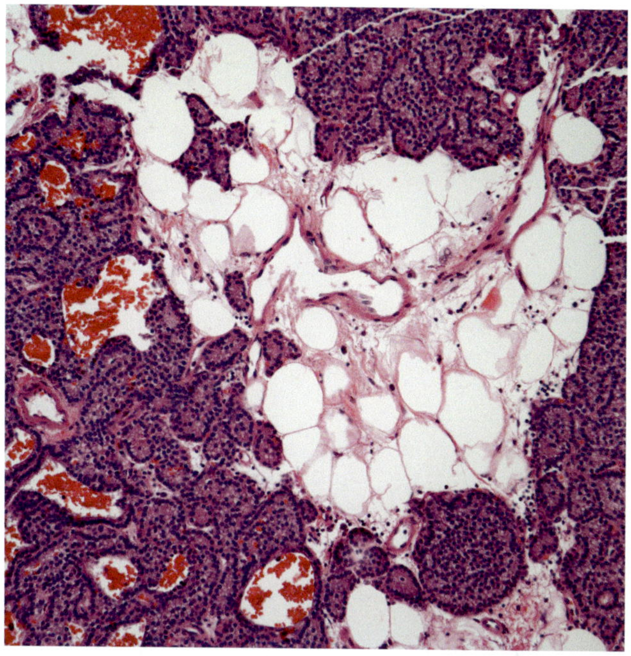

Fig. 9.93 Mediastinal parathyroid adenoma showing focal areas of adipose tissue

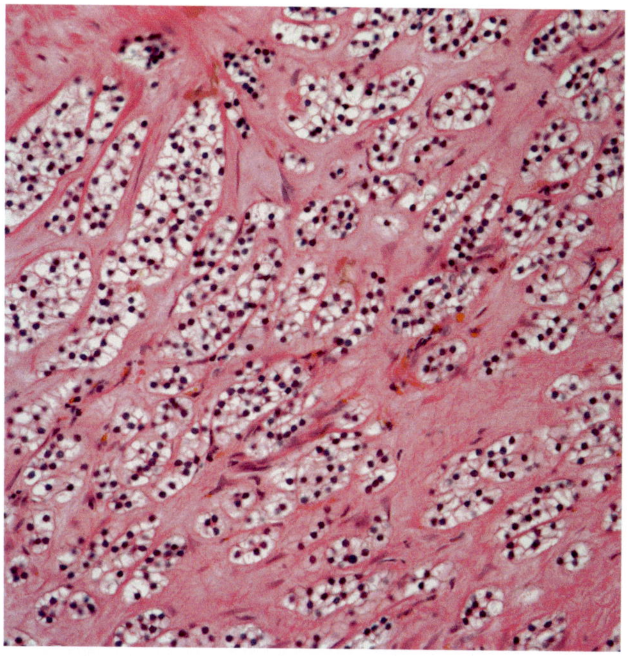

Fig. 9.94 Mediastinal parathyroid adenoma showing cords of clear cells (chief cells) dissecting fibroconnective tissue

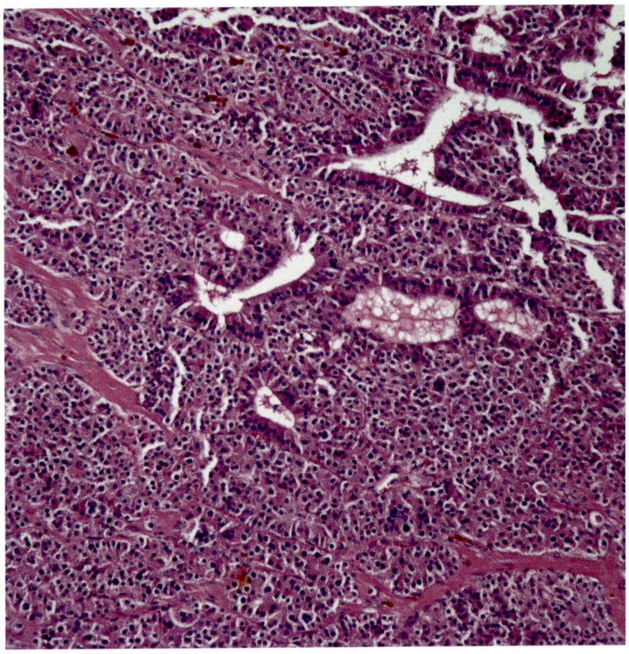

Fig. 9.95 Mediastinal parathyroid adenoma showing diffuse and glandular components

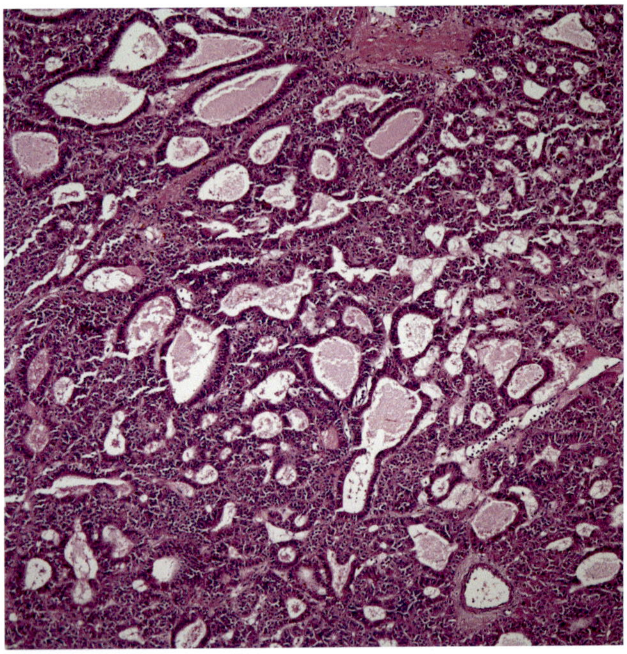

Fig. 9.96 Mediastinal parathyroid adenoma showing glandular like areas similar to those seen in angiectatic neuroendocrine carcinoma

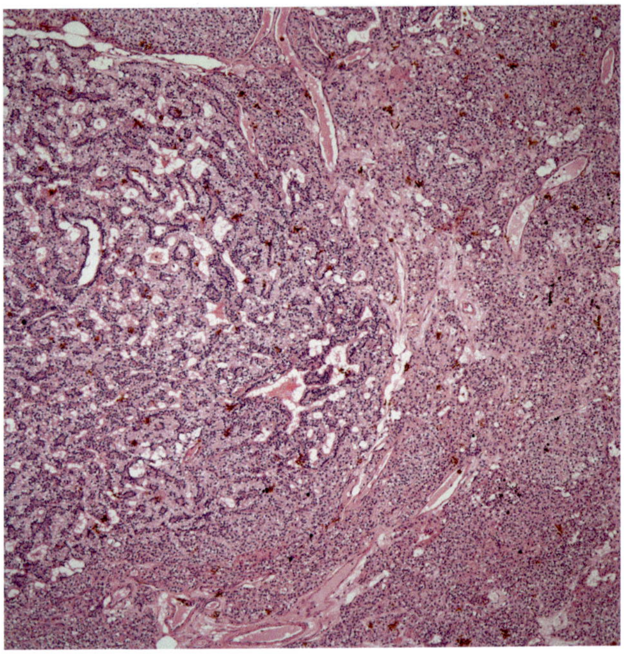

Fig. 9.97 Mediastinal parathyroid adenoma showing a mixture of components one diffuse and the other more glandular

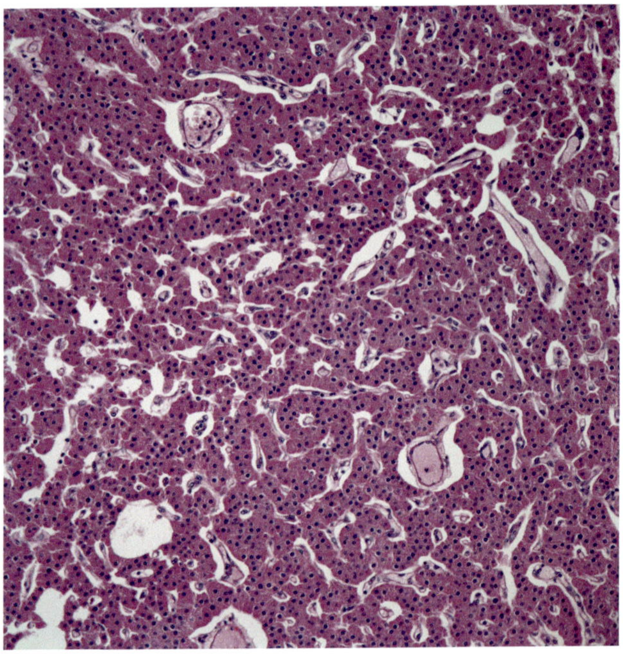

Fig. 9.98 Oncocytic mediastinal parathyroid adenoma. Note the absence of nuclear atypia

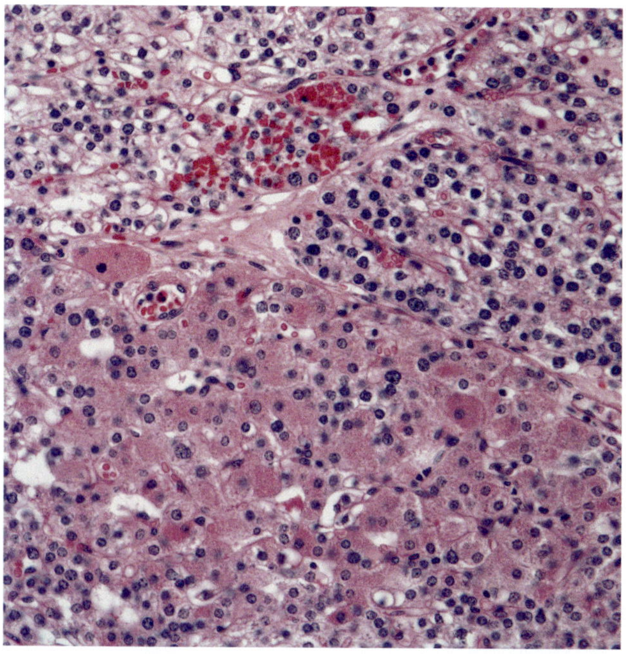

Fig. 9.99 Mediastinal parathyroid adenoma showing a mixture of chief and oncocytic cells

rare mitotic figures may be present. One additional feature that is important to recognize is the presence of extensive areas of sclerosis that are present in either oncocytic or chief cells predominant tumors (Fig. 9.100a–c). In addition, some tumors may show the presence of a combination of oncocytic and chief cell components with similar characteristics as those seen when one of those cell types predominate.

One important parathyroid tumor that has also been described in the mediastinum is parathyroid lipoadenoma [146]. Hargreaves and Wright described such a lesion in the posterior mediastinum. The tumor is characterized by the presence of areas of adipose tissue and parathyroid tissue, which can be arranged in acini, tubules, or simple aggregates. The adipose component may make up to 70% of the tumor mass.

The histopathological features of mediastinal parathyroid carcinoma are similar to those described for those tumors when they occur in the neck. Mainly, the tumor may show a more infiltrative growth pattern with ill-defined borders, presence of fibrous septa of varying thickness, necrosis, and increase mitotic activity. The tumors usually show the presence of a cellular proliferation composed of round to oval cells with oxyphilic and clear cells. Nuclear pleomorphism may be mild, and presence of nucleoli may not be apparent (Fig. 9.101a–c).

Ancillary Studies

The use of histochemical stains in the evaluation of parathyroid tumors may prove to be very useful when compared to other endocrine tumors that may enter in the differential diagnosis of these tumors. Periodic acid-Schiff may show the presence of glycogen in tumors that are composed of chief cells (Fig. 9.102). This particular histochemical stain may not be very useful in tumors that are composed predominantly of oncocytic cells. Mucicarmine is essentially negative in these tumors. Immunohistochemical stains are also of value in the evaluation of parathyroid tumors; however, care must be exercised, as other endocrine tumors may also share similar immunohistochemical phenotypes. Parathyroid tumor may show positive staining for chromogranin, synaptophysin, low molecular weight keratin, neuron-specific enolase, and parathyroid hormone. Because of this immunohistochemical profile, it is highly important to properly analyze these tumors, as other tumors with different clinical behavior may also share similar immunohistochemical features. In addition, the ultrastructural features of these tumors may also disclose the presence of neurosecretory granules that may be indistinguishable from those seen in other endocrine neoplasms.

Differential Diagnosis

By far the most important differential diagnosis of parathyroid tumors is with mediastinal neuroendocrine carcinoma (carcinoid and atypical carcinoid) and paragangliomas. When the parathyroid tumor is composed predominantly of chief cells, it may be slightly easier to reach the appropriate interpretation as neuroendocrine carcinomas with prominent clear cell changes are unusual. In addition, the presence of strong parathyroid hormone immunohistochemical stain may prove useful. In cases in which the tumors shows predominant oncocytic component, the morphological interpretation may be a bit more complicated, as oncocytic neuroendocrine carcinomas are not that unusual. The interpretation may get more complicated when the tumor shows an angiomatoid growth pattern that has been described in both tumors. It is highly important in these cases not only to have a thorough morphological evaluation of the tumor but also to perform a complete immunohistochemical panel that includes parathyroid hormone.

The separation of parathyroid tumor from paragangliomas may be slightly easier if the correct material is available for interpretation. The presence of macronuclei and nuclear atypia with bizarre cells is by far more common in paragan-

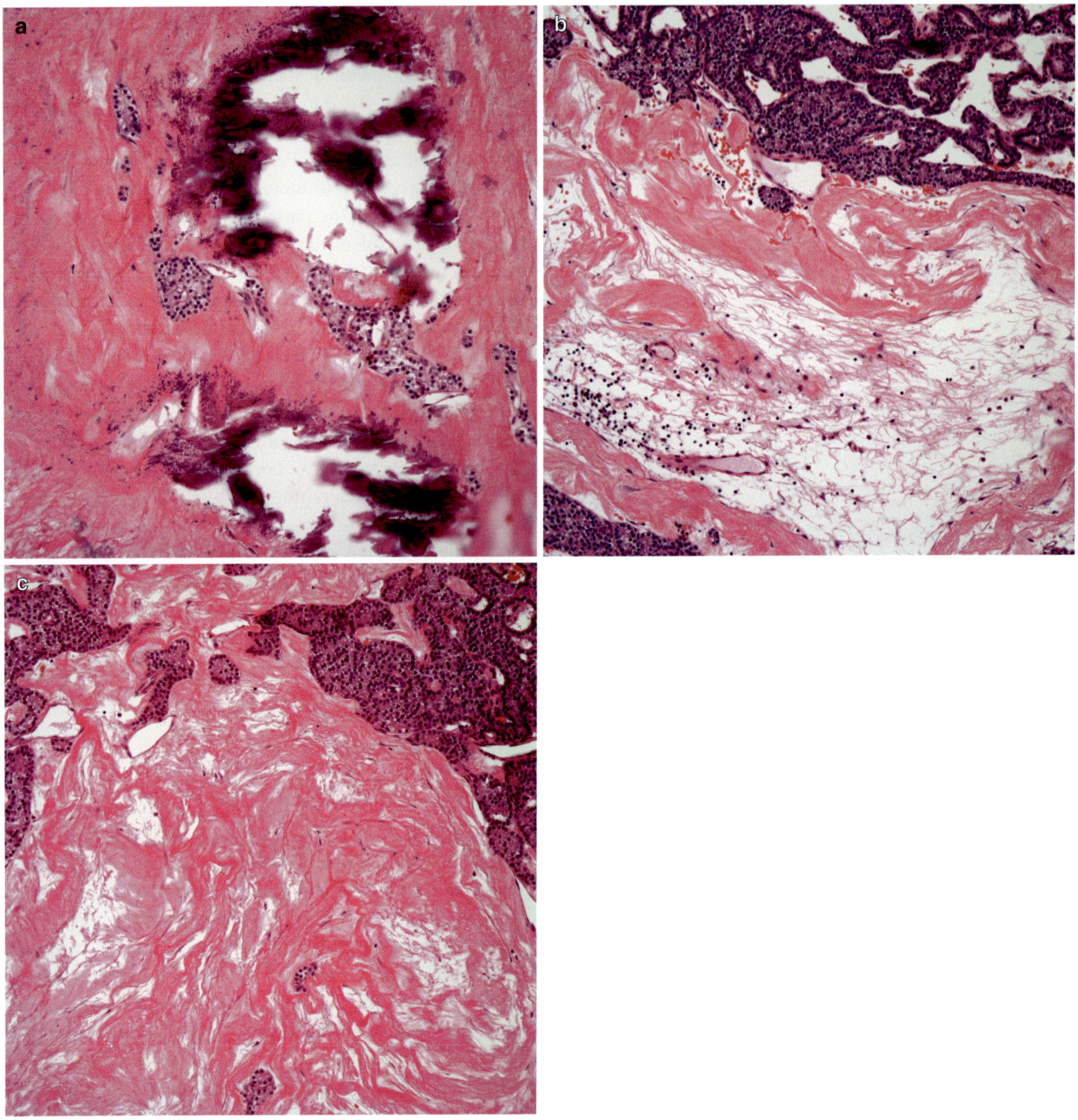

Fig. 9.100 (**a**) Mediastinal parathyroid adenoma with extensive calcification; (**b**) mediastinal parathyroid adenoma showing areas of hyalinization; (**c**) mediastinal parathyroid adenoma with extensive areas of hyalinization

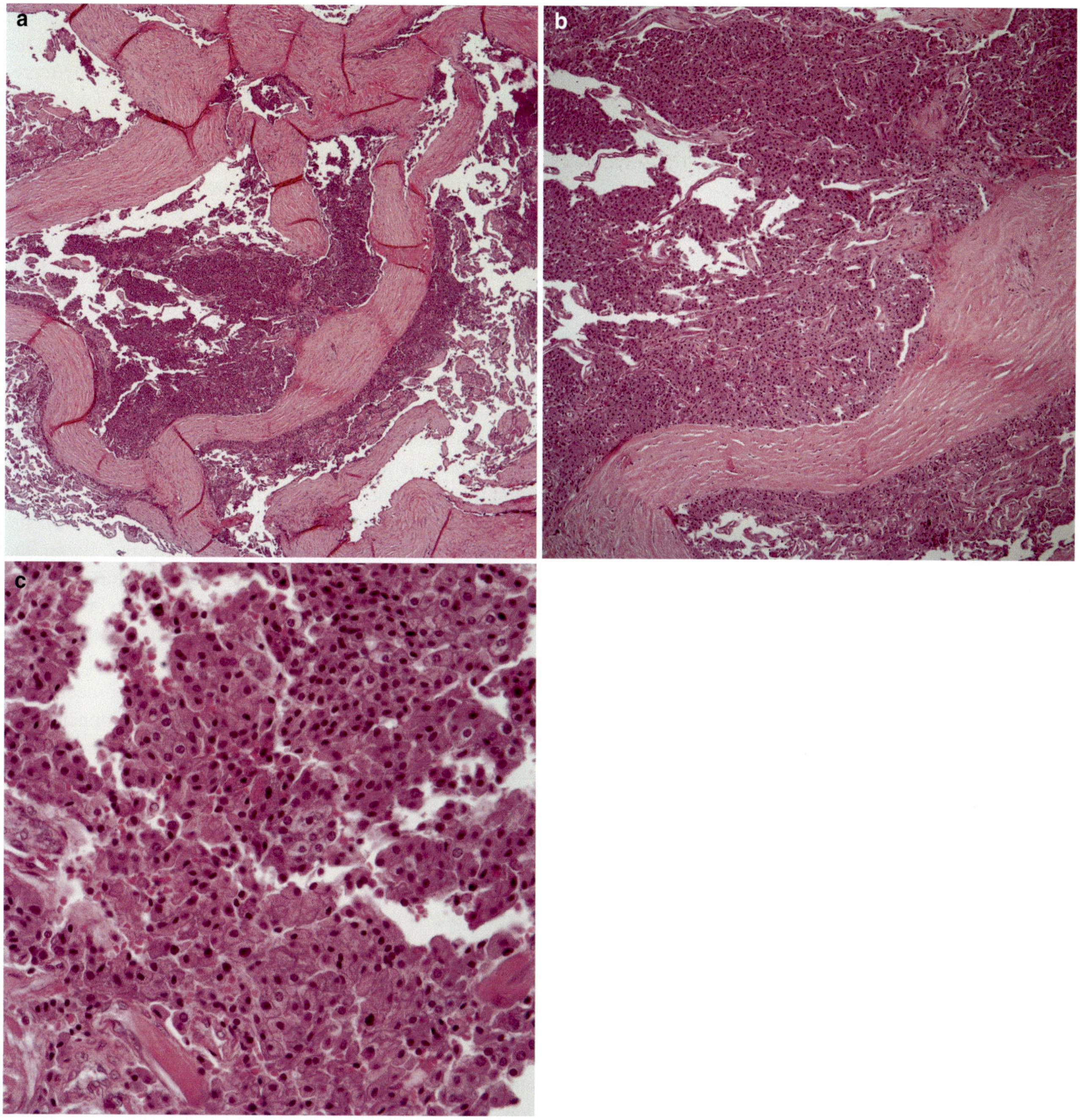

Fig. 9.101 (**a**) Mediastinal parathyroid carcinoma showing thick fibrous bands and a more infiltrate growth pattern; (**b**) Note the tick fibrous bands separating the neoplastic cellular proliferation; (**c**) higher magnification showing cellular and nuclear atypia

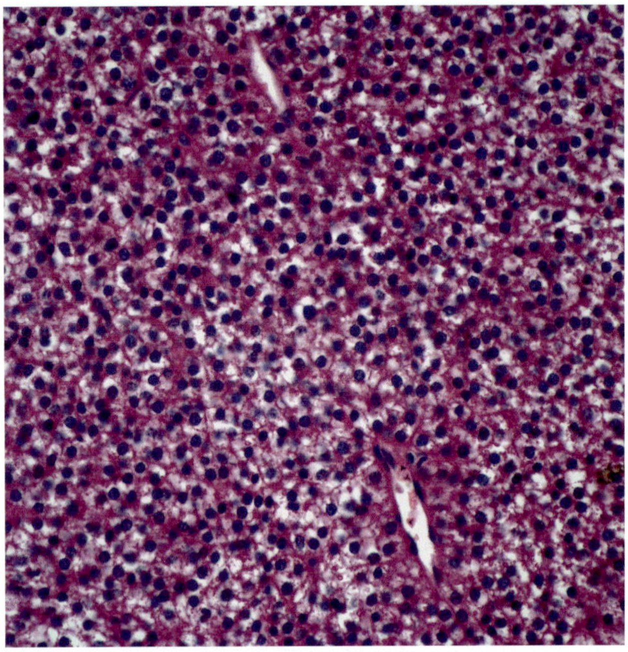

Fig. 9.102 Periodic acid-Schiff (PAS) in a parathyroid adenoma showing abundant glycogen deposition in tumor cells

gliomas than parathyroid tumors. In addition, the presence of positive staining for keratin may be of help in separating the two tumors.

Finally, the separation between mediastinal parathyroid adenoma and parathyroid carcinoma is similar to the histopathological approach for these tumors when they occur in the neck. Mainly, the features of ill-defined tumors with infiltrative borders, necrosis, increased mitotic activity, and fibrous bands of different thickness are more commonly seen in carcinomas.

Thyroid Tumors

Even though the presence of thyroid tumors within the mediastinal compartment may not necessarily belong to the conventional group of neuroendocrine tumors, it is presented in this section, as the thyroid itself is an endocrine gland, thus raising the possibility of developing either benign or malignant tumors of thyroid origin within the mediastinal compartment. Furthermore, the presence of thyroid tissue or thyroid tumors within the mediastinal compartment has been recognized widely in the literature. This occurrence has been reported under different designations including retrosternal, substernal, intrathoracic, and mediastinal [147–155]. Even though the majority of thyroid neoplasms within the mediastinum appear to be of the benign type, mainly represented by mediastinal goiters, it is the definition of what constitutes mediastinal goiter that has been discussed for many years and what at the end determines the incidence of these tumors in the mediastinal cavity. There appears to be at least four definitions regarding mediastinal goiters: (1) any portion of the thyroid below the thoracic inlet, (2) thyroid reaching the level of the aortic arch, (3) thyroid reaching the level of T4 on imaging, and (4) 50% or more of the thyroid below the thoracic inlet. Currently, the last definition of mediastinal goiter is the one that appears more accepted. However, it is essential to recognize that the existence of thyroid in the mediastinal compartment regardless of its definition may be seen in two different forms: (a) primary mediastinal goiter in which there is no connection between the mediastinal thyroid tissue and the cervical thyroid, and (2) secondary mediastinal goiter in which there is a connection between the mediastinal component and the cervical thyroid. By far, the most common is the secondary mediastinal goiter, as true primary mediastinal goiter appears to be a rare occurrence. The possible explanation to account for these two distinct occurrences may be based on the embryological development of the thyroid gland. The true or primary mediastinal goiter may result from autonomic growth of germinal nuclei of the thyroglossal duct, while the secondary mediastinal goiter may develop from the cervical thyroid that becomes disconnected from it. In view of the different definitions of mediastinal goiter, it is difficult to be exact regarding their true incidence; however, it has been estimated that it may vary from 5 to 20%. Erbil and associates [150] reported their experience with substernal goiters and calculated that they occur in approximately 6.4% of the patients. The authors reviewed 2650 patients with thyroid gland disorders between 1990 and 2003, identifying 170 patients (6.4%) with substernal goiter. Raffaelli and associates [149], in a study of substernal goiters using the criteria of 50% or more of the thyroid gland below the thoracic inlet, identified 355 patients out of 2263 patients who underwent thyroidectomy, which represents 15.7% of patients with substernal goiter. Huins and associates [153] reviewed the literature of the subject, and, after analyzing cumulative data of more than 22000 patients with goiter, the authors estimated that retrosternal extension occurs in approximately 6.28% of patients. On the contrary, the occurrence of true "primary" mediastinal goiters appears to be much more uncommon, with estimates of approximately 1% of all mediastinal goiters. One important issue that needs to be highlighted is the fact that malignant thyroid neoplasm may arise in the mediastinum. However, it is very difficult to determine the incidence of thyroid carcinomas developing in a substernal goiter, not only because, in general terms, such development in a cervical thyroid is not common and it is difficult to estimate but also because mediastinal goiters are far less common. Thus, the presence of malignancies developing within an otherwise substernal goiter likely represents an unusual phenomenon. Rios and associates [156] studied 672 patients with multinodular goiters and identified 59 patients with an associated malignancy. Papillary microcarcinomas were the most common malignancies associated in 37 of the 59 patients. The authors stated that the risk factors for carcinoma associated with multinodular goiters include family history of thyroid pathology and history of radiation to the neck among others. Nevertheless, the occurrence of thyroid carcinomas within the mediastinal compartment has been recorded in the literature [4, 157–160]. Similar to the cases described as substernal goiters, the cases described of thyroid carcinoma also followed the same characteristics, as some develop in the background of a substernal goiter, while a minority of cases develop as de novo in possible ectopic thyroid tissue with no connection with the cervical thyroid.

Clinical Features

Based on different reviews that have been presented on substernal goiters or thyroid carcinomas arising in a mediastinal compartment, it appears that the majority of these patients are adult women. In some studies, it has been estimated that these tumors are more common in women in a proportion of 7:1 against men. Clinically, patients may present completely asymptomatic or with a diversity of symptoms, which would include palpable neck mass, dysphagia, dyspnea, hoarseness, cough, chest pain, and hyperthyroidism. Interestingly, in some reviews, a thyroid mass has been present in approximately 88% of patients with substernal goiter. Diagnostic imaging is important to determine the presence of a mediastinal involvement, and the use of chest films or chest CT appears to provide good results. Another procedure that has been performed in some patients is thyroid scintigraphy.

Anatomically, the tumors may be in the anterior or posterior mediastinum. However, the anterior mediastinum is much more common, with some estimates at more than 90% of the tumors in that location. The treatment of choice for these tumors is complete surgical resection of the mediastinal tumor, and the prognosis is excellent for those lesions that are in the spectrum of mediastinal goiters. Because there are not meaningful series of cases of thyroid carcinomas developing in the mediastinal compartment, it is difficult to determine the behavior of those tumors while occurring in the mediastinal compartment. However, it is logical to expect that small papillary carcinomas developing in the background of large mediastinal goiters should also have a good prognosis.

Histopathological Features

The diagnosis of these lesions should not pose a problem in interpretation, and these are often diagnosed as substernal goiter, mediastinal goiter, mediastinal colloid goiter, or nodular hyperplasia. The morphological features present in mediastinal goiters are essentially similar to those described in the cervical thyroid, namely, the presence of distended thyroid follicles with or without colloid, and in areas separated in a nodular pattern by fibroconnective tissue (Figs. 9.103 and 9.104a, b). These tumors do not show much in terms of cytologic atypia or increased mitotic figures.

In cases in which carcinoma is present, the histology of these tumors is also similar to that occurring in cervical thyroid. Papillary thyroid carcinoma appears to be probably the most common histology.

Immunohistochemical Features and Other Ancillary Studies

The use of immunohistochemistry in the diagnosis of mediastinal goiter is essentially limited as, in reality, there is no need for it as the morphological features of the lesion are sufficient enough to make an unequivocal diagnosis. However, in cases in which there may be a malignant neoplasm associated, then the use of immunohistochemical studies such as thyroglobulin, calcitonin, or PAX-8 may be of aid in the diagnosis. Similarly, the use of histochemical stains such as PAS with or without diastase, mucicarmine, and the use of ultrastructural studies have very limited use in the diagnosis of these tumors.

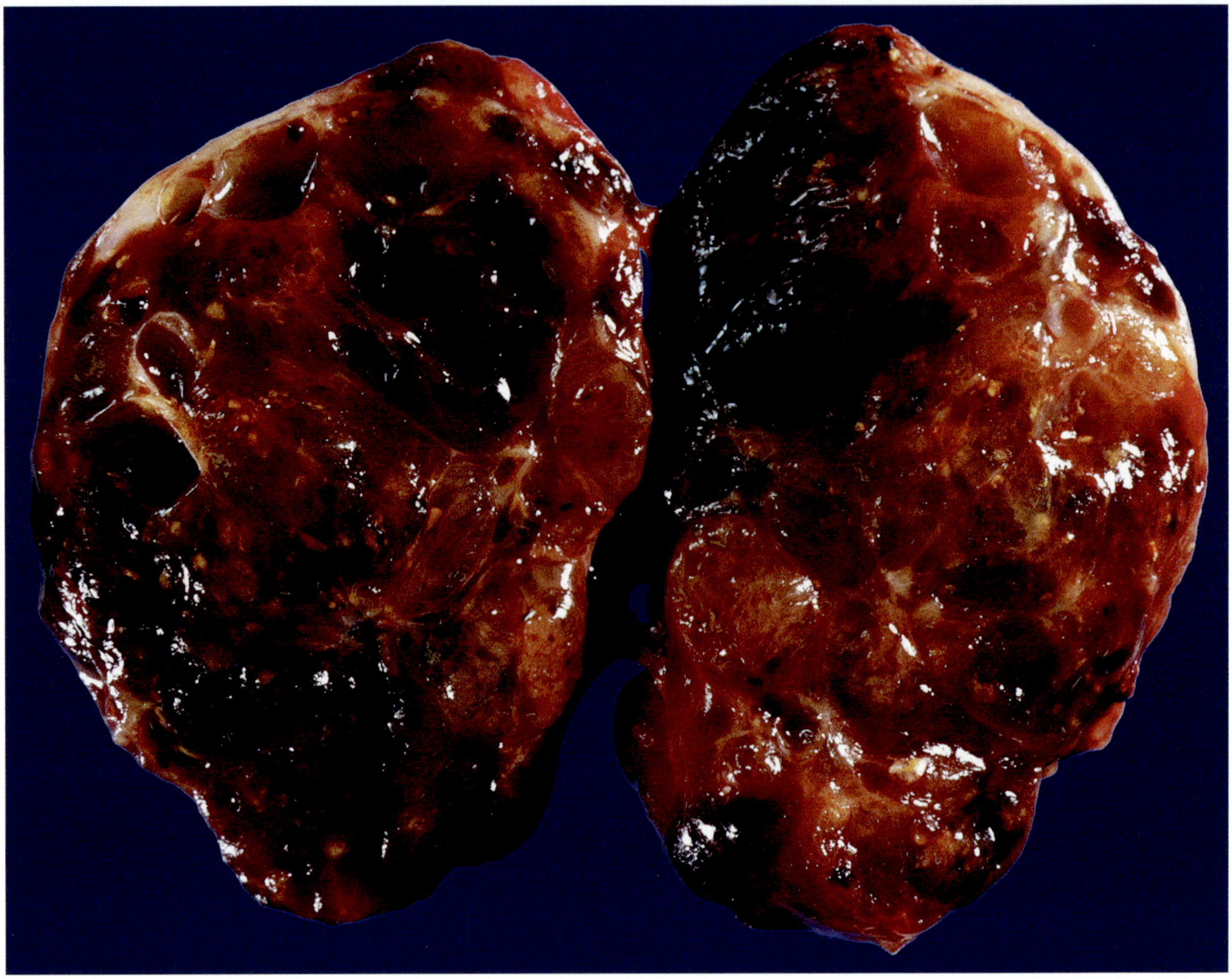

Fig. 9.103 Mediastinal goiter; note the presence a fleshy nodular tumor. Focal areas of hemorrhage are present

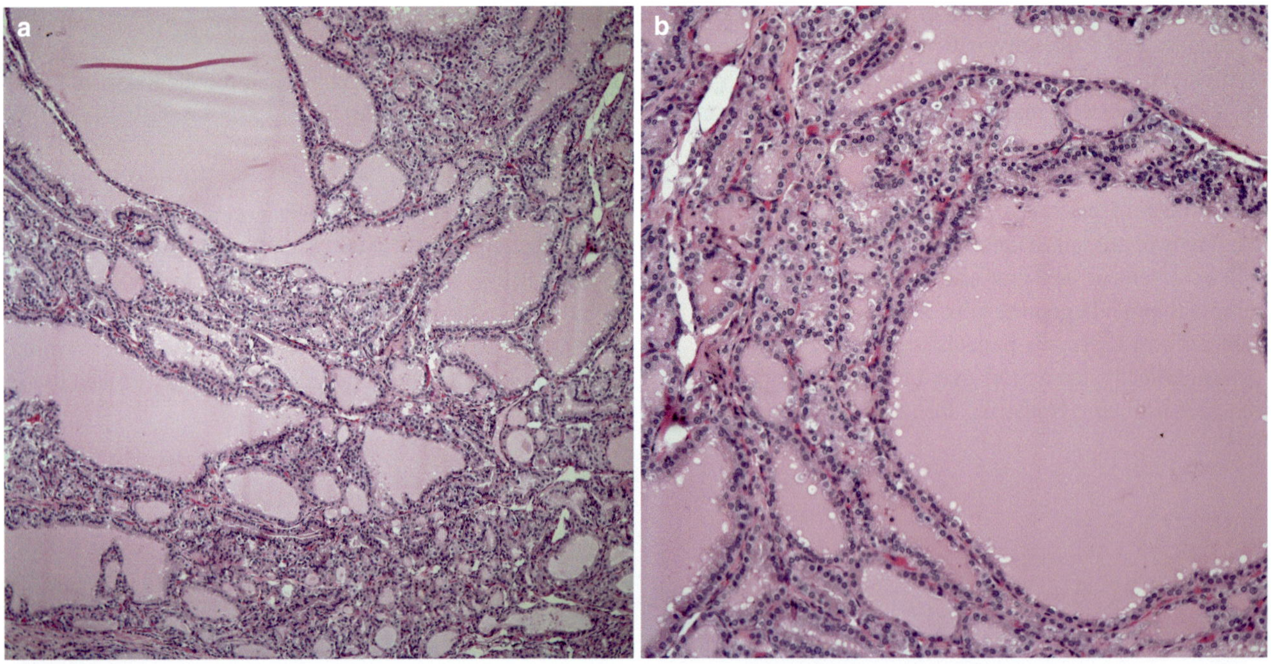

Fig. 9.104 (**a**) Low power view of a mediastinal goiter showing dilated thyroid follicles; (**b**) closer magnification showing thyroid follicles filled with colloid

References

1. Oldham HN, Sabiston DC. Primary tumors and cysts of the mediastinum. Arch Surg. 1968;96:71–5.
2. Wychulis AR, Payne WS, Clagett OT, Woolner LB. Surgical treatment of mediastinal tumors: a 40-year experience. J Thorac Cardiovasc Surg. 1971;62:379–92.
3. Blegvad S, Lippert H, Simper LB, Dybdahl H. Mediastinal tumours. Scand J Thor Cardiovasc Surg. 1990;24:39–42.
4. Hanagiri T, Hatooka S, Oosaki T, Nakanishi R, Mitsudomi T, Shirakusa T. Papillary carcinoma in a huge intrathoracic goiter with tracheal stenosis and invasion. Scand J Thor Cardiovasc Surg. 1993;27:165–8.
5. Adkins PB, Maples MD, Hainsworth JD. Primary malignant mediastinal tumors. Ann Thorac Surg. 1984;38:648–59.
6. Rosai J, Higa E. Mediastinal endocrine neoplasm of probable thymic origin related to carcinoid tumor. Cancer. 1972;29:1061–74.
7. Pachter MR, Lattes R. Uncommon mediastinal tumors. Dis Chest. 1963;43:519–28.
8. Wick MR, Rosai J. Neuroendocrine neoplasms of the mediastinum. Semin Diagn Pathol. 1991;8:35–51.
9. Wick MR. Mediastinal cysts and intrathoracic thyroid tumors. Seminar in Diagnostic Pathology. 1990;7:285–94.
10. Klemm KM, Moran CA. Primary neuroendocrine carcinomas of the thymus. Semin Diagn Pathol. 1999;16:32–41.
11. Moran CA. Primary neuroendocrine carcinomas of the mediastinum: review of current criteria for histopathologic diagnosis and classification. Semin Diagn Pathol. 2005;22:223–9.
12. Moran CA, Suster S. Neuroendocrine carcinomas (carcnoid, atypical carcinoid, small cell carcinoma, and large cell neuroendocrine carcinoma): current concepts. Hematol Oncol Clin North Am. 2007;21:395–407.
13. Rosai J, HIga E, Davie J. Mediastinal endocrine neoplasm in patients with multipke endocrine adenomatosis: a previously unrecognized association. Cancer. 1972;29:1075–83.
14. Manes JL, Taylor HB. Thymic carcnoid in familial multiple endocrine adenomatosis. Arch Pathol. 1973;95:252–5.
15. Lockich JJ, Li F. Carcinoid of the thymus with hereditary hyperparathyroidism. Ann Int Med. 1978;89:364–5.
16. Marchevsky AM, Dikman SH. Mediastinal carcinoid with incomplete Sipple's syndrome. Cancer. 1979;43:2497–501.
17. Stewart CA, Kingston CW. Carcinoid tumour of the thymus with Cushing's syndrome. Pathology. 1980;12:487–94.
18. Floros D, Dosios T, Tsourdis A, Yiatromanolakis N. Carcinoid tumor of the thymus with multiple endocrine adenomatosis. Path Res Pract. 1982;175:404–9.
19. Brown LR, Aughenbaugh GL, Wick MR, Baker BA, Salassa RM. Roentgenologic diagnosis of primary corticotropin-producing carcinoid tumor of the mediastinum. Radiology. 1982;142:143–8.
20. Thorner MO, Martin WH, Ragan GE, MacLeod RM, Feldman PS, Bruni C, et al. A case of ectopic ACTH syndrome: diagnostic difficulties caused by intermittent secretion. Acta Endcorinol. 1982;99:364–70.
21. Birnberg FA, Webb WR, Selch MT, Gamsu G, Goodman PC, et al. Thymic carcinoid tumors with hyperparathyroidism. Am J Radiol. 1982;139:1001–4.
22. Vener JD, Zuckerbraun L, Goodman D. Carcinoid tumor of the thymus associated with a parathyroid adenoma. Arch Otoloryngol. 1982;99:324–6.
23. Huntrakoon M, Lin F, Heitz PU, Tomita T. Thymic carcinoid tumor with Cushing's syndrome: report of a case with electron microscopic and immunoperoxidase studies for neuron-specific enolase and corticotropin. Arch Pathol Lab Med. 1984;108:551–4.
24. Lieske TR, Kincaid J, Sunderrajan JV. Tjhymic carcinoid with cutaneous hyperpigmentation. Ach Int Med. 1985;145:361–3.
25. Gartner LA, Voorhess ML. Adrenocorticotropin hormone-producing thymic carcinoid in a teenager. Cancer. 1993;71:106–11.
26. Kimura N, Ishikawa T, Sasaki Y, Sasano N, Onodera K, Shimizu Y, et al. Expression of prohormone convertase, PC2, in adrenocorticotropin-producing thymic carcinoid with elevated plasma corticotropin-releasing hormone. J Clin Endocrinol Metab. 1996;81:390–5.
27. Baker J, Holdaway IM, Jagush M, Kerr AR, Donald RA, Pullan PT. Ectopic secretion of ACTH and met-enkephalin from a thymic carcinoid. J Endocrinol Investig. 1982;5:33–8.
28. Yamaji I, Iimura O, Mito T, Yoshida S, Shimamoto K, Minase T. An ectopic ACTH producing oncocytic carcinoid tumor of the thymus: report of a case. Jpn J Med. 1984;23:62–6.
29. Zieger MA, Swartz SE, MacGillivray DC, Linnoila I, Shakir M. Thymic carcinoid in association with MEN syndromes. Am Surg. 1992;58:430–4.
30. Wollensak G, Herbst EW, Beck A, Schaefer HE. Primary thymic carcinoid with Cushing's syndrome. Virch Arch A Pathol Anat. 1992;420:191–5.
31. Zahner J, Borchard F, Schmitz U, Schneider W. Thymus carcinoid in multiple endocrine neoplasms type I. Dtsch Med Wochenschr. 1994;119:135–40.
32. Gelfand ET, Basualdo CA, Callagham JC. Carcinoid tumor of the thymus associated with recurrent pericarditis. Chest. 1981;79:350–1.
33. Pimstone BL, Uys CJ, Vogelpoel L. Studies in a case of Cushing's syndrome due to an ACTH-producing thymic tumour. Am J Med. 1972;53:521–8.
34. Lowenthal RM, Gumpel JM, Kreel L, McLaughlin JE, Skeggs BL. Carcinoid tumour of the thymus with systemic manifestations: a radiological and pathological study. Thorax. 1974;29:553–8.
35. Teh BT, McArdle J, Chan SP, Menon J, Hartley L, Pullan P, et al. Clinicopathologic studies of thymic carcinoids in multiple endocrine neoplasia type 1. Medicine. 1997;76:21–9.
36. Wick MR, Scheithauer BW. Thymic carcinoid. A histologic, immunohistochemical, and ultrastructural study of 12 cases. Cancer. 1984;53:475–84.
37. Wick MR, Scott RE, Li CY, Carney JA. Carcinoid tumor of the thyus. A clinicopathologic report of seven cases with a review of the literature. Mayo Clin Proc. 1980;55:246–54.
38. De Montpreville VT, Macchiarini P, Dulmet E. Thymic neuroendocrine carcinoma (carcinoid): a clinicopathologic study of fourteen cases. J Thorac Cardiovasc Surg. 1996;111:134–41.
39. Economopoulos GC, Lewis JW, Lee MW, Silverman NA. Carcinoid tumors of the thymus. Ann Thorac Surg. 1990;50:58–61.
40. Wang DY, Chang DB, Kuo SH, Yang PC, Lee YC, Hsu HC, et al. Carcinoid tumours of the thymus. Thorax. 1994;49:357–60.
41. Cardillo G, Treggiari S, Paul MA, Carleo F, De Massimi AR, Remotti D, et al. Primary neuroendocrine tumours of the thymus: a cllinicopathologic and prognostic study of 19 patients. European J Cardio-thoracic Surgery. 2010;37:814–8.
42. Cardillo G, Rea F, Lucchi M, Paul MA, Margaritora S, Carleo F, et al. Primary neuroendocrine tumors of the thymus: a multicenter experience of 35 patients. Ann Thorac Surg. 2012;94:241–6.
43. Neary NM, Lopez-Chavez A, Abel BS, Boyce AM, Schaub N, Kwong K, et al. Neuroendocrine ACTH-producing tumor of the thymus – experience with 12 patients over 25 years. J Endocrinol Metab. 2012;97:2223–30.
44. Moran CA, Suster S. Neuroendocrine carcinomas (Carcinoid Tumor) of the thymus. A clinicopathologic analysis of 80 cases. Am J Clin Pathol. 2000;114:100–10.
45. World Health Organization (WHO) Classification of Tumours. In: Travis WD, Brambilla E, Muller-Hermelink HK, editors. Patholgy & genetics, tumours of the lung, pleura, thymus, and heart. WHO; Lyon, France. 2004. p. 188–95.

46. Gal AA, Kornstein MJ, Cohen C, Duarte IG, Miller JI, Mansour KA. Neuroendocrine tumors of the thymus: a clinicopathological and prognostic study. Ann Thorac Surg. 2001;72:1179–82.
47. Weissferdt A, Moran CA. thymic carcinoma, part 2: a clinicopathologic correlation of 33 cases with a proposed staging system. Am J Clin Pathol. 2012;138:115–21.
48. Weissferdt A, Moran CA. Staging of primary mediastinal tumors. Adv Anat Pathol. 2013;20(1):1–9.
49. Valli M, Fabris GA, Dewar A, Chikte S, Fisher C, Corrin B, et al. Atypical carcinoid tumour of the thymus: a study of 8 cases. Histopathology. 1994;24:71–375.
50. Rosai J, editor. WHO Histological typing of tumours of the thymus. 2nd ed; Springer-Verlag Berlin. 1999.
51. Travis WD, Brambilla E, Burke AP, Marx A, Nicholson AG, editors. WHO classification of tumours of the lung, pleura, thymus, and heart; Springer-Verlag Berlin. 2015. p. 234–8.
52. Tsuta K, Raso MG, Kalhor N, Liu DD, Wistuba II, Moran CA. Histologic features of low- and intermediate-grade neuroendocrine carcinoma (typical and atypical carcinoid tumors) of the lung. Lung Cancer. 2011;71:34–41.
53. Hughes JP, Ancalmo N, Leonard GL, Ochsner JL. Carcinoid tumour of the thymus gland: report of a case. Thorax. 1975;30:470–5.
54. Tanaka T, Tanaka S, Kimura H, Ito J. Mediastinal tumor of thymic origin and related to carcinoid tumor. Acta Path Jpn. 1974;24:413–26.
55. Sundstrom C, Wilander E. Thymic carcinoid: a case report. Acta Pathol Microbiol Scand Sect A. 1976;84:311–6.
56. Blom P, Johannessen JV. Mediastinal mass in a young male. Ultrastruct Pathol. 1983;4:391–5.
57. Llaverias S, Valls C, Picas E. Carcinoid tumor of the thymus. AJR. 1984;163:478.
58. Kogan J. Carcinoid tumor of the thymus. Postgrad Med. 1984;75:291–6.
59. Chalk S, Donald KJ. Carcinoid tumor of the thymus. A case report including discussion of the morphological diagnosis and the cell or origin. Virchows Arch A Pathol Anat Histol. 1977;377:91–6.
60. Viebahn R, Hiddemann W, Klinke F, Bassewitz DB. Thymus carcinoid. Pathol Res Pract. 1985;180:445–8.
61. Salyer WR, Salyer DC, Eggleston JC. Carcinoid tumors of the thymus. Cancer. 1976;37:958–73.
62. Rao U, Takita H. Carcinoid tumour of possible thymic origin: case report. Thorax. 1977;32:771–6.
63. Paties C, Zangrandi A, Vasallo G, Rinda G, Solcia E. Multidirectional carcinoma of the thymus with neuroendocrine and sarcomatoid components and carcinoid syndrome. Pathol Res Pract. 1991;187:170–7.
64. Kuo TT. Carcinoid tumor of the thymus with divergent sarcomatoid differentiation: report of a case with histogenetic considerations. Hum Pathol. 1994;25:319–23.
65. Mizuno T, Masaoka A, Hashimoto T, Shibata K, Yamakawa Y, Torii K, et al. Coexisting thymic carcinoid tumor and thymoma. Ann Thorac Surg. 1990;50:650–2.
66. Suster S, Moran CA. Thymic carcinoid with prominent mucinous stroma: report of a distinctive morphologic variant of thymic neuroendocrine neoplasm. Am J Surg Pathol. 1995;19:1277–85.
67. Moran CA, Suster S. Angiomatoid neuroendocrine carcinoma of the thymus: report of a distinctive morphological variant of neuroendocrine tumor of te thymus resembling a vascular neoplasm. Hum Pathol. 1999;30:635–9.
68. Lagrange W, Dahm HH, Karstens J, Feichtinger J, Mittermayer C. Melanocytic neuroendocrine carcinoma of the thymus. Cancer. 1987;59:484–8.
69. Ho FCS, Ho JCI. Pigmented carcinoid tumour of the thymus. Histopathology. 1977;1:363–9.
70. Klemm KM, Moran CA, Suster S. Pigmented thymic carcinoids: a clinicopathological and immunohistochemical study of two cases. Mod Pathol. 1999;12:946–8.
71. Moran CA, Suster S. Spindle cell neuroendocrine carcinomas of the thymus: (Spindle cell thymic carcinoid): a clinicopathologic and immunohistochemical study of seven cases. Mod Pathol. 1999;12:587–91.
72. Levine G, Rosai J. A spindle cell variant of thymic carcinoid tumor. A clinical, histologic, and fine structural study with emphasis on its distinction from spindle cell thymoma. Arch Pathol Lab Med. 1976;100:293–300.
73. Moran CA, Suster S. Primary neuroendocrine carcinoma (thymic carcinoid) of the thymus with prominent oncocytic features: a clinicopathologic study of 22 cases. Mod Pathol. 2000;13:489–94.
74. Moran CA, Suster S. Cystic well-differentiated neuroendocrine carcinoma (carcinoid tumor): a clinicopathologic and immunohistochemical study of two cases. Am J Clin Pathol. 2006;126:377–80.
75. Moran CA, Suster S. Thymic neuroendocrine carcinomas with combined features ranging from well differentiated (Carcinoid) to small cell carcinoma. Am J Clin Pathol. 2000;113:345–50.
76. Wick MR, Scheithauer BW. Oat cell carcinoma of the thymus. Cancer. 1982;49:1652–7.
77. Chetty R, Batitang S, Govender D. Large cell neuroendocrine carcinoma of the thymus. Histopathology. 1997;31:274.
78. Miettinen M. Synpatophysin and neurofilament protein as markers for neuroendocrine tumors. Arch Pathol Lab Med. 1987;111:813–8.
79. Herbst WM, Kummer W, Hofmann W, Otto H, Heym C. Carcinoid tumors of the thymus: an immunohistochemical study. Cancer. 1987;60:2465–70.
80. DeLellis RA, Wolfe HJ. Calcitonin in spindle cell thymic carcinoid tumors. Arch Pathol Lab Med. 1976;100:340.
81. Wick MR, Scheithauer BW, Kovacs K. Neuron-specific enolase in neuroendocrine tumors of the thymus, bronchus, and skin. Am J Clin Pathol. 1983;79:703–7.
82. Weissferdt A, Tang X, Wistuba II, Moran CA. Comparative immunohistochemical analysis of pulmonary and thymic neuroendocrine carcinomas using PAX8 and TTF1. Mod Pathol. 2013;26:1554–60.
83. Weissferdt A, Kalhor N, Liu H, Rodriguez J, Fujimoto J, Tang X, et al. Thymic neuroendocrine tumors (paraganglioma and carcinoid tumors): a comparative immunohistochemical study of 46 cases. Hum Pathol. 2014;45:2463–70.
84. Kujari H, Joensuu H, Klemi P, Asola R, Nordman E. A flow cytometridc analysis of 23 carcinoid tumors. Cancer. 1988;61:2517–20.
85. Fetissof F, Boivin F, Jobar P, Arbeille-Brassart B, Romet L, Maillet M. Microfilamentous carcinoid of the thymus: correlation of ultratructural study with Grimelius stain. Ultrastruct Pathol. 1982;3:9–15.
86. Kay S, Willson MA. Ultrastructural studies of an ACTH-secreting thymic tumor. Cancer. 1970 Aug;26(2):445–52.
87. Moran CA, Rush W, Mena H. Primary spinal paragangliomas: a clinicopathological and immunohistochemical study of 30 cases. Histopathology. 1997;31:167–73.
88. Moran CA, Albores-Saavedra J, Wenig BM, Mena H. Pigmented Extradrenal paragangliomas: a clinicopathologic and immunohistochemical study of five cases. Cancer. 1997;79:398–402.
89. Moran CA, Suster S, Fishback N, Koss MN. Mediastinal Paragangliomas: a clinicopathologic and immunohistochemical study of 16 cases. Cancer. 1993;72:2358–64.
90. Phillips B. Intrathoracic pheochromocytoma. Arch Pathol. 1940;30:916–21.
91. Lattes R. Nonchromaffin paraganglioma of ganglion nodosum, carotid body, and aortic arch bodies. Cancer. 1950;3:667–94.
92. Marshall RB, Horn RC. Nonchromaffin paraganglioma: a comparative study. Cancer. 1961;4:779–87.
93. Green WO, Bassett FH. Extrathoracic pheochromocytoma: report of a case. Am J Clin Pathol. 1965;35(2):142–6.

94. Tama L, Ellis H, Hodgson CH, Dockerty MB. Chemodectoma of the mediastinum: report on a patient with superior vena caval obstruction treated by a shunt from the right innominate vein to the right atrium. J Thorac Cardiovasc Surg. 1962;43:585–94.
95. Pachter RM. Mediastinal nonchromaffin paraganglioma: a clinicopathologic study based on eight cases. J Thorac Cardiovasc Surg. 1963;45:152–9.
96. Enquist RW, Tormey DC, Jenis EH, Warkel RL. Malignant chemodectoma of the superior mediastinum with elevated urinary homovanillic acid. Chest. 1974;66:209–11.
97. Victor S, Anand KV, Andappan P, Bharathy S, Rao S, Reddy KC. Malignant mediastinal chemodectoma. Chest. 1975;68(4):583–4.
98. Arom V, Nicoloff DM. Intrathoracic paraganglioma arising from aorticosympathetic paraganglion. Arch Surg. 1976;111:275–9.
99. Lacquet LK, Moulijn AC, Jongerius CM, Rensing JB. Intrathoracic chemodectoma with multiple localisations. Thorax. 1977;32:203–9.
100. Olson JL, Salyer WR. Mediastinal paragangliomas (Aortic Body Tumor): a report of four cases and a review of the literature. Cancer. 1978;41:2405–12.
101. Lack EE, Stillinger RA, Colvin DB, Groves RM, Burnette DG. Aortico-pulmonary paraganglioma: report of a case with ultrastructural study and review of the literature. Cancer. 1979;43:269–78.
102. Gallivan MVE, Chun B, Rowden G, Lack EE. Intrathoracic paravertebral malignant paraganglioma. Arch Pathol Lab Med. 1980;104:46–51.
103. Grace MP, Batist G, Grace WR, Gillooley JF. Aorticopulmonary paraganglioma and gastric leiomyoblastoma in a young woman. Am J Med. 1981;70:1288–92.
104. Evora PRB, Bongiovani HL, Sgarbieri RN, Ribeiro PJ, Pereira LC, Moraes MM, et al. Nonfunctioning paraganglioma of the posterior mediastinum. Scand J Thorac Cardiovasc Surg. 1988;22:295–7.
105. Odze R, Begin LR. Malignant paraganglioma of the posterior mediastinum: a case report and review of the literature. Cancer. 1990;65:564–9.
106. Assaf HM, Al-Momen AA, Martin JG. Aorticopulmonary paraganglioma: a case report with immunohistochemical studies and literature review. Arch Pathol Lab Med. 1992;116:1085–7.
107. Dajee A, Dajee H, Hinrichs S, Lillington G. Pulmonary chondroma, extra-adrenal paraganglioma, and gastric leiomyosarcoma. Carney's tirad. J Thorac Cardiovasc Surg. 1982;84:377–81.
108. Plaza JA, Wakely PE, Moran CA, Fletcher CD, Suster S. Sclerosing paraganglioma: report of 19 cases of an unusual variant of neuroendocrine tumor that may be mistaken for an aggressive malignant neoplasm. Am J Surg Pathol. 2006;30:7–12.
109. Kimani S, Young WF. Hereditary paraganglioma-phechromocytoma syndromes. In: Pagaon RA, et al., editors. GeneReviews [internet]. Seattle: University of Washington, Seattle 1993–2015. 2008 May 21 [updated 2014 Nov 06].
110. Sato H, Shoji S, Kajiwara H, Itoh J, Osamura RY. A novel mutation (P236S) in the succinate dehydrogenase subunit B gene in a Japanese patient with posterior mediastinal paraganglioma. Endocr Pathol. 2013;24:144–8.
111. Garibaldi E, Bresciani S, Panaia R, Delmastro E, Malinverni G, Gabriele P. Hereditary paraganglioma syndrome associated with SDHD gene mutations: a patient with multicentric presentation treated with radiotherapy. Case report. Tumori. 2011;97:214–20.
112. Prodanov T, Havekes B, Nathanson KL, Adams KT, Pacak K. Malignant paraganglioma associated with succinate dehydrogenase subunit B in an 8-year-old child: the age of first screening? Pediatr Nephrol. 2009;24:1239–42.
113. Ortega PF, Sosa LA, Patel M, Zambrano E. Cystic paraganglioma of the anterior mediastinum. Ann Diagn Pathol. 2010;14:341–6.
114. Flieder DB, Moran CA, Suster S. Primary alveolar soft part sarcoma of the mediastinum: a clinicopathological and immunohistochemical study of two cases. Histopathology. 1997;31:469–73.
115. Brewer LA. The occurrence of parathyroid tissue within the thymus: report of four cases. Endocrinology. 1934;18(3):397–408.
116. Cope O. Surgery of hyperparathyroidism: the occurrence of parathryoids in the anterior mediastinum and the division of the operation into two stages. Ann Surg. 1941;114:706–33.
117. Bauer W, Federman DD. Hyperparathryoidism epitomized: the case of captain Charles E. Martell. Metabolism. 1962;XI(1 (January)):21–9.
118. Hardy JD, Snavely JR, Langford HG. Low intrathoracic parathyroid adenoma: large functioning tumor representing fifth parathyroid, opposite eight dorsal vertebra with independent arterial supply and opacified at operation with arteriogram. Ann Surg. 1964;159:310–5.
119. Nathaniels EK, Nathaniels AM, Wang C. Mediastinal parathyroid tumors: a clinical and pathological study of 84 cases. Ann Surg. 1970;171(2):165–70.
120. Thacker WC, Wells VH, Hall ER. Parathryoid cyst of the mediastinum. Ann Surg. 1971;174:969–75.
121. Margolis IB, Wayne R, Organ CH. Parathryoid cysts: functional and mediastinal. Surgery. 1975;77:462–6.
122. Simkin EP. Hyperparathyroidism associated with a parathyroid cyst: an unusual presentation. Br J Surg. 1976;63:927–8.
123. Calandra DB, Shah KH, Prinz RA, Sullivan H, Hofmann C, Oslapas R, et al. Parathyroid cyst: a report of eleven cases including two associated with hyperparathyroid crisis. Surgery. 1983;94:887–92.
124. Ramos-Gabatini A, Mallette LE, Bringhurst FR, Draper MW. Functional mediastinal parathyroid cyst: dynamics of parathyroid hormone secreting during cyst aspirations and surgery. Am J Med. 1985;79:633–9.
125. Linos DA, Schoretsanitis G, Carvounis E. Parathyroid cysts of the neck and mediastinum. Acta Chir Scand. 1989;155:211–6.
126. Petri N, Holten I. Parathyroid cyst: report of case in the mediastinum. J Laryngol Otol. 1990;104:56–7.
127. Downey RJ, Cerfolio RJ, Deschamps C, Grant CS, Pairolero PC. Mediastinal parathyroid cyst. Mayo Clin Proc. 1995;70:946–50.
128. Gurbuz AT, Peetz ME. Giant mediastinal parathyroid cyst: an unusual cause of hypercalcemic crisis—case report and review of the literature. Surgery. 1996;120:795–800.
129. Scholz DA, Purnell DC, Woolner LB, Clagett OT. Mediastinal hyperfunctioning parathyroid tumors. Ann Surg. 1973;178:173–8.
130. Wang C, Mahaffey JE, Axelrod L, Perlman JA. Hyperfunctioning supernumerary parathyroid glands. Surg Gynecol Obstet. 1979;148:711–4.
131. Russell CF, Edis AJ, Scholz DA, Sheedy PF, van Heerden JA. Mediastinal parathyroid tumors: experience with 38 tumors requiring mediastinotomy for removal. Ann Surg. 1981;193:805–9.
132. Clark OH. Mediastinal parathyroid tumors. Arch Surg. 1988;123:1096–100.
133. Conn JM, Goncalves MA, Mansour KA, McGarity WC. The mediastinal parathyroid. Am Surg. 1991;57:62–6.
134. Roslyn JJ, Gordon HE, Mulder DG. Mediastinal parathyroid adenomas: a cause of persistent hyperparathyroidism. Am Surg. 1983;49:523–7.
135. Schlinkert RT, Whitaker MD, Argueta R. Resection of select mediastinal parathyroid adenomas through an anterior mediastinotomy. Mayo Clin Proc. 1991;66:1110–3.
136. Murphy MN, Glennon PG, Diocee MS, Wick MR, Cavers DJ. Nonsecretory parathyroid carcinoma of the mediastinum: light microscopic, immunohistochemical, and ultrastructural features of a case, and review of the literature. Cancer. 1986;58:2468–76.

137. Kastan DJ, Kottamasu SR, Frame B, Greenwald KA. Carcinoma in a mediastinal fifth parathyroid gland. JAMA. 1987;257(9):1218–9.
138. Putnam JB, Schantz SP, Pugh WC, Hickey RC, Samaan NA, Garza R, et al. Extended en bloc resection of a primary mediastinal parathyroid carcinoma. Ann Thorac Surg. 1990;50:138–40.
139. Avramides A, Papamargaritis K, Antoniadis A, Gakis D, Leontsini M. Large parathyroid functioning carcinoma (1,200 g) presenting as substernal goiter. J Endocrinol Investig. 1992;15:39–42.
140. Kelly MD, Sheridan BF, Farnsworth AE, Palfreeman S. Parathyroid carcinoma in a mediastinal sixth parathyroid gland. Aust N Z J Surg. 1994;64:446–9.
141. Yoshiike F, Koizumi T, Yoneyama A, Komatu M, Yamaguchi S, Hanaoka M, et al. Thymic squamous cell carcinoma producing parathyroid hormone-related protein and CYFRA 21-1. Intern Med. 2004;43(6):493–5.
142. Hsiao LT, Chiou TJ, Yu IT, Chen PM. Superior vena cava syndrome and hypercalcaemia in a patient with primary mediastinal B-cell lymphoma secreting parathyroid hormone-related protein. Br J Haematol. 2002;119(1):1.
143. Moran CA, Suster S. Primary parathyroid tumors of the mediastinum: a clinicopathologic and immunohistochemical study of 17 cases. Am J Clin Pathol. 2005;124:749–54.
144. Becker FO, Tausk K. Radiologically evident functioning mediastinal parathyroid adenoma. Chest. 1970;58:79–81.
145. College D, Rohati PK. Mediastinal parathyroid cyst. J Comput Assist Tomogr. 1983;7(1):140–2.
146. Hargreaves HK, Wright TC. A large functioning parathyroid lipoadenoma found in the posterior mediastinum. Am J Clin Pathol. 1981;76:89–93.
147. Hajhosseini B, Montazeri V, Hajhosseini L, Nezami N, Beygui RE. Mediastinal goiter: a comprehensive study of 60 consecutive cases with special emphasis on identifying predictors of malignancy and sternotomy. Am J Surg. 2012;203:442–7.
148. Zapatero J, Baamonde C, Gonzalez F, Orusco E, Gallardo MP, Folque E. Ectopic goiters of the mediastinum: presentation of two cases and review of the literature. Jpn J Surg. 1988;18:105–9.
149. Raffaelli M, De Crea C, Ronti S, Bellantone R, Lombardi CP. Substernal goiters: incidence, surgical approach, and complications in a tertiary care referral center. Head Neck. 2011;33:1420–5.
150. Erbil Y, Bozbora A, Barbaros U, Ozarmagan S, Azezli A, Movalilar S. Surgical management of substernal goiters: clilnical experience of 170 cases. Surg Today. 2004;34:732–4.
151. Gao B, Zhang X, Zhao J, Zhao J, He Y, Wen Y, et al. Surgical treatment of large substernal thyroid goiter: analysis of 12 patients. Int J Clin Exp Med. 2013;6:488–96.
152. Shasha AR. Substernal goiter: what is in a definition? Surgery. 2010;147:239–40.
153. Huins CT, Georgalas C, Mehrzad H, Tolley NS. A new classification system for retrosternal goiter based on a systematic review of its complications and management. Int J Surg. 2008;6:71–6.
154. Barker TA, Daultrey CR, Trotter SE, Kalkat M. Intrathymic primary intrathoracic goiter in a patient with breast malignancy. Ann Thorac Surg. 2012;93:35–6.
155. Landeta F, Hoffmeier A, Fuchs M, Scheld H, Maintz D, Stypmann J, et al. Ectopic thyroid mass in the heart. Lancet. 2012;379:1762.
156. Rios A, Rodriguez JM, Canteras M, Galindo PJ, Balsalobre MD, Parrilla P. Risk factors for malignancy in multinodular goiters. EJSO. 2004;30:58–62.
157. Bellafonte R, Lombardi CP, Bossola M, Fadda G, Salvatori M, Princi P. Posterior mediastinal hyperfunctioning insular thyroid carcinoma. Thorax. 2005;95:358–60.
158. Nervi M, Iacconi P, Spinelli C, Janni A, Miccoli P. Thyroid carcinoma in intrthoracic goiter. Langenbeck's Arch Surg. 1998;383:383–7.
159. Oikonomou A, Astrinakis E, Giatromanolaki A, Karros P, Margaritis D, Prassopoulos P. Intrathoracic papillary thyroid carcinoma from occult primary disease. Gen Thorac Cardiovasc Surg. 2014;62:198–201.
160. Sand J, Pehkonen E, Mattila J, Seppănen S, Salmi J. Pulsating mass at the sternum: a primary carcinoma of ectopic mediastinal thyroid. J Thorac Cardiovasc Surg. 1996;112:833–5.

10 Germ Cell Tumors

Introduction

Mediastinal germ cell tumors (MGCT) are an unusual group of tumors that share similar histopathological features with those occurring in the gonads or along the midline line. By far, germ cell tumors occur more often in the gonads. However, they also can occur in the pineal gland, retroperitoneum, and sacral area [1–4]. In several series [5–8], extragonadal germ cell tumors have accounted for approximately 1–15% of mediastinal tumors in adults and 25% in children.

Because of their putative origin from germ cells and their rarity in extragonadal locations, the very existence of primary GCT outside the gonads has been questioned in the past, and their presence was invariably attributed to metastases from occult or "burned-out" gonadal primary. Nevertheless, the existence of mediastinal germ cell tumors has been known for more than one century. The first description of what is today considered a mediastinal teratoma is attributed to Gordon [9], who, in 1823, described a mediastinal neoplasm containing teeth and hair in an autopsy of a 21-year-old female. Toward the end of the eighteenth century, Hare [10] reviewed the current literature and found ten cases of teratomatous lesions, and Hertzler [11] in 1916 had compiled 72 case reports of teratomatous lesions. It was not until the middle of the twentieth century that other non-teratomatous mediastinal germ cell tumors were recognized [12, 13]. In view of the similarities that germ cell tumors share regardless of the anatomic site, it is essential that a careful clinical evaluation be undertaken prior to diagnosing a tumor as primary in the mediastinum. This will be of importance not only for proper determination of the primary site but also for staging and treatment purposes. Despite the histopathological similarities displayed by both gonadal and extragonadal germ cell tumors, certain subtle differences have been observed, which may carry important diagnostic and prognostic implications. For instance, mediastinal non-seminomatous GCT are often seen in association with Klinefelter's syndrome, hematologic malignancies, and secondary development of high-grade sarcomas. However, in general, mediastinal non-teratomatous GCT have been associated with diverse clinical conditions. Table 10.1 depicts some of the different clinical conditions associated with mediastinal non-teratomatous GCT.

The true incidence of MGCT is difficult to assess. Some estimates consider that in general GCT account for 1–5% in the mediastinum [14], while others estimate that MGCT account for approximately 10–20% of all mediastinal tumors [15, 16]. Mullen and Richardson [7] evaluated 702 adults with primary anterior mediastinal tumors and found that 15% of them corresponded to MGCT. In addition, the authors also evaluated 179 children with primary anterior mediastinal masses and found that 24% of these neoplasms were MGCT. Davis and colleagues [6] reviewed 2399 cases of mediastinal tumors between the years of 1952 and 1973 and found 72 cases (3%) of MGCT. Unfortunately, most available figures are based on relatively short series of cases or from studies that included benign cysts and other types of neoplasms. One important conclusion that can be drawn from previous studies is the fact that MGCT are more common in young men. In our experience with 322 cases of MGCT, we were able to observe a dramatic predominance of men in a proportion of 9:1 [17]. The few cases of MGCT that we were able to see in women were teratomatous lesions. We also noted that teratomatous lesions represent the most common MGCT. Figures 10.1 and 10.2 show the different distributions of mediastinal GCT by age groups and by histological types. Based on those distributions, it is clear that the most common mediastinal GCT is teratoma. Also important to highlight is that among the teratomatous tumors, mature teratomas are more common, while immature teratomas account for less than 5% of all teratomatous tumors (Fig. 10.3). Among the non-teratomatous tumors, seminomas are the most common, while among the non-seminomatous, non-teratomatous tumors; yolk sac tumor is the most common (Fig. 10.4). However, the bulk of mediastinal GCT is made of teratomas and seminomas, leaving the rest of GCT to account for no more than 25% of all mediastinal GCT [17].

© Springer Nature Switzerland AG 2019
N. Kalhor, C. Moran, *Mediastinal Pathology*, https://doi.org/10.1007/978-3-319-98980-8_10

Several theories have been presented in order to explain the presence of GCT in the mediastinum. Although some of these theories are provocative and interesting, the puzzle of the origin of GCT of the mediastinum is still far from solved. Whether the cell or cells of origin are ectopically misplaced or represent an integral normal component of this region, the bulk of the evidence seems to point in the direction of a thymic origin [18–23].

Classification

Although for the most part the classification system used for MGCT is similar to that proposed by the World Health Organization (WHO) [24], we have introduced a few modifications in order to provide more histopathological information on these tumors [17]. Tables 10.2 and 10.3 provide the classification schema devised for these tumors. Those changes are mainly in the area of teratomatous tumors. Terms such as teratocarcinoma and malignant teratoma are rather non-specific and in many circumstances misleading; thus, we have proposed abandoning such terminology. The concept of separating teratomatous lesions based on the presence of specific cellular components with the respective percentage may lead to more specific therapy, which may also be translated into an improve clinical response for these patients.

Table 10.1 Clinical conditions associated with non-teratomatous MGCT

Tumor type	Associated Condition
Seminoma	Ventricular septal defect
	Congenital absence of thoracic hemivertebra
	Pulmonic stenosis
	Gynecomastia
	SVC syndrome
Yolk sac tumor	Klinefelter's syndrome
	Idiopathic thrombocytopenia
	Acute megakaryoblastic leukemia
	Malignant histiocytosis
	SVC syndrome
Embryonal Carcinoma	Idiopathic thrombocytopenia
	Klinefelter's syndrome
Choriocarcinoma	Gynecomastia
	SVC syndrome
	Klinefelter's syndrome

Staging

A staging system has been devised as an attempt to properly identify the anatomic distribution of GCT and also to stratify those patients who may benefit from any additional therapy [17]. This staging system was developed after an analysis of 322 cases of mediastinal GCT including all the different histological types. The staging schema is depicted in Figs. 10.5, 10.6, 10.7, and 10.8, and it is as follows:

- Stage I – well-circumscribed tumor with or without focal adhesion to the pleura or pericardium but without microscopic evidence of invasion into adjacent structures (Fig. 10.5).
- Stage II – tumor confined to the mediastinum with macroscopic and/or microscopic evidence of infiltration into adjacent structures (such as pleura, pericardium, and great vessels) (Fig. 10.6).
- Stage III – Tumor metastases:
  - IIIA – with metastases to intrathoracic organs (lymph nodes, lung, etc.) (Fig. 10.7)
  - IIIB – with extrathoracic metastases (Fig. 10.8)

Following this schema, we encountered that mature and immature teratomas were the only tumors that invariably were in stage I, while the remaining tumors were found in different

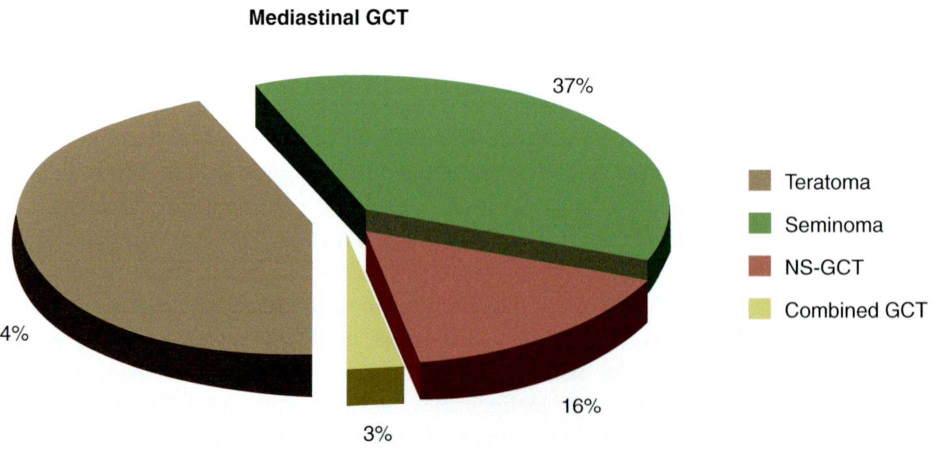

Fig. 10.1 Distribution of mediastinal germ cell tumors by histological type. (Adapted with permission of John Wiley and Sons from Moran and Suster [17])

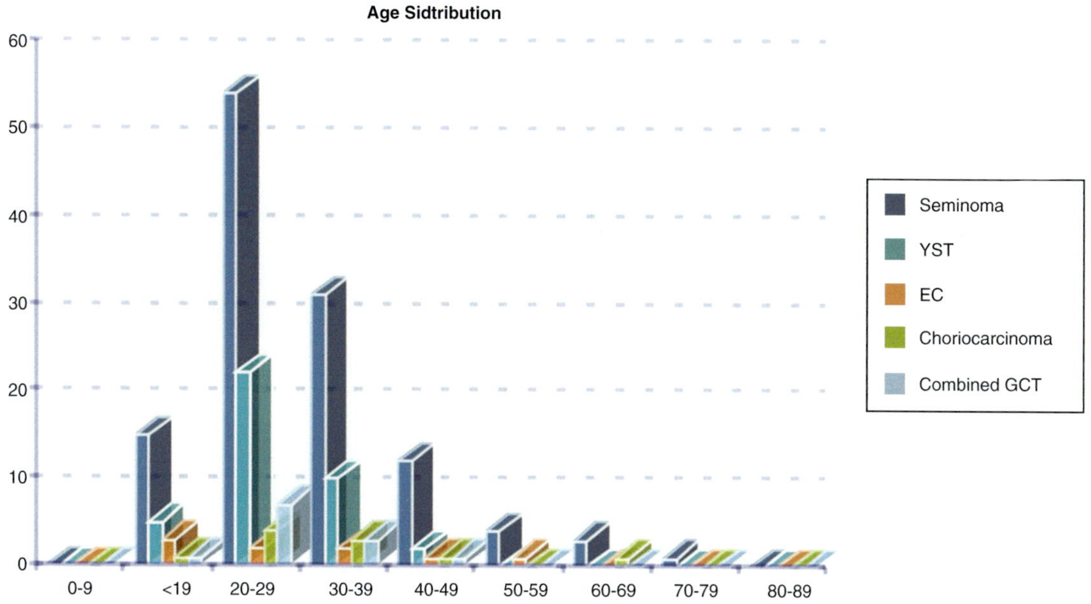

Fig. 10.2 Distribution of mediastinal germ cell tumors by age group. (Adapted with permission of John Wiley and Sons from Moran and Suster [17])

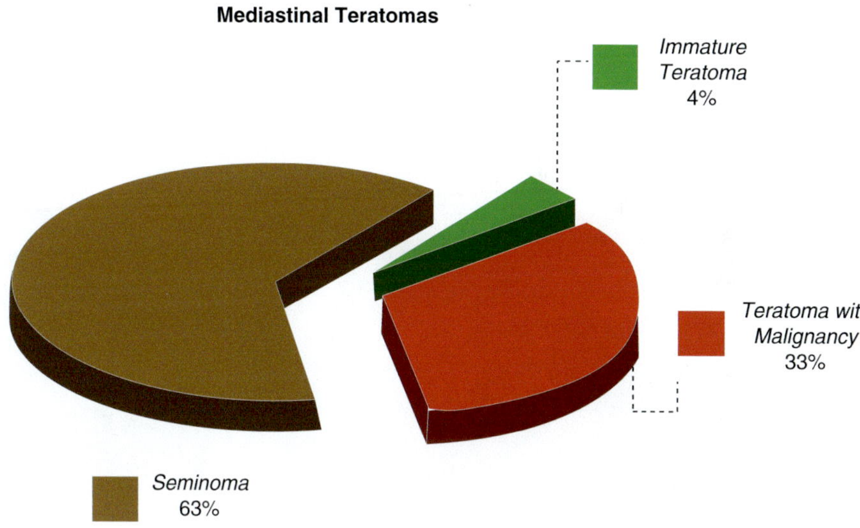

Fig. 10.3 Distribution of mediastinal teratomatous lesions. (Adapted with permission of John Wiley and Sons from Moran and Suster [17])

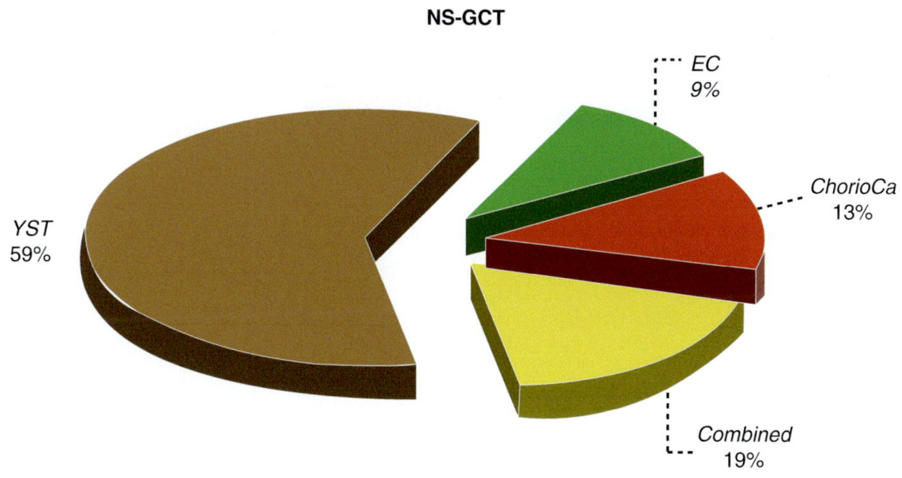

Fig. 10.4 Distribution of mediastinal non-seminomatous germ cell tumors

Table 10.2 Classification of MGCT

Teratoma
Mature
Immature
With Malignant component
Type I: with another GCT, i.e., seminoma, YST, EC, etc.
Type II: with a malignant epithelial neoplasm, i.e., adenocarcinoma, squamous cells carcinoma, etc.
Type III: with a malignant mesenchymal component, i.e., rhabdomyosarcoma, angiosarcoma, etc.
Type IV: with any combination of previous types
Seminoma
Embryonal carcinoma
Yolk sac tumor (endodermal sinus tumor)
Choriocarcinoma
Combined germ cell tumor

A combination of any of the above tumors without teratomatous elements

Adapted with permission of Wiley and Sons from Moran and Suster [17]

Table 10.3 Distribution by histologic type of 138 mediastinal teratomas

Mature teratoma	87 cases	63%
Immature teratoma	6 cases	4%
With malignant component	45 cases	33%

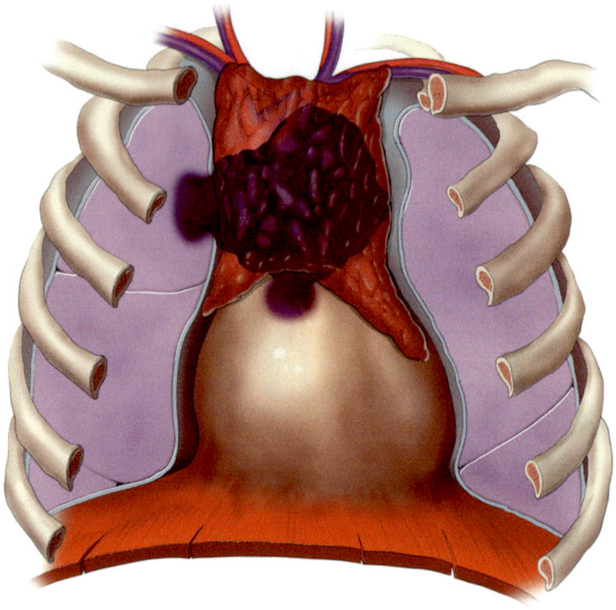

Fig. 10.6 Stage II in mediastinal germ cell tumors. (Copyright © 2012 with permission from Dr. Kalhor and Moran)

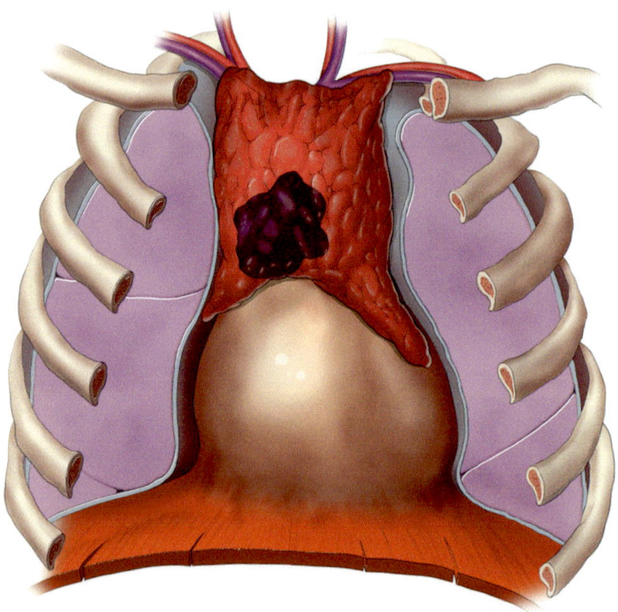

Fig. 10.5 Stage I in mediastinal germ cell tumors. (Copyright © 2012 with permission from Dr. Kalhor and Moran)

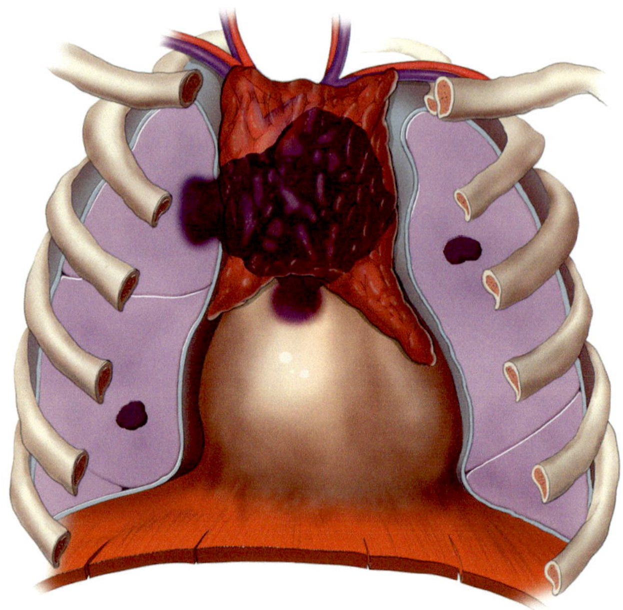

Fig. 10.7 Stage IIIA in mediastinal germ cell tumors. (Copyright © 2012 with permission from Dr. Kalhor and Moran)

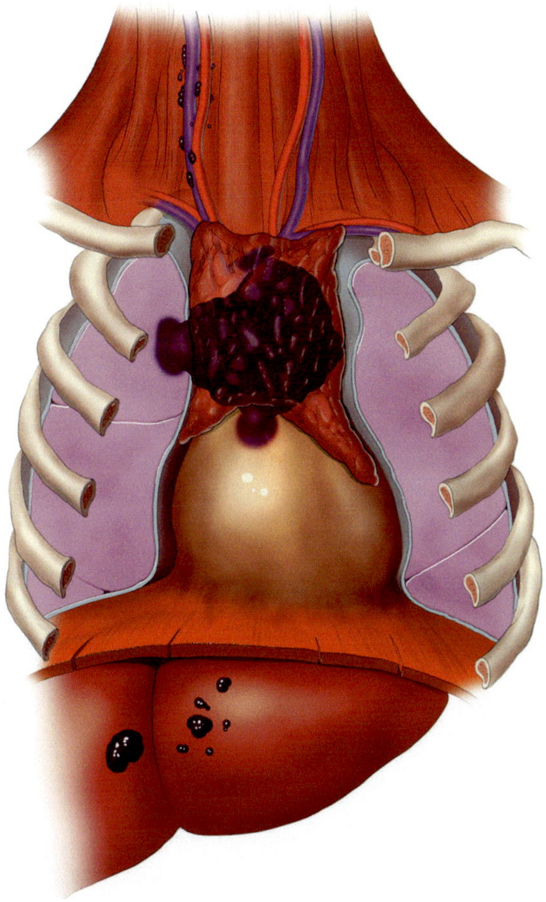

Fig. 10.8 Stage IIIB in mediastinal germ cell tumors. (Copyright © 2012 with permission from Dr. Kalhor and Moran)

stages. It is considered that the stratification of cases following such schema may be used not only to determined additional therapy but also to estimate possible outcome in these patients.

Teratomas

Teratomas are defined as tumors showing tissues derived from all three germ cell layers. However, a tumor may be accepted as teratoma, if at least two of the germ cell layers are represented. Those tumors composed exclusively of tissues derived from ectoderm are often termed "dermoid" cysts and have been variously regarded as monodermal teratomas. Mediastinal teratomas represent the most commonly reported MGCT and have accounted for up to 80% of all primary MGCT in different series [2, 4, 8, 18, 19, 21, 25–65].

Mature Teratoma

Mature teratoma appears to represent the most common MGCT. Undoubtedly, it is the most often reported and also the earliest one to have been recognized in the literature. Short series of cases or large series of cystic tumors of the mediastinum including cystic lesions not related to teratomatous lesions have been commonly presented in the literature [6, 8, 18, 19, 25–29]. Interestingly, in all those published series of cases, the tumors appear to be present in men and women in almost equal proportion, the great majority of patients were treated with surgical resection, and the follow-up was that of an indolent process. Clinically, the reported symptomatology includes cough, chest pain, dyspnea, and hemoptysis. However, in some series, up to 36% of the patients were asymptomatic [28]. More recently, Dulmet and colleagues [15] reviewed a 30-year experience and found 98 cases of MGCT. Fifty were mature teratomas; 38 tumors were in women and 12 in men. All these patients were treated with surgical resection, and the survival rate after 15 years was approximately 95%. On the other hand, teratomas in children appear not to be as common as in adults. In a few large series [30–34], the number of cases reported in children is dramatically less than those in adults. However, the treatment and prognosis appear to be similar as that reported for adult patients.

In our experience with 87 cases of mature teratomas, we found a male/female ratio of approximately 2:1, in contrast to other reported series of 1:1 [18]. Interestingly, when we separate teratomas with malignant component from mature teratomas, there appears to be a high predominance of male patients in the former [17]. Nevertheless, teratomas are more commonly seen in the anterior mediastinum with sporadic cases reported in the posterior mediastinal compartment [35, 36].

Based on our experience and that collected from the literature, one can conclude that the treatment of choice for these tumors is complete surgical resection, and the outcome in these patients appears to be good. However, reported cases of mature teratomas with metastasis showing frank malignant component have been reported [37]. In these cases, it is difficult to determine whether the malignant component was present from the outset. These instances may represent examples of incompletely resected tumors or inadequate sampling.

Clinical Features

The symptomatology in these patients is related to the size of the tumor. In small tumors, the patients may be completely asymptomatic, while in patients with larger tumors, symptoms of cough, chest pain, shortness of breath, etc. may be present. In some cases, Klinefelter's syndrome has been associated [38]. However, the symptomatology present does not allow a separation between mature teratomas and other types of teratomatous tumors. Unusual symptoms including hemoptysis and pericarditis [39, 40] may be present. In this context, mediastinal teratomas should be distinguished from intrapericardial teratomas [41]. Also, endocrine abnormalities such as production of insulin have been reported [42].

Radiologically, mature teratomas may show extension toward one side of the midline. Calcifications can be seen and have been reported in about 20–40% of the cases; teeth and the presence of fat-fluid level are considered specific for teratoma [43]. Nonetheless, there is no radiological characteristic that can separate mature teratoma from teratomatous tumors with malignant component.

Gross Features

The tumors can vary in size from a few centimeters to over 15 cm in greatest diameter. They are usually soft, ill defined, and surrounded by thin membranous tissue. The tumors can show predominantly a cystic appearance with presence of abundant sebaceous material, hair, and teeth. On the other hand, teratomas can present as solid lesions or as combination of solid and cystic areas (Figs. 10.9a, b and 10.10). Because of the large size that these tumors may have, it is highly important to properly sample these lesions in order to fully determine if the components present are mature tissues. Even though there is not a "magic" number of sections that one must take, it is recommended to take a reasonable number of sections equivalent to one section per centimeter of tumor; however, close attention should be paid to suspicious

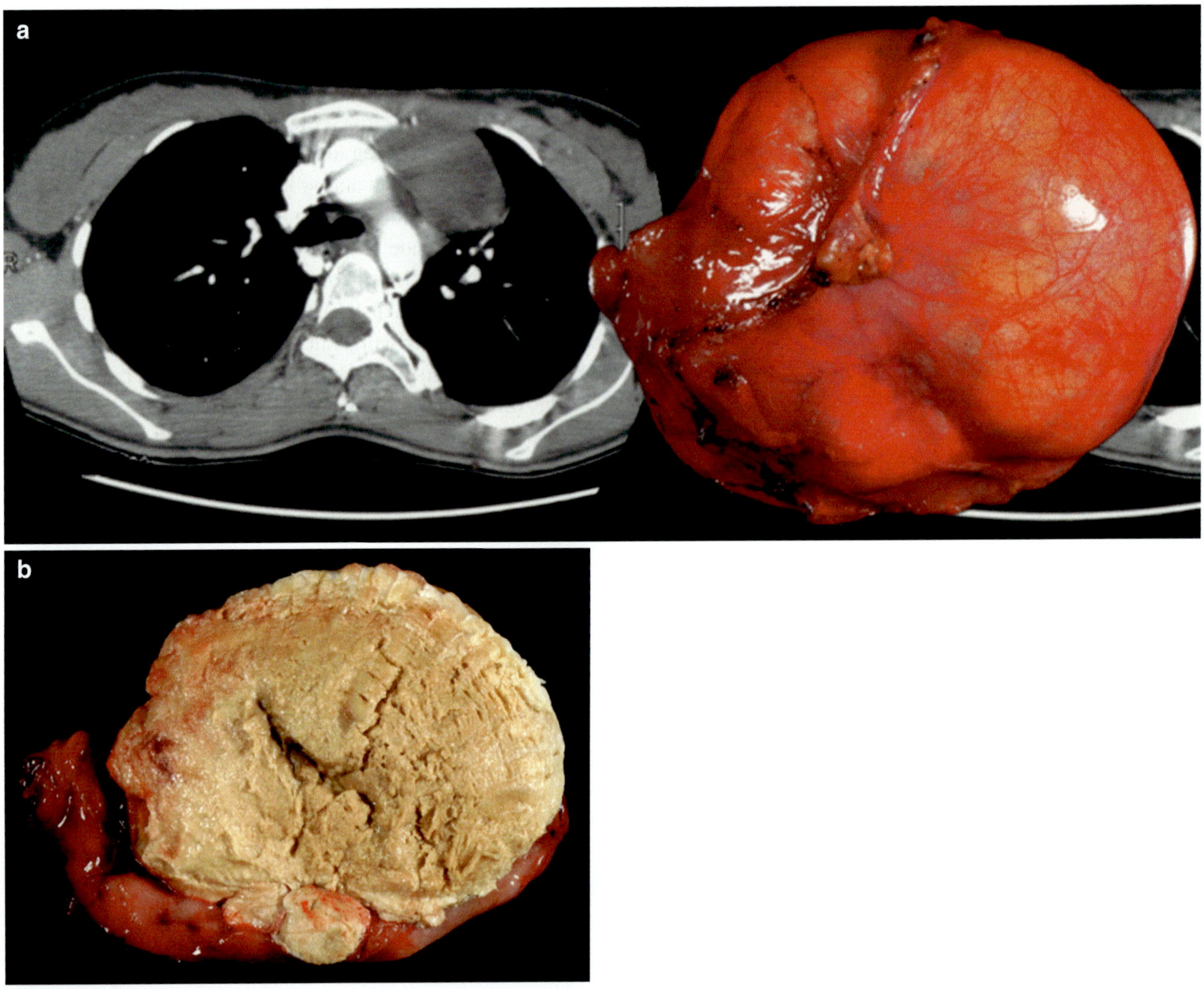

Fig. 10.9 (**a**) Mediastinal mature teratoma compared to the CT image of the tumor. (**b**) Mediastinal teratoma showing sebaceous material

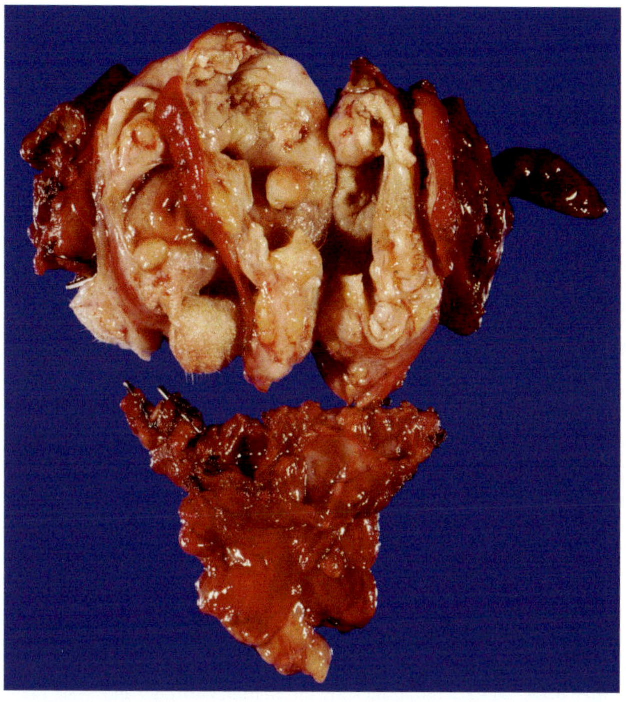

Fig. 10.10 Mediastinal mature teratoma showing classic cystic structures

solid areas of the tumor, and, if needed, extensive sampling should be performed.

Histological Features

The classical features of mature teratoma are the presence of cystic structures lined by columnar epithelium admixed with areas of fibroconnective tissue, cartilage, skin appendages, keratinization, and areas of mature glial tissue. In some areas, cystic structures lined by squamous epithelium are commonly seen. The cystic structures are generally filled with sebaceous or keratinous material. The cysts may occasionally rupture provoking an intense inflammatory reaction that may extend outside the confines of the lesion into the pleura or pericardium, simulating an infiltrative process. A wide variety of mature tissues may be observed in mature teratomas; however, pancreatic tissue appears to be one of the most commonly encountered [44, 45]. Absence of immature elements or malignant component is necessary in order to arrive at the diagnosis of mature teratoma (Figs. 10.11, 10.12, 10.13, 10.14, and 10.15).

Immunohistochemical Features

The use of immunohistochemical markers in the diagnosis of mature teratomas is limited. Essentially, the diagnosis is made on standard H&E sections. The use of neuroendocrine markers may be useful for identification of a variety of neuropeptides in cases in which pancreatic tissue is present and clinically functioning.

Differential Diagnosis

The diagnosis of mature teratoma is in the great majority of cases fairly simple and straightforward. Since the presence of immature neural tissue or foci harboring a malignant component may significantly alter the prognosis, adequate sampling of the tumor is of the utmost importance. Thorough extensive sampling is therefore recommended.

Immature Teratoma

This term is reserved for those tumors in which, in addition to the mature teratomatous elements, the tumor also shows areas of immature neuroepithelium. Because of the lack of a standard nomenclature for teratomas, it is difficult to determine the incidence or prevalence of these tumors in the mediastinum. However, they appear to be quite rare. It is possible that cases of immature teratomas may have been reported along with other cases of teratoma with malignant component in previous studies; conversely, tumors showing the criteria for immature teratoma have been included in reports dealing with other germ cell tumors of the mediastinum. In one study, it was estimated that immature teratomas might account for approximately 1% of all mediastinal teratomas [46]. Different series of MGCT in which immature teratomas have been included have been presented in the literature [5, 15, 32, 33, 46–48]. Most of the cases corresponding to immature teratomas have been described in relatively younger individuals or in children. The documented outcome from those series of cases is variable; however, it is possible that immature teratomas in children have a better outcome than in adults. Nevertheless, the most important element is the sampling process, which needs to be adequate. The determination of the amount (percentage) of immature elements present in a particular tumor needs to be made.

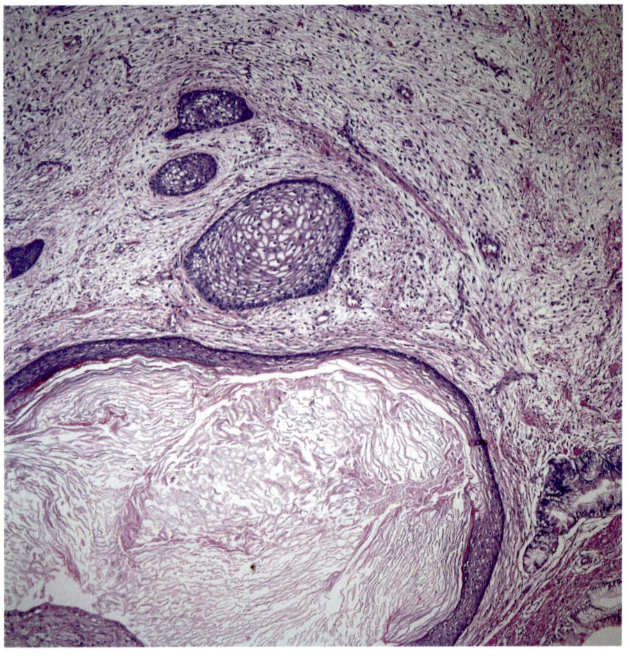

Fig. 10.11 Mediastinal mature teratoma showing dermal appendages and cystic structures

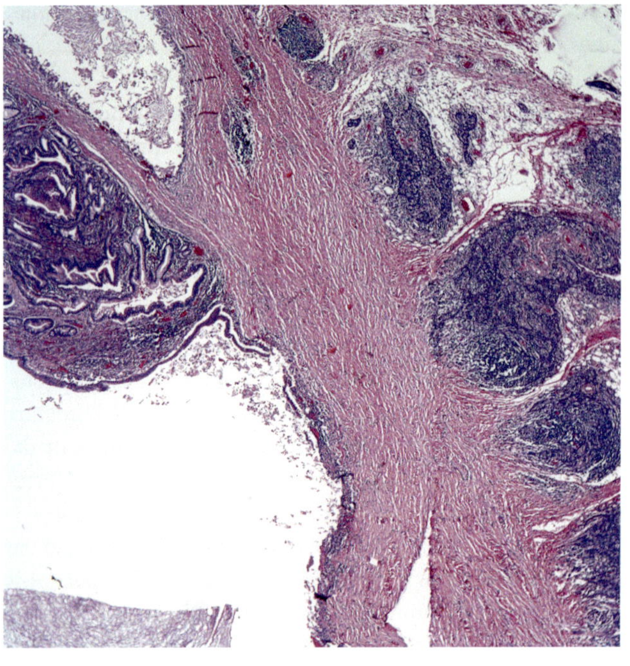

Fig. 10.12 Mediastinal mature teratoma showing remnants of thymic tissue and mature glandular proliferation

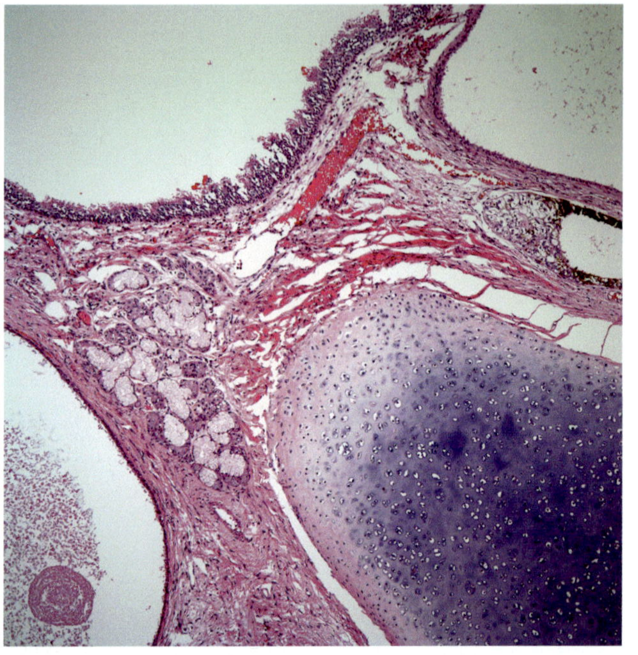

Fig. 10.13 Mature teratoma showing mature cartilage and cysts lined by low columnar epithelium

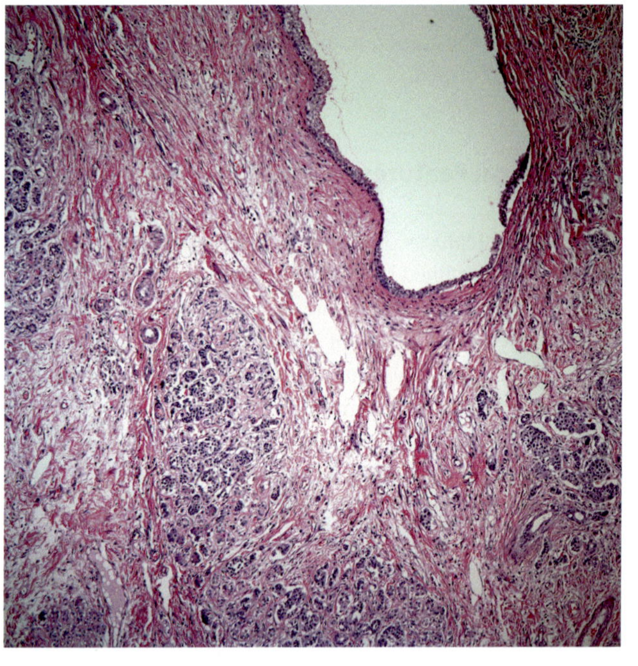

Fig. 10.14 Mediastinal mature teratoma showing pancreatic tissue

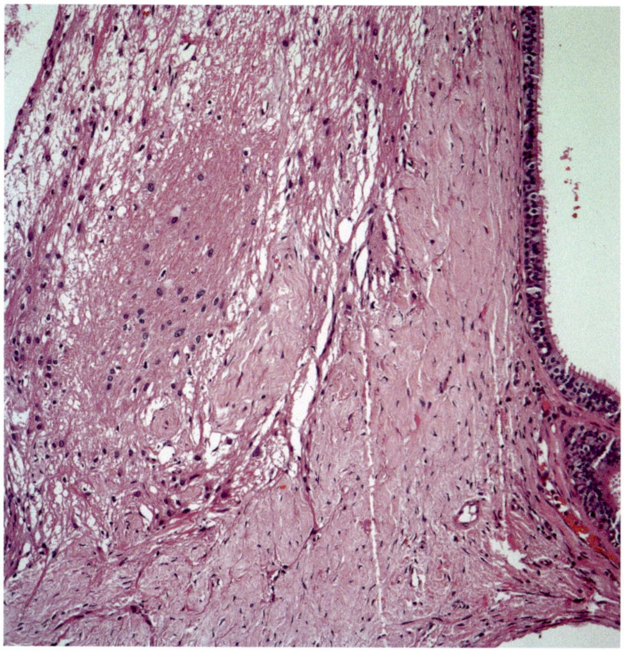

Fig. 10.15 Mediastinal mature teratoma showing mature glial tissue

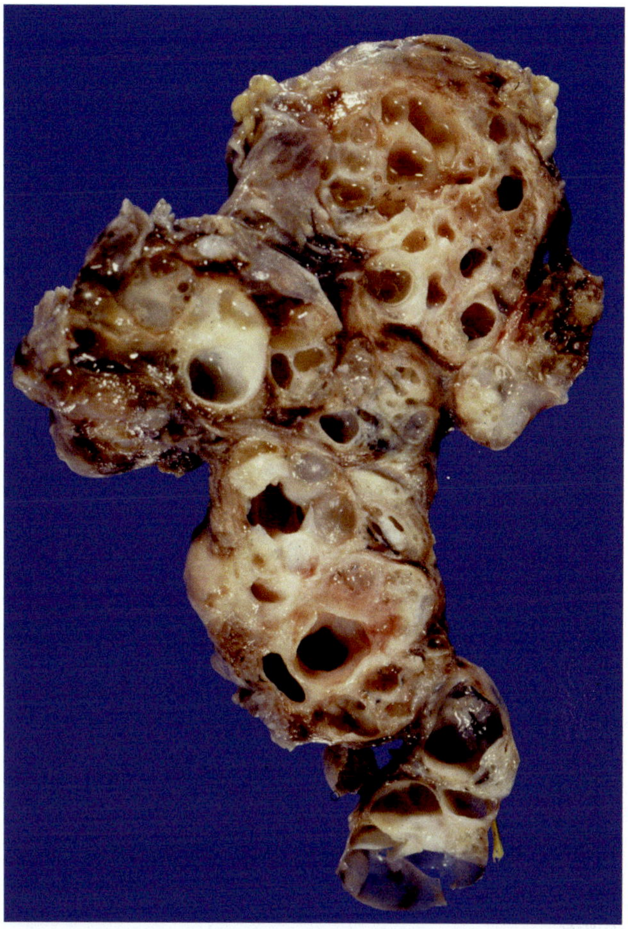

Fig. 10.16 Immature teratoma showing solid and cystic areas

Clinical Features

The clinical manifestations of patients with immature teratomas are essentially indistinguishable from those of mature teratomas. The patients may present with cough, fever, and/or chest pain, or with respiratory distress related to the size of the mass, which can compromise adjacent mediastinal structures.

Gross Features

The tumors can be partially cystic with solid areas. The outer surface is generally lobulated and fairly well delimited. On cut surface, the tumor may show clear fluid or areas of induration within the cyst walls. In the solid component, the tumor may show a soft, tan, and homogeneous appearance. The size of these tumors, the same as that of mature teratoma, can vary from a few centimeters to over 10 cm in greatest diameter (Fig. 10.16).

Histological Features

The classical feature of immature teratoma is the presence of foci of immature neuroepithelium. This latter component may comprise over 80% of the tumor, while in some cases its presence may be limited to focal areas. Morphologically, it is characterized by the presence of neuroepithelial tubules and rosettes. These structures may be embedded in an immature neuroepithelial background (neurophil), while in other areas the neural structures may be admixed with cartilage or other mature elements. Closer view of the cellular proliferation will show spindle or oval cells with dark nuclei, inconspicuous nucleoli, and scant cytoplasm. Mitoses are rare, and the appearance of the cellular proliferation is more reminiscent of an embryonic type of epithelium (Figs. 10.17, 10.18, 10.19, and 10.20a, b).

Immunohistochemical Features

The use of immunohistochemical markers in these tumors is limited to neural markers such as S-100 protein, neurofilaments, glial fibrillary acidic protein (GFAP), and neuron-specific enolase (NSE). In the majority of cases, the diagnosis can be reached on morphological grounds, leaving the use of immunohistochemical stains for cases in which the immature component is not apparent.

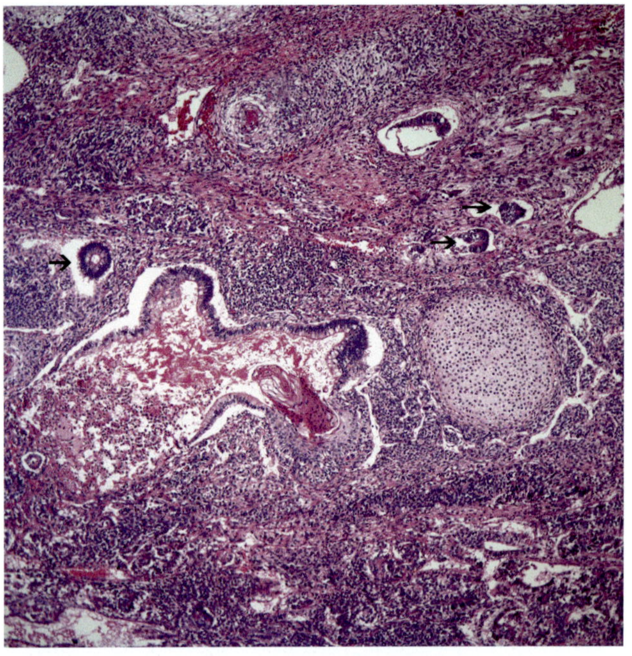

Fig. 10.17 Mediastinal teratoma showing predominantly mature elements with only focal immature component (see arrow)

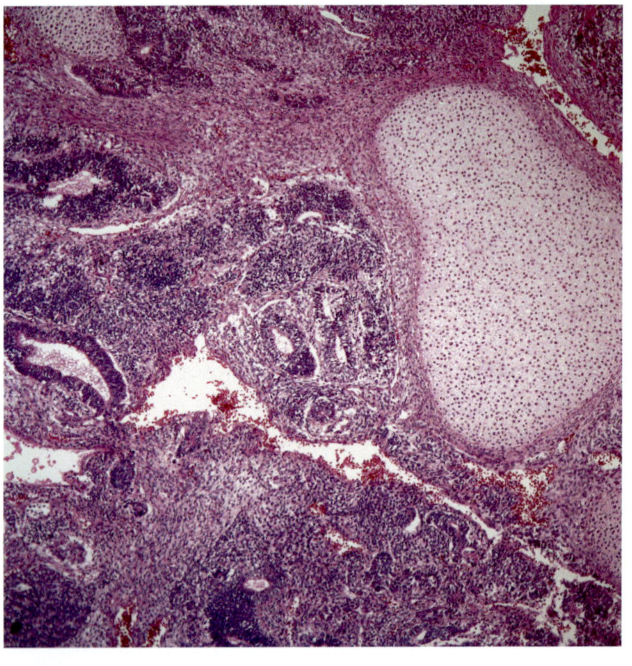

Fig. 10.18 Immature teratoma showing also mature cartilaginous component

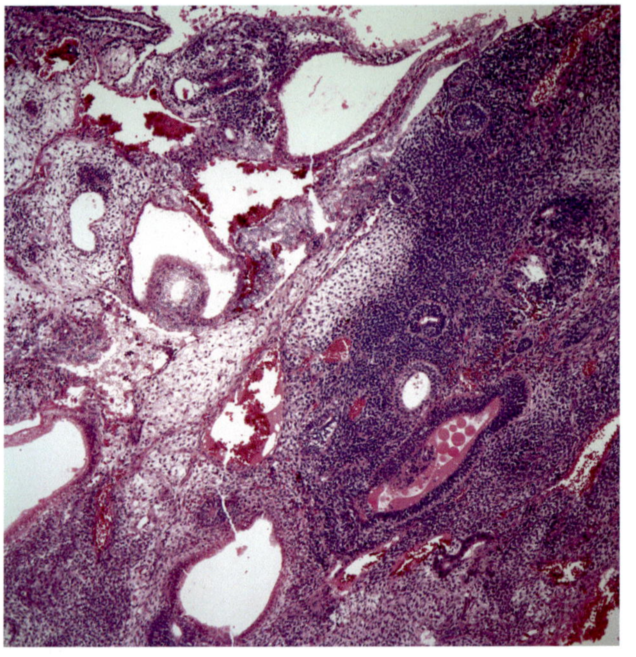

Fig. 10.19 Epithelial cystic mature structures admixed with immature teratoma in the form of neuro-rosettes and solid areas

Differential Diagnosis

The diagnosis of immature teratoma is rather straightforward, if there is enough material available for evaluation. However, in small biopsies, sampling error may obscure the diagnosis. Alternatively, when only neuroepithelium is present, the possibility of other tumors that may show neural differentiation may be entertained. Malignant peripheral nerve sheath tumors, Schwannomas, and extraskeletal Ewing's sarcoma may be a consideration in small biopsies. Correlation with clinical and radiographic findings may be of help in narrowing down the differential diagnosis in such instances.

Teratoma With Malignant Component

This term encompasses several types of teratomatous lesions, which may show a variety of malignant components [4–6, 8, 19, 26, 27, 29, 32, 34, 48–67]. In the past, terms such as teratocarcinoma and malignant teratoma were variously employed for these tumors. Whether the malignant component arises from malignant transformation of the benign mature teratomatous elements, represents a collision tumor, or originates from multidirectional differentiation of primi-

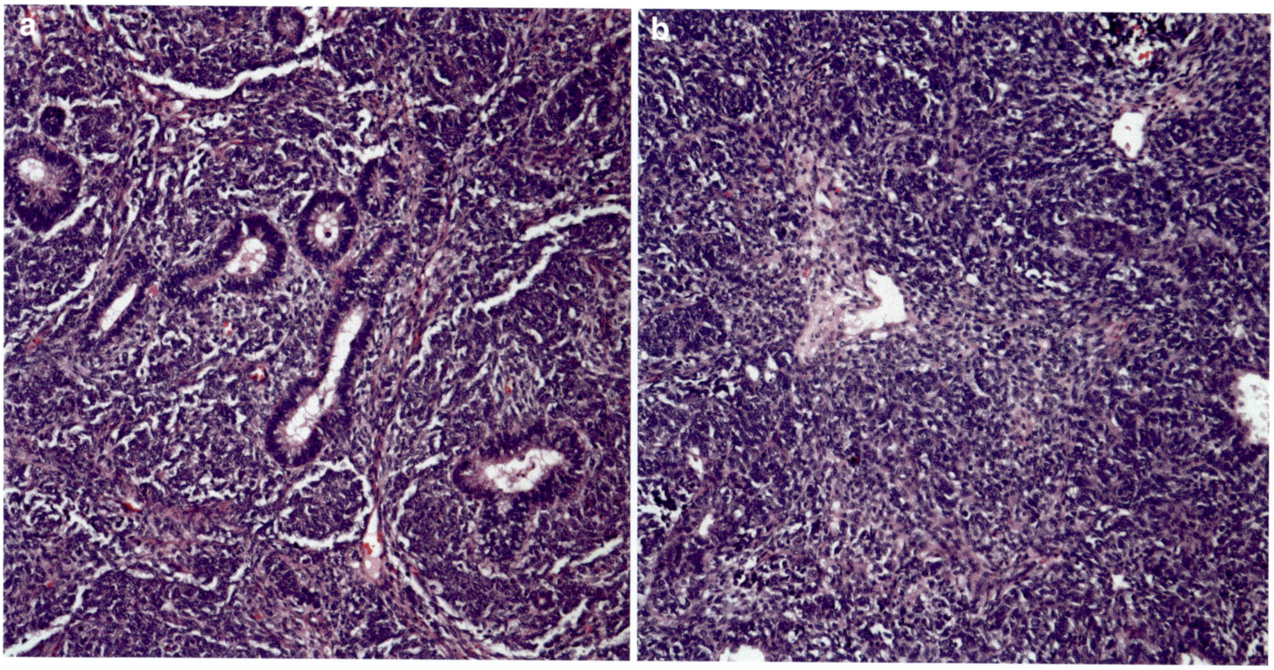

Fig. 10.20 (**a**) Immature teratoma showing classical features of neurotubules embedded in solid immature neural component. (**b**) Immature teratoma showing solid areas of neural component

tive stem cells is a question that remains unanswered. Because of the uncertainty as to the exact pathogenesis of these tumors, we prefer the descriptive term "teratoma with malignant component" to those previous terminologies. We have further subdivided these tumors into four distinct categories:

- Type I – teratoma admixed with another type of MGCT (seminoma, yolk sac tumor, embryonal carcinoma, choriocarcinoma)
- Type II – teratoma admixed with another type of epithelial neoplasm (squamous cell carcinoma, adenocarcinoma, small cell carcinoma, large cell carcinoma, etc.)
- Type III – teratoma admixed with a mesenchymal neoplasm (rhabdomyosarcoma, angiosarcoma, chondrosarcoma, osteosarcoma, etc.)
- Type IV – teratoma admixed with two or more of the above

Although in general the treatment for these patients is surgical resection followed by adjuvant therapy, the prognosis is rather poor in comparison with that of mature teratomas. However, we consider that by providing a more specific diagnosis for the malignant component, therapeutic efforts can be more beneficially tailored toward the different specific types of malignant components present, thereby improving the patients' chances for better survival.

Clinical Features

The symptoms of patients with teratoma with malignant component are similar to those of other teratomas. The symptoms will depend on the size of the lesion and the compromised adjacent structures. The vast majority of patients are asymptomatic, and the tumors are found to be unresectable at the time of exploratory thoracotomy. Teratomas with malignant component ("malignant teratoma," "teratocarcinoma") represent approximately 20% of all mediastinal teratomas [6, 68]. Teratomas with malignant component have been associated with hematological conditions such as lymphoblastic leukemia, megakaryoblastic leukemia, hemophagocytic syndrome, histiocytosis, and other medical conditions such as precocious puberty and Klinefelter's syndrome [58, 69–79]. Chromosomal abnormalities have also been observed in cases of malignant teratomas of the mediastinum. Tricot [80] documented 5q-anomalies in the bone marrow in patients with mediastinal teratoma with malignant transformation.

Although teratomas with malignant component can occur in all age groups, there is a tendency for this tumor to occur in the third and fourth decades of life. We do not know of any case in which a mediastinal teratomatous lesion with malignant component has given rise to mature teratomatous metastases as has been described for testicular tumors [5].

There are no specific radiographic features that can separate mature teratomas from teratomas with malignant component. The diagnosis should be strictly based on histopathological examination.

Gross Features

The gross features of teratomas with malignant component are similar to those of other teratomas (Fig. 10.21). These tumors can show extensive cystic changes as well as more solid areas. The tumors are usually poorly circumscribed and infiltrative and may be surrounded by thin membranous tissue. Their size may vary from a few centimeters to over 12 cm in greatest diameter.

Histopathological Features

- *Type I* – this type may show one or more of the other types of germ cell tumors, including seminoma, yolk sac tumor, embryonal carcinoma, and/or choriocarcinoma. In our experience, this type represents the most common form of teratoma with malignant component. The admixture of mature teratomatous elements such as the hair, skin, bone, and cartilage, with areas showing other types of germ cell tumor such as seminoma, etc., characterizes the histologic features of these tumors (Figs. 10.22a, b and 10.23).
- *Type II* – teratomatous elements are admixed with other differentiated malignant neoplasms of epithelial origin. Adenocarcinoma or squamous cell carcinomas are the most frequent types observed in these lesions. The features of the malignant component observed in this type will be those of conventional adenocarcinoma or keratinizing squamous cell carcinoma. In rare occasions, the malignancy will be of a large cell carcinoma or small cell carcinoma (Fig. 10.24a, b).
- *Type III* – a variety of malignant mesenchymal neoplasms such as rhabdomyosarcoma, liposarcoma, and/or angiosarcoma can be seen in association with mature teratoma. In some cases, the mature teratoma may be associated with an undifferentiated mesenchymal neoplasm. The features of the sarcomatous elements will be those seen in the conventional soft tissue counterparts of these tumors (Fig. 10.25a, b).
- *Type IV* – this is an unusual phenomenon in which a teratoma may show areas of mature or immature teratoma associated with carcinoma, sarcoma, and/or another germ cell tumor. We have documented cases of this unusual phenomenon [17].

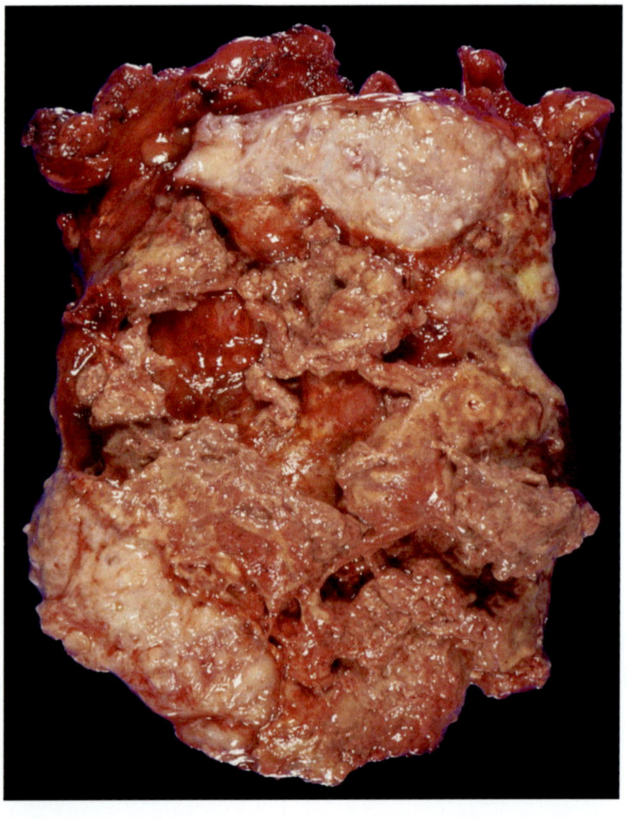

Fig. 10.21 Teratoma with malignant component. At the macroscopic level, there is no pathognomonic feature that will discriminate this tumor from other teratomatous lesion

Histochemical, Immunohistochemical, and Ultrastructural Features

The use of specific markers may be of help for identifying the different neoplastic components of these tumors. Germ cell markers such as placental-like alkaline phosphatase (PLAP), alpha-fetoprotein (AFP), SALL-4, Glypican 4, OCT4, TCL1, and human chorionic gonadotrophin (HCG) may be of aid in separating germ cell elements from other malignant epithelial neoplasms. The use of keratins, vimentin, actin, desmin, and S-100 protein may be of aid in identifying specific features of differentiation in pleomorphic and spindle cell elements in these tumors. The use of these special markers should therefore be guided to identify the different specific components. The role of electron microscopy is more limited due to the sampling difficulties inherent to these tumors. However, ultrastructural examination may be of aid in adequately sampled cases for differentiating sarcomatous from anaplastic carcinomatous and germ cell elements.

Differential Diagnosis

Teratomas are easily recognizable tumors that do not pose a problem for diagnosis. However, because malignant components may be small and focal, caution should be exercised before rendering an unequivocal diagnosis of mature teratoma

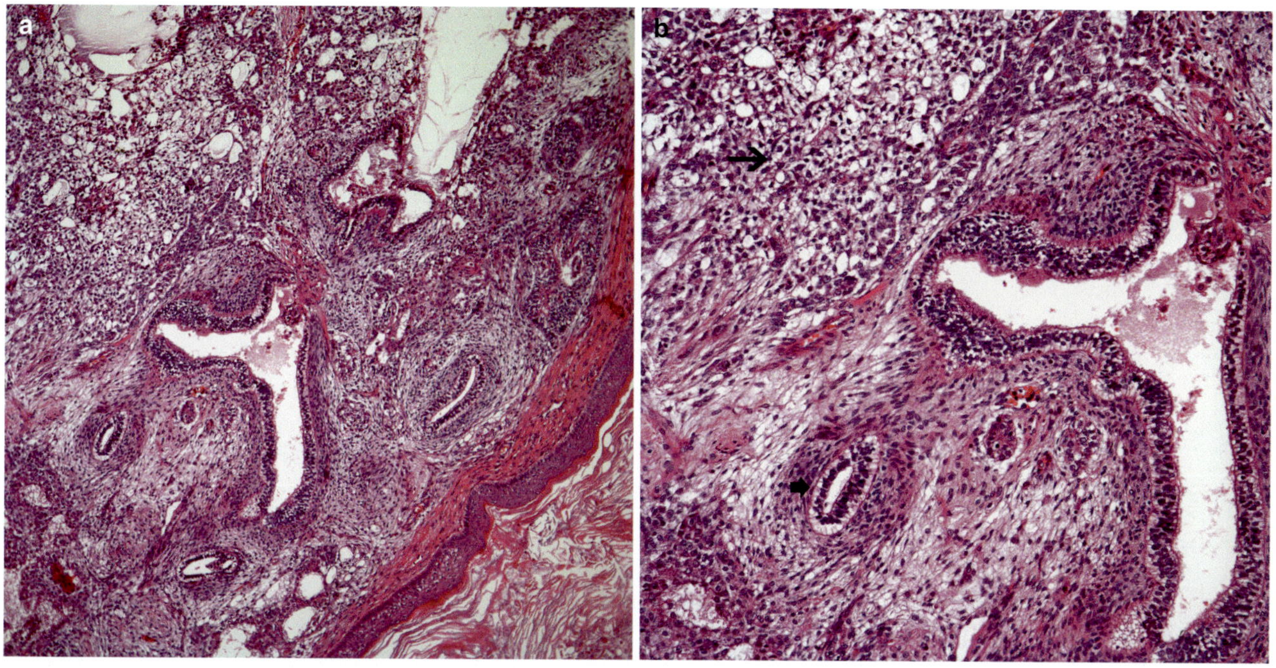

Fig. 10.22 (**a**) Type I mediastinal teratoma displaying mature, immature, and malignant component in the form of yolk sac tumor. (**b**) Close magnification of the immature component (neurotubules and rosettes) and yolk sac tumor (see arrows)

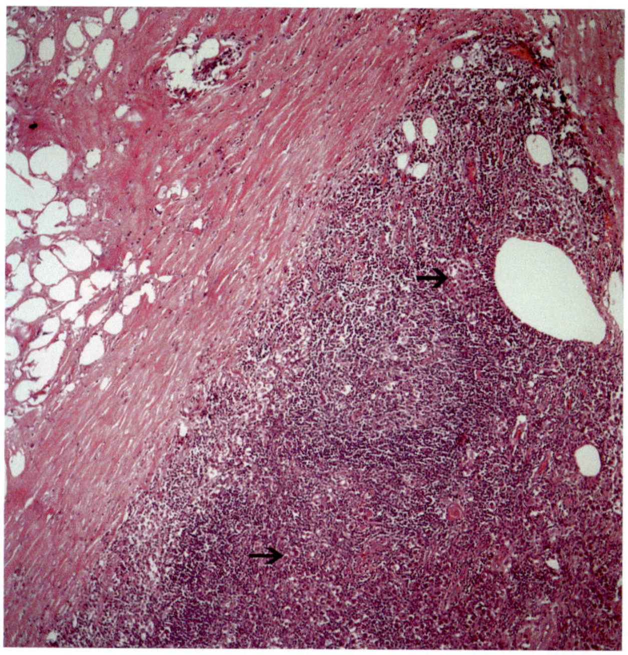

Fig. 10.23 Type I mediastinal teratoma with malignant component in which there is another germ cell tumors associated, in this case seminoma (see arrows)

in small biopsy specimens. By the same token, a small biopsy of an anterior mediastinal mass may show only mesenchymal elements with rhabdomyosarcomatous or liposarcomatous features that may be part of a teratoma. Such cases should be separated from pure mesenchymal tumors, which have also been described in the anterior mediastinum [81, 82]. Because of the possibility that even mature lesions may harbor an additional malignant component, complete excision and extensive sampling of these tumors are recommended for accurate diagnosis.

Seminoma

Primary mediastinal seminomas are neoplasms that have been well recognized for over 50 years [12, 83–86]. The first description of a pure seminoma in the anterior mediastinum is attributed to Woolner and colleagues [12] in 1955, who described two seminomas (germinomas) arising in the anterior mediastinum. It is important to note that previous descriptions of teratomatous germ cell tumors of the mediastinum had already mentioned the presence of seminomatous component [21, 67]. There appears to have been some reluctance in the past to accept the existence of seminomas as primary mediastinal tumors; hence, mediastinal seminomas were designated by other names such as "seminoma-like tumor," "seminomatous thymoma," and "pseudo-seminome, thymome" [85, 86]. In 1962, Lattes [86], in an analysis of 107 cases of thymomas and other tumors of the thymus, alluded to four cases of seminoma-like tumors of the mediastinum in young males and concluded that morphologically the tumors were indistinguishable from those seen in the male and female gonads. However, he cautioned about the danger of lumping together other pathological entities under the term "thymic seminoma" and "pseudo-seminomatous thymoma." Today, the existence of these tumors occurring primarily in the mediastinum is well-established [5, 6, 14, 29, 50, 51, 61, 62, 87–108].

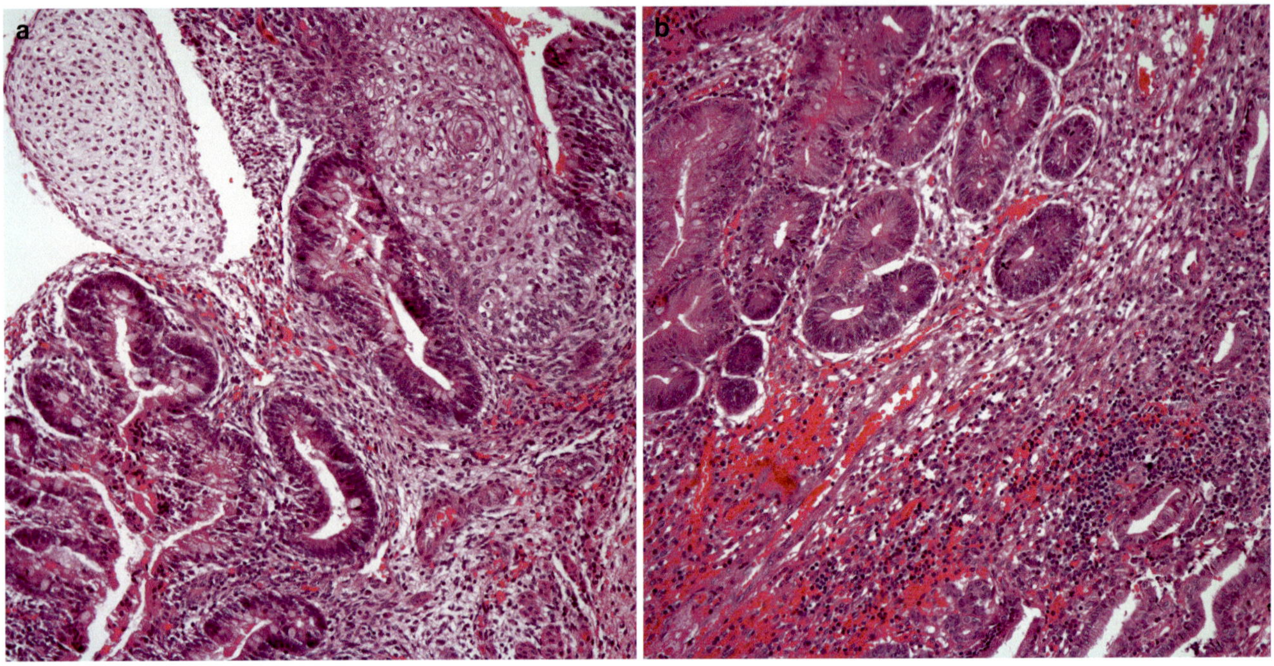

Fig. 10.24 Type II teratoma with malignant component. (**a**) In this case note the presence of cartilage and adenocarcinoma. (**b**) Adenocarcinoma embedded in a fibrous inflammatory stroma

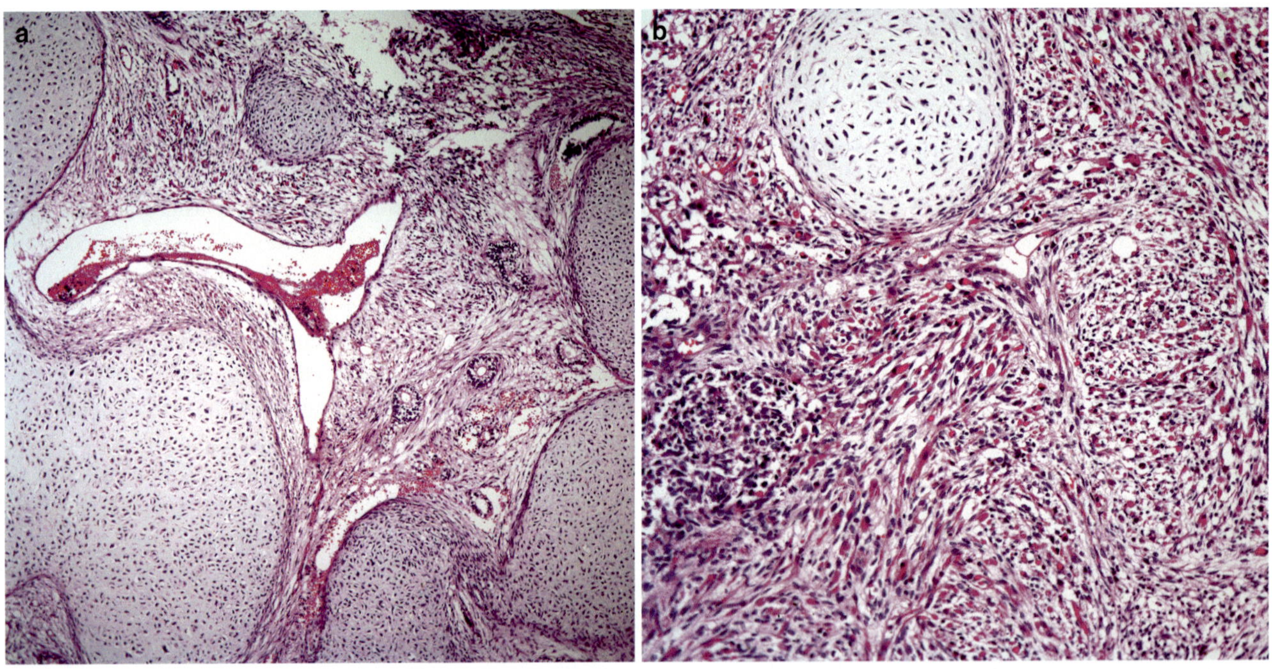

Fig. 10.25 Type III, mediastinal teratoma with malignant component. (**a**) In this case note the presence of cartilage and rhabdomyosarcoma. (**b**) Closer view of the rhabdomyosarcomatous component

Although seminomas occur often in the anterior mediastinum, cases of seminomas in the posterior mediastinal compartment have been also described [88].

Because of the rarity of this neoplasm and the lack of more comprehensive studies of these tumors, it is difficult to determine the exact incidence of mediastinal seminomas in the general population. However, in our experience, pure seminomas of the anterior mediastinum represent the second most common germ cell tumor after teratomatous lesions. Seminomas have been estimated to account for approximately 37% of all mediastinal germ cell tumors [109]. Although in our material we did not find any cases of seminomas occurring in women, such an association has been cited in the literature [62, 83, 100, 107]. It has been stated that seminomas are tumors more commonly seen in young adults. Interestingly, in our review of 120 cases of primary anterior mediastinal seminomas, the ages ranged from 14 to 79 years with an average of 46.5 years. Nevertheless, seminomas are more common in the third and fourth decade of life (Fig. 10.26a, b).

Clinical Features

The symptoms of patients with seminomas of the anterior mediastinum depend largely on the size of the tumor. Symptoms are mostly related to compression of adjacent organs. These symptoms include cough, chest pain, hemoptysis, and/or dyspnea. In some instances, the patients may present with superior vena cava syndrome [50, 83, 94]. The latter symptom has been estimated to occur in approximately 10–25% of the cases of anterior mediastinal seminomas [88, 95, 102, 110]. Interestingly, in some patients, a history of testicular trauma, orchitis, or maldescended testis has been documented [88]. However, a good number of patients with anterior

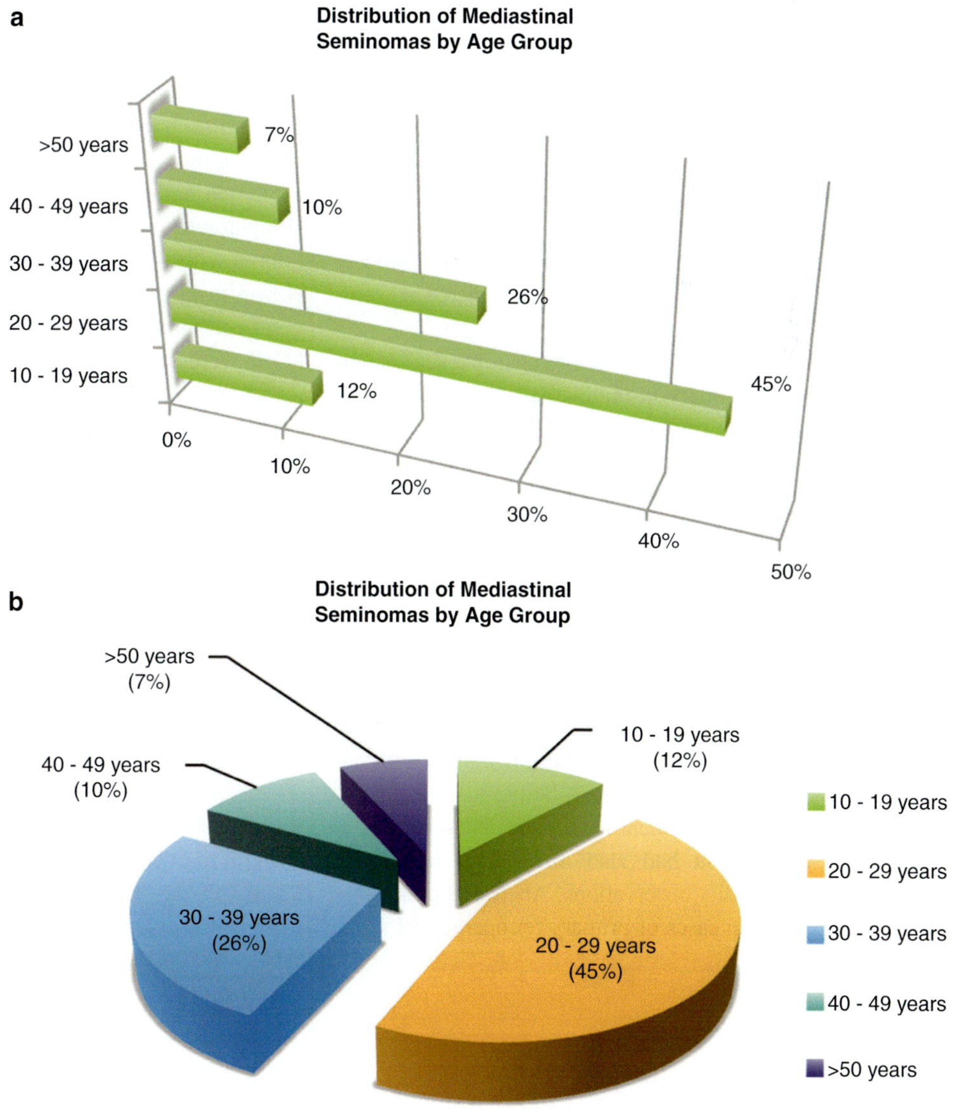

Fig. 10.26 (**a**) Distribution of seminomas per age group. (**b**) It is the respective % of seminomas per age group

Table 10.4 Common and uncommon symptoms in mediastinal seminomas

Symptoms
Chest pain
Shortness of breath
Superior vena cava syndrome
Cough
Dysphagia
Arm pain
Upper respiratory infection
Vocal cord paralysis
Hoarseness
Asymptomatic

mediastinal seminomas are asymptomatic, and the tumor is detected during a routine physical examination or chest radiographs. Table 10.4 depicts some of the common and uncommon symptoms associated with mediastinal seminomas.

Several clinical syndromes and unusual clinical conditions have been observed in association with seminomas. Raghavan and Barret [101] described a 13-year-old boy with mediastinal seminoma in association with ventricular septal defect and congenital absence of thoracic hemivertebra. Kinding and Tavel [98] described a 43-year-old man with acquired pulmonic stenosis due to an anterior mediastinal seminoma, which resolved after resection of the tumor. Nagi and colleagues [87] described a young man who presented with a history of painful gynecomastia and was found to have an anterior mediastinal seminoma with increased serologic levels of β-HCG.

Perhaps the most important question regarding seminomas is whether they are primary in the mediastinum or represent metastases from occult primary testicular tumors. This topic has been debated for quite some time. In the past, due to the reluctance to accept mediastinal seminomas as primary neoplasms, the discovery of such tumors was invariably followed by testicular biopsies. Although the results appear to some extent controversial, important knowledge was obtained from those studies. Azzopardi and Hoffbrand [111] cautioned against the uncritical acceptance of extragonadal germ cell tumor. The authors documented a case of viable metastases from a retrogressed testicular seminoma and reviewed six similar cases from the literature. In addition, the authors concluded that great caution is necessary before making a diagnosis of primary retroperitoneal seminoma; interestingly, in this review, one patient had also mediastinal seminoma. Contrary to Azzopardi's observations, Abell and colleagues [112] documented ten cases of primary retroperitoneal seminomas in patients without evidence of testicular involvement. Buskirk and colleagues [113] in a more recent study described 12 cases of primary seminoma of the retroperitoneum in the absence of testicular involvement. However, there have been some authors who have argued against the acceptance of extragonadal germ cell tumors without proper histologic evaluation of testicular biopsies [114]. In actuality, testicular seminomas rarely metastasize to the anterior mediastinum. In a review of 16 patients with extragonadal germ cell tumors and negative testicular tumor at palpation, Bohle and coworkers [115] found that 10 of 12 patients with retroperitoneal tumors had an occult testicular primary, whereas in four patients with MGCT, none had evidence of an occult testicular primary. Luna and Valenzuela-Tamaris [51] also documented a study of 20 autopsy cases of mediastinal germ cell tumors of various histologies. In all 20 cases, the testes were carefully step-sectioned, and the authors were able to find only two cases in which the testes contained an occult tumor or a well-defined testicular scar. Interestingly, the histology of the mediastinal tumors in those cases was that of a non-seminomatous tumor. The authors cited two studies from large series of testicular germ cell tumors, one by Johnson and coworkers [116], who in a review of 78 autopsies of patients with testicular germ cell tumors found no metastases to the anterior mediastinal region without involvement of mediastinal nodes, and another by Lynch and Blewett [117], who quoted a publication by Houghton of a study of 220 cases of metastasizing testicular tumors with no documented metastases to the mediastinum. However, rare metastases to the mediastinum from testicular germ cell tumors have been described. White and coworkers [118] were able to document pericardial metastasis from a testicular seminoma. Also, Man-Cha [90] reported a case of simultaneous retroperitoneal and mediastinal seminoma in an 18-year-old boy who underwent left orchiectomy without any evidence of a testicular tumor. On the other hand, there are reports of the development of testicular seminomas several years after the patient has been diagnosed and treated for a mediastinal seminoma [28, 88]. In these cases in particular, it may be possible to argue that the testicular tumor had already been present; however, based on the length of appearances of both tumors, a second primary is most likely.

Germ cell tumors (GCT) can display distinctive chromosomal abnormalities. Bosl and coworkers [119] in a study of 29 cases of different primary sites (including mediastinum) found that the isochromosome of chromosome 12[1(12p)] is a useful marker of GCT in males. However, because of similar histologic features displayed by these tumors in either mediastinal or testicular location, there have been attempts to further analyze these tumors for more discriminant features. In this regard, Oosterhuis and coworkers [120] studied the ploidy in 19 primary MGCT, encountering that the ploidy of mediastinal tumors was remarkably different from that of testicular tumors of adults and closer to those of children. MGCT share similar features with childhood testicular GCT in terms of both being diploid; nevertheless, diploid testicular GCT are rare. Seminomas are usually hypertriploid, while non-seminomatous tumors are usually hypotriploid. The authors proposed that the pathogenesis of malignant MGCT is probably different from that of testicular tumors of adults and stated that ploidy studies in questionable cases may be of help in elucidating the site of origin of these tumors when the clinical setting is obscured. More recently, we analyzed the expression of p53 and K-ras-2 oncogene in 13 cases of primary mediastinal seminomas. We found that the k-ras-2 genotype was normal in approximately 92% of the cases, and also identified a single mutation in codon 13. This latter finding may be of help in distinguishing mediastinal from testicular tumors since most testicular tumors show abnormalities of codon 12 rather than codon 13 [121].

The radiological features of these tumors have been well defined. Rosado-de-Christenson and coworkers [43] found that seminomas are typically large and bulky, well-marginated, lobulated masses, which may extend to both sides of the midline. On CT scans, seminomas appear large and coarsely lobulated with a homogeneous attenuation equal to that of soft tissue. Seminomas enhance slightly after the administration of contrast material. Areas of low attenuation may also be detected [122]. Extension of the tumor into the midline and posterior mediastinal compartments can also occur. Ringlike and stippled calcifications within a mediastinal seminoma on CT studies have been reported [123].

Seminomas are eminently radiosensitive tumors [64, 102, 124–127]. However, it is also known that approximately 20–30% of advanced germ cell tumors will fail to achieve a durable complete response to chemotherapy [128]. Medini and coworkers [129] evaluated the follow-up of eight patients with extragonadal seminomas, including five patients in whom the tumors were primary in the mediastinum, and found that 50% of the patients died within a period ranging from 2 months to 16 years; 25% of these patients died of unrelated conditions, and, in one patient, metastases to the brain were documented. The remaining 50% of the patients were alive and well after a period of 5–17 years. Hurt [95] followed 17 patients with primary mediastinal seminoma of whom 16 had received radiation therapy after initial diagnosis, concluding that possible factors that may influence the progression of disease include age (older than 35 years), presentation with fever, superior vena cava syndrome, supraclavicular or cervical adenopathy, and roentgenographic evidence of hilar disease. Hainsworth and coworkers [130] also studied 32 patients with extragonadal GCT (17/32 MGCT; 6/32 seminomas), concluding that extragonadal GCT can be as curable as testicular GCT when treated with intensive chemotherapy and surgical resection. In a study of exclusively MGCT (28 cases; 11/28 seminomas), Economou [63] found 82% of the patients free of tumor after a period ranging from 6 months to 15 years. The primary treatment for these patients was radiation therapy, except in one patient who received chemotherapy for metastatic disease. Green and coworkers [131] encountered similar findings in a study of 17 retroperitoneal seminomas and 1 mediastinal seminoma. However, it is important to note that cardiac disease that may be the source of much morbidity and mortality may appear after mediastinal irradiation for seminoma [132]. In a study of 27 patients with primary MGCT including 13 patients with pure seminomas treated with radiation therapy alone, it was found that the most important factor was the histology of the tumor. The 5-year survival rate for all of the patients with pure seminoma was of 100%, whereas tumors showing non-seminomatous features displayed a worse prognosis. On the other hand, late recurrences have been reported after many years of successful remission [133]. A recent study by Rodney and coworkers [134] addressing the survival outcomes in 34 men with mediastinal GCT including 27 with non-seminomatous GCT (NS-GCT) and 7 with pure seminomas showed that 41% with NS-GCT were alive with a median overall survival of 33.5 months. Patients with seminoma were treated with platinum-based chemotherapy and did invariably well.

Although a good number of seminomas are limited to the anterior mediastinal region without invasion into adjacent structures, metastases of mediastinal seminomas to other organs can occur. In our experience, we have observed metastatic lesions from mediastinal seminomas to the lung, brain, lymph node, pleura, liver, and bone [109]. Serum tumor markers have also been studied to further determine staging and prognosis of GCT. In a study of 111 patients with GCT of the testicle, Scardino and coworkers [135] found that 33% of patients with testicular seminoma had elevated CEA levels; however, CEA levels did not correlate with the course of disease.

Follow-up information obtained in 65 patients with primary mediastinal seminomas studied by us disclosed that 49 patients were alive and well after a period ranging from 1 to 19 years (mean: 10 years). Sixteen patients died during the same period of time. We were not able to find a statistically meaningful correlation between aggressive behavior and any clinical or histopathological feature in these tumors.

Gross Features

Seminomas vary in size from a few centimeters to over 16 cm in greatest diameter (Fig. 10.27). The outer surface may be smooth and glistening or may show a lobulated appearance. The cut surface can show either a coarsely lobular or a discrete nodular pattern. The color may vary from white to light tan, and the consistency is rather soft. In some cases, solid areas may alternate with large cystic areas containing necrotic material, while in other areas the tumor may have the appearance of an entirely cystic mass. In some cystic tumors, it is possible to observe indurated areas within the walls of the cysts.

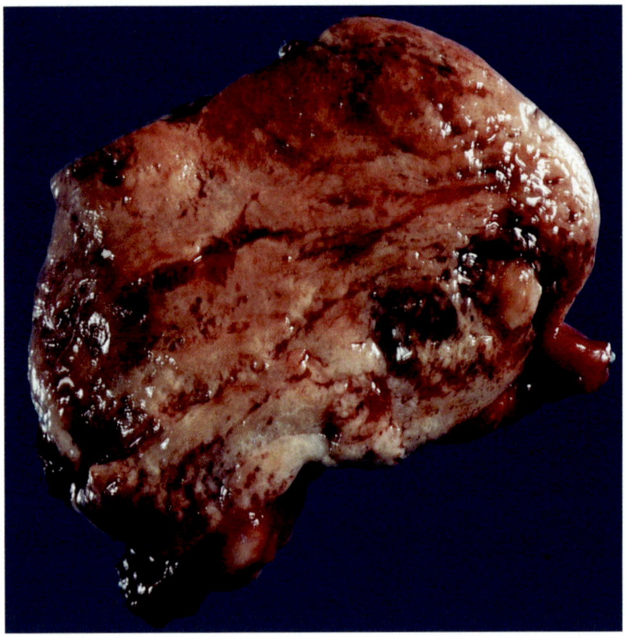

Fig. 10.27 Mediastinal seminoma showing a solid tumor mass

Histologic Features

The histology of primary mediastinal seminomas is similar to those described for their gonadal counterparts. On scanning magnification, the neoplastic cells may be arranged in sheets or forming a discrete nesting pattern-containing uniform round to oval tumor cells (Fig. 10.28a–d). In cases in which the neoplastic cells are arranged in a nesting pattern separated by thin fibrovascular septa, the fibrovascular septa will be characteristically infiltrated by a large number of lymphocytes; however, the presence of lymphocytes may vary as, in some cases, despite the presence of areas of hyalinization, the inflammatory component is not present (Fig. 10.29a–c). In some other cases, the lymphoid component is completely admixed with the neoplastic component (Fig. 10.30). However, this phenomenon may obey to the normal lymphocytic component of the thymus. In some unusual cases, mediastinal seminomas may show focal or extensive areas of "crush artifact," which may obscure the true nature of the neoplasm (Fig. 10.31a, b). On higher magnification, the neoplastic cells are composed of large, round to polygonal cells with pale cytoplasm; round nuclei and prominent nucleoli may or may not be apparent (Fig. 10.32). Mitotic figures are usually present but not in large numbers (Fig. 10.33). Seminomas can also show foci containing large giant cells of syncytiotrophoblast type. In our experience, this feature was observed in less than 5% of the cases. Although most of the cases described in the literature belong to the classical type of seminoma, there are a few reports of anaplastic seminoma in the anterior mediastinum [103]. Other microscopic features that may be associated with mediastinal seminomas include (A) presence of thymic remnants, which can be seen in approximately 27% of the

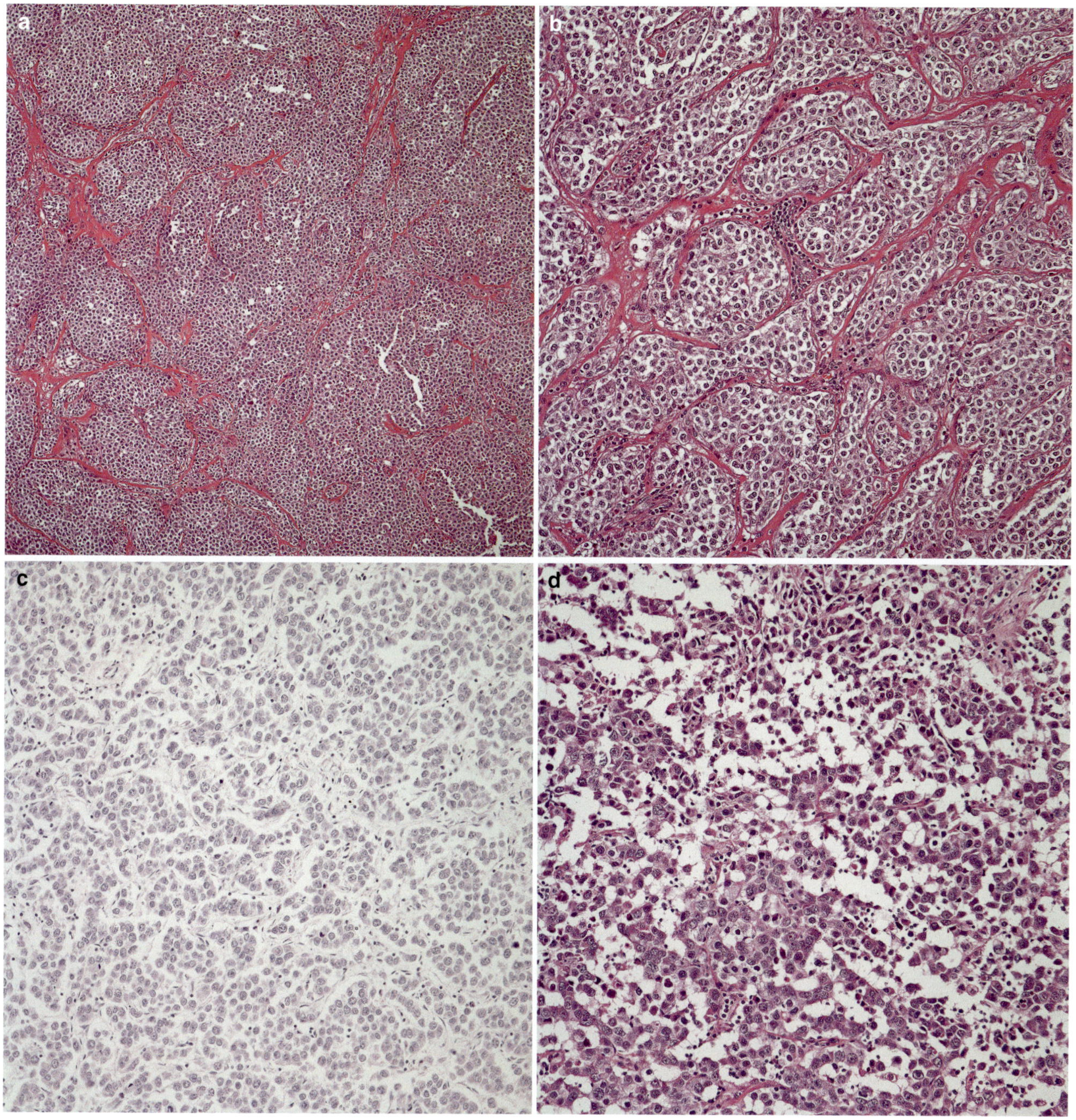

Fig. 10.28 (**a**) Mediastinal "thymic" seminoma showing a discrete nested pattern of growth; (**b**) intermediate magnification showing a subtle nested pattern. (**c**) Seminoma showing ribbons of neoplastic cells. (**d**) Seminoma showing sheets of neoplastic cells

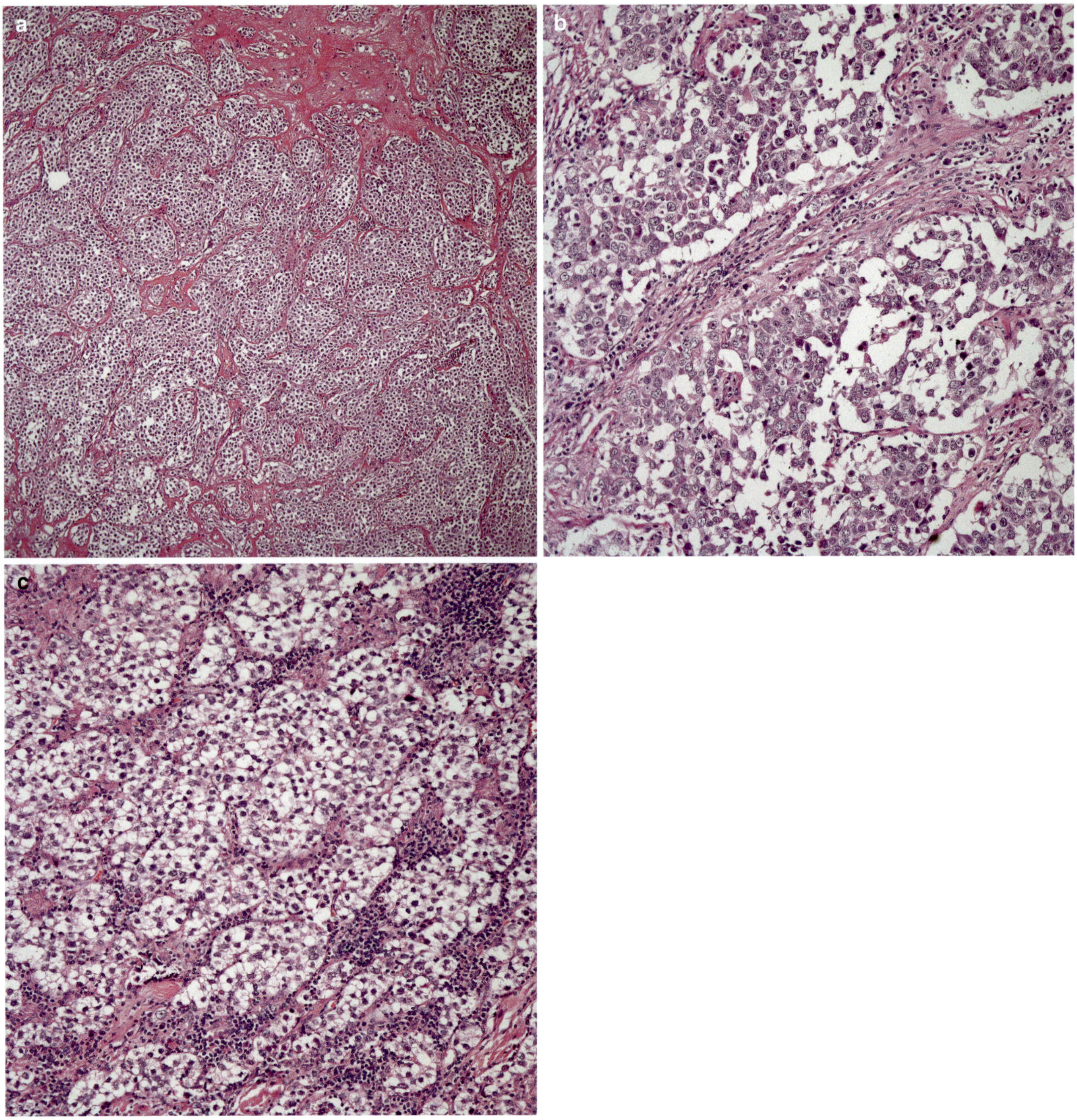

Fig. 10.29 (**a**) Seminoma showing discrete presence of hyalinization with no presence of lymphocytes. (**b**) Seminoma with mild presence of lymphocytes in the fibroconnective tissue. (**c**) Seminoma with more lymphocytic component

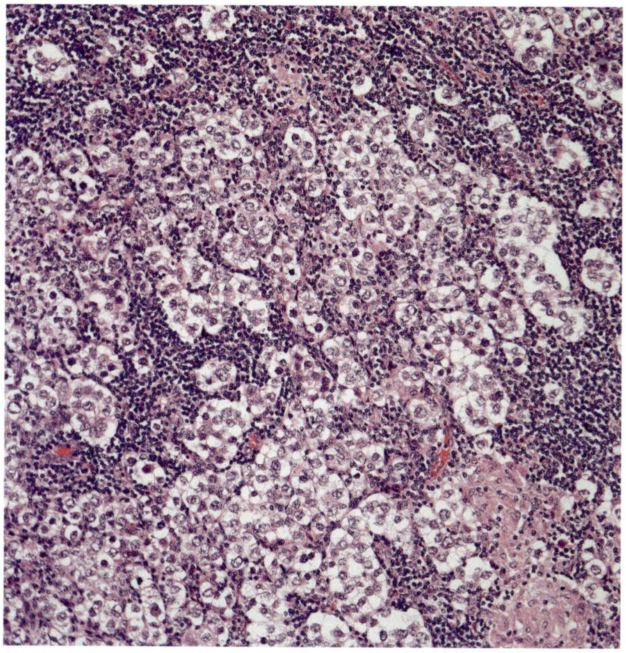

Fig. 10.30 Seminoma admixed with abundant lymphocytic component

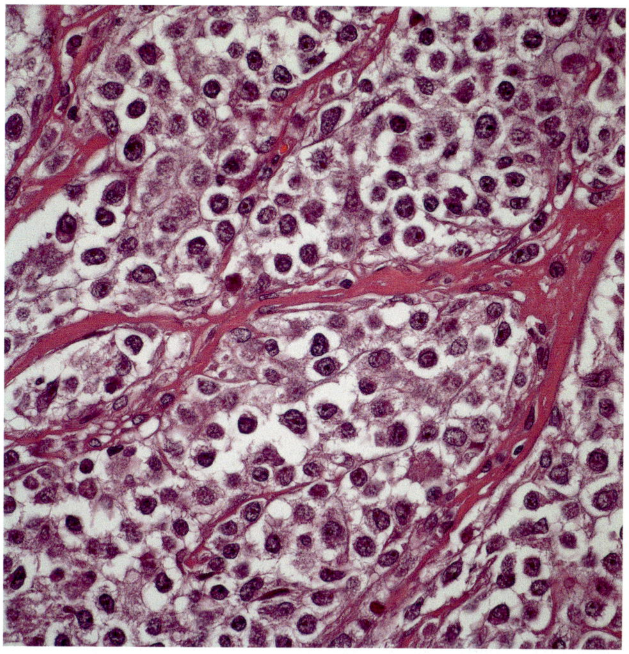

Fig. 10.32 High-power magnification of seminoma showing round to oval tumor cells with distinct cell borders round to oval nuclei, and in some cells prominent nucleoli is present

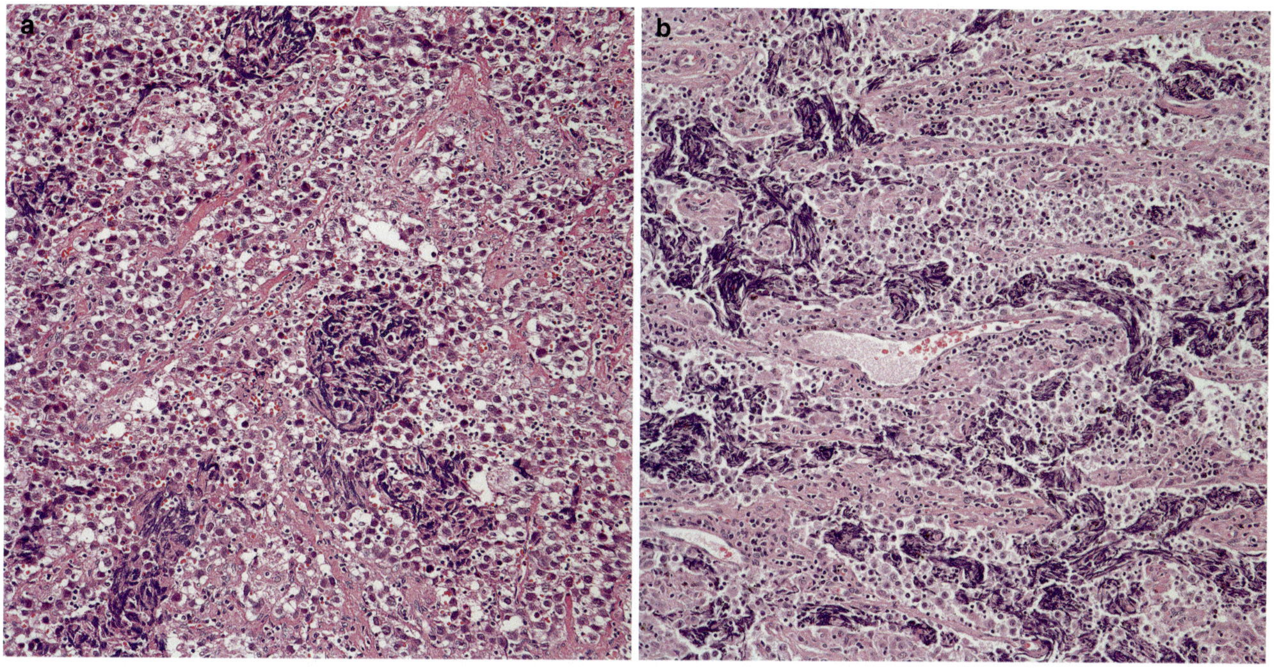

Fig. 10.31 (**a**) Seminoma with focal areas of crush artifact. (**b**) Seminoma with more extensive areas of crush artifact

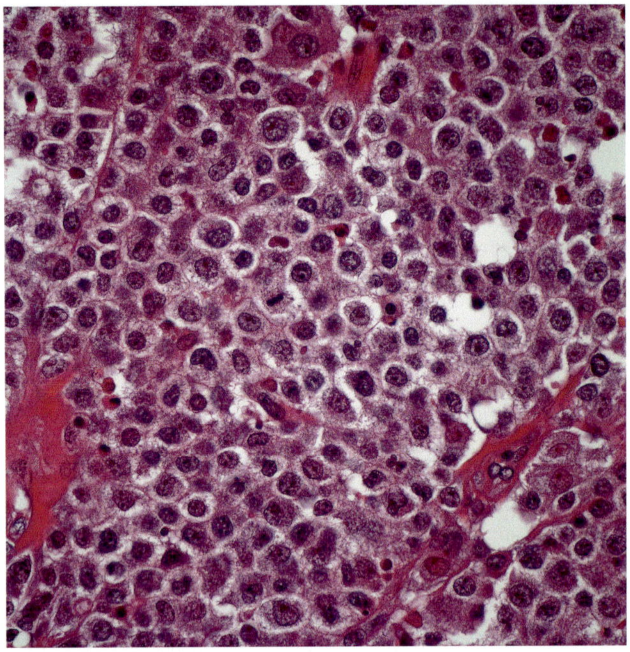

Fig. 10.33 High-power magnification of a seminoma showing scattered mitotic figures

tumors (Fig. 10.34a–c); (B) granulomatous reaction, which can be seen in the form of isolated giant cells admixed with the neoplastic cells to full blown florid non-caseous granulomas inflammation in about 46% of the cases (Fig. 10.35a–e); and (C) necrosis, which can be focal or extensive, making in some cases difficult the identification of neoplastic cells (Fig. 10.36a–c). Mediastinal seminomas may also show other unusual features including lymphoid hyperplasia with the presence of prominent germinal centers and tumors characterized by a predominantly cystic appearance. The two latter features are present in less than 10% of the tumors and have been reported separately as uncommon morphological features associated with these tumors in the mediastinal region.

In our experience with cystic seminomas, the tumors were reported as grossly cystic tumors, and, histopathologically, they mimic multilocular thymic cyst [136]. These tumors characteristically show areas of lymphoid hyperplasia, cysts lined by squamous epithelium and cholesterol cleft granulomas. The seminomatous component is found growing along the cystic walls of the tumor (Fig. 10.37a, b). In cases in which there is a predominantly cystic tumor, extensive sampling becomes necessary in order to determine the presence of seminoma. On the other hand, seminomas may also show extensive florid follicular lymphoid hyperplasia, which may pose a problem in separating this tumor from a lymphoproliferative tumor in the anterior mediastinum. In these cases, seminomas show at low power a striking lymphoid hyperplasia with prominent germinal centers. The tumor cells are placed in between the germinal centers (Fig. 10.38a, b). This unusual histological feature has been described in fewer than 10% of the cases, and the clinical and demographic features of the cases reported are similar to those described for mediastinal seminomas. The reported cases include male patients between the ages of 24 and 31 years who presented with non-specific clinical symptoms, and the presence of florid follicular lymphoid hyperplasia does not appear to influence the outcome of these patients [137].

One other additional unusual feature of seminomas is its association with another non-GCT. We have described the presence of seminoma in a case of primary leiomyosarcoma of the anterior mediastinum [138]. More recently, we described the association of a thymic seminoma with a thymoma [139]. In these two particular scenarios, the final diagnosis is likely to be reached after complete surgical resection has taken place. It is important to highlight that, in a small mediastinoscopic biopsy, it is likely that only one of the tumors in question may be represented, which may lead to important treatment decisions. However, once the surgical resection is available, in cases in which the seminoma may be associated with another mesenchymal neoplasm like in the case of leiomyosarcoma, it is likely that one should be able to distinguish the two processes on morphological grounds. However, in the case that a seminoma is associated with a thymoma, the diagnosis may pose more challenges. In either of these situations, it is prudent to perform additional immunohistochemical stains that may aid in separating the seminomatous component from either leiomyosarcoma or

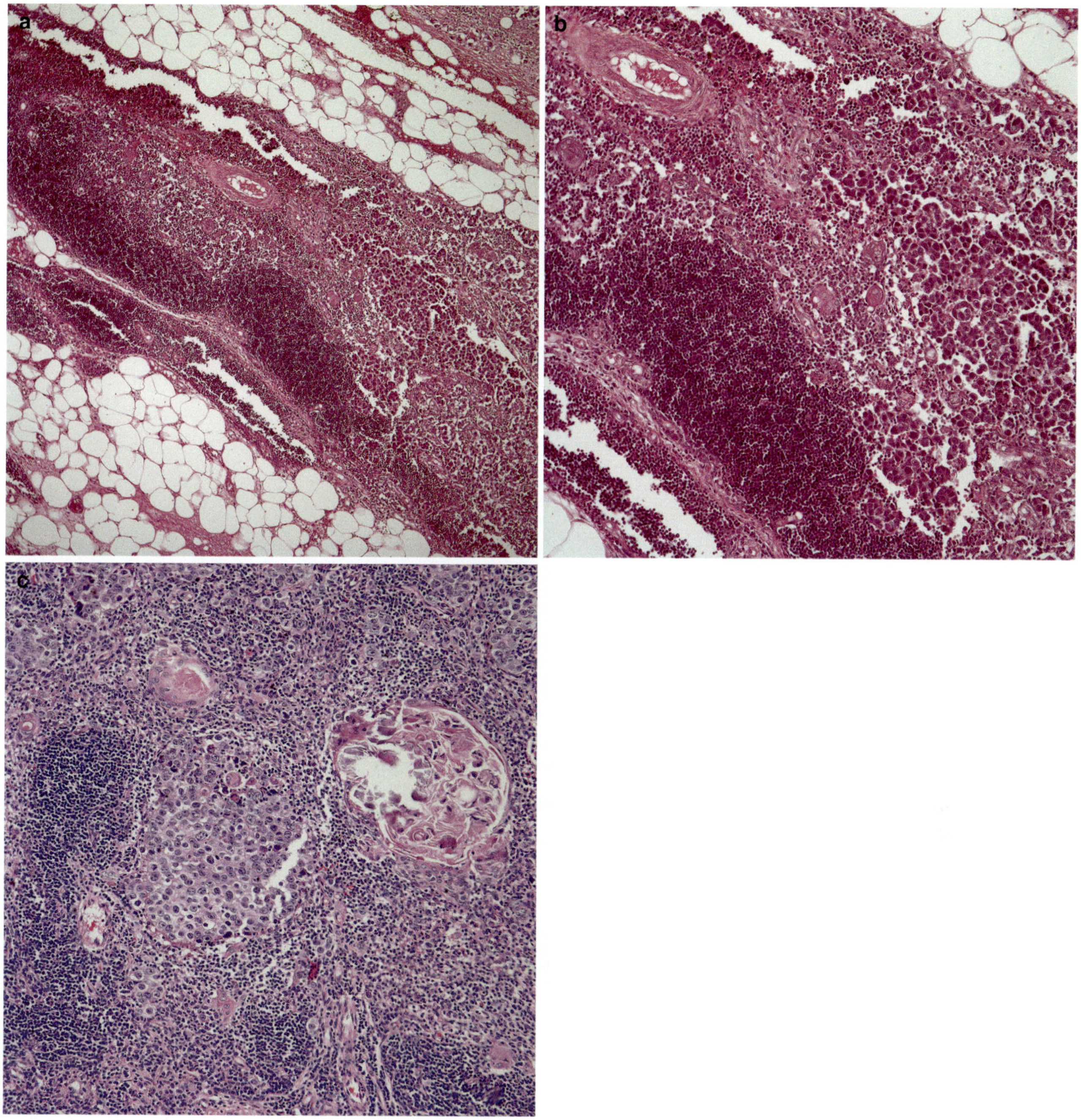

Fig. 10.34 (**a**) Seminoma involving portion of the thymic gland. (**b**) Seminoma adjacent to Hassall's corpuscles. (**c**) Dilated Hassall's corpuscle adjacent to areas of seminoma

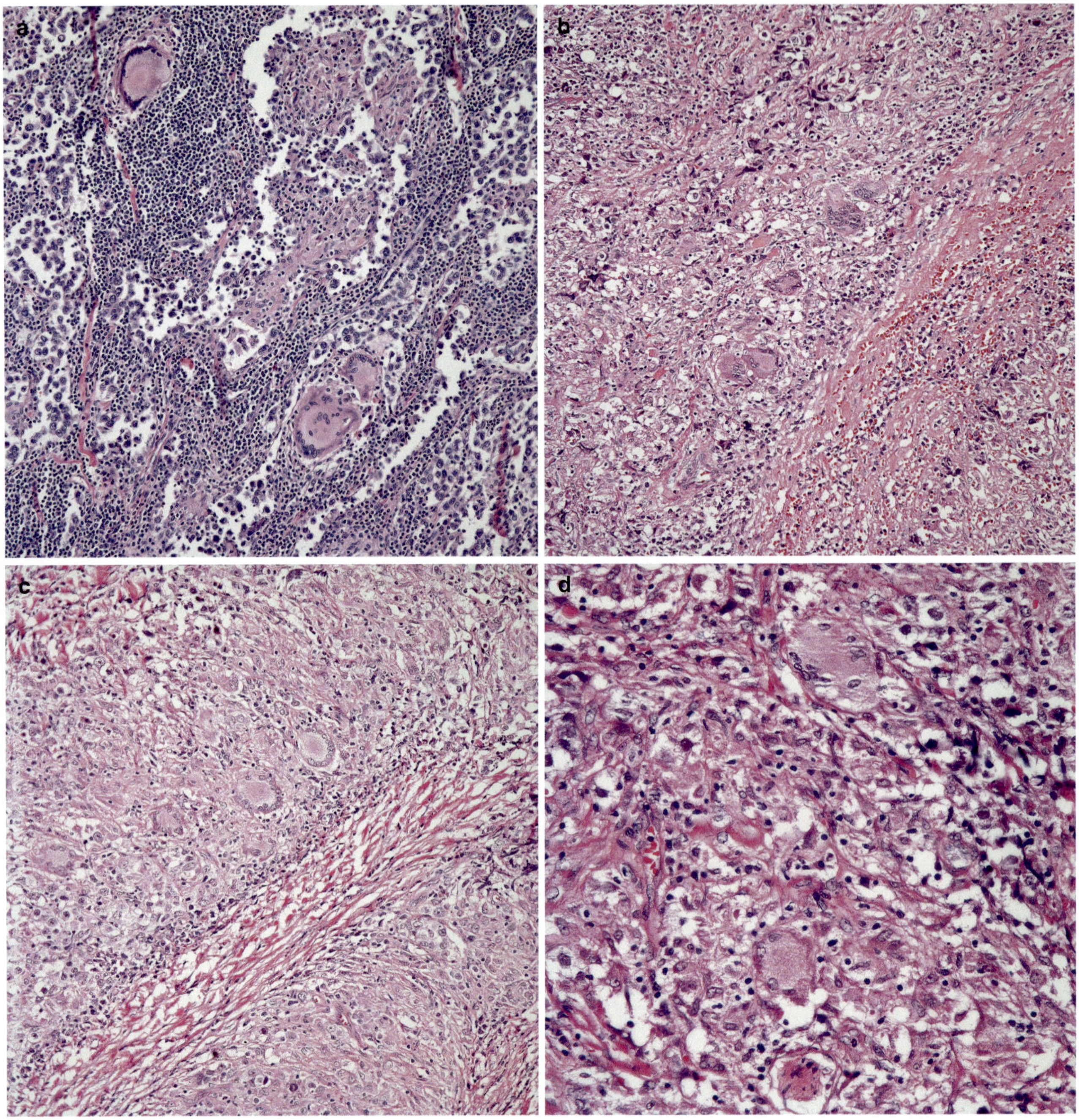

Fig. 10.35 (**a**) Seminoma with presence of scattered giant cells. (**b**) Numerous multinucleated giant cells with some viable tumor cells. (**c**) Florid granulomatous reaction. (**d**) Multinucleated giant cells with only focal viable tumor cells.

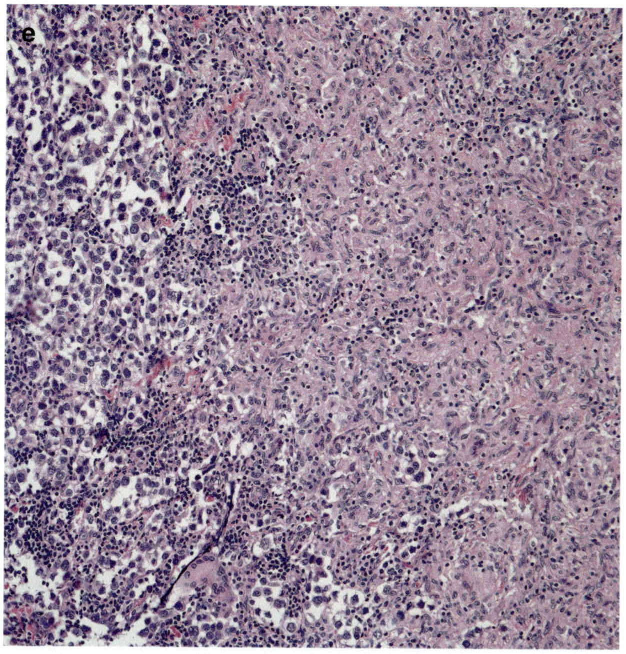

Fig. 10.35 (continued) (**e**) Seminoma with non-caseating granulomatous inflammation

thymoma. The careful use of immunohistochemical stains in these settings is highly advised. Table 10.5 depicts some of the most important histopathological features of mediastinal seminomas.

The most important histochemical stain in seminomas is the use of periodic acid-Schiff (PAS) to demonstrate the presence of glycogen within the neoplastic cells (Fig. 10.39). The neoplastic cells are negative for intracellular mucin using mucicarmine and D-PAS.

Mediastinal seminomas just like any other malignant neoplasm may spread within the thoracic cavity or invade below the diaphragm or above the thoracic inlet (Fig. 10.40a, b). The prognosis of these tumors, although good in general terms, is in great part determined by the stage of the tumor at the time of diagnosis. A common current practice is the medical treatment of these tumors prior to surgical resection. However, once medical treatment has been provided to a patient in whom the biopsy shows the presence of germ cell tumor, the surgical resection may just show extensive areas of necrosis and histiocytic reaction without any remaining viable tumor.

Immunohistochemical Features

Most of what is known about the immunohistochemical features of GCT is drawn from studies in testicular tumors. Beckstead [140] studied 32 cases of gonadal GCT using alkaline phosphatase and found that this antibody showed strong plasma membrane positivity in all 9 cases of seminoma in his study. The author suggested that alkaline phosphatase reaction is a useful adjunct in the diagnosis of GCT. Battifora and associates [97] studied the presence and distribution of keratin in 34 cases of GCT, including 18 seminomas. The authors found that all cases of seminomas gave negative results and suggested that the presence or absence of keratin can be helpful in distinguishing seminoma from other GCT such as embryonal carcinoma, which may show at least focal positive staining. Niehans and associates [141] studied 121 cases of GCT of diverse sites including gonadal and extragonadal primaries, using several antibodies including cytokeratin, vimentin, epithelial membrane antigen (EMA), placental-like alkaline phosphatase (PLAP), S-100 protein, leukocyte common antigen (LCA), CD-45 (T-and B-cell markers), LN-2, carcinoembryonic antigen (CEA), neuron-specific enolase (NSE), chromogranin A, Leu-7, alpha-fetoprotein (AFP), alpha-1-antitrypsin (AAT), and the beta-subunit of HCG. The authors concluded that the presence of PLAP-positive staining and negative EMA appeared to be a staining pattern unique for GCT in general. In addition, the authors also found that cytokeratin was helpful in distinguishing seminomas from non-seminomatous germ cell tumors. However, the authors acknowledged the presence of focal or diffuse-positive reaction for cytokeratin in approximately 10% of seminomas. NSE immunostaining was positive in about 75% of all GCT, while vimentin was found to be positive in approximately 30% of seminomas.

We have studied 50 cases of primary mediastinal seminomas using antibodies against PLAP, CAM 5.2 (low molecular weight keratin), wide-spectrum keratin, HCG, EMA, CEA, and AFP. Our results parallel those of other studies in that positive membrane and cytoplasmic staining for PLAP was observed in 80% of the cases. However, we also observed strong dot-like paranuclear positivity with CAM 5.2 in 75% of the cases using a microwave antigen retrieval technique. In addition, broad-spectrum keratin also showed weak cytoplasmic positivity in approximately 70% of the cases. The discrepancy with previous studies concerning keratin immunoreactivity in these tumors

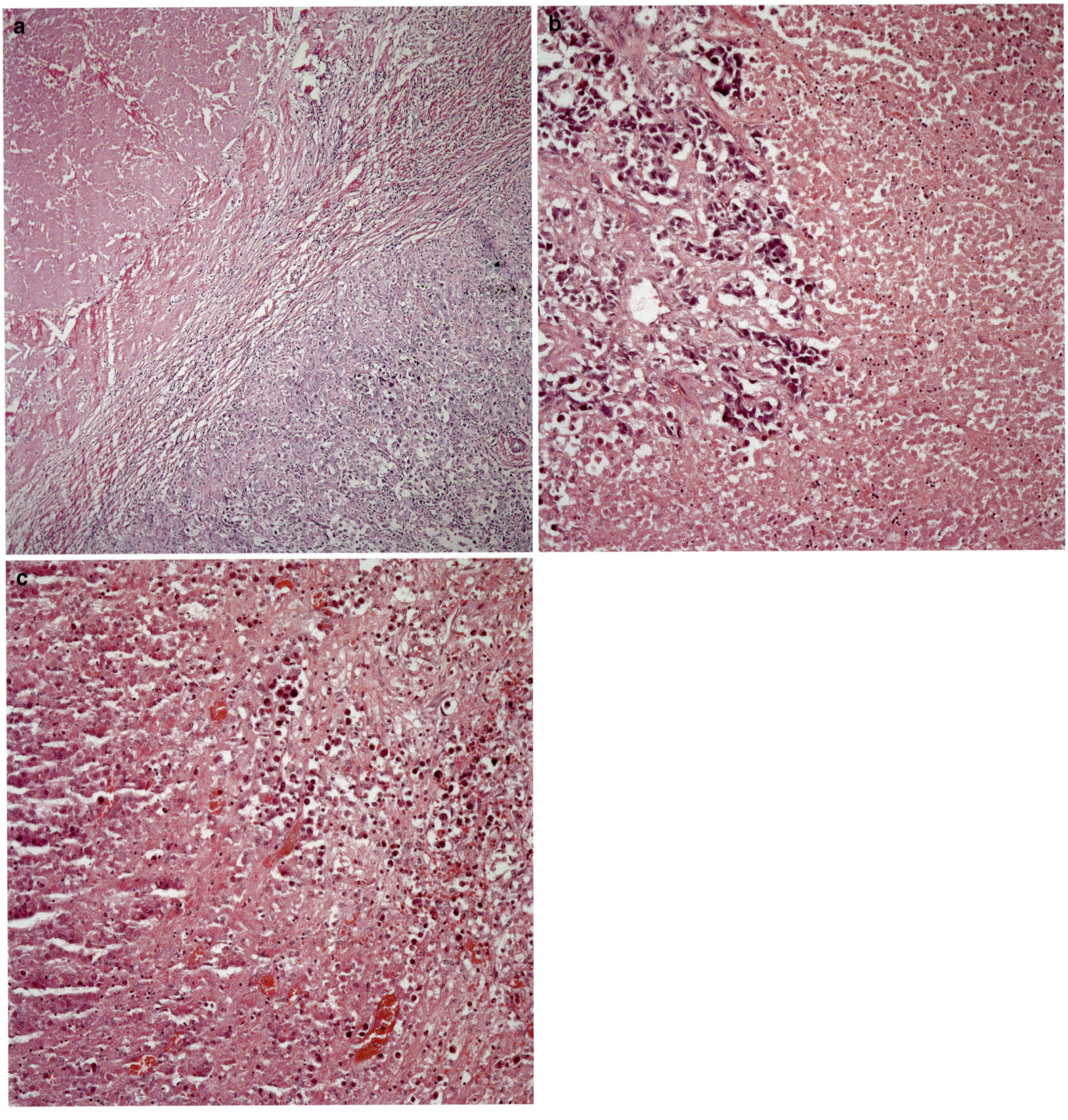

Fig. 10.36 (**a**) Seminoma showing areas of necrosis; however, the tumor cells are easily identified. (**b**) Seminoma with more extensive necrosis and only focal areas of viable tumor cells. (**c**) Extensive necrosis with only scattered tumor cells

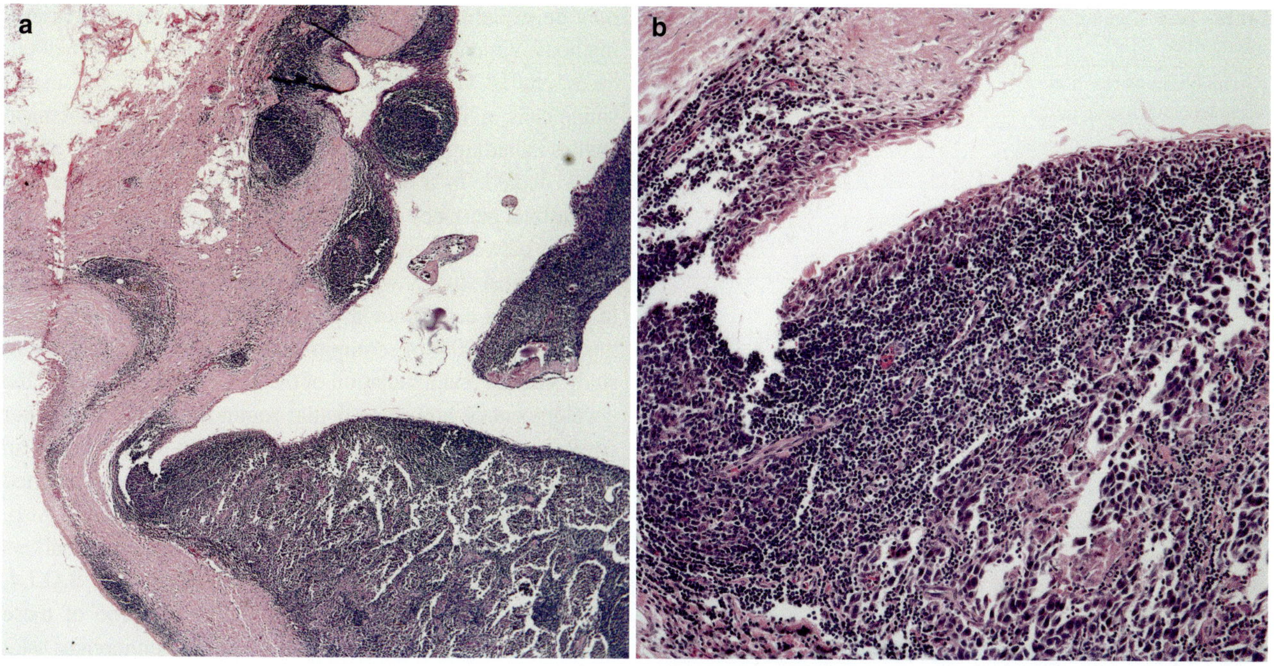

Fig. 10.37 (**a**) Predominantly cystic seminoma. (**b**) Higher magnification of a cystic seminoma showing conventional tumor cells

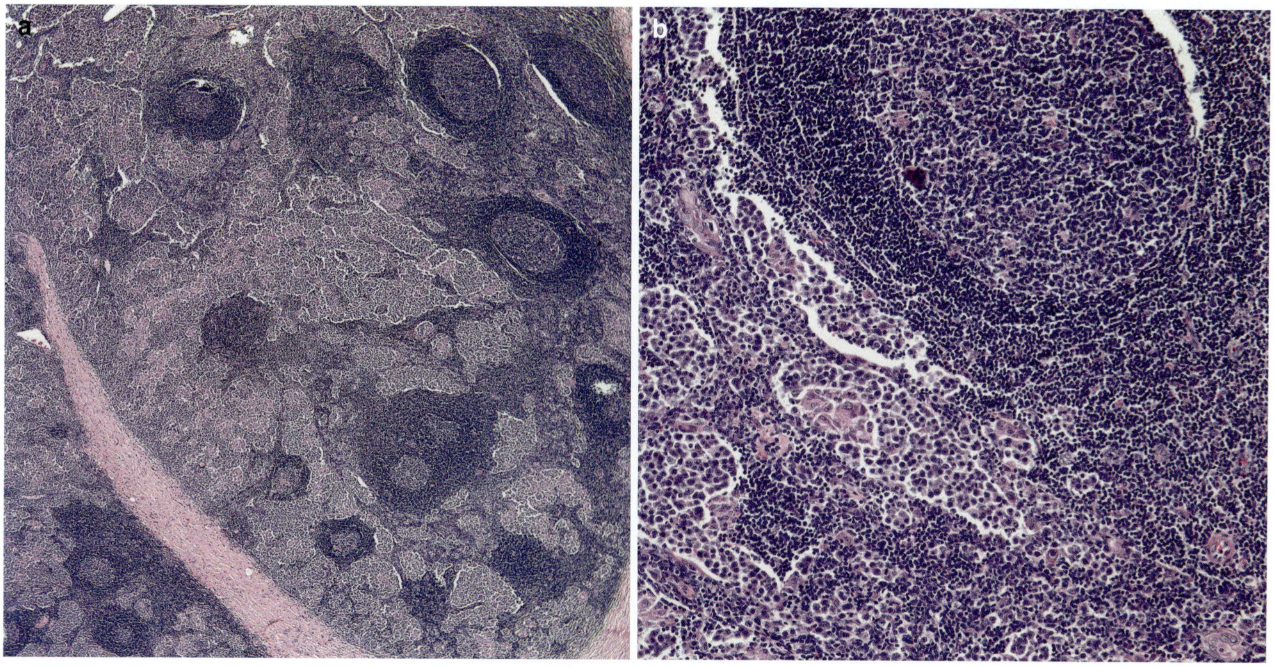

Fig. 10.38 (**a**) Seminoma with prominent lymphoid hyperplasia and presence of germinal centers. (**b**) Seminomatous areas adjacent to a germinal center

Table 10.5 Common histologic findings in 120 mediastinal seminomas

Granulomatous reaction	45%
Remnants of thymic tissue	27%
Necrosis	25%
Scattered giant cells	12%
Lymphoid follicular hyperplasia	<10%
Cystic changes	<10%
Trophoblastic giant cells	<5%

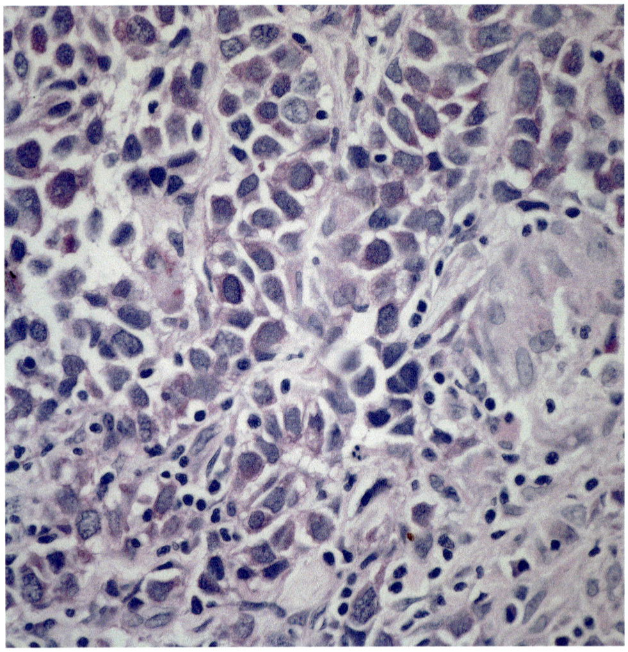

Fig. 10.39 Periodic acid-Schiff histochemical stain showing areas of intracellular glycogen in tumor cells

may be explained on the basis of improved antigen retrieval methods. Vimentin also showed positive staining in 50% of our cases; and HCG showed scattered, focal positivity of isolated single cells in 15% of the cases. Other immunohistochemical studies including CEA, EMA, and AFP were negative in all the cases studied. In a separate study comparing testicular and mediastinal germ cell tumors, we were able to detect some differences between these two groups [142]. In addition, immunohistochemical studies with p53 tumor suppressor gene protein in adult germ cell testicular tumors have shown expression of this protein in 90% of seminomatous tumors [143]. A different study showed that a mutation of the p53 gene is involved in the development of human testicular seminoma [144]. One other development worth mentioning is the recent availability of an anti-seminoma monoclonal antibody, which has been reported to be of value in the diagnosis of these neoplasms [145]. Also, seminomas have been investigated with the use of new markers including c-kit (CD-117) and the stem cell markers SALL4, OCT4, NANOG, UTF1, TCL1, and SOX2. Some of these markers have been reported to stain 100% of seminomas; c-kit may show positive staining in about 74% of the cases, while SOX2 has been consistently negative [146–148]. More recently, we performed an immunohistochemical study of 32 cases of primary mediastinal seminomas with emphasis on novel markers. We identified that 97% of tumor expressed SOX17, 91% showed positive staining for SALL4 and OCT3/4, and 88% stain positively for MAGEC2 and CAM5.2, while only 6% showed positive staining for polyclonal PAX8 and 3% for TCL1 (Fig. 10.41a–d). None of the tumors show positive staining for keratin 5/6, GATA-3, SOX3, and glypican 3 [149]. Table 10.6 depicts the immunohistochemical features more commonly associated with mediastinal seminomas.

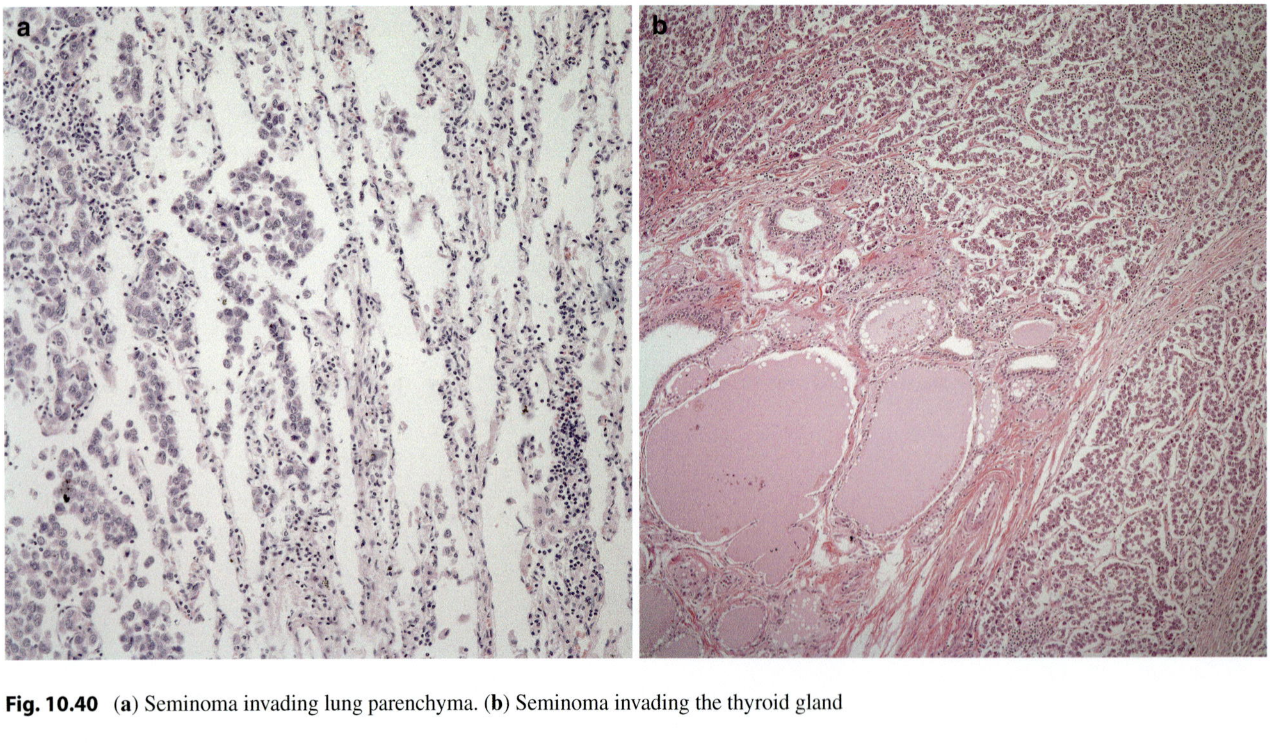

Fig. 10.40 (**a**) Seminoma invading lung parenchyma. (**b**) Seminoma invading the thyroid gland

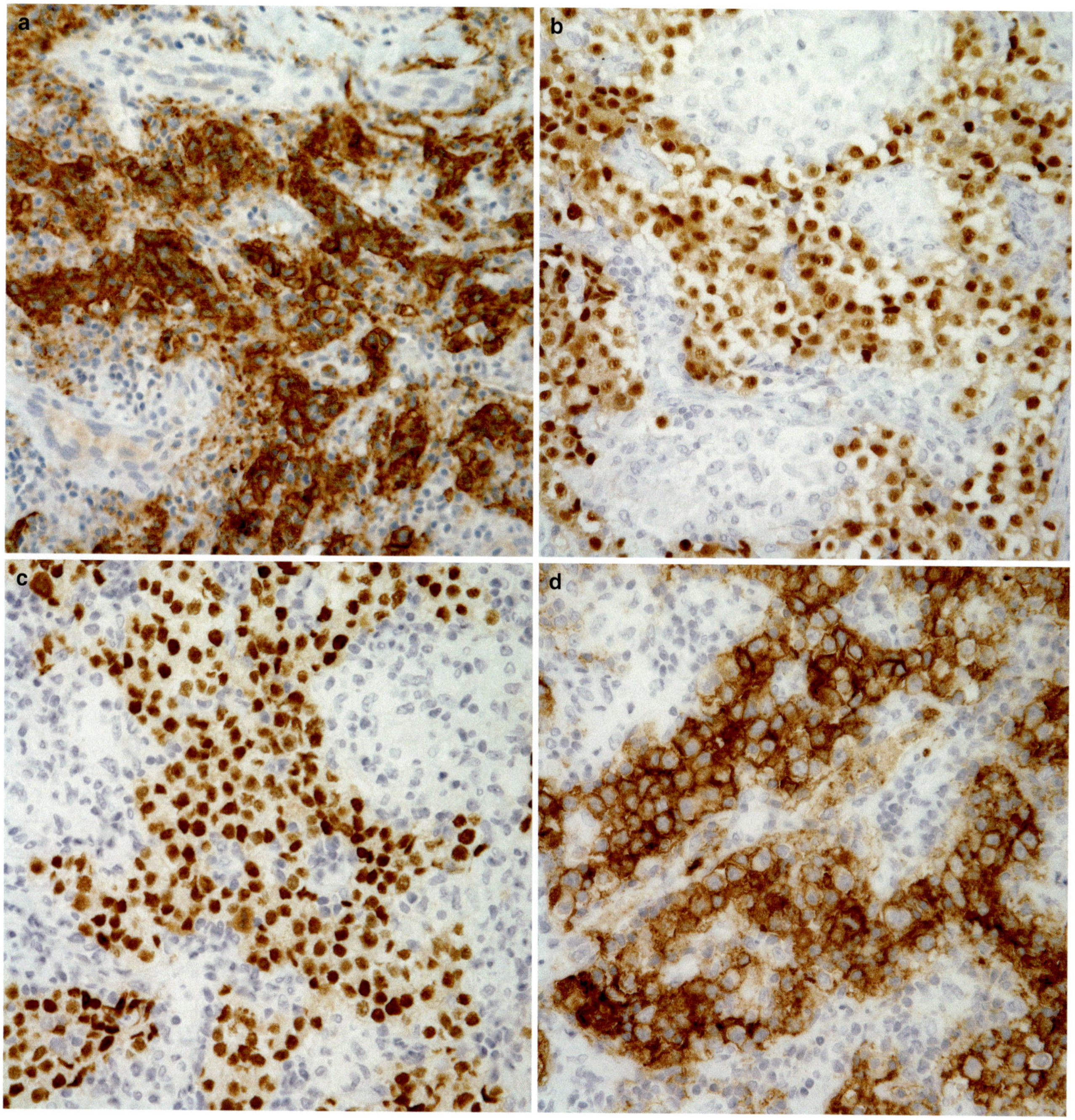

Fig. 10.41 (**a**) Seminoma showing positive staining for CD117. (**b**) Seminoma showing positive reaction in tumor cells for OCT 3/4. (**c**) Seminoma showing positive staining in tumor cells for SALL4. (**d**) Placental-like alkaline phosphatase showing positive reaction in tumor cells

Table 10.6 Immunohistochemical profile of MGCT

Tumor	PLAP	AFP	CAM5.2	HCG	SALL4	Glypican	OCT3/4	CD30	CD117
Seminoma	++	–	++	–	++	–	–/+	–	++
YST	–	++	++	–	++	+	–	–	+
E.C.	–	++	++	–				++	
ChorioCa	–	–	+	++	–	–	–	––	––

Ultrastructural Features

There are a few reports of ultrastructural studies of primary mediastinal seminomas. Levine [106] described the ultrastructural features in a case of primary mediastinal seminoma and concluded that these tumors shared similar features with their gonadal counterpart. The most salient ultrastructural features of mediastinal seminomas include the presence of large, round nuclei with smooth contours and fine, evenly dispersed nuclear chromatin, abundant cytoplasm poor in organelles, and abundant glycogen particles forming small glycogen rosettes or arranged in focal clusters (Fig. 10.42). Another rather distinctive feature in seminoma, although by no means pathognomonic, is the presence of loose, elongated rope-like nucleolonema within the nuclei of the cells. The cell membranes are generally round and smooth and voided of specialized organelles such as microvilli, complex interdigitating, or well-developed cell junctions. Rudimentary junctions and occasional desmosomes may be seen.

Differential Diagnosis

The most important differential diagnosis is with metastatic seminoma from a gonadal primary, even though such occurrence is highly unusual. Nevertheless, a careful clinical history and physical examination is always important. Other tumoral conditions that should be considered in the differential diagnosis include metastatic melanoma, thymic carcinoma, and malignant lymphoma, especially Hodgkin's lymphoma and large cell lymphoma. The use of immunohistochemical studies can help in solving this problem, as melanomas would show positive staining using antibodies for S-100 protein, HMB-45, and Pan Mel. The same applies to lymphoma and thymic carcinoma. In the former studies for LCA, B- and T-cell markers, Leu-M1 (CD-15), and CD-30 can be helpful, while in the latter the use of PLAP can lead to a correct interpretation. Nonetheless, the issue in a small biopsy can be more challenging, and a careful study of the morphology of the tumor becomes of utmost importance. Important to highlight is the unusual association of seminoma with another non-GCT, which may be difficult to diagnose in a small mediastinoscopic biopsy, which in turn may also affect treatment decisions. Some of these tumors' treatment of choice may depend on the initial interpretation of the mediastinal tumor. Finally, in cases of cystic seminomas, judicious sampling is highly important in order to identify diagnosable areas of seminoma.

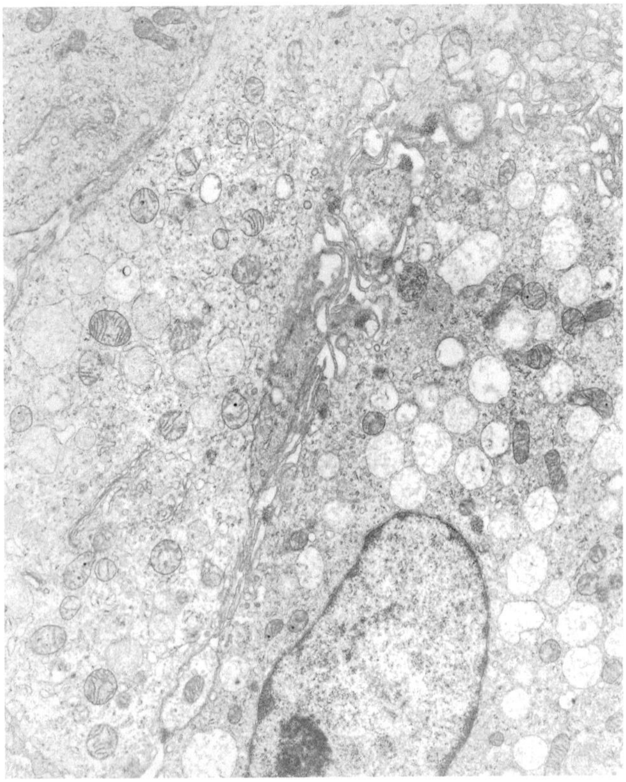

Fig. 10.42 Ultrastructural study of a mediastinal seminoma showing abundant glycogen droplets, classical of seminoma

Non-seminomatous Germ Cell Tumor

The term non-seminomatous germ cell tumor as used in this chapter refers to a group of tumors that encompasses yolk sac tumor (endodermal sinus tumor), embryonal carcinoma, and choriocarcinoma. As a group, non-seminomatous germ cell tumors are still outnumbered by seminoma as primary malignant germ cell tumors of the mediastinum. When NS-GCT occurs in the anterior mediastinum, these tumors show striking predilection for males in the third and fourth decades of life, just the same as seminomas. However, unlike mediastinal seminomas, these neoplasms have a clearly documented association with non-germ cell malignancies and Klinefelter's syndrome. Serum tumor markers for AFP and β-HCG are elevated in over 80% of patients with non-seminomatous germ cell tumors and may be of aid for diagnosis and for monitoring treatment. Elevated serum AFP may be seen with either yolk sac tumor or embryonal carcinoma, whereas marked elevation of β-HCG will be highly suggestive of choriocarcinoma. Antibodies specific for these peptide markers are of great value for histopathologic diagnosis.

Yolk Sac Tumor

Yolk sac tumor (YST) is also known as embryonal carcinoma infantile type or endodermal sinus tumor. YST in the mediastinum is a rare neoplasm. This tumor appears to be a common testicular GCT in childhood, while in adults it is more often associated with other GCT [150]. Teilum [151] in 1959 first described this neoplasm and observed that a mixture of undifferentiated neoplastic "mesoblastic cells" and irregular spaces closely resembling the endodermal sinuses of Duval, characteristic of the rat's placenta, were features of YST. In Teilum's opinion, this tumor represented a proliferation of entirely undifferentiated embryonal cells differentiating toward extraembryonic membrane structures such as the mesoblast and yolk sac endoderm.

In 1967, Teilmann and associates [13] were the first to describe an example of YST in the anterior mediastinum in a 33-year-old man. At autopsy, the tumor showed extensive metastases; however, the testes did not show any evidence of neoplasm. The authors therefore concluded that the mediastinal region was the primary site for this tumor.

YST in extragonadal location and more specifically in the mediastinum is rare [152–164]. Although these tumors occur more frequently in the third and fourth decades of life, YST may also occur in infants [155]. These tumors appear to predominate in males; however, there are a few reports of these tumors in females [152, 155, 162]. To assess a specific incidence is rather difficult in view of their rarity. In our experience, YST is the most common non-seminomatous/non-teratomatous malignant GCT of the mediastinum, and accounts for approximately 12% of all MGCT [17]. In our study, these tumors were more prevalent in the third and fourth decades of life, with only sporadic cases found in the second and fifth decades of life [165]. We did not find any cases of YST in females.

Clinical Features

The clinical presentation of these tumors will be directly related to their size. Larger tumors are likely to compress adjacent structures, and the patients may present with symptoms of dyspnea, cough, chest pain, or superior vena cava syndrome. On the other hand, some patients may be completely asymptomatic [156]. An unusual presentation for YST is mimicking pericardial effusion [154]. The presence of increase levels of alpha-fetoprotein in the serum is a feature highly suggestive of YST [166, 167].

Interestingly, a few other medical conditions have been associated with mediastinal YST. Sogge and associates [168] documented a case of mediastinal YST in a 26-year-old man in association with Klinefelter's syndrome. The patient had a buccal smear with about 20% of Barr bodies, small testes, without palpable masses, and no gynecomastia. Similar findings of YST in association with Klinefelter's syndrome and Klinefelter's syndrome with sexual precocity were described by Nichols and associates and Floret and associates, respectively [169, 170].

Hematologic disturbances have also been associated with YST. Garnick and associates [171] found an association between idiopathic thrombocytopenia and mediastinal non-seminomatous GCT. The authors stated that the presence of thrombocytopenia might be an adverse prognostic feature for patients with extragonadal GCT. Nichols and associates [172] in 1990 reported 16 additional cases of hematologic neoplasms associated with primary mediastinal GCT and reviewed 27 similar cases reported in the literature. The median time between the diagnosis of GCT and the development of hematologic neoplasia was about 5 months. In 13 of the patients, both conditions occurred simultaneously, leading the authors to suggest that the development of hematologic neoplasia in this setting is not the result of chemotherapy for the GCT. The association of hematologic neoplasia and GCT appears to be more intimately related with tumors showing yolk sac elements. The most common lymphoproliferative lesion associated with YST appears to be acute megakaryoblastic leukemia and malignant histiocytosis. It is of interest that, in one patient with this association, a cytogenetic abnormality of the chromosome i12p was found in the GCT and in the leukemic blasts, thus suggesting a common progenitor cell for both processes. Nonetheless, the authors stated that the cytogenetic abnormalities were not consistent. Most recently, Orazi and associates [173] stated that hematopoietic precursor cells within the yolk sac tumor component are the source of secondary hematopoietic malignancies in patients with MGCT.

Another unusual event in these tumors is the secondary development of sarcomatous elements. Some authors have claimed that the pluripotential nature of the mesenchyme-like component of YST may give rise to sarcomas occurring in some patients with treated germ cell neoplasms [174, 175]. Ulbright and associates [176] documented such experience in 14 patients with GCT.

The radiologic findings displayed by YST are by no means pathognomonic of this tumor. The same as with other non-seminomatous GCT, radiographically, the tumor may be smooth or lobulated, well circumscribed, or ill defined. On CT scans, the tumor may show heterogeneous attenuation. Large central regions of low attenuation may occupy up to 50% of the lesion and correspond to areas of necrosis and/or hemorrhage [43].

The treatment and prognosis of non-seminomatous GCT in general have changed over the years. The median survival rate for these tumors in the older literature was about 8 months [152]. However, many patients included in those studies may not have benefited from the more modern treatment protocols presently available. In 1976, Kurman and Norris [177] analyzed 71 cases of yolk sac tumors of the ovary documenting only 9 survivors among 65 patients in whom follow-up was available. The survival rate after 3 years was 13%, while in 93% of the cases the neoplasm recurred within 1 year after diagnosis. Interestingly, about 90% of the deaths occurred within 2 years after diagnosis. The authors concluded that size and stage of the tumor had prognostic significance. In the mediastinal location, it has been estimated that 27% of the patients will have metastatic disease at the time of the presentation [152]. The most common sites for metastases of mediastinal YST include the lymph node, liver, lung, and brain. The apparently high incidence of metastases at presentation suggests a rapid growth of the tumor.

In Hainsworth's experience with 32 patients with extragonadal GCT, the authors concluded that intensive chemotherapy (cis platinum-based) and surgical resection offer the best results in the management of these tumors [130]. In this study, 89% of the patients survived after a follow-up period of 30 months. Economou and associates [63] reported 28 patients with mediastinal GCT, including 17 patients with non-seminomatous tumors showing only 18% survival after a period between 6 months and 15 years. The authors concluded that non-seminomatous GCT treated with cisplatin-bleomycin chemotherapy had a median survival of 14 months, while those treated with different modalities showed a survival rate of 4 months. However, long-term survival can also occur in patients treated with surgery and combination of chemotherapy and radiation therapy [159]. Another useful parameter for evaluating the prognosis of non-seminomatous GCT of the mediastinum is the return to normal of serum levels of tumor markers (AFP, HCG) after cisplatin therapy [178]. Most authors agree that the most adequate treatment needs to be aggressive including surgical resection and chemotherapy [64, 179–183]. In general, the 5-year survival rate for non-seminomatous GCT varies from 8% to 58% in different series [64, 127, 183].

Our experience mirrors that of the literature: out of 38 cases of YST of the mediastinum that we were able to follow, only 13% of the patients survived 2 years after diagnosis, while approximately 45% of them died of tumor within the same period of time. However, most of our cases included patients who were diagnosed and treated prior to the advent of more modern therapeutic modalities. The use of the current more aggressive germ cell treatment protocols should favorably impact on the outcome of these patients.

Gross Features

These tumors tend to be unencapsulated, large, soft tissue masses with a tendency to invade adjacent structures. The size of the tumors varies from a few centimeters to 20 cm in greatest dimension. Areas of hemorrhage and/or necrosis may be evident (Fig. 10.43). However, there are no distinct gross features that allow distinction from seminomas or other non-seminomatous tumors.

Histologic Features

The histopathological features of YST are quite distinctive, and a diagnosis can be made in the majority of instances with relative ease on routine microscopy. However, it is important to highlight that YST is probably the most versatile GCT in

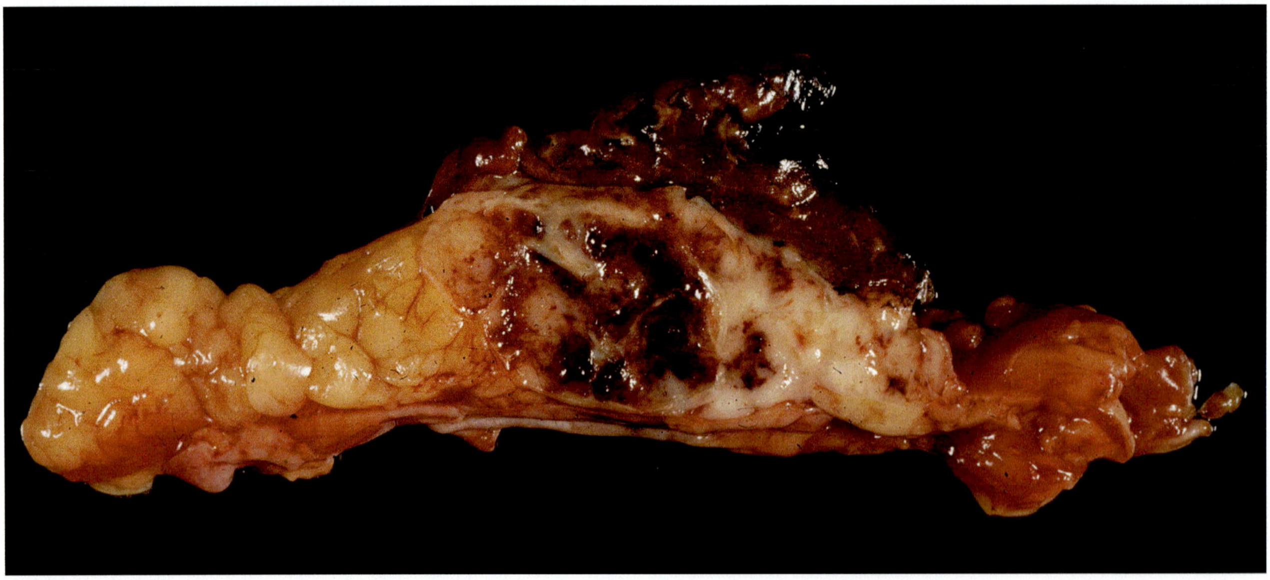

Fig. 10.43 Mediastinal yolk sac tumor showing non-encapsulated, partially hemorrhagic tumor mass

the anterior mediastinum. A variety of growth patterns have been described for these tumors in the gonads, including the reticular, vitelline, pseudo papillary, solid, myxomatous, sarcomatoid, macrocystic, and hepatoid [150]. In our experience, all those histopathologic growth patterns are also recapitulated in mediastinal yolk sac tumors [184–186].

The low-power magnification of these tumors may show different growth patterns, thus the importance to keep this tumor in the differential diagnosis of the different neoplasms that may seed the anterior mediastinum. In some cases, the tumor may be just adjacent to thymic tissue, which lends support to the notion that the tumor is likely to originate from the thymic gland (Fig. 10.44). In some unusual cases, the tumor may be adjacent to areas of thymic tissue showing areas similar to those described as multilocular thymic cyst (Fig. 10.45). The tumor may also show more common growth patterns including reticular, myxoid, glandular, papillary, the so-called intestinal-like growth pattern, solid, hepatoid, pseudovascular, spindle cell, or a combination of them (Fig. 10.46a–j). The most common appearance of these tumors is the reticular pattern, which is characterized by areas containing a loose meshwork of glandular or ductal structures that are lined by low columnar to flattened epithelial cells resulting in microcystic intercellular spaces, separated by basement membrane-like material. In many cases, the neoplastic cellular proliferation may show a prominent myxoid background. However, in other areas, the neoplastic cellular proliferation may adopt a more prominent macrocystic appearance. In some areas, the neoplastic cells may alternate with areas showing an edematous stroma. The neoplastic cells can be disposed in sheets interspersed with cystic areas, while in other areas the tumor may show a papillary configuration alternating with more solid foci. However, in some cases, the neoplastic cells appear to be around sclerotic vessels (Fig. 10.47a–c). The presence of Schiller-Duval bodies characteristic of yolk sac tumors will greatly facilitate the diagnosis. These structures consist of papillary projections lined by primitive epithelial cells that extend into the microcystic spaces and contain a single central blood vessel. Another distinctive feature of YST is the presence of brightly eosinophilic PAS-positive, diastase-resistant hyaline globules scattered within the stroma and intracellularly (Fig. 10.48). These hyaline globules have been shown to be composed of aggregates of alpha-fetoprotein and other plasma proteins. Focal areas in these tumors may show striking cellular atypia with presence of bizarre mitotic figures and large hyperchromatic nuclei. In other areas, the neoplastic cellular proliferation may show a prominent perivascular arrangement. In some tumors, focal areas in which there is a marked spindling of the neoplastic cells can be identified. However, the reticular pattern characterized by ribbons of neoplastic cells, presence of intra and extracellular hyaline droplets, and Schiller-Duval bodies is

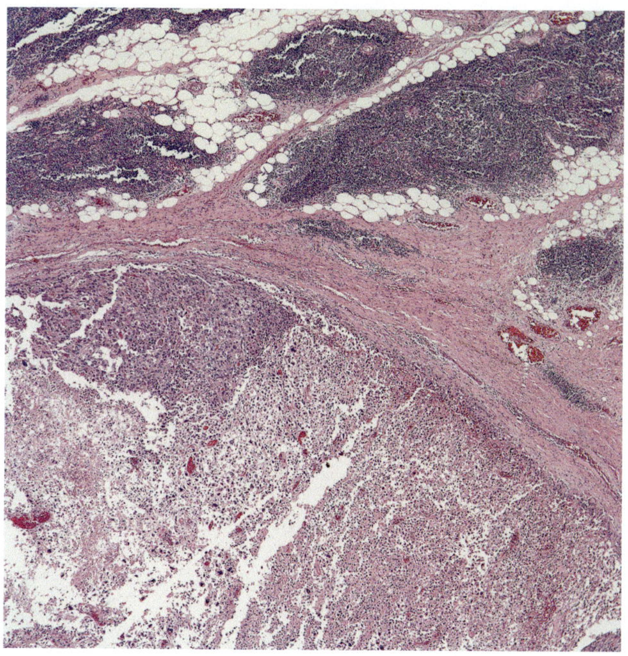

Fig. 10.44 Yolk sac tumor adjacent to thymic gland

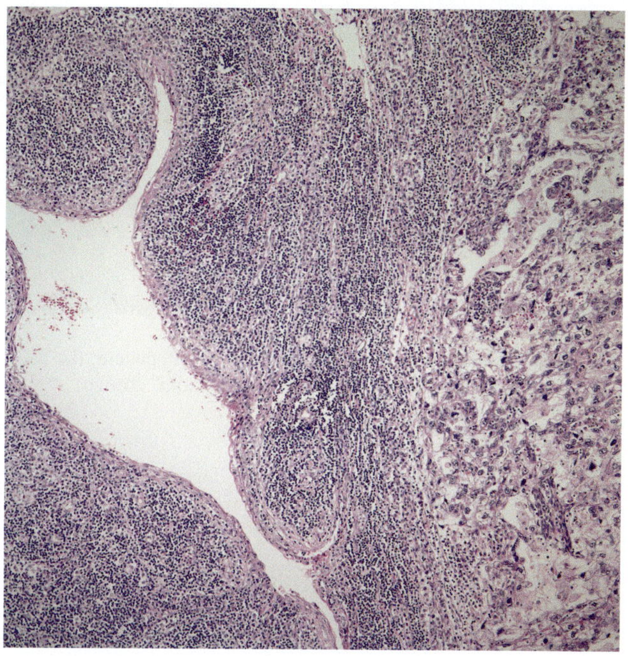

Fig. 10.45 YST adjacent to cystic thymic areas similar to those described in multilocular thymic cyst

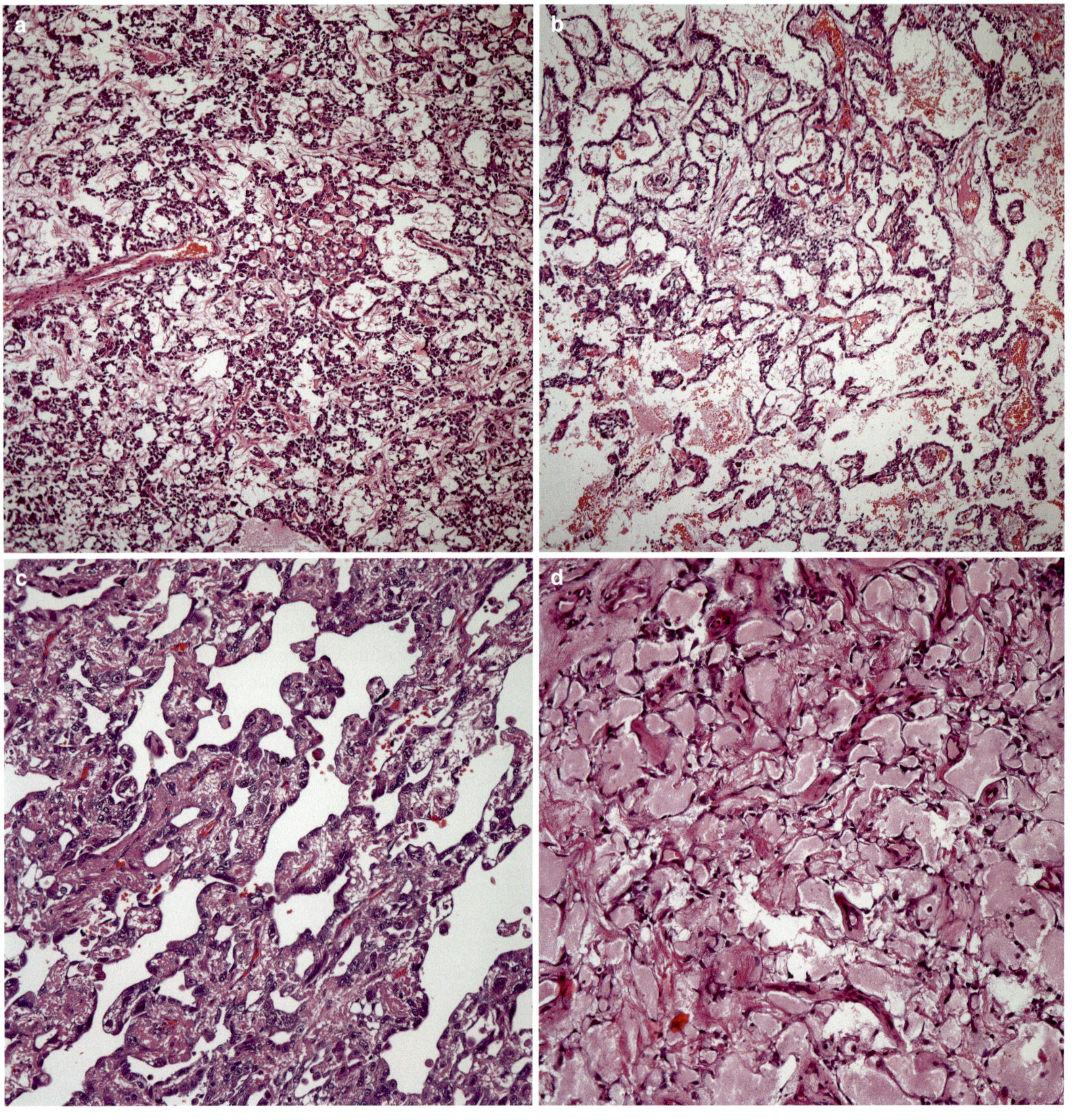

Fig. 10.46 (**a**) YST tumor shows a reticular growth pattern; (**b**) YST showing a microcystic growth pattern; (**c**) YST showing a pseudovascular pattern; (**d**) YST with prominent edematous "myxoid" change

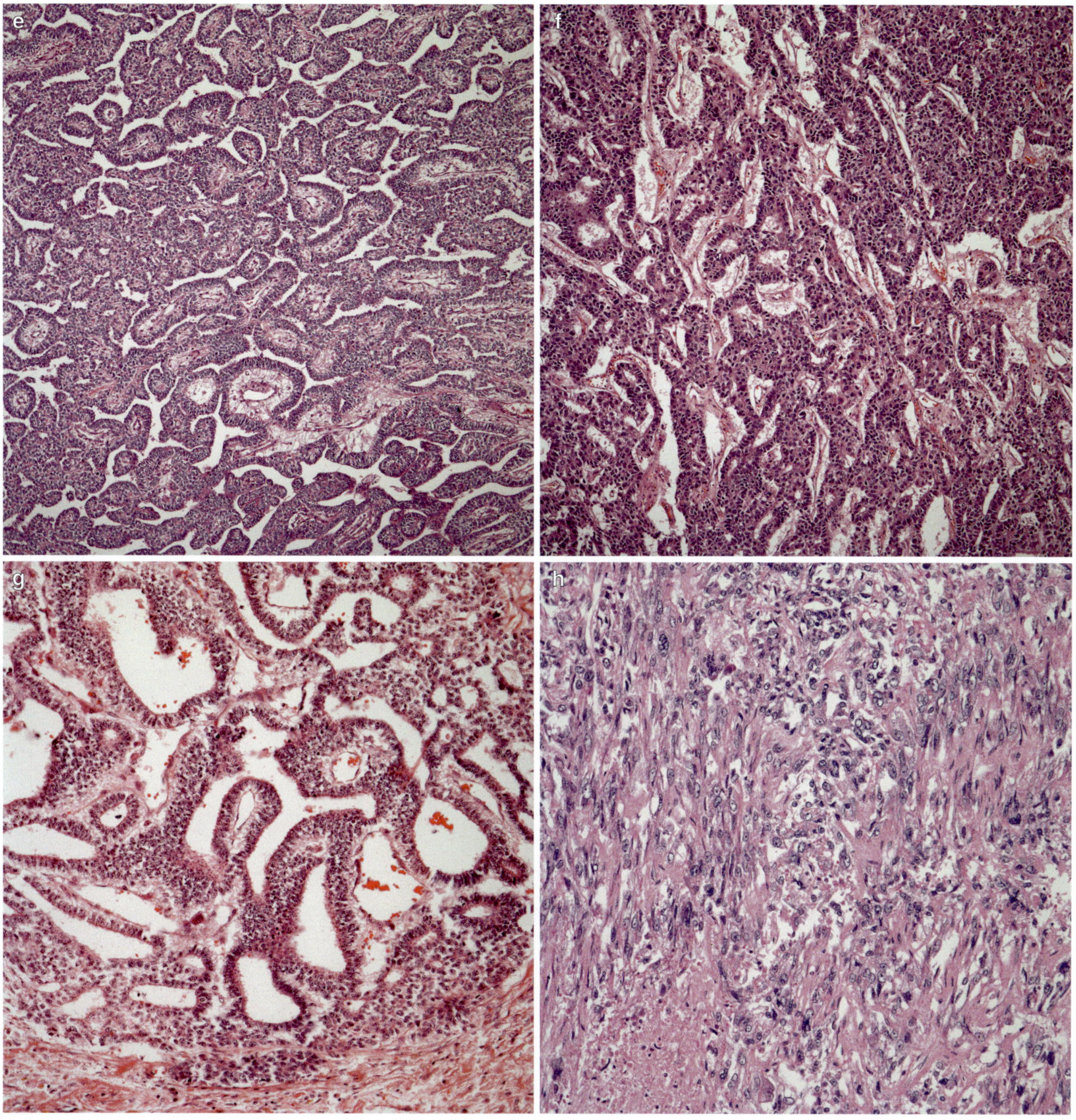

Fig. 10.46 (continued) (**e**) YST with a pseudoglandular appearance; (**f**) YST with glandular-like appearance; (**g**) YST with more "embryonic glandular appearance"; (**h**) YST with spindle cell features

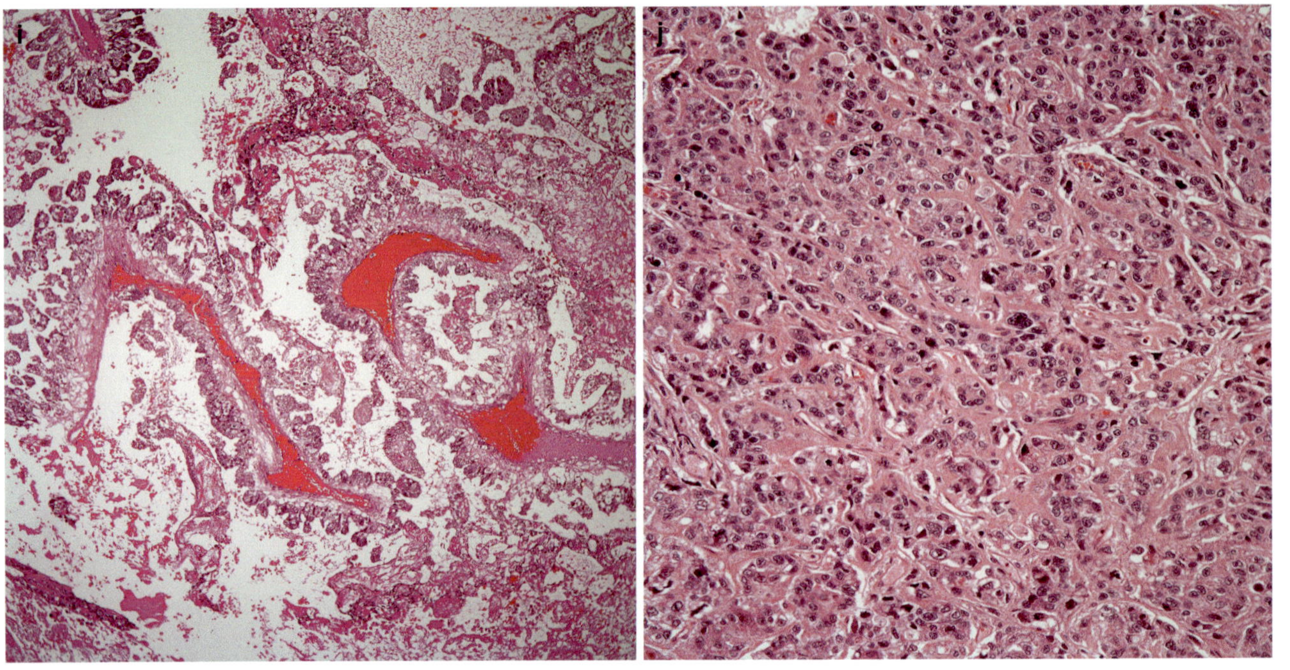

Fig. 10.46 (continued) (**i**) YST with the so-called "intestinal" growth pattern; (**j**) YST with solid growth pattern

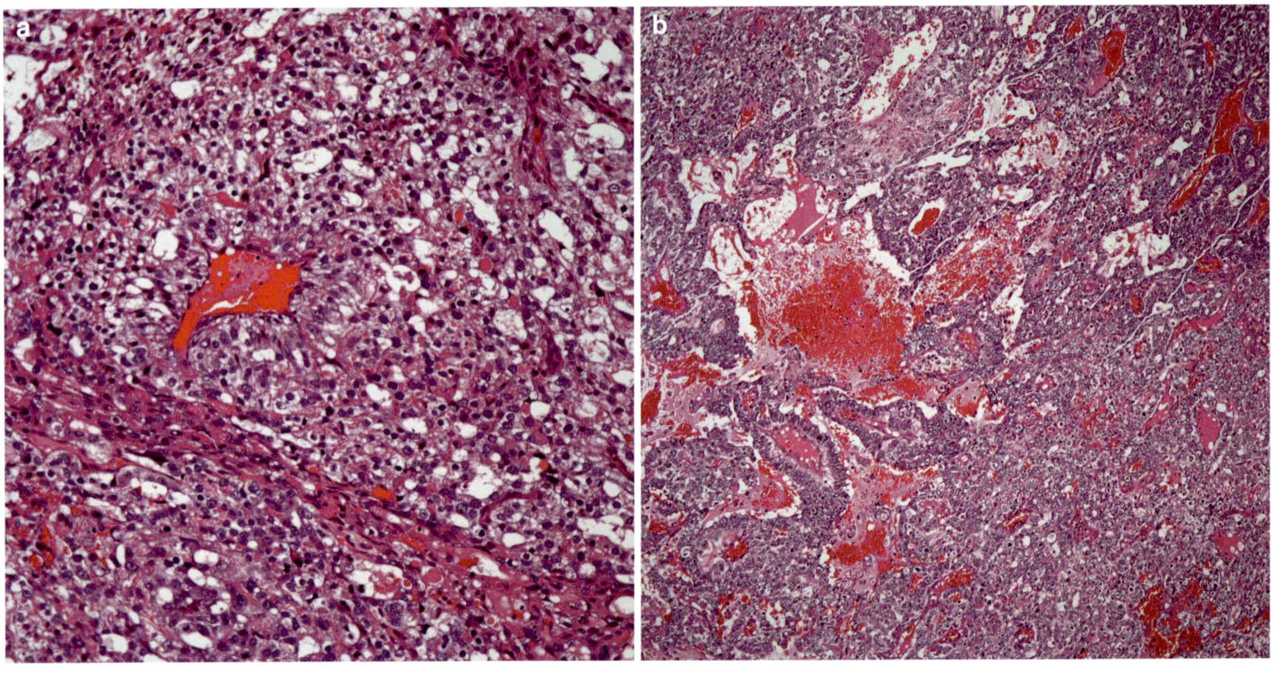

Fig. 10.47 (**a**) YST showing a Schiller-Duval body in a solid clear cell pattern. (**b**) Several Schiller-Duval bodies are present in this rather solid growth pattern

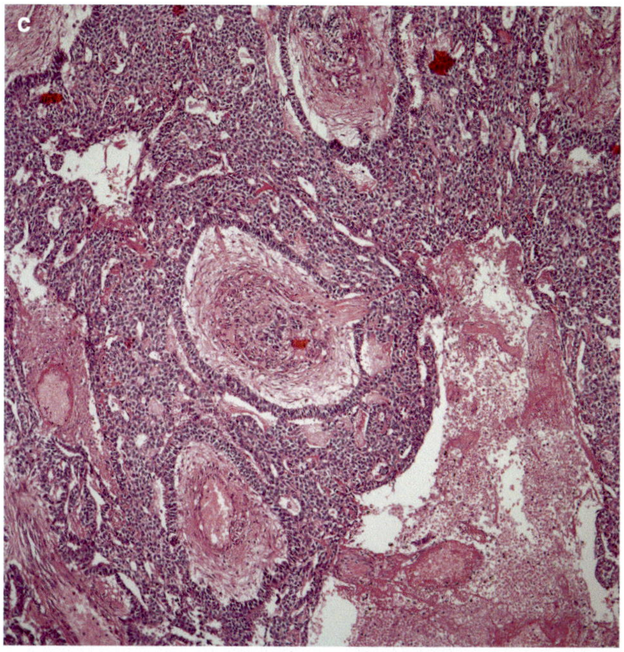

Fig. 10.47 (continued) (**c**) In some cases, the tumor cells are arranged around fibrotic or sclerotic vessels

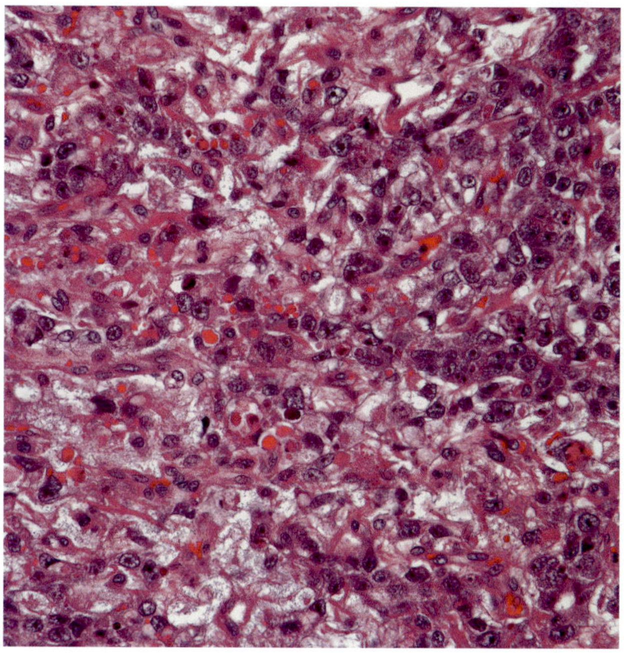

Fig. 10.48 Higher magnification of a YST tumor showing numerous hyaline globules

the most classic presentation of yolk sac tumors. In general, the high cytological features of YST are those of a proliferation of rather small cells, with round to oval nuclei and inconspicuous nucleoli (Fig. 10.49a–d). In some cases, the neoplastic cells may show prominent clear cytoplasm (Fig. 10.50a, b). Mitotic figures and areas of necrosis and hemorrhage may also be present (Fig. 10.51a–d). An unusual histopathologic growth pattern of yolk sac tumors that can be observed in the mediastinum is the so-called hepatoid variant, which is characterized by a tightly cohesive, solid neoplastic proliferation of cells with abundant cytoplasm that resembles liver tissue. In this growth pattern, it is also possible to observe cellular atypia and mitotic figures (Fig. 10.52a–d). Occasionally, more differentiated tissues of endodermal origin may be present in YST, including enteric-like glands or endometrioid-like areas. Another relatively unusual feature of YST that we have observed in the mediastinum is the presence of prominent cystic changes similar to those seen in multilocular thymic cysts and cystic seminomas [136]. In our experience, this unusual presentation accounts for less than 5% of these tumors.

Just like with other malignant neoplasm, the tumor may also invade adjacent organs such as the pleura, pericardium, or lung (Fig. 10.53). Also, the tumor may invade other structures below the diaphragm or above the thoracic inlet.

The current practice of treating patients with MGCT with chemotherapy followed by surgical resection in many cases does not provide enough viable tumor to confidently determine the percentage of tumor that may be present.

Immunohistochemical Features

The use of immunohistochemistry has shown that these tumors may display positive staining for AFP, CEA, keratin, and alpha-1-antitripsin (AAT) [97, 152, 187]. Stains for PLAP, EMA, NSE, Leu-7, and vimentin have also shown some variable positivity [139]. In our experience, in addition to the above mentioned stains, we also noted a strong positive reaction of the tumor cells with low molecular weight keratin CAM 5.2 [165]. Also, we have seen YST showing strong positive reaction for SALL4, while CD117 and Glypican may show only focal positive staining in tumor cells (Fig. 10.54a–e). The most reliable and consistent stain supporting the diagnosis of YST, however, is AFP.

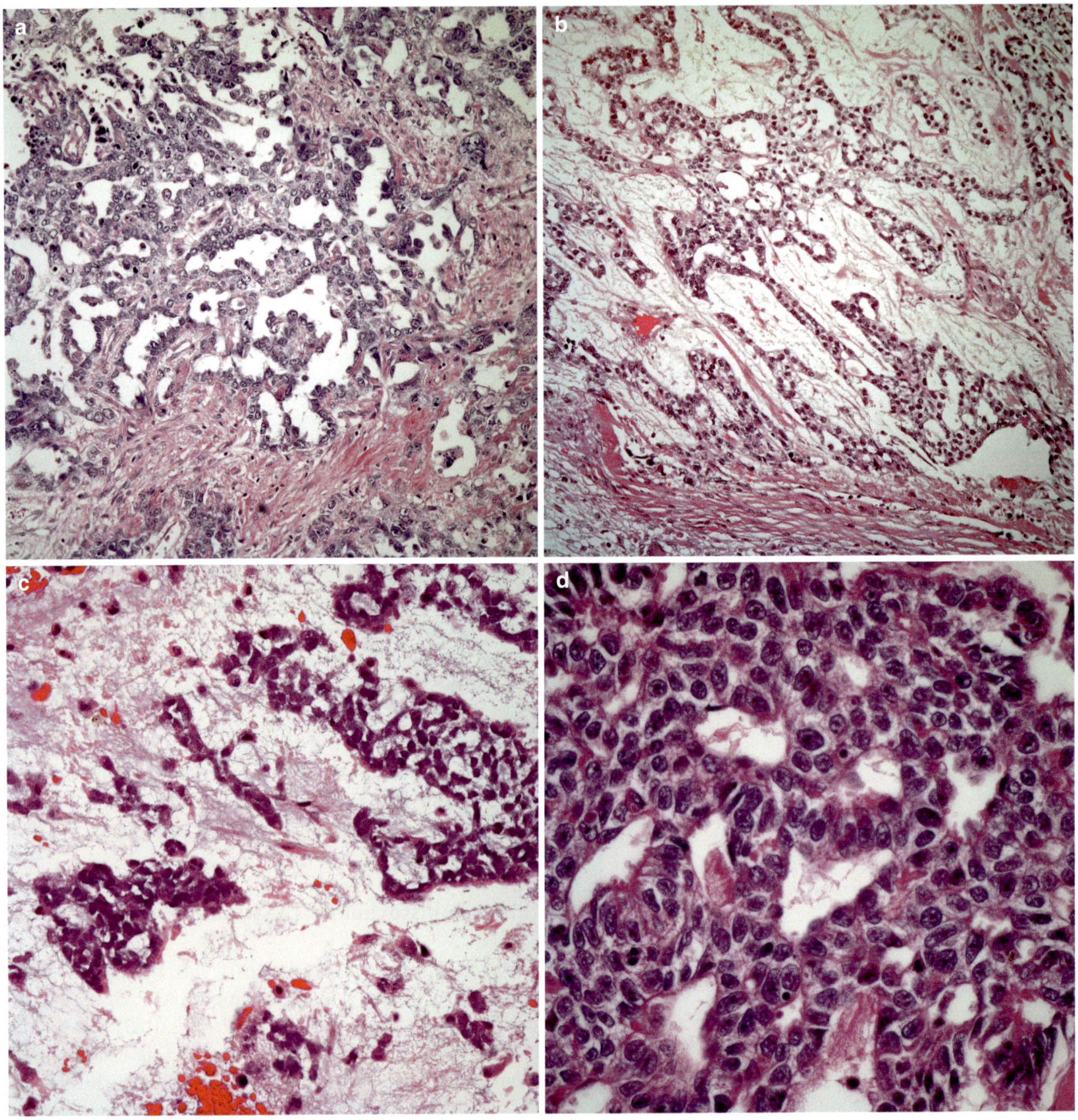

Fig. 10.49 (**a**) YST showing a neoplastic cellular proliferation composed of rather small cells without marked nuclear atypia or mitotic activity. (**b**) Ribbons of neoplastic cells embedded in a myxoid stroma without increased mitotic activity or nuclear atypia. (**c**) Clusters of small cells embedded in a mucinous stroma. Note the absence of increase mitotic activity. (**d**) High-power view of the small cells with round to oval nuclei and inconspicuous nucleoli

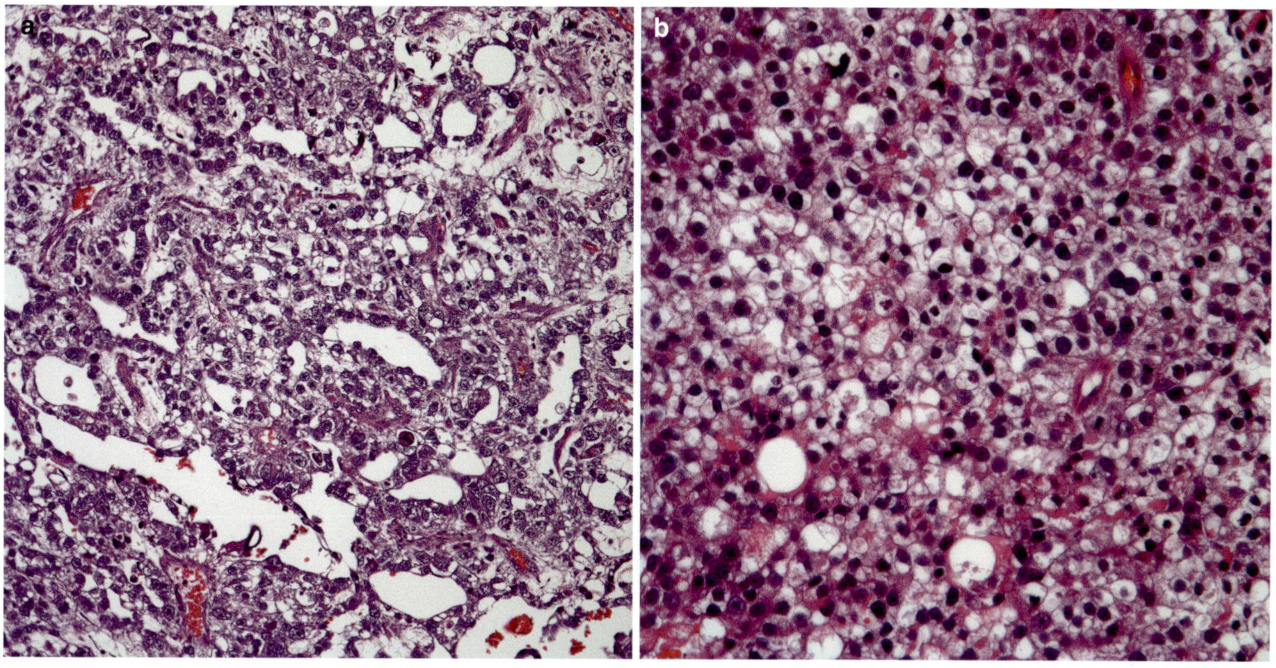

Fig. 10.50 (**a**) YST tumor showing cells with clear cytoplasm. (**b**) High-power magnification showing YST composed of rather small cells with clear cytoplasm

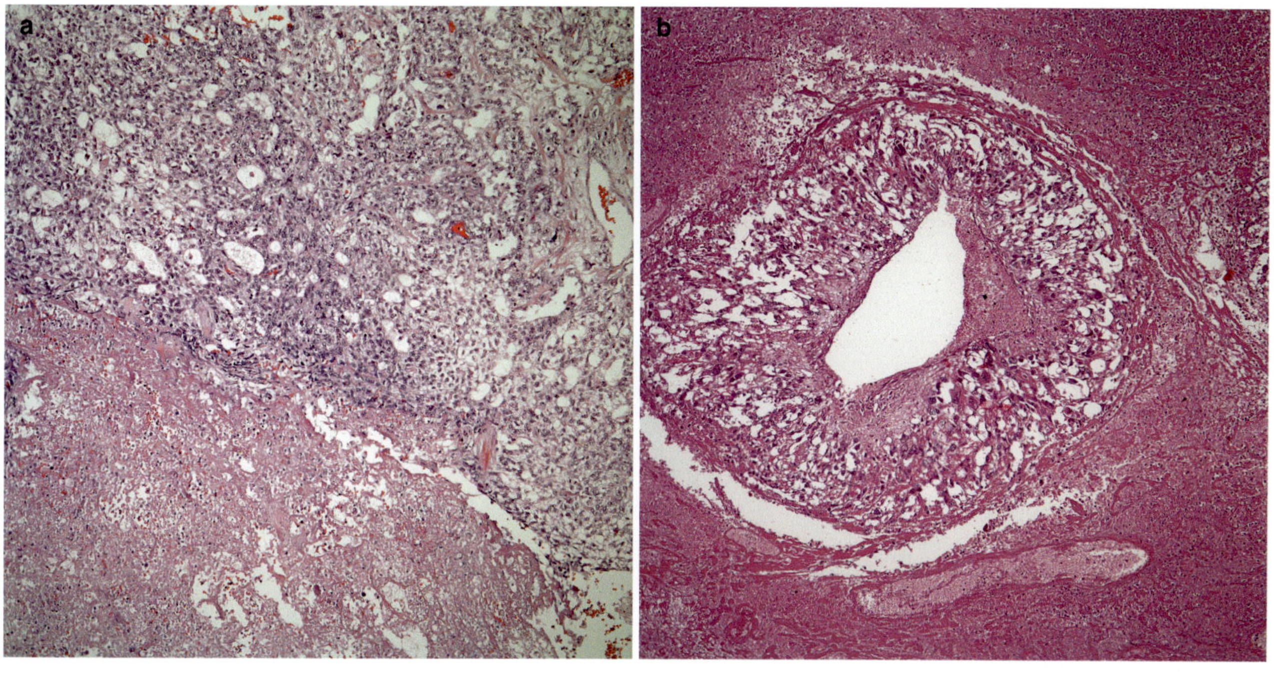

Fig. 10.51 (**a**) YST showing areas of necrosis. (**b**) Extensive necrosis is present with only focal areas of YST; note the Schiller-Duval body

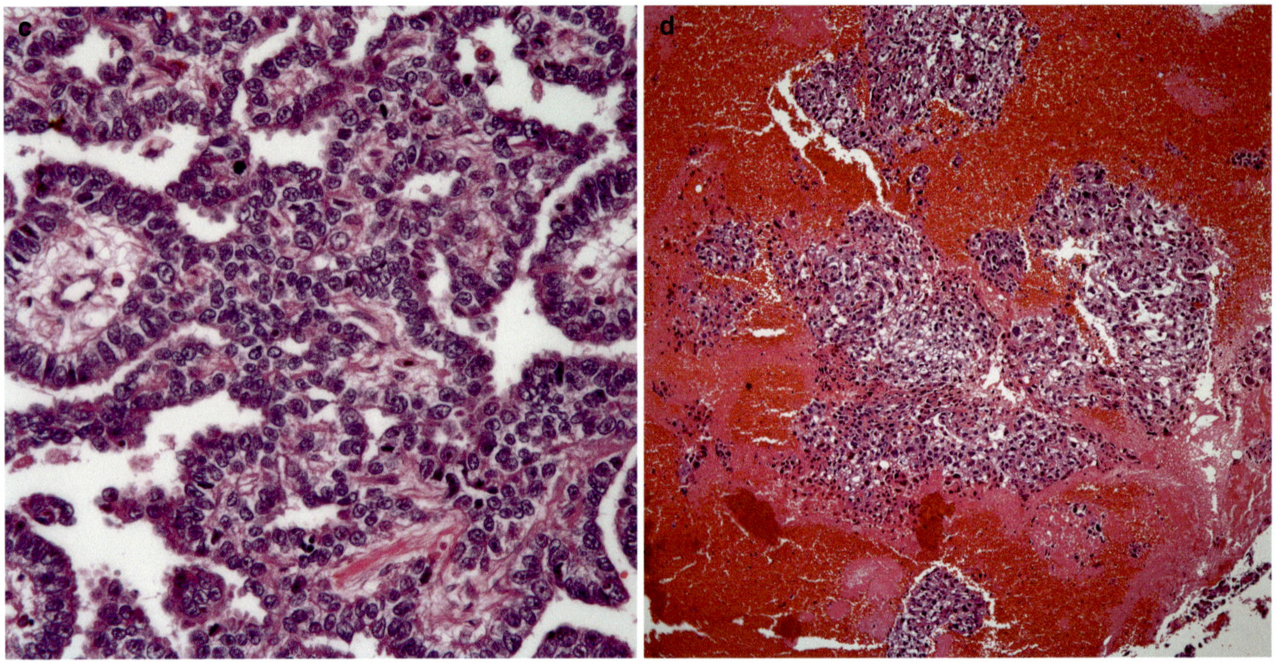

Fig. 10.51 (continued) (**c**) Solid growth pattern of YST showing numerous mitotic figures. (**d**) YST showing areas of hemorrhage

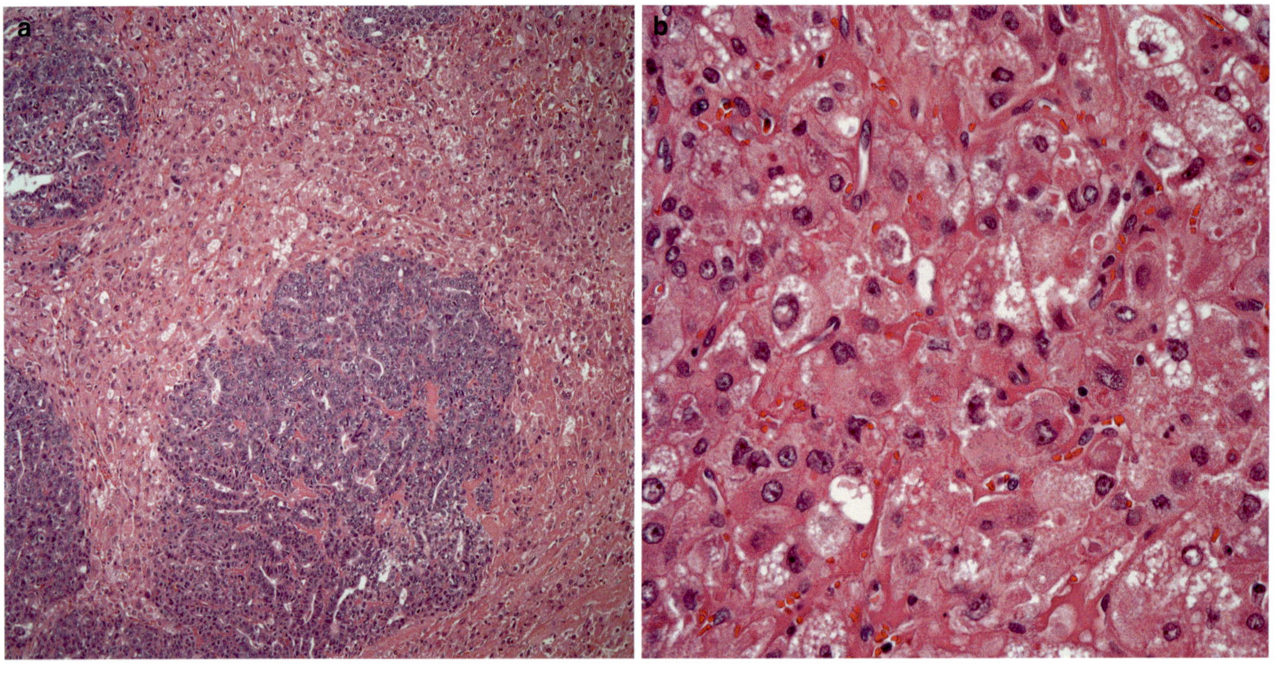

Fig. 10.52 (**a**) YST showing focal conventional areas admixed with hepatoid growth pattern. (**b**) Higher magnification of the hepatoid variant showing large cells with eosinophilic cytoplasm

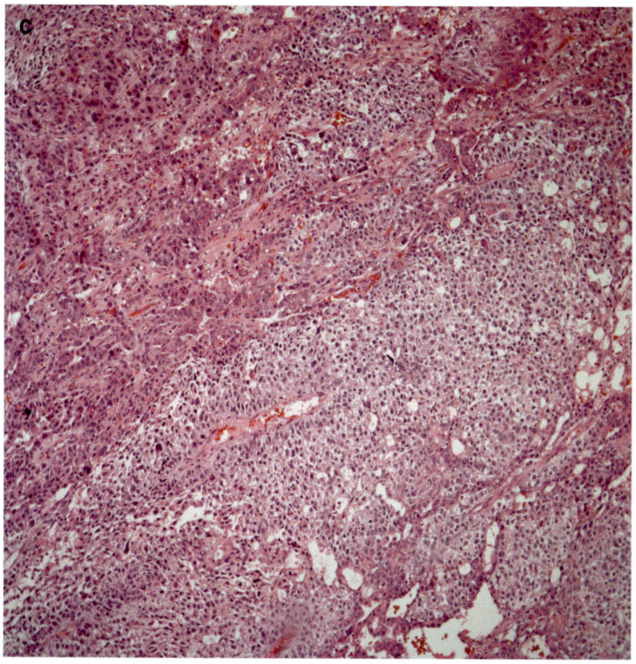

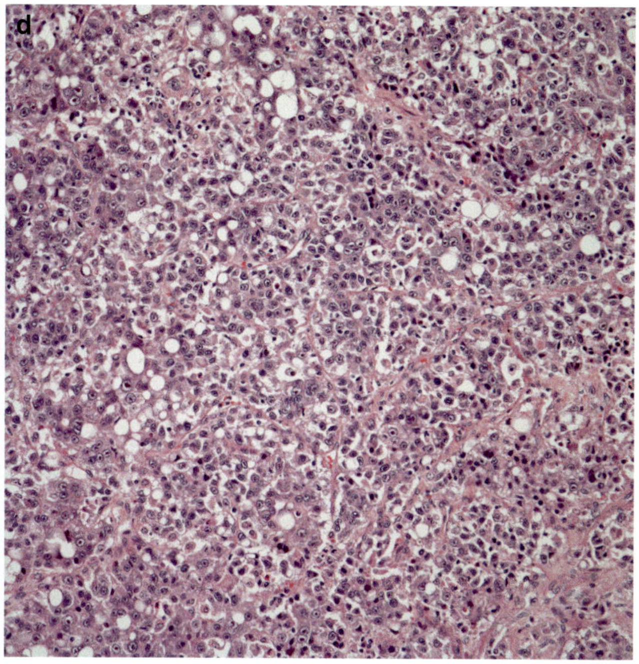

Fig. 10.52 (continued) (**c**) Conventional areas of YST adjacent to areas of hepatoid pattern composed of ribbons of neoplastic cells. (**d**) High magnification of the hepatoid variant showing areas similar to "fat droplets"

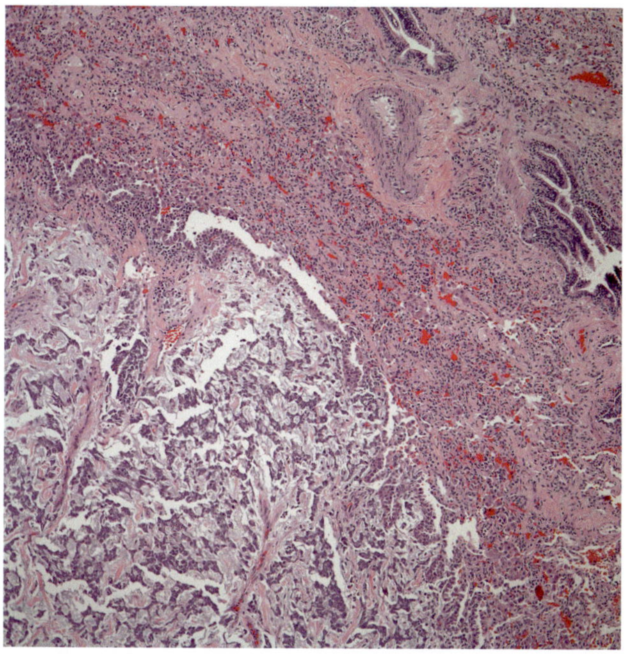

Fig. 10.53 Yolk sac tumor invading lung parenchyma

Ultrastructural Features

YST may show the presence of abundant extracellular electron-dense basement membrane material surrounding the cell membranes and electron-dense spheroidal bodies lying free in the cytosol. The cytoplasm of the cells may contain prominent rough endoplasmic reticulum with dilated cisternae, numerous uniform mitochondria, free ribosomes, and a well-developed Golgi apparatus. Glycogen granules and/or large lysosomes may be present. The cell membranes are joined by frequent small desmosomes, while glandular and ductular structures with true lumens displaying short microvilli may also be present. The electron-dense spheroidal bodies corresponding to the hyaline globules seen by light microscopy may be occasionally found lying free in the cytosol or may be present in extracellular location (Fig. 10.55).

Differential Diagnosis

The diagnosis of YST – when the tumor presents classical microcystic growth pattern, hyaline globules, and Schiller-Duval bodies – is straightforward. However, in some instances, clear separation from embryonal carcinoma may not be quite that simple. Another problem lies with the fact that the two tumors may coexist. Metastatic poorly differentiated carcinoma to the mediastinal region may also be confused with the solid variant of YST, while YST with prominent papillary features may be mistaken for a metastatic papillary neoplasm from other sites. In the latter two cases, the presence of areas displaying more characteristic features such as hyaline globules or Schiller-Duval bodies will be of aid in arriving at a correct interpretation. In addition, the presence of AFP in serum and/or its demonstration in tissue sections represents an added valuable tool for diagnosis.

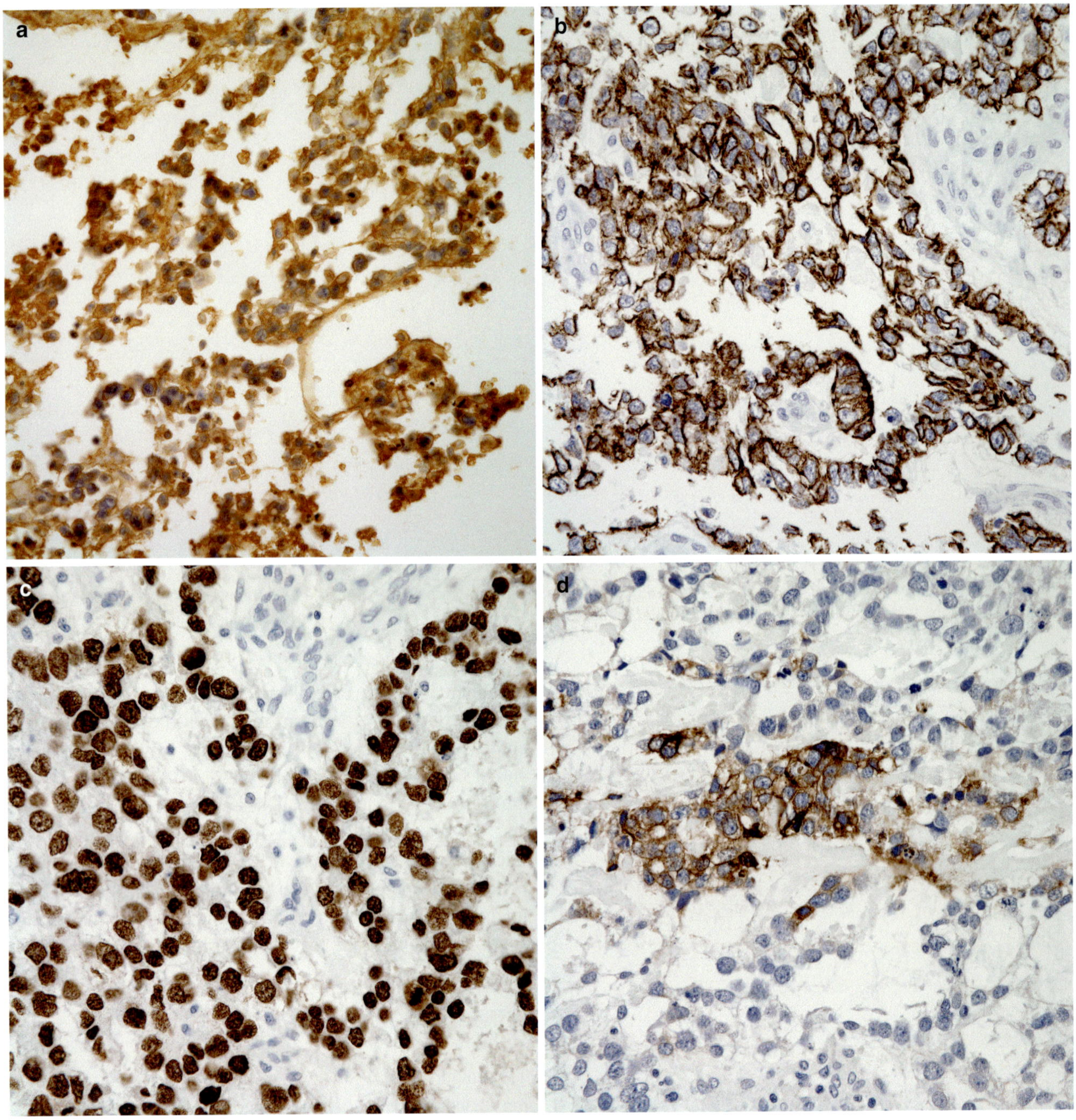

Fig. 10.54 Immunohistochemical stains in YST. (**a**) Positive staining for AFP. (**b**) CAM5.2 shows positive staining in tumor cells. (**c**) SALL4 showing strong nuclear positive staining in YST. (**d**) YST showing focal staining for glypican

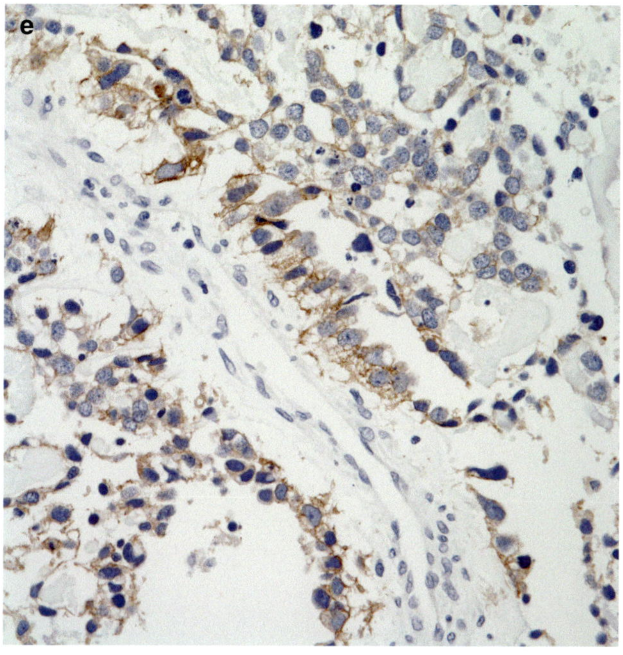

Fig. 10.54 (continued) (**e**) YST showing focal positive staining for CD117

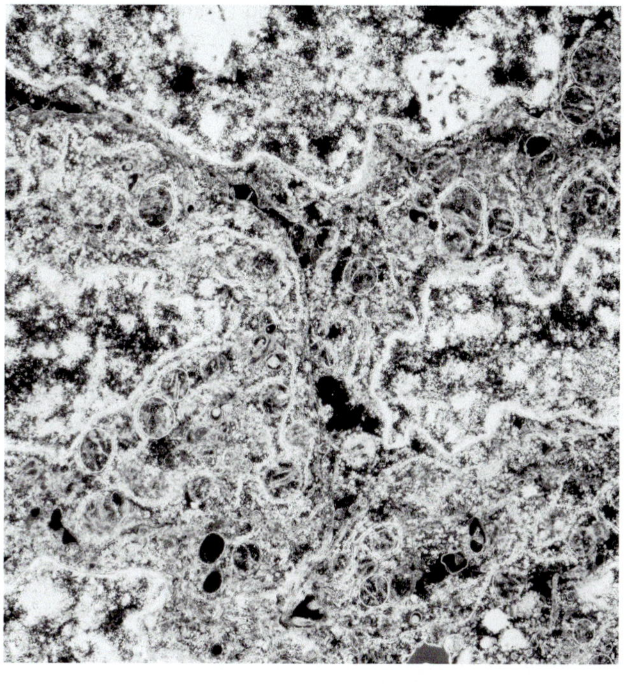

Fig. 10.55 Ultrastructural study of M-YST showing cells with irregular nuclei, tight junctions, numerous mitochondria, and lysosomes

Embryonal Carcinoma

Embryonal carcinoma (EC) is one of the most unusual MGCT. It rarely presents in its pure form [32, 153], and in most instances it is associated with another GCT [188–191]. In the past, these tumors were also known as the "adult type" of embryonal carcinoma to differentiate this tumor from the "infantile type," which is now currently known as YST.

Clinical Features

The true incidence of this tumor in the general population is difficult to estimate due to its rarity in its pure form. In our experience [165], EC accounts for approximately 10% of all MGCT. The same as with YST, embryonal carcinoma is more common in men in the third and fourth decades of life. However, cases of EC in women and in older individuals have been described [32, 188, 190].

The clinical manifestations of primary mediastinal EC are similar to those described for YST. Essentially, the symptomatology is linked to the size of the tumor mass. When these tumors reach a large size, they will compress adjacent structures and produce symptoms including shortness of breath, dyspnea, and chest pain. Similarly to YST, embryonal carcinomas have been associated with hematologic abnormalities such as idiopathic thrombocytopenia [171] and chromosomal abnormalities such as Klinefelter's syndrome [191].

The radiological appearance of EC is similar to that of YST. The most important feature is the presence of a large smooth or lobulated mass, which may be well circumscribed or may have irregular margins that pushes into the adjacent lung parenchyma. Evidence of metastatic tumor in the lung fields is commonly seen. However, there are no radiologic features that will allow distinction between EC and other non-seminomatous GCT.

The treatment for patients with these tumors is similar to that described for YST. Essentially, both neoplasms have been grouped under the heading of non-seminomatous GCT, and have been treated the same way in the majority of studies in the literature. The treatment consists of a cis-platinum-based chemotherapy with or without surgical resection of the tumor [63, 64, 130, 159, 179–183].

Gross Features

The tumors are usually large, ill defined, and soft, with or without extensive areas of necrosis and/or hemorrhage. They can measure from a few centimeters to over 10 cm in greatest dimension (Fig. 10.56). There are no gross features helpful in distinguishing these tumors from any other MGCT.

Histologic Features

On scanning magnification, the tumor may show a solid growth pattern mimicking an undifferentiated epithelial neoplasm (Fig. 10.57a–d). On closer view, the tumor may

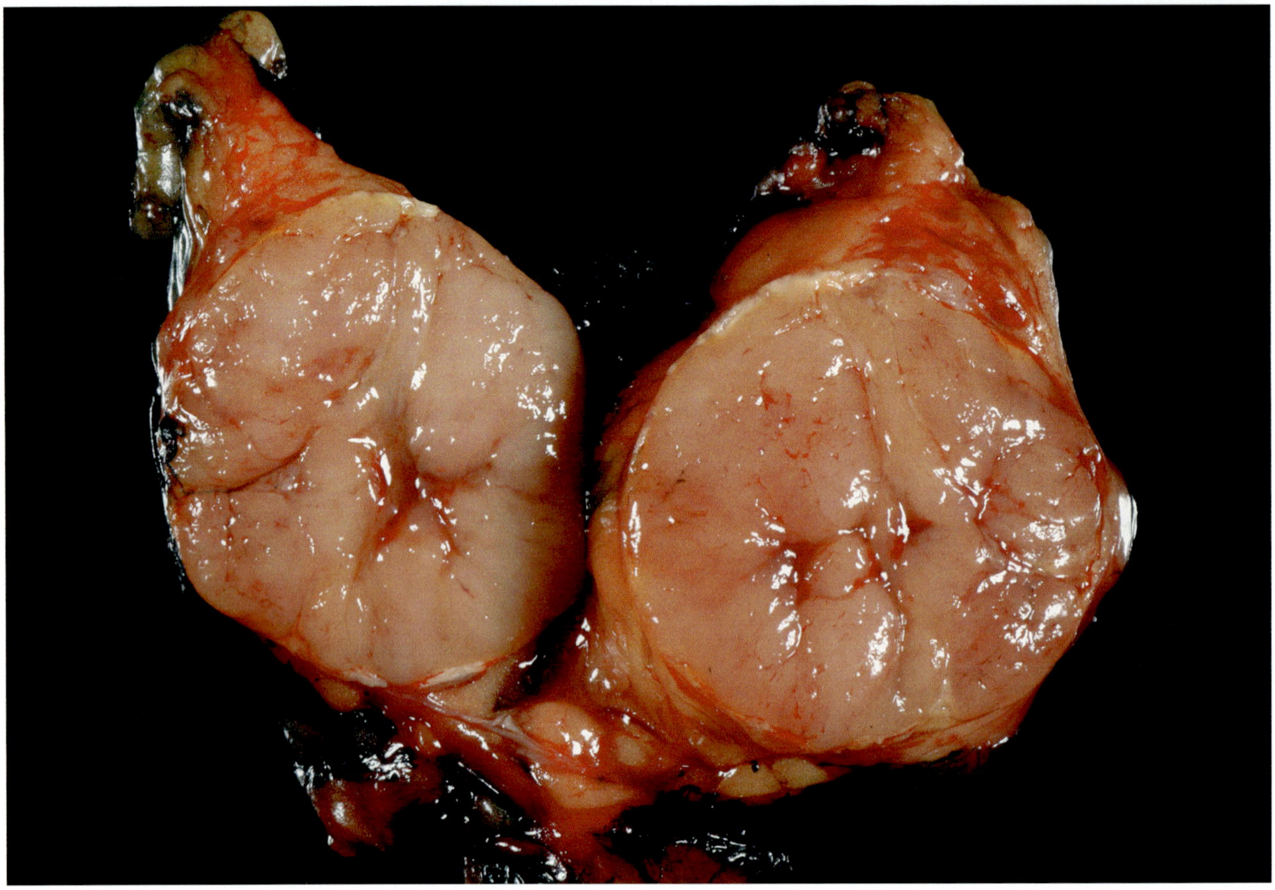

Fig. 10.56 Mediastinal embryonal carcinoma showing an ill-defined tumor mass with focal areas of hemorrhage

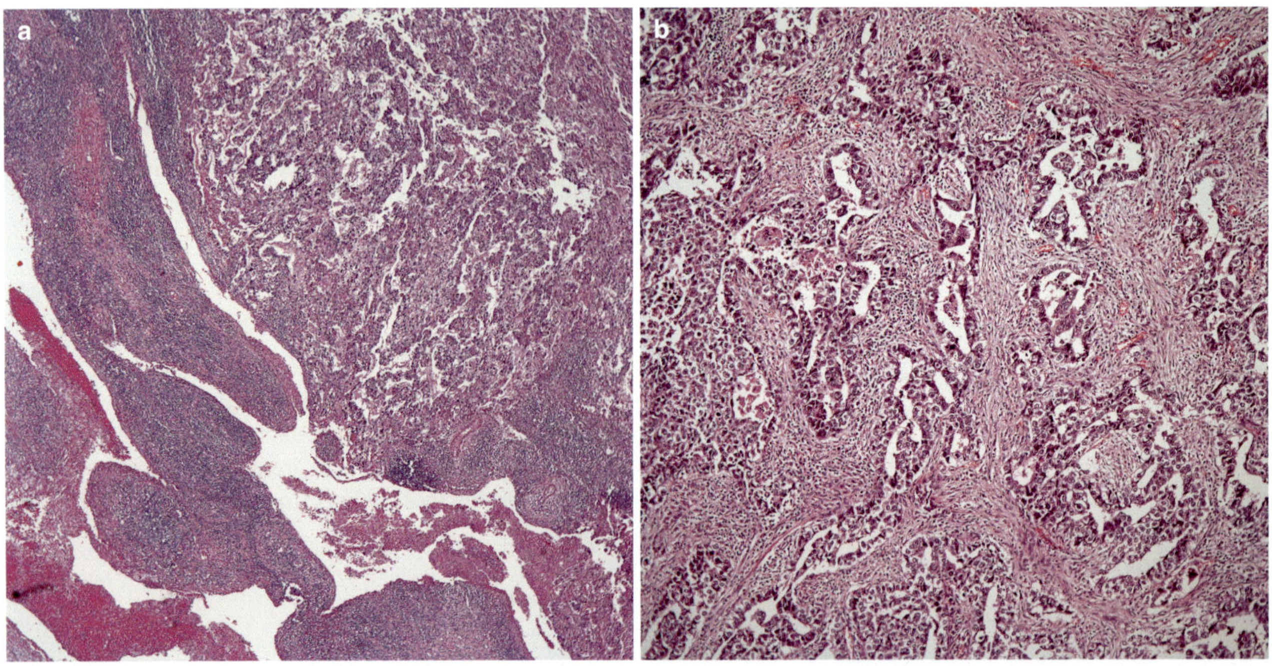

Fig. 10.57 (**a**) Embryonal carcinoma adjacent to areas of thymic tissue. (**b**) Embryonal carcinoma showing glandular component dissecting fibroconnective tissue

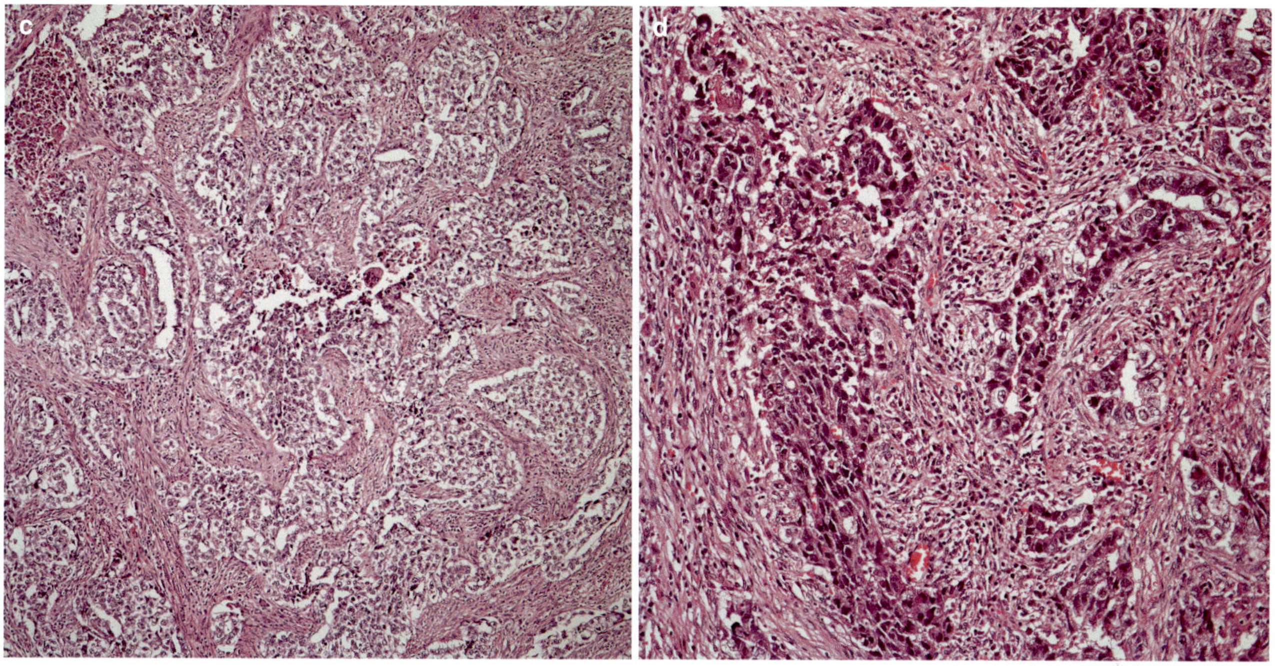

Fig. 10.57 (continued) (**c**) Solid areas alternating with poorly formed glands. (**d**) Poorly formed glands dissecting fibroconnective tissue with mixed inflammatory reaction

disclose a more glandular appearance (Fig. 10.58). However, the tumor may show a solid pattern with haphazard distribution of the neoplastic cells (Fig. 10.59a, b). The neoplastic cellular proliferation is composed of relatively large, primitive-appearing cells with round to oval nuclei and prominent nucleoli (Fig. 10.60a–d). The cytoplasm can be either clear or slightly eosinophilic. In some areas, it is possible to identify ill-defined glandular structures admixed with a more undifferentiated neoplastic cellular proliferation. The tumor may be overshadowed by extensive areas of necrosis in which there may be glandular structures embedded within the necrotic debris (Fig. 10.61a, b). More undifferentiated areas are commonly seen showing an increase number of mitoses and cytologic atypia as well as the presence of scattered syncytiotrophoblast-type multinucleated giant cells. Often, the tumor infiltrates into adjacent organs such as the pericardium and pleura.

The use of histochemical stains is mainly to rule out the possibility of a poorly differentiated adenocarcinoma, in which case the D-PAS and mucicarmine stains will show intracellular mucin, unlike EC in which no intracellular mucin is evident.

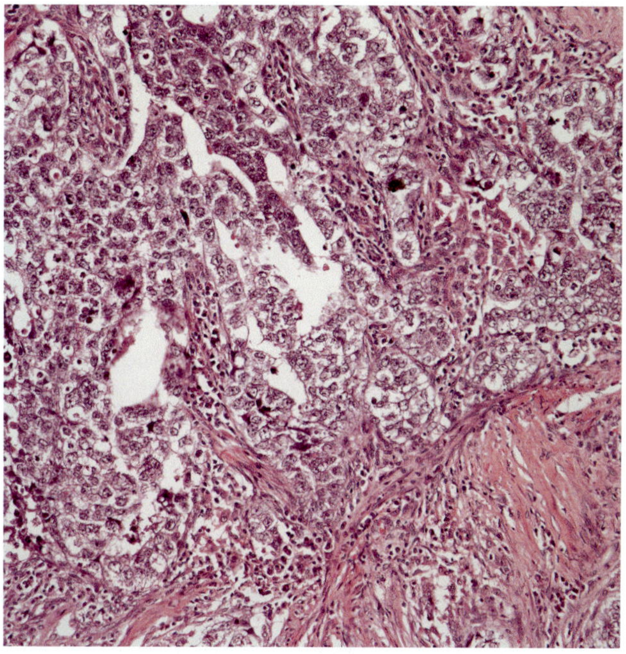

Fig. 10.58 E.C. showing poorly formed glands composed of larger cells with clearing of the nuclei and conspicuous nucleoli

Immunohistochemical Features

EC shares some of the immunohistochemical features with YST. They may show positive staining using antibodies against AFP, PLAP, NSE, Leu-7, Keratin, and vimentin [141]. Unlike AFP immunoreactivity in YST and PLAP immunoreactivity in seminomas, the positivity for these markers in EC will be more patchy and focal. The low molecular weight cytokeratins, such as CAM 5.2, are more often present in these tumors than the broad-spectrum type and will stain strongly and diffusely the neoplastic elements.

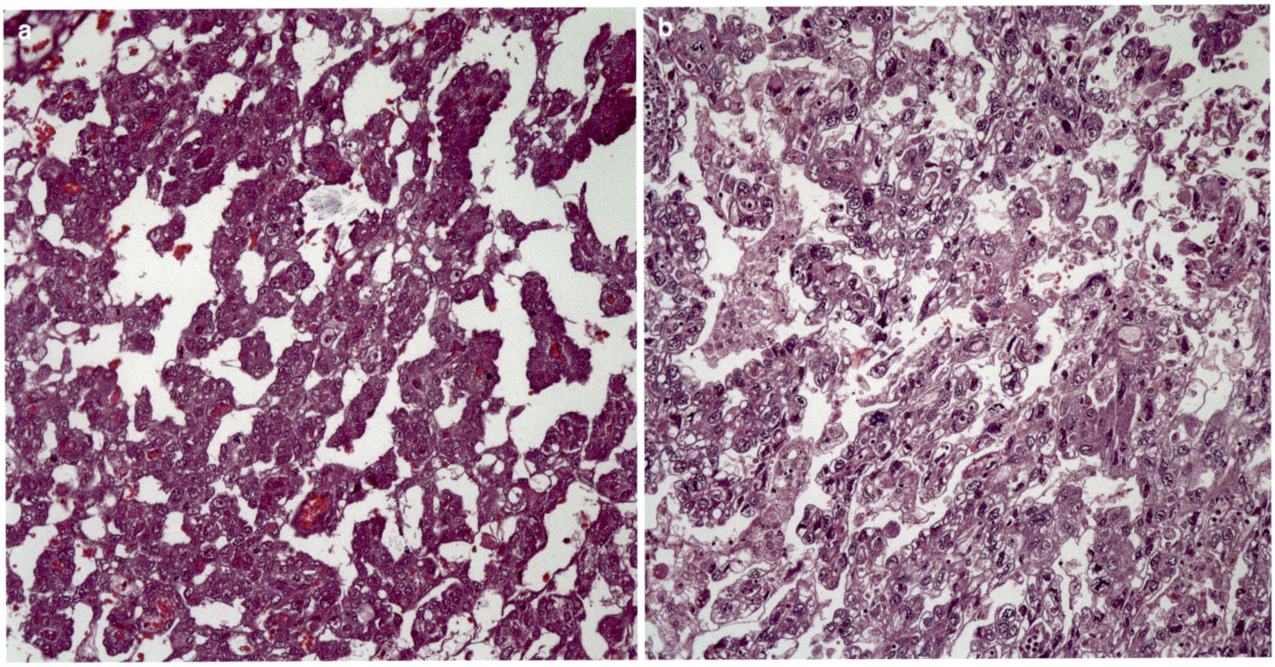

Fig. 10.59 (**a**) E.C. showing sheets of neoplastic cells. (**b**) E.C. composed of larger cells with vacuolization of the cytoplasm, large nuclei with prominent nucleoli

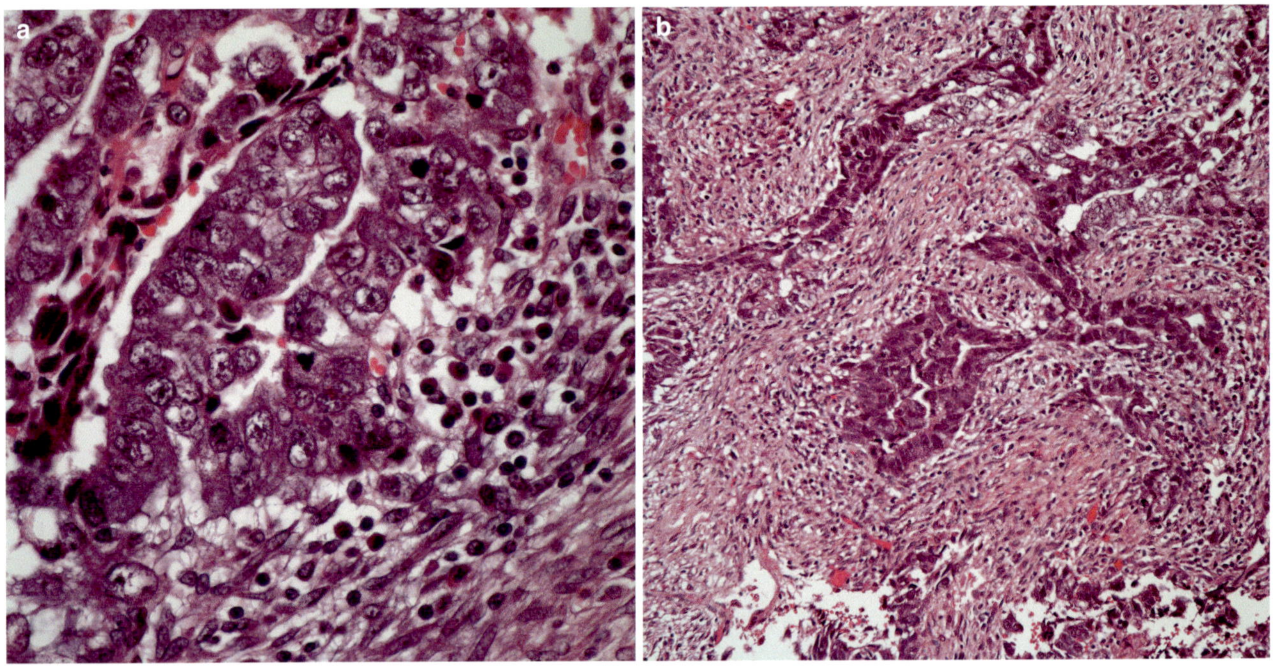

Fig. 10.60 (**a**) Higher magnification of E.C. showing larger cells with clear nuclei and prominent nucleoli; mitotic figures are also present. (**b**) Collapsed glandular structures infiltrating fibroconnective tissue

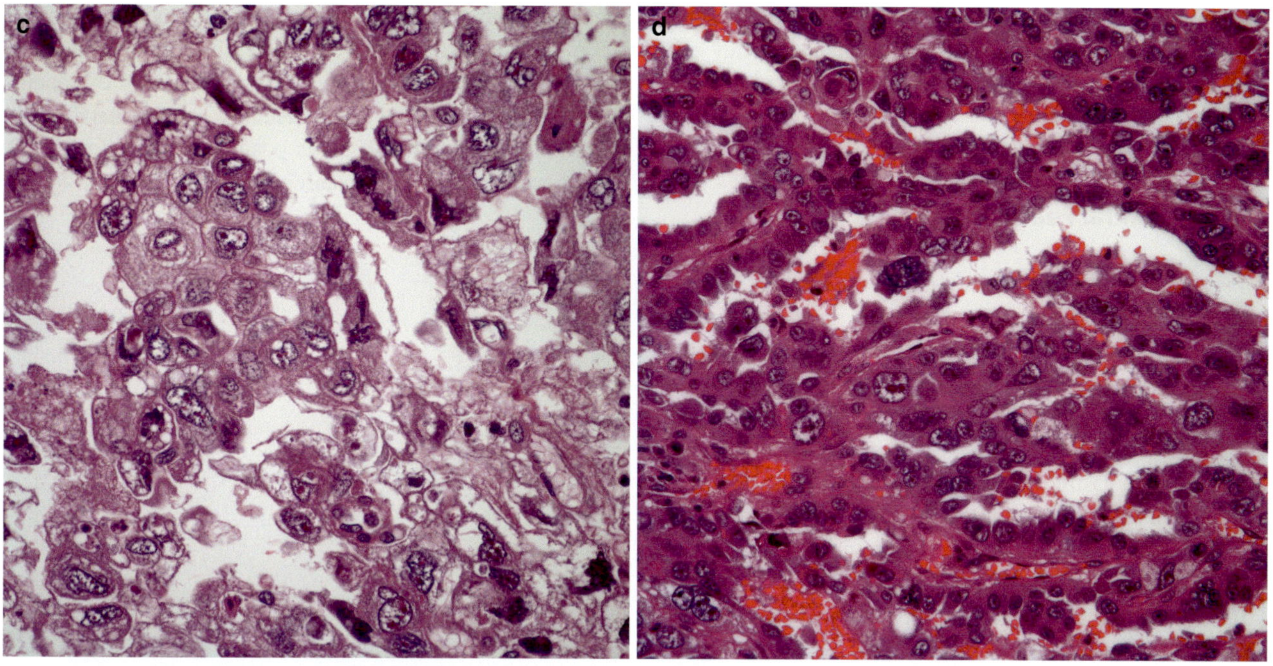

Fig. 10.60 (continued) (**c**) E.C. showing large cells with ample cytoplasm, round to oval nuclei and prominent nucleoli. (**d**) E.C. showing ribbon and glands composed of large cells with eosinophilic cytoplasm, round nuclei, and prominent nucleoli

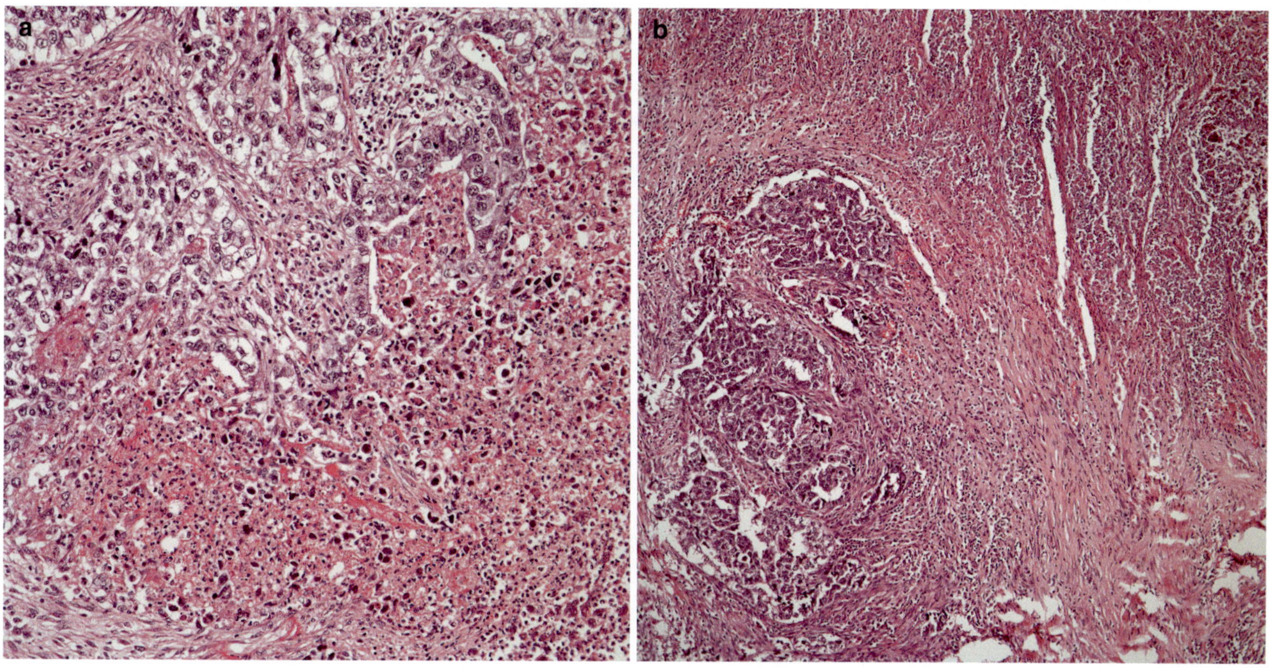

Fig. 10.61 (**a**) E.C. showing discrete areas of necrosis in which neoplastic cells are also evident. (**b**) E.C. with more extensive areas of necrosis and only focal areas of viable tumor

Interestingly, EC also shows positive staining with CD-30 [192]. This latter characteristic is not shared by any other GCT and may be of potential value for differential diagnosis (Fig. 10.62a, b).

Ultrastructural Features

There are no distinctive ultrastructural features for this neoplasm. The tumor is composed of solid sheets of primitive, undifferentiated epithelial cells with large nuclei and prominent electron-dense nucleoli (Fig. 10.63). However, one can observe desmosomal intercellular junctions, bundles of cytokeratin filaments, and occasional lumen formation. The presence of cytoplasmic AFP globules can occasionally be observed in close association with rough endoplasmic reticulum, indicating areas of presumed yolk sac differentiation. In an ultrastructural study reported by Ulbright and associates [193], the authors stated that long-tight junctions and telolysosomes were found in all cases of EC, whereas they were generally less well developed in carcinomas of teratomatous origin.

Differential Diagnosis

The most important issue in the differential diagnosis of embryonal carcinoma is with metastasis from an undifferentiated large cell carcinoma or a poorly differentiated adenocarcinoma. Primary lung carcinomas can often metastasize to the mediastinum. In this setting, a proper clinical and radiological evaluation is essential. The diagnosis is aided by recognition of the primitive, immature appearance of the glands and cellular elements in embryonal carcinoma. Extensive sampling is also important to exclude the possibility of a combined GCT. Two important aspects that can be of help are the fact that the overwhelming majority of patients with EC are young with a bulky anterior mediastinal mass. In addition, EC commonly shows positive staining for CD30, which would be unusual in carcinoma of lung origin.

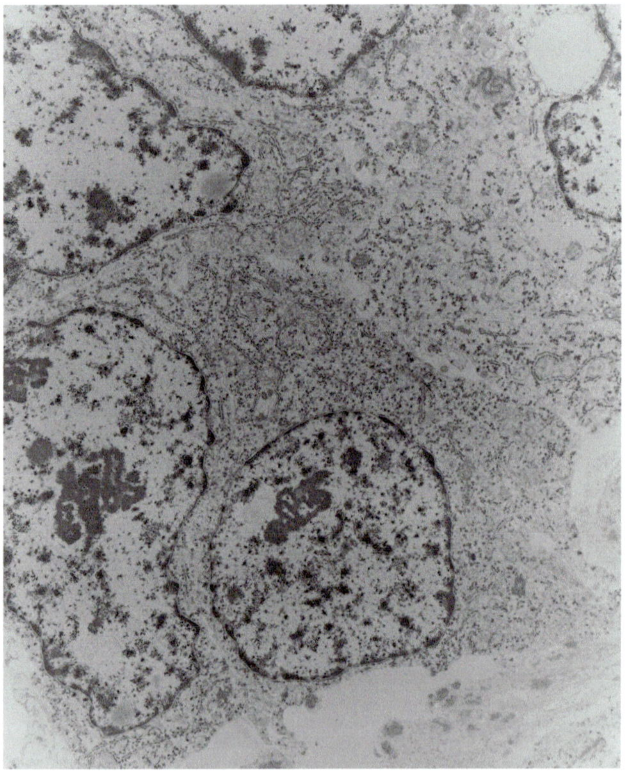

Fig. 10.63 Ultrastructural study of E.C. showing larger cells with round to oval nuclei and dense nucleoli

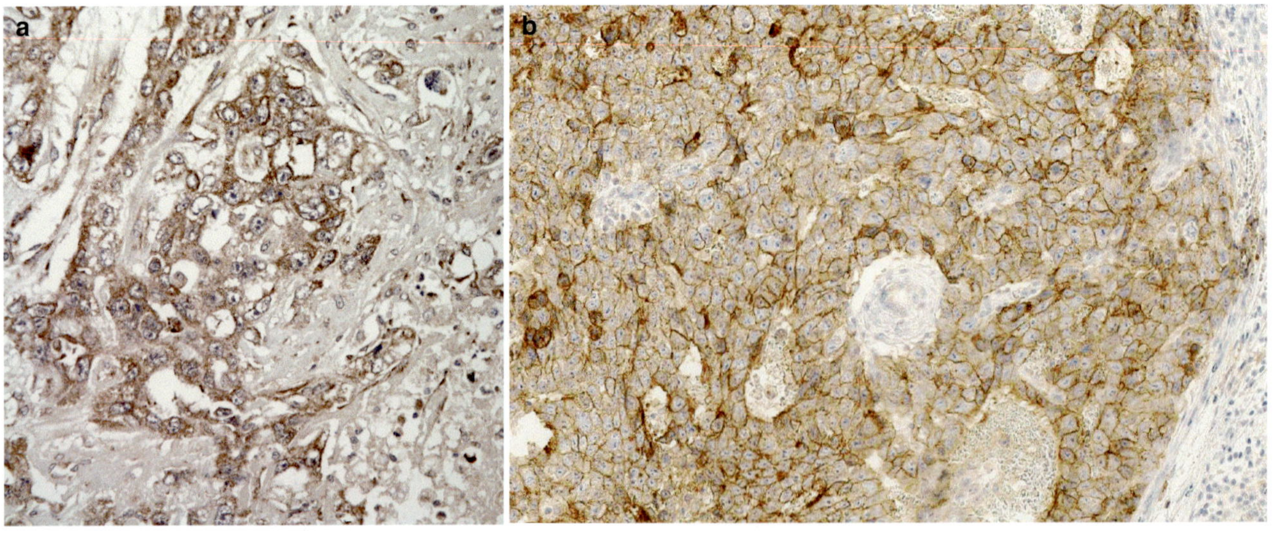

Fig. 10.62 (**a**) E.C. showing strong positive staining for keratin. (**b**) E.C. showing strong positive staining for CD-30

Choriocarcinoma

Extragonadal choriocarcinomas are not only rare but also probably the most debatable GCT to occur outside of the gonads. Part of the controversy surrounding the existence of primary extragonadal choriocarcinomas is the fact that small testicular tumors can give rise to widespread metastatic lesions. On the other hand, it has been stated that in some instances the primary lesion may undergo complete regression, therefore casting doubts over the real existence of primary mediastinal choriocarcinomas.

In 1961, Azzopardi and associates [194] studied 17 patients with widespread metastases of GCT. Eight of the cases were compatible with choriocarcinoma. The authors found that, in all cases, a distinct and well-defined testicular scar was found, which the authors interpreted as the primary site of origin. In addition, in 13 cases, the authors noted the presence of "peculiar amorphous hematoxylin-staining deposits" in dilated seminiferous tubules. These deposits were shown to consist of phospholipid, protein debris, and DNA, as well as mucoid substances and calcium phosphate, which were believed to result from tumor necrosis. The authors concluded that the presence of these deposits was consistent with a "burned-out" primary testicular tumor. Similar findings had already been described in a single case by Prim as cited by Azzopardi [194]. Therefore, it was proposed that before rendering the diagnosis of primary extragonadal choriocarcinoma, a careful search for a testicular scar or microscopic neoplasm must be undertaken. In 1953, Lynch and Blewett [117] reported a case of choriocarcinoma in the mediastinal region and cited Ritchie as the first to describe such a tumor in the anterior mediastinum. The authors analyzed previously reported cases and found great disagreement regarding the concept of primary choriocarcinoma of the mediastinum and concluded that the best manner to establish the diagnosis of primary choriocarcinoma of the mediastinum requires serial sectioning of the testes and hormonal studies of the urine and of the tumor. Based on these criteria, the number of cases accepted as primary choriocarcinoma of the mediastinum is definitely low. Interestingly, the authors noted a tendency to interpret testicular scars as representing the origin of choriocarcinoma without considering that the scar themselves might be secondary reaction. On the other hand, some authors have questioned the so-called spontaneous healing of primary choriocarcinoma. In any event, the issue is merely of academic interest since the finding of a small, burned-out, or regressed primary tumor in the gonads is unlikely to alter the prognosis or clinical behavior of the tumor.

Clinical Features

The true incidence of choriocarcinomas arising primarily in the mediastinum is extremely difficult to assess. Although numerous single cases of choriocarcinomas arising in the mediastinum have been reported [4, 5, 61, 64, 117, 168, 195–202], the presence of an anterior mediastinal mass in the absence of testicular lesion on palpation is not necessarily an indication that the case represents a primary mediastinal choriocarcinoma, and some of the reported cases may have corresponded to metastases to the mediastinum from an occult or regressed primary. These tumors predominantly affect men in the third and fourth decades of life and constitute a small percentage of MGCT. In our experience, this tumor accounts for less than 5% of all MGCT [203].

Choriocarcinomas presenting as anterior mediastinal masses usually produce symptoms of cough, shortness of breath, dyspnea, gynecomastia, chest pain, and/or superior vena cava syndrome [168, 198, 199]. It is of interest to note that, in the great majority of the cases reported, by the time the diagnosis is established, the tumor has already spread outside the mediastinal compartment and is usually found involving the lungs.

There are no radiological characteristics that can help separate choriocarcinoma from other non-seminomatous MGCT. However, in most of the cases reported, the radiological features correspond to those of a more advanced tumor with multiple tumoral nodules in the lungs or in other areas such as the liver. Therefore, the presence of an anterior mediastinal mass suspected clinically of being a GCT, which is already involving lung and/or other viscera, should be highly suggestive of choriocarcinoma.

The prognosis for patients with mediastinal choriocarcinoma as reported in the literature is dismal. In most of the reported cases as well as in our experience, at the time of diagnosis, the tumor had already spread within the thoracic or extrathoracic area. The tumors appear to metastasize widely and rapidly to other organs such as liver and brain. In most of the early cases described in the literature, treatment was ineffectual. However, in a few cases, the patients experienced survival rates of several years after treatment with chemotherapy [168, 200]. Nevertheless, the clinical course is that of rapid deterioration and death within few months.

Gross Features

In the majority of cases, the tumors appear as non-encapsulated masses that may occupy a good portion of the anterior mediastinum involving pericardium, pleura, lungs, and/or heart. However, in a few cases, the tumors appear to be better circumscribed without evidence of involvement of adjacent structures [168, 198, 200].

Histologic Features

At scanning magnification, choriocarcinomas show extensive areas of hemorrhage and/or necrosis (Fig. 10.64). Closer view of the tumor shows areas displaying two different cell types: cytotrophoblastic and syncytiotrophoblastic cells. Large polygonal cells showing abundant clear cytoplasm, central round to oval nuclei, and distinct cell borders characterize the cytotrophoblastic proliferation. On the other hand, large, multinucleated giant cells with abundant eosinophilic cytoplasm characterize the syncytiotrophoblastic component. Mitoses and bizarre cellular features are also common findings (Fig. 10.65a–f).

Histochemical studies may be of value to determine the presence of intra- and extracellular mucin and may serve to rule out the possibility of a primary large cell carcinoma of the lung.

Immunohistochemical Features

The hallmark of choriocarcinoma is the presence of HCG immunoreactivity in the syncytiotrophoblastic component of the tumor (Fig. 10.66). However, antibodies for PLAP, EMA, AFP, CEA, and keratins may also display focal positivity in these tumors [141].

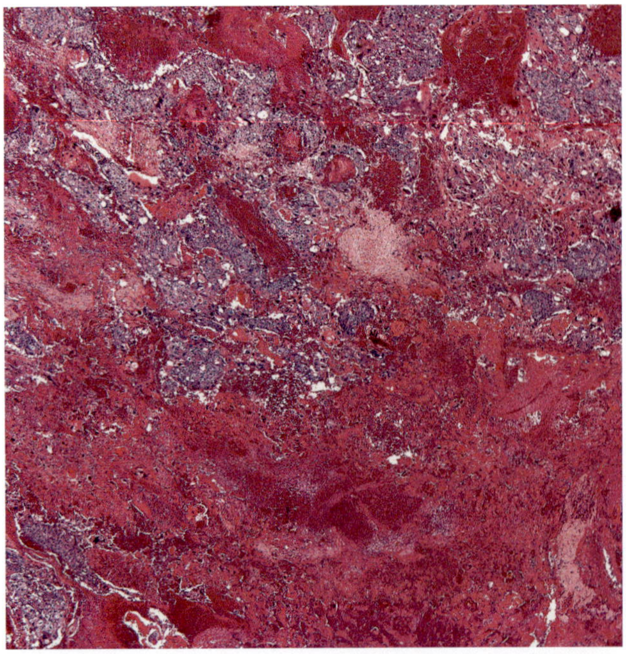

Fig. 10.64 Low-power view of a mediastinal choriocarcinoma showing extensive areas of hemorrhage

Ultrastructural Features

Electron microscopic studies in choriocarcinoma of the mediastinum are not available. However, in those occurring in the testicular region, it has been noted that the cytotrophoblastic component may closely resemble embryonal carcinoma.

Differential Diagnosis

The most important differential diagnosis lies in distinguishing a primary from a metastatic choriocarcinoma. A number of other tumors may show prominent areas composed of multinucleated malignant giant cells that may be confused with syncytiotrophoblastic cells. In particular, primary lung neoplasms such as pleomorphic carcinoma [204] may metastasize to the mediastinum. In addition, pleomorphic carcinomas or large cell carcinomas occurring primarily in the lung may also show ectopic production of HCG, making the distinction from choriocarcinoma a challenge for the pathologist. The presence of a dual cell population comprising both cyto- and syncytiotrophoblast would be more in keeping with a primary choriocarcinoma, whereas the presence of a concomitant, single large intrapulmonary mass would be highly suggestive of a metastasis from a lung primary. Although most cases of primary mediastinal choriocarcinoma involve the lung at the time of diagnosis, such involvement is usually characterized by the presence of multiple pulmonary tumor nodules rather than a single, large solitary mass. In addition, primary mediastinal choriocarcinomas appear to affect more commonly young men while pleomorphic lung carcinomas predominantly affect an older age group.

Combined Germ Cell Tumors

This term is used in this text to describe tumors showing combinations of seminoma, embryonal carcinoma, YST, and/or choriocarcinoma, in the absence of teratomatous components. We prefer such designation instead of the term "mixed tumors" in view not only of the existence of neoplasms in other systems that are known by this designation but also because of its lack of specificity. In addition, we consider that tumors showing teratomatous components should be grouped with teratomas rather than be included under the heading of combined germ cell tumors [205].

Clinical Features

In our experience with 322 cases of MGCT, we were able to identify 12 cases that fulfill these criteria, which we diagnosed as combined GCT. Therefore, these neoplasms represented approximately 5% of all mediastinal GCT. These

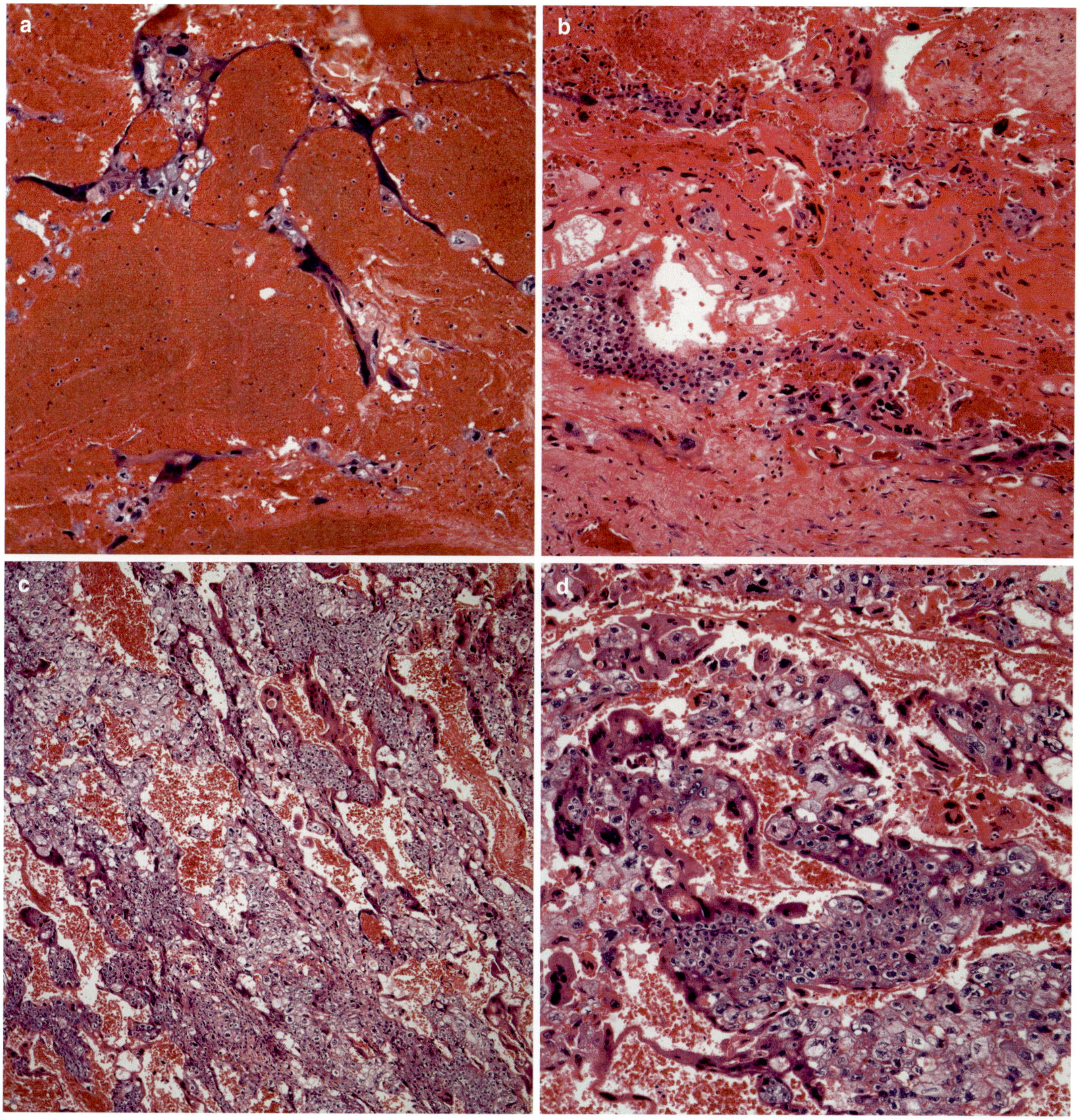

Fig. 10.65 (**a**) Choriocarcinoma with extensive areas of hemorrhage and the outlines of syncytiotrophoblastic cells. (**b**) Syncytiotrophoblastic and cytotrophoblastic cells admixed with hemorrhage. (**c**) Choriocarcinoma with classic cellularity of cyto- and syncytiotrophoblastic cells. (**d**) Dual component formed by multinucleated syncytiotrophoblastic cells and mononuclear cytotrophoblastic cells

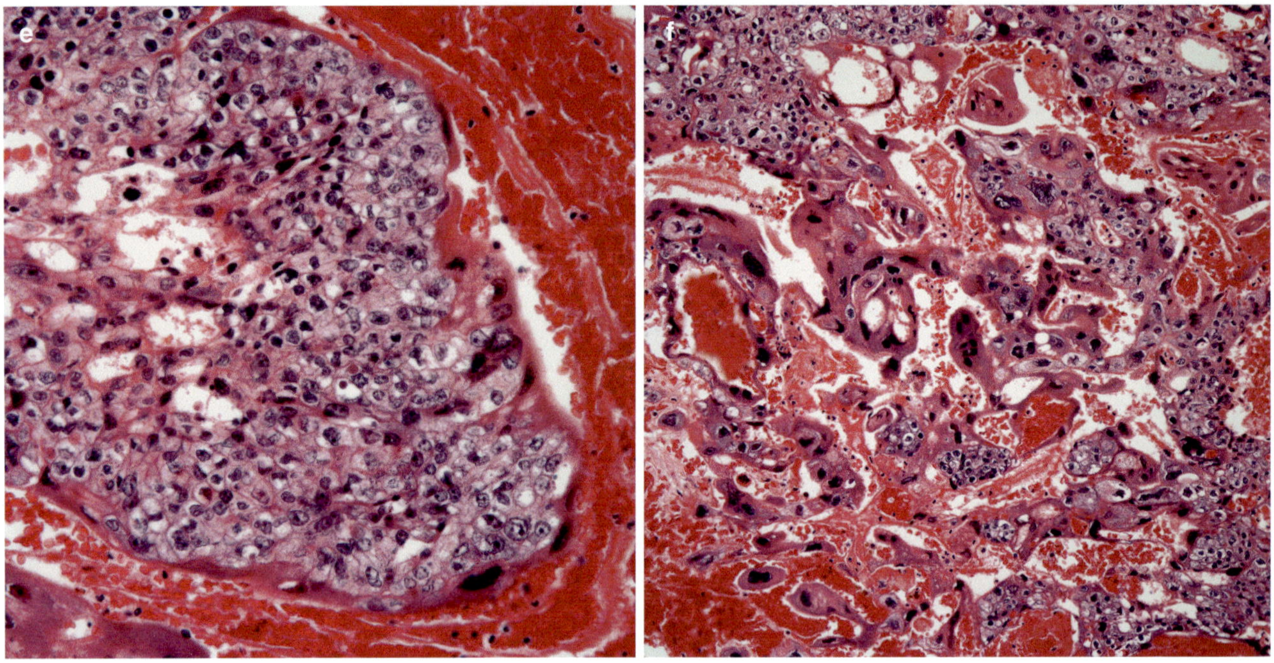

Fig. 10.65 (continued) (**e**) Choriocarcinoma with predominant cytotrophoblastic component. (**f**) Choriocarcinoma with predominant syncytiotrophoblastic component

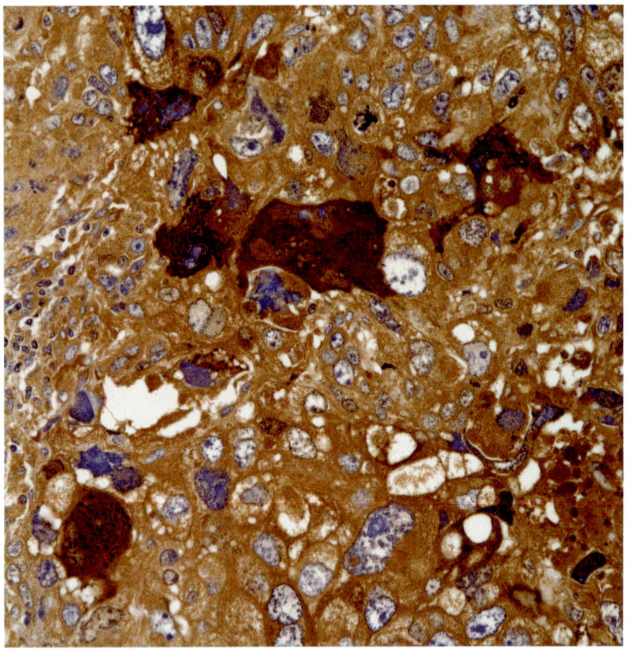

Fig. 10.66 Immunohistochemical stain for HCG showing positive staining in the syncytiotrophoblastic component

tumors predominantly affect males in their third and fourth decades of life. However, female patients with this type of tumor have also been described [188].

The clinical features shown by patients are similar to those described for other GCT, namely, chest pain, cough, and shortness of breath. In our experience, none of these tumors was associated with hematologic or chromosomal abnormalities. Nonetheless, such abnormalities have been previously reported [169, 206]. There is no radiologic feature which can separate combined GCT from other GCT. Therefore, histologic examination is the only way to arrive at a specific diagnosis.

The treatment and prognosis for these tumors will depend on the amount (percentage) of a particular germ cell component and the extent of the disease at the time of diagnosis.

Gross Features

These tumors may vary in size from small to very large tumors (>10 cm in diameter). The outer surface may be glistening and surrounded by membranous tissue. The cut surface shows a firm, slightly nodular tan to whitish appearance. Areas of hemorrhage and/or necrosis may be seen.

Histologic Features

A combination of the different tumors already described may be seen. In essence, these tumors may show any combination among seminoma, YST, EC, and/or choriocarcinoma [32, 188–190]. In our experience, seminomas are the tumor component more often present as part of these tumors (Fig. 10.67a–c). The histologic features of each of those tumors have already been described. The histochemical, immunohistochemical, and ultrastructural features of these tumors will depend on the particular components present.

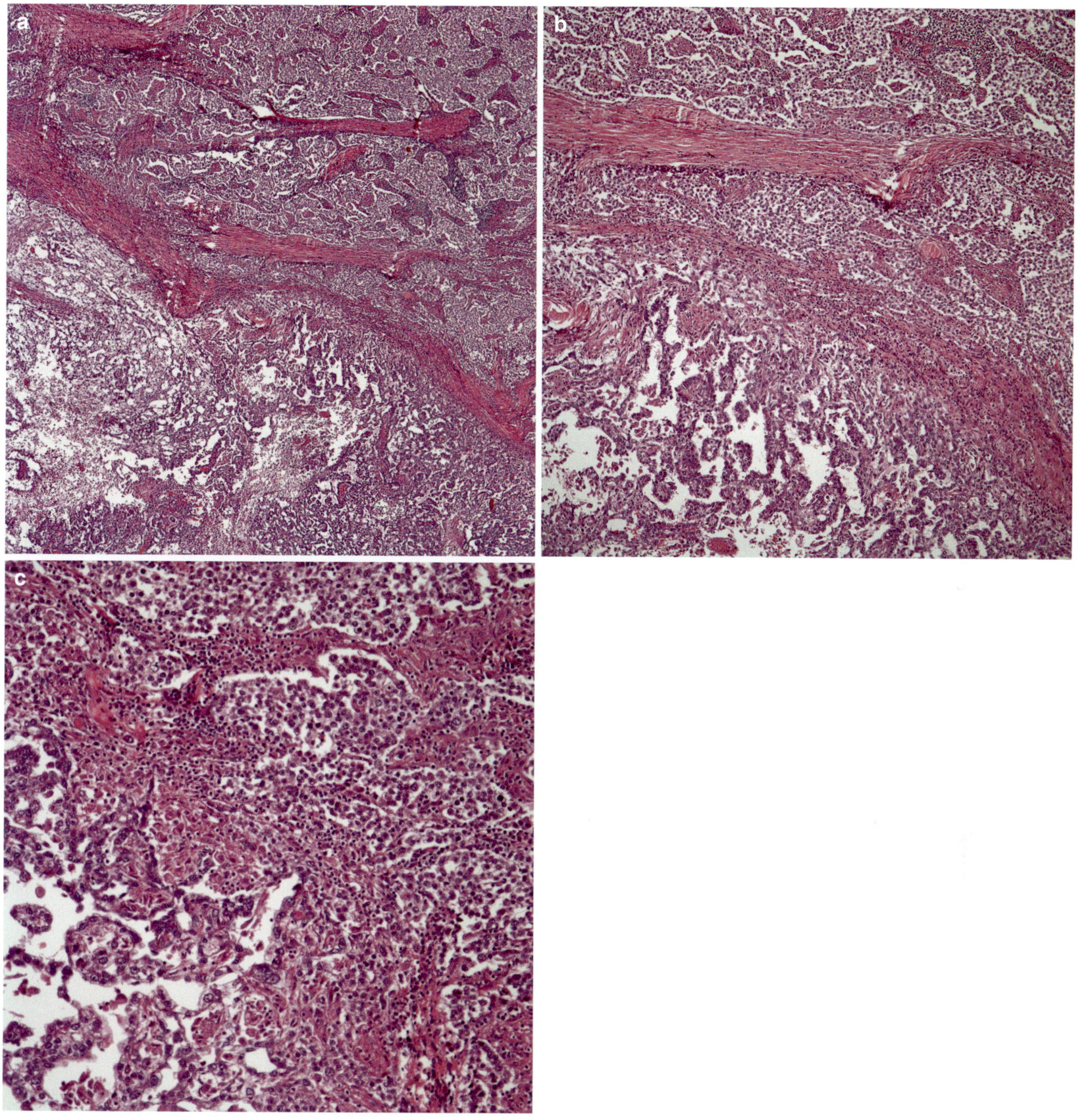

Fig. 10.67 (**a**) Combined GCT showing sharp separation of YST and seminoma. (**b**) YST and seminoma separated by a thin fibroconnective tissue with inflammatory reaction (**c**) YST and seminoma with very discrete transition

Summary

Mediastinal GCT represent an important group of tumors that need to be carefully evaluated, as current therapeutic modalities over the years have made a significant difference in their treatment and prognosis. Even though mature teratomas may represent the most common mediastinal GCT, the need for proper sampling in order to properly exclude other tumors that may need a different approach beyond complete surgical resection should be underscored. Among the non-teratomatous tumors, seminomas are by far the most common, while among the NS-GCT, yolk sac tumor is the more common. Special attention should be given to providing approximate percentages of the different components that may be present in MGCT.

References

1. Bjornsson J, Scheithauer BW, Okazaki H, Leech RW. Intracranial germ cell tumors: Pathological and immunohistochemical aspects of 70 cases. J Neuropathol Exp Neurol. 1985;44:32–46.
2. Gonzales-Crussi F, Winkler RF, Mirkin DL. Sacrococcygeal teratomas in infants and children. Arch Pathol Lab Med. 1978;102:420–5.
3. Engel RM, Elkins RC, Fletcher BD. Retroperitoneal teratoma: review of the literature and presentation of an unusual case. Cancer. 1968;5:1068–73.
4. Johnson DE, Laneri JP, Mountain CF, Luna M. Extragonadal germ cell tumors. Surgery. 1973;73:85–90.
5. Knapp RH, Hurt RD, Payne WS, Farrow GM, Lewis BD, Hahn RG, et al. Malignant germ cell tumors of the mediastinum. J Thorac Cardiovasc Surg. 1985;89:82–9.
6. Davis RD, Oldham NH, Sabiston DC. Primary cysts and neoplasms of the mediastinum: recent changes in clinical presentation, methods of diagnosis. Management, and results. Ann Thorac Surg. 1987;44:229–37.
7. Mullen B, Richardson DJ. Primary anterior mediastinal tumors in children and adults. Ann Thorac Surg. 1986;42:338–45.
8. Wychulis AR, Payne WS, Clagett OT, Woolner LB. Surgical treatment of mediastinal tumors: a 40 year experience. J Thorac Cardiovasc Surg. 1971;62:379–92.
9. Gordon JA. Tumor in the anterior mediastinum containing bone and teeth. Med Chir Trans. 1827;13:12–6.
10. Hare HA. Clinical history and diagnosis of affections of the mediastinum. Philadelphia: P. Blakiston's Son & Co; 1889.
11. Hertzler AE. Dermoids of the anterior mediastinum. Am J Med Sci. 1916;152:165–73.
12. Woolner LB, Jamplis RW, Kirklin JW. Seminoma (germinoma) of the anterior mediastinum. New Engl J Med. 1955;252:653–7.
13. Teilmann I, Kassis H, Pietra G. Primary germ cell tumor of the anterior mediastinum with features of endodermal sinus tumor (mesoblastoma vitellinum). Acta Pathol Microbiol Scand. 1967;70:267–78.
14. Hainsworth JD, Greco FA. Extragonadal germ cell tumors and unrecognized germ cell tumors. Semin Oncol. 1992;19:119–27.
15. Dulmet EM, Macchiarini P, Suc B, Verley JM. Germ cell tumors of the mediastinum. Cancer. 1993;72:1894–901.
16. Dehner LP. Germ cell tumors of the mediastinum. Semin Diagn Pathol. 1990;7:266–84.
17. Moran CA, Suster S. Primary germ cell tumors of the mediastinum: I. Analysis of 322 cases with special emphasis on teratomatous lesions and a proposal for histopathologic classification and clinical staging. Cancer. 1997;80:681–90.
18. Laipply TC. Cysts and cystic tumors of the mediastinum. Arch Pathol. 1945;39:153–61.
19. Schlumberger HG. Teratoma of the mediastinum in the group of military age: a study of sixteen cases, and a review of theories of genesis. Arch Pathol. 1946;41:398–444.
20. Gonzales-Crussi F. The human yolk sac and yolk sac (endodermal sinus) tumors. A review. Perspect Pediatr Pathol. 1979;5:179–215.
21. Friedman NB. The comparative morphogenesis of extragenital and gonadal teratoid tumors. Cancer. 1951;4(2):265–76.
22. Friedman NB. The function of the primordial germ cell extragonadal tissues. Int J Androl. 1987;10:43–9.
23. Rosai J, Parkash V, Reuter VE. On the origin of mediastinal germ cell tumors in males. Int J Surg Pathol. 1995;2:73–8.
24. Travis WD, Brambilla E, Muller-Hermelink HK, et al. WHO Classification of Tumours: pathology and genetics of tumours of the lung, pleura, thymus and heart. Lyon: IARC; 2004.
25. Rusby NL. Dermoid cyst and teratoma of the mediastinum. J Thorac Surg. 1944;13:169–222.
26. Ringertz N, Lidholm SO. Mediastinal tumors and cyst. J Thoracic Surg. 1956;31:458–87.
27. Hodge J, Aponte G, McLaughlin E. Primary mediastinal tumors. J Thorac Surg. 1959;37:730–44.
28. Lewis BD, Hurt RD, Payne WS, Farrow GM, Knapp RH, Muhm JR. Benign teratomas of the mediastinum. J Thorac Cardiovasc Surg. 1983;86:727–31.
29. Bergh NP, Gatzinnsky P, Larsson S, Lundin P, Ridell B. Tumors of the thymus and thymic region: III. Clinicopathologic studies on teratomas and tumors of germ cell type. Ann Thorac Surg. 1978;25:107–11.
30. Whittaker LD, Lynn HB. Mediastinal tumors and cysts in the pediatric patient. Surg Clin North Am. 1973;53:893–904.
31. Pokorny WJ, Sherman JO, Idriss FS. Mediastinal masses in infants and children. J Thorac Cardiovasc Surg. 1974;68:869–75.
32. Lack EE, Weinstein HJ, Welch KJ. Mediastinal germ cell tumors in childhood: a clinical and pathological study of 21 cases. J Thorac Cardiovasc Surg. 1985;89:826–35.
33. Berry CL, Keeling J, Hilton C. Teratoma in infancy and childhood: a review of 91 cases. J Path. 1969;98:241–52.
34. Mahour GH, Woolley MM, Trivedi SN, Landing BH. Teratomas in infancy and childhood: experience with 81 cases. Surgery. 1974;76:309–18.
35. Karl S, Dunn J. Posterior mediastinal teratomas. J Pediatr Surg. 1985;20:508–10.
36. Wilms G, Thijs M. Posterior mediastinal teratoma. RoFo. 1986;145:112–3.
37. Canty TG, Siemens R. Malignant mediastinal teratoma in a 15-year-old girl. Cancer. 1978;41:1623–6.
38. Lachman MF, Kim K, Koo BC. Mediastinal teratoma associated with klinefelter's syndrome. Arch Pathol Lab Med. 1986;110:1067–71.
39. Aravanis C, Papasteriades E, Steriotis J. Recurrent pericarditis due to cystic teratoma of the mediastinum. Angiology. 1980;31:427–30.
40. Robertson JM, Fee HJ, Mulder DG. Mediastinal teratoma causing life-threatening hemoptysis. Am J Dis Child. 1981;135:148–50.
41. Deenadayalu RP, Tuuri D, Dewall RA, Johnson FG. Intrapericardial teratoma and bronchogenic cyst. J Thorac Cardiovasc Surg. 1974;67:945–52.
42. Honicky RE, dePapp EW. Mediastinal teratoma with endocrine function. Am J Dis Child. 1973;126:650–3.
43. Rosado-de-Christenson ML, Templeton P, Moran CA. Mediastinal germ cell tumors: Radiologic and Pathologic correlation. Radiographics. 1992;12:1013–30.
44. Bordi C, De Vita O, Pollice L. Full pancreatic endocrine differentiation in amediastinal teratoma. Hum Pathol. 1985;16:961–4.

45. Suda K, Mizuguchi K, Hebisawa A, Wakabayashi T, Saito S. Pancreatic tissue in teratoma. Arch Pathol Lab Med. 1984;108:835–7.
46. Carter D, Bibro MC, Touloukian RJ. Benign clinical behavior of immature mediastinal teratoma in infancy and childhood: report of two cases. Cancer. 1982;49:398–402.
47. Pate JW, Buker R, Korones SB. Mediastinal teratoma in the newborn. Pediatr Surg. 1963;54:533–5.
48. Oberman HA, Libcke JH. Malignant germinal neoplasms of the mediastinum. Cancer. 1964;17:498–507.
49. Rubush JL, Gardner IR, Boyd WC, Ehrenhaft JL. Mediastinal tumors: review of 186 cases. J Thorac Cardiovasc Surg. 1973;65:216–22.
50. Recondo J, Libshitz HI. Mediastinal extragonadal germ cell tumors. Urology. 1978;11:369–75.
51. Luna MA, Valenzuela-Tamaris J. Germ cell tumors of the mediastinum, postmortem findings. Am J Clin Pathol. 1976;65:450–4.
52. Daniel RA, Diveley WL, Edwards WH, Chamberlain N. Mediastinal tumors. Ann Surg. 1960;151:783–95.
53. Wirtanen GW, Stephenson JA, Wiley AL. Primary anterior mediastinal malignant teratoma: a case report with long-term survival. Cancer. 1989;63:1823–5.
54. Morinaga S, Nomori H, Kobayashi R, Atsumi Y. Well-differentiated adenocarcinoma arising from mature cystic teratoma of the mediastinum (teratoma with malignant transformation). Am J Clin Pathol. 1994;101:531–4.
55. Parker D, Holford CP, Begent RHJ, Newlands ES, Rustin GJS, Makey AR. Effective treatment for malignant mediastinal teratoma. Thorax. 1983;38:897–902.
56. Manivel C, Wick MR, Abenoza P, Rosai J. The occurrence of sarcomatous components in primary mediastinal germ cell tumors. Am J Surg Pathol. 1986;10:711–7.
57. Ahmed T, Bosl GJ, Hajdu SI. Teratoma with malignant transformation in germ cell tumors in men. Cancer. 1985;56:860–3.
58. Beasley SW, Tiedermann K, Howat A. Precocious puberty associated with malignant thoracic teratoma and malignant histiocytosis in child with Klinefelter's syndrome. Med Pediatr Oncol. 1987;15:277–80.
59. Ulbright TM, Clark SA, Einhorn LH. Angiosarcoma associated with germ cell tumors. Hum Pathol. 1985;16:268–72.
60. Cushing B, Bhanot PK, Watts FB, Herztler JH, Brough AJ. Rhabdomyosarcoma and benign teratoma. Pediatr Pathol. 1983;1:345–8.
61. Cox JD. Primary malignant germinal tumors of the mediastinum: a study of 24 cases. Cancer. 1975;36:1162–8.
62. Kiffer JD, Sandeman TF. Primary malignant mediastinal germ cell tumors: a study of eleven cases and a review of the literature. Int J Radiat Oncol Biol Phys. 1989;17:835–41.
63. Economou JS, Trump DL, Holmes EC, Eggleston JE. Management of primary germ cell tumors of the mediastinum. J Thorac Cardiovasc Surg. 1982;83:643–9.
64. Kersh RC, Constable WC, Hahn SS, Spaulding CA, Eisert DR, Jenrette JM, et al. Primary malignant extragonadal germ cell tumors: an analysis of the effect of radiotherapy. Cancer. 1990;65:2681–5.
65. Aliotta PJ, Castillo J, Englander LS, Nseyo UO, Huben RP. Primary mediastinal germ cell tumors: Histologic patterns of treatment failures at autopsy. Cancer. 1988;62:982–4.
66. Hawkins EP, Finegold MJ, Hawkins HK, Krischer JP, Starling KA, Weinberger A. Nongerminomatous malignant germ cell tumors in children. Cancer. 1986;58:2579–84.
67. Pugsley WS, Carleton RL. Germinal nature of teratoid tumors of the thymus. Arch Pathol. 1953;56:341–7.
68. Saabye J, Elbirk A, Andersen K. Teratomas of the mediastinum. Scand J Thorac Cardiovasc Surg. 1987;21:271–2.
69. DeMent SH, Eggleston JC, Spivak JL. Association between mediastinal germ cell tumors and hematologic malignancies. Am J Surg Pathol. 1985;9:23–9.
70. Dexeus FH, Logothetis CJ, Chong C, Sell A, Ogden S. Genetic abnormalities in men with germ cell tumors. J Urol. 1988;140:80–4.
71. Larsen M, Evans WK, Shepherd FA, Phillips MJ, Bailey D, Messner H. Acute lymphoblastic leukemia: possible origin from a mediastinal germ cell tumor. Cancer. 1984;53:441–4.
72. Hoekman K, Ten Bokkel WW, Egbers-Bogaards MA, Mc Vie JG, Somers R. Acute leukemia following therapy for teratoma. Eur J Cancer Clin Oncol. 1984;20:501–2.
73. Hagberg H, Gustavson KH, Sundstrom C, Gerdes U. Blastic phase of myeloproliferative syndrome coexisting with a malignant teratoma. Scand J Haematol. 1983;30:36–40.
74. Domingo A, Romagosa V, Callis M, Vivancos P, Guionnet N, Soler J. Mediastinal germ cell tumor and acute megakaryoblastic leukemia. Ann Intern Med. 1989;111:539.
75. Curry WA, McKay CE, Richardson RL, Greco FA. Klinefelter's syndrome and mediastinal germ cell neoplasms. J Urol. 1981;125:127–9.
76. Myers TJ, Kessimian N, Schwartz S. Mediastinal Germ cell tumors associated with the hemophagocytic syndrome. Ann Int Med. 1988;109(6):504–5.
77. Redman JR, Vugrin D, Arlin ZA, Gee TS, Kempin SJ, Godbold JH, et al. Leukemia following treatment of germ cell tumors in men. J Clin Oncol. 1984;2:1080–7.
78. Penchansky L, Krause JR. Acute leukemia following a malignant teratoma in a child with klinefelter's syndrome: case report and review of secondary leukemias in children following treatment of a primary neoplasm. Cancer. 1982;50:684–9.
79. Landanyi M, Roy I. Mediastinal germ cell tumors and histiocytosis. Hum Pathol. 1988;19:586–90.
80. Tricot G, Fryns JP, Thomas J, Moerman P, Broeckaert-Van Orshoven A, Vermaelen K, et al. 5q-Anomaly in a patient with disseminated teratoma. Cancer Genet Cytogenet. 1983;9:239–44.
81. Suster S, Moran CA, Koss MN. Rhabdomyosarcomas of the anterior mediastinum: report of four cases unassociated with germ cell, teratomatous, or thymic carcinomatous components. Hum Pathol. 1994;25:349–56.
82. Klimstra DS, Moran CA, Perino G, Koss MN, Rosai J. Liposarcoma of the anterior mediastinum and thymus: a clinicopathologic study of 28 cases. Am J Surg Pathol. 1995;19:782–91.
83. el-Domeiri AA, Hutter RV, Pool JL, Foote FW Jr. Primary seminoma of the anterior mediastinum. Ann Thorac Surg. 1968;6:513–21.
84. Kleitsch WP, Taricco A, Haslam GJ. Primary seminoma (germinoma) of the mediastinum. Ann Thorac Surg. 1967;4:249–55.
85. Nazari A, Gagnon ED. Seminoma-like tumor of the mediastinum. A case report with 7 year follow-up. J Thorac Cardiovasc Surg. 1966;51:751–4.
86. Lattes R. Thymoma and other tumors of the thymus: an analysis of 107 cases. Cancer. 1962;15:1224–60.
87. Nagi DK, Jones WG, Belchetz PE. Gynaecomastia caused by a primary mediastinal seminoma. Clin Endocrinol. 1994;40:545–8.
88. Bush SE, Martinez A, Bagshaw MA. Primary mediastinal seminoma. Cancer. 1981;48:1877–82.
89. Sterchi M, Cordell AR. Seminoma of the anterior mediastinum. Ann Thorac Surg. 1975;19:371–7.
90. Cha EM. Ectopic seminoma (germinoma) in the retroperitoneum and mediastinum: with emphasis on the lymphangiogram. J Urol. 1973;110:47–9.
91. Nickels J, Franssila K. Primary seminoma of the anterior mediastinum. A case report with 10-year follow-up. Acta Pathol Microbiol Scand A. 1972;80:260–2.

92. Lajos TZ, Charrette EJ, Farr JA. Primary mediastinal seminoma. Chest. 1971;59:575–8.
93. Martini N, Golbet RB, Hajdu SI, Whitmore WF, Beattie EJ. Primary mediastinal germ cell tumors. Cancer. 1974;33:763–9.
94. Schantz A, Sewall W, Castleman B. Mediastinal seminoma: a study of 21 cases with an excellent prognosis. Cancer. 1972;30:1189–94.
95. Hurt RD, Bruckman JE, Farrow GM, Bernatz PE, Hahn RG, Earle JD. Primary anterior mediastinal seminoma. Cancer. 1982;49:1658–63.
96. Aygun C, Slawson RG, Bajaj K, Salazar OM. Primary mediastinal seminoma. Urology. 1984;23:109–17.
97. Battifora H, Sheibani K, Tubbs RR, Kopinski MI, Tung-Tien S. Antikeratin antibodies in tumor diagnosis: distinction between seminoma and embryonal carcinoma. Cancer. 1984;54:843–8.
98. Kinding JR, Tavel ME. Clinical problems in cardiopulmonary disease: acquired pulmonic stenosis due to mediastinal seminoma. Chest. 1980;78:493–5.
99. Burns BF, McCaughey WTE. Unusual thymic seminomas. Arch Pathol Lab Med. 1986;110:539–41.
100. Polansky SM, Barwick KW, Ravin CE. Primary mediastinal seminoma. Am J Roentgenol. 1979;132:17–21.
101. Raghavan D, Barrett A. Mediastinal seminoma. Cancer. 1980;46:1187–91.
102. Lee YM, Jackson SM. Primary seminoma of the mediastinum. Cancer. 1985;55:450–2.
103. Friedman SJ, Belbel RL, Martin NJ. Extragonadal mediastinal seminoma. Mil Med. 1988;153:32–4.
104. Cefaro GA, Turriziani LA, Salvi G, Marmiroli L. Primary mediastinal seminoma. Br J Urol. 1988;62:461–4.
105. Janssen M, Johnston WH. Anaplastic seminoma of the testis: ultrastructural analysis of three cases. Cancer. 1978;41:538–44.
106. Levine GD. Primary seminoma- a neoplasm ultrastructurally similar to testicular seminoma and distinct from epithelial thymoma. Cancer. 1973;31:729–41.
107. Brown K, Collins JD, Batra P. Mediastinal germ cell tumor in a young woman. Med Pediatr Oncol. 1989;17:164–7.
108. Takahashi N, Chifu S, Matsuo K, Nakao S, Noguchi K, Kohno T, et al. Primary mediastinal seminoma - a case report. Gan No Rinsho. 1988;34:331–41.
109. Moran CA, Suster S, Przygodski RM, Koss MN. Primary germ cell tumors of the mediastinum. II. Mediastinal seminomas - a clinicopathologic and immunohistochemical study of 120 cases. Cancer. 1997;80:691–8.
110. Polansky SM, Barwick KW, Ravin CE. Primary mediastinal seminoma. AJR. 1979;62:179–82.
111. Azzopardi JG, Hoffbrand AV. Retrogression in testicular seminoma with viable metastases. J Clin Pathol. 1965;18:135–41.
112. Abell MR, Fayos JV, Lampe I. Retroperitoneal germinomas (seminomas) without evidence of testicular involvement. Cancer. 1965;18:273–90.
113. Buskirk SJ, Evans RG, Farrow GM, Earle JD. Primary retroperitoneal seminoma. Cancer. 1982;49:1934–6.
114. Daugaard G, Olsen J, von der Maase H, Rorth M, Skakkebaek NE. Carcinoma in-situ testis in patients with assumed extragonadal germ-cell tumours. Lancet. 1987;330:528–9.
115. Bohle A, Studer UE, Sonntag RW, Scheidegger JR. Primary or secondary extragonadal germ cell tumors? J Urol. 1986; 135:939–43.
116. Johnson DE, Appelt G, Samuels ML, Luna M. Metastases from testicular carcinoma: study of 78 autopsied cases. Urology. 1976;3:234–9.
117. Lynch MJG, Blewett GL. Choriocarcinoma arising in the male mediastinum. Thorax. 1953;8:157–61.
118. White JE, Fincher RM, D'Cruz IA. Pericardial metastasis from testicular seminoma: appearance and disappearance by echocardiography. Am J Med Sci. 1991;301:182–5.
119. Bosl GJ, Dmitrovsky E, Reuter VE, Samaniego F, Rodriguez E, Geller NL, et al. Isochromosome of chromosome 12: clinically useful marker for male germ cell tumors. J Natl Cancer Inst. 1989;81:1874–8.
120. Oosterhuis JW, Rammeloo RHU, Cornellisse CJ, de Jong B, Dam A, Sleijfer DT. Ploidy of malignant mediastinal germ cell tumors. Hum Pathol. 1990;21:729–32.
121. Przygodzki RM, Moran CA, Suster S, Khan MA, Swalsky PA, Bakker A, et al. Primary mediastinal and testicular seminomas: a comparison of K-ras-2 gene sequence and p53 immunoperoxidase analysis of 26 cases. Hum Pathol. 1996;27:975–9.
122. Lee KS, Im JG, Han CH, Han MC, Kim CW, Kim WS. Malignant primary germ cell tumors of the mediastinum. AJR. 1989;153:947–51.
123. Shin MS, Odrezin GT, Van Dyke JA, Ho KJ. Unusual initial calcifications of primary and metastatic seminomas: detection by computed tomography. Chest. 1991;99:1543–5.
124. Smalley SR, Earle JD, Evans RG, Richardson RL. Modern radiotherapy results with bulky stages II and III seminoma. J Urol. 1990;144:685–9.
125. Sagerman RH, Kotlove DJ, Regine WF, Chung CT, King GA, Dalal PS. Stage II seminoma: results of postorchiectomy irradiation. Radiology. 1989;172:565–8.
126. Jose B, Perkins LP, Kays H, Chu AM, Sharma SC. Is mediastinal irradiation necessary for stage I testicular seminoma? J Surg Oncol. 1984;25:250–1.
127. Kersh CR, Eisert DR, Constable WC. Primary malignant mediastinal germ-cell tumors and the contribution of radiotherapy: a southeastern multi-institutional study. Am J Clin Oncol. 1987;10:302–6.
128. Motzer RJ, Bajorin DF, Bosl GJ. "Poor Risk" germ cell tumors: current progress and future directions. Semin Oncol. 1992;19:206–14.
129. Medini E, Levitt SH, Jones TK, Tao Y. The management of extratesticular seminoma without gonadal involvement. Cancer. 1979;44:2032–8.
130. Hainsworth JD, Einhorn LH, Williams SD, Stewart M, Greco FA. Advanced extragonadal germ-cell tumors: successful treatment with combination chemotherapy. Ann Intern Med. 1982; 97:7–11.
131. Green N, Broth E, George FW, Kaplan R, Lombardo L, Skaist L, et al. Radiation therapy in bulky seminoma. Urology. 1983;21:467–9.
132. Lederman GS, Sheldon TA, Chaffey JT, Herman TS, Gelman RS, Coleman CN. Cardiac disease after mediastinal irradiation for seminoma. Cancer. 1987;60:772–6.
133. Biester RJ, Lippert MC, Mills SE. Late recurrence of a seminoma. J Urol. 1987;137:749–50.
134. Rodney AJ, Tannir NM, Siefer-Radtke AO, Liu P, Walsh GL, Millikan RE, et al. Survival outcomes for men with mediastinal germ cell tumors: the University of Texas M. D. Anderson Cancer Center experience. Urol Oncol. 2012;30(6):879–85.
135. Scardino PT, Cos DH, Waldmann TA, Mcintire RK, Mittemeyer B, Javadpour N. The value of serum tumor markers in the staging and prognosis of germ cell tumors of the testis. J Urol. 1977;118:994–9.
136. Moran CA, Suster S. Mediastinal seminomas with prominent cystic changes: a clinicopathologic study of 10 cases. Am J Surg Pathol. 1995;19:1047–53.
137. Weissferdt A, Moran CA. Mediastinal seminoma with florid follicular hyperplasia: a clinicopathological and immunohistochemical study of six cases. Virchows Arch. 2015;466:209–15.
138. Moran CA, Suster S, Perino G, Kaneko M, Koss MN. Malignant smooth muscle tumors presenting as mediastinal soft tissue masses. Cancer. 1994;74:2251–60.
139. Weissferdt A, Kalhor N, Moran CA. Combined thymoma-thymic seminoma. Report of 2 cases of a heretofore unreported association. Hum Pathol. 2014;45:2168–72.

140. Beckstead JH. Alkaline phosphatase histochemistry in human germ cell neoplasms. Am J Surg Pathol. 1983;7:341–9.
141. Niehans GA, Manivel C, Copland GT, Scheithauer BW, Wick MR. Immunohistochemistry of germ cell and trophoblastic neoplasms. Cancer. 1988;62:1113–23.
142. Suster S, Moran CA, Dominguez-Malagon H, Quevedo-Blanco P. Germ cell tumors of the mediastinum and testis: a comparative immunohistochemical study of 120 cases. Hum Pathol. 1998;29(7):737–42.
143. Lewis DJ, Sesterhenn IA, McCarthy WF, Moul JW. Immunohistochemical expression of P53 tumor suppressor gene protein in adult germ cell testis tumors: clinical correlation in stage I disease. J Urol. 1994;152:418–23.
144. Wei YD, Jiafu Z, Xi QS, Yongjiang M, Xiulong Z, Daizong L, et al. P53 gene mutations in chinese human testicular seminoma. J Urol. 1993;150:884–6.
145. Baily D, Baumal R, Marks A. Use of anti-seminoma monoclonal antibody to confirm the diagnosis of mediastinal seminoma. APMIS. 1988;96:206–10.
146. Weissferdt A, Moran CA. Primary mediastinal "thymic" seminomas. Adv Anat Pathol. 2012;19:75–80.
147. Jung SM, Chu PH, Shiu TF, Wu HH, Kuo TT, Chu JJ, et al. Expression of OCT4 in primary germ cell tumors and thymoma in the mediastinum. Appl Immunohistochem Mol Morphol. 2006;14:273–5.
148. Liu A, Cheng L, Du J, Peng Y, Allan RW, Wei L, et al. Diagnostic utility of novel stem cell markers SALL4, OCT4, NANOG, SOX2, UTF1, and TCL1 in primary mediastinal germ cell tumors. Am J Surg Pathol. 2010;34:697–706.
149. Weissferdt A, Rodriguez J, Liu H, Fujimoto J, Wistuba II, Moran CA. Primary mediastinal seminomas: a comprehensive immunohistochemical study with focus on novel markers. Hum Pathol. 2015;46:376–83.
150. Ulbright TM. Germ cell neoplasms of the testis. Am J Surg Pathol. 1993;17:1075–91.
151. Teilum G. Endodermal sinus tumor of the ovary and testes; comparative morphogenesis of so-called mesonephroma ovarii (Schiller) and extraembryonic (yolk-sac allantoid) structures of rat's placenta. Cancer. 1959;12:1092–105.
152. Truong LD, Harris L, Mattioli C, Lee A, Wheeler T, Lane M. Endodermal sinus tumor of the mediastinum. Cancer. 1986;58:730–9.
153. Burt ME, Javadpour N. Germ cell tumors in patients with apparently normal testes. Cancer. 1981;47:1911–5.
154. Chamsi-Pasha M, Bernstein A. Mediastinal yolk sac tumor mimicking pericardial effusion. Thorax. 1988;43:339–40.
155. Gooneratne S, Keh P, Sreekanth S, Recant W, Talerman A. Anterior mediastinal endodermal sinus (Yolk sac) tumor in a female infant. Cancer. 1985;56:1430–3.
156. Mukai K, Adams WR. Yolk sac tumor of the anterior mediastinum: case report. Am J Surg Pathol. 1979;3:77–83.
157. Fox MA, Vix VA. Endodermal sinus (Yolk sac) tumors of the anterior mediastinum. Am J Roentgenol. 1980;135:291–4.
158. Huntington RW, Bullock WK. Yolk sac tumors of extragonadal origin. Cancer. 1970;25:1368–76.
159. Kuzur ME, Cobleigh MA, Greco FA, Einhorn LH, Oldham RK. Endodermal sinus tumor of the mediastinum. Cancer. 1982;50:766–74.
160. Nogales-Fernandez F, Silverberg SG, Bloustein PA, Martinez-Hernandez A, Pierce GB. Yolk sac carcinoma (endodermal sinus tumor). Cancer. 1977;39:1462–74.
161. Roth LM, Panganiban WG. Gonadal and extragonadal yolk sac carcinomas: a clinicopathologic study of 14 cases. Cancer. 1976;37:812–20.
162. Brown NJ. Teratomas and yolk sac tumours. J Clin Pathol. 1976;29:1021–5.
163. Vuletin JC, Rosen Y, Brigati DJ, Gourin A. Endodermal sinus tumor of the mediastinum. Chest. 1977;72:112–4.
164. DeSmet AA, Silver TM, Hart WR. Endodermal sinus tumor of the anterior mediastinum. South Med J. 1977;70:757–8.
165. Moran CA, Suster S, Koss MN. Primary germ cell tumors of the mediastinum. III Yolk sac tumor, embryonal carcinoma, choriocarcinoma, and combined nonteratomatous germ cell tumors of the mediastinum - a clinicopathologic and immunohistochemical study of 64 cases. Cancer. 1997;80:699–707.
166. Pedersen-Norgaard P, Albrechtsen R, Teilum G. Serum alphafoetoprotein as a marker for endodermal sinus tumour (yolk sac tumour) or a vitelline component of "teratocarcinoma". Acta Pathol Microbiol Scand. 1975;83:573–89.
167. Talerman A, Haije WG, Baggerman L. Serum alphafetoprotein (AFP) in patients with germ cell tumors of the gonads and extragonadal sites: correlation between endodermal sinus (yolk sac) tumor and raised serum AFP. Cancer. 1980;46:380–5.
168. Sogge MR, McDonald SD, Cofold PB. The malignant potential of the dysgenetic germ cell in klinefelter's syndrome. Am J Med. 1979;66:515.
169. Nichols CR, Heerema NA, Palmer C, Loehrer PJ, Williams SD, Einhorn LH. Klinefelter's syndrome associated with mediastinal germ cell neoplasm. J Clin Oncol. 1987;5:1290–4.
170. Floret D, Renaud H, Monnet P. Sexual precocity and thoracic polyembryoma: klinefelter's syndrome? J Pediatr. 1979;94:163.
171. Garnick MB, Griffin JD. Idiopathic thrombocytopenia in association with extragonadal germ cell cancer. Ann Intern Med. 1983;98:926–7.
172. Nichols CR, Roth BJ, Heerema N, Griep J, Tricot G. Hematologic neoplasia associated with primary mediastinal germ cell tumors. N Engl J Med. 1990;322:1425–9.
173. Orazi A, Neiman RS, Ulbright TM, Heerema NA, John K, Nichols CR. Hematopoietic precursor cells within the yolk sac tumor component are the source of secondary hematopoietic malignancies in patients with mediastinal germ cell tumors. Cancer. 1993;71:3873–81.
174. Michael H, Ulbright TM, Brodhecker CA. The pluripotential nature of the mesenchyme-like component of yolk sac tumor. Arch Pathol Lab Med. 1989;113:1115–9.
175. Dehner LP. Yet another face on the yolk sac tumor. Arch Pathol Lab Med. 1989;113:1113–4.
176. Ulbright TM, Michael H, Loehrer PJ, Donohue JP. Spindle cell tumors resected from male patients with germ cell tumors: a clinicopathologic study of 14 cases. Cancer. 1990;65:148–56.
177. Kurman RJ, Norris HJ. Endodermal sinus tumors of the ovary. Cancer. 1976;38:2404–19.
178. Kay PH, Wells FC, Goldstraw P. A multidisciplinary approach to primary nonseminomatous germ cell tumors of the mediastinum. Ann Thorac Surg. 1987;44:578–82.
179. Wright CD, Kesler KA, Nichols CR, Mahomed Y, Einhorn LH, Miller ME, et al. Primary mediastinal nonseminomatous germ cell tumors. J Thorac Cardiovasc Surg. 1990;99:210–7.
180. McLeod DG, Grant TH, Skoog SJ, Dawson NA, Waxman JA. Extragonadal germ cell tumors: clinicopathologic findings and treatment experience in 12 patients. Cancer. 1988;61:1187–91.
181. Sham JST, Fu KH, Chiu CSW, Lau WH, Choi PHK, Khin AM, et al. Experience with the management of primary endodermal sinus tumor of the mediastinum. Cancer. 1989;64:756–61.
182. Broun ER, Nichols CR, Einhorn LH, Tricot GJK. Salvage therapy with high-dose chemotherapy and autologous bone marrow support in the treatment of primary nonseminomatous mediastinal germ cell tumors. Cancer. 1991;68:1513–5.
183. Nichols CR, Saxman S, Williams SD, Loehrer PJ, Miller ME, Wright C, et al. Primary mediastinal nonseminomatous germ cell tumors. Cancer. 1990;65:1641–6.

184. Moran CA, Suster S. Yolk sac tumors of the mediastinum with prominent spindle cell features. Am J Surg Pathol. 1997;21:1173–7.
185. Moran CA, Suster S. Mediastinal yolk sac tumors associated with prominent multilocular cystic changes of thymic epithelium: a clinicopathologic and immunohistochemical study of five cases. Mod Pathol. 1997;10(8):800–3.
186. Moran CA, Suster S. Primary yolk sac tumors of the mediastinum prominent hepatoid features: a clinicopathologic and immunohistochemical study of 4 cases. Am J Surg Pathol. 1997;21:1210–4.
187. Kurman RJ, Scardino PT, McIntire KR, Waldmann TA, Javadpour N. Cellular localization of alpha-fetoprotein and human chorionic gonadotrophin in germ cell tumors of the testis using an indirect immunoperoxidase technique. Cancer. 1977;40:2136–51.
188. Sandhaus L, Strom R, Mukai K. Malignant germ cell tumor of the mediastinum in a female. Lab Investig. 1980;42:147.
189. Sangalli G, Livraghi T, Giordano F, Tavani E, Schiaffino E. Primary mediastinal embryonal carcinoma and choriocarcinoma: a case report. Acta Cytol. 1986;30:543–6.
190. Knapp RH, Fritz SR, Reiman HM. Primary embryonal carcinoma and choriocarcinoma of the mediastinum: a case report. Arch Pathol Lab Med. 1982;106:507–9.
191. McNeil MM, Leong AS-E, Sage RE. Primary mediastinal embryonal carcinoma in association with klinefelter's syndrome. Cancer. 1981;47:343–5.
192. Pallesen G, Hamilton-Dutoit SJ. Ki-1 (CD30) antigen is regularly expressed by tumor cells of embryonal carcinoma. Am J Pathol. 1988;133:446–50.
193. Ulbright TM, Goheen MP, Roth LM, Gillespie JJ. The differentiation of carcinomas of teratomatous origin from embryonal carcinoma. A light and electron microscopic study. Cancer. 1986;57:257–63.
194. Azzopardi JG, Mostofi FK, Theiss EA. Lesions of testes observed in certain patients with widespread choriocarcinoma and related tumors. Am J Pathol. 1961;38:207–25.
195. Wenger ME, Dines DE, Ahmann DL, Good CA. Primary mediastinal choriocarcinoma. Mayo Clin Proc. 1968;43:570–5.
196. Sickles EA, Belliveau RE, Wiernik PH. Primary mediastinal choriocarcinoma in the male. Cancer. 1974;33:1196–203.
197. Greenwood SM, Goodman JR, Schneider G, Forman BH, Kress SC, Gelb AF. Choriocarcinoma in a man. Am J Med. 1971;51:416–22.
198. Storm PB, Fallon B, Bunge RG. Mediastinal choriocarcinoma in a chromatin-positive boy. J Urol. 1976;116:838–40.
199. Hsueh YS, Tsung SH, Shamsai R, Chang HH. Primary mediastinal choriocarcinoma in a man with an abnormal chromosome. South Med J. 1984;77:1466–9.
200. Kathuria S, Jablokov VR. Primary choriocarcinoma of mediastinum with immunohistochemical study and review of the literature. J Surg Oncol. 1987;34:39–42.
201. Connolly CE, Gillan J, Maguire R, Hitchcock H. Primary choriocarcinoma of the mediastinum. Ir J Med Sci. 1979;148:20–2.
202. Candes FP, Ajinkya MS. Primary mediastinal choriocarcinoma (case report). J Postgrad Med. 1987;33:219–21.
203. Moran CA, Suster S. Primary mediastinal choriocarcinomas: a clinicopathologic and immunohistochemical study of eight cases. Am J Surg Pathol. 1997;21:1007–12.
204. Fishback NF, Travis WD, Moran CA, Guinee DG, McCarthy WF, Koss MN. Pleomorphic (Spindle/Giant cell) carcinoma of the lung. Cancer. 1994;73:2936–45.
205. Taccagni GL, Parafioriti A, Dell'Antonio G, Crespi G. Mixed germ cell tumors of the mediastinum (seminoma, embryonal carcinoma, choriocarcinoma and teratoma). Pathol Res Pract. 1989;185:506–10.
206. Nichols CR, Hoffman R, Einhorn LH, Williams SD, Wheeler LA, Garnick MB. Hematologic malignancies associated with primary mediastinal germ cell tumors. Ann Intern Med. 1985;102:603–9.

11 Neurogenic Tumors

Introduction

Primary mediastinal neurogenic tumors in general are rare and can be present in children and adults as well. Even though for the most part the most common tumors are generally of the benign type in the adult population (ganglioneuroma, schwannoma, neurofibroma), that may not be the case in the pediatric age group (ganglioneuroblastoma, neuroblastoma). However, the gamut of these tumors in the mediastinal location is wide and can pose problems in interpretation when limited material is available for evaluation. Even though the posterior mediastinal compartment is the most common location for these tumors, it is not unusual to see any one of these tumors occurring in the anterior mediastinal compartment. Regardless of the anatomic location, for practical purposes, one can separate mediastinal neurogenic tumors into benign and malignant, which in turn may help not only in terms of diagnosis but also in terms of the follow-up that patients with these tumors may obtain.

A simple practical schema based on the occurrence of these tumors would include the following neoplasms:

- Benign neurogenic tumors
  - Neurofibroma
  - Ganglioneuroma
  - Schwannoma
  - Granular cell tumor
- Malignant neurogenic tumors
  - Neuroblastoma/ganglioneuroblastoma
  - Malignant peripheral nerve sheath tumor (MPNST)
  - Peripheral neuroectodermal tumor (PNET/Ewing Sarcoma)
  - Pigmented neuroectodermal tumor of infancy (melanotic progonoma, retinal anlage tumor): considered benign but with the potential to metastatize in a small percentage of cases
  - Ependymoma
  - Meningioma
  - Malignant granular cell tumor

Following this schema, it is likely that the vast majority of tumors may be approachable following morphological, immunohistochemical, ultrastructural, and molecular biological features.

However, it is important to highlight that neurogenic tumors may also be divided into those originating from nerve sheaths and those originating from nerve cells (paraganglia, parasympathetic ganglia). Those originating from nerve sheath are supposed to arise from differentiated adult Schwann cell, thus its name Schwannoma, and these represent one of the most common benign tumors in the posterior mediastinum. The nerve cell tumors are represented by another common neoplasm: ganglioneuroma. It is important to highlight that either nerve sheath or nerve cell tumors may range from benign to their malignant counterparts. Thus, for the nerve sheath tumors, the benign tumor is represented by schwannoma, while the malignant counterpart will be represented by "malignant schwannoma" or "malignant peripheral nerve sheath tumor" (MPNST). Tumors from nerve cells also range from the mature and differentiated ganglioneuroma to the more immature and undifferentiated neuroblastoma. One tumor that may share features of both mature and immature elements is ganglioneuroblastoma. In addition, it is important to recognize that all nerve elements – axons, sheath cells, and connective tissue – form tumors like neurofibromas. Those neurofibromas that show plexiform features are commonly associated with neurofibromatosis. It is of interest to mention that it has been suggested that all these tumors have a neural crest origin, and the term "thoracic neurolophomas" has been advanced [1].

In this chapter, there will not be an attempt to specifically separate by clinical means the different types of neurogenic tumors, except when indicated and appropriate. The clinical features of these tumors, including their radiological features, will be conjointly discussed, and appropriate observations will be made when specifically indicated to separate a benign neoplasm from a malignant one or a specific tumor from others.

© Springer Nature Switzerland AG 2019
N. Kalhor, C. Moran, *Mediastinal Pathology*, https://doi.org/10.1007/978-3-319-98980-8_11

In 1949, Blades [2], in reference to the practice of routine roentgenologic examination of the chest, stated that such practice would uncover that mediastinal tumors are not as rare as it is commonly believed. Blades [2] also stated that successful treatment of mediastinal tumors depends on their detection before clinical signs are apparent, and a discovery of any mediastinal mass demands positive diagnosis. Furthermore, he stated that the mediastinum could harbor any type of tumor, and it would be convenient to classify mediastinal tumors into two groups (anterior and posterior mediastinal tumors); he also stated that posterior mediastinal tumors are chiefly of one common variety: neurogenic. More than 70 years later, one can only agree with what has been proven by many who have studied the mediastinum. Needless to say, sporadic exceptions are not unusual as nothing can be completely fool-proof regarding the location of these tumors.

In 1958, Richards and Reeves [3], in a study of mediastinal tumors and cysts in children, stated that their occurrence in children is rare. The authors made reference to a single case of a 2-year-old child who was diagnosed with neuroblastoma of the posterior mediastinum. The authors stated that there are three other tumors that may occur in this anatomic location: (1) neurinoma, (2) sympathogonioma, and (3) ganglioneuroma. They added that these tumors are often associated with vertebral body or neural arch erosion, which translates into "back pain." In 1960, Carey and colleagues [4] presented a study of 140 cases of what the author called extrapleural mediastinal neurogenic tumors. The patients' ages spanned between 0 and 69 years, and there does not appear to be a gender predilection. The vast majority of tumors belonged to schwannomas and ganglioneuromas, with only six malignant tumors, one "malignant schwannoma" in a patient with neurofibromatosis, and five neuroblastomas. The malignant tumors were seen in patients less than 20 years of age, while the majority of benign tumors were seen in patients older than 20 years. More than half of the patients were asymptomatic, and the frequent complaint was that of "thoracic pain." Horner's syndrome was associated in three cases. What is interesting in this report is that the authors arbitrarily separated all these tumors anatomically into five different compartments: superior, superior and middle, middle, middle and inferior, and inferior. In a study of 50 cases, Pachter and Lattes [5] divided these tumors into two types: (1) tumors of nerve sheath origin, neurilemmoma, neurofibroma, and malignant schwannoma; and (2) tumors of the sympathetic nervous system, ganglioneuroma, ganglioneuroblastoma, and neuroblastoma. Of the 50 cases described, 12 were malignant, while 47 were located in the posterior mediastinum. Three of these neurogenic tumors were located in the anterior mediastinum. The majority of the tumors appear in adult individuals, while the malignant tumors (neuroblastoma, ganglioneuroblastoma) appear to be more common in children. Interestingly, in the two cases of malignant schwannoma, there was no history of von Recklinghausen's disease. Meyer and Ochsner [6] also reported their experience with intrathoracic neurogenic tumors in 32 cases from 1942 to 1965. Four of the reported cases were not located in the posterior mediastinum. The reported patients ranged in age from 3 to 72 years, and the gender distribution was similar between men and women (18 women and 14 men). One third of the cases reported were malignant: five with neurogenic sarcomas (two patients with history of von Recklinghausen's disease) and five patients with neuroblastomas (one adult patient over 50 years of age). Whittaker and Lynn [7] reported 105 mediastinal tumors in children under 16 years of age during the period from 1935 to 1968 and found 37 cases of neurogenic tumors; the majority was basically represented by 16 ganglioneuromas and 11 neuroblastomas. The authors concluded that, in general, mediastinal masses in children may not cause symptoms and that the lack of symptoms should not be interpreted as the lesion being benign. Pokorny and colleagues [8] reported their experience with mediastinal tumors in infants and children: 109 cases between 1954 and 1972. The ages ranged from 2 h to 16 years; 35 of the 109 cases were neurogenic tumors, and the majority of the cases were neuroblastomas (18 cases) followed by ganglioneuroblastoma (8 cases). King and colleagues [9], in a review of benign and malignant mediastinal tumors in children, identified 27 out of 52 tumors in children as benign neurogenic tumors (ganglioneuroma, neurilemmoma, and neurofibroma), while 20 tumors out of 136 were identified as malignant (neuroblastoma, ganglioneuroblastoma). Vidne and Levy [10] reported on 45 patients between 1964 and 1970 (24 males and 21 females between the ages of 7 months and 74 years) and encountered only nine cases corresponding to neurogenic tumors with only one of the nine cases being malignant (neuroblastoma). Davison and colleagues [11] also reported 55 cases of intrathoracic neural tumors over a 25-year period of time. The patients' ages ranged from 7 months to 63 years; 41 patients were asymptomatic, 52 tumors were in the posterior mediastinum, and only 3 tumors were malignant (neuroblastoma). In a more focused study, Akwari and colleagues [12] reported on 69 patients with mediastinal neurogenic tumors, with extension through an intervertebral foramen "dumbbell-shaped" mass. The cases represented 9.8% of all mediastinal neurogenic tumors (706 cases in total). The authors stated that the majority of these patients present with neurologic symptoms of spinal cord compression and that about 10% of these tumors are malignant. In a larger series of mediastinal tumors in the period from 1954 to 1973, Luosto and coworkers [13] reported 208 cases in patients between the ages of 2 and 74 years, of which only 39 belonged to neurogenic tumors. The majority of the tumors were benign (neurilemmoma, neurofibroma, ganglioneuroma), with only two malignant tumors (neurofibrosarcoma and ganglioneuroblastoma). In a study of 160 thoracic neural tumors from the radiological point of view, Reed and coworkers [14] argued that radiologists may suggest a specific preoperative diagnosis by combining radiographic appearance and age of the patient, and stated that a posterior mediastinal mass in a young child is most likely a neuroblastoma or ganglioneuroblastoma, while the same presentation in an adult patient would be most likely a ganglioneuroma, schwannoma, or neurofibroma. Harjula and coworkers [15], in a study on mediastinal neurogenic tumors with emphasis on early and late results of surgical treatment, identified 66 cases with a mean follow-up of 12 years. The patients' ages ranged from 13 to 72 years of age (only one 2-year-old child). The vast majority of cases were benign tumors with only a couple of malignant neoplasms. Three patients were identified to have recurrence of a benign tumor (neurilemmoma and neurinoma). Malignant transformation was identified in two of eight neurofibromas 5 and 13 years postoperatively. Blegvad and coworkers [16] reported on 129 mediastinal tumors in 72 men and 57 women over a period from 1971 to 1987; the patients' ages ranged from 3 months to 81 years, and the mean age was 44 years. Twenty-seven tumors were identified as neurogenic, and, of those, 12 were in children. Of the 27 cases identified as neurogenic, 5 were malignant and all were in children. Saenz and coworkers [17], in a study of 63 patients with focus on posterior mediastinal tumors, described 63 patients between the ages of 1 day and 26 years; the median age was 6 years. While 89% of the tumors were categorized as neurogenic, the symptomatology presented included respiratory symptoms or chest pain 45% and neurologic symptoms 13% (half related to spinal cord compression). Palpable masses were discovered in 5% of the patients. In 32% of the patients, the discovery of the posterior mediastinal mass was an incidental finding. Neuroblastoma was the most common malignant neoplasm, and malignancy was identified in 60% of all patients. Follow-up in patients with neuroblastoma showed that 4 out of 32 patients had died after a period of 7–289 months; the median was 73 months. The authors stated that patients in whom the diagnosis of neuroblastoma was made during the first year of life had better prognosis than older patients. In addition, the authors stated that MRI is superior to CT in the evaluation of posterior mediastinal tumors. In that regard, Sakai and coworkers [18], in a study of nine patients with intrathoracic neurogenic tumor using MRI, stated that some of these tumors have a characteristic appearance that may be helpful in the differential diagnosis. Also, Strollo and coworkers [19], in a review of middle and posterior mediastinal tumors, stated that on MRI schwannoma and neurofibroma typically have low to intermediate signal intensity on T1-weighted images and may have areas of intermediate to high signal intensity on T2-weighted sequences. The authors also added that MRI should be performed preoperatively in all patients with suspected neurogenic tumors to definitely exclude intraspinal tumor extension. Tanaka and coworkers [20] made similar observations in a study of neurogenic mediastinal tumors using MRI. Carachi and coworkers [21], in a study of 145 children with neuroblastoma over a 20-year period of time (1961–1980), identified 30 children with thoracic neuroblastoma with a mortality rate of 16%. In a similar study of 196 infants and children, Grosfeld and coworkers [22] found that 72% of the mediastinal tumors in this group were malignant. Despite this, lymphoma was the most common malignancy, and neuroblastoma was the second most common malignancy in this group. Ganglioneuroma, schwannoma, and neurofibroma together represented 21 of the 196 tumoral cases. From the anatomic point of view, Sugio and colleagues [23] reported 39 cases of neurogenic tumors of the mediastinum, specifically identifying two neurilemmomas originating from the vagus nerve. Takeda and colleagues [24] reviewed 50 years of experience from a single institution in Japan and accounted for 146 patients (74 male and 72 female, 60 children and 86 adults). The posterior mediastinum was the most common location, with 136 tumors located in that anatomic area with 118 tumors belonging to ganglioneuromas, schwannomas, and neurofibromas. Only 23 cases were identified as neuroblastomas and ganglioneuroblastomas. Most patients were asymptomatic: 84% of adults and 60% of children. Overall, about 20% of the tumors were malignant, and most of them occurred in the first 5 years of life. In a more general study of mediastinal tumors from patients ranging from 6 months to 62 years, Shrivastava and colleagues [25] documented 106 patients with mediastinal tumors, with only 16% of these tumors located in the posterior mediastinum. Other authors have also found a similar trend when all mediastinal tumors are put together [26], determining that the presence of neurogenic tumors in the posterior mediastinum still is not a common occurrence. Other authors have focused mainly on the most adequate surgical procedure for the treatment of benign neurogenic tumors, stating that video-assisted thoracoscopic surgery (VATS) is the procedure of choice [27]. In a more recent review of intrathoracic neurogenic tumors, Bicakcioglu [28] reported on 149 patients (including 4 patients with paragangliomas): 90 females and 59 males between the ages of 7 months and 77 years (average, 24.5 years), comprised of 29 infants and children and 120 adults. Of the 149 patients reported, 113 had benign neurogenic tumors (schwannoma, neurofibroma, ganglioneuroma), while 13 had ganglioneuroblastoma/neuroblastoma, and 10 patients had malignant schwannoma. The majority of these tumors was located in the posterior mediastinum (131 cases), while 3 were in the anterior mediastinum. The rest of the tumors were distributed in other parts of the thoracic cavity. Seven patients had a history of von Recklinghausen's disease. The authors concluded that complete surgical resection is the treatment of choice for malignant and benign thoracic neurogenic tumors, and that after histopathologic analysis other treatment options should be considered.

Based on the published literature on intrathoracic tumors, it is likely that benign neurogenic tumors are more common than their malignant counterparts. However, it is also likely that malignant neurogenic tumors are more common in the pediatric age group. Also important to highlight is the fact that benign neurogenic tumors – ganglioneuroma, neurofibroma, and schwannoma – are likely to be treated with complete surgical resection alone, while malignant neoplasms may also be treated with complete surgical resection plus additional medical therapy.

Benign Tumors

Ganglioneuroma

In 1947, Stout [29] presented 10 cases of his own and reviewed previous literature, which included 233 additional cases of what the author called ganglioneuroma of the sympathetic nervous system. In this review, Stout [29] gave credit to Loretz who, in 1870, described a similar tumor in the mediastinum. In Stout's review of 243 cases, 62 occurred in the mediastinum. In addition, Stout suggested that it is possible to divide ganglioneuromas into three groups: (1) fully differentiated, (2) ganglioneuromas with diffusely scattered cells of a lesser degree of differentiation, and (3) composite tumors made up of two or more parts, one being ganglioneuroma and the other neuroblastoma. Based on that categorization, 146 tumors reported would belong to the fully differentiated tumors, 23 to those showing diffusely scattered cells of a lesser degree of differentiation and 20 to the composite group. He also added that the fully differentiated tumor should be considered benign contrary to the other two groups. It is important to highlight that the occurrence of ganglioneuromas has been hypothesized as possibly occurring by spontaneous maturation of neuroblasts [30].

Clinically, ganglioneuromas are often asymptomatic, and their presence is discovered as an incidental finding [31–33]. In general, ganglioneuromas in the mediastinum are more common in the posterior compartment. Spinelli and colleagues [31] reported 14 surgical cases of ganglioneuromas in which their original diagnosis was an incidental finding; these were treated by complete surgical resection. In this report, only two cases were located in the costovertebral space, while the rest of the tumors were in extrathoracic location. However, in a review of reported cases of ganglioneuromas by specific site, the authors [31] stated that the mediastinum might be involved in about 22% of the cases. In addition, it is also stated that cough, back pain, and dyspnea may be seen in those tumors occurring in the mediastinum. Interestingly, Shea and Abshire [34] reported a case of thoracic ganglioneuroma in a previously healthy 11-year-old child with an associated Philadelphia chromosome-positive chronic myeloid leukemia, an occurrence that is unusual. Another association that has been described is the presence of a mediastinal ganglioneuroma and retroperitoneal non-functioning pheochromocytoma in a 52-year-old woman [35].

From the radiological point of view, Guan and colleagues [36], in a study of 23 cases of thoracic ganglioneuromas, concluded that ganglioneuromas show hypodensity in plain CT, while on CT and MRI, non-enhancement or slight enhancement in artery phase and progressive mild enhancement in delay phase are features of this tumor. Ozawa and colleagues [37] study the morphological differences between schwannomas and ganglioneuromas in the mediastinum in 22 cases using craniocaudal length (CC) to major axis ratio (CC/M R) using CT/MRI. The authors found that ganglioneuromas show higher mean CC/M R than schwannomas, which the authors concluded as being important in separating those tumors by such means.

Because ganglioneuromas are considered benign neoplasms, complete surgical resection is the treatment of choice and offers the best alternative. Although recurrences have been reported, it is likely that this rare occurrence may take place in tumors that are incompletely removed.

Pathological Features

Ganglioneuromas appear to be well defined but not encapsulated tumors that may range in size from a couple of centimeters to more than 10 cm in greatest diameter. Usually, the tumors are tan in color with a smooth surface (Fig. 11.1). Areas of necrosis and hemorrhage are not common.

Histologically, the tumor is composed of a mixture of ganglion cells characterized by larger cells with eosinophilic cytoplasm, round eccentrically placed nuclei and prominent nucleoli. In some of these ganglion cells, it is possible to identify basophilic granules, which represent Nissl substance (granules). In addition to the ganglion cells, the tumor also shows a spindle cell proliferation characterized by elongated cells with scant cytoplasm, fusiform nuclei, and inconspicuous nucleoli. These components are commonly arranged in a tightly or loose growth pattern. Mitotic activity is not common, and areas of necrosis and hemorrhage are rare. In some cases, the tumor may show areas of calcifications and myxoid change (Figs. 11.2, 11.3, 11.4, 11.5, 11.6, and 11.7).

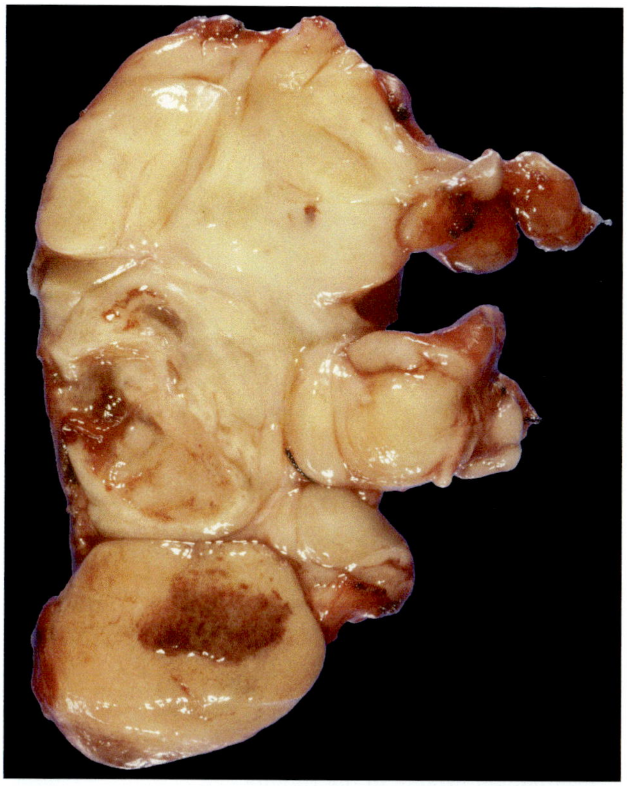

Fig. 11.1 Gross image of a ganglioneuroma showing a light tan, solid tumor without areas of necrosis or hemorrhage

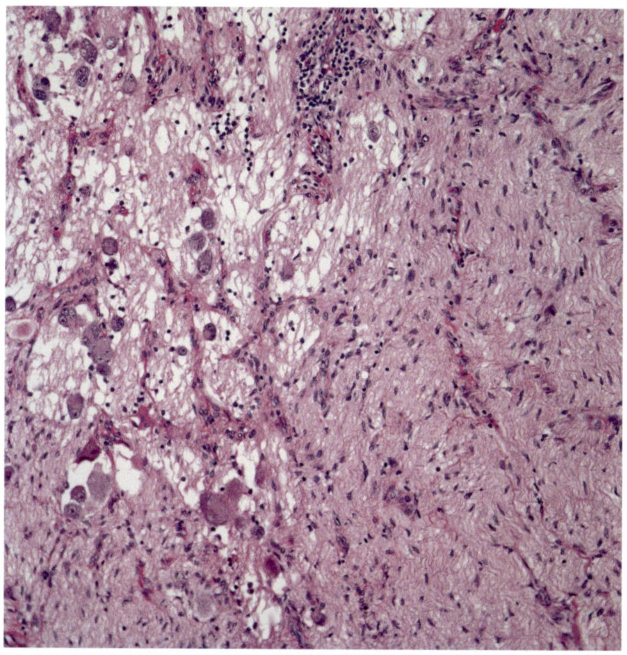

Fig. 11.2 Ganglioneuroma showing a loose fibroconnective tissue with numerous mature ganglion cells

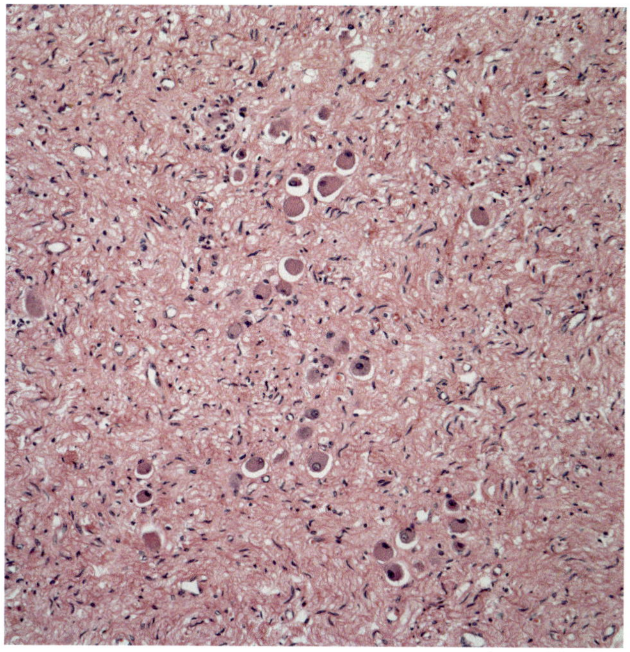

Fig. 11.3 Ganglioneuroma showing areas of a more solid component in which the ganglion cells are haphazardly displayed

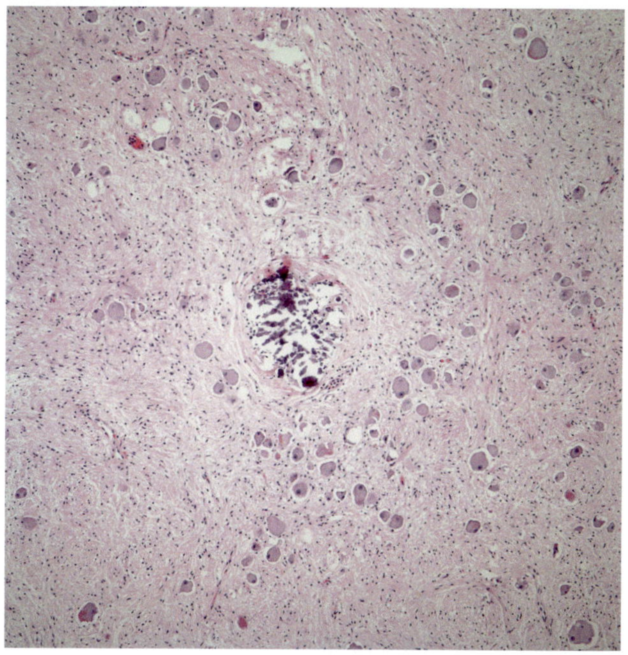

Fig. 11.4 Ganglioneuroma with focal calcification and numerous mature ganglion cells

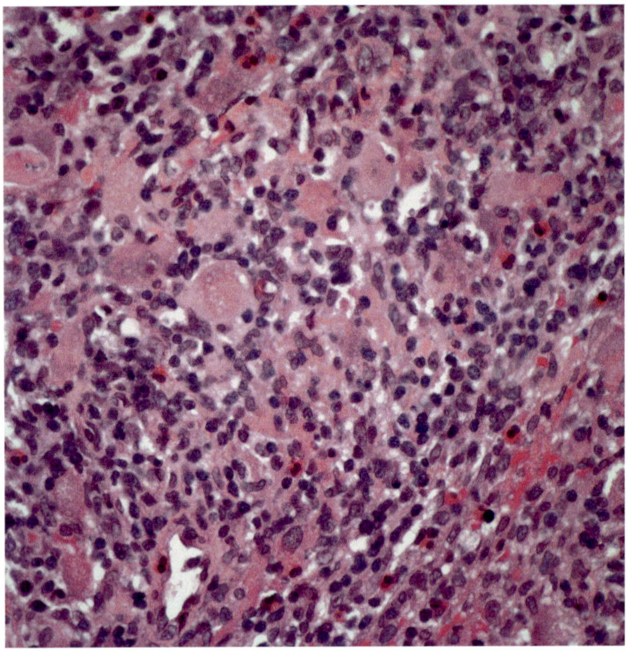

Fig. 11.5 Ganglioneuroma with prominent inflammatory reaction in which the ganglion cells are more difficult to identified

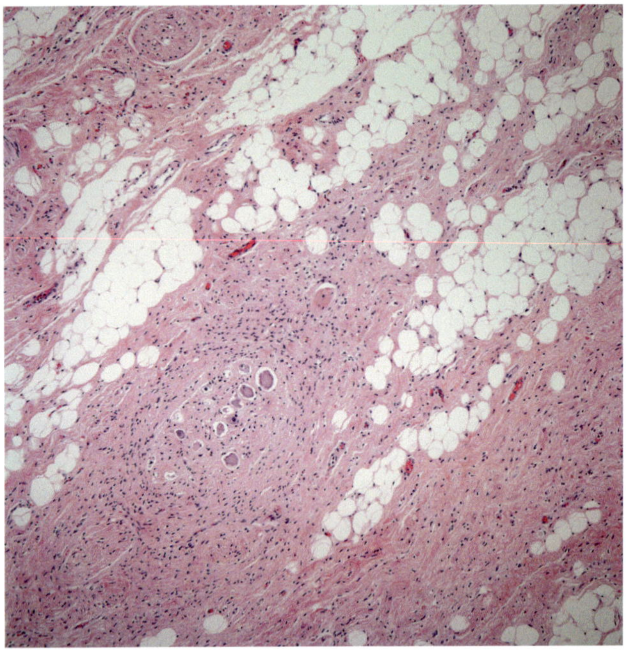

Fig. 11.6 Ganglioneuroma showing areas of adipose tissue and mature ganglion cells

Ancillary Diagnostic Tools

Even though the diagnosis of ganglioneuromas is rather straightforward by morphological means, the use of electron microscopic studies in these tumors has shown the presence of neurofilaments, microtubules, and dense-core vesicles. On the other hand, immunohistochemical studies may show immunoreactivity for S-100 protein and

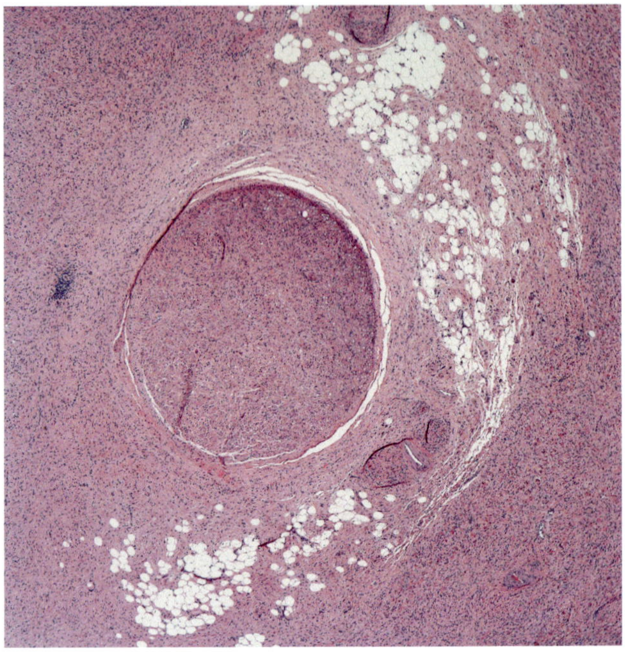

Fig. 11.7 Ganglioneuroma with more solid proliferation involving adipose tissue and encircling a nerve trunk

neurofilament protein in the spindle cell component, while the ganglion cell component may show some reactivity for synaptophysin and NeuN.

Differential Diagnosis

Because ganglioneuromas occur in the posterior mediastinum more often, it is often logical to include other neurogenic tumors in the differential diagnosis. In small biopsy samples in which the presence of ganglion cells may not be apparent, other spindle cell lesions such as neurofibromas or schwannomas are usually considered in the differential diagnosis. Important to consider is the fact that both of those lesions may also show positive staining for S-100 protein and possibly with neurofilament protein, thus making an unequivocal interpretation more challenging. One other consideration would be with a smooth muscle neoplasm; however, in this setting, the use of immunohistochemistry, namely, S-100 protein, would aid in arriving at a correct interpretation.

Neurofibromas

As stated earlier in this chapter, neurofibromas are tumors that have a mixture of all nerve elements (axons, sheath cells, and connective tissue). In general, similar to ganglioneuromas, these tumors in the mediastinum are more common in the posterior compartment. A common association for neurofibromas is the presence of von Recklinghausen's disease or neurofibromatosis type 1 (NF1). NF1 disease is an autosomal dominant disorder with an approximate incidence of 1 in 3000 patients with no specific gender predilection [38]. However, it is also important to highlight that neurofibromatosis may be associated with other conditions including mental retardation, Bourneville's syndrome, Morquio's syndrome, and Batten's type of lipofuscinosis, among others [39].

Clinically, patients may present with upper respiratory symptoms, tracheal compression, or scoliosis [38]. Ueda and colleagues [40], in a computed tomography (CT) study of 88 patients with NF1, identified 13 patients with mediastinal masses of which 3 were neurofibromas and 7 other lesions were considered to be neurofibromas. However, it is also important to highlight that, even though the occurrence of neurofibromas is more common in the posterior mediastinum, sporadic cases can also be present in the anterior mediastinum. Yano and colleagues [41], in a study of 43 patients with "small-size" anterior mediastinal tumors, detected one case of neurofibroma in the anterior mediastinum. One other unusual association that has been described in the literature includes an intrathoracic meningocele in a 43-year-old man with multiple neurofibromatosis [42]. In addition, in some unusual cases, the coexistence of ganglioneuroma and neurofibroma in the background of NF1 has been reported [43]. Reports of unusual occurrences such as intrathoracic neurofibromas of the phrenic nerve, bilateral mediastinal neurofibromas of the vagus nerve, and giant intrathoracic neurofibroma with mediastinal shift have been reported [44–46].

Just as with other benign neurogenic tumors of the mediastinum, complete surgical resection is the treatment of choice for these neoplasms and is considered curative.

Pathological Features

These tumors are usually well circumscribed with no capsule. They are whitish in color and of soft consistency (Fig. 11.8). Neurofibromas usually track along the nerve giving the appearance of an elongated tumor rather than a spherical lesion. In patients with neurofibromatosis, the plexiform neurofibroma appearance is that of an elongated and nodular tumor that may extend along a nerve.

Histologically, neurofibromas are not encapsulated tumors; characteristically, the tumors show a spindle cellular proliferation composed of cells with scant cytoplasm, fusiform nuclei with a wavy appearance, and inconspicuous nuclei. This cellular proliferation is often embedded in a loose fibroconnective tissue, which may show myxoid or edematous changes. In some areas, the tumor may show inflammatory changes that may vary from area to area (Figs. 11.9, 11.10, 11.11, 11.12, 11.13, 11.14, 11.15, 11.16, 11.17, 11.18, and 11.19). In general, neurofibromas do not

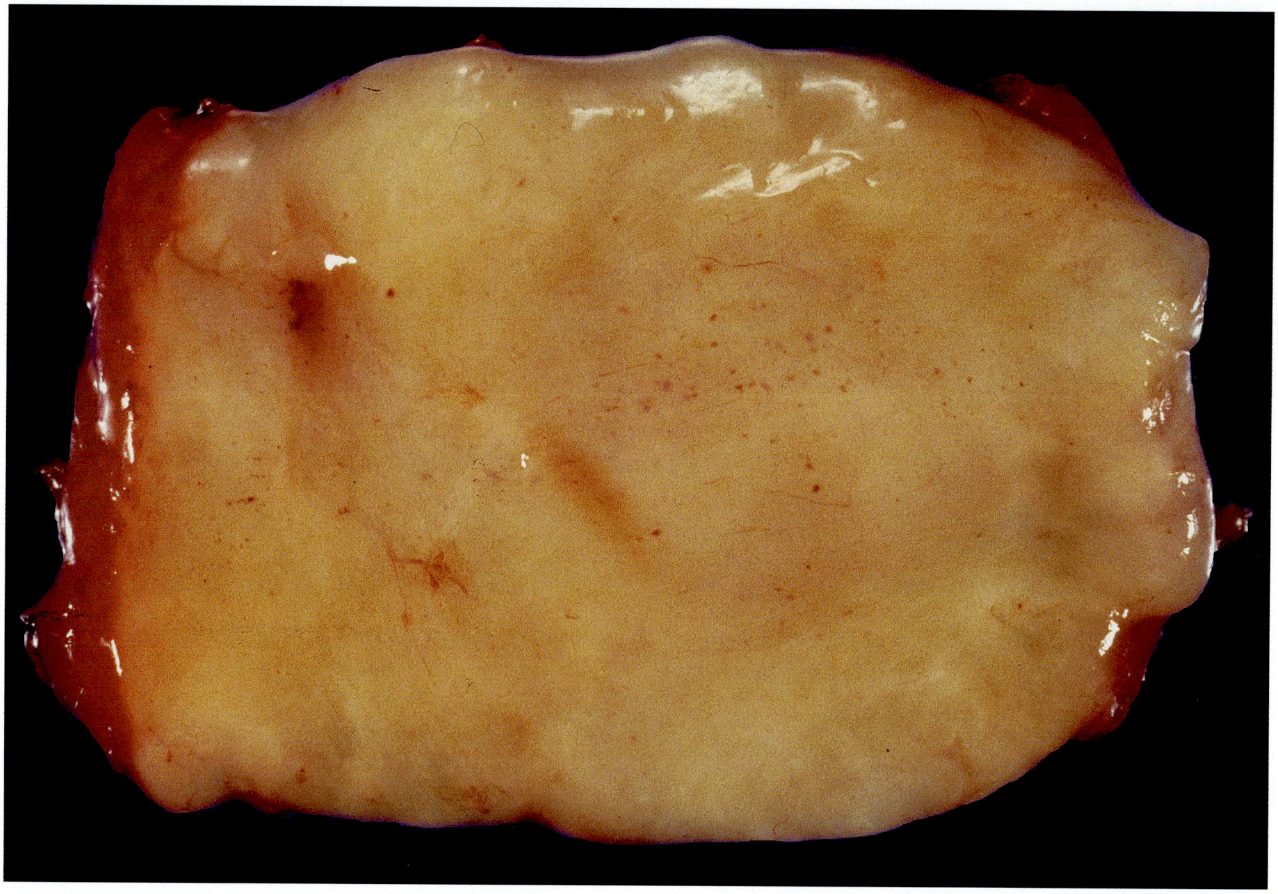

Fig. 11.8 Neurofibroma showing a tumor yellowish in color, well circumscribed and with no areas of necrosis and hemorrhage

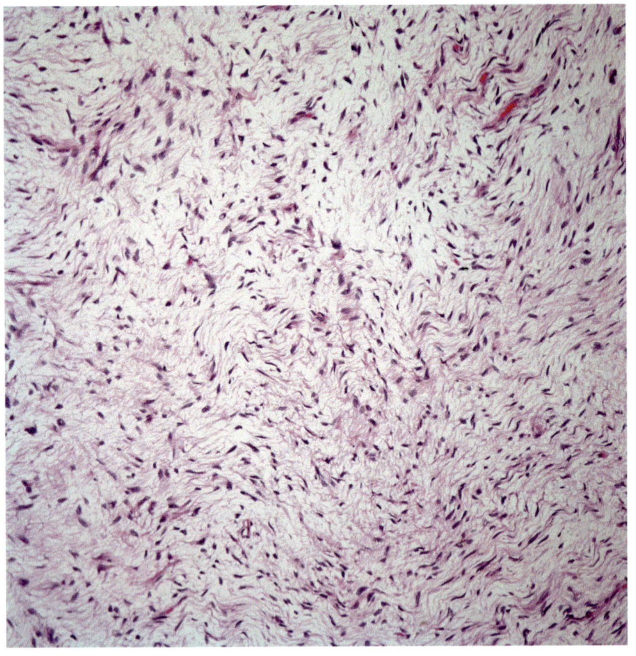

Fig. 11.9 Neurofibroma showing spindle cell proliferation in a loose fibroconnective tissue stroma

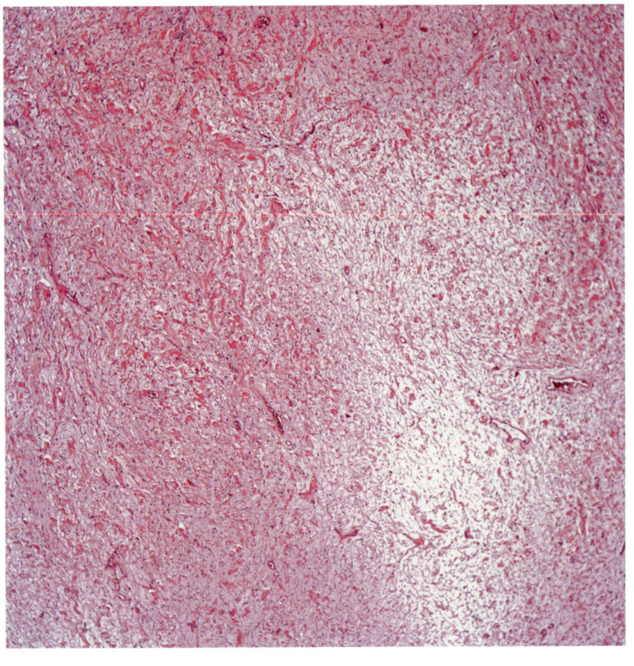

Fig. 11.10 Neurofibroma showing more loose fibroconnective tissue areas and focal myxoid changes

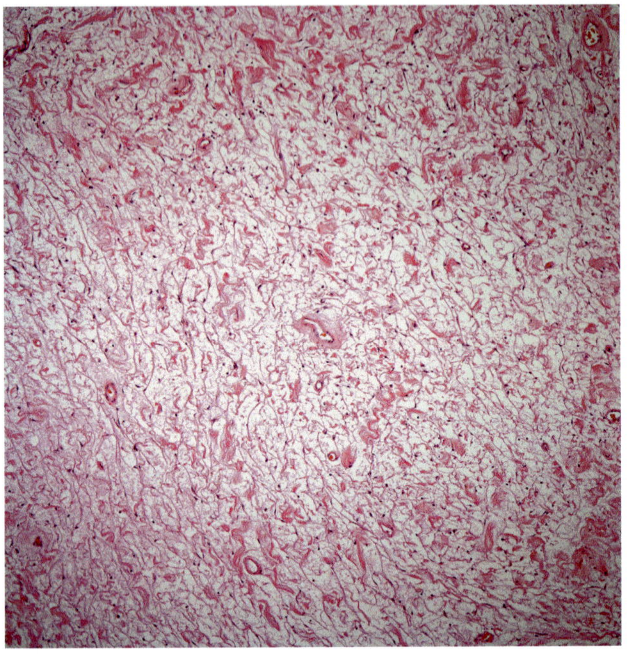

Fig. 11.11 Neurofibroma composed almost exclusively of loose fibroconnective tissue in which the spindle cell proliferation is more subtle

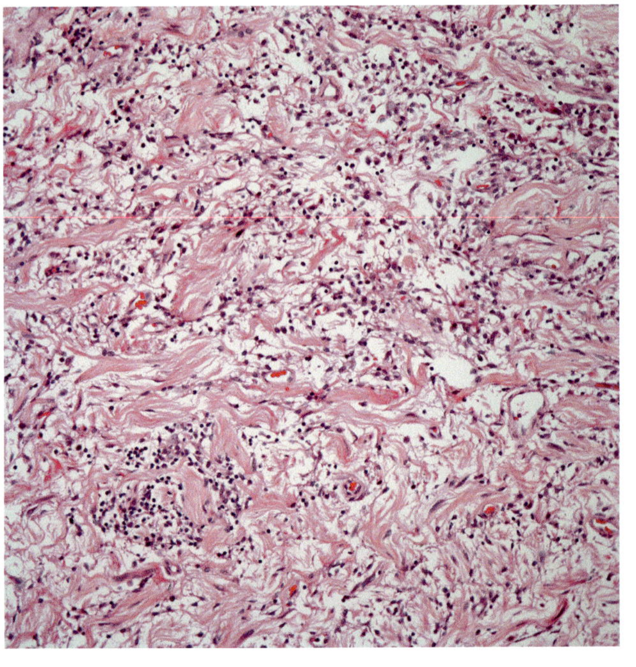

Fig. 11.12 Neurofibroma with inflammatory component

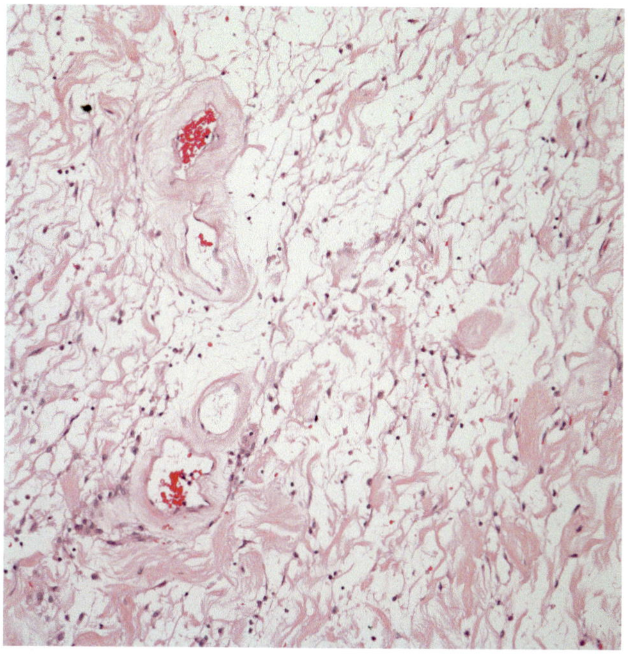

Fig. 11.13 Higher magnification of a neurofibroma with degenerative changes

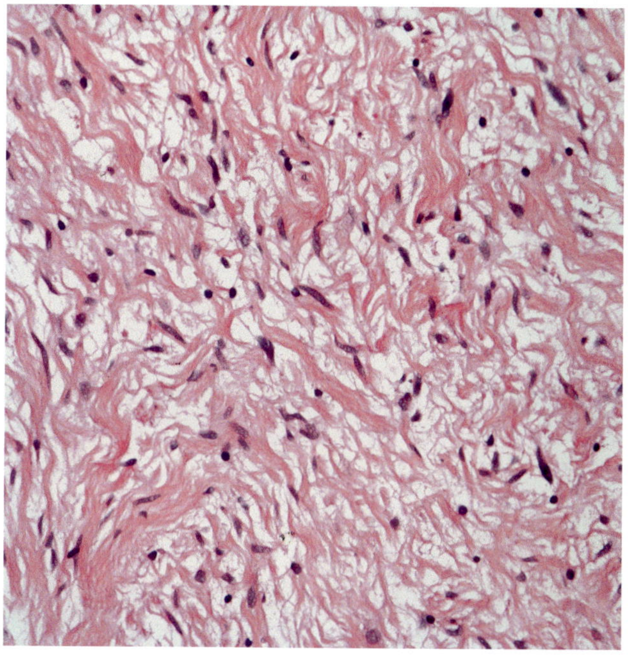

Fig. 11.14 Higher magnification of a neurofibroma showing a tumor with no cellular atypia

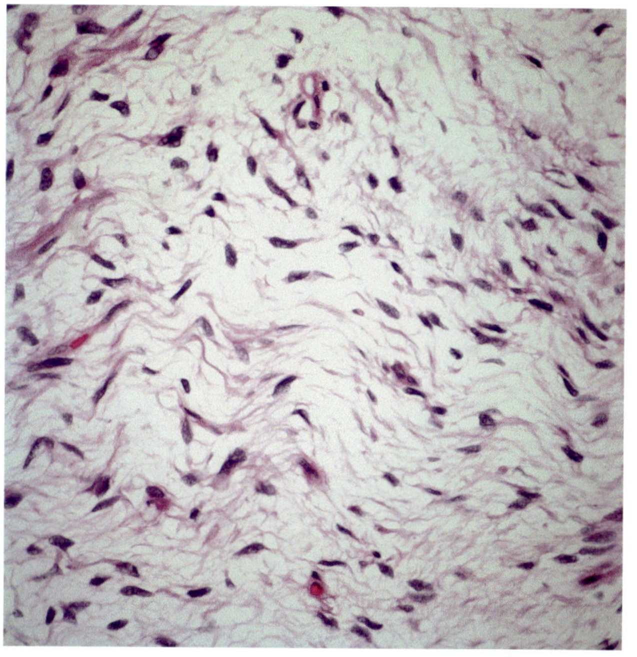

Fig. 11.15 Higher magnification of a neurofibroma showing spindle cells with elongated nuclei and inconspicuous nucleoli. No mitotic activity or nuclear atypia are present

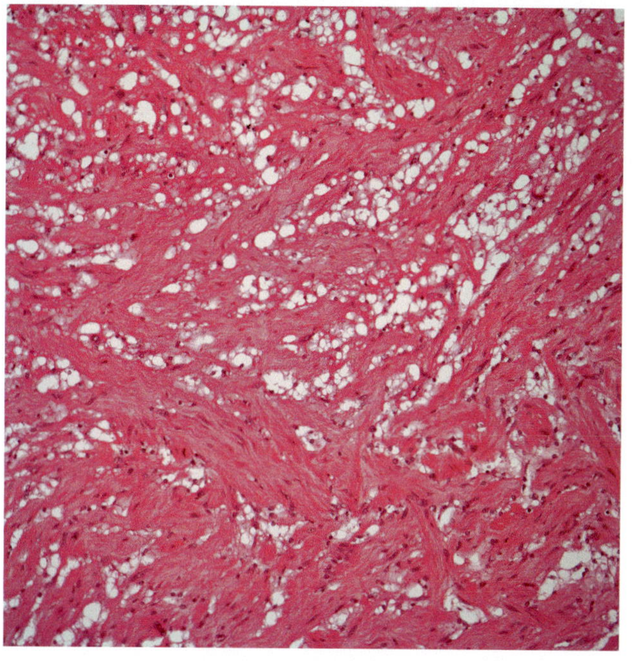

Fig. 11.16 Neurofibroma with extensive vacuolization of the cells giving an appearance of clear cell component

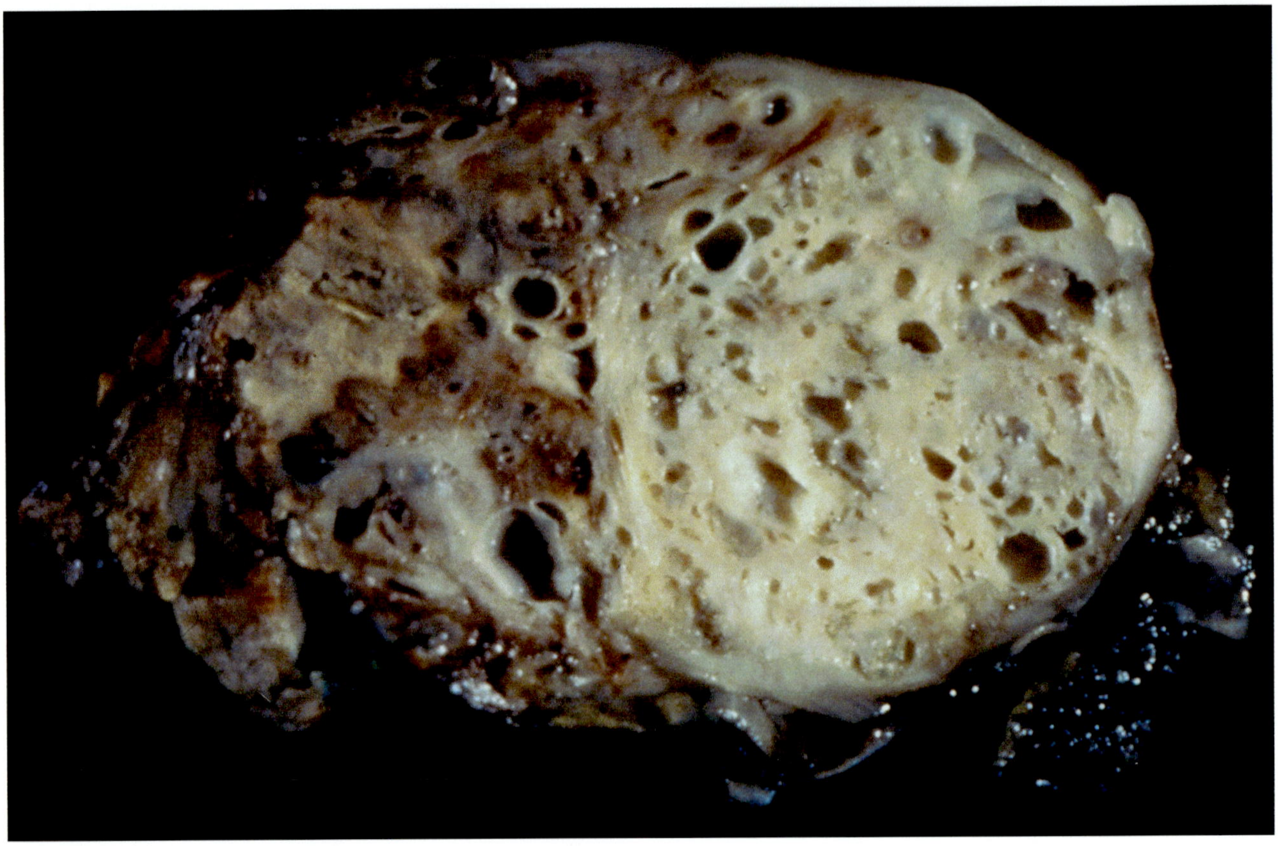

Fig. 11.17 Gross image of a mediastinal schwannoma with cystic changes

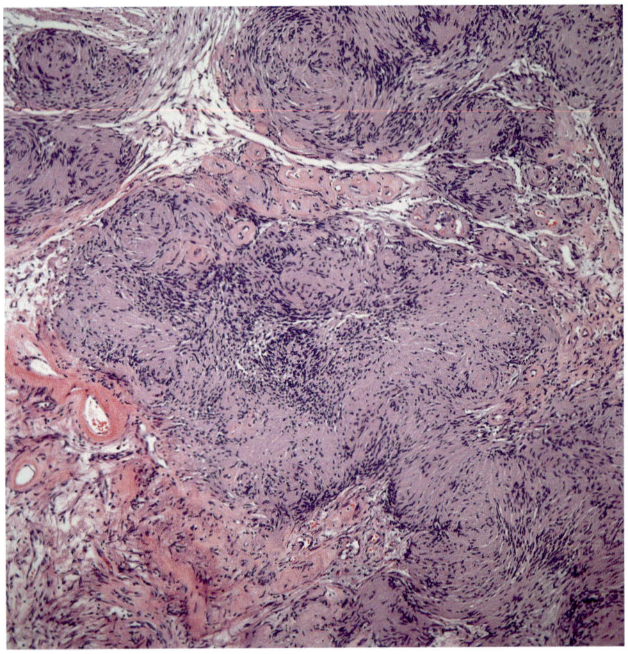

Fig. 11.18 Low power view of a conventional schwannoma showing the classical features of hypo and hyper cellular areas

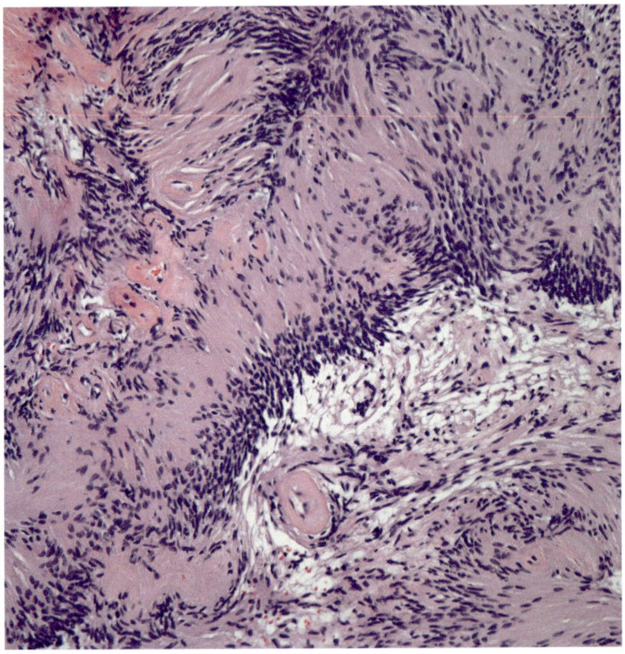

Fig. 11.19 Schwannoma showing palisading of the nuclei

show marked cellular atypia, necrosis, or increase mitotic activity. However, in some tumors in which there is the background of neurofibromatosis, the tumors may show more cellularity and nuclear atypia, which should in some cases raise a suspicion for sarcomatous transformation. It has been stated that malignant transformation may occur in approximately 2–10% of the cases. In such cases, reasonable sampling with careful evaluation of the histology plays an important role. Other unusual features that have been associated with neurofibromas include the presence of Pacini's corpuscles, Wagner-Meissner bodies, pigment, and gland formation [47, 48].

Ancillary Diagnostic Tools

Just like with ganglioneuroma, the diagnosis of neurofibroma is straightforward on morphological grounds. However, the use of immunohistochemical stains for its diagnosis may be reserved for small biopsies in which the morphological features may not be so apparent. Immunohistochemical studies that may aid in the diagnosis of neurofibromas are rather limited. S-100 protein may be helpful, but it is usually weakly positive or negative in many cases. Neurofilament protein also may show positive staining, but again it is usually a weak positivity, and many cases are negative. Ultrastructural studies have shown cytoplasmic processes interspersed with occasional myelinated and unmyelinated axons in an extensive collagenous stroma with a well-defined basement membrane coating the plasmalemma [49].

Differential Diagnosis

The differential diagnosis of neurofibromas logically will include other neurogenic posterior mediastinal neoplasms such as schwannoma, ganglioneuroma, perineurioma, and neurothekeoma. However, other neoplasms of non-neurogenic origin such as liposarcomas and myxomas may also enter in the differential diagnosis. In small biopsies, the challenge of separating any of these entities may prove difficult as there may not only be an overlap in some histological features but there may also be an overlap in the immunohistochemical profile. From the morphological point of view, ganglioneuromas would show the presence of ganglion cells, which can facilitate the separation from neurofibromas. Schwannomas may also show classical features such as the presence of Verocay bodies and strong positive staining for S-100 protein. Perineuriomas may show positive staining for EMA, which will also lead to the correct interpretation. Neurothekeomas may show more myxoid component, which may help in arriving at a more correct interpretation. Myxomas and liposarcomas will not originate from a nerve, which may help in arriving at a more correct interpretation. Needless to say, those considerations may be more common in a small biopsy; surgical resection of the tumor with enough tissue to evaluate should rarely pose a serious difficulty in the diagnosis.

Schwannoma

This tumor has also been known as neurilemmoma and neuroma. The tumors originate from the nerve sheath and are supposed to arise from differentiated adult Schwann cells. These tumors are more common in the third and fourth decade of life, and there does not appear to be gender predilection for their occurrence. They may also occur in the background of neurofibromatosis (NF1/von Recklinghausen's disease). It is likely that the size of the tumor plays an important role in the symptomatology that these patients may have. Small tumors are often diagnosed during routine radiographic films, while large tumors may compress adjacent structure, and the patients may develop symptoms related to the structures involved. Despite the fact that it is well known that these tumors occur in the posterior mediastinal compartment, there are no large series of these tumors in this locations, and most of what is known about schwannomas is derived from the experience of these tumors in other locations where they may occur more often. For instance, in a review of 75 cases of intrathoracic peripheral nerve sheath tumors, Boland and colleagues [50] documented only 13 cases of schwannomas, even though the authors stated that the most common peripheral nerve sheath tumors are of the benign type. Based on this finding, we can estimate the occurrence of schwannomas in the thoracic cavity at approximately 15–20% of all of this family of tumors.

Clinically, these tumors do not appear to have any predilection for gender or age, although most cases are seen in adult individuals. Just like with other nerve sheath tumors, schwannomas may be associated with neurofibromatosis (von Recklinghausen disease). However, intrathoracic schwannomas have also been associated with other conditions such as Horner's syndrome [51, 52]. Horner's syndrome is characterized by miosis, blepharoptosis, enophthalmos, and anhidrosis due to blocking of the sympathetic pathway at any point. Miura and colleagues [51] documented a 48-year-old woman with a dumbbell-shaped tumor discovered during routine chest radiography. Apparently, the patient had noticed some of the symptoms of right-sided Horner's syndrome, which improved after the tumor was resected. Mathew and colleagues [52] also documented another unusual case of a mediastinal schwannoma with Horner's syndrome. In Mathew's case, a 21-year-old man was found to have a superior mediastinal sympathetic chain benign schwannoma 7 years after the onset of

Horner's syndrome and unilateral headaches. In general, outside of the specific association of schwannomas with specific conditions and syndromes, a large number of patients will present with non-specific symptomatology, which in many patients will be caused by the size of the tumors and by the anatomic structures that may be compromised due to the size of the neoplasm. Therefore, non-specific symptoms such as cough, chest pain, dyspnea, and neuralgia are commonly seen in association with these tumors. Nevertheless, it is important to highlight that, even though the majority of schwannomas occur in the posterior mediastinum, there is a small number of cases that may present in the anterior mediastinum; thus, such an occurrence needs to be kept in mind. One such case is the one described by Tajima and colleagues [53], who documented a case of a 23-year-old man with no symptoms of von Recklinghausen's disease, asymptomatic, and in whom diagnostic imaging – CT and MRI – demonstrated an anterior mediastinal tumor.

Regardless of the clinical association that schwannomas may have, the treatment of choice for these tumors is complete surgical resection, which apparently can be accomplished via minimally invasive approach [54].

Pathological Features

Schwannomas are usually well-circumscribed neoplasms with round or oval shape. The tumors may have extensive calcifications and cystic changes (Fig. 11.17). They are usually light tan, and areas of necrosis and hemorrhage are not common. They may vary in size from a few centimeters to more than 10 cm in greatest diameter. In some cases, it is possible to identify their attachment to a nerve.

Histologically, the majority of schwannomas have a very characteristic growth pattern, which allows for an easy morphological diagnosis. The tumors may show a well-defined fibrous capsule, and the tumor is composed of a proliferation of spindle cells with a fusiform nuclei, eosinophilic cytoplasm, and indistinct cell borders. The spindle cell proliferation is arranged to form hypercellular and hypocellular areas, also known as Antoni A and B, respectively (Figs. 11.18, 11.19, 11.20, 11.21, and 11.22). In addition, the tumor usually shows the presence of Verocay bodies, which are represented by the palisading of nuclei in the Antoni A areas. This latter feature is commonly associated with the benign schwannomas. The spindle cells do not show nuclear atypia, and mitotic activity is generally absent or minimal. Other commonly observed features in schwannomas are the presence of edematous areas, calcifications, cystic changes, and thick blood vessels (Figs. 11.23, 11.24, 11.25, 11.26, 11.27, and 11.28). However, areas of necrosis and hemorrhage are generally absent.

Even though the majority of schwannomas will not pose a difficulty for arriving at a correct interpretation, some cases of schwannomas may show unusual histological features that may pose a challenge in the diagnosis. Among those cases are cases of pigmented schwannomas and the so-called cellular schwannomas; these require special attention.

Pigmented Schwannoma

Essentially, the presence of melanin pigment in these tumors may be seen in either benign or malignant schwannomas. The presence of melanin pigment may be only a minor component of the tumor, while in other tumors, it may be prominent enough to pose a challenge in arriving at a definitive separation between schwannoma and melanoma. One important issue to highlight is that even though this particular histopathological feature of schwannomas may be seen with some frequency in tumors of the soft tissue, the occurrence of pigmented or melanotic "melanocytic" schwannomas in the mediastinal compartment is not common [55–59]. Paris and colleagues [55], in 1979, described a single case in a 49-year-old woman who presented with right arm pain in the distribution of the eighth cervical nerve root. Radiographic evaluation disclosed a right upper mediastinal mass, while spinal films showed widening of the intervertebral foramen between the seventh cervical and first thoracic vertebrae. Histologically, the tumor was described as a cellular schwannoma with no mitotic activity, and the cells were filled with variable amounts of small black pigment granules. Histochemical stain for Fontana showed the melanin nature of the pigment. Abbott and colleagues [56] reported two cases of this occurrence in two patients, one a 20-year-old man with a posterior mediastinal tumor and the other a 30-year-old woman with a right paravertebral tumor. The posterior mediastinal tumor was described as a tumor with rare mitoses and variable amount of melanin pigment in the cells. Prieto-Rodriguez and associates [57] also described a similar case of a posterior mediastinal tumor that the authors were able to diagnose by fine needle aspiration cytology. The tumor was not only pigmented but in addition it was also described as psammomatous. More recently, Zhang and associates [58] described 13 melanotic schwannomas in diverse anatomic locations; only one of these 13 cases was in a patient with a mediastinal tumor, which raises the possibility that these tumors in the mediastinum account for approximately 5–10% of all these particular neoplasms. Even though these tumors may involve the spinal canal, the majority of tumors appear to have a relatively small size of under 10 cm.

Pathological Features

The pathological features of these tumors are similar to tumors without pigment. Grossly, the tumor is well circumscribed. Histologically, the tumors are composed of a spindle cellular proliferation of elongated cells, with small oval nuclei, and inconspicuous nucleoli. Areas of Antoni A and B are present. The cells have a moderate amount of eosinophilic cytoplasm. Mitotic activity is rare or nonexistent.

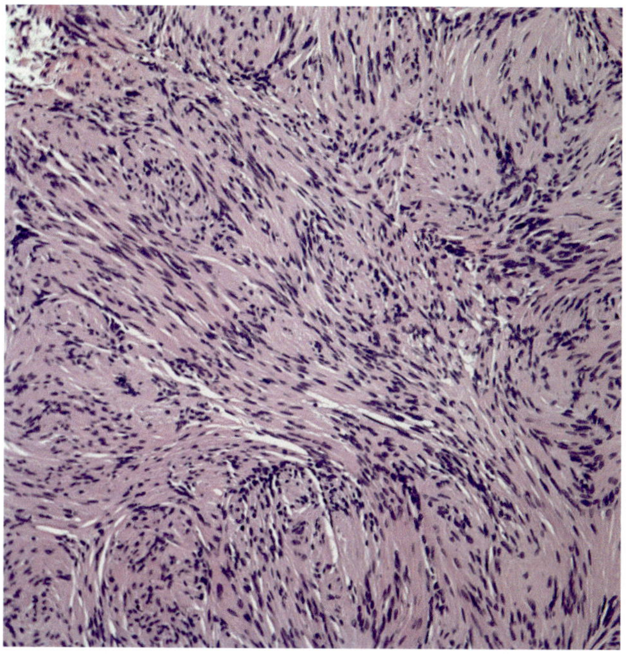

Fig. 11.20 Schwannoma showing spindle cell proliferation without areas of necrosis or hemorrhage

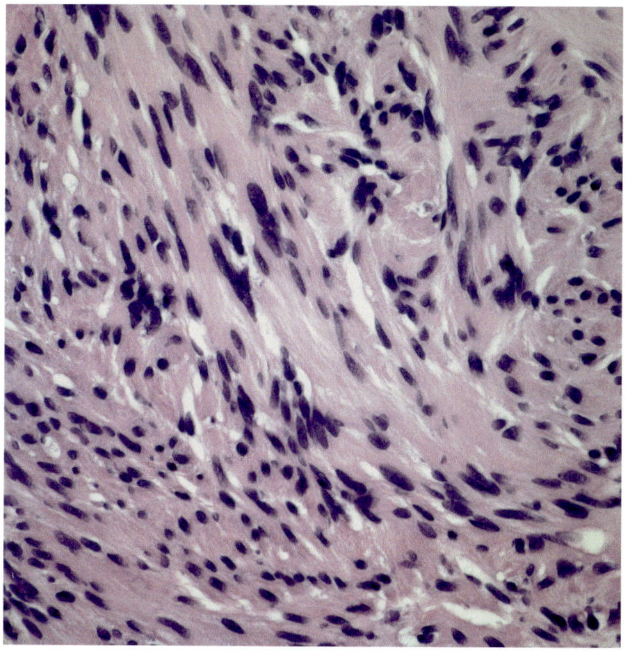

Fig. 11.21 In focal areas, conventional schwannomas may show nuclear atypia

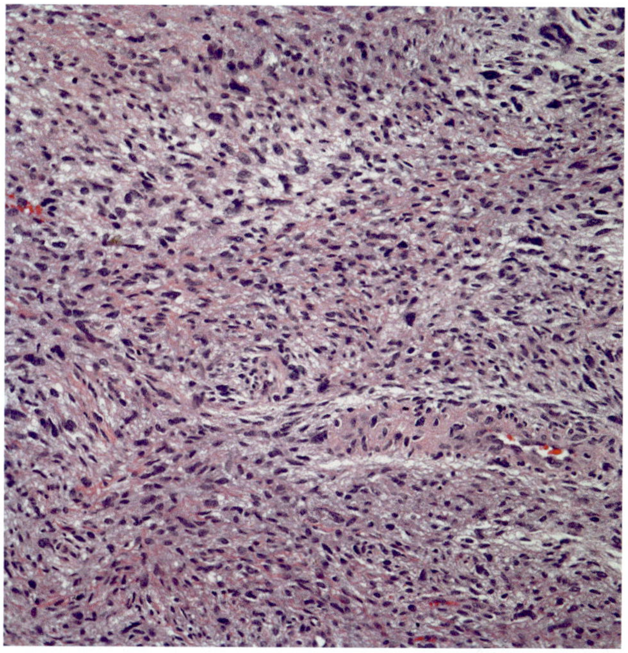

Fig. 11.22 Schwannoma with focal epithelioid features

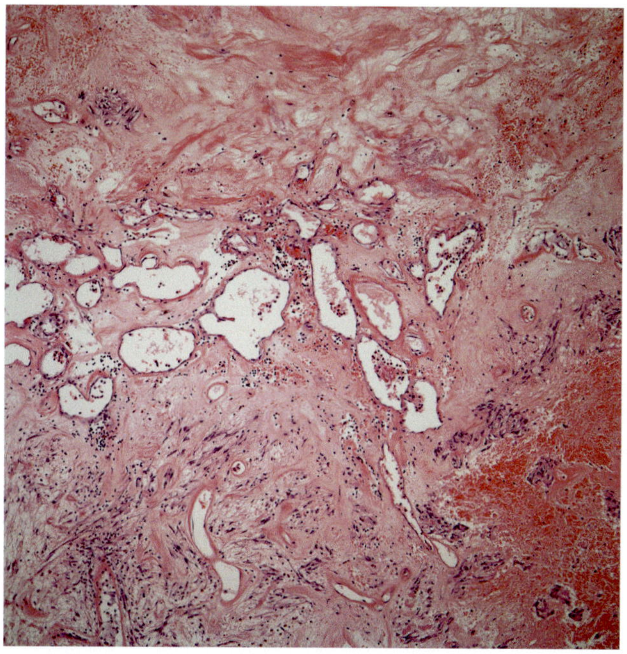

Fig. 11.23 Schwannoma with extensive hyalinization and vascular proliferation

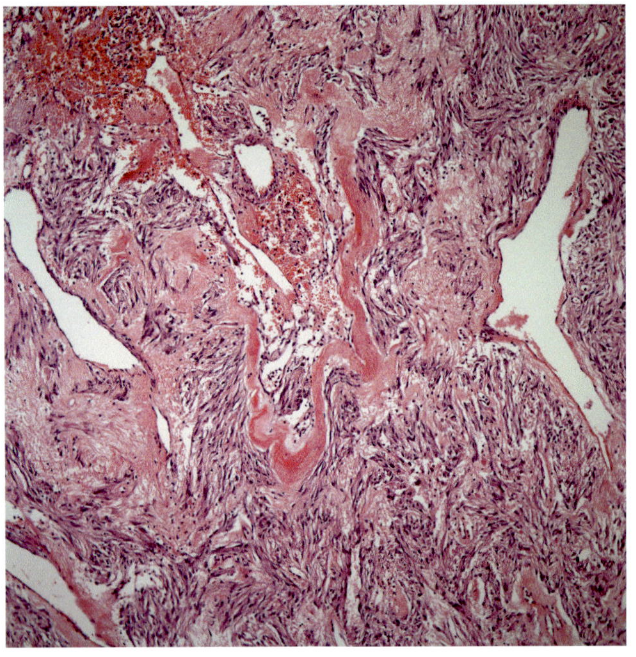

Fig. 11.24 Schwannoma with numerous ectatic blood vessels

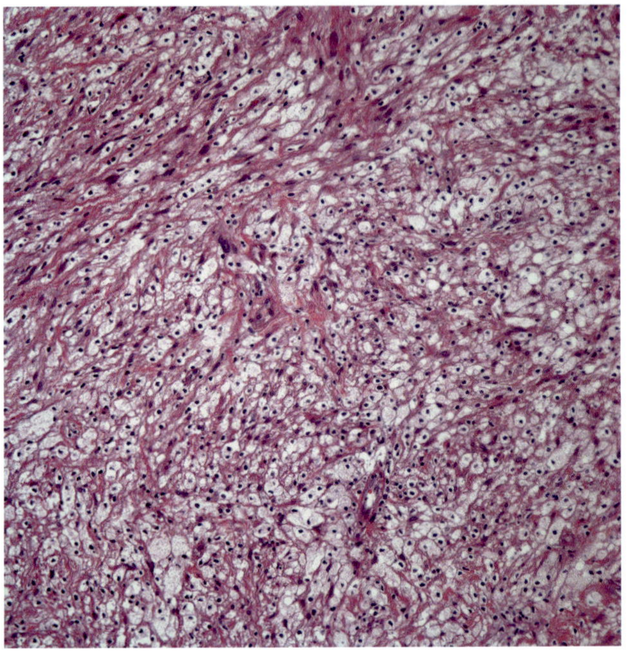

Fig. 11.26 Schwannoma with collections of macrophages

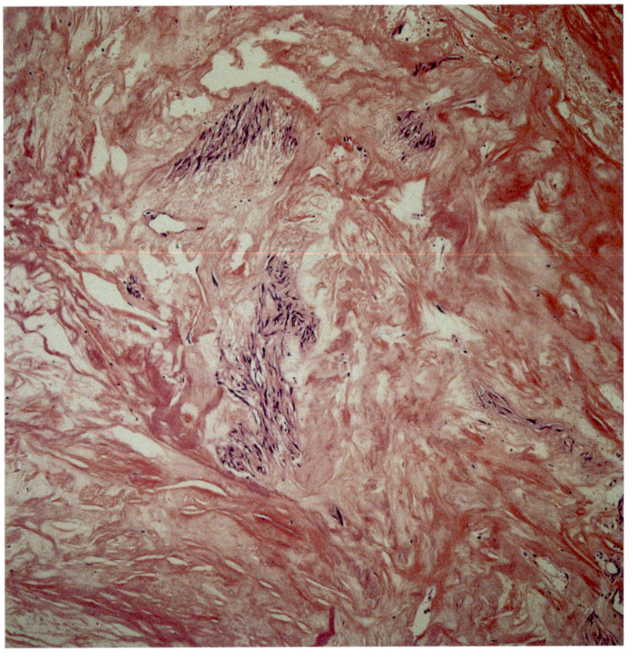

Fig. 11.25 Schwannoma with extensive hyalinization and only focal areas of spindle cells

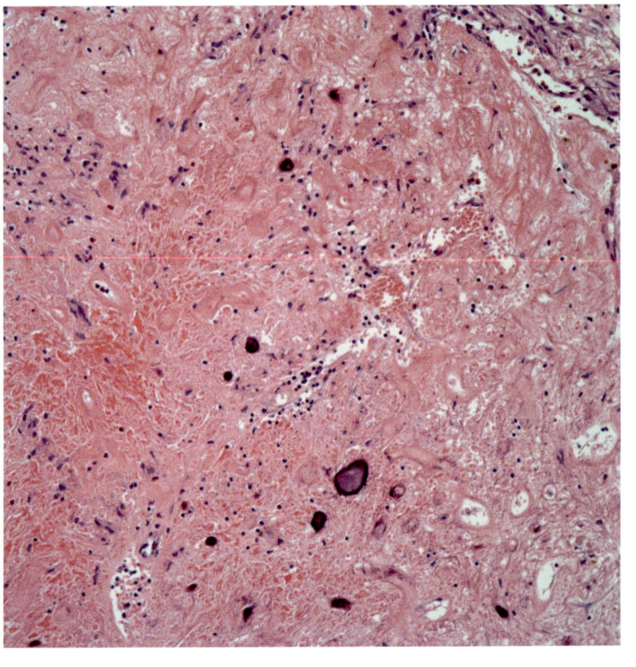

Fig. 11.27 Schwannoma with focal calcifications

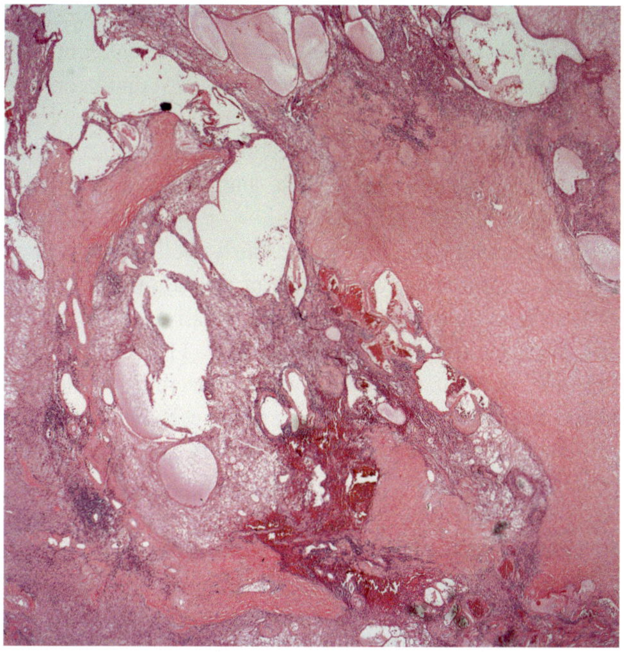

Fig. 11.28 Schwannoma with extensive cystic changes

Areas of necrosis and hemorrhage are generally not present. The tumors may show variable amounts of melanin pigment in some cases; the presence of pigment may be marked while in others it is subtler.

Cellular Schwannoma

The original description of this type of schwannoma is credited to Woodruff and associates [59], who, in 1981, described 14 cases of such a tumor, which histologically could be confused with malignant neoplasms. The authors stated that this type of tumor has no gender predilection; the patients' ages ranged from 25 to 81 years of age, and the tumors appeared to be more common in the neck, posterior mediastinum, and pelvis. In 1990, White and associates [60] described 57 patients with this tumor to reemphasize the benign nature of these neoplasms. In the cases described, there was a slight female predominance, with 63% of the tumors described in female patients. Anatomically, the tumors were more common in the paravertebral area of the retroperitoneum, pelvis, and mediastinum. Interestingly, the author stated that, in 28% of these tumors, a malignant diagnosis had been made. However, follow-up in those patients, which ranged from 1 to 24 years, revealed that three patients had recurrence, while none of the patients had developed metastatic disease. Also, Lodding and associates [61] described their experience by reporting on 29 cases of a similar tumor. In this particular series of cases, there was a female predominance of 82% with an age range of between 15 and 79 years. Twenty tumors were located in the mediastinum, which accounts for over half of the tumors described. One of the patients described had von Recklinghausen's neurofibromatosis. Follow-up information with a median duration of 7 years showed that no deaths, local recurrences, or metastatic disease were documented in any of the patients presented.

Pathological Features

Grossly, these tumors, similarly to the conventional schwannomas, have been described as well demarcated or encapsulated neoplasms, which at cut surface may show a homogenous light tan color, firm consistency, and some may have cystic changes. Areas of necrosis and hemorrhage are commonly absent. Histologically, since the initial description by Woodruff [59], the tumors have been characterized by the absence of Verocay bodies and the presence of fascicles of spindle cells (which can be arranged in a storiform or herringbone pattern), mitotic activity (usually fewer than 5 × 10 hpf), nuclear atypia, and in some cases microscopic focus of necrosis. Areas of collections of foamy histiocytes and inflammatory reaction composed of lymphocytes may be present. In other areas, the presence of thick wall vessels can be prominent. The tumors may erode bony structures.

Ancillary Diagnostic Tools

In general, the immunohistochemical features of conventional schwannomas are those of a tumor that shows strong positivity for S-100 protein and vimentin. However, the tumor may also show focal positive staining for glial fibrillary acid protein, while showing usually negative staining for neuroendocrine markers, neurofilament protein, and epithelial markers such as keratin and epithelial membrane antigen. In addition, the tumor also shows negative staining for CD-34, STAT6, and muscle markers (smooth muscle actin, desmin, caldesmon, myoglobin, Myo-D). Cellular schwannomas may show similar immunohistochemical profile to conventional schwannomas; however, in these particular variants, an immunohistochemical stain for Ki-67 may show an increased labeling of tumor cells, which may also represent a diagnostic pitfall in the interpretation. In this setting, careful evaluation of the histopathological features of the tumor may lead to a correct interpretation. By far the most challenging interpretation of immunohistochemical stains is with the pigmented schwannomas, as these tumors have been reported to be positive for S-100 protein, HMB-45, Leu 7, Melan-A, and vimentin. Thus, it is highly important to separate these tumors from malignant melanoma, which could elicit similar immunophenotype. Perhaps the real problem is not with the conventional schwannoma but rather with the malignant schwannoma (MPNT), which may show nuclear atypia, mitotic activity, and other morphological features similar to those of melanoma. One additional feature that may be considered in difficult cases is the use of electron microscopy, which could show the presence of basement membrane, a feature that is common in schwannomas [49], and the absence of pre-melanosomes, which would be more consistent with melanoma.

Differential Diagnosis

In conventional schwannomas, the most common differential diagnosis is that with smooth muscle tumors, namely, leiomyomas. In this setting, the use of S-100 protein and muscle markers should lead to the correct interpretation. One other possibility includes solitary fibrous tumor, which may show different histopathological patterns and may present as a mediastinal tumor. Once again, in this setting the use of CD-34 and STAT6 should clarify the true nature of the neoplasm. In small biopsies, neurofibroma may enter in the differential diagnosis; however, in this setting, the strong positive reaction for S-100 protein may be more in keeping with schwannoma.

In cellular schwannoma, the tumor may pose a challenge in the separation with a malignant schwannoma based on the cellular atypia and mitotic activity. In this setting, the use of immunohistochemical stains is of limited value as both tumors may share similar immunophenotype. In this setting, the morphological characteristics of the tumor – namely, the absence of an increase mitotic activity, marked nuclear atypia, necrosis, and hemorrhage – will lead to a more correct interpretation. By far the most challenging differential diagnosis may be with pigmented schwannoma; however, conventional schwannomas with pigment will lack increased mitotic activity and nuclear atypia. Even though S-100 protein may sow positive staining in both tumors, the use of other stains such as Mel A and MITF may be of help.

Granular Cell Tumor

Granular cell tumors are neoplasms of ubiquitous distribution; however, they are more common in the head and neck area and in the soft tissues. In the past, it was believed that these tumors had a relation to muscle, thus the previous name of myoblastoma or granular cell myoma. However, more recently, it is believed that granular cell tumors have a probable Schwann cell origin, and this is the reason why they are presented in this section.

The occurrence of these tumors in the mediastinal region is rare, with only few reports in the literature, and all of them in case reports [62–66]. These reported cases have been in patients between 16 and 43 year of age without any gender predilection. Clinically, patients with granular cell tumor may be asymptomatic, and the discovery of their tumors is either during a follow-up evaluation of a different condition or during a routine physical evaluation. However, the case described by Shikatani and associates [63] was that of a 19-year-old woman who presented with left ptosis and miosis (Horner's syndrome), and in whom a CT and MRI revealed the presence of a posterior mediastinal mass.

Pathological Features

Grossly, these tumors have been described as small tumors measuring approximately 1–5 cm in greatest diameter. The tumors are round to oval, and at cut surface, they are yellow-white, soft, with a whorled or smooth surface. Areas of hemorrhage may be present, but necrosis is usually absent.

Histologically, the tumors are fairly well circumscribed but not encapsulated, with sheets of round, oval to spindle cells with ample granular cytoplasm, small eccentric nuclei, and inconspicuous nucleoli (Figs. 11.29, 11.30, and 11.31). In some areas, the tumor may have discrete presence of fibrocollagenous bands separating tumor cells, with presence of ectatic blood vessels. Mitotic activity and necrosis are generally absent.

Ancillary Diagnostic Tools

The morphological appearance of granular cell tumors is characteristic enough to make a morphological diagnosis not a difficult task. However, in some cases, the use of immunohistochemical stains may aid in the diagnosis. Granular cell tumors are commonly positive for S-100 protein and neuron-specific enolase. However, the tumor is generally negative for epithelial markers (keratin, epithelial membrane antigen), for neuroendocrine markers (chromogranin and synaptophysin), and for muscle markers (desmin, muscle-specific actin, and smooth muscle actin). Ultrastructural features of granular cell tumors include the presence of abundant lysosomes.

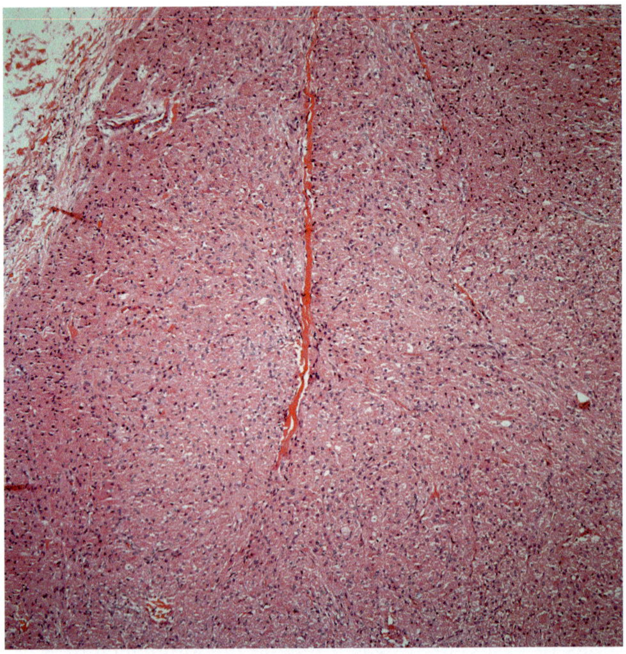

Fig. 11.29 Low power magnification of a granular cell tumor showing a well-defined neoplasm but not encapsulated

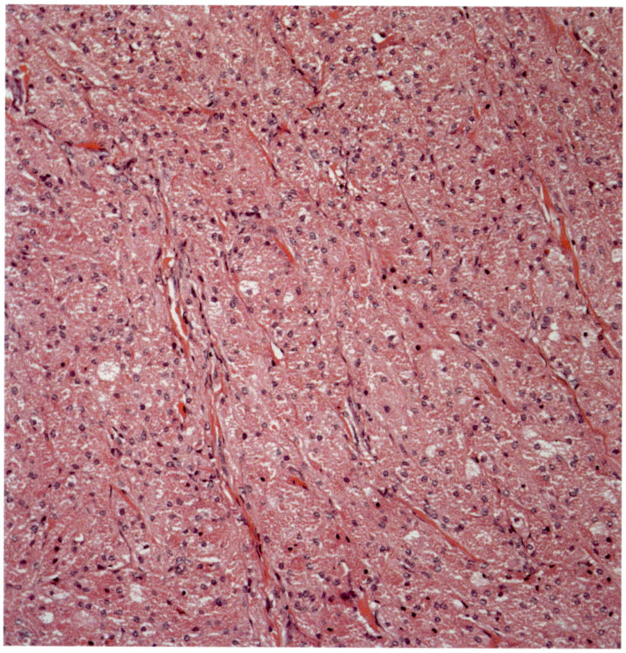

Fig. 11.30 Granular cell tumor showing a subtle nested pattern composed of cells with prominent oncocytic changes

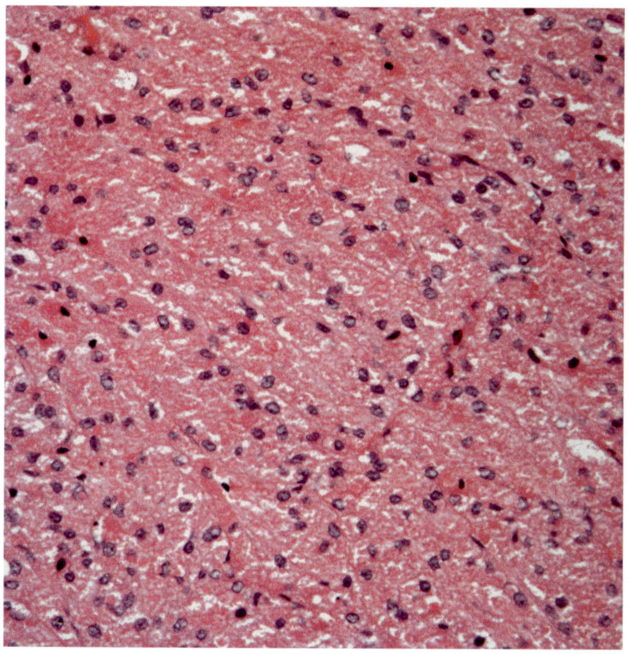

Fig. 11.31 High power view of a granular cell tumor showing cells with ample granular eosinophilic cytoplasm. Note the absence of nuclear atypia or mitotic activity

Differential Diagnosis

Even though the diagnosis of granular cell tumor is rather straightforward, other tumors that may be confused with this tumor, mainly in the mediastinum, include paraganglioma and neuroendocrine neoplasms. In either of these particular settings, the use of neuroendocrine markers including chromogranin and synaptophysin will aid in the diagnosis. Also, the use of keratin will be valuable as neuroendocrine carcinomas are positive for keratin. In addition, in cases of paragangliomas, even though S-100 may show positive staining, such staining is in sustentacular cells, while the positivity in granular cell tumor is in the cytoplasm of the tumor cells.

Malignant Tumors

As stated earlier in this chapter, the occurrence of malignant neurogenic tumors is much more common in the pediatric age group than in the adult population. In addition, even though these tumors are more commonly seen in the posterior mediastinum, occasionally they can also occur in the anterior mediastinum. Almost every benign neurogenic tumor has its malignant counterpart; thus, it is important to adhere to specific histopathological features in order to make such determinations in tumors that may share similar features or in tumors that may show mature and immature elements.

Neuroblastoma/Ganglioneuroblastoma

These two malignant neoplasms will be discussed in this section in a parallel form as the two tumors share some histopathological features: one has complete lack of maturation, while the other has an incomplete maturation. Both tumors originate from the neural crest, and a depiction of their maturation process is presented in Fig. 11.32a–c.

In 1910, Wright [67] analyzed five cases with the idea of highlighting the occurrence of a tumor that at that particular juncture had escaped recognition. Wright considered the tumor cells more or less undifferentiated nerve cells, or neurocytes, or neuroblasts, thus the names neurocytoma or neuroblastoma. Prior to this description, it is likely that most of these tumors now known as neuroblastomas had been called gliomas, sarcomas, or lymphoma. In 1927, Cushing and Wolbach [68] described a 2-year-old child with a paravertebral sympathicoblastoma (neuroblastoma), histologically proven, and 10 years later the recurrence of the tumor was that of a histologically proven ganglioneuroma. The authors interpreted such change as mature differentiation. Such description gave rise to the identification of cases that fall under the designation of ganglioneuroblastoma.

In 1957, Stowens [69], in a review of 236 cases of neuroblastoma and related tumors (ganglioneuroma and ganglioneuroblastoma) from the files of the Armed Forces Institute of Pathology, identified 110 cases coded as neuroblastoma, while only 17 cases belong to ganglioneuroblastoma. The balance of the other tumors corresponded to the mature ganglioneuroma. The vast majority of the neuroblastomas occurred in the

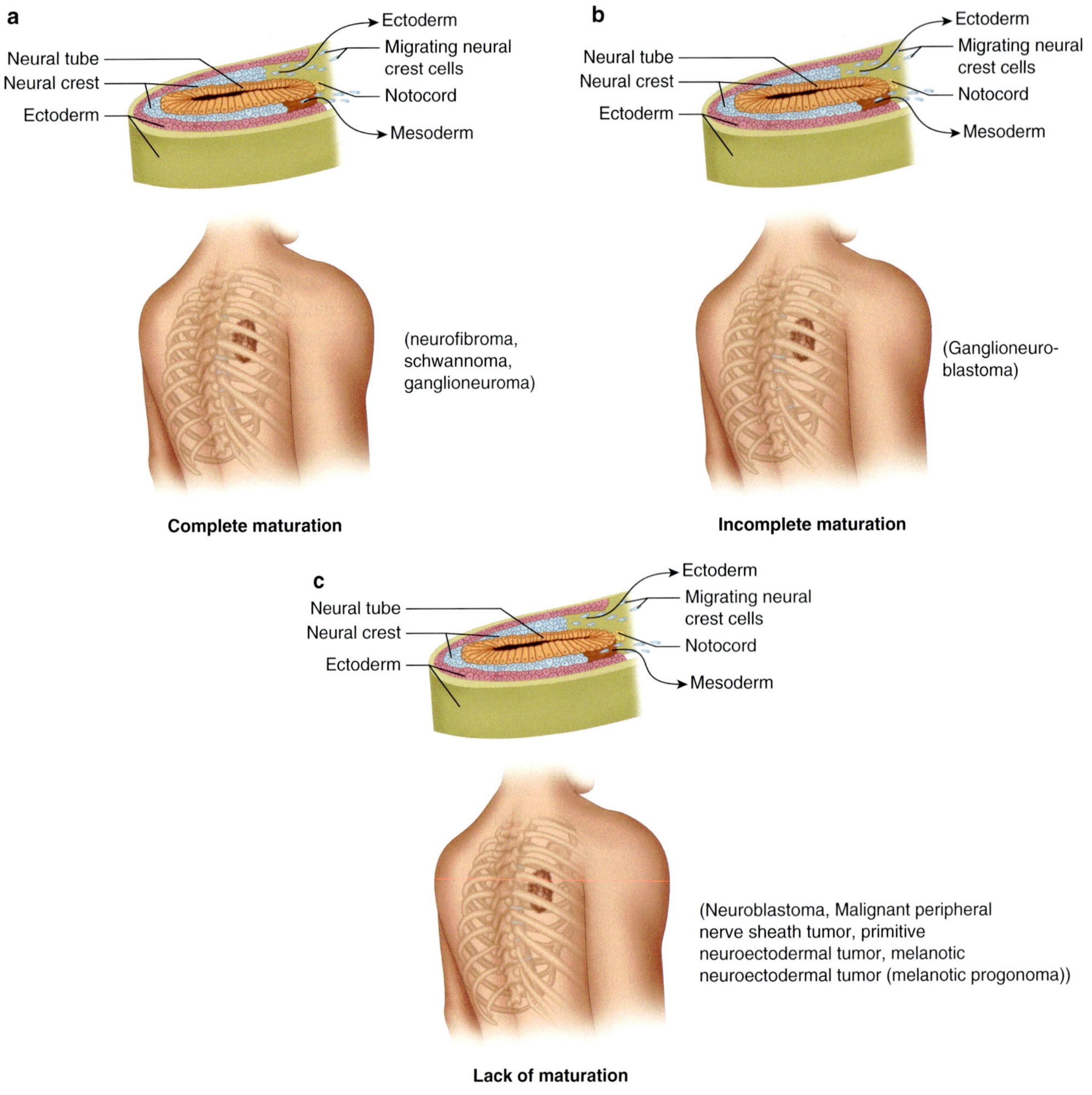

Fig. 11.32 (**a**–**c**) Diagramatic possibility of the development of different neurogenic tumors in the mediastinum

pediatric age group in children under 4 years of age, predominantly before 1 year of age, with only rare cases in older patients. Similar occurrence was also identified in cases designated as ganglioneuroblastomas. In addition, the majority of neuroblastomas and ganglioneuroblastomas predominantly occurred in the abdominal cavity (adrenal and retroperitoneum), while only 16 cases were identified in the mediastinal compartment. The author stated that neuroblastoma is primarily a disease of early childhood, with approximately 70% of the cases occurring in the first 4 years of life, and also adding that some of these tumors may be congenital in origin, whereas ganglioneuroma is predominantly a disease of adult life. Interestingly, Stowens [69], in order to explain the occurrence of ganglioneuroblastoma, advanced the idea of "partial differentiation," which the authors called "pseudodifferential embryogenesis." It is important to highlight that, in publications prior to the 1970s, the terminology of these tumors was somewhat more cumbersome. Oberman [70], for instance, even though acknowledging that these tumors are collectively designated as neuroblastomas, preferred to separate these tumors into "sympathicogoniomas" (the least differentiated of these tumors and composed of small cells the size of a lymphocyte with dark nuclei and indistinct cytoplasm) and "sympathicoblastoma"(greater differentiation, larger cells, thin rim of cytoplasm, and fibrillar stroma). In addition, the preferred nomenclature for ganglioneuromas was that of mature and partially differentiated (ganglioneuroblastoma). Even though it is well known that the occurrence of neurogenic tumors is by far more common in the posterior mediastinum, Buthker and associates [71] described a "sympathicoblastoma" in the anterior mediastinum in a 67-year-old woman. The authors reviewed previous literature on the subject and encountered 15 neurogenic tumors that apparently were in the anterior mediastinal location, but only three of those were "sympathicoblastomas," two of them in patients older than 60 years. In a separate description of a "sympathicoblastoma" of the anterior mediastinum, Oberman [72] alluded to the possibility of ganglionic tissue overlying the heart as a possible origin for this tumor in such location. Hutchinson [73] also described a neuroblastoma of the anterior mediastinum in a 51-year-old man who clinically was thought to have an aneurysm. Due to the unusual occurrence of neuroblastomas in the adult, a few small series of cases have been presented in the literature. Mackay and associates [74] described nine patients between the ages of 18 and 72; however, none of the cases presented had a thoracic origin. Other authors have focused more on the occurrence of ganglioneuroblastoma by reporting such occurrence in adult patients with either primary thoracic or abdominal primaries [75].

In 1981, Adam and Hochholzer presented the largest series of ganglioneuroblastomas of the posterior mediastinum [76]. The authors described 80 such cases in 38 male and 42 female patients; in one third of the patients, the tumor was diagnosed during the first 2 years of life, one half during the first 3 years of life and fourth-fifths during the first 10 years of life. Ten of the 80 patients were between 12 and 20 years and 3 over 20 years of age. Clinically, none of the patients had a history of neurofibromatosis. In half of the patients, the discovery of the tumor was during routine chest films, while 15 patients had some respiratory symptoms. Interestingly, other clinical presentations included Horner's syndrome and chronic diarrhea. Clinical follow-up was obtained in 72 patients; 55 were followed for 2–23 years. The 5-year survival rate was of 88%, and their prognosis was related to the stage of the tumor at the time of diagnosis. Fatal outcome was observed in patients with stage IV disease, while for those patients in stage I surgical resection appeared to be curable. The authors stated that the prognosis for this group of patients is far better than for neuroblastomas or intra-abdominal ganglioneuroblastomas. Even though the vast majority of these tumors occur in the posterior mediastinal location, it is also important to highlight that neuroblastomas and ganglioneuroblastomas in the anterior mediastinum have also been reported. Talerman and Gratma [77] described a 61-year-old woman with an anterior mediastinal ganglioneuroblastoma whose tumor was found incidentally at autopsy. Nagashima and associates [78] also described a ganglioneuroblastoma of the anterior mediastinum in a 79-year-old man who complained of chest pain. Complete surgical resection was performed followed by chemotherapy, and at 5 years the patients had no evidence of recurrence or metastasis. Asada and associates [79] described a case of adult ganglioneuroblastoma in a 61-year-old woman with syndrome of inappropriate secretion of antidiuretic hormone. The symptomatology of the patient was related to the endocrine abnormality, and MRI showed the presence of an anterior mediastinal tumor, which was surgically removed. Similar case of an adult neuroblastoma in the anterior mediastinum was also recorded by Kaye and associates [80] who described among three adult patients with neuroblastoma a 26-year-old woman who also had the syndrome of inappropriate antidiuretic hormone and hypercortisolism due to ectopic production of ACTH. More recently, Jrebi and associates [81] evaluated their collective experience by reviewing all adult cases of neuroblastoma and ganglioneuroblastoma in patients 18 years or older, corresponding to the years 1980–2009. The authors found 15 patients ages 19–66 years, corresponding to six men and nine women, and in five patients the tumor was found incidentally. Anatomically, four tumors were in the pelvis, three in the mediastinum, two in the abdomen, two in the adrenal gland, two in the retroperitoneum, and two were labeled as "mixed locations." The authors concluded that complete surgical resection might lead to long-term disease free survival in patients in stage I.

Regarding the occurrence of ganglioneuroblastoma in children, Bove and McAdams [82] reported their experience with 19 cases, which the authors designated as "composite ganglioneuroblastoma." The authors review 30-year period (1948–1978) at the Children's Hospital Medical Center in Cincinnati, identifying 19 such cases in children ranging in ages from 56 to 108 months. Eleven of these cases were in stage I, eight cases were in the mediastinum, and six patients followed a fatal outcome. Two patients with tumor in the mediastinum followed a fatal course. In a larger cohort of patients, Adams and associates [83] from the pediatric oncology group evaluated 96 patients with thoracic neuroblastoma. The median age at presentation of the tumor was 9 months. In 49% of the cases in which the tumor was in the posterior mediastinum, the tumor was found incidentally by radiographic films; 16% presented with neurological symptoms, and 16% presented with respiratory distress. Urinary catecholamines were elevated in 76% of the cases. Only 47% of the patients were treated with complete surgical resection. The overall survival was 88% at 4 years. The authors stated that the basic biology of thoracic neuroblastomas appears to be different from other locations in that the majority of patients present at a younger age with localized disease or regional lymph node metastases. In a different study by Demir and associates [84] between the years 1973 and 2007, 87 children with thoracic neuroblastic tumors were identified. Eighty-six of these tumors were located in the posterior mediastinum; the median age was 2.1 years of age. Histologically, 46 were neuroblastomas, 26 ganglioneuroblastomas, and 15 ganglioneuromas. The highest percentage of cases was in stage IV (38.2%), followed by stage III (22.1%). Clinically, the tumor was found incidentally in 20 patients, while the rest showed some symptomatology including Horner's syndrome. Clinical follow-up showed that 10-year overall and event-free survival rates were 71.2% and 67.4%, respectively. The survival of these patients appears to correlate with the stage of the tumor as the 10-year overall survival for stages I and II was 88.8%. An interesting association of ganglioneuroma and ganglioneuroblastoma has been reported by Geraci and associates [85] in three patients between the ages of 4 and 23 years with histories of neurofibromatosis type I. Two patients developed ganglioneuromas (adrenal and parapharyngeal), while one patient developed a ganglioneuroblastoma (posterior mediastinum).

Regarding diagnostic imaging in neuroblastomas and ganglioneuroblastomas, Lonergan and associates [86], in a review of these tumors, stated that the results depend on the modality employed. Plain radiographs may show the presence of a mediastinal, retroperitoneal, or neck mass, which may reveal the presence of calcifications in about 30% of the cases. Upon ultrasonography, these tumors are heterogeneously echogenic. Computerized tomography (CT) may be the most commonly used modality as it can reveal the extent of tumor, organ of origin, invasion, adenopathy, and calcification. Magnetic resonance imaging (MRI) commonly shows a heterogeneous, variably enhancing, and relatively low signal intensity on T1 and high signal intensity in T2-weighted images.

Different studies on the prognosis of neuroblastoma and ganglioneuroblastoma have been presented in the literature. Brook and associates [87] studied 41 neuroblastomas using several immunohistochemical stains including neuron-specific enolase (NSE), protein gene product (PGP) 9.5, and S-100 protein and concluded that there was no significant correlation between immunohistochemical staining and prognosis. Hachitanda and Hata [88], in a more focused analysis of 45 stage IVS neuroblastomas, concluded that most stage IVS neuroblastomas have favorable histology and may have a good prognosis. However, the authors also stated that a poor prognosis group does exist and could be identified on histopathology. Gutierrez and colleagues [89], in a 30-year analysis of 1646 patients with neuroblastoma, estimated an annual incidence of 0.9 per 100,000, with a median age of 1 year. The majority of tumors occurred in the retroperitoneum, accounting for 75.6%, while mediastinal tumors account for 15.3%. Disease-specific survival at 1, 2, 5, and 20 years for the entire cohort was 81, 70, 61, and 59%, respectively. The authors also stated that tumors in the mediastinum and pelvis have a better prognosis, while high-grade tumors with 10 cm or more in greatest dimension have worse prognosis. Kubota and colleagues [90], in a study on prognostic factors related to better clinical outcome in ganglioneuroblastoma, concluded that the better prognosis is related to the absence of N-*myc* amplification.

Clinical Staging

In 1971, Evans and colleagues [91], in an analysis of 100 children with neuroblastoma, proposed a clinical staging system for patients with this tumor. This staging system is also known as Children's Cancer Study Group (CCSG):

- Stage I: Tumor confined to the organ or structure of origin.
- Stage II: Tumors extending in continuity beyond the organ or structure of origin but not crossing the midline. Regional lymph nodes on the homolateral side may be involved.
- Stage III: Tumors extending in continuity beyond the midline. Regional lymph nodes may be involved bilaterally.
- Stage IV: Remote disease involving skeleton, organs, soft tissues, or distant lymph nodes groups.
- Stage IV-S: Patients who would otherwise be stage I or II but who have remote disease confined only to one or more of the following sites: the skin, liver, or bone marrow (without radiographic evidence of bone metastases on complete skeletal survey).

In 1980, Evans [92], in a review of the staging and treatment of neuroblastoma, stated that patients with local resectable tumors probably do not require irradiation or chemotherapy, while patients with residual disease (stage III) benefit from radiation therapy. For patients with stage IV, surgical resection may not be required as chemotherapy assumes a major role. Also, Evans and colleagues [93], in an analysis of 124 children with neuroblastoma, estimated an overall survival rate of 60% at 2 years. In addition, the authors suggested that a combination of age, stage, serum ferritin, and histologic type might play a role as prognostic factors in neuroblastoma. However, Hata and colleagues [94], in a study of neuroblastoma comparing the Evans system and the International Union Against Cancer (UICC) system (which is essentially a TNM system that includes separate clinical stages (CS) and postsurgical histopathological stages (PS), suggested that, for predicting the prognosis for advanced cases, the UICC staging system and especially the PS staging system may be more rational than the Evans staging system. This TNM system can be summarized as follows:

T 0 = tumor not detected	**N 0** = normal LN	**M 0** = no metastasis
T 1 = tumor <5 cm	**N 1** = abnormal regional LN	**M 1** = metastasis
T 2 = tumor 5–10 cm	**N x** = not available	
T 3 = tumor >10 cm		
T 4 = multicentric tumor		

It is important to highlight that there are two additional staging systems for neuroblastomas in addition to the one proposed by Evans (CCSG) and the TNM system by the UICC. These are the St Jude Children's Research Hospital [95] and the one used by the Pediatric Oncology Group (POG) [96]. These systems can be summarized as follows:

St Jude Staging System

Stage I: Localized disease completely removed; regional nodes and liver negative.

Stage IIA: Microscopic residual primary disease; incorporated lymph nodes may be positive. Regional lymph nodes and liver negative.

Stage IIB: Gross residual primary disease; regional lymph nodes and liver negative.

Stage IIIA (N): Regional spread with positive regional lymph nodes; liver negative.

Pediatric Oncology Group (POG) System

Stage A: Complete gross resection of primary tumor with or without microscopic residual disease. Attached lymph nodes may be positive. Distant liver and nodes negative.

Stage B: Grossly unresected tumor. Nodes and liver same as stage A.

Stage C: Complete or incomplete resection. Unattached nodes positive.

In that regard, Evans and colleagues [97] evaluated the accuracy of the four staging systems in a retrospective study of 251 neuroblastoma patients. The authors concluded that all four systems had value for prognostication, and all identified with accuracy the low-stage patient who fares well. However, the authors also concluded that the CCSG staging system most accurately identifies patients with regional tumor who have a poor prognosis. In view of the different staging systems suggested, however, the international neuroblastoma staging system (INSS) proposed an internationally accepted staging system [98]. This system is as follows:

International Neuroblastoma Staging System (INSS)

Stage 1: Localized tumor with complete gross excision, with or without microscopic residual disease; representative ipsilateral lymph nodes negative for tumor microscopically; nodes attached to and removed with the primary tumor may be positive.

Stage 2A: Localized tumor with incomplete gross excision; representative ipsilateral nonadherent lymph nodes negative for tumor microscopically.

Stage 2B: Localized tumor with or without complete gross excision, with ipsilateral nonadherent lymph nodes positive for tumor. Enlarged contralateral lymph nodes must be negative microscopically.

Stage 3: Unresectable unilateral tumor infiltrating across the midline with or without regional lymph node involvement; or localized unilateral tumor with contralateral regional lymph node involvement; or midline tumor with bilateral extension by infiltration (unresectable) or by lymph node involvement.

Stage 4: Any primary tumor with dissemination to distant lymph nodes, bone, bone marrow, liver, skin, and/or other organs (except as defined for stage 4S).

Stage 4S: Localized tumor (as defined for stage 1, 2A, or 2B) with dissemination limited to the skin, liver, and/or bone marrow (limited to infants <1 year of age).

Shortly after this staging system was proposed, essentially the same group revised some of the definitions to the stages proposed [99]. Essentially, for stage 1, the clarification was made that "adherent nodes in direct continuity and removed with the primary tumor may be positive for tumor." For stage 3, a redefinition of the midline was introduced to basically consider the vertebral column as the midline.

Pathologic Classification

In 1999, the International Neuroblastoma Pathology Committee (INPC) convened to produce a classification system with terminology and morphologic criteria [100, 101]. The proposed terminology and morphologic criteria was adopted after reviewing 227 cases, using a morphologic approach. Essentially, the INPC adopted the Shimada system, which is based on the differentiation of the tumor, their cellular turnover index, and the presence or absence of Schwannian stromal development. Based on such criteria, neuroblastomas were divided into four categories:

1. Neuroblastoma (Schwannian stroma-poor), undifferentiated, poorly differentiated, and differentiating (Figs. 11.33, 11.34, 11.35, 11.36, 11.37, 11.38, 11.39, 11.40, 11.41, 11.42, 11.43, 11.44, 11.45, 11.46, 11.47, and 11.48)
2. Ganglioneuroblastoma, intermixed (Schwannian stroma-rich)
3. Ganglioneuroma (Schwannian stroma-dominant), maturing and mature
4. Ganglioneuroblastoma, nodular (composite, Schwannian stroma-rich/stroma-dominant, and stroma-poor)

Specific Histological Features

- Mitosis-karyorrhexis index (MKI) is defined as the number of tumor cells in mitosis and in the process of karyorrhexis.
- Mitotic rate (MR) is counted at ten contiguous high-power fields (hpf) at x400 magnification.
  - Tumors with fewer than ten mitoses in 10 hpf belong to the low MR class.
  - Tumors with greater than ten mitoses in 10 hpf belong to the high MR class.
- Calcification – No quantification is required; however, its presence is associated with favorable prognosis.

In 2001, the INPC further defined four categories of tumor, this time by association with the MYCN status and the histology of the tumor [102]. The committee evaluated 535 neuroblastomas, 21 ganglioneuroblastomas (intermixed), 9 ganglioneuromas, and 63 ganglioneuroblastoma (nodular). The tumors were separated into tumor with favorable histology and tumors with unfavorable histology, with their corresponding MYCN amplification or non-amplification. Based on this study, the authors found that favorable histology with non-amplified tumors had a 5-year event-free survival of 92.1%, while 8 tumors with favorable histology and amplified tumor had a 5-year event-free survival of 37.5%. Regarding the tumor with unfavorable histology and non-amplified tumors, the 5-year event-free survival was 40.9%, while similar tumors with amplified tumors had 15.0%. The authors concluded that histopathologic evaluation and MYC status appear to correlate with prognosis. In addition, the authors, in a separate publication, stressed the importance of the histopathology of these tumors and the importance of separating these tumors into favorable and unfavorable histology [103].

A few years after these proposals had been presented, the INPC revised their classification by confirming categories of favorable and unfavorable prognostic subsets for ganglioneuroblastoma, nodular type [104, 105]. Essentially, the evaluation of ganglioneuroblastomas will also involve the macroscopic appearance of the tumor. Thus, the following features:

- Ganglioneuroma – maturing (Schwannian stroma-dominant): essentially a ganglioneuromatous tumor with scattered neuroblasts and/or maturing ganglion cells. Favorable histology.
- Ganglioneuroblastoma-intermixed (Schwannian stroma-rich) (Figs. 11.49, 11.50, 11.51, and 11.52): transitional tumor between neuroblastoma and ganglioneuroma. Microscopic residual foci of neuroblastoma containing neurophil and neuroblasts. The proportion of ganglioneuromatous component to neuroblastomatous component should exceed 50%. Favorable histology.
- Ganglioneuroblastoma-nodular (composite, Schwannian stroma-rich/stroma-dominant, and stroma-poor) (Figs. 11.53, 11.54, 11.55, 11.56, and 11.57): Macroscopic neuroblastomatous nodule(s). The proportion of neuroblastomatous and ganglioneuromatous component varies from case to case. This particular subtype can be further subclassified into favorable and unfavorable histology based on age-linked evaluation, grade of neuroblastic differentiation, and mitosis-karyorrhexis index of the neuroblastomatous nodule.

Histochemical, Ultrastructural, Immunohistochemical, and Molecular Features

Even though the majority of neuroblastomas are purported to be negative for the presence of glycogen, which in turn helps distinguish these tumors from other small round cell tumors such as primitive neuroectodermal tumor (Ewing sarcoma) or rhabdomyosarcoma, there is a group of neuroblastomas that may show the presence of glycogen by staining the tumor with periodic acid-Schiff (PAS) histochemical stain or by ultrastructural studies. Yunis and colleagues [106], in 1979 in a study of 40 cases, encountered the presence of glycogen in four cases of neuroblastomas; at least two of those cases were confirmed neuroblastomas by morphology and electron microscopy. In a separate study of nine patients of adult neuroblastoma, Mackay and colleagues [74] stated that one constant feature of neuroblastomas that reflects the neural crest derivation is the presence of cytoplasmic processes, while the presence of electron-dense granules with limiting membranes is a significant feature. By immunohistochemistry, there is not a specific immunohistochemical profile that is pathognomonic for neuroblastoma. The tumor may show positive staining for NSE (neuron-specific enolase), CD99, PGP 9.5, and S-100 protein, while negative for keratins, EMA, GFAP, chromogranin, and synaptophysin (except in the neutrophil

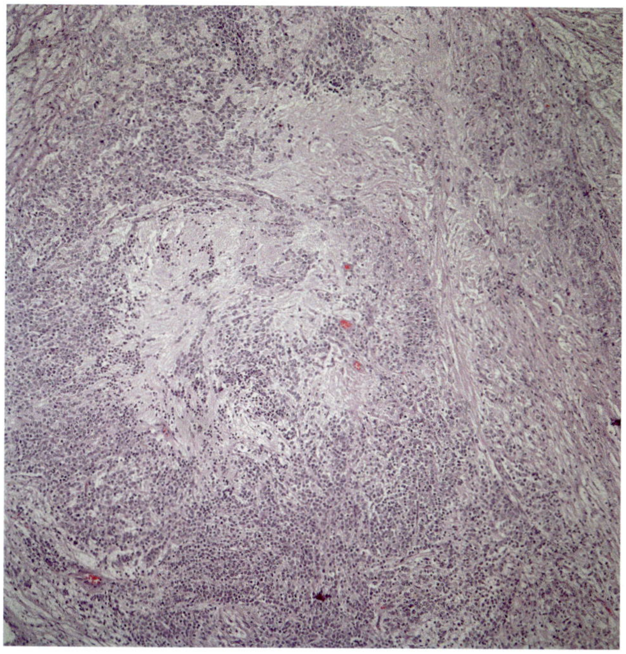

Fig. 11.33 Low power view of a neuroblastoma showing extensive areas of neurophil and sheets of small cells

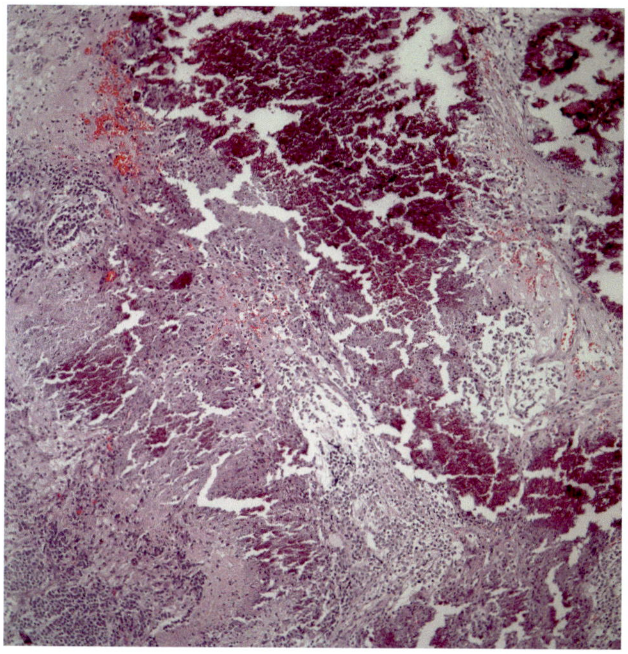

Fig. 11.34 Neuroblastoma with extensive calcification and only focal areas of viable tumor

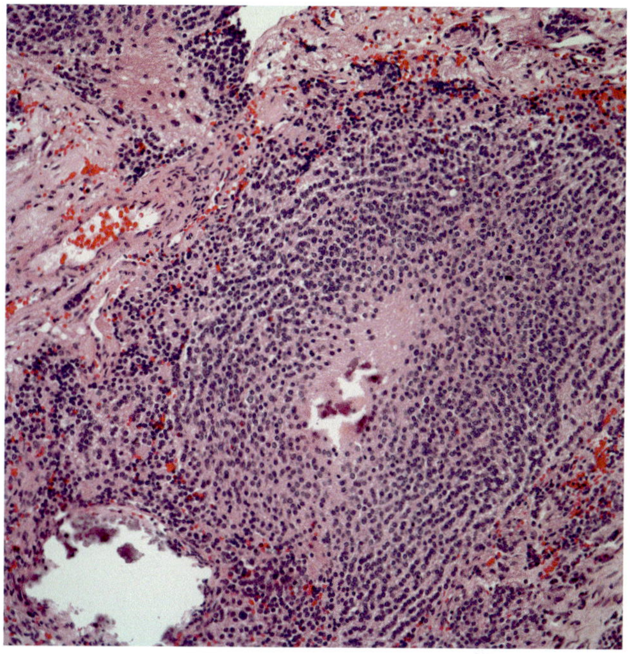

Fig. 11.35 Closer view of a neuroblastoma showing central calcification and areas of neurophil. Note the fairly homogeneous cellular proliferation composed of small cells

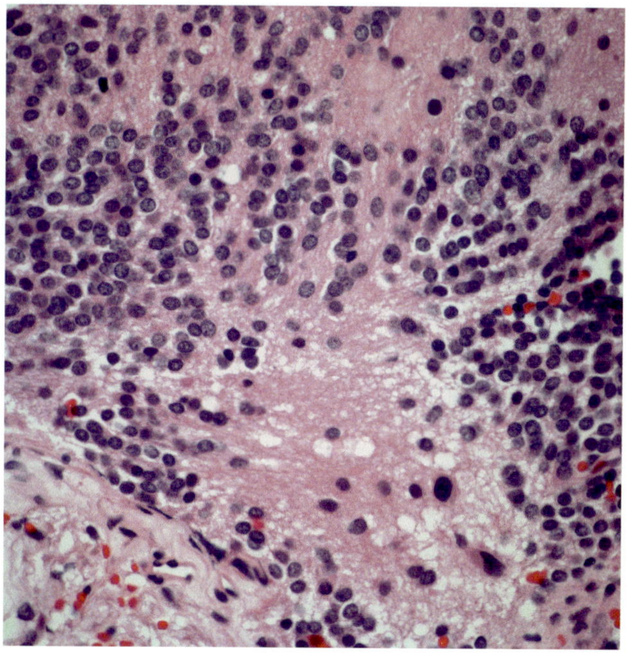

Fig. 11.36 Higher magnification of a neuroblastoma showing the cellular proliferation composed of small cells with scant cytoplasm, round nuclei, and inconspicuous nucleoli embedded in neurophil. No mitotic activity is present

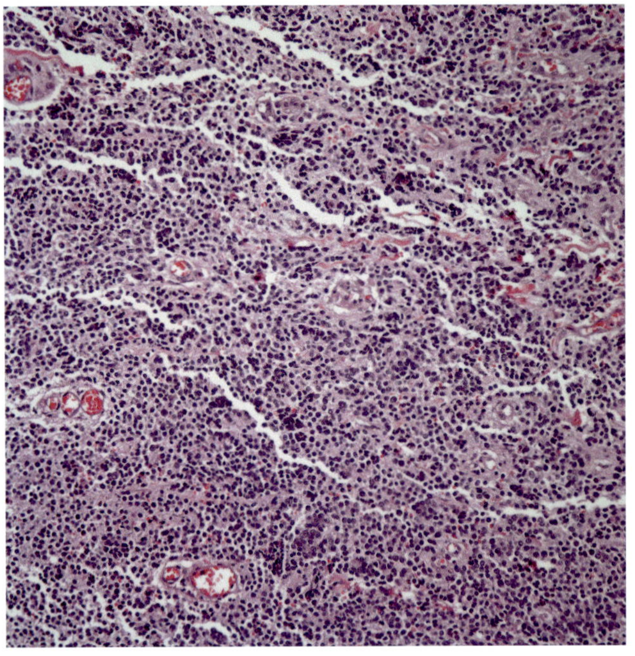

Fig. 11.37 A different view of a less differentiated neuroblastoma showing sheets of small neoplastic cells

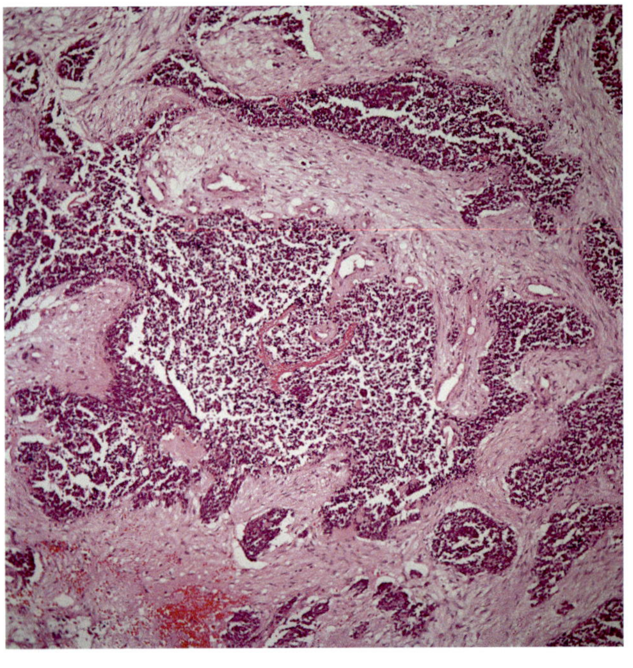

Fig. 11.38 Neuroblastoma with extensive areas of fibrocollagenous tissue and nested areas of tumors cells

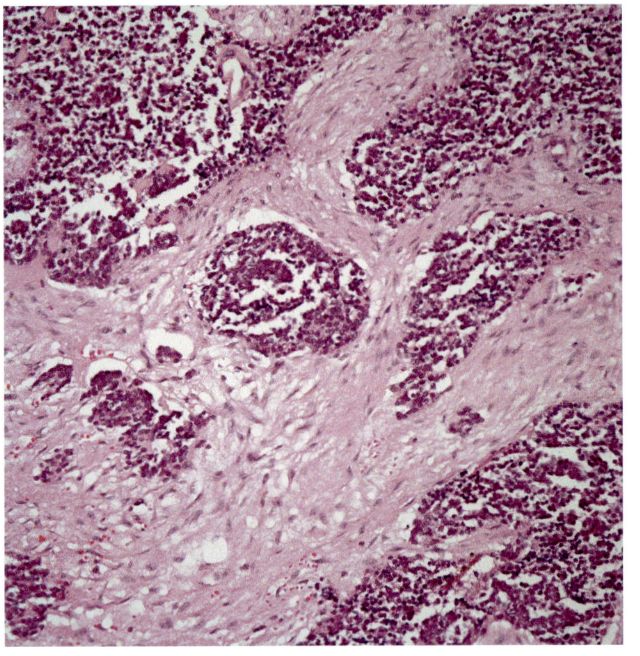

Fig. 11.39 Closer view of the neoplastic cells in this less differentiated neuroblastoma showing small cells arranged in nests and separated by fibrocollagenous tissue

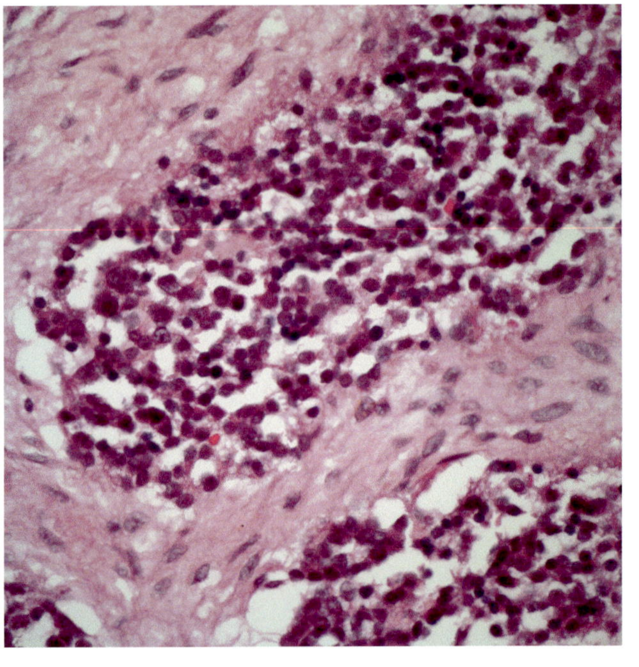

Fig. 11.40 High power view of a less differentiated neuroblastoma showing small cells with round vesicular nuclei and in some cells nucleoli is identified. The tumor does not show areas with neurophil

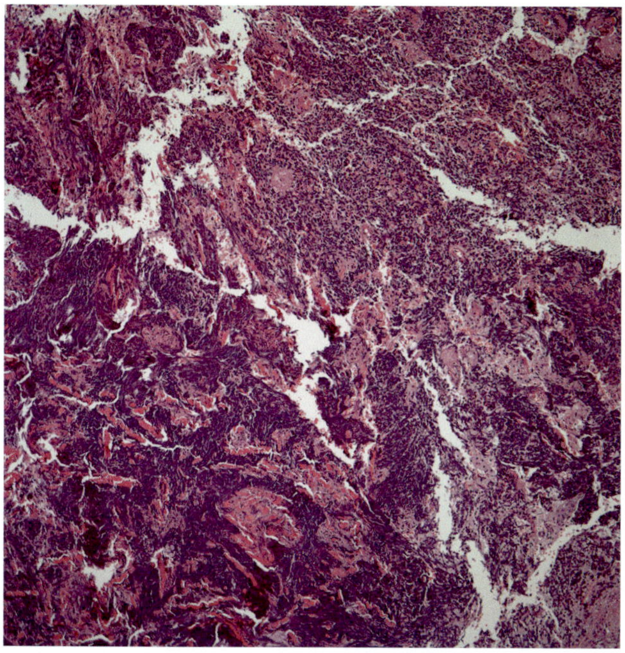

Fig. 11.41 Poorly differentiated neuroblastoma showing extensive crush artifact

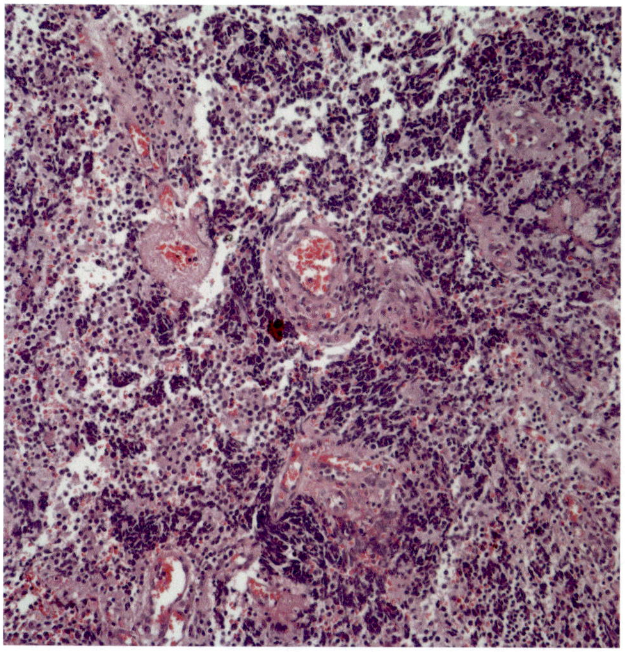

Fig. 11.42 Poorly differentiated neuroblastoma showing small cell proliferation around vessels

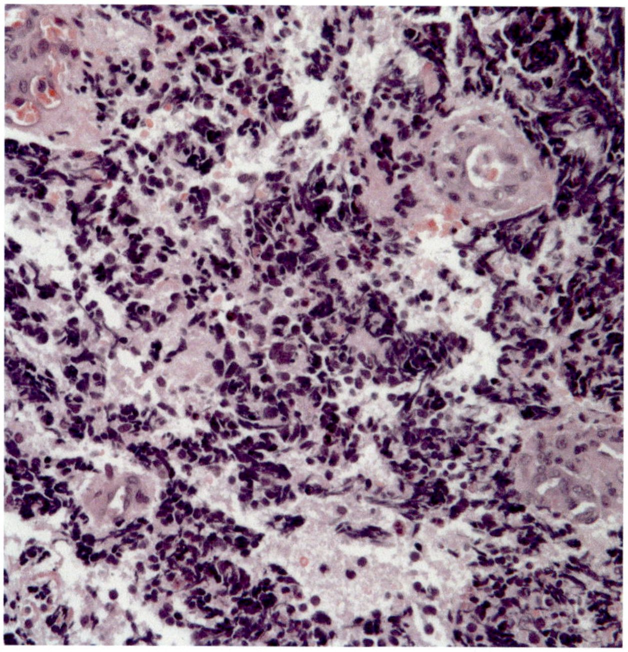

Fig. 11.43 Neuroblastoma with features mimicking small cell carcinoma

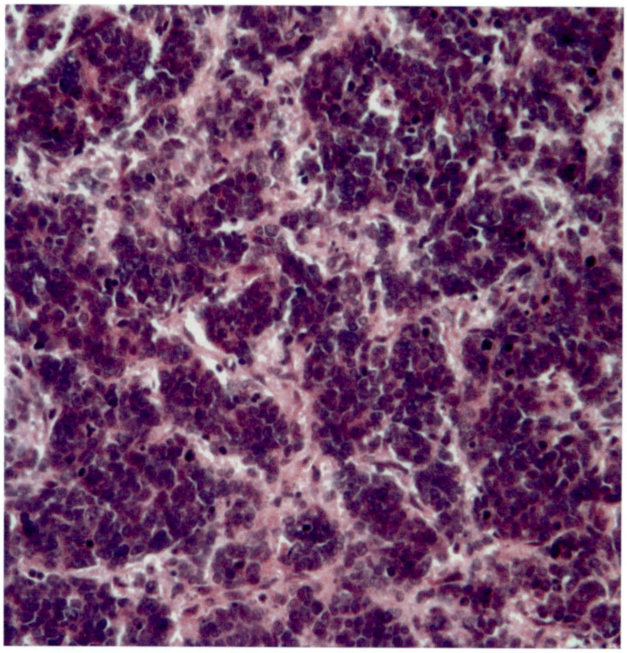

Fig. 11.44 Neuroblastoma showing increased mitotic activity

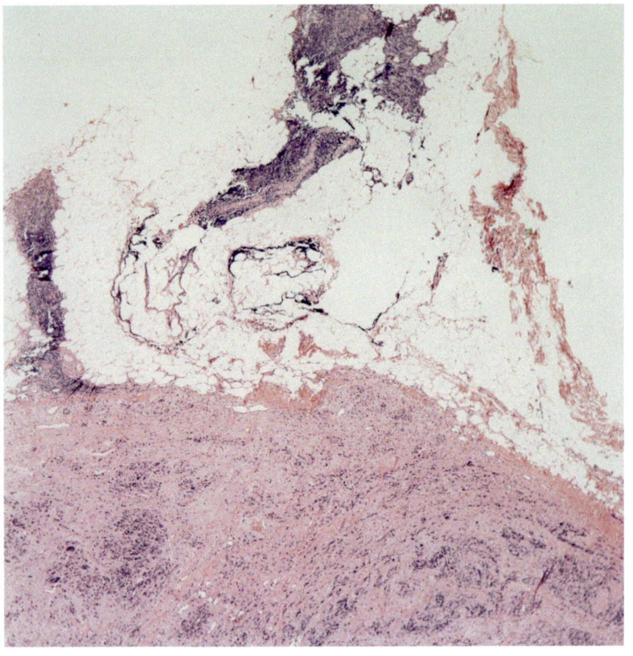

Fig. 11.45 Anterior mediastinal neuroblastoma. Note the presence of remnants of thymic tissue in the periphery

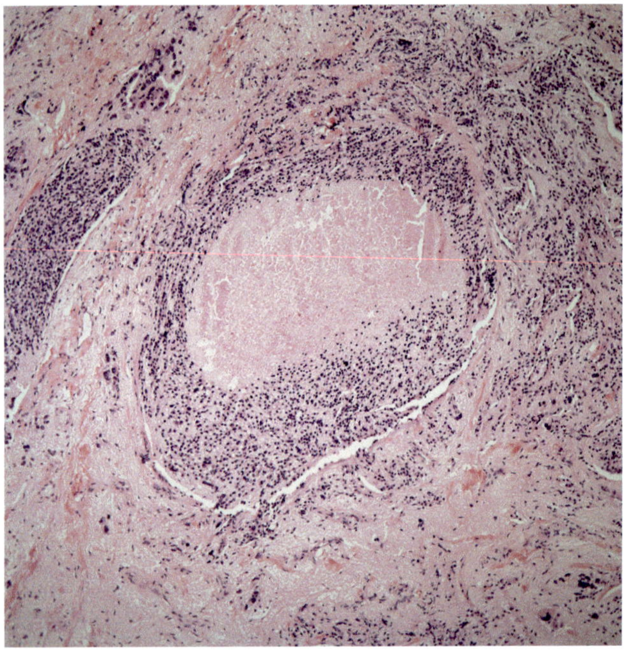

Fig. 11.46 Thymic neuroblastoma showing areas of comedo-like necrosis

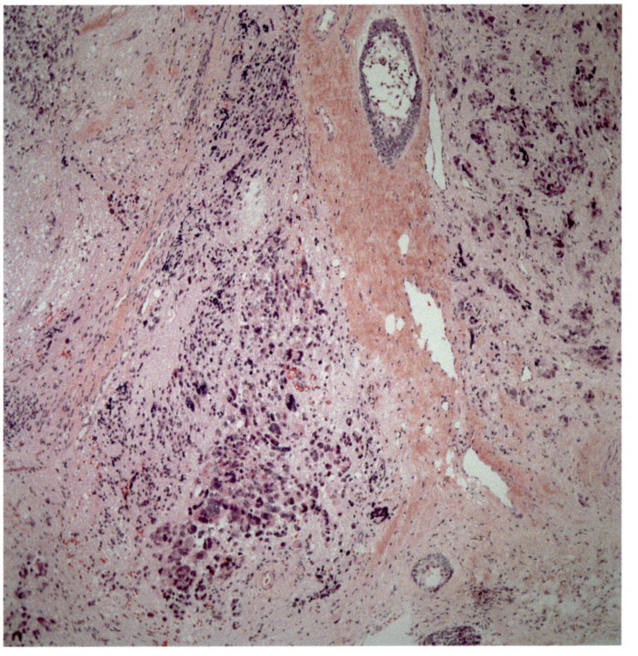

Fig. 11.47 Thymic neuroblastoma showing cellular atypia. Note the remnants of thymic epithelium

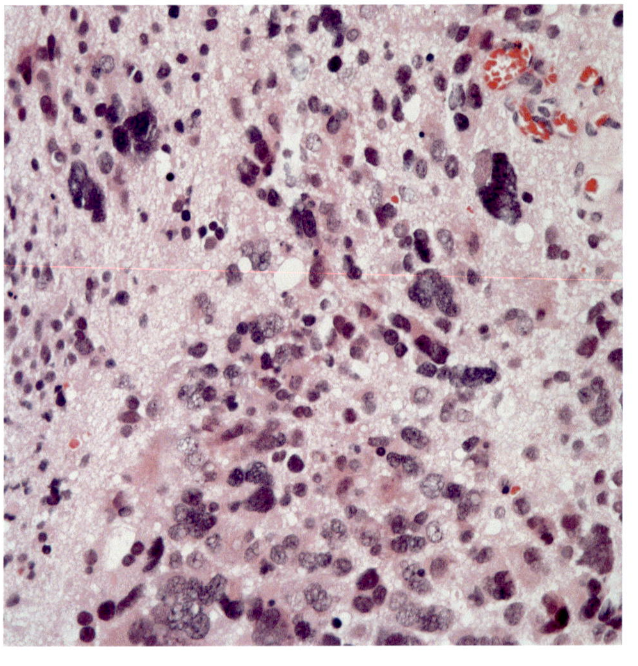

Fig. 11.48 Higher magnification of a thymic neuroblastoma with marked cellular and nuclear atypia

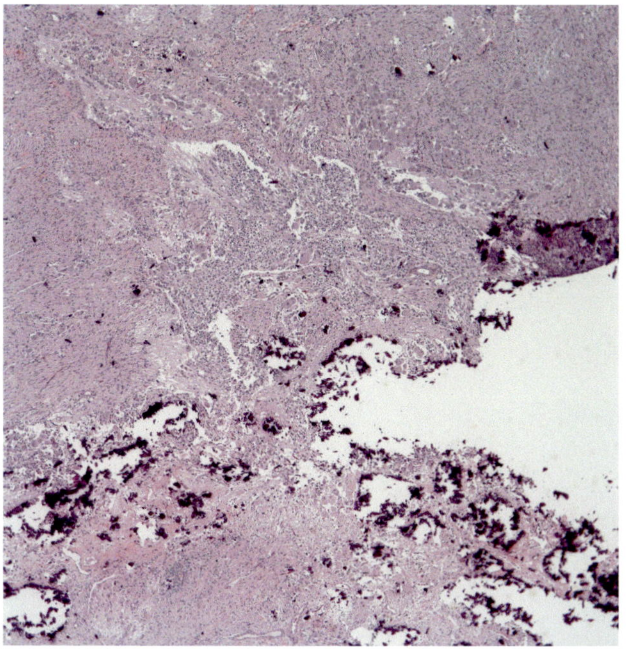

Fig. 11.49 Predominantly ganglioneuromatous component with focus of neuroblastoma and calcifications

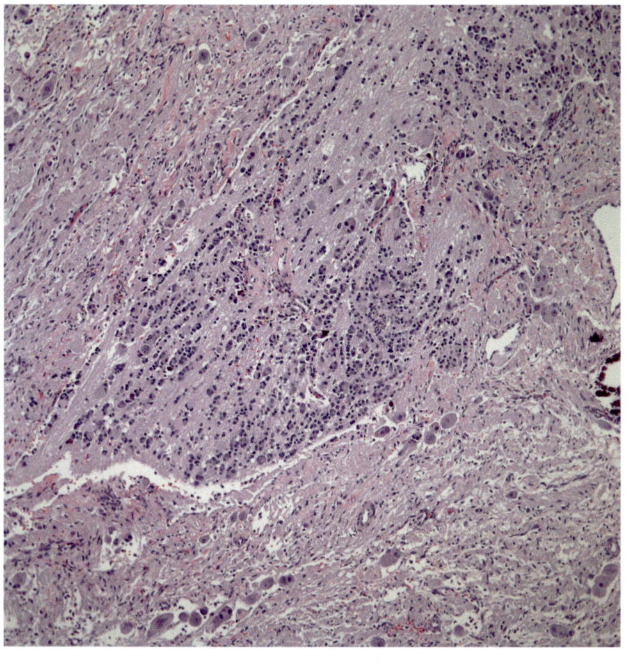

Fig. 11.50 Small nodule of neuroblastoma embedded in a ganglioneuromatous component

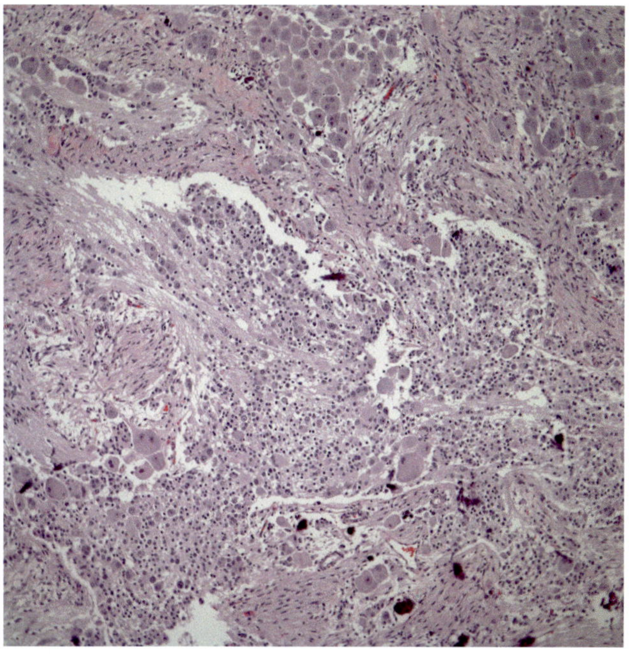

Fig. 11.51 Closer view of a ganglioneuroblastoma showing a microscopic nodule of neuroblastoma. Note the presence of numerous ganglion cells

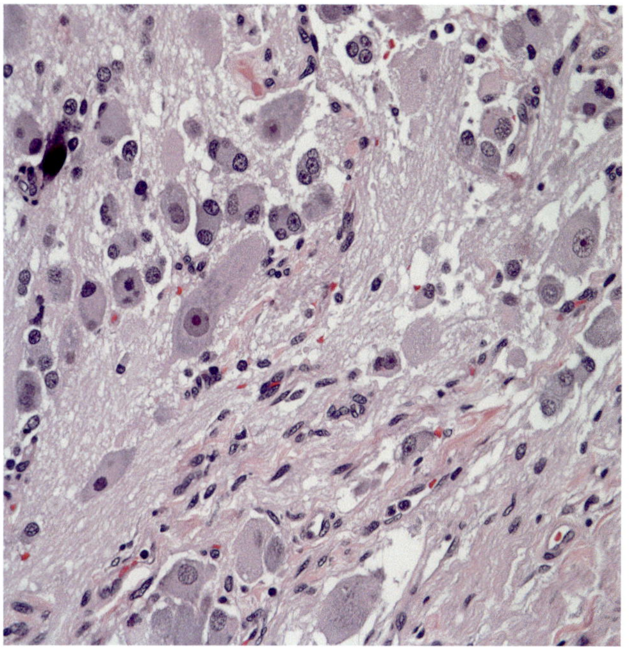

Fig. 11.52 Higher magnification of a ganglioneuroblastoma showing predominantly ganglion cells with scattered neuroblastoma cells

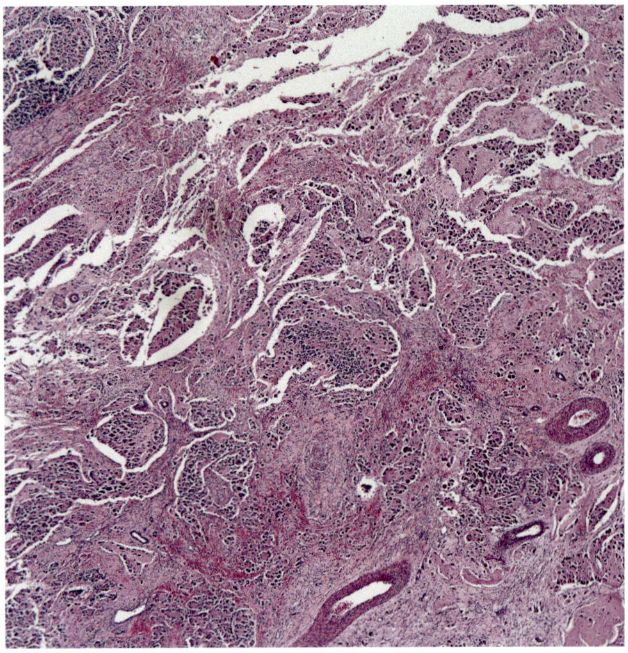

Fig. 11.53 Low power view of a ganglioneuroblastoma showing extensive areas of tumor

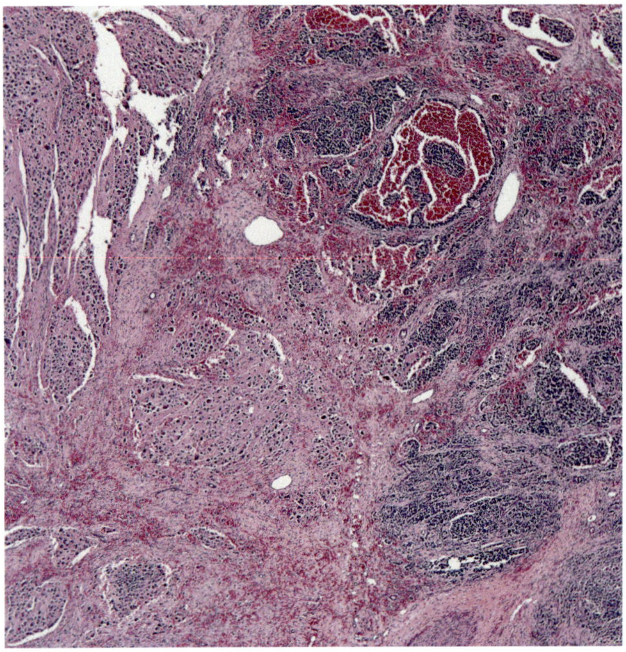

Fig. 11.54 Low power view of a ganglioneuroblastoma showing two populations of cells (larger and smaller cells)

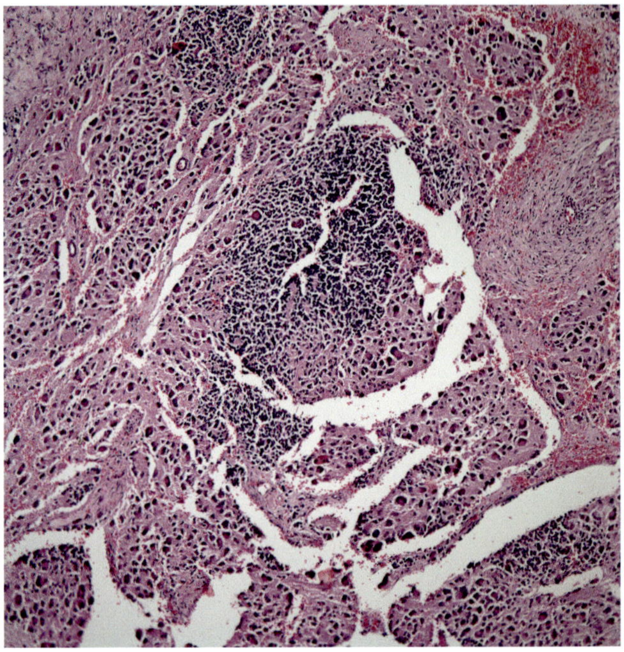

Fig. 11.55 Higher magnification of a ganglioneuroblastoma showing a population of larger cells and a small focus of small dark cells

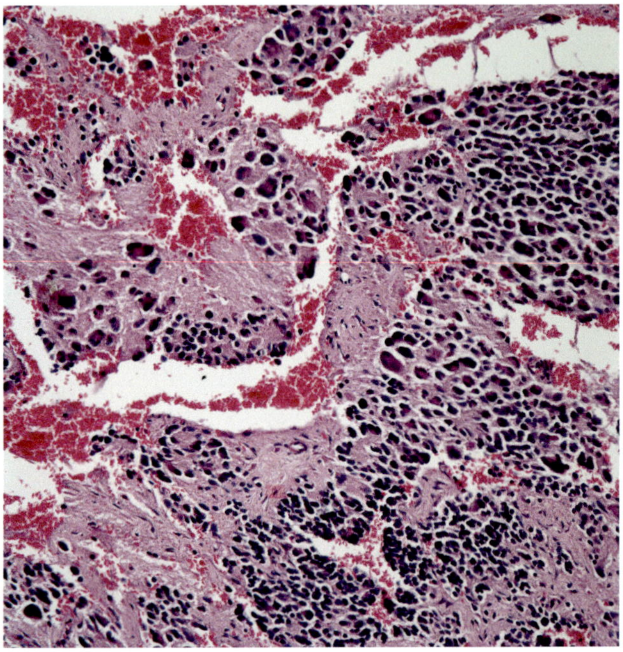

Fig. 11.56 Higher magnification of a ganglioneuroblastoma showing two populations of cells

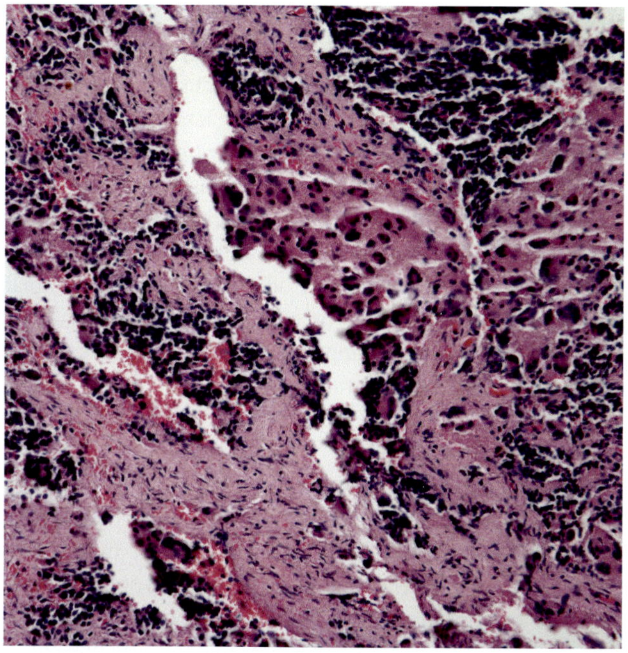

Fig. 11.57 Higher magnification of a ganglioneuroblastoma showing less differentiated neuroblastomatous component (dark cells)

areas), desmin, myoD, or other muscle markers. Favrot and colleagues [107], in a study of 45 neuroblastomas with focus in the expression of integrin receptors, encountered that none of the tumors expressed α-5 chain of the integrins; the majority of tumors expressed α-1 and α-3 chain of the integrins. All the tumors expressed β-1 chain. The authors concluded that the role of integrins in the malignant behavior of the cells is more complex than is usually predicted by experimental models. In a more sophisticated study to determine genomic damage in neuroblastic tumors, Munoz and colleagues [108] did not find an association between genomic damage fraction and tumor location, proliferation index, diagnosis, or age of the patient. However, the authors stated that tumors with MYCN amplification have a higher genomic damage fraction, which may contribute to the genomic instability of neuroblastomas. More recently, Angelini and colleagues [109], in a study of nodular ganglioneuroblastoma in eight children to determine the clonality of the neuroblasts, ganglion cells, and Schwann cells, concluded that the ganglion cells and neuroblasts are genetically related and may arise from the same clone, while the Schwann cells have a different origin and may be derived from a nonneoplastic neural crest precursor.

Differential Diagnosis

Neuroblastomas belong to the generic category of small round cell tumors; thus, the differential diagnosis of these tumors will include similar other tumors that belong to this category, namely, rhabdomyosarcoma and PNET. Since these tumors occur in childhood, it is essential to arrive to a particular diagnosis in order to properly establish treatment and prognosis for these children. Even though, as has been stated earlier, neuroblastomas occur more often in very early childhood, it is still important to keep other small round cell tumors in the differential diagnosis. Similarly, since all these tumors are uncommon in older patients, the same differential is maintained. However, the use of immunohistochemistry in this setting may prove beneficial as rhabdomyosarcomas may show reactivity against some or all muscle markers including Myo-D, desmin, myoglobin, and Caldesmon, which would not be the case in neuroblastomas. Regarding PNET, the use of immunohistochemistry may have some overlapping features with neuroblastoma in terms of positive staining for CD99; however, molecular analysis of PNET would show the proper molecular alteration in cases that are not clear by morphological or immunohistochemical analysis. One more consideration in unusual cases when these tumors occur in the adult population would be small cell carcinoma; however, small cell carcinomas commonly show positive staining for keratin, chromogranin, and synaptophysin. In addition, the clinical presentation and anatomic site of the tumor should lead to the correct interpretation.

In cases of ganglioneuroblastoma, the most important differential consideration would be with a conventional ganglioneuroma, mainly in cases in which the neuroblastomatous component is that of small microscopic nodules. In this setting, careful analysis of the morphological features should prompt the consideration of ganglioneuroblastoma. In addition, the use of *myc* amplification may be of help not only in the diagnosis but also in the prognosis of the tumor.

Malignant Peripheral Nerve Sheath Tumor (MPNST)

The term MPNST as it is used in this section refers to tumors that over the years have been called neurofibrosarcomas or malignant schwannomas [110–112]. It is also important to note that, contrary to the occurrence of other neural tumors, MPNST are more common in the adult population in contrast to neuroblastomas or ganglioneuroblastomas, which are more commonly observed in the pediatric age group [17]. At the same time, it is difficult to determine their exact occurrence as, in the majority of cases, all these tumors have been grouped with other neural tumors, and, in that sense, their occurrence would vary from 10 to more than 25% [113]. However, the exact occurrence of MPNST in the mediastinum is not only rare but also difficult to estimate. It is important to highlight that, in early literature, tumors that were classified as "neurofibrosarcoma" may in current standards be classified differently. For instance, the case described by Rossman [110] as neurofibrosarcoma causing hypoglycemia in a 51-year-old woman with a posterior mediastinal mass likely may correspond to what we know now as solitary fibrous tumor, which commonly has as a clinical symptomatology hypoglycemia, and tumors that histologically show a variety of growth patterns [114]. Interestingly, even in early literature, cases of anterior mediastinal tumors have already been described [112]. In 1951, Ackerman and Taylor [115] reported 48 neurogenous tumors within the thorax and included four cases of what the author called "malignant schwannoma." The four cases were in adult patients, and all were located in the posterior mediastinum.

Sordillo and colleagues [116], in a study of 165 patients with malignant schwannoma, divided patients into those with solitary malignant schwannoma and those with von Recklinghausen's disease (VRD)-associated malignant schwannoma. The authors encountered that 40% of these patients had evidence of neurofibromatosis on physical examination, with a median age of 32 years in those with associated von Recklinghausen's disease (VRD), while those without it had a median age of 48 years. The tumor appeared to affect both genders equally in patients without VRD, while in those patients with VRD, the tumor was more frequent in females. The clinical course in both groups follows multiple local recurrences even though such occurrences had more aggressive course in patients with VRD. In addition, the authors noted that 8.5% of patients developed malignant schwannoma in an area of prior radiation. Follow-up information provided in this study shows that patients with VRD have shorter survival than those without VRD. In a different study on long-term follow-up of von Recklinghausen neurofibromatosis, Sorensen and colleagues [117] followed 212 affected patients and families; they encountered that survival rates were diminished in relatives with neurofibromatosis, worse in probands and worst in female probands. The authors concluded that patients with severe neurofibromatosis requiring hospital admission often have a poor prognosis. Of interest in this study is the association of different types of tumors in these patients. According to the table presented, four cases were classified as neurofibrosarcomas, one as neuromyxoma, one as acoustic neuroma, two as sarcoma fusocellular, one as fibrosarcoma, and one as fibromyxosarcoma, among many other epithelial and mesenchymal tumors.

As documented by Sordillo and colleagues [116], Ducatman and Scheithauer [118] analyzed 109 patients with neurofibrosarcoma in the period from 1912 to 1981, also documenting 12 patients in whom the tumor arose from an area previously irradiated. Seven of these 12 patients had evidence of neurofibromatosis. The authors determined that the latency period between the radiation and the occurrence of the tumor was 15.6 years (range 5–26 years). More recently, in a study of 75 cases of intrathoracic peripheral nerve sheath tumors, Boland and colleagues [50] found only five cases of MPNST, four of those tumors in a pleuropulmonary location and one in the anterior mediastinum. Based on these publications, it is likely that the occurrence of MPNST in the mediastinal location represents less than 1% of all tumors. However, the clinical history of von Recklinghausen neurofibromatosis and a posterior mediastinal mass should alert to the possibility of MPNST, especially when there is a history of previous radiation in that area.

As it has been noted with other posterior mediastinal tumors, these patients may be completely asymptomatic or have other non-specific symptoms related to the compression of the tumor in adjacent structures.

Pathological Features

Macroscopically, MPNST are usually larger tumors of more than 5–8 cm in greatest dimension. Even though a nerve may be grossly identified, in many cases that feature may not be possible to observe. The tumors are round to ovoid, solid, tan in color, and usually will show areas of hemorrhage and/or necrosis (Fig. 11.58). Cystic changes may also be present in some tumors, while in others that are heavily pigmented, dark areas may be observed.

Histologically, the tumors are characterized by the presence of a spindle cell proliferation that may be arranged in interlacing fascicles. The tumor may display several growth patterns including a "herringbone" pattern that commonly is ascribed to fibrosarcomas; thus, earlier publications use such nomenclature. However, for the most part, the spindle cellular proliferation is solid, which in some areas may show nuclear palisading and tactoid differentiation. Areas of hyalinization, necrosis, and/or hemorrhage are commonly encountered. At higher magnification, the malignant cells have a wavy appearance with a comma-shaped nuclei, easily identifiable mitotic activity, apoptotic cells, and cellular pleomorphism. One important feature commonly seen in MPNST is the presence of perivascular hyalinization (Figs. 11.59, 11.60, 11.61, 11.62, 11.63, 11.64, 11.65, 11.66, and 11.67). In addition, the tumors may show focal areas of muscle, cartilage, and bone elements.

Important variants of MPNST that have been described include epithelioid [119], pigmented [120–123], malignant Triton tumor [124–127], glandular [128], and tumors with small round cells type and pleomorphic spindle cell sarcomatous areas [129].

Epithelioid PMNST

These tumors are characterized by the presence of a cellular neoplasm composed of large epithelioid, round to oval cells with abundant amounts of cytoplasm, round nuclei, and prominent nucleoli. The tumor may have a subtle nodular appearance and also the presence of focal myxoid areas. Nuclear atypia and mitotic activity are commonly seen (Figs. 11.68, 11.69, and 11.70).

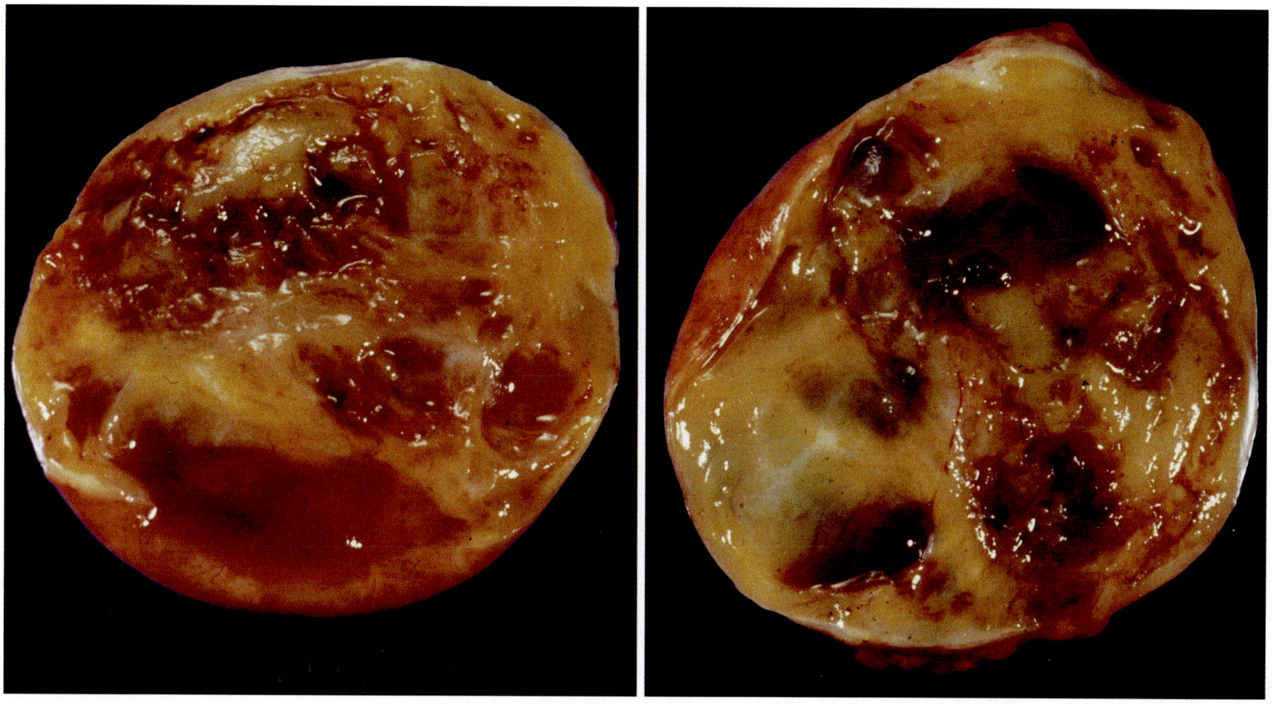

Fig. 11.58 Gross illustration of a MPNST showing a round to oval tumor with focal areas of necrosis and hemorrhage

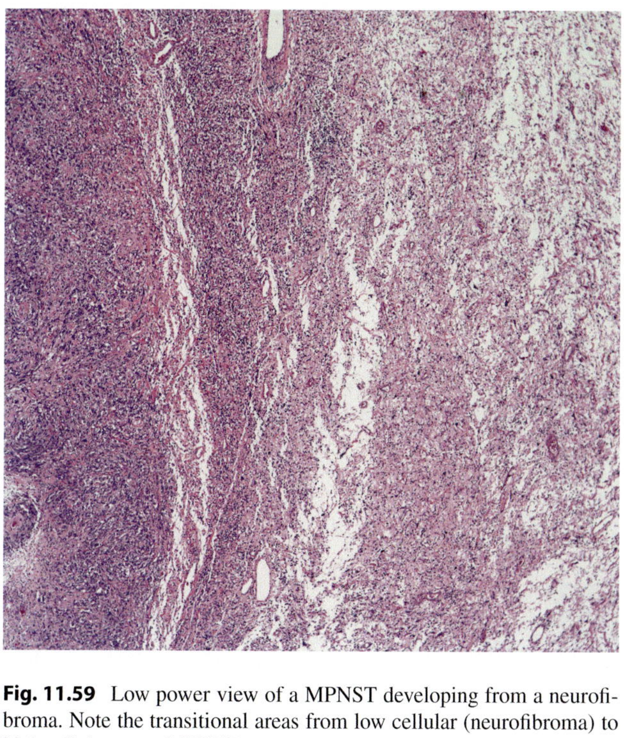

Fig. 11.59 Low power view of a MPNST developing from a neurofibroma. Note the transitional areas from low cellular (neurofibroma) to high cellular areas MPNST

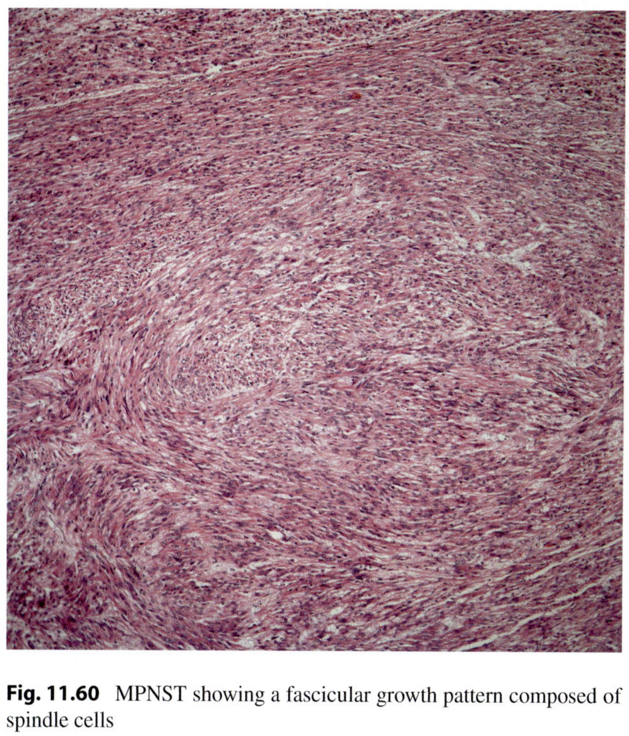

Fig. 11.60 MPNST showing a fascicular growth pattern composed of spindle cells

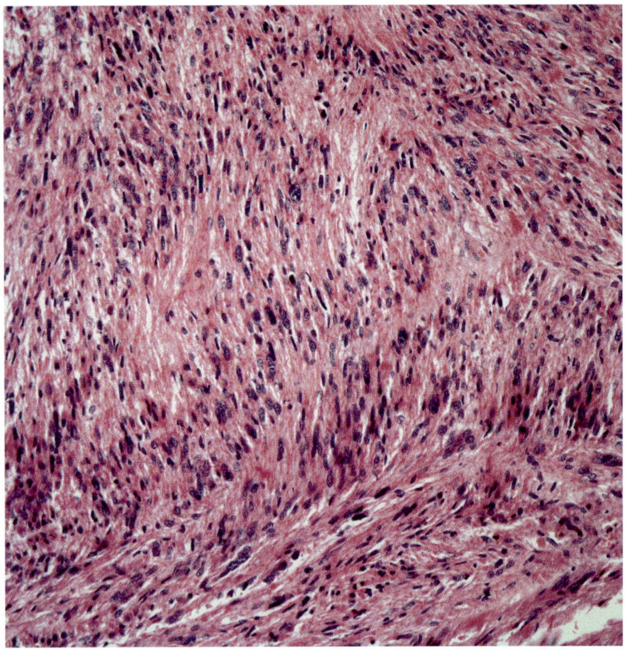

Fig. 11.61 MPNST showing focal and subtle areas in which there is a hint of nuclear palisading

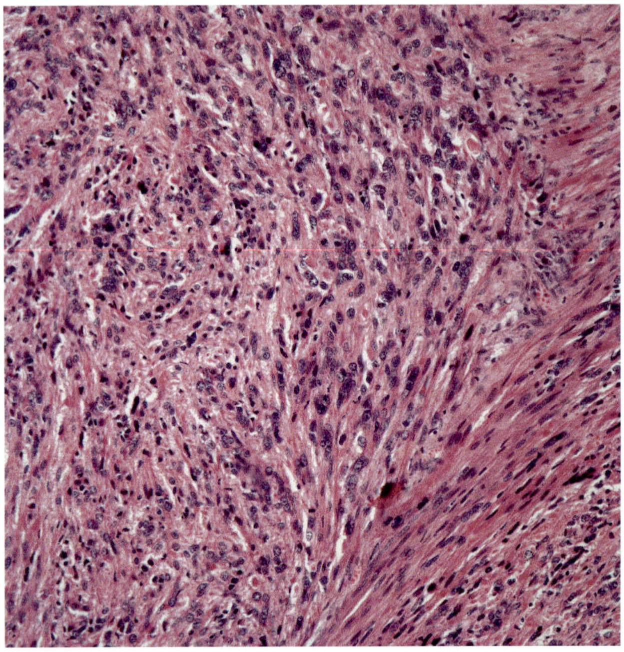

Fig. 11.62 Intermediate magnification of MPNST showing nuclear atypia and apoptotic cells

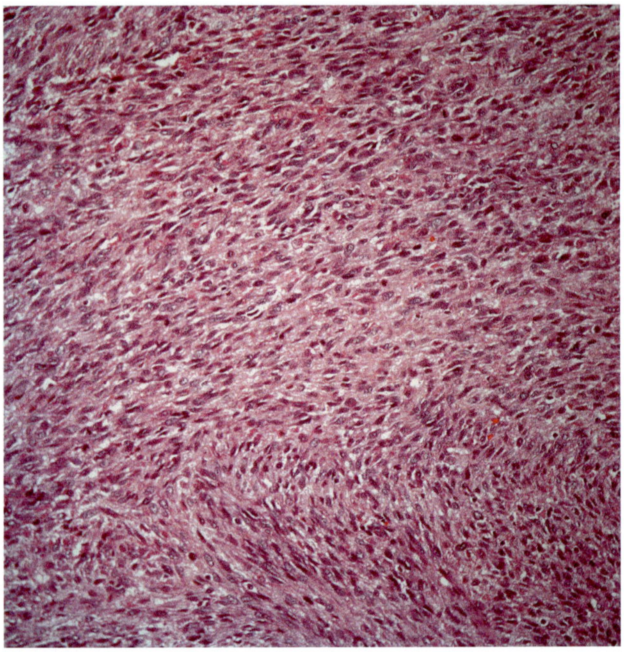

Fig. 11.63 MPNST showing solid areas of atypical spindle cells

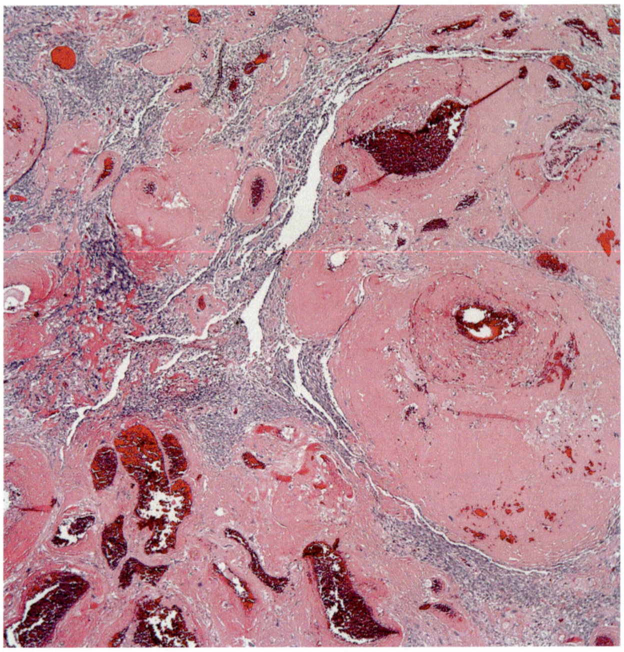

Fig. 11.64 MPNST showing extensive hyalinization of blood vessels

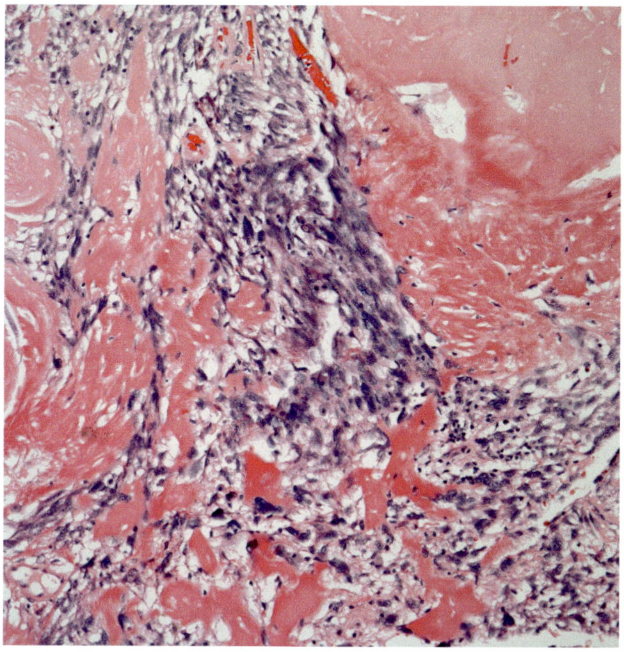

Fig. 11.65 MPNST showing focal areas of extensive hyalinization

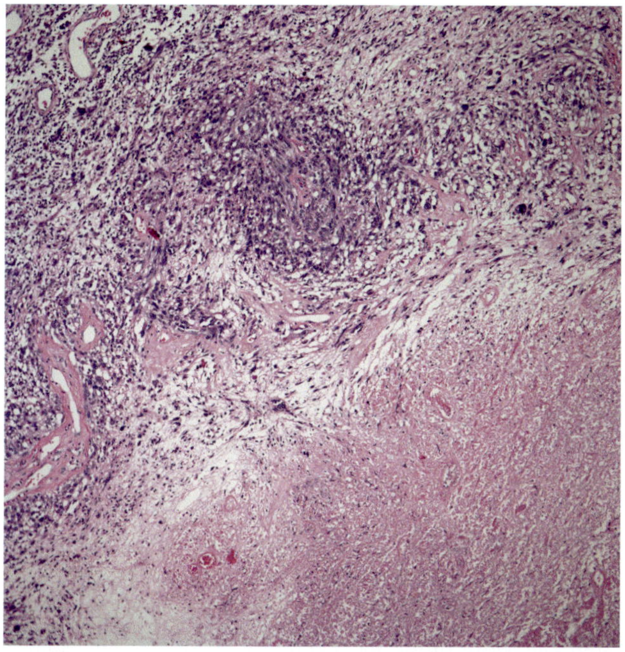

Fig. 11.66 MPNST showing malignant spindle cells and areas of necrosis

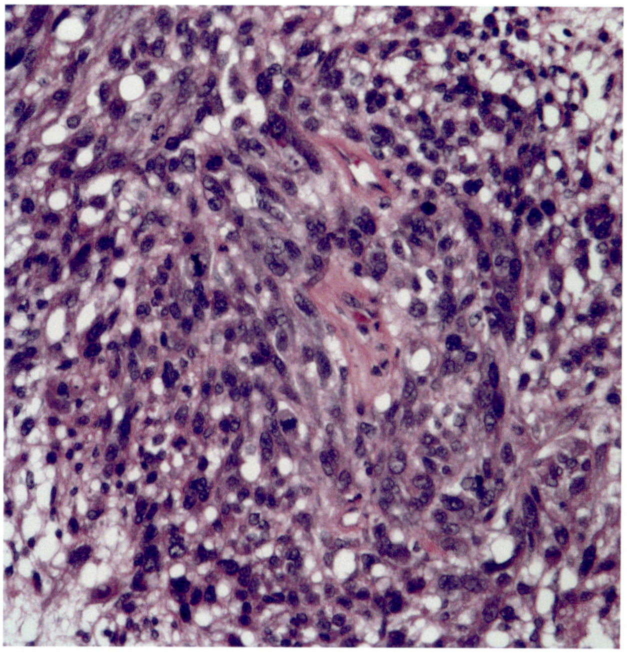

Fig. 11.67 MPNST showing nuclear atypia and increase mitotic activity

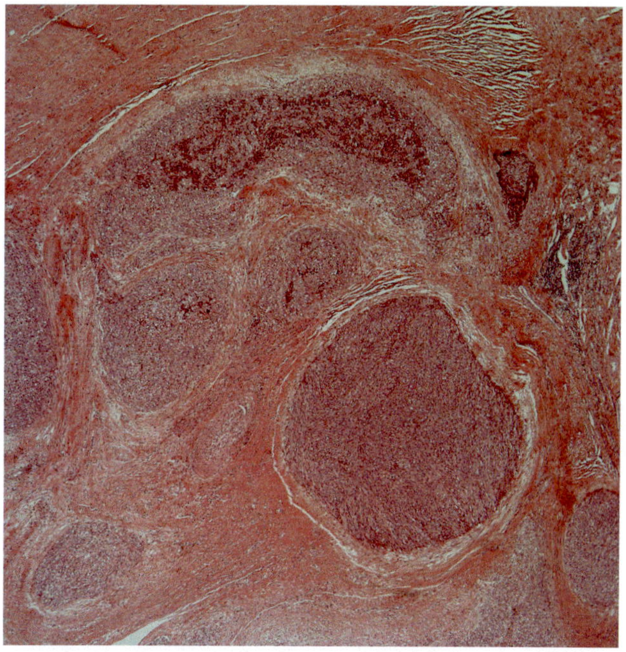

Fig. 11.68 Low power view of an epithelioid MPNST. Note the nodular growth pattern of the tumor

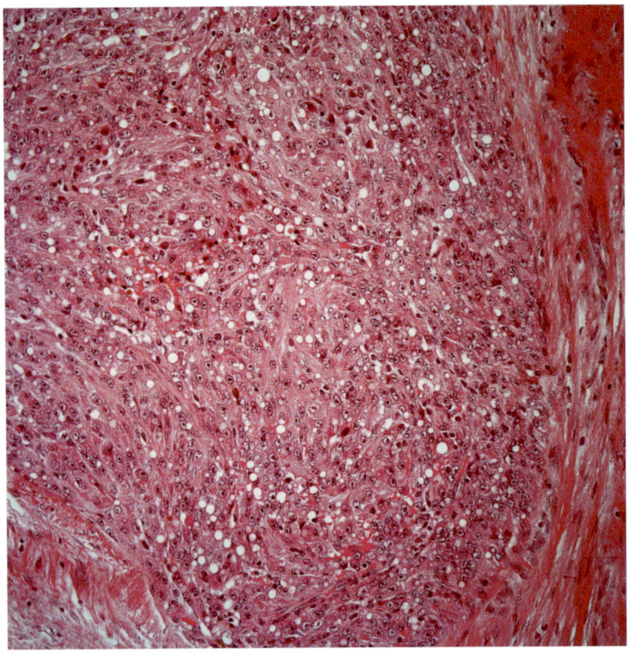

Fig. 11.69 Epithelioid MPNST showing oval cells with prominent nucleoli

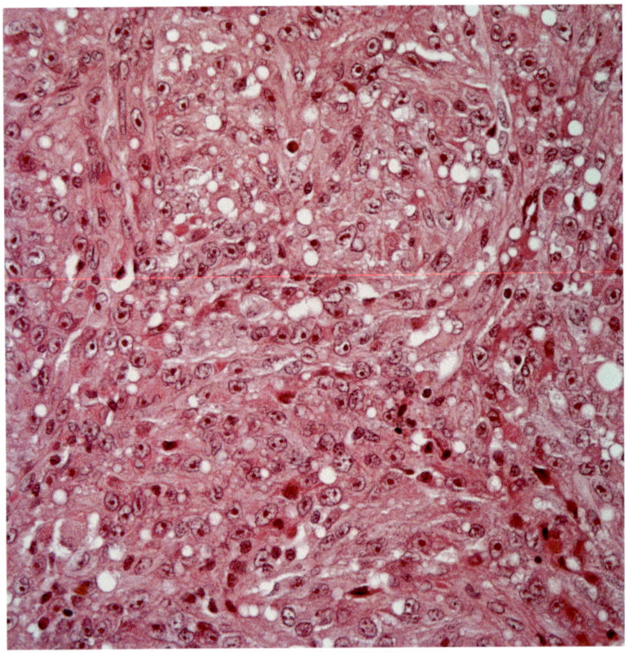

Fig. 11.70 Higher magnification of an epithelioid MPNST showing slightly elongated cells with round to oval nuclei and prominent nucleoli

Pigmented MPNST

The basic histological features are similar to those described with conventional cases or those with epithelioid morphology. However, the tumor is characterized by the presence of melanin pigment, which can be present in subtle form or in easily identifiable dark pigment on low power evaluation of the tumor. In cases in which the tumor shows more subtle pigmented areas, the melanin is present in intracytoplasmic cells that may be in groups or alternating with cells without melanin pigment. However, in some cases, the presence of melanin is extensive, which can easily obscure the true nature of the neoplasm and raise the possibility of malignant melanoma (Figs. 11.71 and 11.72). Tumoral areas containing psammoma bodies may be seen in some tumors. In the reported series of 40 cases by Torres-Mora and colleagues [122], 3 of the 40 cases were in mediastinal location. However, in general, the authors documented local recurrences in 35% of cases and metastases in 44%. In a period spanning from 1 to 300 months, seven patients had died of tumor.

MPNST with Rhabdomyosarcomatous Differentiation: "Malignant Triton Tumor"

The basic histological features of a MPNST are the presence of a solid spindle cell proliferation with areas of focal palisading of the nuclei, cellular and nuclear atypia, mitotic activity, perivascular hyalinization, and areas of necrosis and/or hemorrhage. However, associated with this spindle cell proliferation, one can identify the presence of larger cells with moderate amounts of eosinophilic cytoplasm and nuclei displaced toward the periphery, representing the rhabdomyoblastic differentiation (Figs. 11.73, 11.74, and 11.75). This tumor has been described in the anterior and posterior mediastinum. In addition, malignant Triton tumors with glandular differentiation, although uncommon, can also pose a significant problem in diagnosis. These tumors, in addition to showing the conventional neural and rhabdomyoblastic differentiation, also show the presence of a glandular component, which can be either focal or extensive. The glands are formed by columnar epithelium with well-formed lumen, and these glands can be of different sizes. The glands are haphazardly embedded in the spindle cell component (Figs. 11.76, 11.77, and 11.78).

Glandular MPNST

These tumors are characterized by the presence of haphazard glandular structures composed of low cuboidal to tall columnar cells lining the glandular elements. The glands are of different sizes and shapes and may contain intraluminal mucinous material. These glandular elements are separated by the spindle cell proliferation as described in conventional cases of MPNST. The presence of the glandular component may be focal or more prominent in some cases (Figs. 11.79, 11.80, and 11.81). Contrary to glandular Triton tumor, in this particular growth, the tumor does not show rhabdomyoblastic differentiation. In addition, the glandular component to some extent is histopathologically somewhat different. However, the differentiation of these

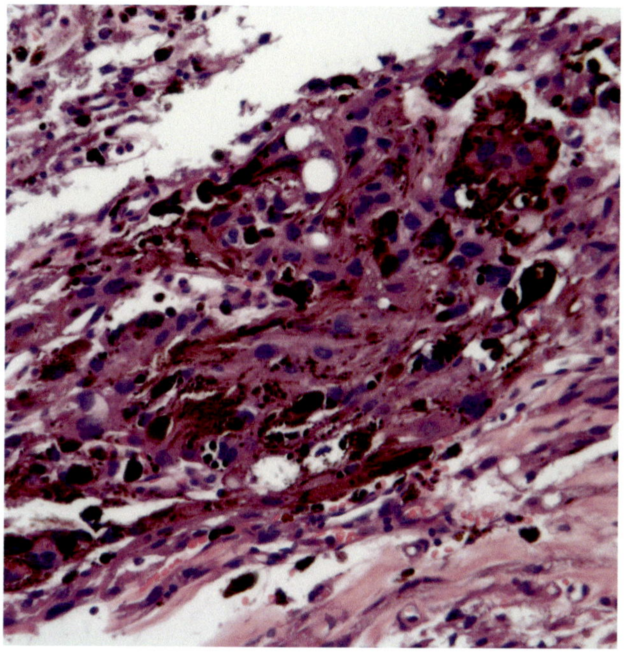

Fig. 11.71 Pigmented MPNST showing extensive areas of melanin pigment. Note the presence of spindle cells admixed with the pigment

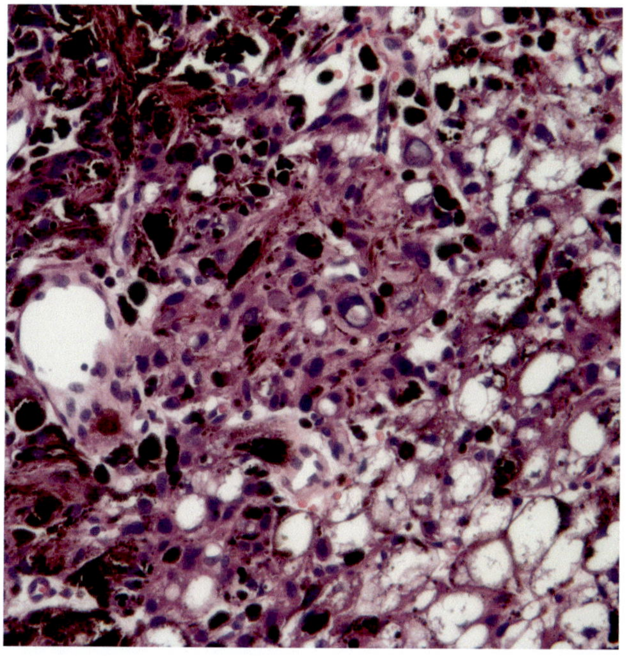

Fig. 11.72 Pigmented MPNST showing malignant cells with nuclear vacuolization and marked nuclear atypia. Note the presence of extensive melanin pigment deposition

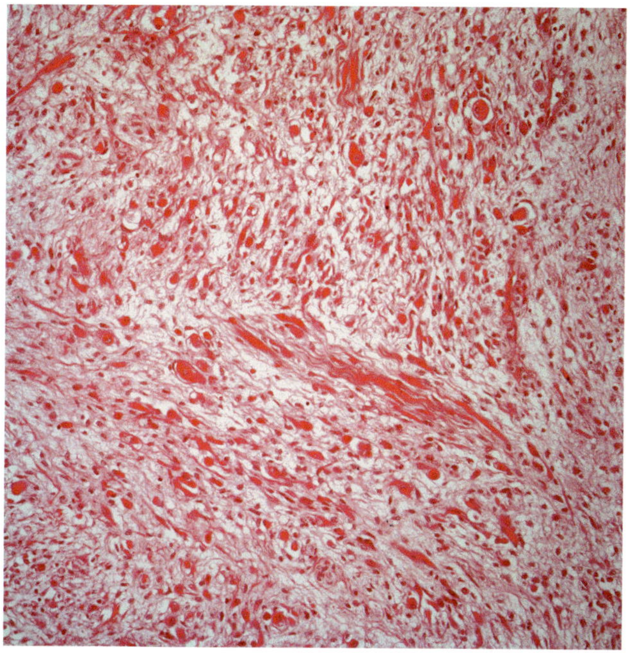

Fig. 11.73 MPNST with areas of rhabdomyoblastic differentiation (Triton Tumor). Note the presence of scattered rhabdomyoblastic cells

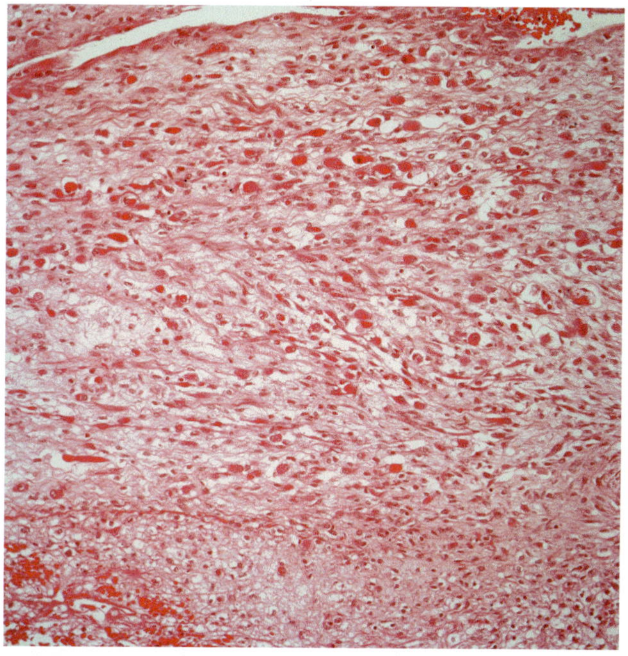

Fig. 11.74 Malignant Triton Tumor showing two distinct populations of cells. The larger cells representing rhabdomyoblasts

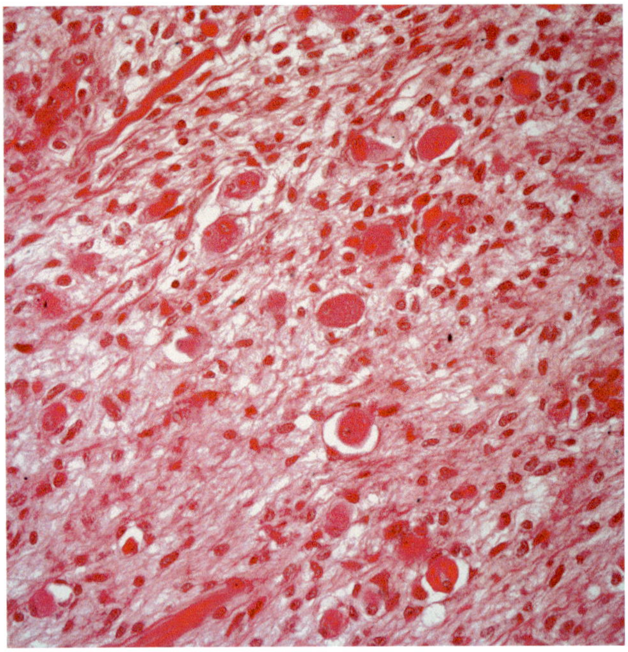

Fig. 11.75 Higher magnification of a Triton tumor showing the presence of rhabdomyoblasts separated by spindle neural component

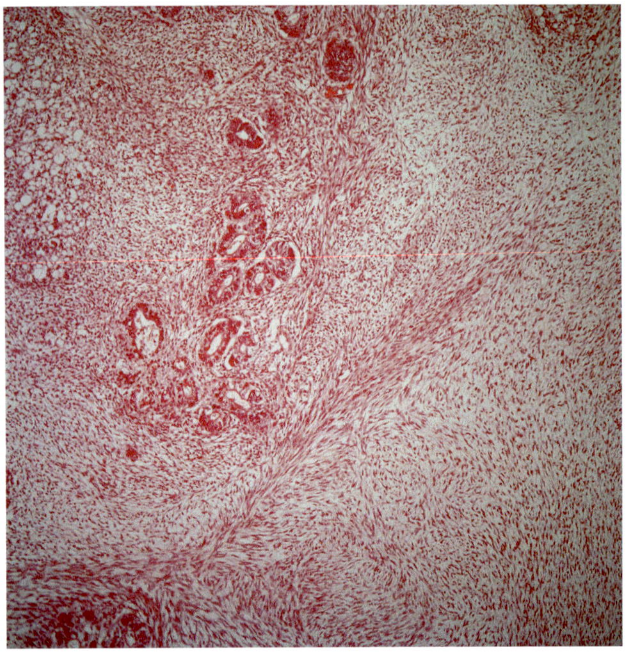

Fig. 11.76 Glandular Triton tumor showing well-defined glandular component embedded in spindle cells

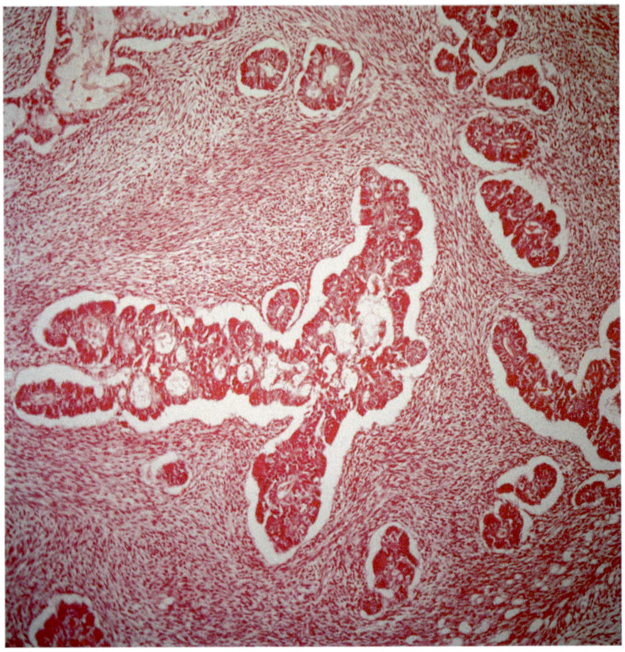

Fig. 11.77 Glandular Triton tumor showing closer view of the glandular component, mimicking adenocarcinomatous component

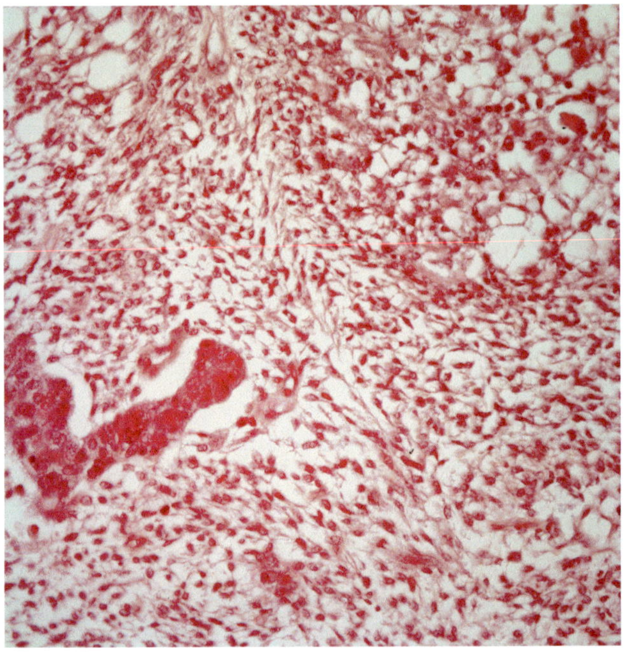

Fig. 11.78 Higher magnification of a glandular Triton tumor showing the three components -glands, neural, and rhabdomyoblastic differentiation

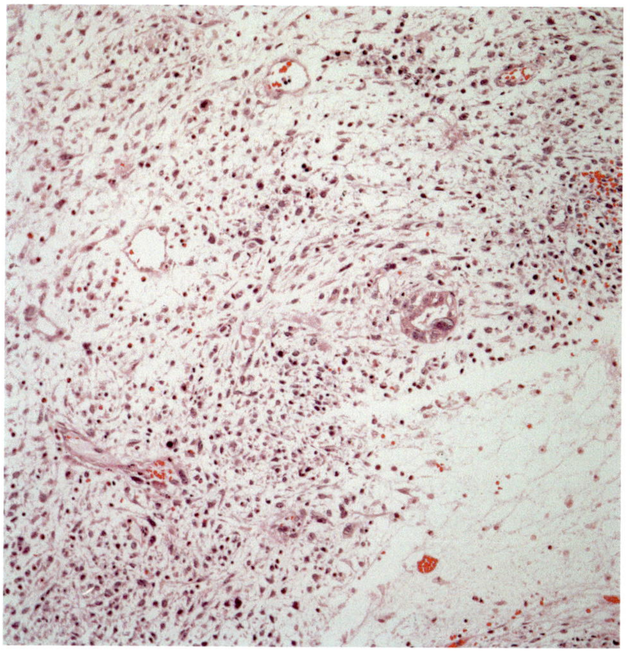

Fig. 11.79 Glandular MPNST showing predominantly neural component with only a focal area of glandular component

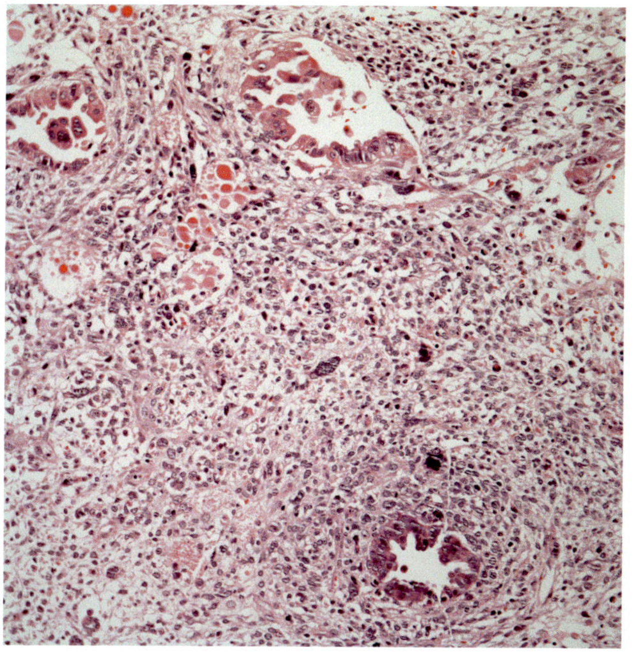

Fig. 11.81 Glandular MPNST showing the glandular component, which is composed of small glands with cylindrical type of epithelium. The neural component shows some epithelioid features

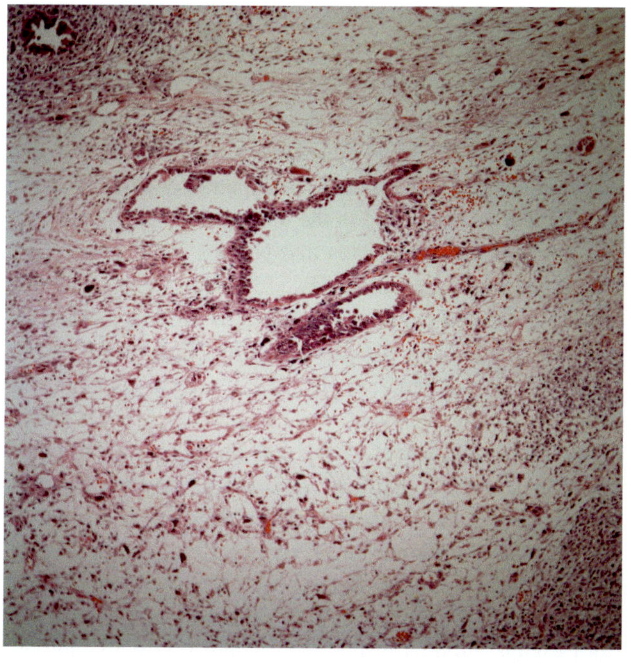

Fig. 11.80 Glandular MPNST in which the glandular component is more obvious

two tumors is based on the presence or absence of rhabdomyoblastic differentiation.

MPNST with Sarcomatous Areas and Small Round Cells

This growth pattern in MPNST is unusual and is characterized by the presence of the basic histological features of MPNST; however, the tumor also shows areas composed of small cells that can be arranged in tubular-like structures, and in some cases with rosette formation. In addition, in some areas the tumor may also show the presence of larger cells with ample cytoplasm and pleomorphic cells.

Immunohistochemical, Ultrastructural, and Molecular Features

The essential work-up of MPNST is done by ruling out other malignant spindle cell tumors that may show similar morphological features. Furthermore, the use of S-100 protein, even though helpful, may show negative results in about 50% of cases. Therefore, the use of other immunohistochemical markers to properly rule out other spindle cell sarcomas is recommended. Other immunostains that may show positive staining and yet are not specific include NSE, vimentin, and neurofilament protein (NFP). The problem may be much more complicated when these tumors show different growth patterns. For instance, in a series of pigmented MPNST, the tumors in addition to S-100 positivity have also shown positive staining for Melan A, HMB45, and tyrosinase [122], which has led some authors to suggest a different name for these tumors: "malignant melanotic schwannian tumors." For tumors with glandular elements, the glandular structures will show positive staining for epithelial markers such as keratin and EMA. Also, in cases with rhabdomyoblastic differentiation, the tumor may show positive staining for MyoD, myoglobin, desmin, and/or caldesmon.

Ultrastructure studies often may show the presence of abundant rER, well-developed Golgi apparatus, microtubules, lysosomes, and cell processes coated with lamina. All these features suggest Schwannian differentiation. At the molecular level, NF1 mutation may be present in some cases, while some other cases may show PTEN overexpression.

Differential Diagnosis

The differential diagnosis of MPNST will include other spindle cell sarcomas of non-neural origin such as leiomyosarcoma, rhabdomyosarcoma, and solitary fibrous tumor. Also important to include is the benign schwannoma in the differential diagnosis. In cases in which the tumor shows extensive pigmented areas, the most difficult differential diagnosis is with malignant melanoma. In cases in which the tumor shows an epithelioid morphology, the most important differential diagnosis is with carcinoma or melanoma, while in cases in which the tumor shows glandular component, the most important differential diagnosis is with carcinosarcoma.

In tumors of non-neural origin such as leiomyosarcoma and rhabdomyosarcoma, the presence of positive staining for desmin, MyoD, myoglobin, and/or caldesmon will lead to the correct interpretation. However, it is also important to know that malignant triton tumor may also show rhabdomyoblastic differentiation. Leiomyosarcomas will unlikely show positive staining for S-100 protein, and the same applies for pure rhabdomyosarcomas. In the setting of epithelioid MPNST, if the consideration is carcinoma, the use of epithelial markers such as keratins and EMA would lead to the correct interpretation. In cases of pigmented MPNST, the interpretation of immunohistochemistry may be much more difficult, as it has been stated that pigmented MPNST may also show positive staining for markers such as Melan A and HMB45. In such cases, the use of electron microscopy may be of aid. Glandular MPNST may be confused with carcinosarcomas; however, by definition, carcinosarcomas should show the presence of malignant epithelial component (squamous cell carcinoma or adenocarcinoma) in addition to the malignant mesenchymal component. Perhaps the most important differential in many cases is with a cellular schwannoma. In this setting, the presence of necrosis and/or hemorrhage and high mitotic activity would lead to a more correct interpretation. Because solitary fibrous tumor is much more common in the thoracic location and because of its stated wide spectrum of growth patterns, this tumor should be very carefully included in the differential diagnosis. In this setting, the use of CD34 and STAT6 would be of great aid in ruling in or out such a possibility.

In essence, the diagnosis of MPNST may be facilitated using good clinical information such as the clinical diagnosis of von Recklinghausen's disease, a reasonable biopsy, the use of a wide panel of immunohistochemical stains, and the use if necessary of ultrastructural studies. The global interpretation of these findings would be of great help in arriving at a proper diagnosis.

Peripheral Neuroectodermal Tumor (PNET)/ Extraskeletal Ewing Sarcoma

For consistency, the term PNET will be used in this section to refer to this entire category, of course noting that often both of these tumors are considered in the same spectrum. However, throughout history, many other names have been used to describe this particular tumor including neuroepithelioma, small round cells tumor of thoracopulmonary region, Askin Tumor, and malignant small round cell tumor.

It is very likely that the existence of these peripheral neuroectodermal tumors had been recognized more than a century ago. However, the specific designation of PNET had not been properly recognized in the literature [130]. However, it was not until the mid-1970s that Nesbitt and Vidone [131] and Seemayer and colleagues [132] documented similar tumors as the one described by Stout in 1918 in the peripheral soft tissues. The case described by Nesbitt and Vidone [131] was in a 6-year-old boy with a sciatic nerve tumor, which the authors designated as "primitive neuroectodermal tumor (Neuroblastoma)." The authors acknowledged that few similar tumors had been reported in the literature and considered that these tumors are best classified as "primitive neuroectodermal neoplasms." Also in 1975, Angervall and Enzinger [133] reported 39 cases of a "small, round, or oval cell sarcoma" of soft tissue, histologically indistinguishable from Ewing sarcoma of the bone. Interestingly, the authors stated "it is impossible to prove or disprove whether the tumors described as Ewing's sarcoma share similar histogenesis."

Despite the fact that the existence of these tumors in the soft tissue was becoming more evident, the occurrence of these tumors in the thoracic cavity had not been properly determined, even though early publications alluding to the occurrence of similar tumors in the paravertebral region had been mentioned. Tefft and colleagues [134] described the radiographic features of five children with what the authors described as "unusual histologic characteristics" and designated these tumors as "paravertebral round cell tumors." However, it was not until Askin in 1979 [135] reported 20 cases in children and adolescents of a malignant tumor that the authors coined as "malignant small cell tumor of the thoracopulmonary region," which subsequently also became known as "Askin tumor." The tumors described were more common in female patients, and the tumor originated from the soft tissues of the chest wall or the peripheral lung. The median survival in these patients was 8 months. Interestingly, ultrastructural studies performed in some of these cases suggested a "neuroepithelial derivation"; however, the authors concluded that the histogenesis remained uncertain. Perhaps more important to mention is that in 1979, the basis to separate Ewing sarcoma from this new entity – "small round cell tumor of the thoracopulmonary region"– was the presence of PAS positive material in the tumor cells (negative in all the cases reported by Askin). In 1989, Marina and colleagues [136] reported 26 cases of what the authors called "peripheral primitive neuroectodermal tumor (peripheral neuroepithelioma) in children." Of these 26 cases, 6 were located in the chest wall, similar to those described by Askin [135]; the remaining cases were in different soft tissue locations. All the patients were children and young adolescents, and, after a median follow-up of 109 months, 9 of the 26 reported patients were alive. Interestingly, in a report of ten of these tumors, Llombart-Bosch and colleagues [137] described a mean age of 32.6 of the patients reported, with a male predominance. In a different report of 54 patients, Kushner and coworkers [138] described patients ranging in ages from 1 to 81 years, with a median of 17 years; of the 54 cases described, 25 were in the thoracopulmonary region while the remaining were in different soft tissue locations. The authors also stated that radiation therapy induced tumor shrinking but was not curative. The progression-free survival in 43 patients with localized tumor was 25% at 24 months, while patients with localized tumor who had complete surgical resection within 3 months of diagnosis had significant longer progression-free survival. The authors also concluded that the possible way to treat these patients is with complete surgical resection, radiation therapy, and chemotherapy.

In general, the occurrence of PNET in the lung or mediastinum is rather rare [139–143]. In the mediastinal compartment, all the tumors described have been in adults and in either anterior or posterior mediastinal location. The patients have presented with diverse clinical findings including superior vena cava compression. Even though one can only assume that the clinical course in the mediastinal location is similar to that described in other locations, due to the limited number of cases described in the literature, it is impossible to come to meaningful conclusions about PNET in the mediastinal compartment.

Pathological Features

Macroscopically, the tumors in the anterior or posterior mediastinal compartment may reach a size of over 10 cm in greatest dimension. The tumors are ill-defined and may involve adjacent structures. The tumors are light tan in color with areas of hemorrhage and/or necrosis.

Histologically, the tumors are characterized by a uniform cellular proliferation composed of small, round to oval cells, with small round nuclei and inconspicuous nucleoli. The neoplastic cells contain scant eosinophilic cytoplasm. Even though the tumors may show different growth patterns, usually the neoplastic cellular proliferation may be arranged in sheets or cords of neoplastic cells. The presence of pseudorosettes or rosettes of the Homer-Wright type may be seen in these tumors, but their presence is not always found. Mitotic activity is variable in these tumors and may be increased in some tumors, while in others it appears more subdued. Areas of necrosis and/or hemorrhage are easily identified in these tumors, and their presence is also variable and depends on the type of material available for evaluation (Figs. 11.82, 11.83, 11.84, 11.85, 11.86, and 11.87).

Histochemical, Immunohistochemical, Ultrastructural, and Molecular Features

At the initial publication of these tumors in the thoracopulmonary region, Askin and coworkers [135] discussed extensively the absence of PAS material in these tumors and used such feature to separate PNET from Ewing sarcoma. However, focal positive reaction for PAS may be seen in some cases. Other histochemical stains including mucicarmine are generally negative. The use of immunohistochemical stains, although important, may also have some limitations; even though the tumor appears to commonly express CD99 and focally synaptophysin, chromogranin, and CD56, these immunohistochemical stains may also show positive staining in other tumors that are not related to PNET, and that may mimic its morphology. Other immunostains that have shown positive staining include S-100 protein, NSE, and HNK-1. On the other hand, the tumor is commonly negative for muscle and epithelial markers as well as other markers including HMB-45, MelanA, and Sox-10. Ultrastructurally, PNET may show the presence of interdigitating processes, primitive intercellular attachments, and membrane bound granules. However, in current practice, the use of molecular analysis may prove to aid further in the diagnosis. Ambros and coworkers in 1991 [144] reported what the authors considered the specific expression of MIC2 gene in Ewing sarcoma and PNET as evidence for a common histogenesis for both tumors. In addition, Selleri

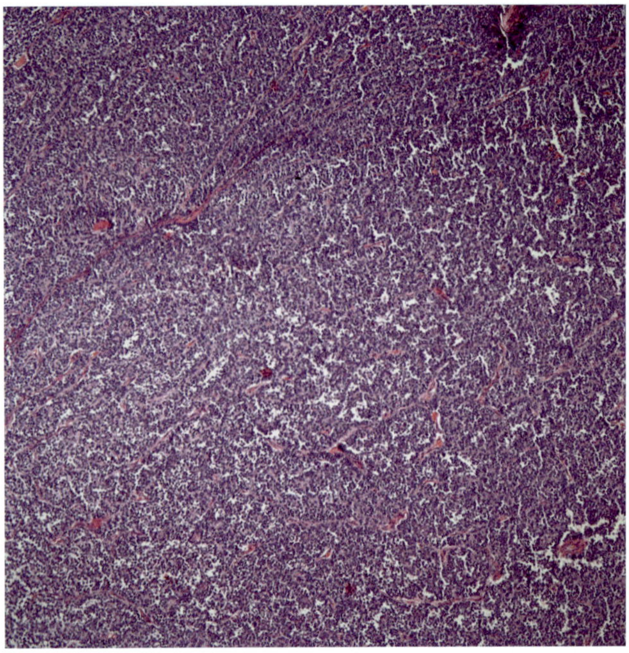

Fig. 11.82 Low power view of a PNET showing a solid neoplastic cellular proliferation

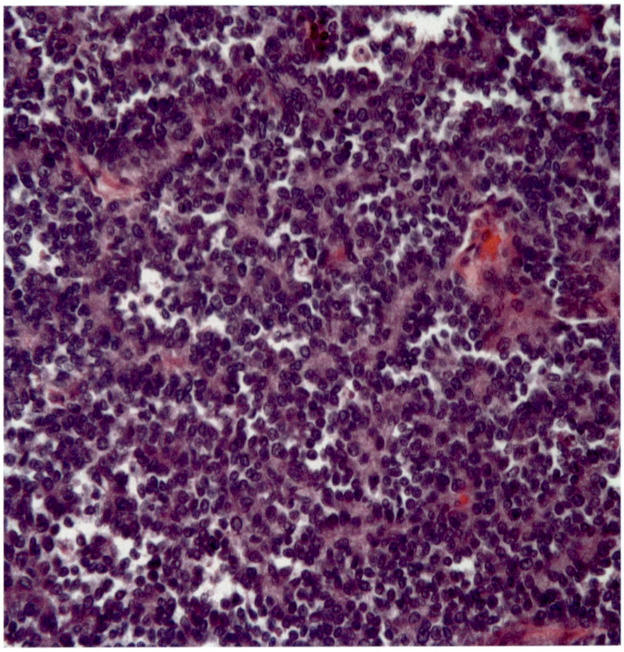

Fig. 11.84 Higher magnification of a PNET showing pseudorosettes. The tumor is composed of small cells with round to val nuclei and inconspicuous nucleoli. No mitotic activity is present

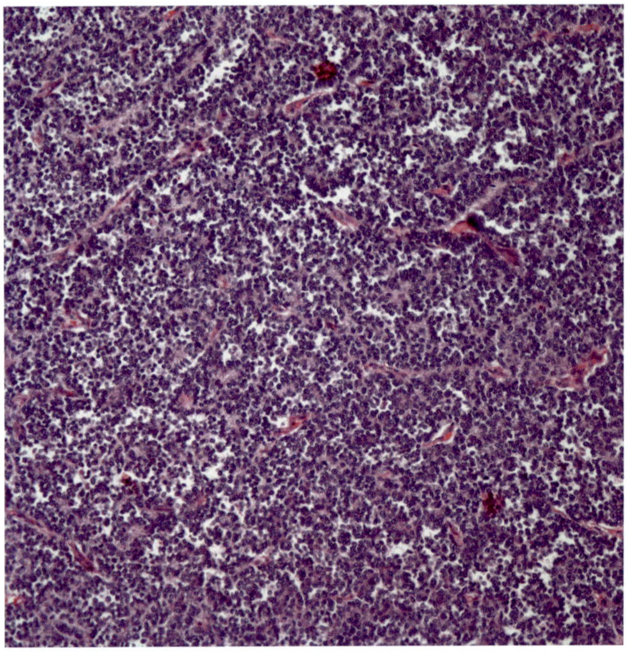

Fig. 11.83 PNET showing numerous pseudorosettes. Note the fairly homogeneous cellular proliferation

and coworkers [145] analyzed the molecular localization of the t(11;22)(q24;q12) translocation, which essentially occurs in Ewing sarcoma and PNET. Turc-Carel and coworkers [146] encountered similar findings in a study of 85 cases in which the authors identified similar translocation in Ewing sarcoma.

Differential Diagnosis

The differential diagnosis of PNET in the mediastinal compartment will include not only tumors within the ranged of "small round cells neoplasms" but also other tumors that potentially mimic PNET in the mediastinum. By far, since these tumors occur predominantly in young patients, the consideration of rhabdomyosarcoma and neuroblastoma is highly important. In cases of rhabdomyosarcoma, the use of muscle markers will lead to a correct interpretation as PNET invariably show negative staining for those antibodies. In cases of neuroblastoma, mainly in the poorly differentiated tumors in which there is absence of neutrophil, the diagnosis can be much more difficult, as neuroblastomas may also show positive staining for CD99. However, in this setting in the difficult cases, the molecular analysis and the identification of the common translocation will lead to a correct interpretation. One important consideration will include a tumor that may occur in the pleural region and that may pose a significant challenge – desmoplastic small round cell tumor (DSRCT). This latter neoplastic process also occurs in young patients and may present as a thoracic bulky mass. In addition, the tumor may also show similar immunohistochemical profile as PNET. However, it is important to mention that DSRCT may show positive staining for desmin, keratin, EMA, and WT1, while about 20% of the cases show positive staining for CD99. Molecular analysis of DSRCT shows that site on chromosome 11 is WT1, while for Ewing sarcoma it is FLI1 gene, thus the translocation for Ewing sarcoma t(11;22)(q24;q12) and that of DSRCT t(11;12)(q13;q12)

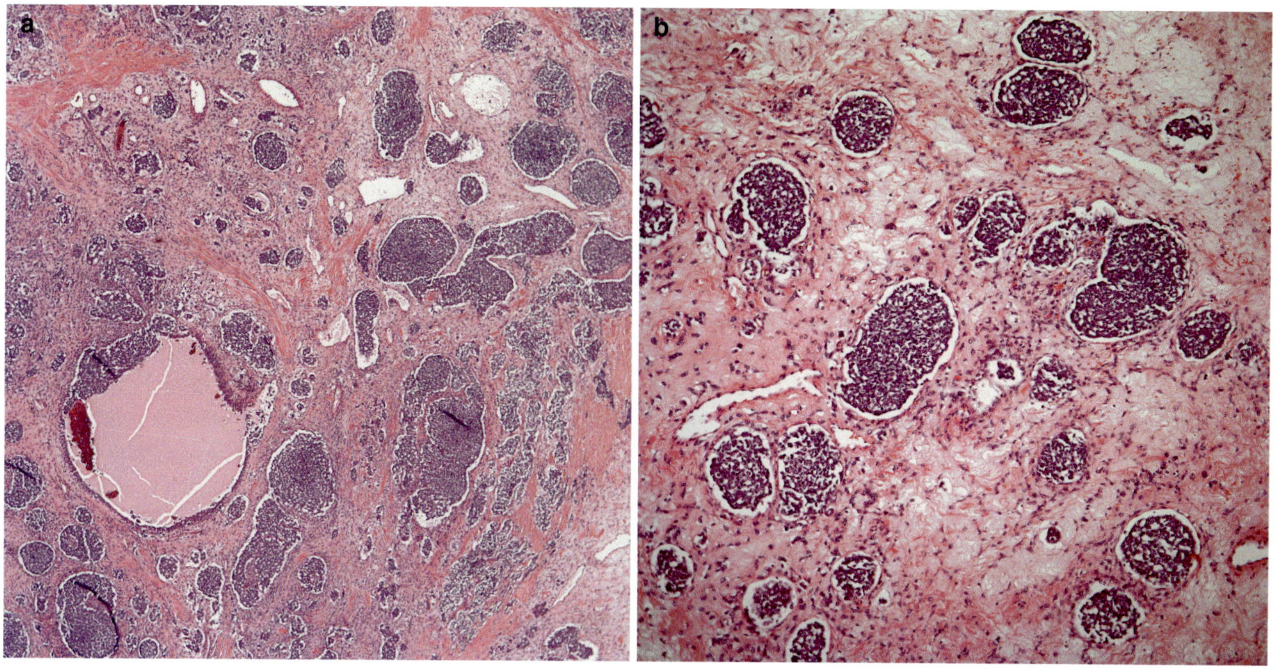

Fig. 11.85 (**a**) PNET showing a pseudo-alveolar growth pattern composed of nests of tumor cells. (**b**) Higher magnification showing lymphatic permeation by tumor and in other areas retraction of the fibroconnective tissue

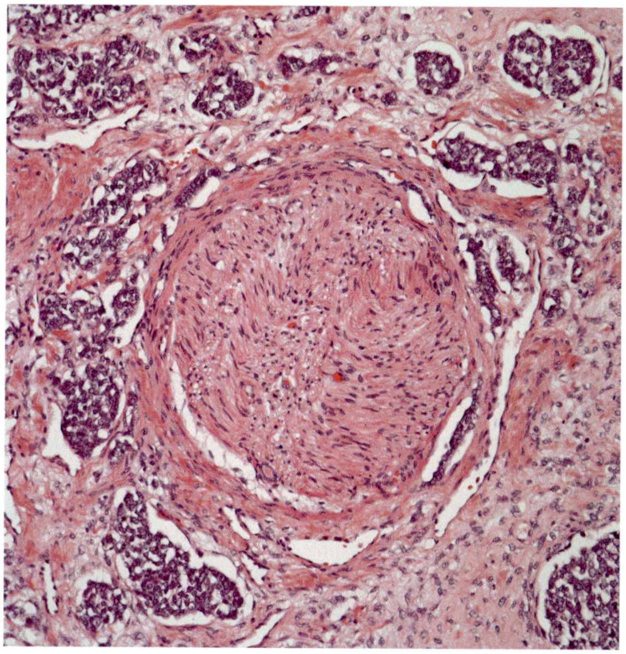

Fig. 11.86 PNET showing perineural invasion

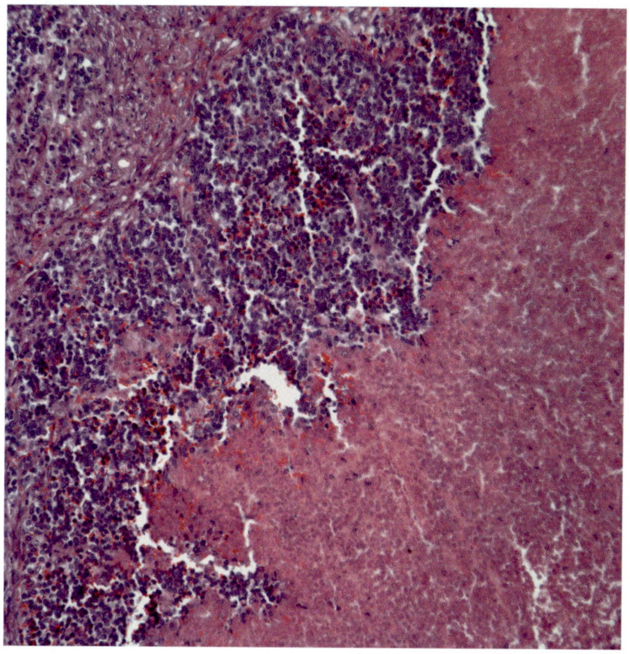

Fig. 11.87 PNET showing extensive necrosis

[147]. Even though this tumor in large resections may show histopathological features, which may aid in the diagnosis such as the presence of extensive desmoplasia, the challenge in small biopsies cannot be overemphasized.

Pigmented Neuroectodermal Tumor of Infancy (Melanotic Progonoma, Retinal Anlage Tumor)

This tumor is a very rare occurrence in the mediastinal region [148]. The tumor is commonly observed in infants during the first year of life and anatomically affects more often the head and neck area with preference for the maxillary region [149]. However, the tumor has been reported in numerous other locations. The only case that has been published of this particular tumor in the mediastinal region is credited to Misugi and coworkers [148], who, in 1965, described a 7-month-old child with a posterior mediastinal mass. The child underwent a right posterolateral thoracotomy with initial partial resection of a tumor that extended from the right costovertebral sulcus to the left, across the thoracic spine, posterior to the aorta and from the level of D4 to the esophageal hiatus. The tumor was described as compressing the trachea and right stem bronchus, displacing the heart anteriorly, and the esophagus to the left. Due to the initial unresectability of the tumor, the child received radiation therapy with subsequent further thoracotomy, and the authors provided a follow-up of 6 months in which the child remained alive. Even though in general terms, this tumor is considered benign, the tumor can be aggressive, and in a small proportion of patients, it may metastasize. However, it is difficult to determine whether these tumors in the mediastinal location will follow an indolent or aggressive clinical behavior. It is possible that the initial treatment of these tumors in the mediastinum should have the goal of complete surgical resection whenever possible. Important to highlight is that due to the infrequent occurrence of these tumors in the mediastinum, a more precise clinical behavior is not possible.

Pathological Features

In the report by Misugi [148], even though the mass was initially incompletely resected, the resected tumor mass measured 7 cm in greatest dimension and weighed 65 grs; the tumor was slightly lobulated, grayish-black, and solid.

Histologically, the tumor shows similar features as those tumors in the more conventional location, namely, the presence of extensive areas of fibrous tissue with a neoplastic cellular proliferation composed of cuboidal cells, while in other areas, the tumors cells appear more undifferentiated. The neoplastic cells may be arranged in small clusters, while in other areas, the tumor cells appear to be forming small glandular structures with a subtle alveolar growth pattern. In addition, one of the most important features is the occurrence of pigmented cells, which can be seen in the glandular-like areas in the cluster of neoplastic cells. The cells appear to be rather small, with round nuclei, and inconspicuous nucleoli (Figs. 11.88, 11.89, 11.90, 11.91, and 11.92). Mitotic activity is not high, but, in some cases, mitotic activity can be easily identified. Areas of necrosis and hemorrhage are usually not common.

Immunohistochemical, Ultrastructural, and Molecular Features

The use of immunohistochemical stains plays an important role in the diagnosis of these tumors, as these tumors may also show some features that may be seen in other small round cell neoplasms. However, in general terms, as the name (retinal anlage tumor) implies, this particular neoplasm shows similar immunohistochemical phenotype as the normal retina, namely, the presence of positive staining for keratin as well as for S-100 protein. In general, the tumor does not show positive staining for muscle marker, mainly desmin, Myo D, Myoglobin, smooth muscle actin, or caldesmon. The ultrastructural findings in the case described by Misugi and coworkers [148] showed two different types of pigmented cells: (1) large spindle cells with abundant cytoplasm, well-developed granular endoplasmic reticulum, and prominent Golgi complex; and (2) small cells filled with numerous pigment granules of varying electron density. More recently, Barnes and coworkers [150] reported a case in which by molecular means, the authors identified that the tumor showed a germline mutation of CDKN2A and a novel RPL1-C19MC fusion.

Differential Diagnosis

By far the most important differential diagnosis will be with other small round cell tumors of infancy. The histopathological features of retinal anlage tumors may be confused with rhabdomyosarcomas, and, in this setting, the use of immunohistochemical stains for muscle markers, including desmin, myoglobin, MyoD, and caldesmon, would lead to the correct interpretation. One other important differential diagnosis would be with neuroblastoma, as the tumor also occurs in infants and young children. In this setting, the positive staining using keratin and S-100 protein will lead to the interpretation of retinal anlage tumor. Even though the age group for the occurrence of melanoma is highly unusual, the histology of the tumor – mainly the presence of pigment – may mimic melanoma. One other tumor to consider, even though it would be unusual in young children, is the desmoplastic small round cell tumor. This latter tumor not only may show a small round cell tumor but also will show extensive areas of hyalinization and fibrous tissue, somewhat similar to that display of the retinal anlage tumor. However, even though desmoplastic small round cell tumor may show in some cases positive staining for S-100 protein, it may also show positive staining for desmin and negative staining for keratin.

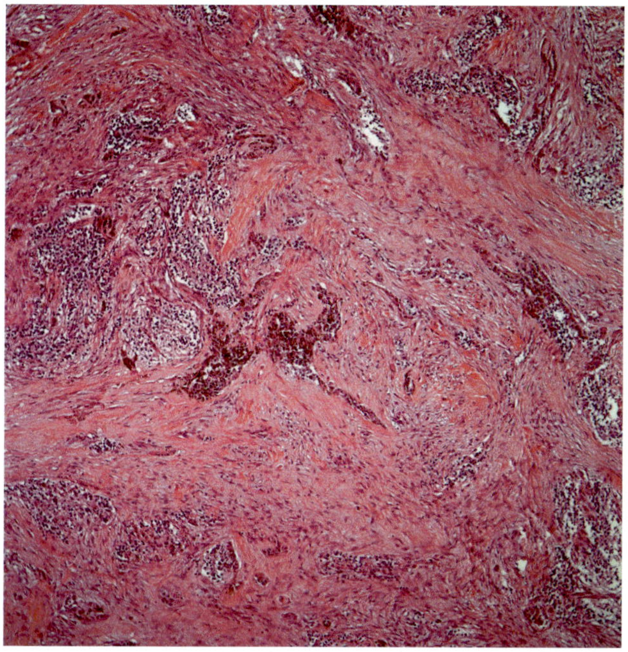

Fig. 11.88 Retinal anlage tumor showing extensive areas of fibrosis. Note the presence of a small tumor cells admixed with focal areas of pigmented cells

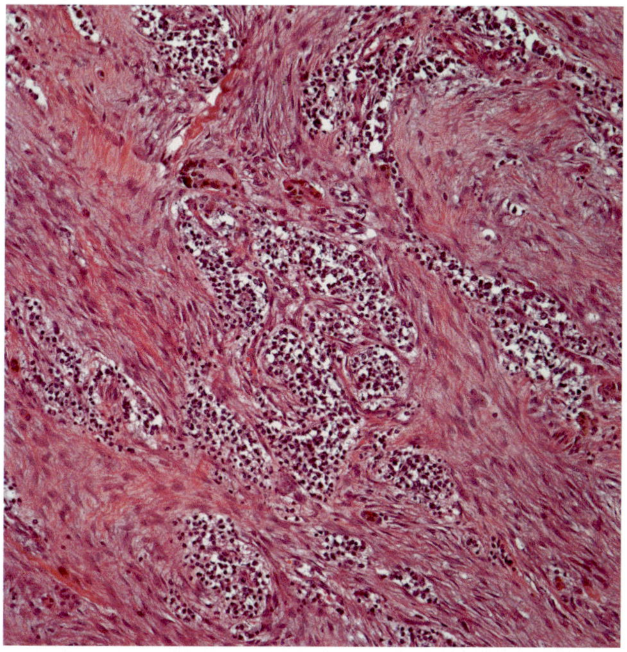

Fig. 11.89 In some areas the presence of pigmented cells in retinal anlage tumor may be focal

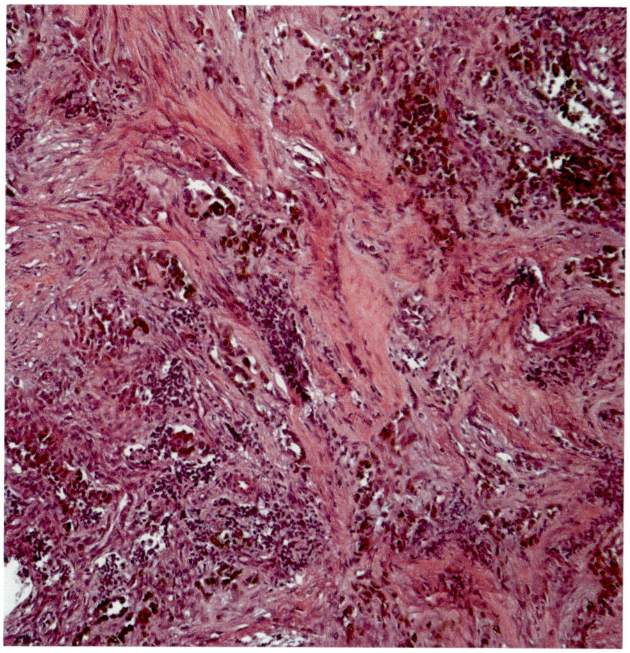

Fig. 11.90 Retinal anlage tumor showing areas of obvious pigmented cells

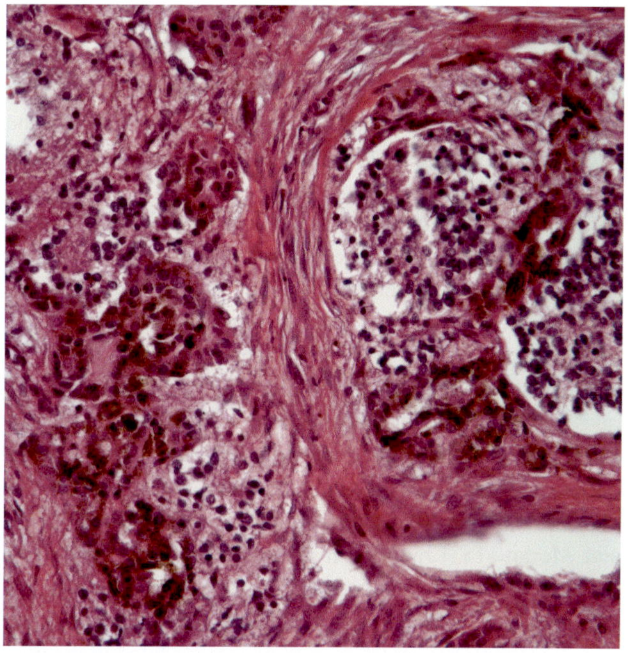

Fig. 11.91 Dual cellular proliferation – one composed of small cells with no pigment while others are arranged in a glandular appearance with cuboidal cells and melanin pigment

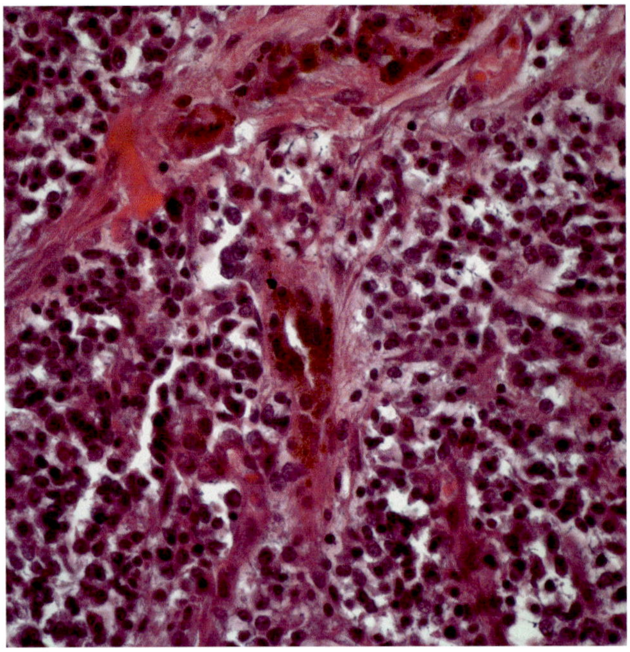

Fig. 11.92 High power view of a retinal anlage tumor showing small pigmented glands admixed with a cellular proliferation composed of small cells. Mitotic activity is not present

Ependymoma

The occurrence of these tumors in the mediastinal region is rare, but it has been well documented in the literature [151–153]. It is possible that Doglioni and coworkers [152] are the ones who first reported a primary ependymoma occurring in the mediastinal region. The authors reported a 51-year-old asymptomatic woman with a posterior mediastinal tumor. Thoracotomy was performed, and the tumor did not show any connection with nerve trunks. The patient died 4 months after surgical resection due to complications. The case described by Nobles and coworkers [151] was that of a 35-year-old woman who presented with chest pain, diaphoresis, and lightheadedness. The tumor was located in the posterior mediastinum with no continuity with the spinal canal. Surgical resection of the tumor was performed. The authors did not document specific follow-up for this patient. Wilson and Moran [153] reported three additional cases; the three patients were women between 36 and 71 years of age (mean age, 50 years). Clinically, the patients presented with non-specific symptoms, and their tumors were located in the posterior mediastinum without any connection to the spinal canal. Surgical resection took place in all these patients. Interestingly, in one of the cases reported, lymph node metastasis was documented; however, after a follow-up (mean, 64 months), none of the patients had recurrence of disease or metastasis.

Based on the reported cases, it appears that these tumors have a predilection for the posterior mediastinum, in middle-aged women who may present with non-specific symptoms or asymptomatic. In addition, it appears that complete surgical resection is the best alternative for long-term survival despite the presence in some cases of lymph node metastasis.

Pathologic Features

Macroscopically, the tumors appear to range in size from 5 to 9 cm in greatest diameter. The tumors have been described as tan in color, solid but some have shown cystic changes. Areas of necrosis and/or hemorrhage may be seen.

Histologically, the tumors are characterized by the presence of a solid, uniform cellular proliferation with mild to moderate atypia. The neoplastic cells are round to oval with round nuclei and inconspicuous nucleoli, and stipple to vesicular chromatin. The cells may be arranged in inter-anastomosing ependymal tubules, presence of pseudorosettes, with true ependymal rosettes and canals with ciliated cells. In some areas, the tumor may show a pseudopapillary configuration with occasional psammoma bodies. Mitotic activity is variable and may range from one to five mitotic figures per high-power field. Areas of necrosis and/or hemorrhage may also be variable from focal to extensive (Figs. 11.93, 11.94, 11.95, 11.96, 11.97, 11.98, 11.99, 11.100, 11.101, and 11.102).

Immunohistochemical and Ultrastructural Features

Mediastinal ependymomas, like their counterpart in the central nervous system, will show similar immunophenotype. The tumors are positive for glial fibrillary acid protein (GFAP) while negative for S-100 protein, chromogranin, synaptophysin, and HMB-45. Some tumors may show focal weakly positive stain for keratin. Ultrastructurally, in the cases described by Wilson [153], the tumors showed the presence of multipart junctional complexes, intracytoplasmic lumina containing microvilli, and occasional apical cilia. Ciliary basal bodies were also present, while no neurosecretory granules or premelanosomes were identified.

Differential Diagnosis

The most important differential diagnosis is with metastatic ependymoma; however, in this setting a proper clinical history should lead to the correct interpretation. Once that is clear, the tumor may be confused with schwannoma, neuroendocrine carcinoma, or melanoma. In these cases, the use of immunohistochemical stains will be of aid as none of those tumors will show positive staining for GFAP, while some of these tumors will show positive staining for S-100 protein, epithelial, and/or neuroendocrine markers.

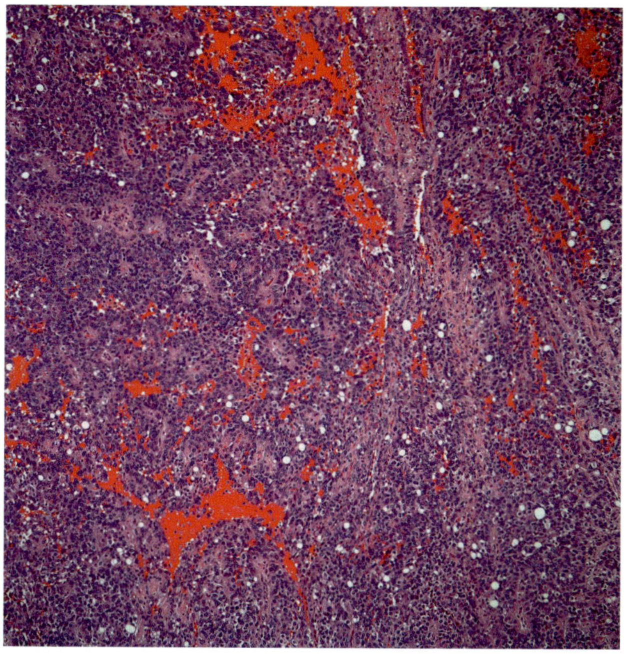

Fig. 11.93 Low power view of a mediastinal ependymoma showing a rather solid cellular proliferation with rosette formation

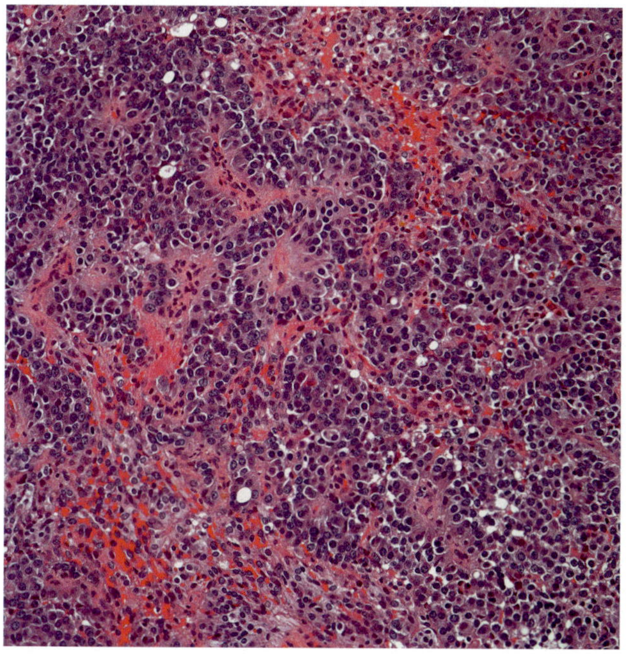

Fig. 11.94 Mediastinal ependymoma showing rosettes and pseudorosettes

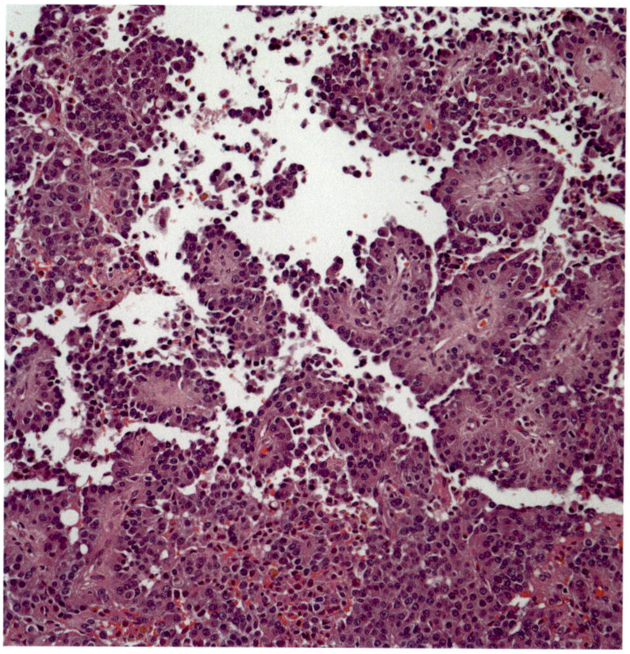

Fig. 11.95 Mediastinal ependymoma with prominent rosette formation giving the appearance of a papillary neoplasm

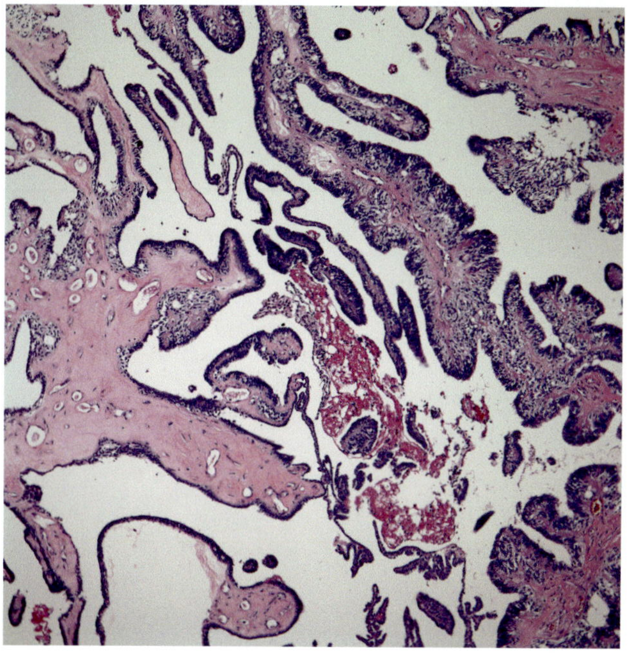

Fig. 11.96 Ependymoma with prominent papillary growth pattern

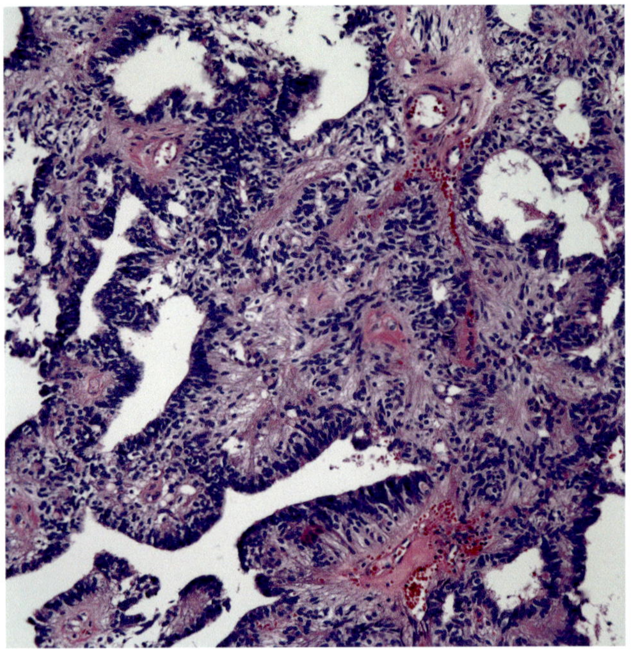

Fig. 11.97 Ependymoma with solid and papillary features

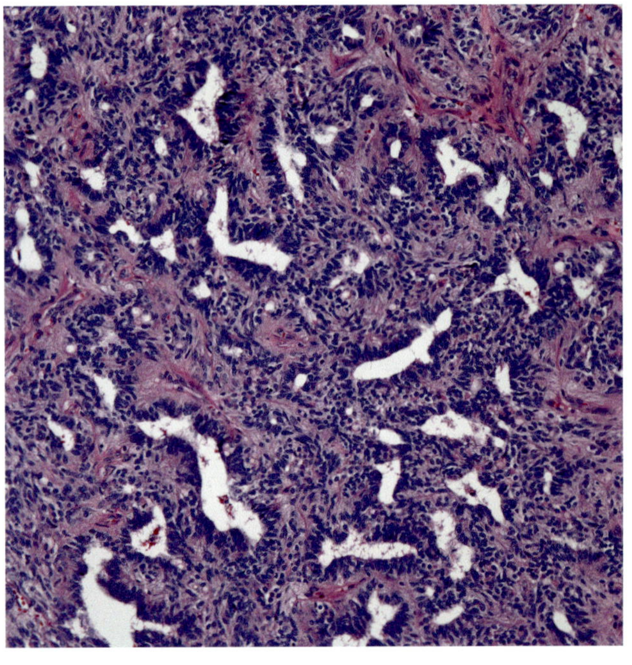

Fig. 11.98 Ependymoma with pseudo-glandular formation

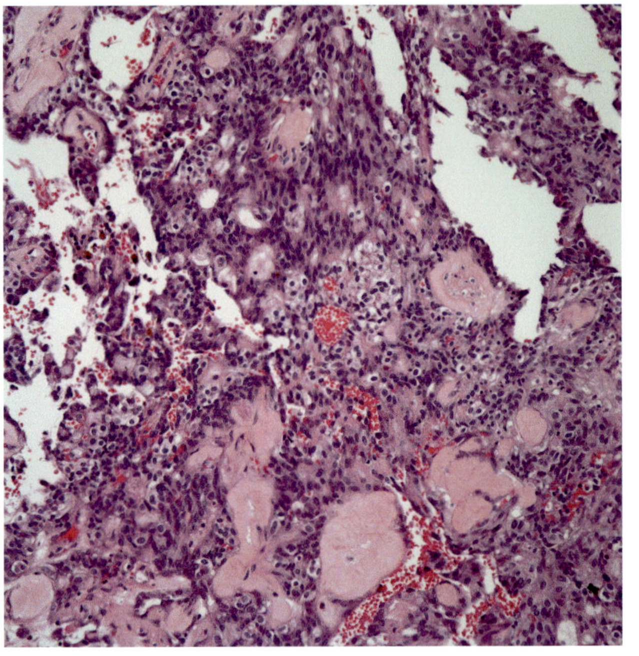

Fig. 11.99 Ependymoma with areas of hyalinization

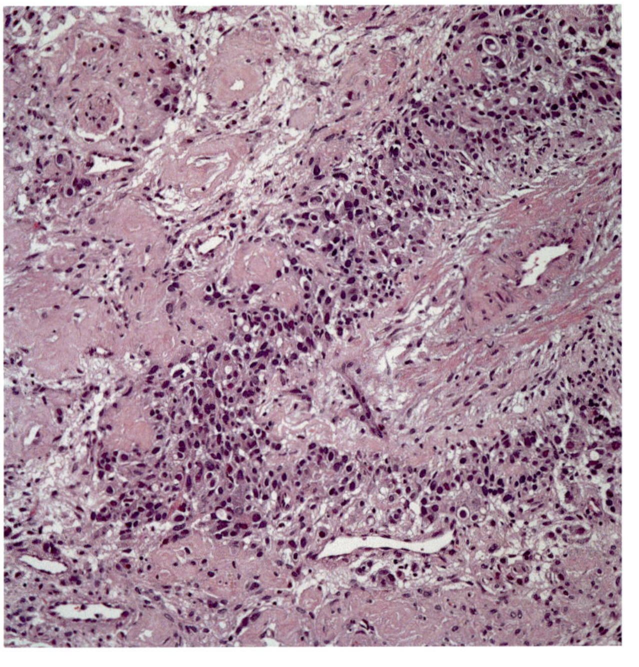

Fig. 11.100 Extensive hyalinization in blood vessels in a mediastinal ependymoma

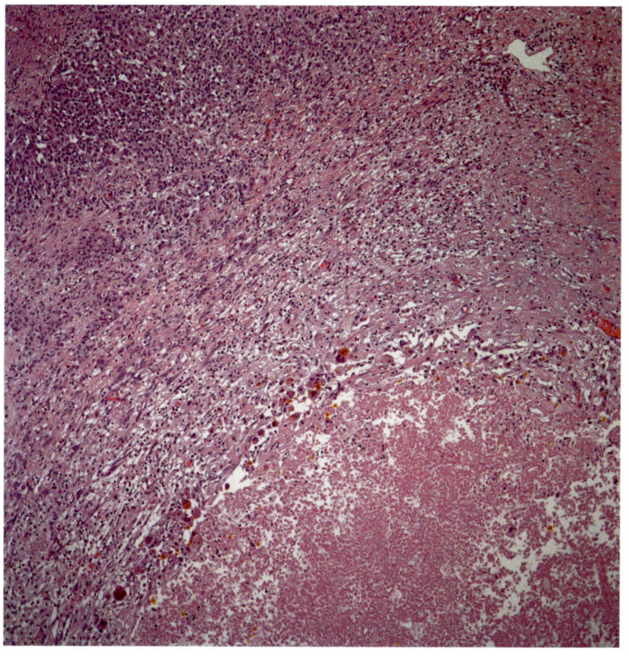

Fig. 11.101 Ependymoma with areas of necrosis

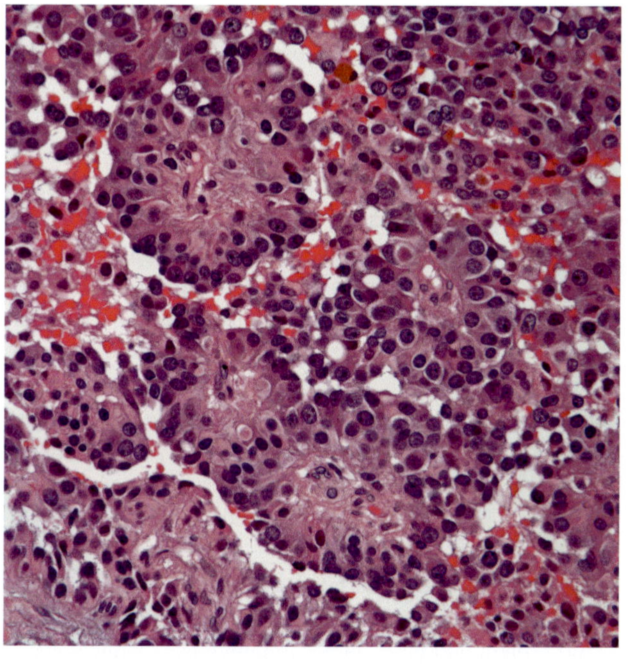

Fig. 11.102 High power magnification of a mediastinal ependymoma showing rosettes. Note the absence of mark cellular atypia or mitotic activity

Meningioma

This is another neural tumor of unusual occurrence in the mediastinal compartment, even though the knowledge of the occurrence of these tumors in the mediastinal compartment dates back more than 30 years. In 1979, Wilson and coworkers [154] reported a case in a patient with Horner's syndrome and absence of intracranial tumor. Since then, the tumor has been reported mainly as case reports [155–159]. Palimento and Picchio [155] reported a case in a 45-year-old woman who presented with spontaneous pneumothorax. A CT scan showed the presence of a left paravertebral mass. Surgical resection took place, and the patient was alive and well 1-month postsurgical resection. Interestingly, despite the description of increase mitotic activity, the diagnosis of malignant or atypical was not provided in this case. Yang and coworkers [157] reported a case of a 41-year-old woman who presented with chest distress and cough and, who on CT scan, showed the presence of an anterior mediastinal mass. Surgical resection of the mass was undertaken followed by radiation therapy. Follow-up after 7 months showed no evidence of tumor recurrence. Even though the authors labeled this tumor as "malignant meningioma" in which focal necrosis was described, the authors did not provide any histological description of mitotic activity. Mogi and coworkers [158] described an anterior mediastinal meningioma in a 64-year-old man who presented with thoracic pain. In this particular case, the tumor appeared to infiltrate lung parenchyma, and, histologically, the tumor showed focal necrosis and mitotic activity of four mitotic figures per 10 hpf. Based on the overall features of this neoplasm, the authors labeled the meningioma as "atypical." Follow-up provided showed the patients alive and well 12 months postsurgical resection. More recently, Lu and associates [159] described a posterior mediastinal meningioma in a 42-year-old man who presented with dysphagia. Surgical resection of the tumor was performed, and the histological description provided was that of a tumor without mitotic activity or necrosis. Follow-up provided stated that the patient was without evidence of recurrence of metastatic disease 24 months postsurgical resection.

Based on the cases reported, it appears that mediastinal meningiomas are tumors that may occur in the anterior or posterior mediastinum. The tumors described have been in adult individuals with diverse symptomatology. Histologically, the tumors may range from the conventional meningioma to the atypical or malignant tumor. Surgical resection appears to be the treatment of choice for these tumors, and, even though the follow-up in the cases described was not long enough, well-documented metastatic disease has not been reported.

Pathological Features

Macroscopically, the tumor may reach a size of more than 10 cm in greatest dimension and infiltrate adjacent organs. The tumor is solid, tan to yellowish with a homogeneous surface. Areas of necrosis and/or hemorrhage may be present.

Histologically, similar to its counterparts in the CNS, the tumor may show the conventional features of epithelioid or spindle cell proliferation; in some cases, one can observe both of these components. In tumors in which the predominant cells are the epithelioid-like cellular proliferation, the tumor is arranged in whorls with scattered presence of psammoma bodies. In focal areas, the tumor may show the presence of foamy macrophages entrapped within the neoplastic cells. When the tumor is composed of spindle cells, the growth pattern may mimic other spindle cell neoplasms. The tumor is arranged in a subtle storiform growth pattern in which the spindle cell bundles are separated by thin fibrocollagenous material with ectatic hyalinized blood vessels. Even in tumors which are predominantly spindle, there may be focal areas in which the tumor shows round cells and focal calcifications (Figs. 11.103, 11.104, 11.105, 11.106, 11.107, and 11.108). In general, conventional meningiomas do not show mitotic activity, necrosis, or hemorrhage. The presence of any necrosis and mitotic activity are features to upgrade the tumor to an atypical or malignant meningioma (Figs. 11.109, 11.110, and 11.111).

Immunohistochemical and Molecular Features

The immunohistochemical features of mediastinal meningiomas are similar to those described for CNS meningiomas or pulmonary meningiomas. Essentially, the tumor may show positive staining for EMA and vimentin. In some cases, CD34 and keratin have been reported to show positive staining in tumor cells. In addition, some tumor may also show positive staining for estrogen receptors. However, in general, the tumor is negative for keratin 5/6, STAT6, P40, P63, and other muscle and vascular markers. Recently, a study of pleuropulmonary meningiomas comparing to those of the CNS, suggested a common histogenesis for these tumors, as some of these tumors show loss of the NF2 gene on chromosome 22 [160]. Such findings suggest that all these tumors arise from the same precursor cell. Even though mediastinal meningiomas have not been investigated for the loss of the NF2 gene, it is possible that the findings would be similar, thus providing further explanation for the occurrence of these tumors in the thoracic cavity.

Differential Diagnosis

By far the most important interpretation would be that of a primary versus a metastatic meningioma. In this setting, obtaining an unequivocal history of previous CNS tumor is highly important in order to arrive at a more definitive interpretation. Other tumors that enter in the differential diagnosis of meningiomas would depend not only on the histology of the tumor but also on the location of the tumor. For instance, tumors that occur in the anterior mediastinum may be easily confused with thymoma. Thymomas are well-known neoplasms that show high versatility in tumor growth and pattern, and some thymomas may show areas that can easily mimic the transitional meningioma, while some tumors showing spindle cells and desmoplastic features may be confused with spindle cell meningiomas. However, if thymoma is a consideration, the use of immunohistochemical stains may aid, as it is known that thymomas are generally negative for EMA and positive for keratin 5/6. Another tumor that may enter in the differential diagnosis, mainly in tumors composed of epithelioid cells (transitional meningiomas), would be a neuroendocrine carcinoma (carcinoid tumor). In this setting, once again the use of immunohistochemical stains such as keratin and neuroendocrine markers should lead to the correct interpretation. Tumors composed of spindle cells, whether in the anterior or posterior mediastinum, can mimic solitary fibrous tumor. In this setting, the use of STAT6 should lead to the correct interpretation.

Malignant Granular Tumor

This tumor is of unusual occurrence in the mediastinum; however, it has been reported [161–164]. Interestingly, the majority of reported cases have been in adult individuals and in the posterior mediastinum. Clinically, the patients reported have either been asymptomatic or with non-specific symptoms, and their tumor has been found during radiographic studies. It appears that surgical resection has been performed in those cases reported, and, in at least one, patient recurrence and death were documented, while in a different patient metastatic disease to the liver was documented. It is likely that these tumors in the mediastinal locations may follow the same clinical behavior as those malignant granular cell tumors of the soft tissues.

Pathological Features

Macroscopically, these tumors have been reported to reach more than 10 cm in greatest dimension. They are tan to yellow in color, solid, and necrosis may or may not be present.

Histologically, the tumor shows a malignant cellular proliferation composed of large cells with ample granular eosinophilic cytoplasm, round nuclei, and prominent nucleoli. Cellular pleomorphism and mitotic activity are easily identifiable, while areas of necrosis may be variable from focal to extensive areas. The neoplastic cellular proliferation is arranged in sheets of cells without any particular growth pattern (Figs. 11.112, 11.113, 11.114, and 11.115).

Immunohistochemical Features

Malignant granular cell tumors are essentially positive for S-100 protein and NSE. Other immunohistochemical stains that have shown positive staining in tumor cells include CD56 and Vimentin. However, the tumor is negative for muscle markers including desmin, caldesmon, MyoD, myoglobin, and smooth muscle actin. In addition, epithelial markers such as keratin and EMA are negative in these tumors. The tumor is negative for HMB45 and Melan A.

Differential Diagnosis

The differential diagnosis of malignant granular cell tumor may encompass different tumors of different histogenesis,

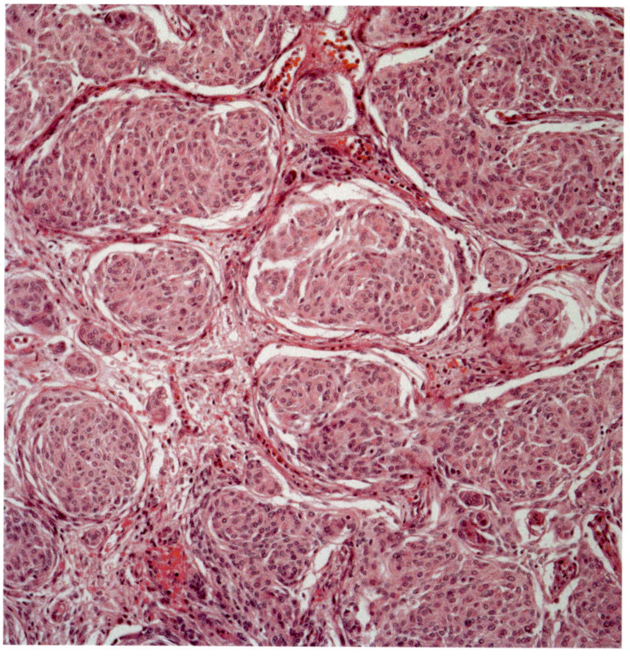

Fig. 11.103 Low power view of a mediastinal meningioma showing the classic whorling pattern

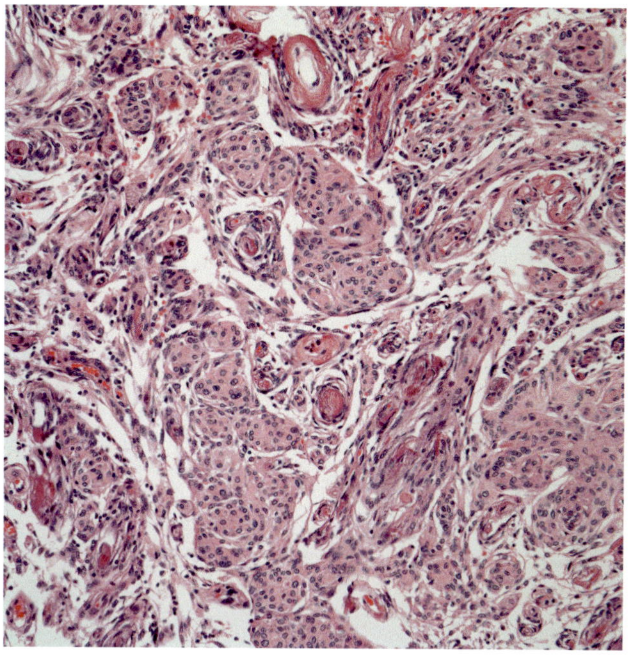

Fig. 11.105 Mediastinal meningioma showing numerous hyalinized ectatic vessels

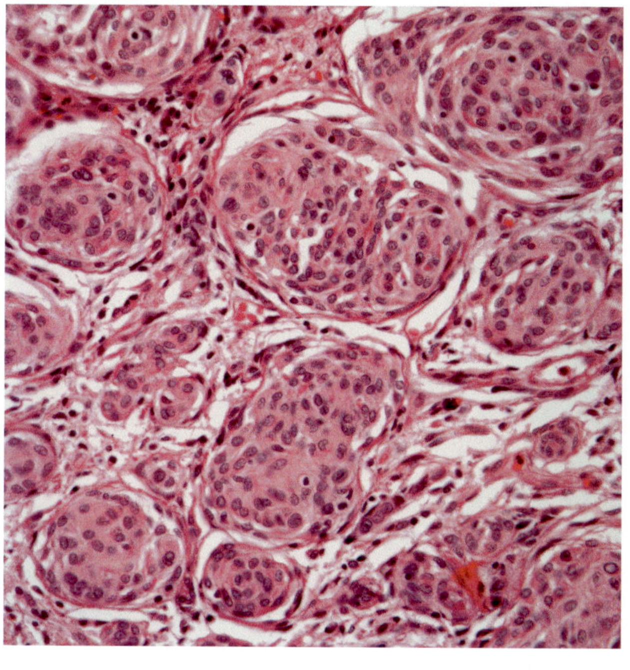

Fig. 11.104 Closer view showing whorls of cells arranged in small nests and separated by thin fibroconnective tissue. No mitotic activity is present

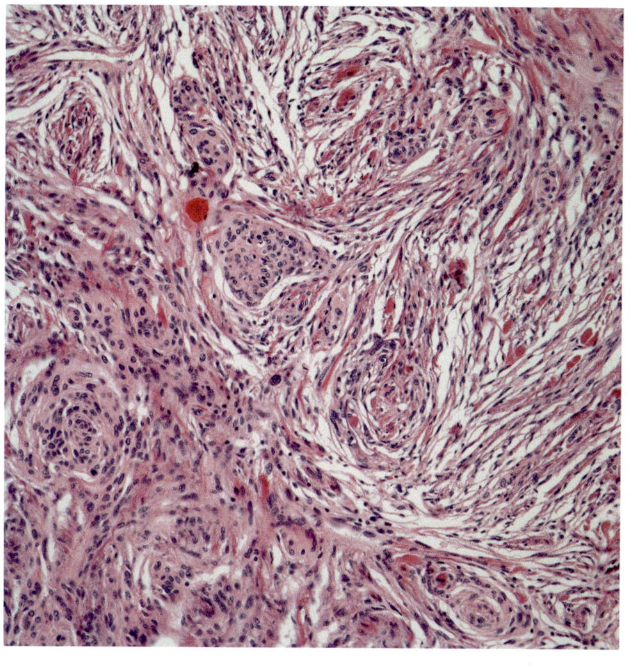

Fig. 11.106 Meningioma with features of both transitional (epithelioid cells) and fibroblastic (spindle cells)

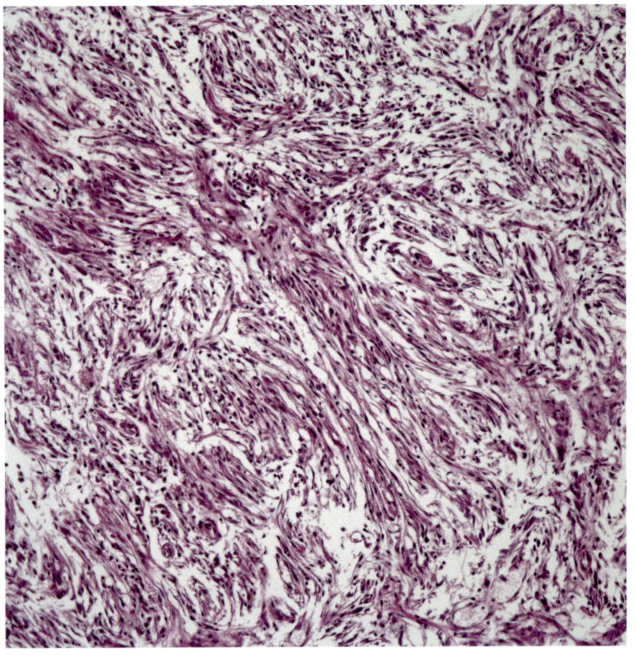

Fig. 11.107 Predominantly fibroblastic meningioma composed of fascicles of spindle cells

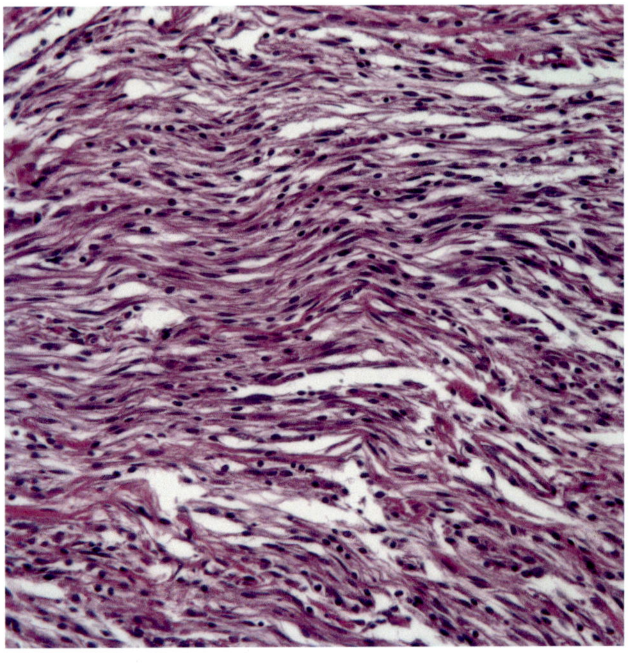

Fig. 11.108 Higher magnification of a fibroblastic meningioma showing spindle cells with lack of nuclear atypia or mitotic activity

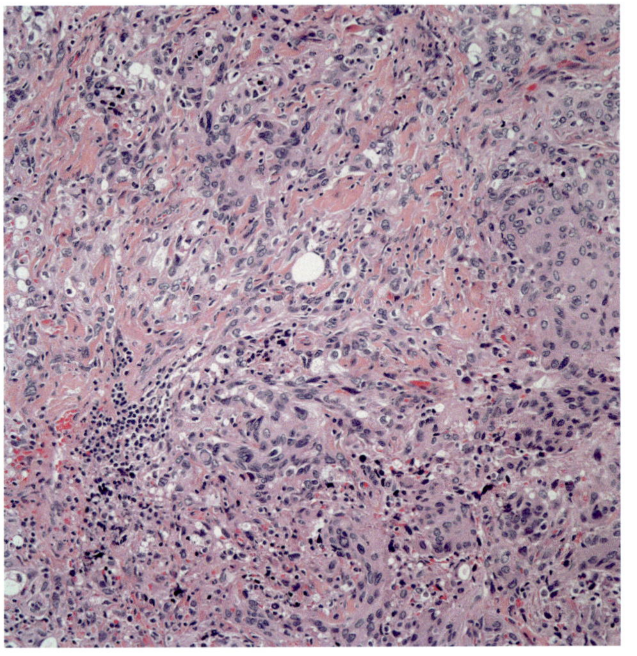

Fig. 11.109 Malignant meningioma showing nuclear atypia

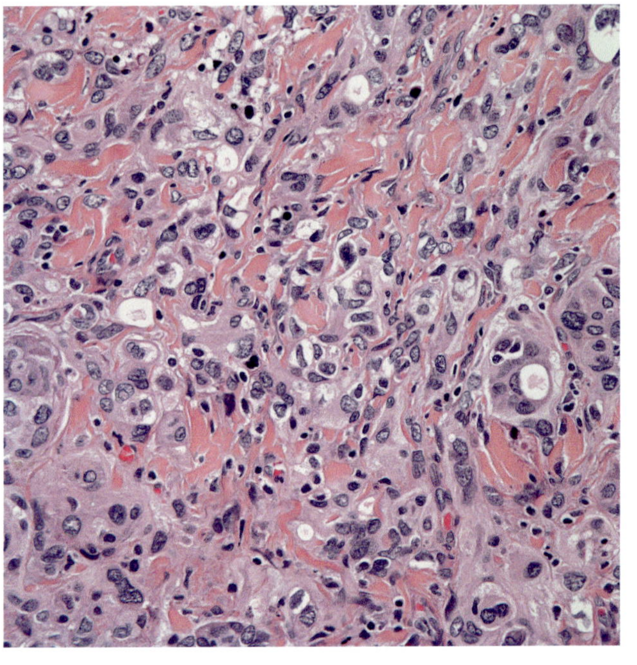

Fig. 11.110 Malignant meningioma showing mitotic activity

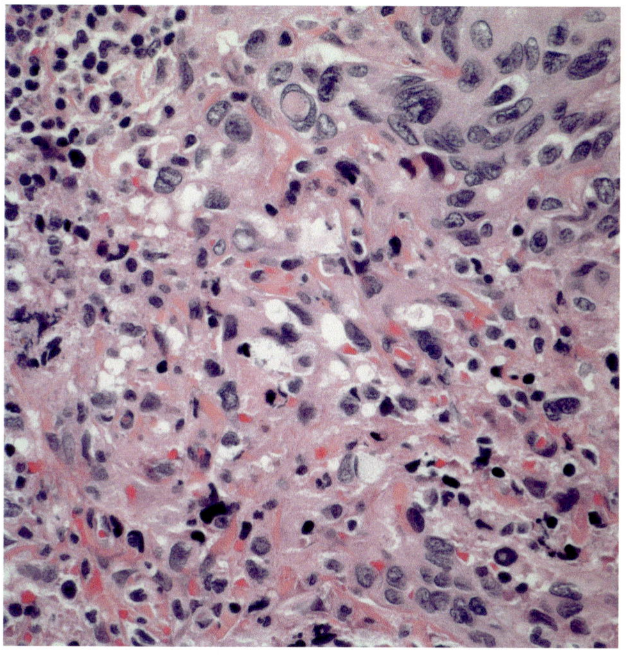

Fig. 11.111 Nuclear atypia with intranuclear inclusion and mitotic activity in a malignant meningioma

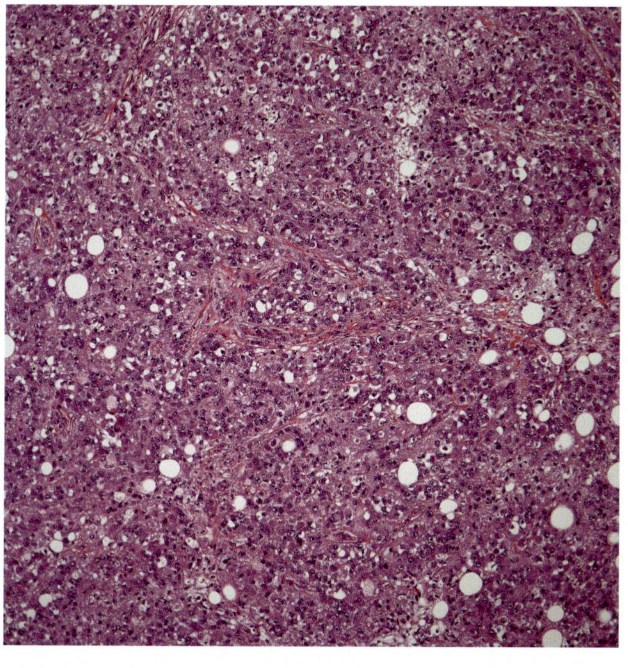

Fig. 11.112 Malignant granular cell tumor showing sheets of malignant cells

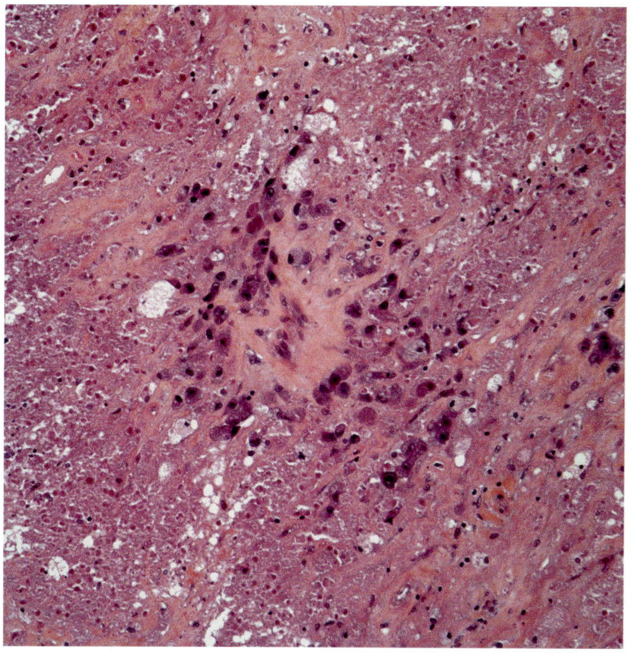

Fig. 11.113 Extensive areas of necrosis with only focal areas of viable tumor in malignant granular cell tumor

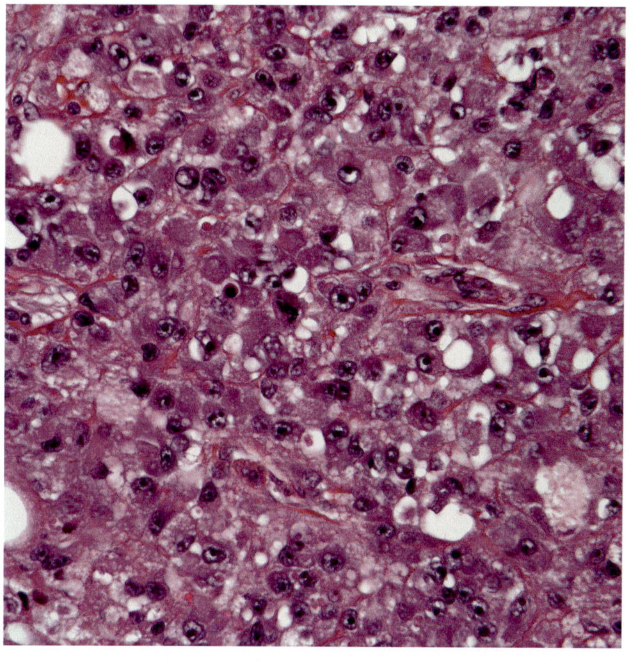

Fig. 11.114 Nuclear atypia and mitotic activity in malignant granular cell tumor

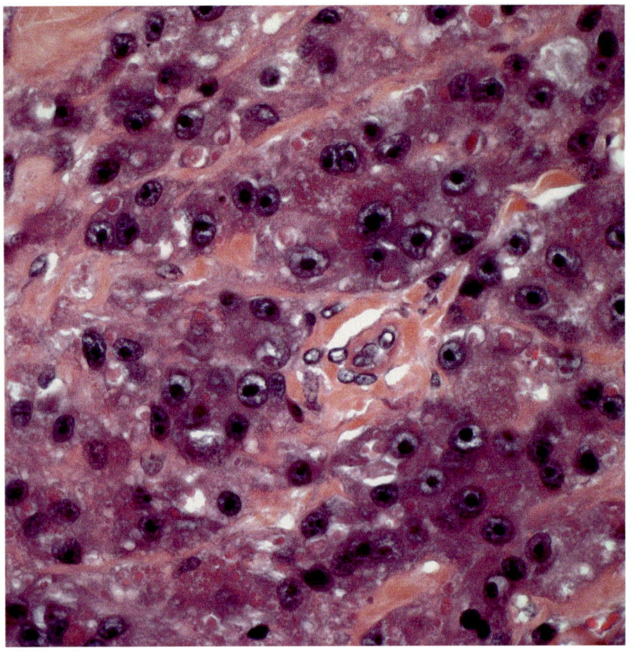

Fig. 11.115 High power view of a malignant granular cell tumor showing cells with granular eosinophilic cytoplasm, round to oval nuclei, and prominent nucleoli

mainly when the tumor occurs in the mediastinal region. Poorly differentiated carcinoma and melanoma would be the leading differential diagnosis. In the former, the negative staining in tumor cells for epithelial markers such as keratins or EMA should alert against that possibility. In the setting of melanoma, the issue may be more challenging, as both tumors will show positive staining for S-100 protein. Granular cell tumor would show negative staining for HMB-45 and Melan A. In addition, negative clinical history of previous cutaneous melanoma and the characteristic cellular features of the tumor, mainly the presence of abundant granular cytoplasm, would be helpful. Ultimately, the ultrastructural features of both tumors are different, and the presence or absence of premelanosomes should lead to the correct interpretation.

References

1. Smith LH. Thoracic neurolophomas. Ann Thorac Surg. 1977;23:586–92.
2. Blades B. Mediastinal tumors. Surg Gynecol Obstet. 1949;88:131–3.
3. Richards GJ, Reeves RJ. Mediastinal tumors and cysts in children. AMA J Dis Child. 1958;95:284–91.
4. Carey LS, Ellis FH, Good CA, Woolner LB. Neurogenic tumors of the mediastinum: a clinicopathologic study. Am J Roentgenol. 1960;84:189–205.
5. Pachter MR, Lattes R. Neurogenous tumors of the mediastinum: a clinicopathologic study based on 50 cases. Dis Chest. 1963;44:79–87.
6. Meyer KK, Ochsner JL. Intrathoracic neurogenic tumors. Surg Clin North Am. 1966;46:1427–36.
7. Whitataker LD, Lynn HB. Mediastinal tumors and cysts in the pediatric patient. Surg Clin North Am. 1973;53:893–904.
8. Pokorny WJ, Sherman JO. Mediastinal masses in infants and children. J Thorac Cardiovasc Surg. 1974;68:869–75.
9. King RM, Telander RL, Smithson WA, Banks PM, Han MT. Primary mediastinal tumors in children. J Pediatr Surg. 1982;17:12–520.
10. Vidne B, Levy MJ. Mediastinal tumours. Surgical treatment in forty-five consecutive cases. Scand J Thorac Cardiovasc Surg. 1973;7:59–65.
11. Davison KG, Walbaum PR, McCormack JM. Intrathoracic neural tumours. Thorax. 1978;33:359–67.
12. Akwari OE, Payne WS, Onofrio BM, Dines DE, Muhm JR. Dumbbell neurogenic tumors of the mediastinum. Mayo Clin Proc. 1978;53:353–8.
13. Luosto R, Koikkalainen K, Jyrala A, Franssila K. Mediastinal tumors: a follow-up study of 208 patients. Scand J Thorac Cardiovasc Surg. 1978;12:253–9.
14. Reed JC, Hallet KK, Feigin DS. Neural tumors of the thorax: subject review from the AFIP. Radiology. 1978;126:9–17.
15. Harjula A, Matilla S, Luosto R, Kostiainen S, Mattila I. Mediastinal neurogenic tumours: early and late results of surgical treatment. Scand J Thorac Cardiovasc Surg. 1986;20:115–8.
16. Blegvad S, Lippert H, Simper LB, Dybdahl H. Mediastinal tumours. A report of 129 cases. Scand J Thorac Cardiovasc Surg. 1990;24:39–42.
17. Saenz N, Schnitzer JJ, Eraklis AE, Hendren WH, Grier HE, Macklis RM, et al. Posterior mediastinal masses. J Pediatr Surg. 1993;28:172–6.
18. Sakai F, Sone S, Kiyono K, Ueda H, Aoki J, Kawai T, et al. Intrathoracic neurogenic tumors: MR-pathologic correlation. AJR. 1992;159:272–83.
19. Strollo DC, Rosado-de-Christenson ML, Jett JR. Primary mediastinal tumors. Part II. Tumors of the middle and posterior mediastinum. Chest. 1997;112:1344–57.
20. Tanaka O, Kiryu T, Hirose Y, Iwata H, Hoshi H. Neurogenic tumors of the mediastinum and chest wall. MR imaging appearance. J Thorac Imaging. 2005;20:316–20.
21. Carachi R, Campbell PE, Kent M. Thoracic neural crest tumors. Cancer. 1983;51:949–54.
22. Grosfeld JL, Skinner MA, Rescorla FJ, West KW, Scherer LR 3rd. Mediastinal tumors in children: experience with 196 cases. Ann Surg Oncol. 1994;1:121–7.
23. Sugio K, Inoue T, Inoue K, Tateishi M, Ishida T, Sugimachi K. Neurogenic tumors of the mediastinum originated from the vagus nerve. Eur J Surg Oncol. 1995;21:214–6.
24. Takeda S, Miyoshi S, Minami M, Matsuda H. Intrathoracic neurogenic tumors – 50 years' experience in Japanese institution. Eur J Cardiothorac Surg. 2004;26:807–12.
25. Shrivastava CP, Devgarha S, Ahlawat V. Mediastinal tumors: a clinicopathological analysis. Asian Cardiovasc Thorac Ann. 2006;14:102–4.
26. Alizzi AM, Hemli JM, Diqer AM, Bidstrup B. Primary solitary mediastinal mass lesions: a review of 37 cases. Heart Lung Circ. 2006;15:310–3.
27. Cardillo G, Carleo F, Khalil MW, Carbone L, Treggiari S, Salvadori L, et al. Surgical treatment of benign neurogenic tumours of the mediastinum: a single institution report. Eur J Cardiothorac Surg. 2008;34:1210–4.
28. Bicakcioglu P, Demirag F, Yazcioglu A, Aydogdu K, Kaya S, Karaoglanoglu N. Intrathoracic neurogenic tumors. Thorac Cardiovasc Surg. 2014;62:147–52.
29. Stout AP. Ganglioneuroma of the sympathetic nervous system. Surg Gynecol Obstet. 1947;84:101–10.
30. Geoerger B, Hero B, Harms D, Grebe J, Scheidhauer K, Berthold F. Metabolic activity and clinical features of primary ganglioneuroma. Cancer. 2001;91:1905–13.
31. Spinelli C, Rossi L, Barbetta A, Ugolini C, Strambi S. Incidental ganglioneuromas: a presentation of 14 surgical cases and review of the literature. J Endocrinol Investig. 2015;38:547–54.

32. Sanal M, Meister B, Kreczy A, Unsinn K, Hager J. Intrathoracic ganglioneuroma and ganglioneuroblastoma: report of four cases. Eur Surg. 2005;37/5:317–20.
33. Forsythe A, Volpe J, Muller R. Posterior mediastinal ganglioneuroma. Radiographics. 2004;24:594–7.
34. Shea MP, Abshire TC. Philadelphia chromosome-positive chronic myeloid leukemia and thoracic ganglioneuroma. Am J Pediatr Hematol Oncol. 1993;15:111–4.
35. Takeda S, Minami M, Inoue Y, Matsuda H. Synchronous mediastinal ganglioneuroma and retroperitoneal pheochromocytoma. Ann Thorac Surg. 2005;80:1525–7.
36. Guan YB, Zhang WD, Zeng QS, Chen GQ, He JX. CT and MRI findings of thoracic ganglioneuroma. Br J Radiol. 2012;85:e365–72.
37. Ozawa Y, Kobayashi S, Hara M, Shibamoto Y. Morphological differences between schwannomas and ganglioneuromas in the mediastinum: utility of the craniocaudal length to major axis ratio. Br J Radiol. 2014;87:20130777.
38. Petroze R, McGahren ED. Pediatric chest II: benign tumors and cysts. Surg Clin N Am. 2012;92:645–58.
39. Castroviejo P, Casas-Fernandez C, Lopez-Martin V. Complicaciones y secuelas de la neurofibromatosis en el nino. An Esp Pediatr. 1976;9:290–9.
40. Ueda K, Honda O, Satoh Y, Kawai M, Gyobu T, Kanazawa T, et al. Computed tomography (CT) findings in 88 neurofibromatosis 1 (NF1) patients: prevalence rates and correlations of thoracic findings. Eur J Radiol. 2015;84:1191–5.
41. Yano M, Sasaki H, Moriyama S, Hikosaka Y, Okuda K, Shitara M, et al. Clinicopathological analysis of small-size anterior mediastinal tumors. Surg Today. 2014;44:1817–22.
42. Perera N, Lynn RB. Intrathoracic meningocele associated with multiple neurofibromatosis: a rare cause of mediastinal tumor. Can J Med. 1974;17:208–9.
43. Lee YH, Shieh SJ. Concomitant mediastinal ganglioneuroma and sciatic neurofibroma in a patient with neurofibromatosis. J Plast Reconstr Aesthet Surg. 2009;62:e645–7.
44. Smahi M, Lakranbi M, Ouadnouni Y, Bouarhroum A, Sbai H, Znati K, et al. Intrathoracic phrenic nerve neurofibroma. Ann Thorac Surg. 2011;91:e57–8.
45. Kanzaki R, Inoue M, Minami M, Sawabata N, Shintani Y, Nakagiri T, et al. Bilateral mediastinal neurofibroma of the vagus nerves in a patient with neurofibromatosis type 1. Ann Thorac Cardiovasc Surg. 2013;19:293–6.
46. Kesieme E, Dongo AE, Affusim C, Prisadov G, Okonta K, Imoloamen C. Late presentation of giant intrathoracic neurofibroma with significant mediastinal shift: a case report and review of the literature. Case Rep Pulmonol. 2013;2013:ID619729.
47. Marchevsky AM. Mediastinal tumors of peripheral nervous system origin. Semin Diagn Pathol. 1999;16:65–78.
48. Watabe K, Kumanishi T, Ikuta F, Oyake Y. Tactile-like corpuscles in Neurofibromas: immunohistochemical demonstration of S-100 protein. Acta Neuropathol. 1983;61:173–7.
49. Razzuk MA, Urschel HC, Martin JA, Kingsley WB, Paulson DL. Electron microscopic observations on mediastinal neurilemmoma, neurofibroma, and ganglioneuroma. Ann Thorac Surg. 1973;15:73–83.
50. Boland JM, Colby TV, Folpe AL. Intrathoracic peripheral nerve sheath tumors – a clinicopathological study of 75 cases. Hum Pathol. 2015;46:419–25.
51. Miura J, Doita M, Miyata K, Yoshiya S, Kurosaka M, Yamamoto H. Horner's syndrome caused by a thoracic dumbbell-shaped schwannoma: sympathetic chain reconstruction after a one-stage removal of the tumor. Spine. 2003;28:E23–36.
52. Mathew BG, Jones RM, Campbell MJ. Horner's syndrome due to superior mediastinal schwannoma. J Neurol Neurosurg Psychiatry. 1988;51:1460–1.
53. Tajima H, Tajima N, Yamamoto K, Maeda S, Koizumi K, Kumazaki T, et al. Anterior mediastinal schwannoma: a case report. Radiat Med. 1995;13:175–7.
54. Smail H, Baste JM, Melki J, Peillon C. Challenging posterior mediastinal mass resection via a minimally invasive approach with neurological monitoring. Eur J Cardiothorac Surg. 2013;43:e44–6.
55. Paris F, Cabanes J, Munoz C, Tamarit L. Melanotic spinothoracic schwannoma. Thorax. 1979;34:243–6.
56. Abbott AE, Hill RC, Flynn MA, McClure S, Murray GF. Melanotic schwannoma of the sympathetic ganglia: pathological and clinical characteristics. Ann Thorac Surg. 1990;49:1006–8.
57. Prieto-Rodriguez M, Camanas-Sanz A, Bas T, Cortés B, Vera-Sempere FJ. Psammomatous melanotic schwannoma localized in the mediastinum: diagnosis by fine-needle aspiration cytology. Diagn Cytopathol. 1998;19:298–302.
58. Zhang H, Yang G, Chen H, Wei B, Ke Q, Guo H, et al. Clinicopathological, immunohistochemical, and ultrastructural study of 13 cases of melanotic schwannoma. Chin Med J. 2005;118:1451–61.
59. Woodruff JM, Goddwin TA, Erlandson RA, Susin M, Martini N. Cellular schwannoma: a variety of schwannoma sometimes mistaken for a malignant tumor. Am J Surg Pathol. 1981;5:733–44.
60. White W, Shiu MH, Rosenblum MK, Erlandson RA, Woodruff JM. Cellular schwannoma: a clinicopathologic study of 57 patients and 58 tumors. Cancer. 1990;66:1266–75.
61. Lodding P, Kindblom LG, Angervall L, Stenmman G. Cellular schwannoma: a clinicopathologic study of 29 cases. Virchows Arch A Pathol Anat Histopathol. 1990;416:237–48.
62. Machida E, Haniuda M, Eguchi T, Kurai M, Yamanda T, Amano J, et al. Granular cell tumor of the mediastinum. Intern Med. 2003;42:178–81.
63. Shikatani Y, Okazaki M, Sakao N, Yukumi S, Shigematsu H, Kitazawa S, et al. A case of mediastinal granular cell tumor with Horner's syndrome. Ann Thorac Cardiovasc Surg. 2015;21:567–9.
64. Angeles RM, Papari M, Malecki Z. Pathologic quiz case: a 43-year-old woman with an incidentally detected posterior mediastinal mass. Arch Pathol Lab Med. 2005;129:e27–8.
65. Kim DY, Jeon HW, Kim KS, Park SK, Sung SW. A rare case of mediastinal granular cell tumor. Korean J Thorac Cardiovasc Surg. 2014;47:494–6.
66. Winchester LM, Pucket Y, Greenspon J, Vogler CA. Mediastinal granular cell tumor in a 16-year-old boy: a surgical and pathologic perspective. Pediatr Dev Pathol. 2016;19:64–8.
67. Wright JH. Neurocytoma or neuroblastoma, a kind of tumor not generally recognized. J Exp Med. 1910;12:556–61.
68. Cushing H, Wolbach SB. The transformation of a malignant paravertebral sympathicoblastoma into a benign ganglioneuroma. Am J Pathol. 1927;3:203–16.
69. Stowens D. Neuroblastoma and related tumors. Am J Pathol. 1957;63:451–9.
70. Oberman HA, Abell MR. Neurogenous neoplasms of the mediastinum. Cancer. 1960;13:882–98.
71. Buthker W, Feltkamp-Vroom T, Groen AS, Wieberdink J. Sympathicoblastoma in the anterior mediastinum. Dis Chest. 1964;46:531–6.
72. Oberman HA. Sympathicoblastoma of the anterior mediastinum. Dis Chest. 1963;43:314–6.
73. Hutchinson JE, Nash AD, McCord CW. Neuroblastoma of the anterior mediastinum in an adult. J Thorac Cardiovasc Surg. 1968;56:147–52.
74. Mackay B, Luna MA, Butler JJ. Adult neuroblastoma: electron microscopic observations in nine cases. Cancer. 1976;37:1334–51.
75. Kilton LJ, Aschenbrener C, Burns CP. Ganglioneuroblastoma in adults. Cancer. 1976;37:974–83.
76. Adam A, Hoccholzer L. Ganglioneuroblastoma of the posterior mediastinum: a clinicopathologic review of 80 cases. Cancer. 1981;47:373–81.
77. Talerman A, Gratma S. Primary ganglioneuroblastoma of the anterior mediastinum in a 61-year-old woman. Histopathology. 1983;7:967–75.

78. Nagashima Y, Miyagi Y, Tanaka Y, Miyashita M, Shigematsu S, Aoki I, et al. Adult ganglioneuroblastoma of the anterior mediastinum. Pathol Res Pract. 1997;193:727–32.
79. Asada Y, Marutsuka K, Mitsukawa T, Kuribayashi T, Taniguchi S, Sumiyoshi A. Ganglioneuroblastoma of the thymus: an adult case with the syndrome of inappropriate secretion of antidiuretic hormone. Hum Pathol. 1996;27:506–9.
80. Kaye JA, Warhol MJ, Kretschmar C, Landsberg L, Frei E 3rd. Neuroblastoma in adults: three case reports and review of the literature. Cancer. 1986;58:1149–57.
81. Jrebi NY, Iqbal CW, Joliat GR, Sebo TJ, Farley DR. Review of our experience with neuroblastoma and ganglioneuroblastoma in adults. World J Surg. 2014;38:2871–8.
82. Bove KE, McAdams J. Composite ganglioneuroblastoma: an assessment of the significance of histological maturation in neuroblastoma diagnosed beyond infancy. Arch Pathol Lab Med. 1981;105:325–30.
83. Adams BA, Shochat SJ, Smith EI, Shuster JJ, Joshi VV, Altshuler G, et al. Thoracic neuroblastoma: a pediatric oncology group study. J Pediatr Surg. 1993;28:372–8.
84. Demir HA, Yalcin B, Buyukpamukcu N, Kale G, Varan A, Akyüz C, et al. Thoracic neuroblastic tumors in childhood. Pediatr Blood Cancer. 2010;54:885–9.
85. Geraci AP, De Csepel J, Shlasko E, Wallace SA. Ganglioneuroblastoma and ganglioneuroma in association with neurofibromatosis type I: report of three cases. J Child Neurol. 1998;13:356–8.
86. Lonergan GF, Schwab CM, Suarez ES, Carlson CL. Neuroblastoma, ganglioneuroblastoma, and ganglioneuroma: radiologic-pathologic correlation. Radiographics. 2002;22:911–34.
87. Brook FB, Raafat F, Eldeeb BB, Mann JR. Histologic and immunohistochemical investigation of neuroblastomas and correlation with prognosis. Hum Pathol. 1988;19:879–88.
88. Hachitanda Y, Hata J. Stage IVS neuroblastoma: a clinical, histological, and biological analysis of 45 cases. Hum Pathol. 1996;27:1135–8.
89. Gutierres JC, Fischer AC, Sola JE, Perez EA, Koniaris LG. Markedly improving survival of neuroblastoma: a 30-year analysis of 1646 patients. Pediatr Surg Int. 2007;23:637–46.
90. Kubota M, Suita S, Tajiri T, Shono K, Fujii Y. Analysis of the prognostic factors relating to better clinical outcome in ganglioneuroblastoma. J Pediatr Surg. 2000;35:92–5.
91. Evans AE, D'Angio GJ, Randolph J. A proposed staging for children with neuroblastoma: Children's Cancer Study Group A. Cancer. 1971;27:374–8.
92. Evans AE. Staging and treatment of neuroblastoma. Cancer. 1980;45:1799–802.
93. Evans AE, D'Angio GJ, Propert K, Anderson J, Hann HW. Prognostic factors in neuroblastoma. Cancer. 1987;59:1853–9.
94. Hata Y, Naito H, Sasaki F, Ohkawa M, Takeda T, Sasaki M, et al. Fifteen years' experience of neuroblastoma: a prognostic evaluation according to the Evans and UICC staging systems. J Pediatr Surg. 1990;25:326–9.
95. Hayes FA, Green A, Hustu O, Kumar M. Surgical pathologic staging of neuroblastoma: prognostic significance or regional lymph node metastases. J Pediatr. 1983;102:59–62.
96. Nitschke R, Smith EI, Shochat S, Altshuler G, Travers H, Shuster JJ, et al. Localized neuroblastoma treated by surgery: A Pediatric Oncology Group study. J Clin Oncol. 1988;6:1271–9.
97. Evans AE, D'Angio GJ, Sather HN, de Lorimier AA, Dalton A, Ungerleider RS, et al. A comparison of four staging systems for localized and regional neuroblastoma: a report from the childrens cancer study group. J Clin Oncol. 1990;8:678–88.
98. Brodeur GM, Pritchard J, Berthold F, Carlsen NL, Castel V, Castelberry RP, et al. Revisions of the international criteria for neuroblastoma diagnosis, staging, and response to treatment. J Clin Oncol. 1993;11:1466–77.
99. Brodeur GM, Pritchard J, Berthold F, et al. Revisions to the international criteria for neuroblastoma diagnosis, staging, and response to treatment. Prog Clin Biol Res. 1994;385:363–9.
100. Shimada H, Ambros IM, Dehner LP, Carlsen NL, Castel V, Castelberry RP, et al. Terminology and morphologic criteria of neuroblastic tumors. Cancer. 1999;86:349–63.
101. Shimada H, Ambros IM, Dehner LP, Hata J, Joshi VV, Roald B, et al. The international neuroblastoma pathology classification (the Shimada System). Cancer. 1999;86:364–72.
102. Goto S, Umehara S, Gerbing RB, Stram DO, Brodeur GM, Seeger RC, et al. Histopathology (International Neuroblastoma Pathology Classification) and MYCN status in patients with peripheral neuroblastic tumors. Cancer. 2001;92:2699–708.
103. Shimada H, Umehara S, Monobe Y, Hachitanda Y, Nakagawa A, Goto S, et al. International neuroblastoma pathology classification for prognostic evaluation of patients with peripheral neuroblastic tumors: a report from the children's cancer group. Cancer. 2001;92:2451–61.
104. Peuchmaur M, d'Amore ESG, Joshi VV, Hata J, Roald B, Dehner LP, et al. Revision of the international neuroblastoma pathology classification: confirmation of favorable and unfavorable prognostic subsets in ganglioneuroblastoma nodular. Cancer. 2003;98:2274–81.
105. Okamatsu C, London WB, Naranjo A, Hogarty MD, Gastier-Foster JM, Look AT, et al. Clinicopathological characteristics of ganglioneuroma and ganglioneuroblastoma: a report from the CCG and COG. Pediatr Blood Cancer. 2009;53:563–9.
106. Yunis EJ, Agostini RM, Walpuk JA, Hubbard JD. Glycogen in neuroblastomas: a light and electron microscopic study of 40 cases. Am J Surg Pathol. 1979;3:313–23.
107. Favrot MC, Combaret V, Goillot E, Lutz P, Frappaz D, Thiesse P, et al. Expression of integrin receptors on 45 clinical neuroblastoma specimens. Int J Cancer. 1991;49:347–55.
108. Munoz J, Vendrell E, Aiza G, Nistal M, Pestaña A, Peinado MA, et al. Determination of genomic damage in neuroblastic tumors by arbitrarily primed PCR: MYCN amplification as a marker for genomic instability in neuroblastoma. Neuropathology. 2006;26:165–9.
109. Angelini P, Baruchel S, Marrano P, Irwin MS, Thorner PS, et al. The neuroblastoma and ganglion components of nodular ganglioneuroblastoma are genetically similar: evidence against separate clonal origins. Mod Pathol. 2015;28:166–76.
110. Rossman EM. Mediastinal Neurofibrosarcoma causing hypoglycemia. Arch Int Med. 1959;104:640–2.
111. Bambirra EA, Miranda C. Spontaneous aortic rupture in a malignant schwannoma. South Med J. 1980;73:1534–5.
112. Verma RN, Hassan MI. Malignant schwannoma of the mediastinum. Indian J Cancer. 1984;21:110–2.
113. Shields TW, Reynolds M. Neurogenic tumors of the thorax. Surg Clin N Am. 1988;68:645–68.
114. Moran CA, Suster S, Koss MN. The spectrum of histologic growth pattern in benign and malignant fibrous tumors of the pleura. Semin Diag Pathol. 1992;9:169–80.
115. Ackerman LV, Taylor FH. Neurogenous tumors within the thorax: a clinicopathological evaluation of forty-eight cases. Cancer. 1951;4:669–91.
116. Sordillo PP, Helson L, Hajdu SI, Magill GB, Kosloff C, Golbey RB, et al. Malignant schwannoma – clinical characteristics, survival, and response to therapy. Cancer. 1981;47:2503–9.
117. Sorensen SA, Mulvihill JJ, Nielsen A. Long-term follow-up of von Recklinghausen neurofibromatosis: survival and malignant neoplasms. NEJM. 1986;314:1010–5.
118. Ducatman BS, Scheithauer BW. Postirradiation neurofibromatosis. Cancer. 1983;51:1028–33.
119. Fukai I, Masaoka A, Yamakawa Y, Niwa H, Eimoto T. Mediastinal malignant epithelioid schwannoma. Chest. 1995;108:574–5.

120. Rothenburger M, Semik M, Schmidt C, Hoffmeier A, August C, Scheld HH. Primary pigmented malignant schwannoma in the posterior mediastinum. Thorac Cardiovasc Surg. 2001;49:306–8.
121. Lioulias AG, Foroulis CN, Fotinou M, Lazopoulos G. Malignant melanocytic schwannoma, a rare tumor of the posterior mediastinum. Eur J Cardiothorac Surg. 2003;23:105.
122. Torres-Mora J, Dry S, Li X, Binder S, Amin M, Folpe AL. Malignant melanotic schwannian tumor: a clinicopathologic, Immunohistochemical, and gene expression profiling study of 40 cases, with a proposal for the reclassification of "melanotic schwannomas.". Am J Surg Pathol. 2014;38:94–105.
123. Lowman RM, Livolsi VA. Pigmented (Melanotic) schwannomas of the spinal canal. Cancer. 1980;46:391–7.
124. Lang-Lazdunski L, Pons F, Jancovici R. Malignant "triton" tumor of the posterior mediastinum: prolonged survival after staged resection. Ann Thorac Surg. 2003;75:1645–8.
125. Ren W, Xu X, Yan J, Qian X, Liu B. Malignant triton tumor of the anterior mediastinum: a case report. Oncol Lett. 2014;7:807–10.
126. Thway K, Hamarneh W, Miah AB, Fisher C. Malignant peripheral nerve sheath tumor with rhabdomyosarcomatous and glandular elements: rare epithelial differentiation in a triton tumor. Int J Surg Pathol. 2015;23:377–83.
127. Daimaru Y, Hashimoto H, Enjoji M. Malignant "triton" tumors: a clinicopathologic and Immunohistochemical study of nine cases. Hum Pathol. 1984;15:768–78.
128. Krumerman MS, Stingle W. Synchronous malignant glandular schwannomas in congenital neurofibromatosis. Cancer. 1978;41:2444–51.
129. Shintaku M, Nakade M, Hirose T. Malignant peripheral nerve sheath tumor of small round cell type with pleomorphic spindle sarcomatous areas. Pathol Int. 2003;53:478–82.
130. Stout AP. A tumor of the ulnar nerve. Proc NY Pathol Soc. 1918;18:2–11.
131. Nesbitt KA, Vidone RA. Primitive neuroectodermal tumor (Neuroblastoma) arising in sciatic nerve of a child. Cancer. 1976;37:1562–70.
132. Seemayer TA, Thelmo WL, Bolande RP, Wiglesworth FW. Peripheral neuroectodermal tumors. Perspect Pediatr Pathol. 1975;2:151–72.
133. Angervall L, Enzinger FM. Extraskeletal neoplasms resembling Ewing's sarcoma. Cancer. 1975;36:240–51.
134. Tefft M, Vawter GF, Mitus A. Paravertebral "round cell" tumors in children. Radiology. 1969;92:1501–9.
135. Askin FB, Rosai J, Sibley RK, Dehner LP, McAlister WH. Malignant small cell tumor of the thoracopulmonary region in childhood: a distinctive clinicopathologic entity of uncertain histogenesis. Cancer. 1979;43:2438–51.
136. Marina NM, Etcubanas E, Parham DM, Bowman LC, Green A. Peripheral primitive neuroectodermal tumor (peripheral neuroepithelioma) in children: a review of the St Jude experience and controversies in diagnosis and management. Cancer. 1989;64:1952–60.
137. Llombart-Bosch A, Terrier-Lacombe MJ, Olaya P, Contesso G. Peripheral neuroectodermal sarcoma of soft tissue (peripheral neuroepithelioma): a pathologic study of ten cases with differential diagnosis regarding other small, round-cell sarcomas. Hum Pathol. 1989;20:273–80.
138. Kushner BH, Hajdu SI, Gulati SC, Erlandson RA, Exelby PR, Lieberman PH. Extracranial primitive neuroectodermal tumors. The memorial slon-kettering cancer center experience. Cancer. 1991;67:1825–9.
139. Weissferdt A, Moran CA. Primary primitive neuroectodermal tumor (PNET): a clinicopathological and Immunohistochemical study of six cases. Lung. 2012;190:677–83.
140. Reali A, Mortellaro G, Allis S, Trevisiol E, Anglesio SM, Bartoncini S, et al. A case of primary mediastinal Ewing's sarcoma/primitive neuroectodermal tumor presenting with initial compression of superior vena cava. Ann Thorac Med. 2013;8:121–3.
141. Bae SH, Hwang JH, Nam BD, Kim HJ, Kim KU, Kim DW, et al. Multiple Ewing sarcoma/primitive neuroectodermal tumors in the mediastinum. Medicine. 2016;95:e2725.
142. Schweigert M, Meyer C, Wolf F, Stein HJ. Peripheral primitive neuroectodermal tumor of the thymus. Interact Cardiovasc Thorac Surg. 2011;12:303–5.
143. Manduch M, Dexter DF, Ellis PM, Reid K, Isotalo PA. Extraskeletal Ewing's sarcoma/primitive neuroectodermal tumor of the posterior mediastinum with t(11;22)(q24;q12). Tumori. 2008;94:888–91.
144. Ambros IM, Ambros PF, Strehl S, Kovar H, Gadner H, Salzer-Kuntschik M. MIC2 is a specific marker for Ewing's sarcoma and peripheral primitive neuroectodermal tumors: evidence for a common histogenesis of Ewing's sarcoma and peripheral primitive neuroectodermal tumors from MIC2 expression and specific chromosome aberration. Cancer. 1991;67:1886–93.
145. Selleri L, Hermanson GG, Eubanks JH, Lewis KA, Evans GA. Molecular localization of the t(11;22)(q24;q12) translocation of Ewing sarcoma by chromosomal in-situ suppression hybridization. Proc Natl Acad Sci. 1991;88:887–91.
146. Turc-Carel C, Aurias A, Mugneret F, Lizard S, Sidaner I, Volk C, et al. Chromosomes in Ewing's sarcoma. I. An evaluation of 85 cases of remarkable consistency of t(11;22)q24;q12. Cancer Genet Cytogenet. 1988;32:229–38.
147. Machado I, Navarro L, Pellin A, Navarro S, Agaimy A, Tardío JC, et al. Defining Ewing and Ewing-like small round cell tumors (SRCT): the need for molecular techniques in their categorization and differential diagnosis. A study of 200 cases. Ann Diagn Pathol. 2016;22:25–32.
148. Misugi K, Okajima H, Newton WA, Kmetz DR, Delorimier AA. Mediastinal origin of a melanotic progonoma or retinal anlage tumor. Cancer. 1965;19:477–84.
149. Elli M, Aydin O, Pinarli FG, Dagdemir A, Dabak N, Selcuk MB, et al. Melanotic neuroectodermal tumor of infancy of the femur. Pediatr Hematol Oncol. 2006;23:579–86.
150. Barnes DJ, Hookway E, Athanasou N, Kashima T, Oppermann U, Hughes S, et al. A germline mutation of CDK2A and a novel PRLP1-C1919MC fusion detected in a rare melanotic neuroectodermal tumor of infancy: a case report. BMC Cancer. 2016;16:629–42.
151. Nobles E, Lee R, Kircher T. Mediastinal ependymoma. Hum Pathol. 1991;22:94–6.
152. Doglioni C, Bontempini L, Iuzzolino P, Furlan G, Rosai J. Ependymoma of the mediastinum. Arch Pathol Lab Med. 1988;112:194–6.
153. Wilson RW, Moran CA. Primary ependymoma of the mediastinum: a clinicopathologic correlation of three cases. Ann Diagn Pathol. 1998;2:293–300.
154. Wilson AJ, Ratliff JL, Lagios MD, Aguilar MJ. Mediastinal meningioma. Am J Surg Pathol. 1979;3:557–62.
155. Palimento D, Picchio M. Meningioma of the mediastinum causing spontaneous hemothorax. Ann Thorac Surg. 2006;81:1903–4.
156. Chen F, Zhang S. Diagnosis and treatment of the primary malignant meningioma in mediastinum: case report. South Med J. 2009;102:1164–6.
157. Yang X, Gao X, Wang S. Primary mediastinal malignant meningioma. Case report. Eur J Cardiothorac Surg. 2009;36:217–8.
158. Mogi A, Kirato J, Kosaka T, Yamaki E, Kuwao H. Primary mediastinal atypical meningioma: report of a case and literature review. World J Surg Oncol. 2012;10:17–21.

159. Lu C, Hu X, Xu M, Mao W, Yang H, Wang Z, et al. Posterior mediastinal ectopic meningioma: a case report. World J Surg Oncol. 2015;13:156–9.
160. Weissferdt A, Tang X, Suster S, Wistuba II, Moran CA. Pleuropulmonary meningothelial proliferations: evidence for a common histogenesis. Am J Surg Pathol. 2015;39:1673–8.
161. Harrer WV, Patchefsky AS. Malignant granular-cell myoblastoma of the posterior mediastinum. Chest. 1972;61:95–6.
162. Soh WM, Yeong ML, Wong KP. Malignant granular cell tumour of the mediastinum. Malaysian J Pathol. 2014;36:149–51.
163. De Luca G, Luciano A, Benincasa G, Sessa R, Petteruti F. Giant malignant granular cell tumor (GCT) of the posterior mediastinum. J Thorac Oncol. 2013;8:1107–8.
164. Nakao M, Hishida T, Ishii G, Yoshida J, Nishimura M, Nagai K. Malignant granular cell tumor of the posterior mediastinum with dissemination. Asian Cardiovasc Thorac Ann. 2012;20:71–3.

12 Mesenchymal Tumors

Introduction

Primary mesenchymal tumors arising in the mediastinal compartment are rare. The occurrence of such tumors is by no means limited to a specific compartment, as these tumors have been described in the anterior and posterior mediastinum. In addition, in terms of the variety of these tumors in the mediastinal compartment, the gamut of soft tissue neoplasms in the mediastinum is similar to that observed in the soft tissues, with some minor differences that are intrinsic to this particular anatomic location.

In 1963, Pachter and Lattes [1] provided possibly the first account of the occurrence of these tumors in the mediastinum and, in reviewing earlier literature, encountered poorly documented reports in terms of histology and type of tumor, among other details. In addition, the authors encountered the use of some terms that may encompass different tumors, indicating possibly that different tumors may have also been recorded among this group of tumors (mesenchymal neoplasms). Also, the authors stated that the terminology used might in fact had obscure the true occurrence of these neoplasms, rendering an accurate account of their occurrence almost an impossible task. Furthermore, the authors advanced their own opinion regarding the low incidence of mesenchymal tumors in the mediastinal compartment, and stated that, once one is able to remove the organs encountered in this area, the remaining mesenchymal tissues, such as adipose tissue connective tissue and vascular elements, represent only a small amount in contrast with other areas such as the retroperitoneum, where these elements are encountered in large amounts. Following strict criteria for inclusion, the authors identified 22 such tumors excluding tumors from the chest wall, esophagus, lung, chest wall, diaphragm, heart, spinal column, and vascular tumors. In addition, cases with inadequate follow-up and diagnostic material were excluded. The 22 cases corresponded to fibromatosis (3 cases), lipomas (4 cases), xanthogranulomas (3 cases), liposarcomas (2 cases), malignant mesenchymoma (2 cases), benign mesenchymoma (2 cases), rhabdomyosarcoma (3 cases), and fibrosarcoma and leiomyoma, one case each. Interestingly, the authors also included one case of mesothelioma in this series of cases. Based on this experience, even though the authors clearly stated that their study might not reflect the true incidence of these tumors in the mediastinum, one can still argue not only that these tumors are rare but also, in light of newer classification and nomenclature, that some of these tumors likely would be reclassified, highlighting once more the difficulty of identifying a true incidence of these tumors. In 1991, Swanson [2] reviewed the occurrence of soft tissue neoplasms of the mediastinum and stated that such account is a "daunting task" because "virtually any lesion of somatic soft tissues may arise in the mediastinum." This review encompassed all types of neoplasms including neurogenic tumors, noting however that these tumors in general are uncommon. More recently, den Bakker and colleagues [3] reviewed the literature on mesenchymal tumors of the mediastinum and quoted earlier literature on the subject; these tumors have accounted for a possible incidence of 2–6% of mediastinal neoplasms. However, it is important to highlight what Pachter and Lattes stated in 1963 [1] with respect to earlier literature: the poorly documented cases render a true account of the incidence of these tumors a very difficult task.

Based on earlier and more current literature, the true occurrence and incidence of mesenchymal tumors in the mediastinum are difficult to analyze. We can all agree that the tumors are rare and likely underreported; thus, one is left with current case reports, small series, and relatively larger series of these tumors to draw upon for some insights on the occurrence of a particular type of tumor. Therefore, in this chapter, we have divided tumors based on the type of tissue present or the specific differentiation of the neoplasm, as far as our current knowledge permits, and have provided an analysis of these tumors in the mediastinum. Since we have separated neurogenic tumors in a separate chapter, this chapter will highlight the following neoplasms:

- Adipose tissue tumors
- Vascular tumors

© Springer Nature Switzerland AG 2019
N. Kalhor, C. Moran, *Mediastinal Pathology*, https://doi.org/10.1007/978-3-319-98980-8_12

- Smooth and skeletal muscle tumors
- Fibroblastic, myofibroblastic, and fibrohistiocytic tumors
- Biphasic (epithelial/mesenchymal) tumors
- Chondroid and osseous tumors
- Other mesenchymal neoplasms

We consider that such organization of these unusual tumors will facilitate their study and understanding. Important to highlight is that the description of such tumors will also be limited to tumors of mediastinal location and will not include tumors that may originate in the esophagus, lung, heart, or chest wall.

Adipose Tissue Tumors

The spectrum of tumors in the mediastinum that can show the presence of adipose tissue may vary depending on what one is able to include as part of these tumors. However, in the strict sense, one can essentially limit this occurrence to two main categories: benign and malignant.

- Benign lipomatous tumors
  1. Thymolipomas/lipomas
  2. Angiomyolipomas
- Malignant lipomatous tumors
  1. Liposarcomas

Benign Lipomatous Tumors

As stated in the outline of lipomatous tumors, the range of tumors showing different components is diverse, and, in some instances, such as in the case of thymolipoma, variants or specific histological features have been associated, which render this particular tumor as the one with more versatility in terms of histopathological characteristics.

It is important to highlight that previous literature on the subject of lipomatous tumors of the mediastinum may not be entirely accurate as tumors designated as "lipomas" may in fact represent examples of thymolipoma. It is known that, with increasing age, the thymus is represented more by adipose tissue than by thymic tissue, thus explaining the possible interpretation of mediastinal lipoma when the tumor may likely have been a thymolipoma. Thus, even though credit is given to Lange [4] for the first description of an adipose tissue tumor in the thymus, the most accurate description and introduction of the term "thymolipoma" came much later in the literature. In 1937, Andrus and Foot [5] described a large anterior mediastinal tumor in a 13-year-old young boy, which the authors recorded as weighing more than 2,000 grams, and histologically resembling "lipoma" with areas of thymic tissue, which the authors designated as "benign thymoma." In 1949, Hall [6] described a similar tumor to the one described by Andrus and Foot [5], in a 47-year-old man who had died of head trauma and who, during an autopsy procedure, was found to have an anterior mediastinal mass. The tumor was described as large, pedunculated, arising from the anterior mediastinum, and lying almost entirely in the right pleural cavity. The tumor was composed of mature adipose tissue and thymic tissue. Based on those findings, Hall [6] considered this tumor a definite entity, suggesting the term "thymolipoma." Interestingly, Hall [6] provided two possibilities to account for this occurrence: one, that the adipose tissue represents a true tumor with a multiplication of thymic tissue, and two, that the growth is primarily a large simple tumor of the thymus, most of which has been replaced by fat. However, the author favored the former explanation, arguing that the latter explanation seems highly unlikely. In addition, Hall [6] suggested that previous descriptions of lipomata might be in fact examples of thymolipoma. He also argued that, in many instances, the presence of thymic tissue may be minimal and easily overlooked, thus prompting the diagnosis of "lipoma." In more modern literature, other authors have lumped different entities like lipoma and involuted thymic hyperplasia into the same spectrum of thymolipomas. Toyama and colleagues [7] described three cases under the designation of "thymolipoma," including one case of lipoma and another of involuted thymic hyperplasia. Interestingly, the authors stated that, in one of the cases described, only one histological section was available for evaluation. Such descriptions hark back the observations of Hall [6], who stated in 1949 that in some cases the presence of thymic tissue may be minimal and can be easily overlooked, thus rendering a different interpretation, as exemplified by the cases reported by Toyama and colleagues [7]. Nevertheless, it is very likely that those two entities represent the same clinicopathological condition that we call "thymolipoma" and that in those cases in which no apparent thymic tissue is present, either the tissue has been overlooked or perhaps the tumor has not been sampled properly.

In general terms, whether we consider these entities of thymolipoma and lipoma together or separately, they remain unusual neoplasms that may represent a small component of all mediastinal neoplasms, possibly representing no more than 10% of all thymic neoplasms. Clinically, thymolipomas have been associated with myasthenia gravis (MG). In this regard, Rieker and colleagues [8] reported nine cases emphasizing its association with MG in five men and four women between the ages of 36 and 76 years. The authors also emphasize that approximately 50% of patients with these tumors may also have another associated autoimmune condition such as aplastic anemia, hypogammaglobulinemia, lichen planus, and Grave's disease. In Rieker's [8] description of nine cases, seven of those patients presented initially with MG. In addition, the authors stated that in one patient the symptoms of MG improved after resection of the mediastinal tumor. Also, Damadoglu and colleagues [9] reported ten cases of thymolipoma in six women and four men between the ages of 16 and 67 years. In this report of ten patients, five patients also had associated MG. It is important to note that the great majority of cases reported in the literature have come via single case reports in which the authors have found either a specific histological feature or a specific clinical condition associated with the tumor [10–16]. Radiologically, Rosado-de-Christenson [17] reported the experience with 27 cases of thymolipoma in which diagnostic imaging was available. The authors encountered 15 male and 12 female patients between the ages of 2–66 years and a mean age of 26.7 years. All the tumors were located in the anterior mediastinum: 12 tumors simulated cardiomegaly and 12 tumors draped over the ipsilateral diaphragm, simulating diaphragmatic elevation. By computed tomographic scans, ten tumors demonstrated a mixture of fat and soft tissue attenuation, which microscopically corresponded to thymic and adipose tissue (Figs. 12.1 and 12.2). Magnetic resonance images in two cases demonstrated fat and soft tissue signal intensity characteristics. In the largest series reported today of 33 cases from the Armed Forces Institute of Pathology in 1995 [18], the authors described 18 male and 15 female patients between the ages of 2 and 64 years. Clinically, none of the patients had a history of myasthenia gravis, and their symptoms were non-specific, including upper respiratory symptoms and chest pain. Important to highlight is that the majority of the patients described were asymptomatic. In addition, the age group most commonly affected appeared to be between 10 and 30 years of age, with fewer cases in either extreme. All the tumors were located in the anterior mediastinum, and complete surgical resection was accomplished in all the cases.

Based on the published cases thus far, it is apparent that thymolipomas (lipothymomas or lipomas) are tumors of the anterior mediastinum (Fig. 12.1) that can affect any age group without specific gender predilection. However, the tumors in children appear to be uncommon. Important to highlight is that complete surgical resection is the treatment of choice in these tumors, and that, if it is accomplished, the patients are cured with no need to additional therapy. Thus far, no recurrence or metastatic disease has been reported in these cases.

Pathological Features

Macroscopically, these tumors have been described as well demarcated, lobulated, soft, and yellowish in color (Fig. 12.3). Solid areas also can be admixed with the adipose tissue. These tumors can reach a fairly large size of more than 30 cm in greatest dimension and can weigh more than 2 thousand grams. Areas of necrosis, hemorrhage, or marked cystic degeneration are not a characteristic of these tumors.

Histologically, the tumors, as their name implies, are composed of variable amounts of thymic and adipose tissue; while in some cases, the amounts can be fairly equal in proportion, in other cases the presence of thymic tissue is more minimal. In some areas, the tumors preserved some of the architectural features of the thymic gland, while in other areas, there is more haphazard distribution of adipose and thymic tissue. The thymic tissue shows the conventional dual population of lymphocytes and epithelial cells with or without Hassall's corpuscles. In some cases, the Hassall's corpuscles appear to have undergone calcification, while in other areas the thymic tissue appears to have undergone atrophy. The adipose tissue does not show any atypical features, and it is composed of mature adipose tissue. Essentially, thymolipomas are composed of normal thymic tissue admixed with mature adipose tissue (Figs. 12.4, 12.5, 12.6, 12.7, 12.8, 12.9, and 12.10).

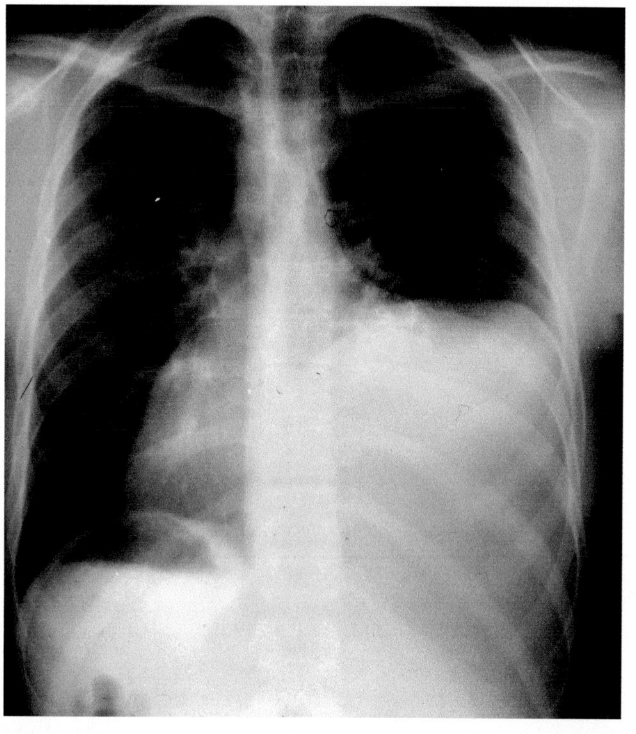

Fig. 12.1 Plain films of the thorax show a large anterior mediastinal mass

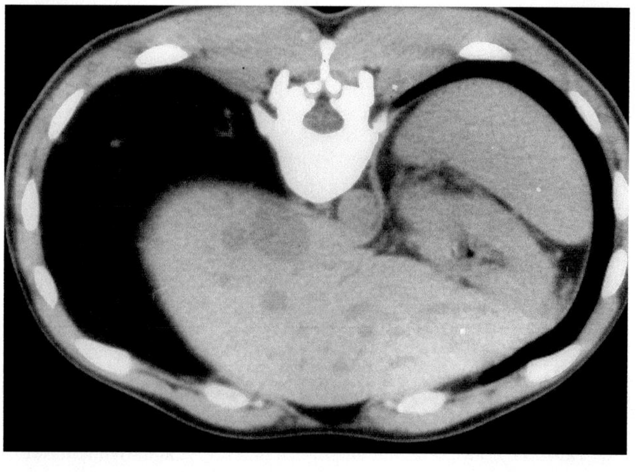

Fig. 12.2 CT scan of the thorax shows a large anterior mediastinal mass

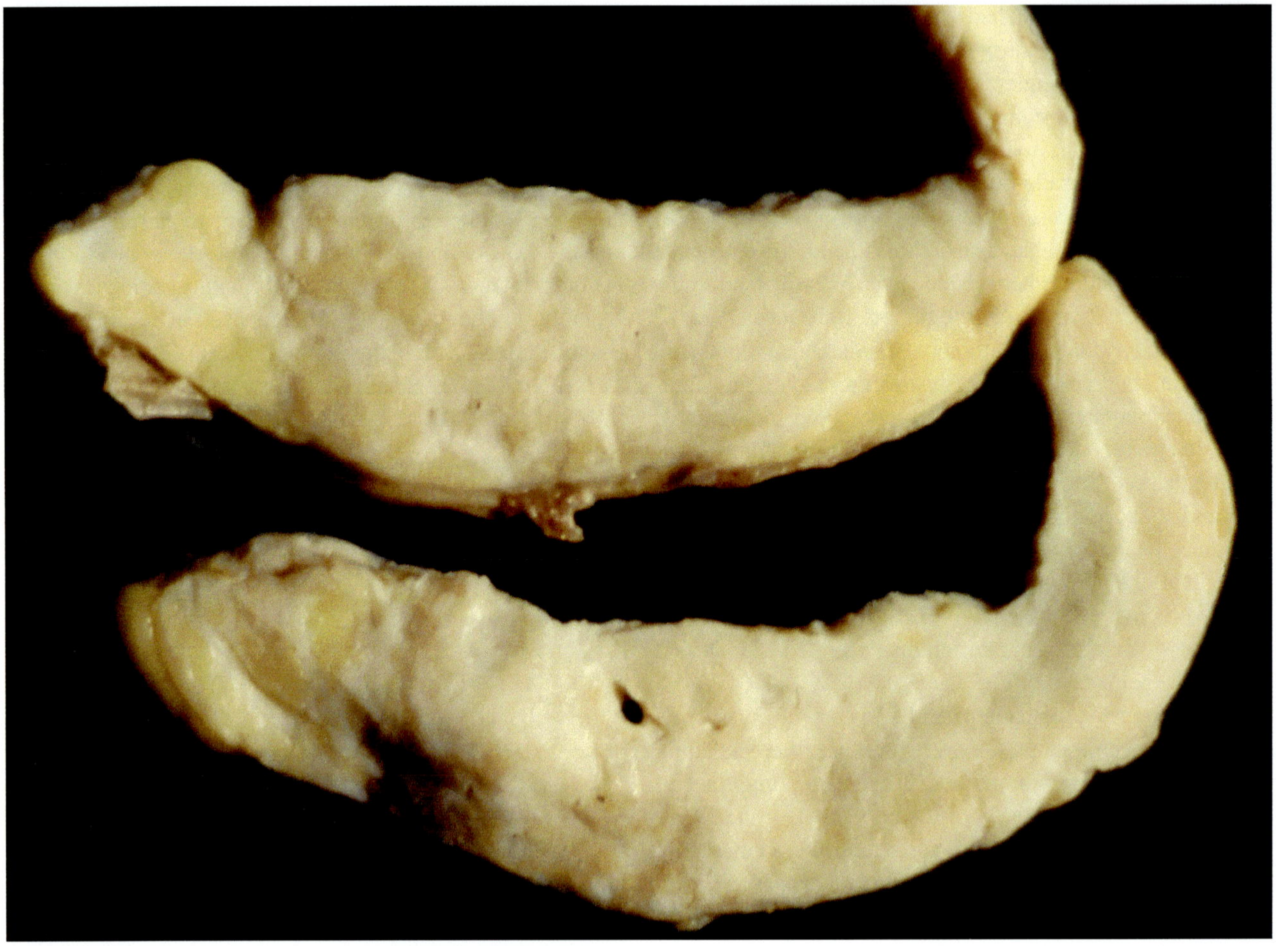

Fig. 12.3 Thymolipoma shows a fleshy yellowish and lobular appearance

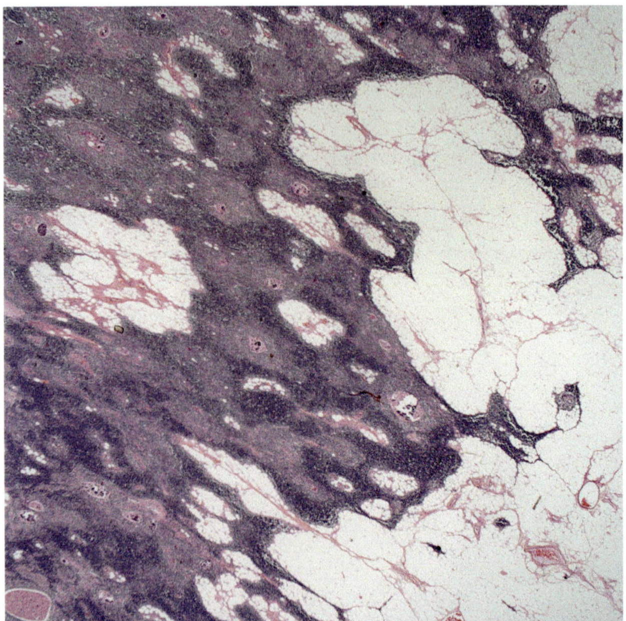

Fig. 12.4 Thymolipoma showing areas of adipose and thymic tissue

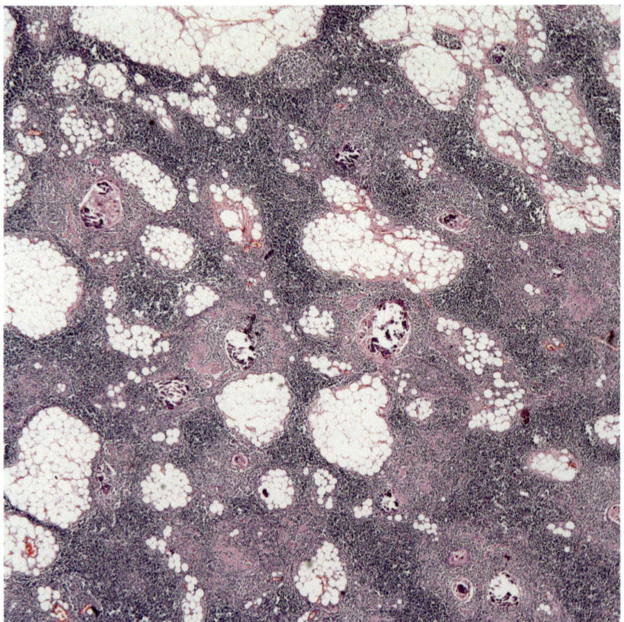

Fig. 12.5 Thymolipoma showing areas of thymic tissue with numerous calcifications and minor component of adipose tissue

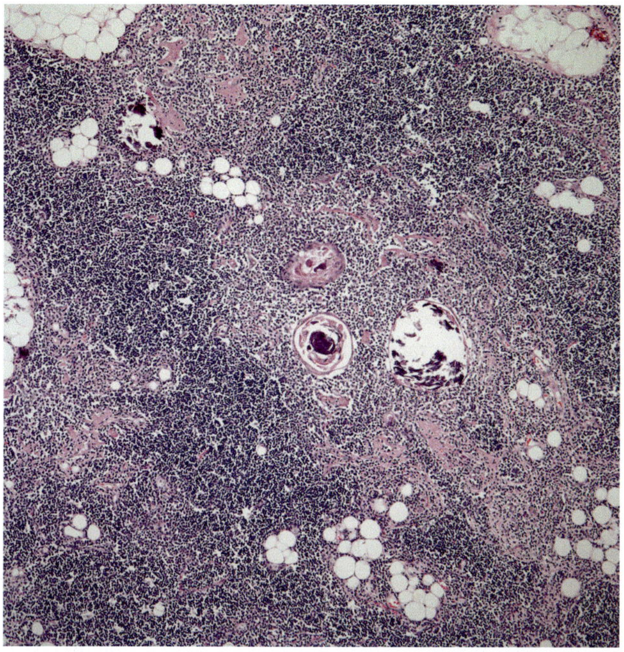

Fig. 12.6 Thymic tissue in thymolipoma with calcified Hassall's corpuscles

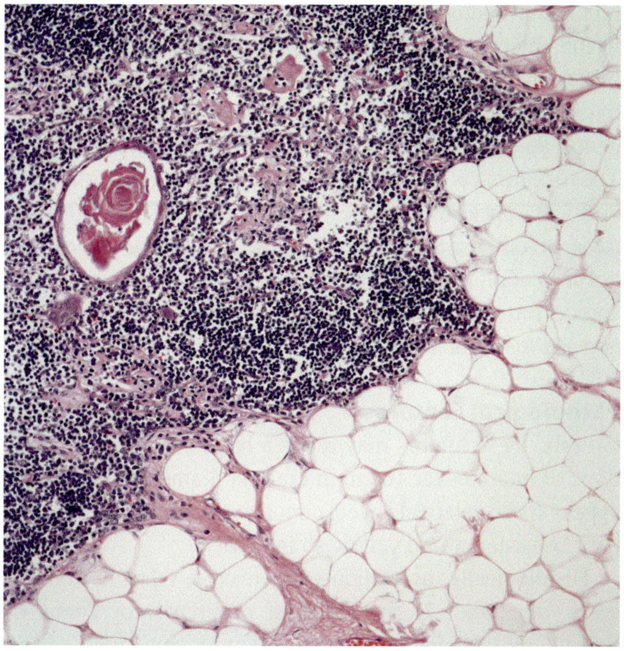

Fig. 12.7 Thymolipoma with almost equal component of thymic and adipose tissue

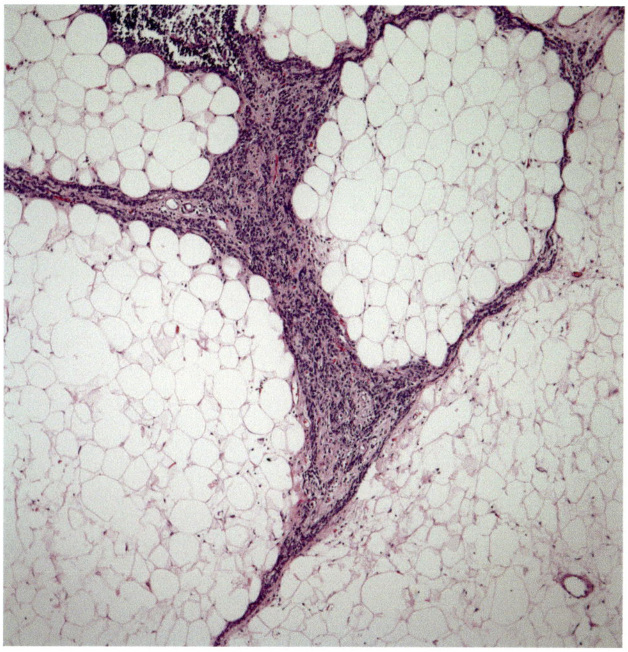

Fig. 12.8 Thymolipoma predominantly composed of adipose tissue

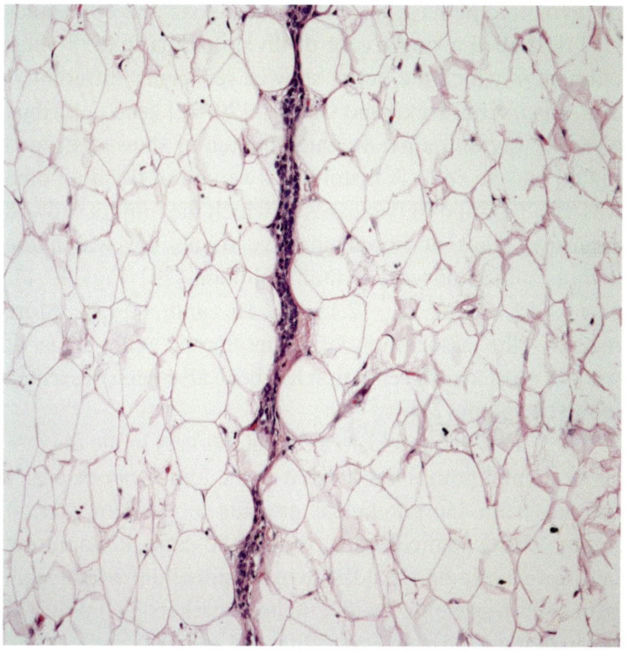

Fig. 12.9 Thymolipoma showing only a strand of residual thymic tissue

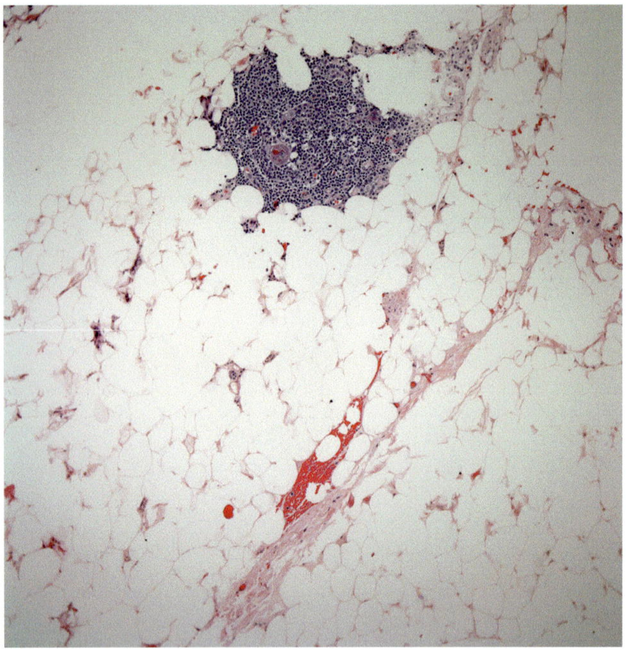

Fig. 12.10 Thymolipoma with a focal remnant of thymic tissue

It is important to mention that some histological variants of thymolipoma have been described. Ajaz and colleagues [19] described a single case of thymolipoma in a 58-year-old man in which the tumor showed sebaceous differentiation. Also, Kim, Iseki, and Gannon [20–22] each described a case of thymolipoma in which the tumor showed striated myoid muscle cells. A histological variant of thymolipoma was also reported in two cases in which the tumors showed extensive areas of fibroconnective tissue, for which the authors coined the term thymofibrolipoma [23] (Figs. 12.11, 12.12, 12.13, 12.14, 12.15, 12.16, and 12.17). More recently, the association of thymolipoma with areas of smooth muscle differentiation has been also been described in the literature [24].

The use of immunohistochemical markers in the diagnosis of thymolipomas has no role as the tumor can be easily diagnosed on morphological grounds alone. However, if immunohistochemical stains were to be done, it would not be surprising to find that the thymic epithelium would stain with keratin as well as with lymphoid markers including Tdt for immature lymphocytes, while the adipose tissue would show possible staining for S-100 protein. In cases in which the tumors may also show different components – whether those components are skeletal muscle, smooth muscle, sebaceous differentiation, or another type of component that is not the conventional thymic and adipose tissue – then the use of the proper immunohistochemical stains may be warranted.

Differential Diagnosis

Although the diagnosis of thymolipomas in resected material is rather straightforward, the fact is that the diagnosis is rarely accomplished in small mediastinoscopic biopsies. In this regard, it is very likely that the tissue sampled may be either represented by adipose tissue or thymic tissue. In those cases in which the two components may be present, the challenge is to separate thymolipoma from thymic hyperplasia, thymoma, or any other tumor in which these two components may be present. Then, final diagnosis for thymolipomas can be accurately done on resected specimens. In addition, even though some of the radiographic findings may suggest such possibility, the final diagnosis remains a histopathological interpretation.

Angiomyolipoma

The occurrence of this tumor in the mediastinal compartment is rare. It is possible that the description of the first case reported in the mediastinum is in the French literature by Bertrand and colleagues [25] in 1984. Essentially, after this description, there have been several more cases described, mainly in the form of case reports [26–31]. Most of these reports have attested to the occurrence of this type of tumor in the anterior mediastinum, with only a single case in the posterior mediastinum. Many of the cases reported that the finding of the anterior mediastinal mass has been rather incidental during a routine imaging study for different reasons. The occurrence of anterior mediastinal angiomyolipomas does not appear to be closely associated with tuberous sclerosis or other types of syndromes. The tumor appears to occur in adult patients. Surgical resection is the treatment of choice for these patients, and complete surgical resection appears to be curative.

Pathological Features

Grossly, these tumors may reach a large size, with descriptions of tumors over 10 cm in greatest diameter. The tumors appear to be relatively well circumscribed with a soft rubbery consistency and yellowish in color.

Histologically, as angiomyolipomas in other anatomical areas, the tumor is composed of different proportions of smooth muscle and adipose tissue with numerous ectatic blood vessels (Figs. 12.18, 12.19, and 12.20). In some areas, the tumor may acquire an epithelioid appearance, showing a more solid cellular proliferation with ectatic vessels and little intervening adipose tissue, mimicking a hemangiopericytoma. Residual thymic tissue has been reported surrounding the angiomyolipoma in some cases. The tumor characteristically does not show mitotic activity, necrosis, and/or hemorrhage.

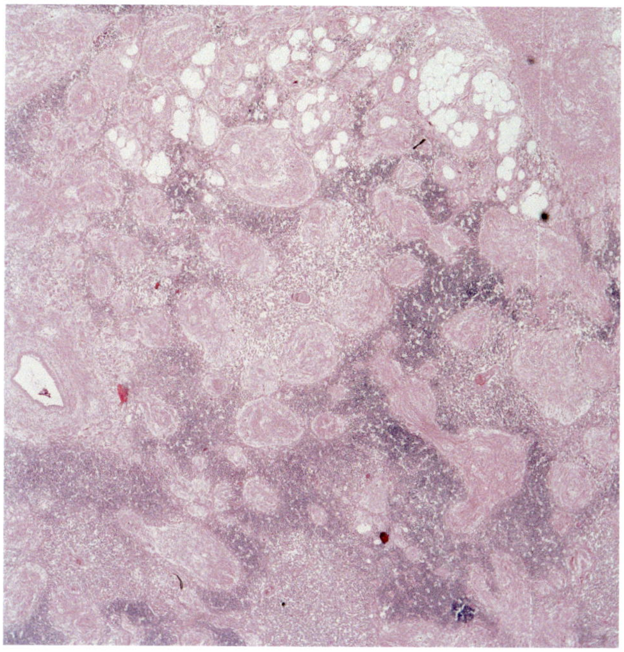

Fig. 12.11 Thymofibrolipoma showing areas of fibrosis

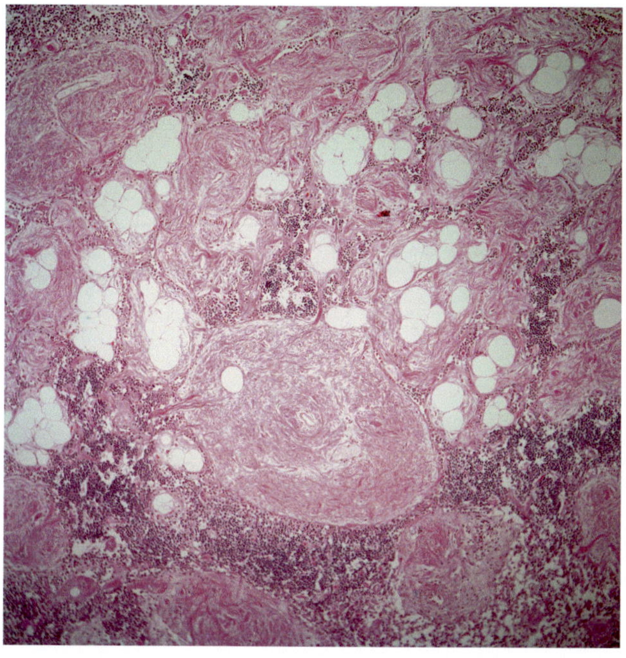

Fig. 12.12 Thymofibrolipoma with more discrete presence of adipose tissue

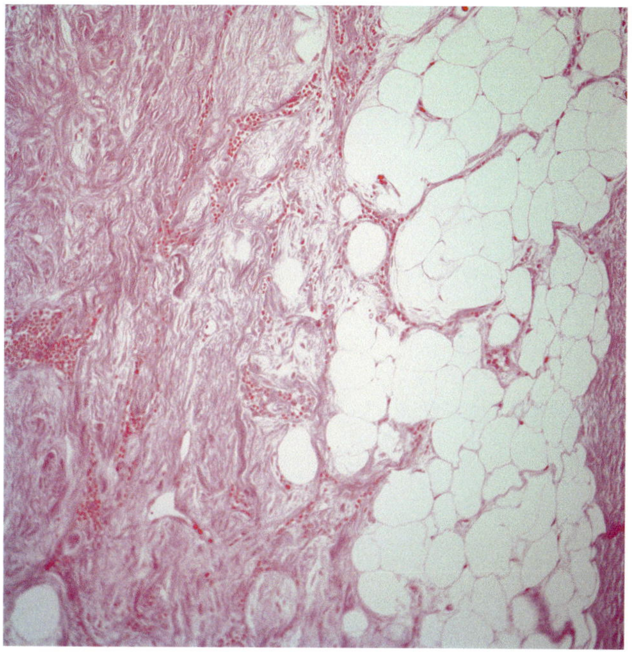

Fig. 12.13 Thymofibrolipoma showing more extensive areas of fibrosis and mature adipose tissue

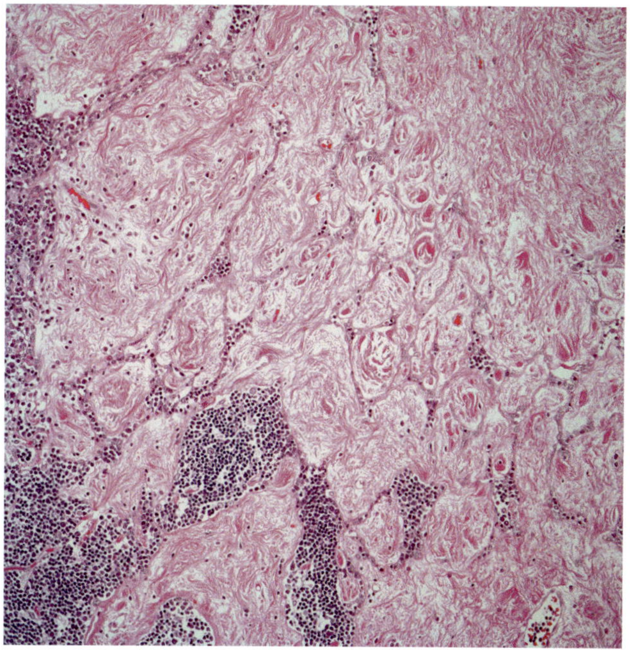

Fig. 12.14 Thymofibrolipoma with only focal areas of residual thymic tissue

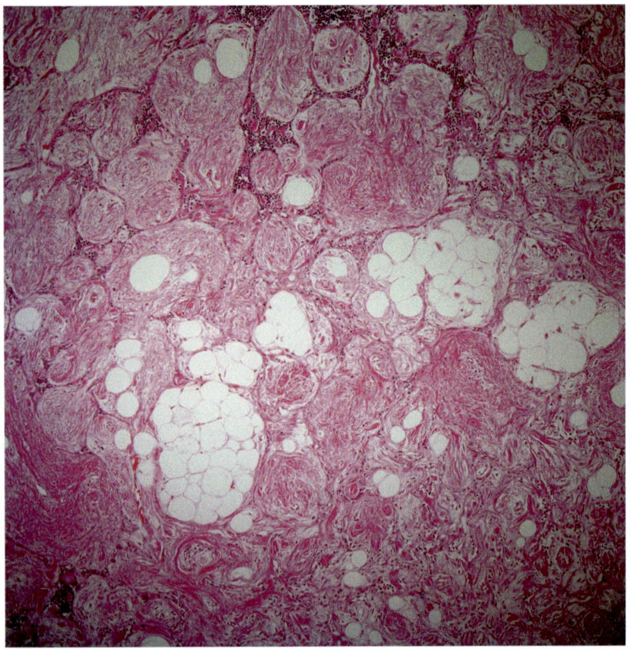

Fig. 12.15 Thymofibrolipoma with well-defined areas of adipose tissue

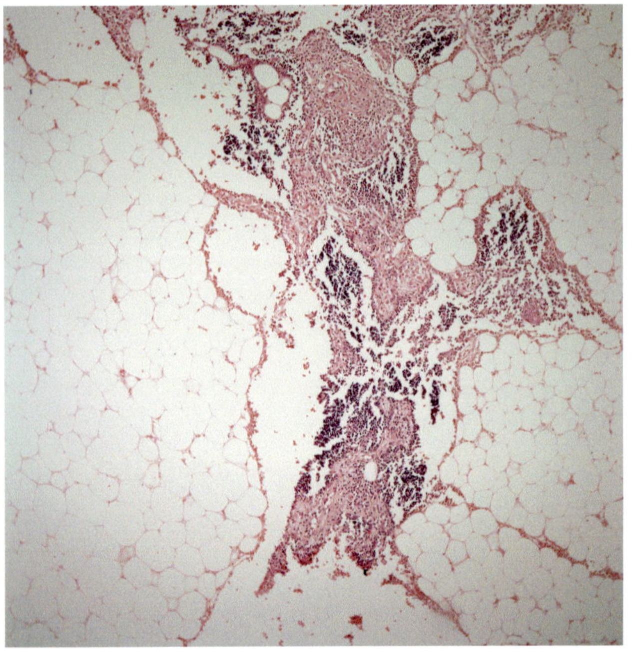

Fig. 12.16 Thymolipoma with focal areas of residual thymic tissue and myoid cells

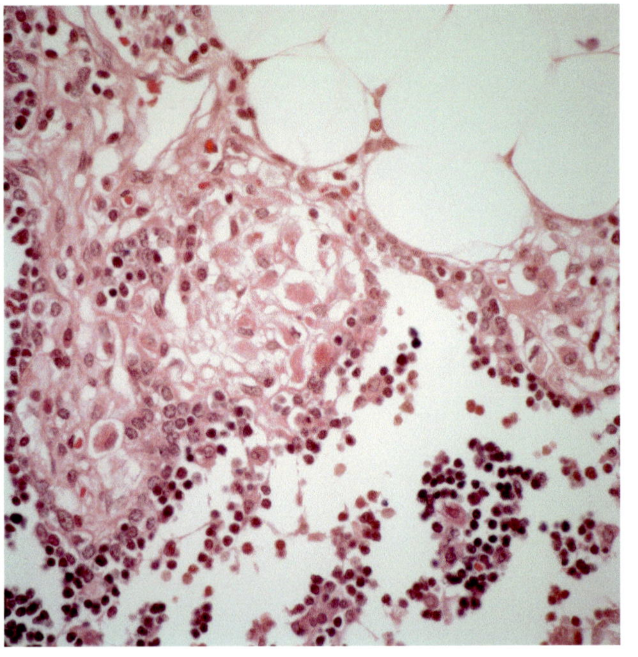

Fig. 12.17 Higher magnification of a thymolipoma with myoid component

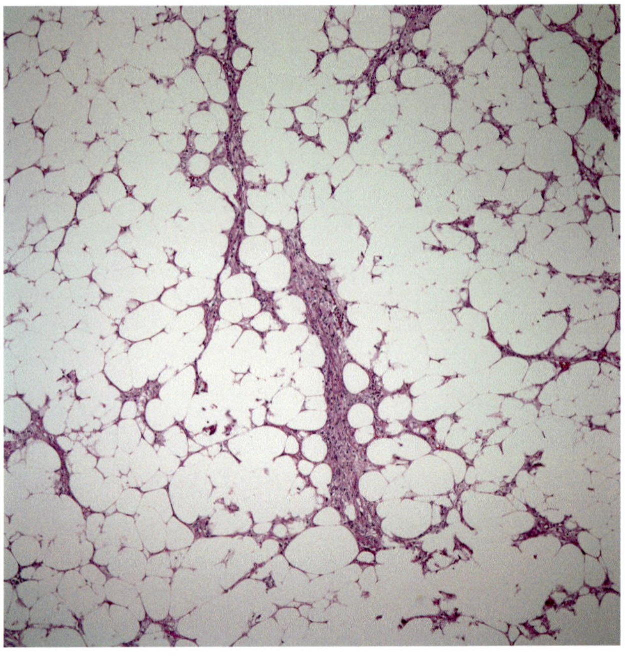

Fig. 12.18 Anterior mediastinal angiomyolipoma showing predominantly mature adipose tissue and strands of smooth muscle

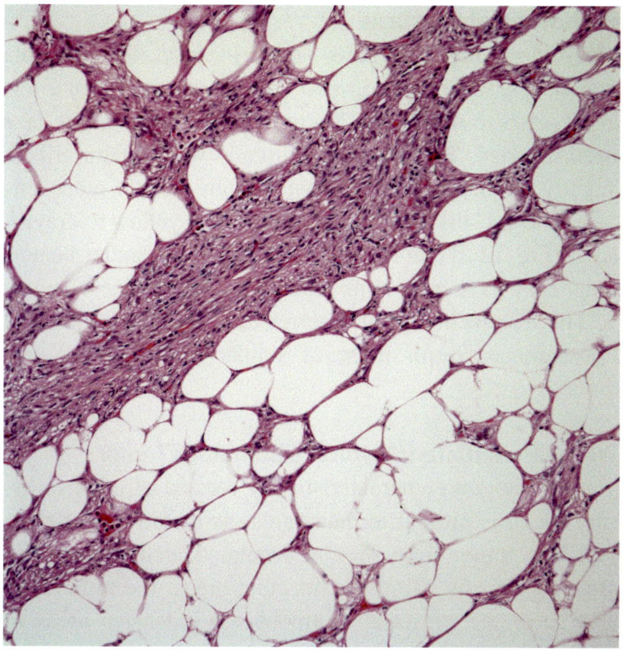

Fig. 12.19 Anterior mediastinal angiomyolipoma showing easily identifiable smooth muscle admixed with adipose tissue

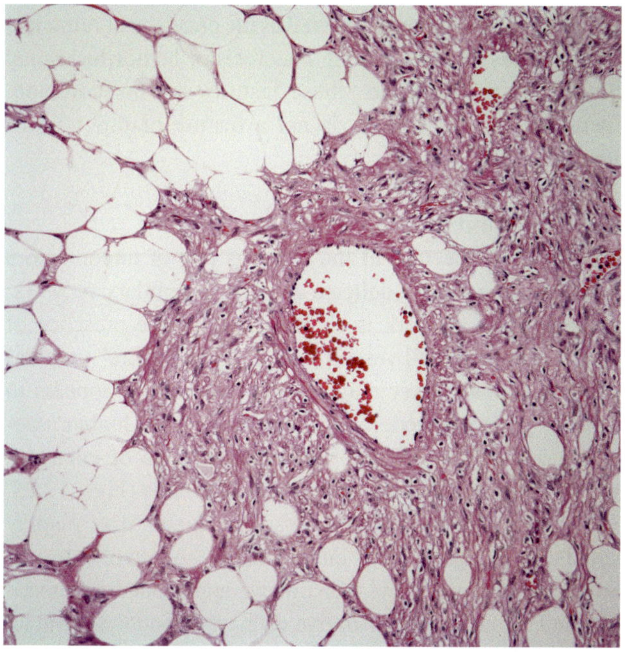

Fig. 12.20 Typical features of angiomyolipoma showing adipose tissue, smooth muscle, and ectatic vessels

Immunohistochemical stains have been reported mirroring similar tumors in other anatomic areas, mainly positive staining for HMB-45, CD34, and smooth muscle actin.

Differential Diagnosis

In small mediastinoscopic biopsies, the diagnostics of angiomyolipoma may be challenging. Due to sampling issues, tumors that will need to be considered in the differential diagnosis include thymolipoma, liposarcoma, or a smooth muscle neoplasm, depending of the tissue sampled. In a surgical resection, the diagnosis may become more apparent; however, similar conditions will enter in the differential diagnosis. In cases in which there is marked presence of smooth muscle component, the possibility of a well-differentiated liposarcoma with muscle component needs to be carefully ruled out.

Liposarcomas

It is well known that the occurrence of liposarcomas in the human body is much more common in deep soft tissue areas such as the extremities, and in adult individuals. The histopathological spectrum of these tumors in the soft tissues is well recognized. In contrast to benign adipose tissue tumors in the mediastinum, mediastinal liposarcomas appear to be more common or at least more commonly reported. Nevertheless, similar spectrum as the one that has been reported in soft tissues seems to mirror tumors occurring in the mediastinal compartment. Important to recognize is that, even though in the mediastinum the anterior compartment appears to be more commonly affected, the tumor may also occur in the posterior compartment.

In general terms, liposarcomas may account for approximately 9 to 16% of all soft tissue sarcomas. This percentage will be dramatically lower for the occurrence of these tumors in the mediastinum. For instance, in a recent review of 19 cases of pleomorphic liposarcomas, Downes and colleagues [32] identified only a single case of such a tumor in the mediastinal compartment. Alaggio and colleagues [33], in a study of 82 liposarcomas occurring in patients younger than 22 years of age, encountered 6 such tumors in the mediastinum. In a more focused report of intrathoracic liposarcomas, Chen and colleagues [34] reported 23 cases of which 10 were in the mediastinum, while the remaining were in the lung and pleura. It is evident that the occurrence of liposarcomas in the thoracic cavity is more common in the mediastinum in contrast to such tumors occurring in the lung parenchyma or pleura. Important to highlight is that the histopathologic criteria for the diagnosis of mediastinal liposarcomas are the same as for tumors in the soft tissue. In addition, the histopathologic spectrum of tumors in the soft tissue also mirrors that encountered in the mediastinal compartment. In essence, the mediastinal liposarcomas may also be divided into three important categories: well-differentiated, myxoid/round cell, and pleomorphic. In some of these categories, there may be histological variants. Also important to highlight is the immunohistochemical profile and molecular analysis of such tumors in the mediastinum, which is essentially the same as those reported in the soft tissues. As it would be expected, the majority of reports of mediastinal liposarcomas have been made via single case reports [35–39], with only a few relatively large series of cases [40–43].

Clinically, mediastinal liposarcomas affect predominantly adult individuals; however, the spectrum of ages in which these tumors have been observed in the mediastinum is wide and includes children under 5 years of age and adults over 70 years of age. The symptomatology that these patients may present is also diverse and includes non-specific symptoms such as cough, dyspnea, and chest pain. In some cases, the presence of superior vena cava syndrome has been reported as the presenting symptom. The anterior mediastinal mass also can be discovered during a routine chest radiographic evaluation. Diagnostic imaging usually discloses the presence of a large anterior mediastinal mass. In one of the first relatively large series of anterior mediastinal liposarcomas, Klimstra and colleagues [40] reported 28 cases in 16 males and 12 females, ranging in ages from 14 to 72 years. In this particular series of mediastinal liposarcomas, routine chest films in approximately 40% of the patients incidentally detected the tumor. In addition, the histology of the majority of the cases (25/28) was of the low-grade liposarcoma. Follow-up information obtained in 23 patients showed that 7 patients had recurrence in a mean interval of 3 years, while 8 patients died in a mean interval of 2.6 years. Fifteen patients were reported alive in a mean interval of 2 years. The authors stated that myxoid tumors exhibited more aggressive behavior than well-differentiated tumors. However, metastatic disease was not documented in any of the patients. Hahn and Fletcher [41] also reported a similar number of cases in 13 males and 11 females; however, 3 patients in this report were children under 15 year of age. Histologically, ten cases corresponded to well-differentiated tumors, eight were dedifferentiated, four were pleomorphic, and two were myxoid. Recurrence and distant metastasis were documented in this group of patients. The authors concluded that mediastinal liposarcomas share similar clinicopathologic features with similar tumors in the retroperitoneum. More recently, Ortega and coworkers [43] reported a specific study of 18 cases of liposarcomas of the posterior mediastinum. The authors reported 11 males and 8 females between the ages of 29 and 87 years. Clinically, the symptoms were non-specific similar to those reported for anterior mediastinal tumors. Histologically, the majority of cases were of the well-differentiated type (55%). In this group of cases, two patients with myxoid/round cell liposarcomas died within 3 years with disseminated metastatic disease. One patient with well-differentiated neoplasm was also reported with metastasis to the liver.

Based on the available literature, it appears that complete surgical resection is the treatment of choice for mediastinal liposarcomas. However, for tumors which are not amenable for complete surgical resection or for higher-grade histological types, it is possible that additional therapy in the form of radiation therapy can be used.

Pathological Features

Macroscopically, regardless of the location, these tumors may have a wide range in size. Tumors ranging from a few centimeters to more than 30 cm in greatest dimension have been reported. The tumors are usually well-circumscribed, slightly lobulated, soft, yellowish, with smooth outer surface. The cut surface may show lobulated, yellow to grayish areas (Fig. 12.21). Focal solid areas, necrosis, and/or hemorrhage may be seen in some cases.

The histopathological features described in mediastinal liposarcomas mirror those of similar tumors in the soft tissues.

Well-Differentiated/Atypical Lipomatous Tumor

These tumors are characteristically formed of adipose tissue, which is present in many areas as mature adipose tissue. The tumor may show a lobulated architecture with areas of fibrosis. However, in other areas, the tumor will also show the presence of lipoblasts. Extensive areas of sclerosis with fibrous septa of varying thickness may be present. At higher magnification, the tumor will show the presence of lipoblastic atypical mononucleated or multinucleated cells (Figs. 12.22, 12.23, 12.24, 12.25, 12.26, and 12.27). The tumor may also display the presence of an inflammatory component as well as the presence of remnants of thymic tissue. Even though necrosis or hemorrhage may be seen in these tumors, these features are not common. Increased mitotic activity is not a feature of this type of liposarcoma.

Myxoid/Round Cell

The basic architecture of the tumor is that of tumor with a myxoid stroma and a delicate arborizing capillary network. This capillary network is characterized by the presence of thin, branching small vessels with a "chicken wire" vascular pattern. At low power magnification, the tumor appears to show a "pulmonary edema-like appearance." At higher magnification, the tumor may show the presence of enlarged, vacuolated cells, and signet ring cell lipoblasts (Figs. 12.28, 12.29, and 12.30). In some areas, the tumor may display spindle or elongated cells embedded in the myxoid stroma. Some tumors may show a distinctive appearance composed of small round to oval primitive cells with vacuolated nuclei (Figs. 12.31, 12.32, and 12.33). Focal areas of necrosis and/or hemorrhage may be seen in these cases, while increase mitotic activity is not common.

Pleomorphic

These tumors, as their name implies, show areas in which the adipose tissue component may not be easily identifiable, as the tumor characteristically shows enlarged mononucleated or multinucleated cells with enlarge pleomorphic nuclei (Figs. 12.34, 12.35, 12.36, and 12.37). Areas of

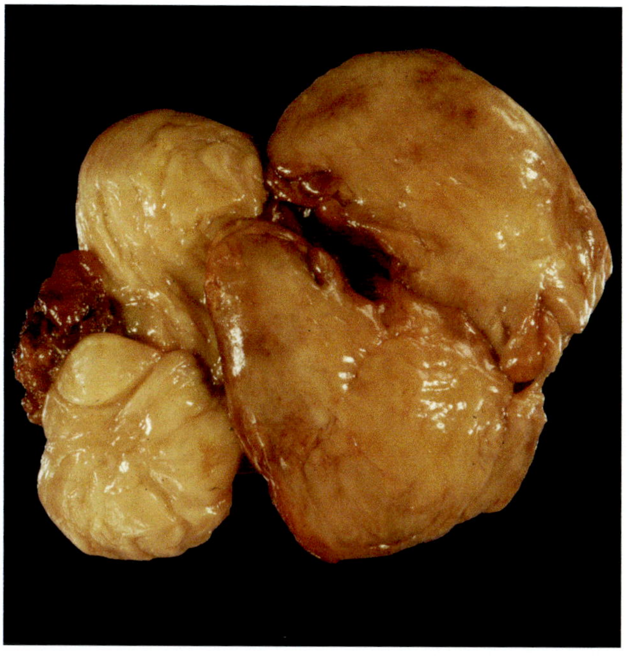

Fig. 12.21 Large anterior mediastinal liposarcoma showing a yellowish lobulated mass

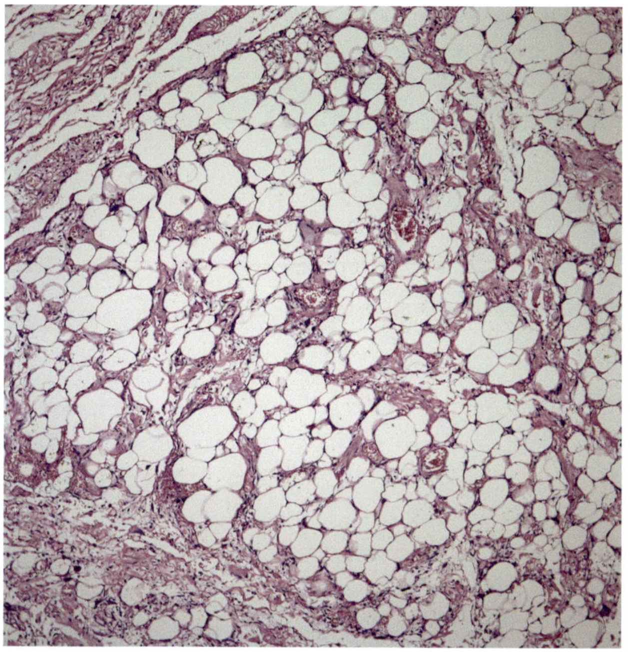

Fig. 12.22 Anterior mediastinal well-differentiated liposarcoma showing lobulation and adipose tissue

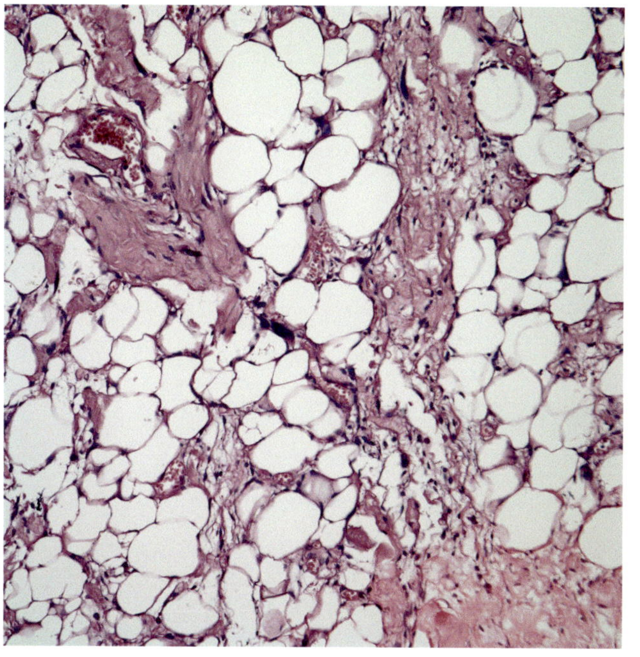

Fig. 12.23 Well-differentiated liposarcoma showing adipose tissue and cytologic atypia with strands of fibroconnective tissue

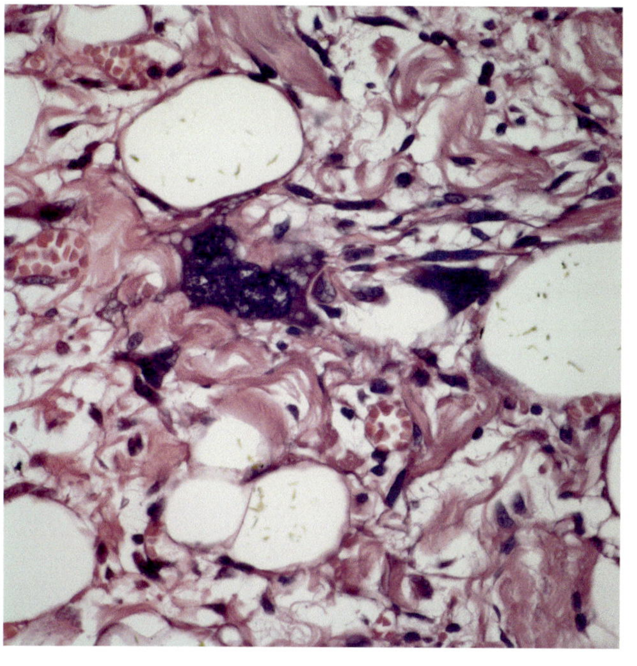

Fig. 12.24 Higher magnification of a well-differentiated liposarcoma showing cellular atypia and multinucleated cells

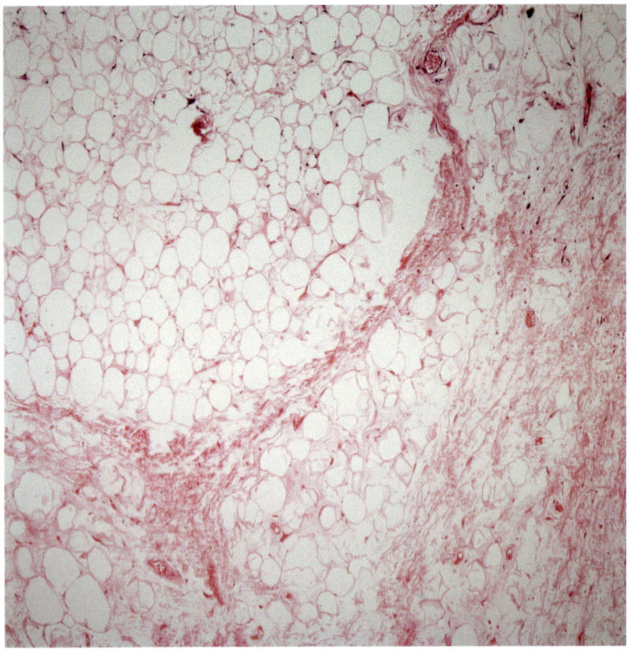

Fig. 12.25 Well-differentiated liposarcoma showing alternating areas of adipose tissue and sclerosis

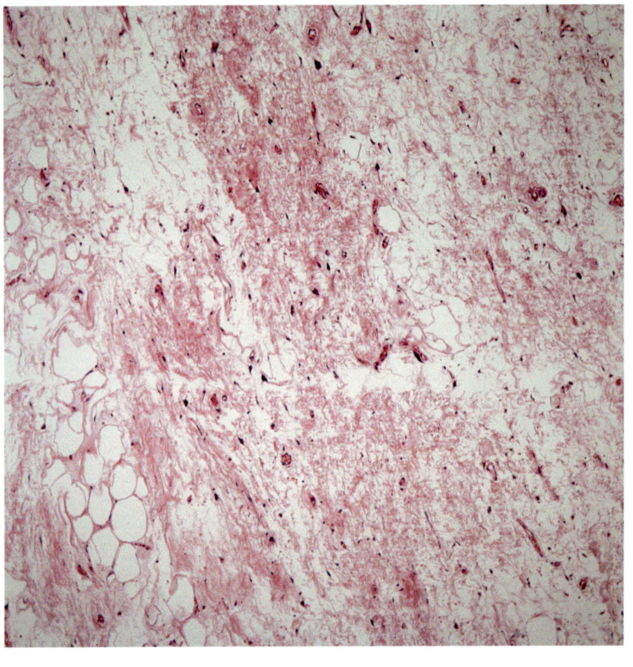

Fig. 12.26 Sclerotic areas showing cellular atypia and focal adipose tissue

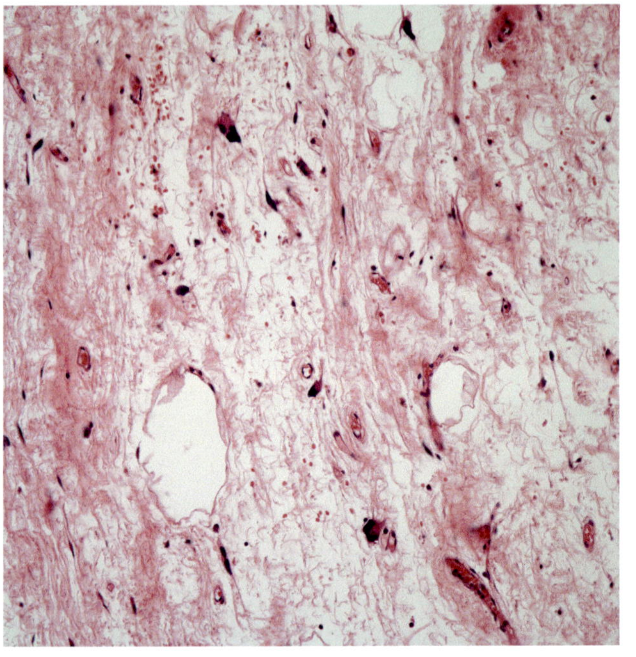

Fig. 12.27 Closer view showing cellular atypia and multinucleated cells

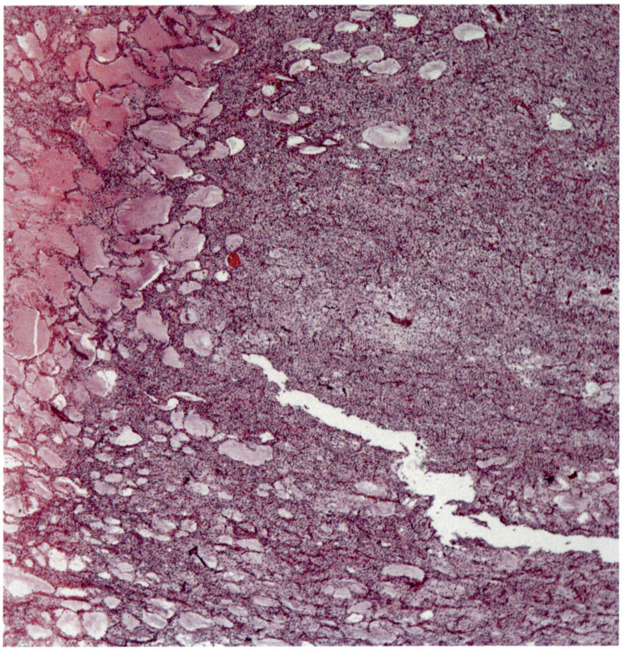

Fig. 12.28 Myxoid liposarcoma showing the characteristic low power view of pulmonary edema-like pattern

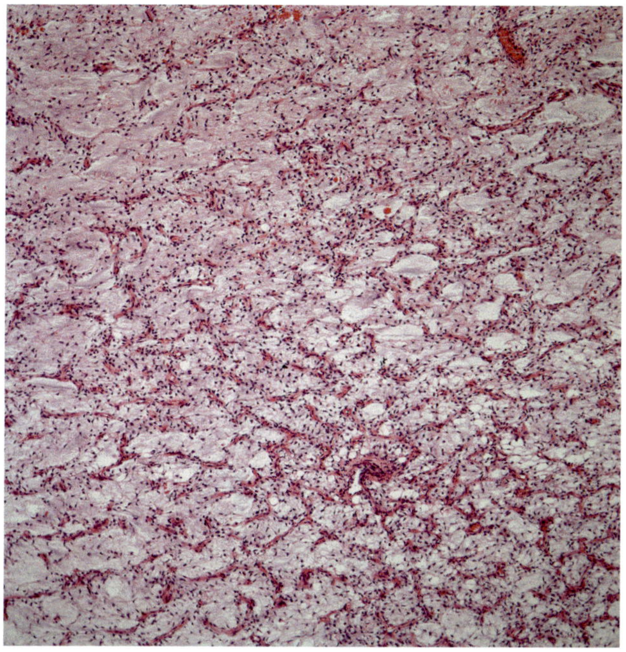

Fig. 12.29 Myxoid liposarcoma showing cellular areas embedded in a myxoid background

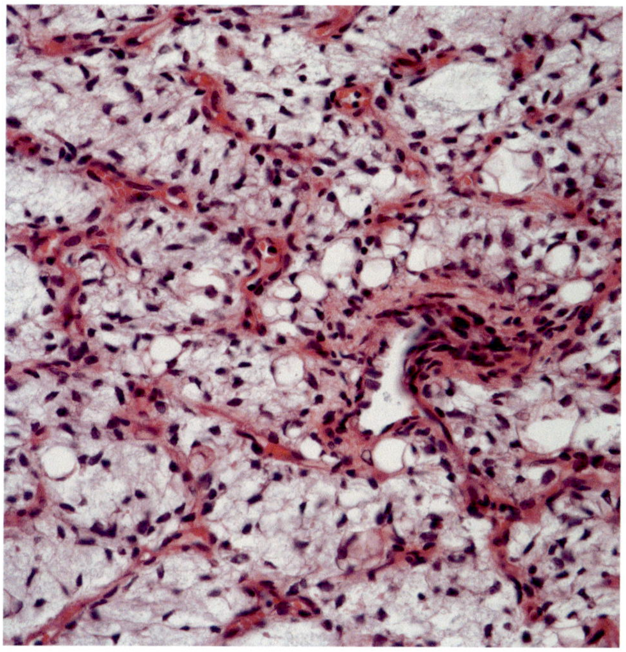

Fig. 12.30 Higher magnification of a myxoid liposarcoma showing cellular areas with a discrete fibrovascular next work

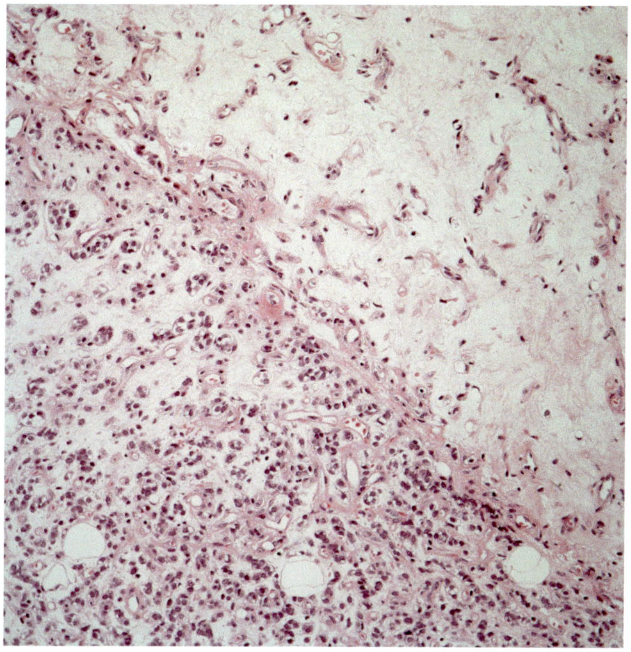

Fig. 12.31 Liposarcoma showing transitional areas of myxoid and round cell liposarcoma

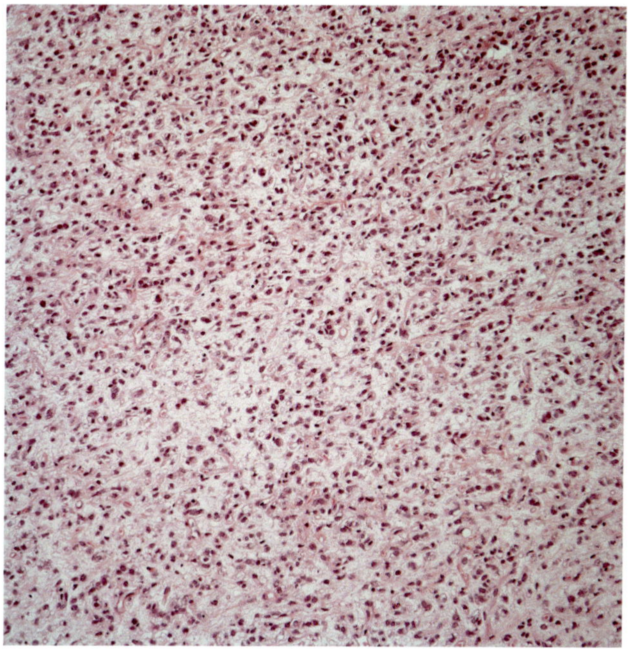

Fig. 12.32 Round cell liposarcoma composed of primitive small cells

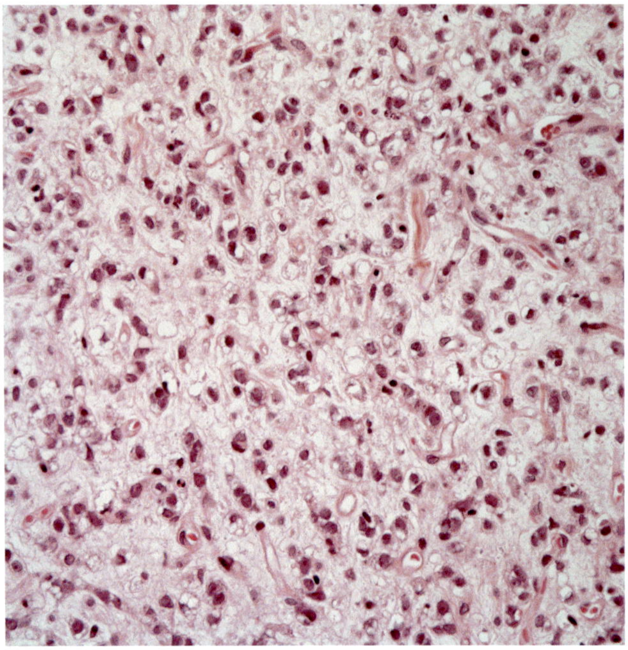

Fig. 12.33 Higher magnification of a round cell liposarcoma showing neoplastic round cells

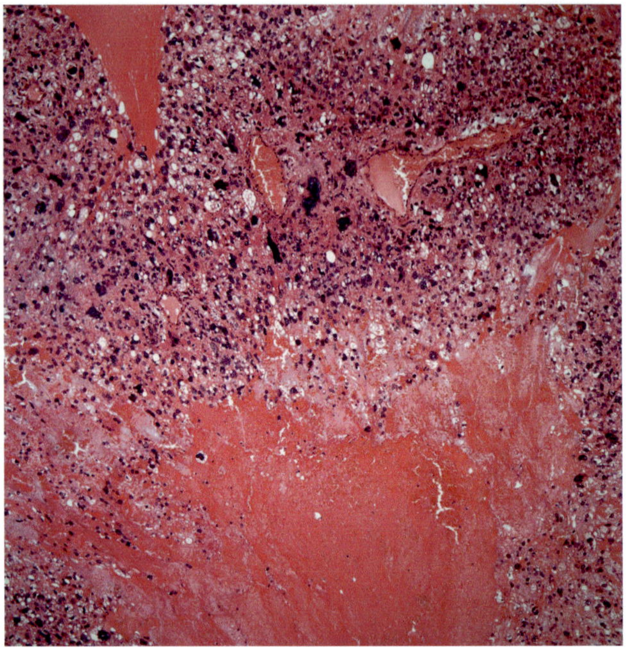

Fig. 12.35 Pleomorphic liposarcoma with areas of hemorrhage

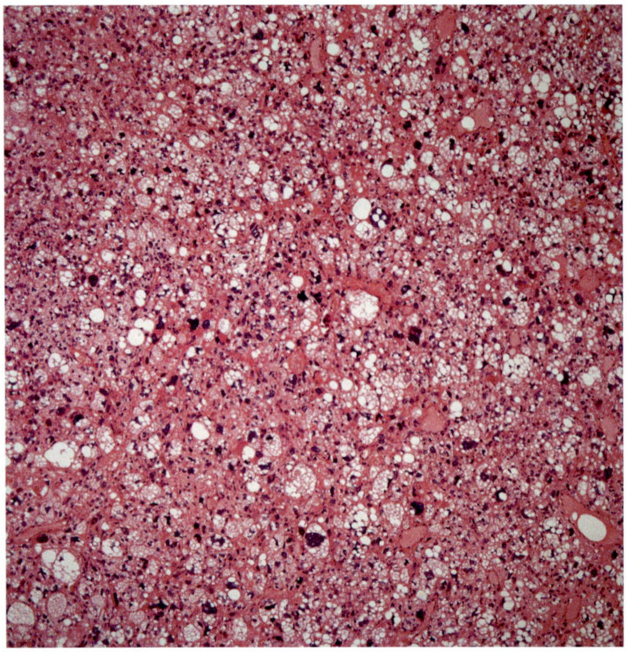

Fig. 12.34 Pleomorphic liposarcoma showing high cellularity and atypia

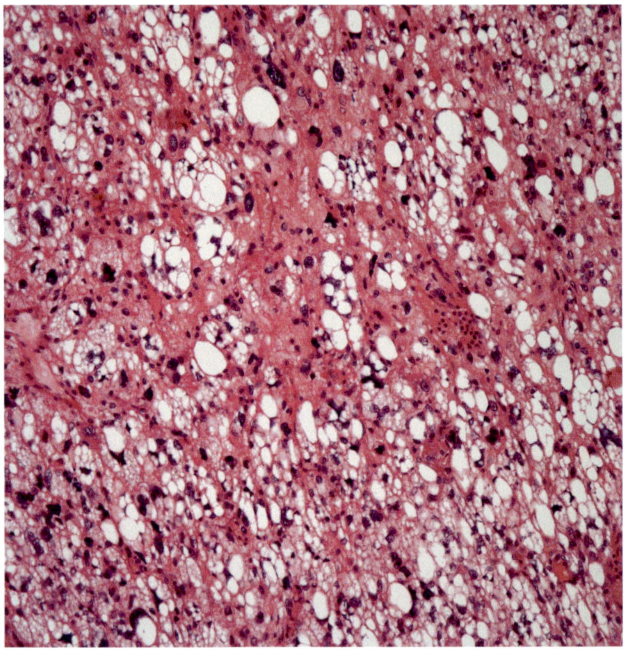

Fig. 12.36 Pleomorphic liposarcoma showing areas in which adipose tissue is still identifiable

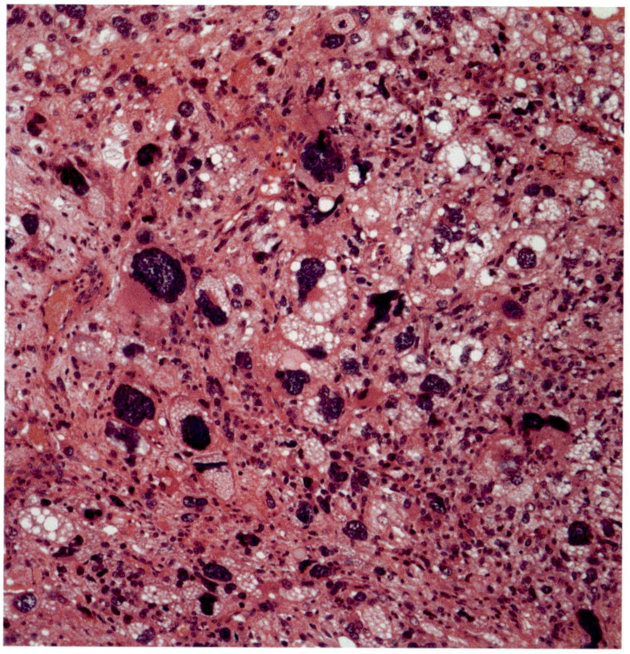

Fig. 12.37 High magnification of a pleomorphic liposarcoma showing prominent cellular atypia

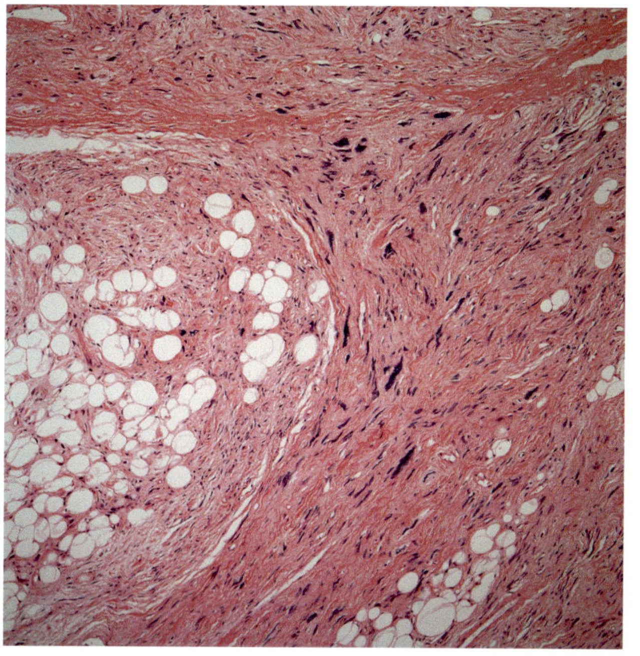

Fig. 12.38 Dedifferentiated liposarcoma showing focal areas of liposarcoma admixed with another non-lipogenic spindle cells sarcoma

necrosis and/or hemorrhage are common in these tumors, and mitotic activity is easily identifiable. The identification of lipoblasts in these tumors is not easily accomplished.

Histological Variants

Dedifferentiated Liposarcoma

This variant is characterized by the presence of areas of well-differentiated liposarcoma with transition to a higher-grade sarcoma. The associated dedifferentiated component (non-lipogenic component) is usually composed of a sarcomatous malignancy in which the presence of nuclear atypia and mitotic activity is easily identifiable (Figs. 12.38, 12.39, and 12.40). The dedifferentiated component of these tumors may be in the form of rhabdomyosarcoma, osteosarcoma, leiomyosarcoma, or angiosarcoma [44].

Smooth Muscle Component

The presence of a smooth muscle component in lipomatous tumors has been well recognized for many years (Figs. 12.41 and 12.42). In 1990, Evan [45] reported three cases of "atypical lipomatous tumor" in three different anatomic areas including the mediastinum. The author stated that the presence of smooth muscle did not appear to influence the behavior of the tumor. Important to highlight is that the occurrence of liposarcoma and leiomyosarcoma or rhabdomyosarcoma has also been predominantly recorded in other tumors outside of the mediastinal compartment [46–49]. The occurrence of this phenomenon in the mediastinum is rare. Gomez-Roman [50] reported a mediastinal tumor in a 72-year-old man, which the authors termed "lipoleiomyosarcoma." Folpe and Weiss [51], in a report of nine cases of "lipoleiomyosarcoma," identified only one case in the mediastinum, while, in a more focused description of this type of association, a report of three cases arising in the mediastinum was reported [52]. It appears that, based on the current report of this type of tumor, anterior mediastinal liposarcomas may be associated with skeletal muscle, smooth muscle, or full-blown leiomyosarcoma.

Epithelioid Liposarcoma

This is a very unusual form of liposarcoma in the mediastinal compartment. This variant of liposarcoma was initially reported by Miettinen and Enzinger [53] in 1999, who encountered 12 cases of a distinctive variant of high-grade liposarcoma which morphologically was reminiscent of a poorly differentiated carcinoma. Even though in the original description of the tumor none of the cases corresponded to the mediastinum, this variant of liposarcoma has also been reported in the mediastinum [54]. The tumor may show similar features to a poorly differentiated carcinoma in which the cellular proliferation may be composed of cords, sheets, or trabeculae of neoplastic cells with ample eosinophilic cytoplasm, round nuclei, and prominent nucleoli (Figs. 12.43, 12.44, 12.45, and 12.46). Even though mitotic activity is not increased, nuclear atypia and mitotic activity are identified. Areas of necrosis may be seen. The tumor may also show focal areas containing lipoblasts and more conventional areas of liposarcoma.

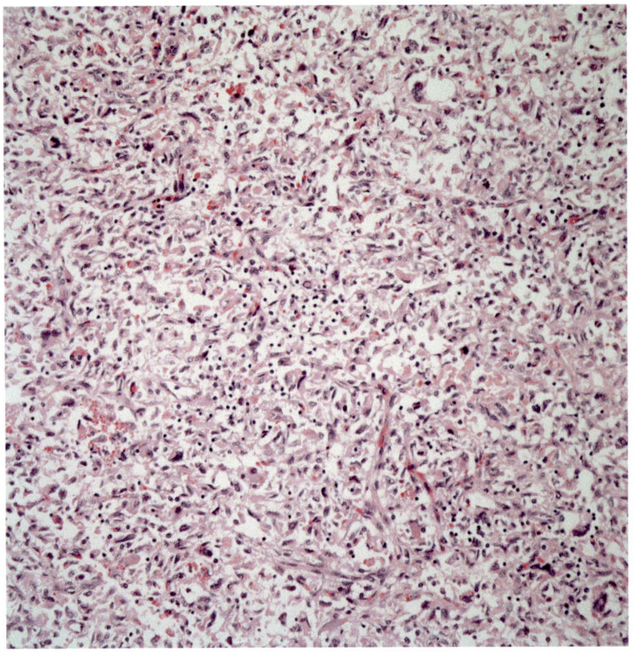

Fig. 12.39 Dedifferentiated liposarcoma showing areas of high-grade sarcoma with features of malignant fibrous histiocytoma

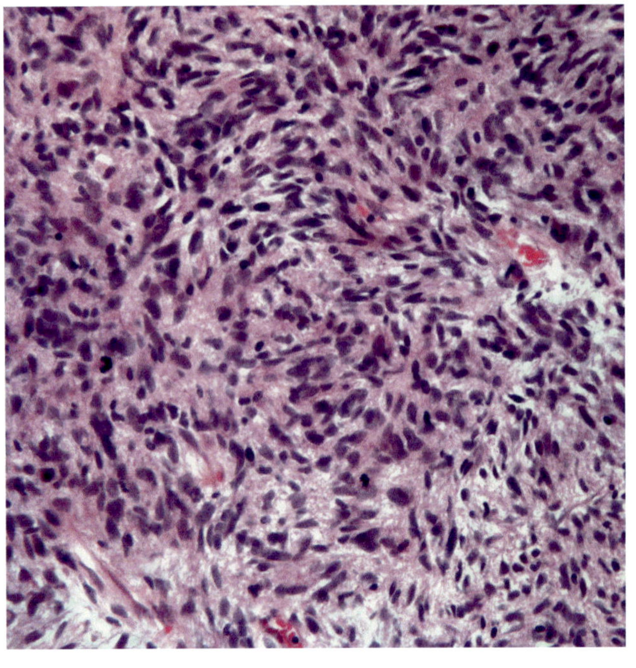

Fig. 12.40 Spindle cell sarcoma in a dedifferentiated liposarcoma. Note the presence of numerous mitotic figures

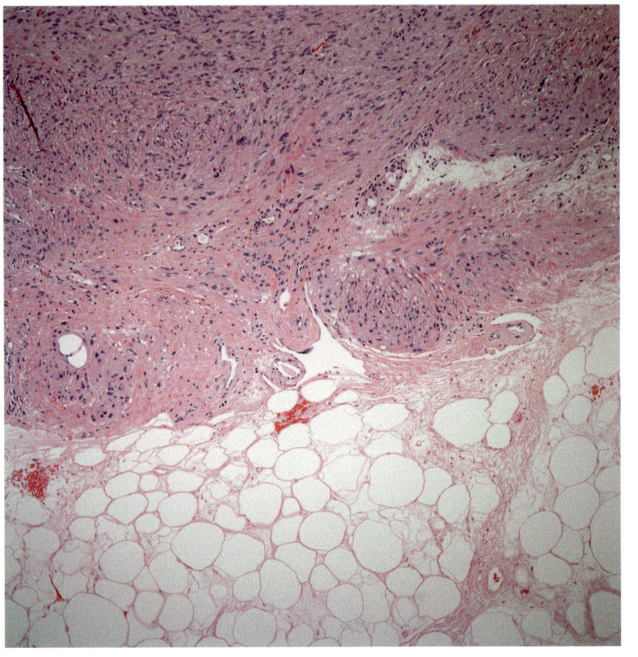

Fig. 12.41 Lowe power view of a lipomatous tumor showing merging areas with smooth muscle component

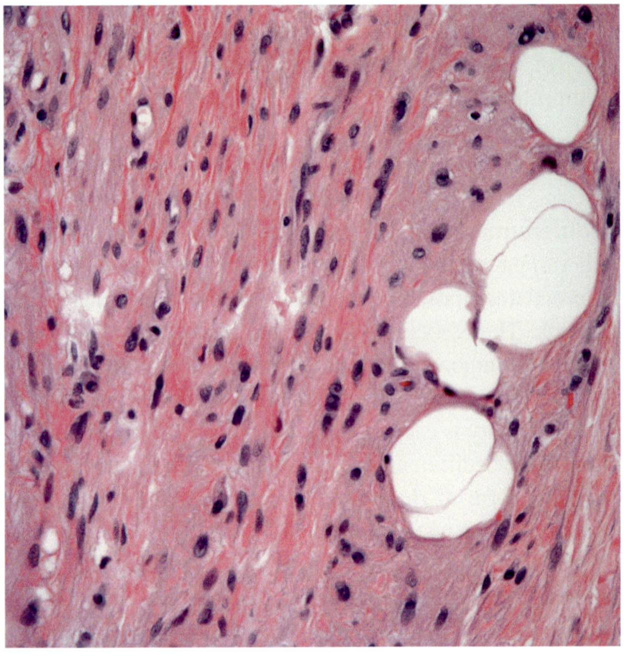

Fig. 12.42 Higher magnification of the smooth muscle component and focal adipose tissue

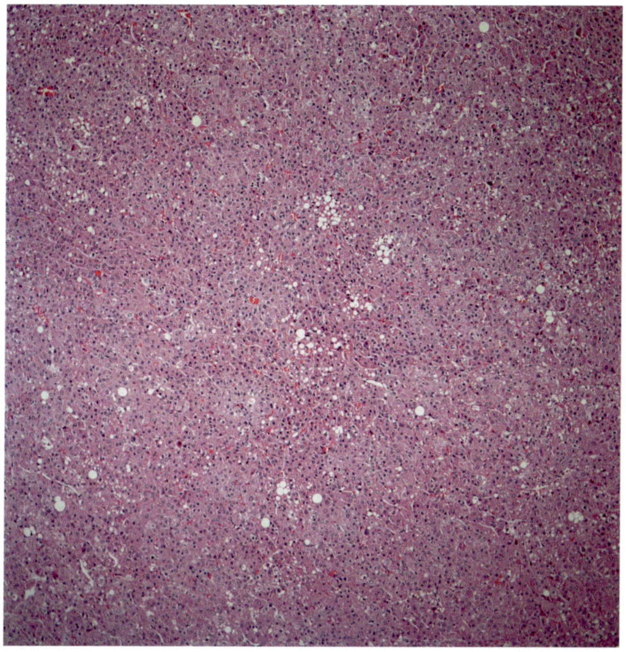

Fig. 12.43 Epithelioid liposarcoma showing a more solid cellular proliferation

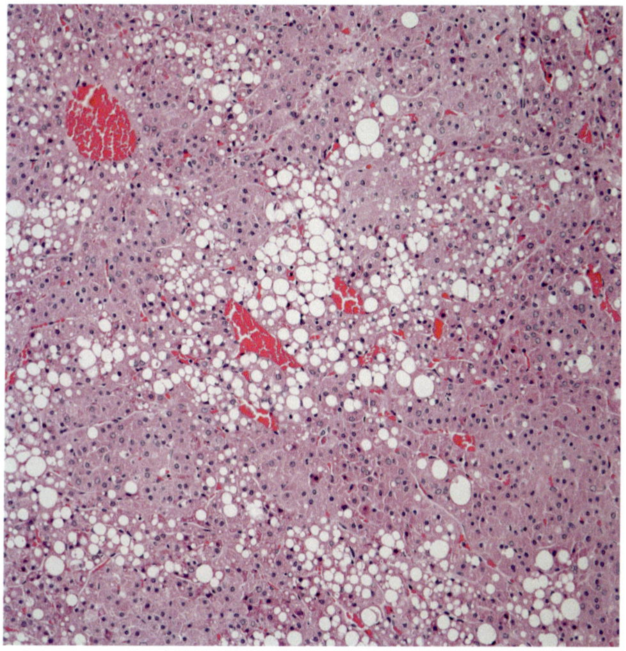

Fig. 12.44 Epithelioid liposarcoma showing epithelioid areas with more conventional adipose component

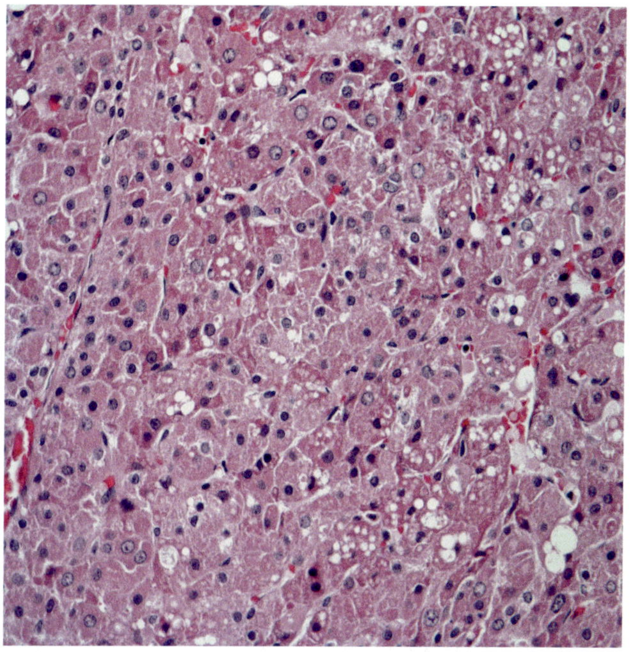

Fig. 12.45 Closer magnification of epithelioid areas showing a subtle "oncocytic" cellular proliferation

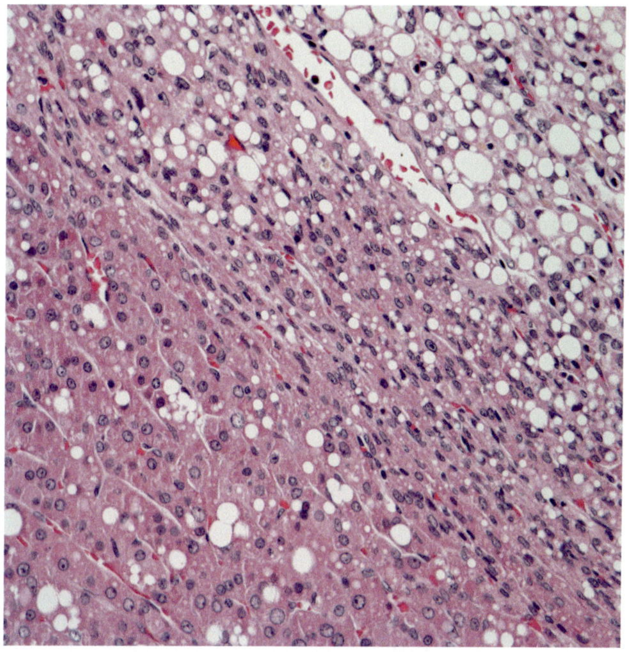

Fig. 12.46 Epithelioid areas merging with more conventional areas of liposarcoma

Immunohistochemical and Molecular Features

Even though in a good number of cases the diagnosis of liposarcoma can be accomplished on morphological grounds, the use of immunohistochemical markers has become part of the routine in evaluating these tumors, mainly in a high-grade tumor in which it is important to be more specific due to the possible treatment options and prognosis. Wang and coworkers [55], in a study of 32 cases of pleomorphic liposarcoma, encountered that 2 of 15 cases showed focal staining with alpha smooth muscle actin, while S-100 protein showed variable staining in the pleomorphic lipoblasts in 20 of 22 cases tested. Ki-67 nuclear staining also was found to be variable, between 10 and 40% labeling. Other stains – including keratin, epithelial membrane antigen, and desmin – were negative. In addition, the authors reported that ten cases were evaluated for MDM2 gene amplification by interphase FISH analysis, and none of the cases showed positive signals. However, MDM2 expression has been reported in some liposarcomas, but it is important to mention that MDM2 and CDK4 immunohistochemistry may be positive in other soft tissue neoplasms. Positive immunohistochemical stains will need confirmation by molecular analysis. Doyle and coworkers [56] have demonstrated by FISH analysis that a subset of dedifferentiated liposarcomas expresses STAT6. These tumors also show expression of STAT6 by immunohistochemistry. In the same report, four cases that were STAT6 negative by immunohistochemistry were tested by FISH analysis, and the four cases did not show amplification.

In general, one can summarize the cytogenetical features of liposarcomas based on the grade of differentiation. For instance, well-differentiated liposarcomas and dedifferentiated liposarcomas are characterized cytogenetically by 12q13–15, noting of course that dedifferentiated tumors also may show other abnormalities. Myxoid/round cell liposarcoma shared the t(12;16). The larger problem is pleomorphic liposarcoma, which appears to be different. Molecular cytogenetics in some cases has shown negative results for DDIT3, EWSR1, and FUS rearrangements.

Differential Diagnosis

In small mediastinoscopic biopsies, the diagnosis of well-differentiated liposarcoma may pose a significant challenge, and the presence of adipose tissue will inevitably lead to the consideration of an adipose tissue tumor such as thymolipoma, angiomyolipoma, or liposarcoma. On the contrary, in high-grade liposarcomas, the challenge may be attempting to separate high-grade liposarcoma from another high-grade sarcoma. Thus, the final interpretation for the diagnosis of liposarcoma is preferably done after complete surgical resection. In some cases of myxoid liposarcoma, the mediastinoscopic biopsy may show enough histopathological features to raise that possibility or to make a definitive diagnosis.

Vascular Neoplasms

The spectrum of vascular neoplasms primarily occurring in the mediastinal compartment ranges from benign to malignant. Nevertheless, the occurrence of these tumors in the mediastinum is rare. In 1949, Seybold and coworkers [57], in a review of approximately 200 surgically resected mediastinal tumors, encountered only 3 cases of vascular origin, which were labeled as either hemangioma or hemangioendothelioma. The authors reviewed the current literature and found only 14 cases which had enough information to be considered. By 1960, Pachter and Lattes [58] presented their own experience, reviewed the current literature, and attested to 78 of these tumors, most of them benign; they also raised some concerns about some of the validity of those reports. Important to highlight is that the authors found the majority of these tumors to occur in the anterior mediastinum, with a minority in the posterior compartment. Pachter and Lattes [58] presented their own experience, describing 11 cases which were categorized as 7 hemangiopericytomas, 2 hemangioendotheliomas, 1 cavernous hemangioma, and 1 hamartomatous angioma. The age distribution of these tumors in the mediastinum is wide, and these tumors may be seen in children as well as in adults. The authors stated that the clinical and diagnostic imaging findings could not be correlated with the histological nature of these tumors, also adding that the criteria of anatomic distribution cannot be applied to these tumors as they may occur in the anterior or posterior mediastinum. The authors noted that those tumors categorized as malignant were more infiltrative and less circumscribed than those that were benign. In a different publication, Pachter and Lattes [59] reported their own experience and reviewed the current literature up to 1960 on the subject of mediastinal lymphangiomas and on 40 such cases described in the literature. The authors presented three additional cases of their own and classified them as one lymphangiomyoma and two as lymphangiopericytomas. Once again, the authors stated that, even though most reported cases are in the anterior mediastinum, some other cases are located in the posterior compartment. In addition, similar to other vascular neoplasms, lymphangiomas can also occur in a wide spectrum of ages ranging from early childhood to older individuals. Clinically, just like other vascular neoplasms, the symptoms are rather non-specific, and in general, may be related to the size of the tumor and its impingement over other thoracic structures. Important to note is that, in previous larger series of mediastinal tumors, the occurrence of lymphangiomas has been rather unusual, and in many instances its occurrence has been the subject of case reports [60–62].

In general terms, one can conclude that vascular tumors of the mediastinal compartment are rare and can be present in either anterior or posterior location. The tumors may be seen in any age group, and the symptomatology is varied and non-specific. Benign vascular tumors are more common than malignant ones, and surgical resection appears to be the treatment of choice for these tumors. However, in those tumors with malignant histological features, the use of radiation or chemotherapy may play a role. Clearly, the separation between benign and malignant tumors plays a role not only in the treatment options but also in the clinical outcome for these patients.

Based on the histological features of these tumors, we can divide them into:

- Benign
  - Hemangioma/lymphangioma
- Malignant
  - Epithelioid hemangioendothelioma
  - Angiosarcoma

Mediastinal Hemangiomas

By far, mediastinal hemangiomas appear to be much more commonly reported than lymphangiomas. It is possible that hemangiomas are also more common than lymphangiomas, and, because of the large size that those tumors may show in the mediastinal compartment, the clinical differential diagnosis may also raise different possibilities. Thus, this may be the possible reason behind the fact that they are more commonly reported. In any case, large series of mediastinal lymphangiomas are lacking, and only few relatively large series of mediastinal hemangiomas have been published in the literature.

Credit for the first description of a "benign" vascular tumor arising in the mediastinum is given to Shennan [63], who, in 1914, described a patient with what the author considered "numerous metastases." In 1978, Davis and coworkers [64] reported four cases of mediastinal hemangiomas and reviewed 77 previously reported cases. The authors stated that approximately 75% of these tumors occur in patients under 40 years of age, while approximately 70% occur in the anterior mediastinum. Interestingly, the authors also indicated that extrathoracic extension might be seen in about 2% of cases, and they reported a similar percentage for lesions involving multiple sites. In the four cases reported by Davis [64], the patients presented with non-specific symptomatology, which included generalized weakness and chest pain. However, patients who are asymptomatic and in whom the tumor was discovered either in the anterior or posterior mediastinum during a routine evaluation have been described [64–66]. Cohen and coworkers [67] reported 15 patients with mediastinal hemangiomas in whom total or partial resection of the tumor was accomplished. The authors stated that, in those patients in whom partial resection was performed, the tumor did not spread, became asymptomatic, or showed evidence of malignant transformation. Based on that experience, the authors stated that these patients would benefit from at least partial resection of the tumor. More recently, John and Folpe [68] described their experience with anastomosing hemangiomas in unusual locations, reporting 17 such cases. The ages of the patients ranged from 2 to 85 years, and, even though 13 cases were described near the vertebral column including the paravertebral region, only one case was described arising in the anterior mediastinum. In one of the largest series of mediastinal hemangiomas, describing 18 cases [69] with emphasis on morphological spectrum, the patients described included nine women and nine men ranging in age from newborn to 74 years. In eight patients, the clinical symptoms were those of chest pain, cough, and dyspnea. Three patients were completely asymptomatic. Two patients presented with heart problems and neck pain, while, in one case, the tumor was found at autopsy where it was also discovered that the individual had gastric hemangioma and facial telangiectasis. The latter case illustrates the issue of multicentricity with these tumors. Fourteen tumors were located in the anterior mediastinum, while only 4 were in the posterior compartment. At least in 17 of these patients, a complete surgical resection was performed, while in 1 patient the tumor appeared to have been partially resected. Follow-up information ranged from 1 to 48 months in 11 patients and showed no recurrence or metastatic disease.

From the radiological point of view, the largest series of mediastinal hemangiomas is the one reported by McAdams and coworkers [70]. In this report, the authors described the radiographic and CT findings of 14 patients with mediastinal hemangiomas, showing that these tumors are well-marginated masses at CT and that calcifications and phleboliths can be identified. About 90% of these tumors show heterogeneous attenuation at contrast material-enhanced CT, with some patients showing mixed central and peripheral non-specific attenuation.

Pathological Features

Macroscopically, mediastinal hemangiomas are tumors that may show variable size. The tumors have been described from 2 to more than 20 cm in greatest diameter. It is possible that those tumors arising in the anterior mediastinum may reach larger sizes than those arising in the posterior compartment. The tumors appear to be well circumscribed, although in a few cases, the tumor may be adherent or infiltrating adjacent structures. The tumors show cystic as well as solid areas, and characteristically are described as hemorrhagic. However, areas of necrosis are not present.

Histologically, mediastinal hemangiomas can be separated into two different categories: cavernous and capillary hemangiomas. The capillary hemangioma is characterized by a lobular growth pattern separated by thin fibrous connective tissue. The lobules are composed of a solid cellular proliferation composed of round to oval cells with indistinct cell borders, peripheral margination of the chromatin, small eccentric nucleoli, and eosinophilic cytoplasm (Figs. 12.47, 12.48, and 12.49). This cellular proliferation in some areas shows compressed vascular lumens. Also, the tumor in other

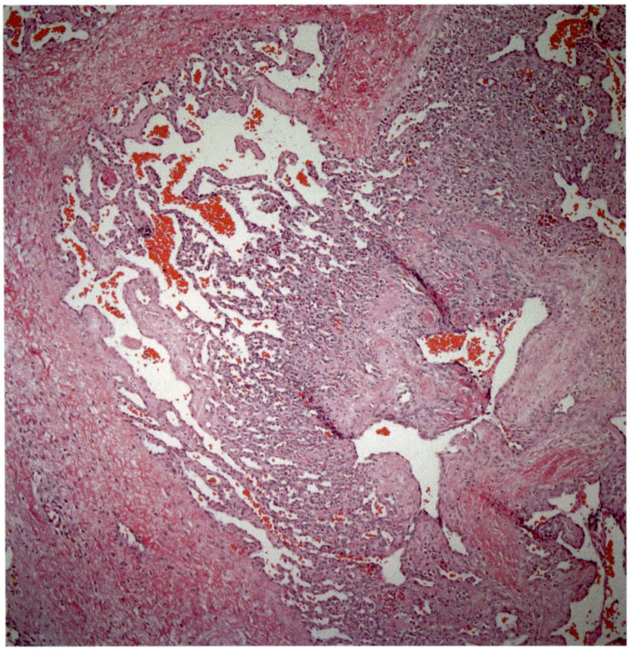

Fig. 12.47 Mediastinal capillary hemangioma showing a benign vascular proliferation admixed with fibroconnective tissue

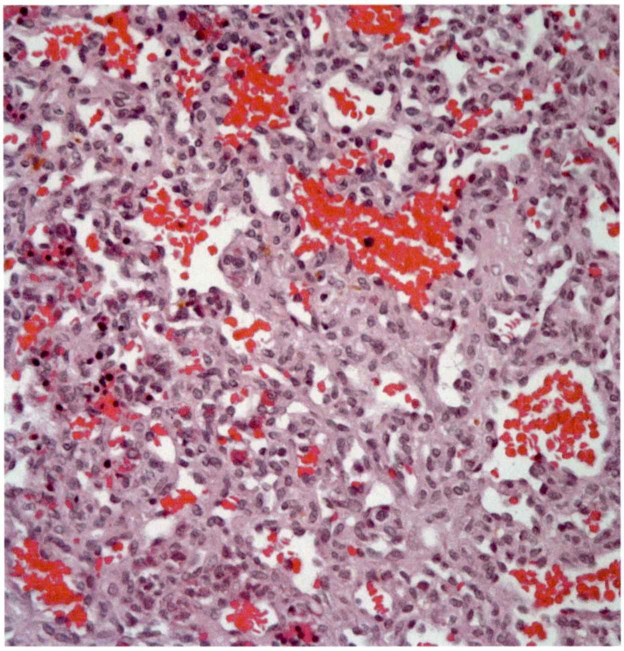

Fig. 12.49 Higher magnification of a capillary hemangioma with bland cytologic appearance

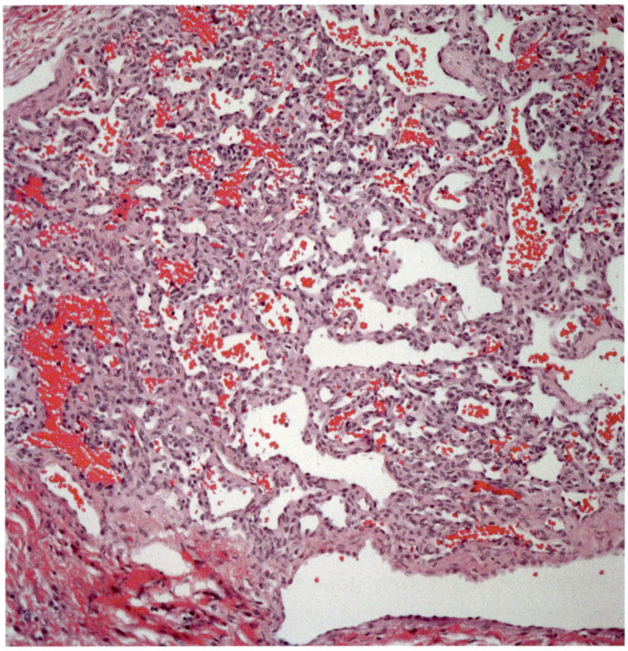

Fig. 12.48 Capillary hemangioma showing anastomotic vascular spaces

areas may show ectatic vessels with blood in its lumen. Even though mitotic figures may be seen occasionally, no cellular atypia is present. In some areas, the tumor may appear as dissecting fibrous connective or adipose tissue, or abutting lymph nodes, giving the impression of invasion. Areas of extensive hyalinization, myxoid changes, or cystic degeneration may be seen in some cases. On the other hand, cavernous hemangiomas characteristically showed prominent ectatic blood vessels filled with varying amounts of blood (Figs. 12.50, 12.51, and 12.52). These ectatic blood vessels are separated by prominent fibrous connective tissue, while in some areas prominent smooth muscle component may be observed. The tumor may show a mixture of ectatic blood vessels with smooth muscle, fibrous connective tissue, and adipose tissue in some areas. Inflammatory changes composed of plasma cells and lymphocytes are observed in many cases. However, contrary to capillary hemangiomas, cavernous hemangiomas are less cellular but with the peculiarity of prominent fibrous connective or smooth muscle tissue. Also, in cavernous hemangiomas, extensive areas of hyalinization may be seen. However, cellular atypia or mitotic activity is not commonly seen.

On the contrary, lymphangiomas show somewhat different histopathological features. The lesions at low power show prominent fibroconnective tissue with a subtle cystic appearance (Figs. 12.53 and 12.54). Endothelial cells lined these cystic-like spaces, and, in some of these dilated spaces, the lumen is filled with chylous fluid. Areas of inflammatory reaction may be seen, but the tumor lacks cellular atypia, increased cellularity, or mitotic activity.

Immunohistochemical Features

The use of vascular markers such as Factor VIII, CD34, CD31, and D2–40 may help in the evaluation of these neoplasms. However, the positive staining in these tumors cannot determine whether a vascular lesion is malignant or benign. In addition, the use of D2–40 may be more helpful in

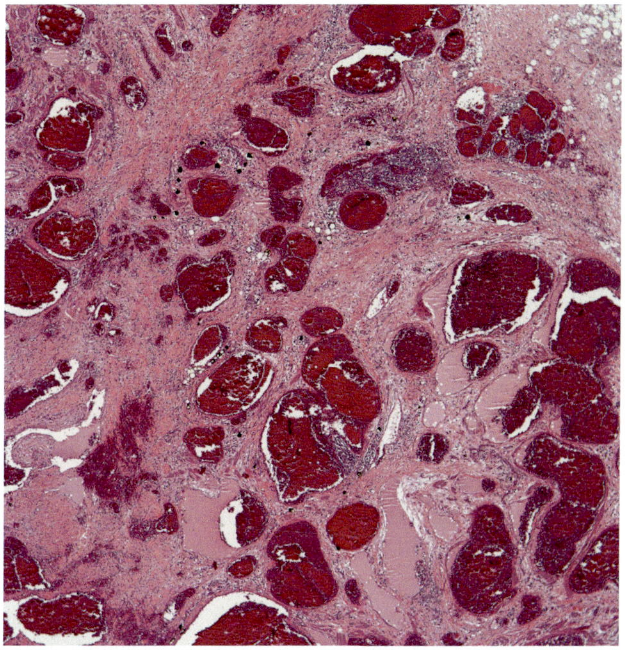

Fig. 12.50 Low power view of a mediastinal cavernous hemangioma, note the presence of dilated vascular spaces filled with blood

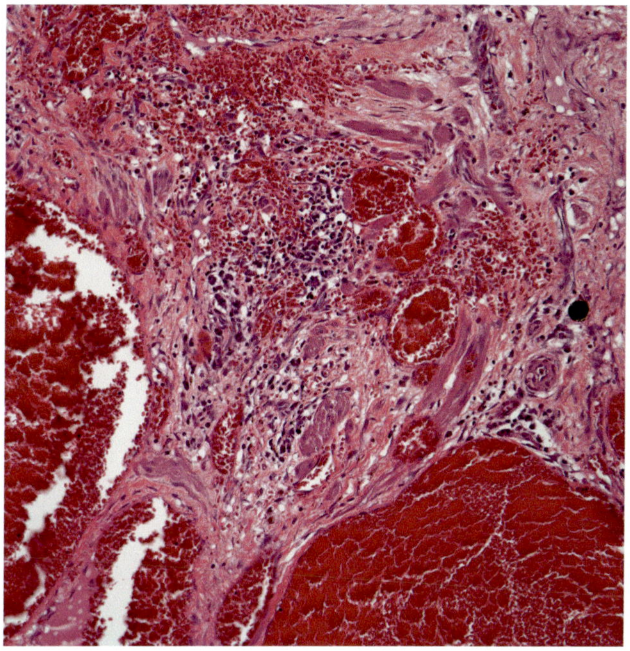

Fig. 12.52 Dilated vascular spaces filled with blood, note the presence of strands of smooth muscle

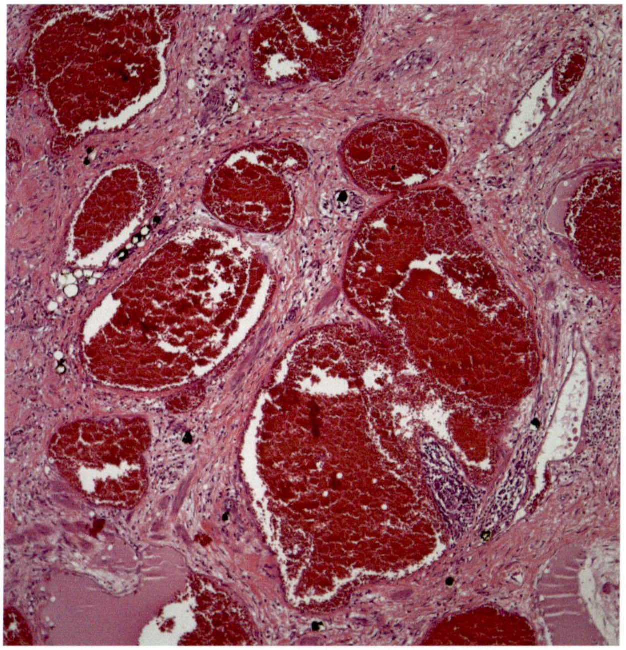

Fig. 12.51 Dilated vascular spaces filled with blood and separated by fibroconnective tissue

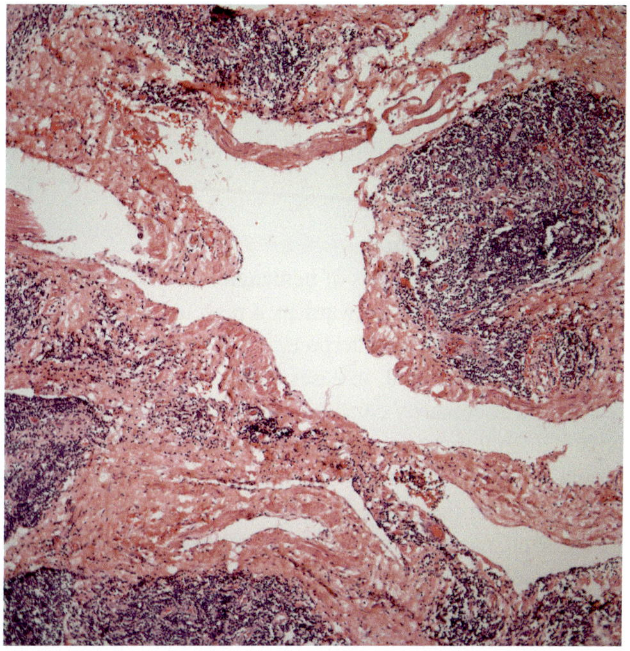

Fig. 12.53 Mediastinal lymphangioma showing the typical appearance of dilated lymphatic spaces

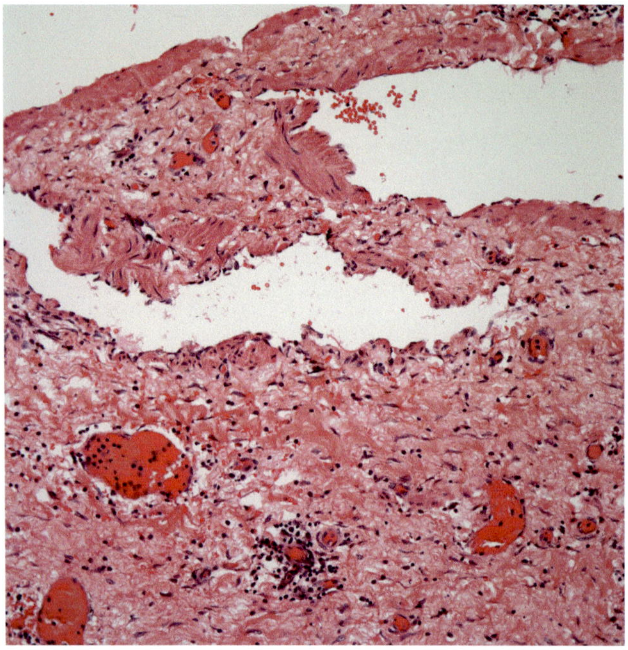

Fig. 12.54 Dilated lymphatic spaces in a background of fibroconnective tissue

the evaluation of lymphangiomas rather than hemangiomas. In some cases, focal staining with epithelial membrane antigen may be seen. However, in general terms, epithelial markers are negative. In cases of cavernous hemangiomas with prominent smooth muscle component, smooth muscle actin and muscle-specific actin would show positive staining in those areas.

Differential Diagnosis

Even though the diagnosis of hemangiomas and lymphangiomas is rather straightforward in a resected specimen, the challenge may be in the interpretation of small thoracoscopic biopsies. In this regard, in cases of capillary hemangiomas, one would necessarily consider the possibility of epithelioid hemangioendothelioma, while in cases of cavernous hemangioma in which the sampling shows smooth muscle, one would consider the possibility of a smooth muscle neoplasm. In resected cases with prominent ectatic vessels, smooth muscle, adipose tissue, and fibrous connective tissue proliferation, the possibility of a hamartomatous lesion or mediastinal angiomyolipoma would be considered. However, in general, the diagnosis of hemangioma, whether capillary or cavernous, can be made on morphologic grounds.

Epithelioid Hemangioendothelioma

Mediastinal epithelioid hemangioendotheliomas are tumors of rare occurrence. There has been some debate about considering this tumor a borderline malignancy or a low-grade angiosarcoma. The vast majority of these tumors occur in soft tissue. Deyrup and coworkers [71] analyzed 49 cases of epithelioid hemangioendothelioma of soft tissue with the idea of defining potential risk for these patients, as some tumors are associated with low mortality. In this particular study [71], the age range of patients with these tumors was of 9–93 years of age, with female predominance. Only four of the tumors described were located in the mediastinum. The authors concluded that the presence of more than 3 mitotic figures per 50 high-power fields and size of more than 3 cm had poor prognosis, while the presence of cytologic atypia, necrosis, and spindle cell component did not correlate with prognosis. Interestingly, patients with the high risk had a 5-year disease-specific survival of 59%, while patients with low risk had no mortality. In a different study by Anderson and coworkers [72], the authors studied 52 cases of what they called "thoracic epithelioid malignant vascular tumors." The authors stratified these cases into low-grade epithelioid hemangioendothelioma, intermediate epithelioid hemangioendothelioma, and angiosarcoma. Based on the description provided, it seems that five of those tumors had exclusive mediastinal involvement, while two additional cases may have had another anatomic structured involved. Interestingly, the authors concluded that higher-grade tumors, tumors in the lung, tumors in the pleura, and pulmonary and pleural involvement by the tumor correlate with poor prognosis. However, there is not much analysis of mediastinal tumors per se. Regarding this particular issue of epithelioid hemangioendothelioma of the mediastinum, most of what is reported is based on case reports [73–77]. In the largest series presented today in the literature [78], 12 cases of epithelioid hemangioendothelioma were described, all originating in the anterior mediastinum. The patients were three women and nine men ranging in age from 19 to 62 years. Clinically, seven patients presented with compression of adjacent structures, while five patients were asymptomatic. The histology of these tumors was that of a low-grade epithelioid hemangioendothelioma, and the follow-up observed in nine patients disclosed that seven patients were alive and well during a period ranging from 2 to 21 years, while one patient had recurrence and died due to surgical complications, and one additional patient died due to undetermined causes. The authors concluded that epithelioid hemangioendothelioma in the mediastinal compartment may be treated with surgery alone and appears to have a good prognosis.

It is important to highlight in the diagnosis of mediastinal epithelioid hemangioendothelioma that the tumor is indeed a mediastinal tumor, and not one that involves the mediastinum and originates in the pleura, lung, or extrathoracic origin. Thus, this highlights the importance of proper radiological evaluation (Fig. 12.55a, b).

Pathological Features

Macroscopically, the tumors appear to be well circumscribed and with well-defined borders in most cases (Fig. 12.56). However, in some cases, the tumor may show infiltrative bor-

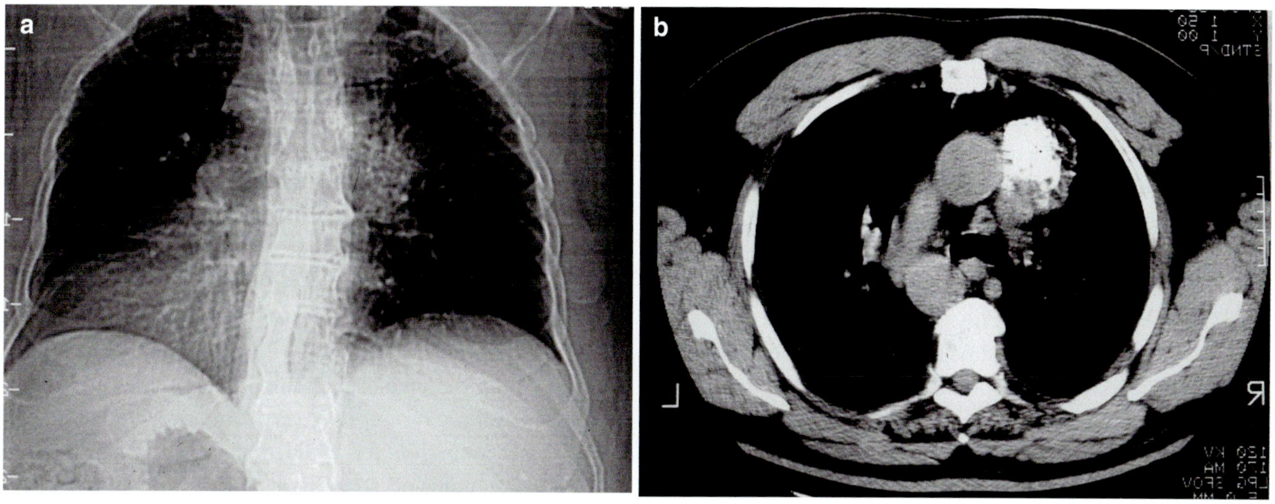

Fig. 12.55 (**a**) Plain chest film of the thorax showing an anterior mediastinal mass(epithelioid hemangioendothelioma), (**b**) CT scan of the chest showing a mediastinal mass (epithelioid hemangioendothelioma)

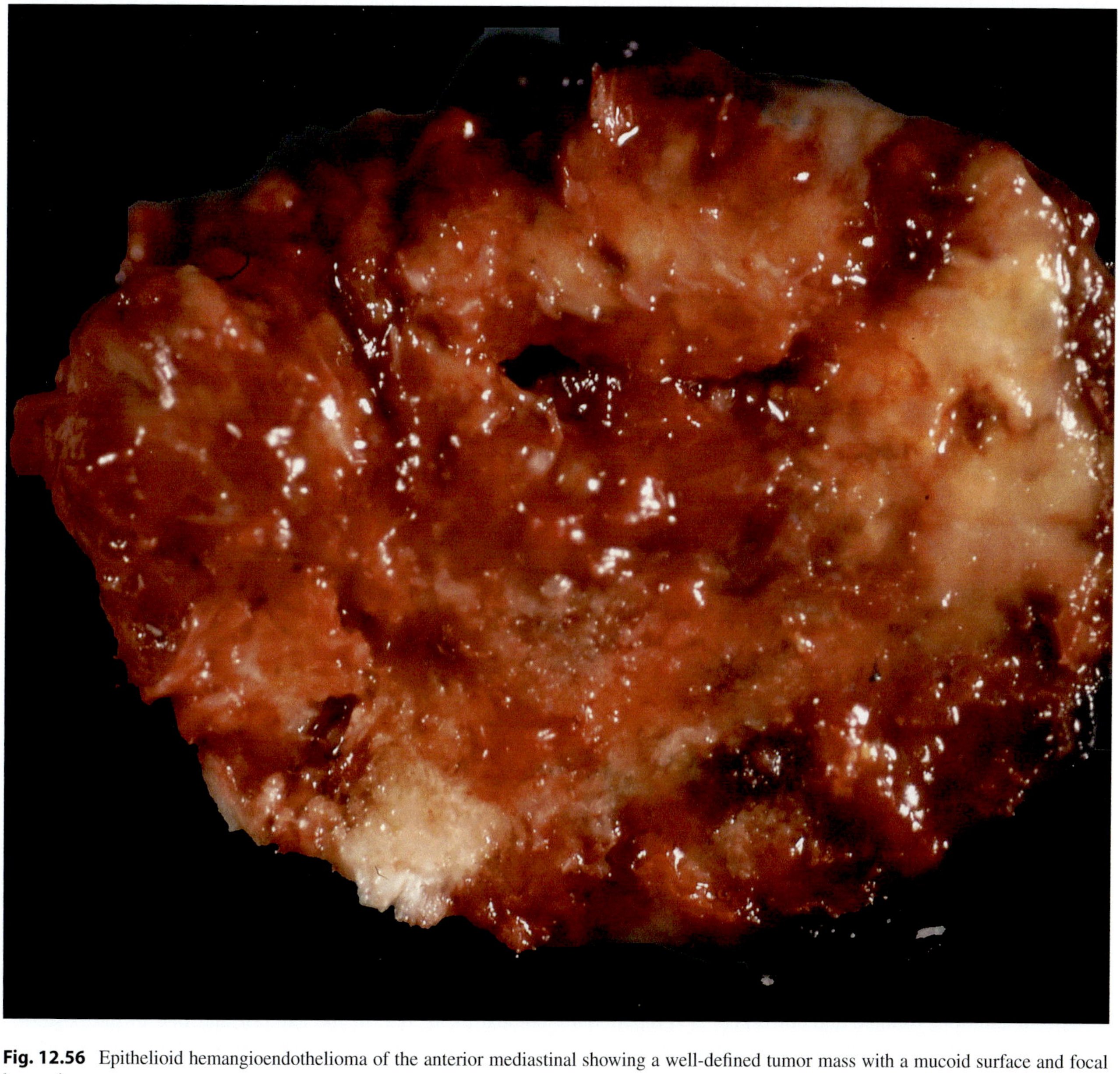

Fig. 12.56 Epithelioid hemangioendothelioma of the anterior mediastinal showing a well-defined tumor mass with a mucoid surface and focal hemorrhage

ders. The tumors may be attached to the pleura, pericardium, or diaphragm by membranous adhesions. In some cases, the tumor may be surrounding major vessels. The tumors size can vary from 4 to more than 10 cm in greatest dimension. The cut surface shows a tumor that is tan-white, rubbery with myxoid consistency, and areas of hemorrhage. Palpable calcifications may be encountered in some cases.

Histologically, epithelioid hemangioendothelioma in the mediastinum recapitulates the features that these tumors show in the soft tissue (Figs. 12.57, 12.58, 12.59, 12.60, 12.61, 12.62, 12.63, and 12.64). The tumor cellularity may vary from round to oval to spindle cellular proliferation growing in cords or nests. The cellular proliferation may lack cytologic atypia, or in focal areas may show moderate cytologic atypia. The cellular proliferation is embedded in a light basophilic myxoid matrix, which may resemble hyaline cartilage, while in other areas the cellular proliferation is surrounded by dense collagenized stroma. High power view of the cellular proliferation shows large, round, centrally placed nuclei with inconspicuous nucleoli. The cytoplasm contains variable amounts of glycogen, and cytoplasmic vacuolization may be prominent in some cases. Anastomosing vascular channels can be identified, while, in other cases, the presence of osteoclast-like giant cell and metaplastic bone formation may be seen. Mitotic activity may be seen in some cases, but it will not be more than three mitotic figures per 10-high-power fields. Areas of necrosis may be present but usually focal.

Histochemical, Ultrastructural, Immunohistochemical, and Molecular Features

Even though the use of histochemical stains in the diagnosis of epithelioid hemangioendothelioma is not a common practice, mucicarmine and periodic acid-Schiff (PAS) with and without diastase can be used. PAS histochemical stains may show the presence of intracytoplasmic glycogen in the cells of this tumor.

Ultrastructural analysis of epithelioid hemangioendotheliomas may also prove to be helpful in diagnosing these tumors. The presence of cells with abundant cytoplasm surrounded by a continuous layer of basal lamina material, pinocytotic activity, immature cell junctions, and abundant intracytoplasmic intermediate filaments appears to be the common finding in these tumors [78]. The presence of Weibel-Palade bodies has been associated with this tumor.

On the contrary, the use of immunohistochemical studies plays an important role in the diagnosis of these tumors in order to separate this neoplasm from other more common thymic tumors of different histogenesis. In this regard, the use of vascular markers such as Factor VIII, CD34, CD31 may show positive staining in tumor cells with some variability. Other immunohistochemical stains that may show positive staining include vimentin, ERG, and D2–40. In some cases, the tumor may also show positive staining for keratin. In addition, Weinreb and coworkers [79] reported a study of nine cases of epithelioid hemangioendothelioma and found that seven of nine cases showed positive staining for CD10.

Anderson and coworkers [72], in a study of 52 thoracic vascular tumors, performed FISH analysis in 30 cases classified as epithelioid hemangioendotheliomas, identifying gene rearrangement involving both WWTR1 and CAMTA1 in 3 of 7 cases of low grade, while similar findings were found in 23/23 intermediate-grade tumors.

Differential Diagnosis

Due to the infrequent occurrence of epithelioid hemangioendothelioma in the mediastinal compartment, the differential diagnosis of these tumors may vary depending upon the type of material available for evaluation. In mediastinoscopic biopsies, the tumor needs to be separated from atypical thymoma or spindle cell thymoma. The use of keratin 5/6 in this setting would be helpful as thymomas are commonly positive for this marker. In addition, positive staining for vascular markers such as Factor VIII, CD31, CD34, ERG, or D2–40 would be more in keeping with a vascular neoplasm. In cases in which the tumor shows prominent myxoid changes and round to oval cells, the possibility of a yolk sac tumor needs consideration; however, the use of markers such as SALL4 and vascular markers would lead to a correct interpretation. Much more difficult would be the separation in a small mediastinoscopic biopsy between epithelioid hemangioendothelioma and angiosarcoma. Such distinction may prove very difficult and may require either an open biopsy or tumor resection. It is possible that the use of molecular techniques such as FISH for the identification of gene rearrangement for CAMTA 1 may help, as this feature is more often encountered in epithelioid hemangioendotheliomas than in angiosarcomas. Of course, in a complete surgical resection, the presence of increased mitotic activity, necrosis, and prominent cellular atypia may be more in keeping with angiosarcoma. The use of vascular markers may show an overlap between these two tumors.

Angiosarcoma

As it is the case with epithelioid hemangioendotheliomas, the existence of primary mediastinal angiosarcomas has been recorded in the literature. However, these tumors are rare, and every effort should be made to properly rule out the possibility of metastatic disease from anatomic areas in which these tumors are more common, whether from the thorax, such as the heart or lung, or from soft tissue tumors. Most of what has been published in the literature regarding mediastinal angiosarcomas derives from single case reports [80–82]. In a study of 15 cases of angiosarcomas arising in viscera and soft tissue in young adults, Deyrup and coworkers [83] encountered two tumors arising in the mediastinal compartment: one in the anterior and one in the posterior mediastinum. The two patients were one boy and one girl, 10

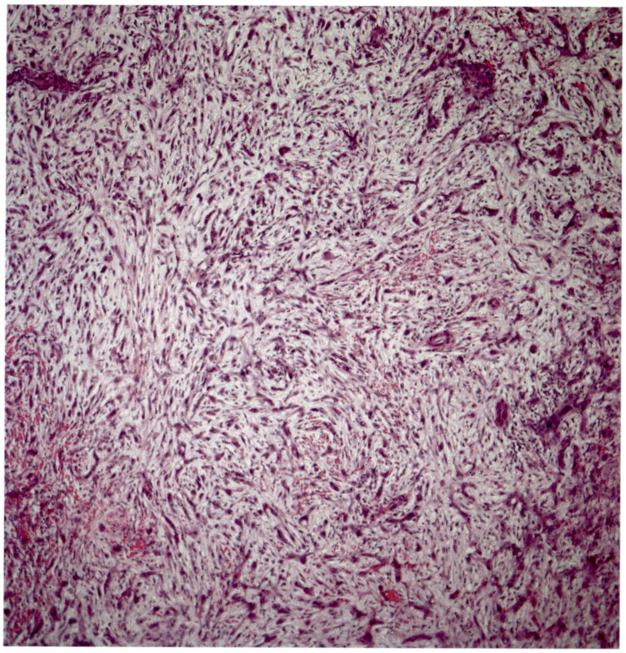

Fig. 12.57 Epithelioid hemangioendothelioma sowing a cellular proliferation embedded in a rather loose stroma

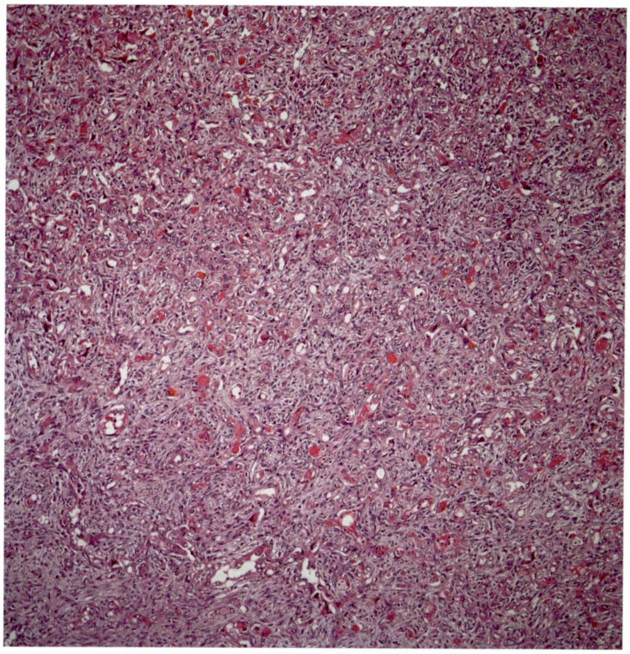

Fig. 12.59 Epithelioid hemangioendothelioma with a more solid cellular proliferation

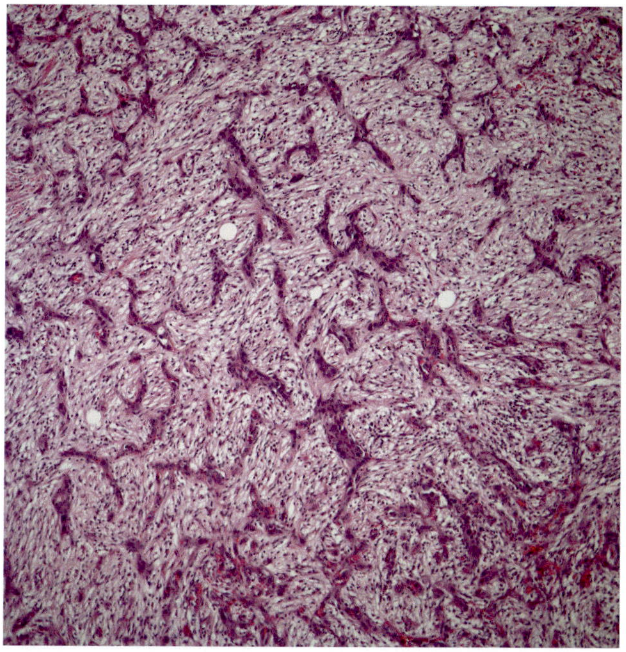

Fig. 12.58 Epithelioid hemangioendothelioma showing islands of epithelioid cells embedded in fibroconnective tissue

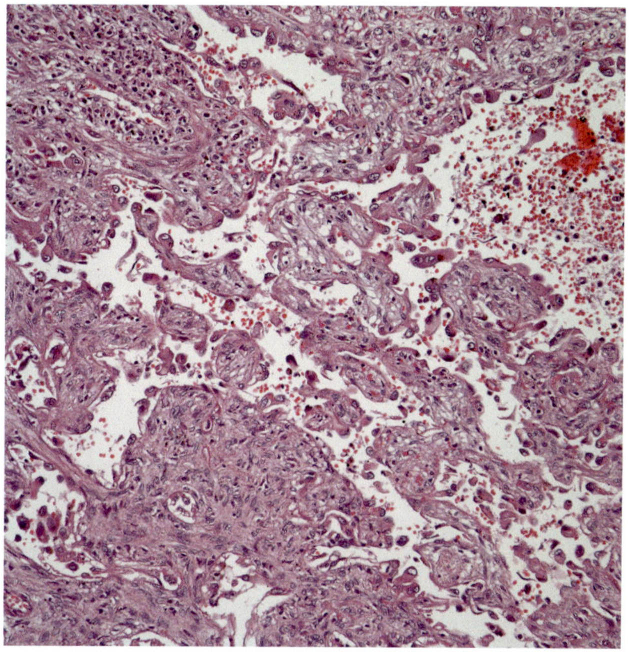

Fig. 12.60 Epithelioid hemangioendothelioma showing areas of more conventional vascular channels

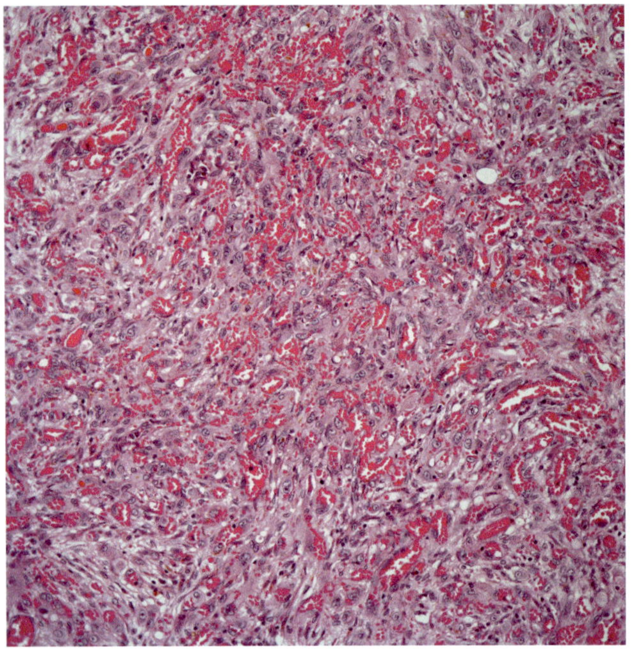

Fig. 12.61 Epithelioid hemangioendothelioma with numerous extravasated red cells

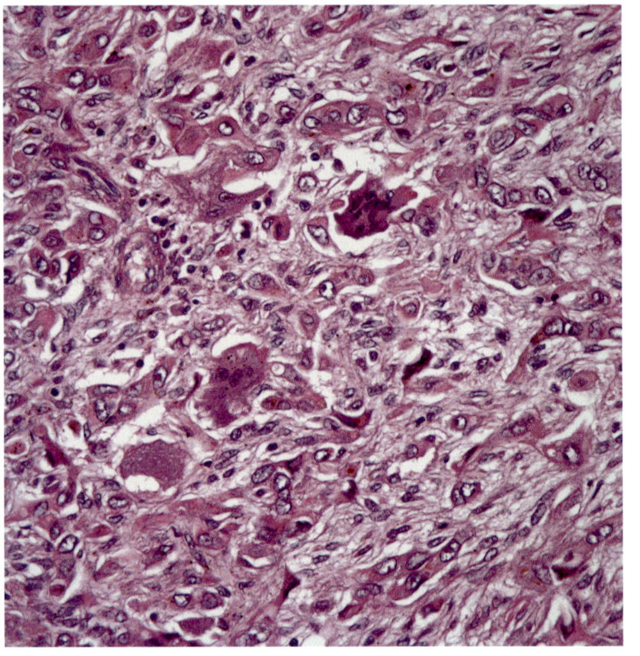

Fig. 12.63 Multinucleated giant cells can be seen in epithelioid hemangioendothelioma

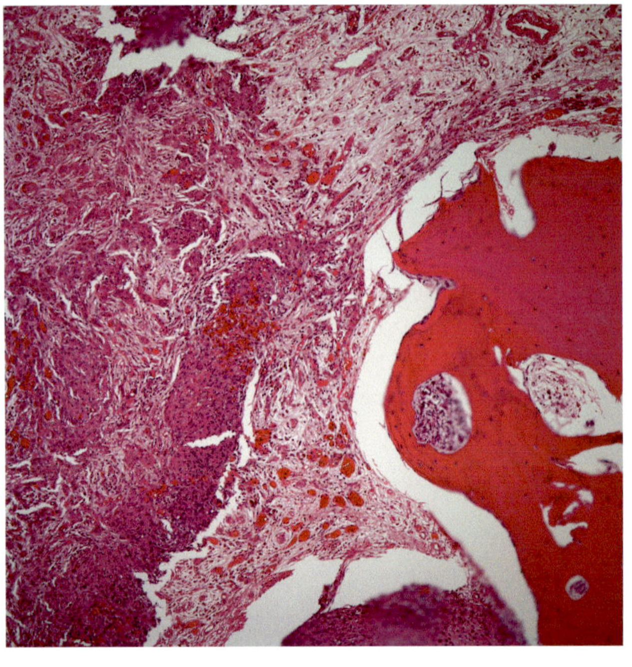

Fig. 12.62 Metaplastic bone formation in epitheloid hemangioendothelioma

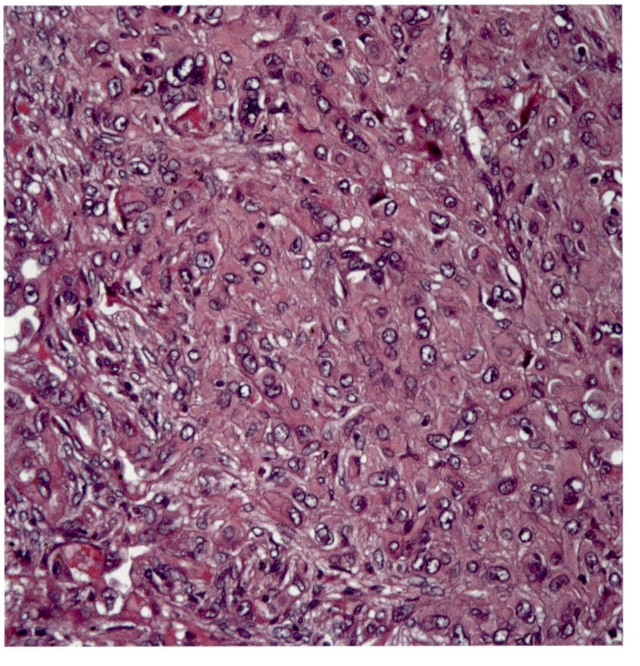

Fig. 12.64 Higher magnification of epitheloid hemangioendothelioma showing medium size cells with round to oval nuclei and lacking mitotic activity

and 5 years of age, respectively. Both patients died of the tumor within 15 months. In a larger series of 80 cases of angiosarcomas of soft tissues, Meis-Kindblom [84] identified 3 cases arising in the mediastinum. Even though the authors provided follow-up information in 49 patients with a median follow-up of 20 months, identifying 53% of those patients who died due to tumor, there is no specific mention of those tumors arising in the mediastinum. Up to now, the largest series focused on primary angiosarcomas of the anterior mediastinum reported nine patients: five men and four women between the ages of 25 and 62 years [85]. Clinically, these patients presented with varied symptomatology including chest pain, dyspnea, hemorrhagic pericarditis, swelling of the neck, pneumonia, dizziness, cough, and fever. Diagnostic imaging detected all tumors in the anterior mediastinum. All patients underwent surgical resection of the tumor followed by adjuvant chemotherapy. Follow-up information was provided in six patients showing that four patients were alive between 6 and 36 months; one patient was alive with recurrence after 48 months, and one patient died due to the tumor 10 months after initial diagnosis.

Even though the diagnosis of mediastinal angiosarcoma may not pose a problem, it is important to reserve such diagnosis to patients in whom the surgical resection of the tumor shows angiosarcoma only. In mediastinoscopic biopsies, the possibility of having an angiosarcoma associated with other neoplasms is probably more common than primary angiosarcoma. For instance, angiosarcomatous components have been described in numerous cases of germ cell tumors [86, 87].

Pathological Features

Macroscopically, mediastinal angiosarcomas may vary in size from 3 to more than 10 cm in greatest dimension. The tumors are described as hemorrhagic and not well circumscribed. Solid and cystic areas may be present, and necrosis is not a common finding.

Histologically, the tumors may show low-, high-, and mixed-grade (low and high grade) histological features. The spectrum of differentiation that may be seen in these tumors include large ectatic areas filled with blood admixed with areas of anastomosing channels of varying size, solid areas or capillary-like proliferation, and slit-like spaces lined by atypical endothelial cells. The cytology is that of medium size cells with hyperchromatic nuclei with a hobnail pattern. Focal areas of papillary endothelial hyperplasia, solid epithelioid cellular proliferation, pleomorphic giant cells, and myxoid areas may be seen in some cases. In addition, hemorrhage, extravasation of red cells, hemosiderin deposition, calcifications, ossification, and cystic changes are commonly seen. Necrosis is commonly encountered in these tumors in more than 75% of the cases. The mitotic activity in these tumors will depend on the material available for evaluation and may vary from two to more than five mitoses per ten high-power fields. Important to identify is that angiosarcomas are commonly infiltrative tumors that extend into the adipose tissue (Figs. 12.65, 12.66, 12.67, 12.68, 12.69, and 12.70).

Immunohistochemical and Molecular Features

Just like other vascular neoplasm, mediastinal angiosarcomas may react positively to vascular markers, namely, Factor VIII-related antigen, CD31, and CD34. Other markers including keratin, desmin, smooth muscle actin, and S-100 protein are commonly negative.

As it has been reported, FISH gene rearrangement for CAMTA1 is commonly negative in angiosarcomas and more often positive in epithelioid hemangioendotheliomas [72].

Differential Diagnosis

The most important differential diagnosis is primarily the separation between a low-grade angiosarcoma and epithelioid hemangioendothelioma. In a small biopsy, such differentiation may be challenging; however, in a surgical resection, the histological features of epithelioid hemangioendothelioma and low-grade angiosarcoma are somewhat different, which may allow for leaning toward one diagnosis over the other. In addition, the use of molecular studies may help in separating both tumors in some cases. In the high-grade angiosarcomas, the presence of increased mitotic activity, necrosis, extensive hemorrhage, cellular atypia, and infiltrative growth pattern of the tumor should lead to the correct interpretation. In addition, other neoplasms that may be considered in the differential diagnosis may include atypical thymoma or unusual variant of thymoma, thymic carcinoma, and yolk sac tumor. In this setting, the use of immunohistochemical vascular markers should lead to the correct interpretation. One important consideration in the diagnosis of angiosarcoma is the limiting factor of a small biopsy. As it has already been mentioned, the fact that angiosarcomas are commonly associated with germ cell tumors [86, 87] poses a significant problem in interpretation. Therefore, the final diagnosis of angiosarcoma may be best after surgical resection of the tumor, with ample sampling in order to rule out the possibility of germ cell tumor.

Muscle Tumors

The existence of tumors originating from muscle in the mediastinum has been recorded in the literature. However, it is important to highlight that such occurrence is rare. Whether the tumor is of smooth muscle or of skeletal muscle origin, the occurrence of these tumors in the mediastinal compartment is rather rare. In addition, based on what has been published in the literature, these tumors also occur in either anterior or posterior mediastinal compartment. The origin of these neoplasms in the mediastinal compartment remains speculative. Important to recognize is that, in many circumstances, smooth muscle neoplasms originating from the

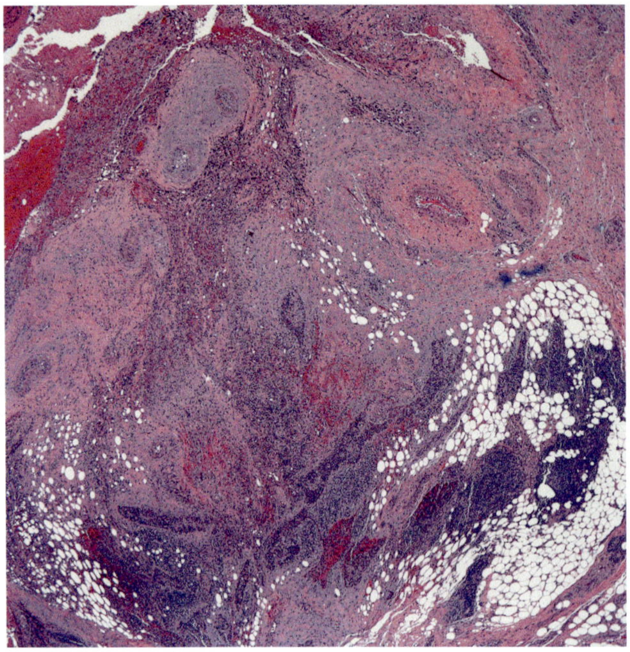

Fig. 12.65 Mediastinal angiosarcoma, note the presence of residual thymic epithelium

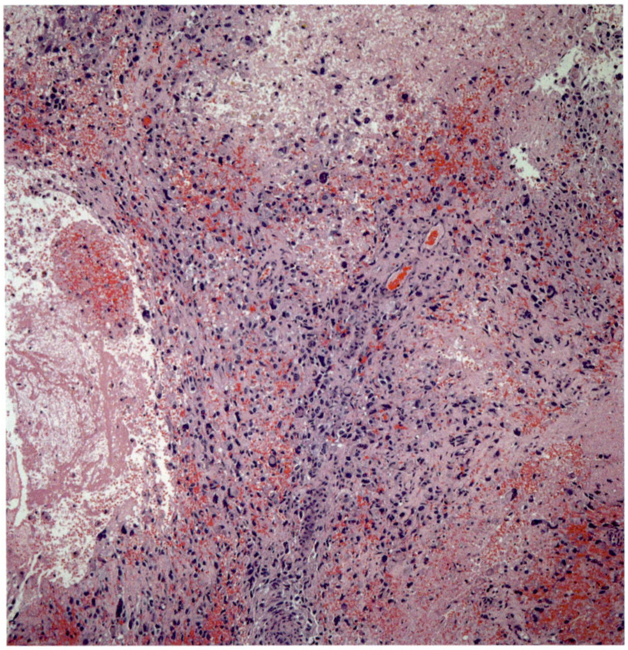

Fig. 12.66 Hemorrhagic areas admixed with an atypical cellular proliferation

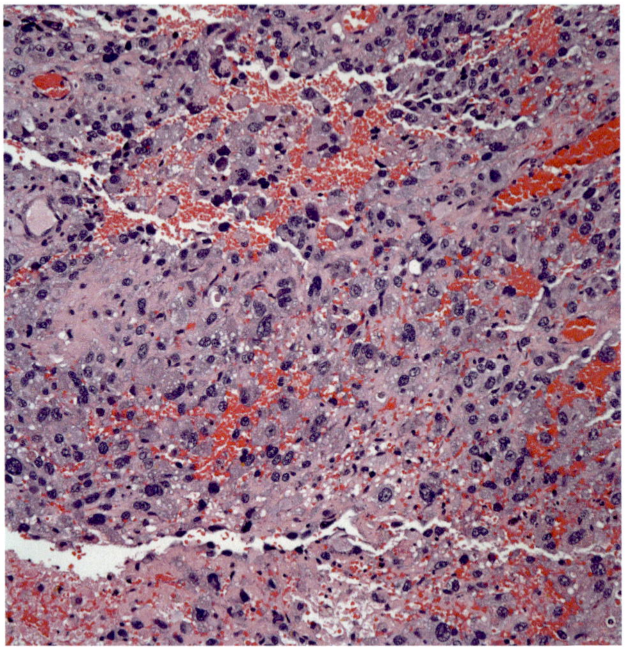

Fig. 12.67 Neoplastic cellular proliferation composed of round to oval cells with eosinophilic cytoplasm and round nuclei

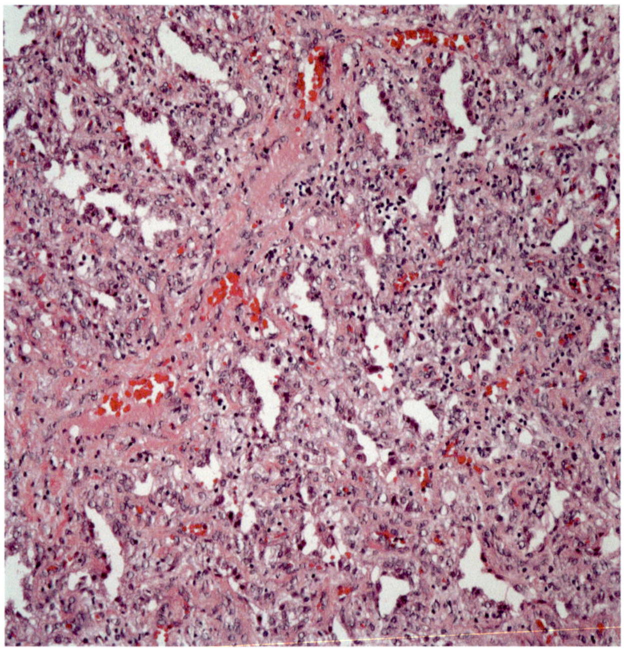

Fig. 12.68 More conventional areas of angiosarcoma showing slits representing vascular spaces lined by neoplastic cells

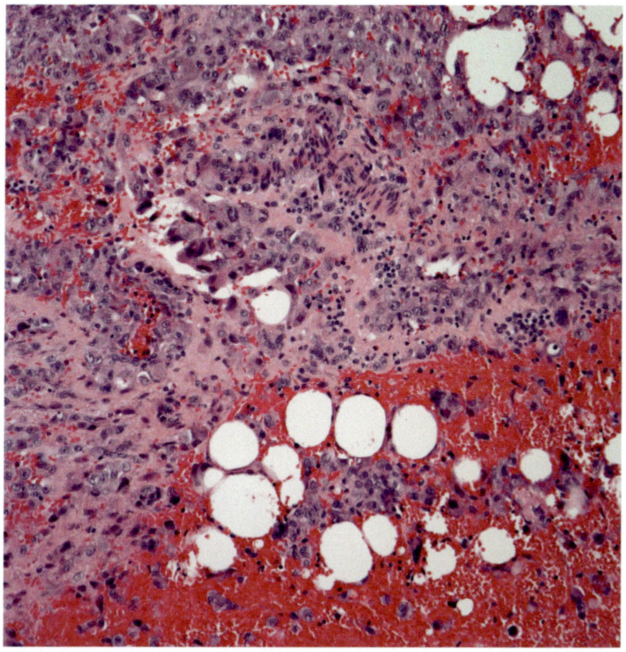

Fig. 12.69 Angiosarcoma infiltrating adipose tissue

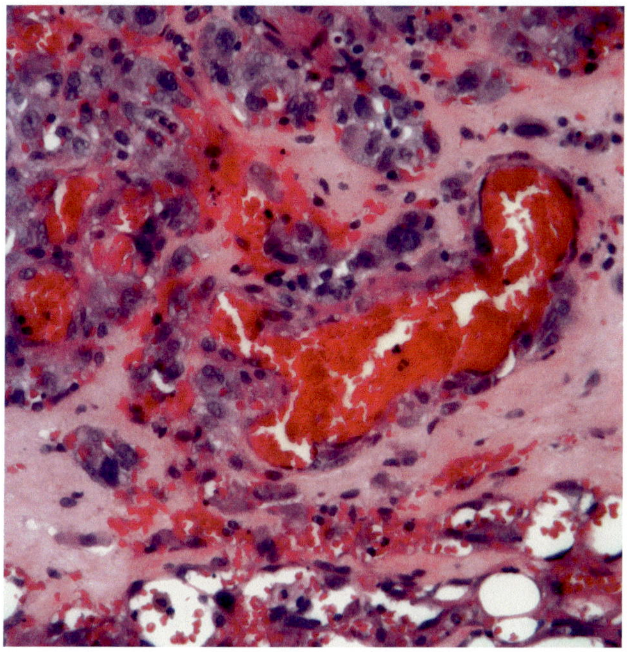

Fig. 12.70 Angiosarcoma showing vascular structures lined by malignant cells; note the prominent cellular atypia

walls of the esophagus may present as mediastinal tumors; however, in reality those tumors should not be accounted for "true" mediastinal neoplasms. Also, the fact that smooth muscle neoplasms may originate from the walls of blood vessels should designate the tumor as not a "true" mediastinal neoplasm. In this regard, the use of diagnostic imaging techniques may provide important information to properly designate the true origin of these tumors. Even though this issue may seem to be an academic exercise, the fact is that a tumor that arises in the wall of a major vessel or from the wall of the esophagus may be treated differently from one arising from the soft tissue of the mediastinum. In addition, it is likely that the prognosis of those patients may be different as well. Having excluded tumors originating from the wall of the esophagus or the wall of a major vessel, then the only explanation for the occurrence of these tumors in the mediastinal compartment, one is left with the only hypothesis regarding the origin of these tumors as originating from the soft tissues of the anterior or posterior mediastinum.

Reports of the occurrence of leiomyosarcomas in the mediastinum, recorded for the most part through individual case reports that have included tumors originating from the wall of the esophagus and wall of a major vessel [88, 89], show only a few cases in which the occurrence of such tumors did not involve those structures [90–96]. Interestingly, it appears that the occurrence of leiomyosarcomas is more common than the occurrence of leiomyomas [94, 97]. Mediastinal leiomyomas have been described in adult patients with rather non-specific symptoms or in asymptomatic patients. Diagnostic imaging in some of the cases described has shown that the tumor is not attached to the wall of the esophagus or any major vessel. Surgical resection has been the treatment of choice in those patients, and their follow-up has been uneventful.

The largest series of mediastinal leiomyosarcoma [98] up to now described ten patients: seven men and three women between the ages of 26 and 71 years. Three tumors were located in the anterior mediastinum, while seven were in the posterior mediastinum. The spectrum of differentiation in the tumors reported ranged from low-, moderate-, and high-grade leiomyosarcomas. Clinically, the patients had non-specific symptomatology, and some patients were asymptomatic. Diagnostic imaging revealed that the sarcomas did not involve the esophagus or a major vessel. Surgical resection was performed in all the patients. Follow-up information ranging from 2 to 7 years was documented in six patients; two patients were alive at 4 and 6 years, respectively; three patients had died of tumor in a period of 2 to 7 years; and two patients had documented recurrences within 2 years and subsequently died of tumor. The authors concluded that histologic grade and extent or lack of invasiveness represent important parameters in assessing prognosis for these patients.

Pathological Features

Macroscopically, mediastinal leiomyosarcomas may vary in size from 5 to more than 10 cm in greatest diameter. The tumors appear to be well circumscribed but not encapsulated, firm to rubbery with a smooth or nodular surface. The tumors are tan to gray in color, and areas of hemorrhage and/or necrosis may be seen (Fig. 12.71). Cystic and myxoid changes have been reported in some cases.

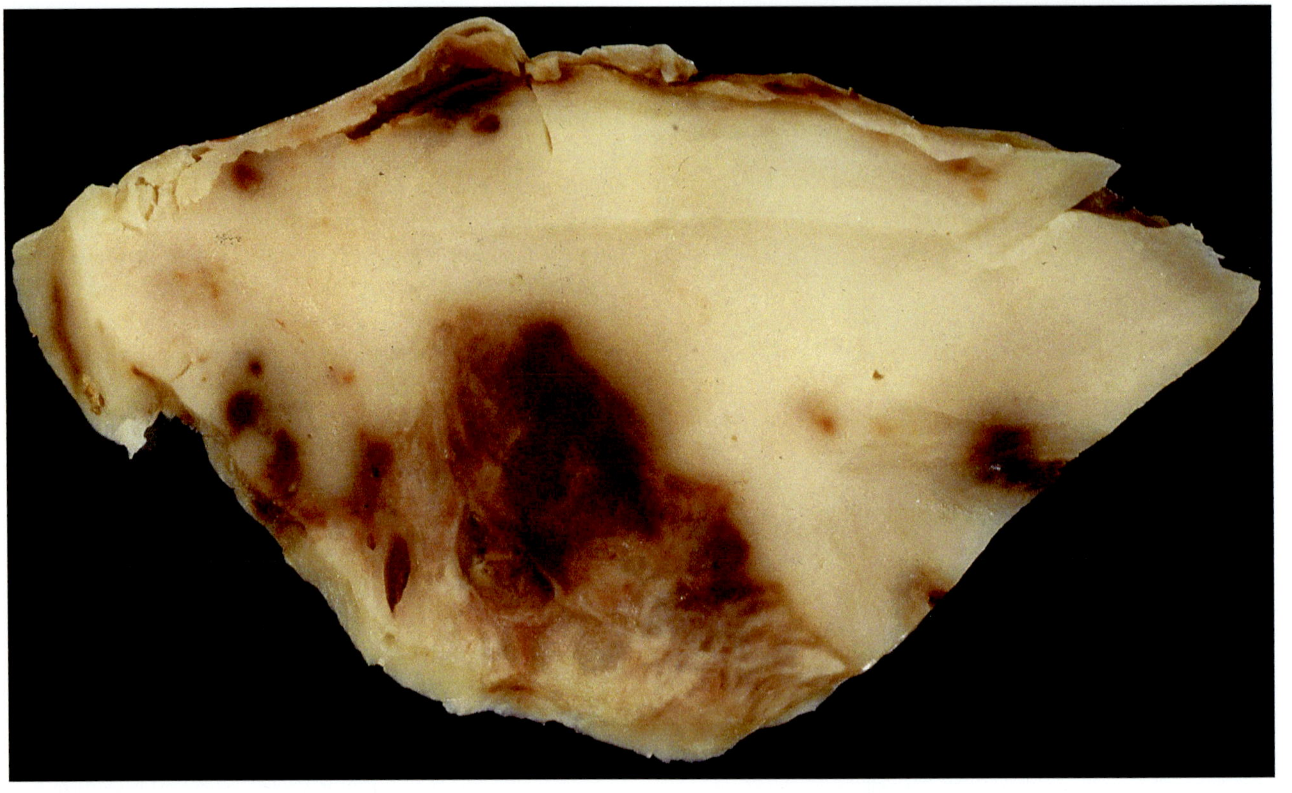

Fig. 12.71 Anterior mediastinal leiomyosarcoma showing areas of necrosis and hemorrhage

Histologically, the tumors may range from conventional leiomyoma to leiomyosarcomas of low- to high-grade sarcomas.

Leiomyoma

This tumor is characterized by the presence of a spindle cell proliferation arranged in fascicles. The tumors cells are elongated with a cigar-shaped nuclei and finely dispersed chromatin. The growth pattern is rather organized, and the tumors do not display nuclear atypia or mitotic activity (Figs. 12.72 and 12.73). Areas of necrosis and/or hemorrhage are not components of these tumors.

Low-Grade Leiomyosarcoma

These tumors are characterized by fascicles of spindle cells showing mild nuclear pleomorphism; scattered atypical or giant cells may be seen. In these tumors, the mitotic activity is of 1 or 2 mitotic figures per 10 hpf (Figs. 12.74 and 12.75).

Intermediate-Grade Leiomyosarcoma

These tumors show similar growth pattern as the low-grade tumors. However, atypical cells with hyperchromatic nuclei are commonly seen. Focal areas of necrosis or hemorrhage may be identified, while the mitotic activity in these tumors is between 3 and 5 mitotic figure per 10 hpf (Figs. 12.76 and 12.77).

High-Grade Leiomyosarcoma

In these tumors, the presence of marked cytologic atypia is obvious and composed of a dense proliferation of atypical spindle cells. Tumors with prominent epithelioid morphology can be seen. In addition, areas of myxoid degeneration, hyalinization, and stromal degeneration are common. The presence of atypical, pleomorphic tumor cells with bizarre nuclei is a common finding. The mitotic activity in these tumors is easily identified and commonly is over ten mitoses per 10 hpf (Figs. 12.78, 12.79, 12.80, and 12.81). These tumors are also commonly seen to be more infiltrative into adjacent adipose tissue.

Immunohistochemical and Molecular Features

The use of muscle markers as a diagnostic aid in the evaluation of smooth muscle tumors is important in order to separate these neoplasms from other more common spindle cell tumors of the mediastinum. Therefore, the use of smooth muscle actin, muscle-specific actin, desmin, and caldesmon (Fig. 12.82a–c) may prove helpful as these tumors may show variable positive staining in tumor cells. However, it is important to highlight that some smooth muscle tumors may show positive staining for epithelial markers, namely, keratin. The tumors, however, are generally negative for keratin

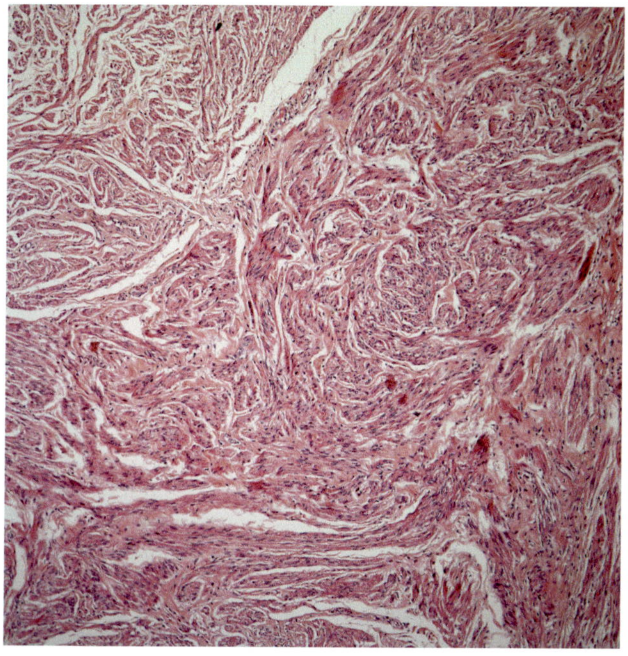

Fig. 12.72 Anterior mediastinal leiomyoma showing spindle cells in a fairly organized pattern

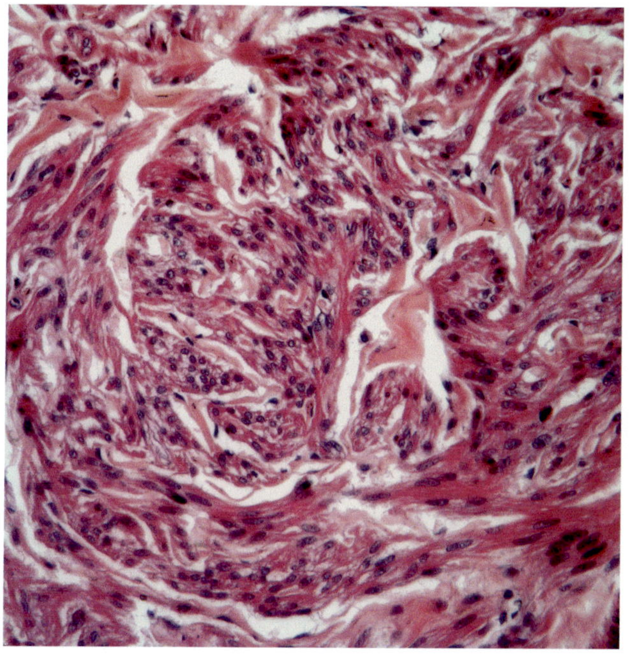

Fig. 12.73 Leiomyoma showing spindle cell proliferation lacking cellular atypia and mitotic activity

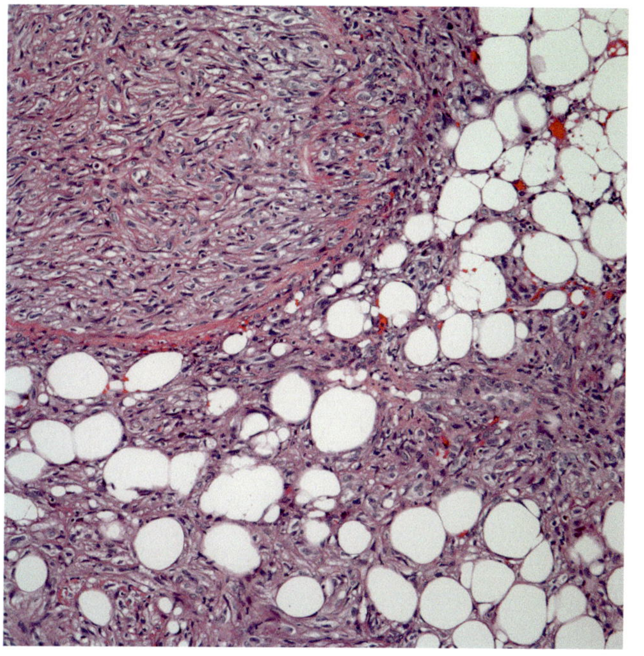

Fig. 12.74 Low-grade leiomyosarcoma infiltrating mediastinal adipose tissue

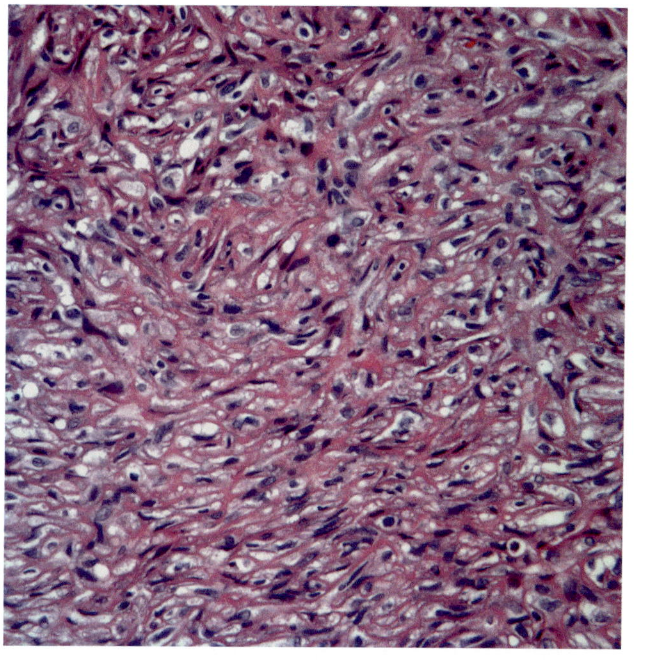

Fig. 12.75 Low-grade leiomyosarcoma showing scattered mitotic figures

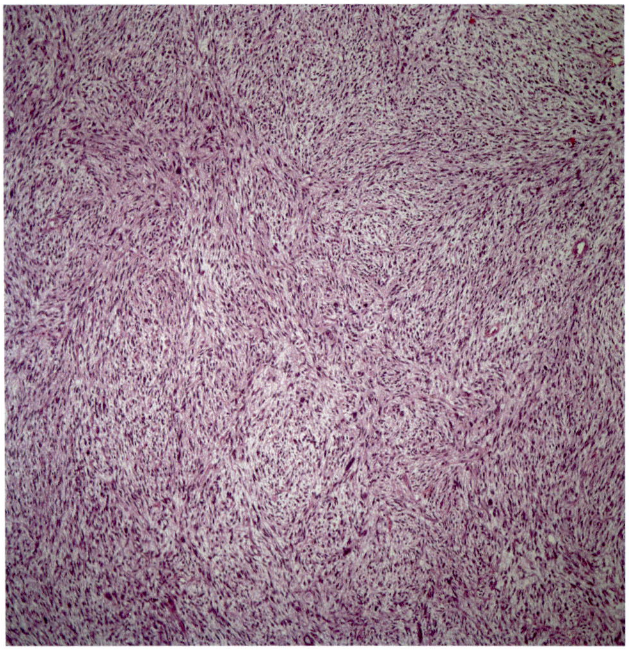

Fig. 12.76 Intermediate-grade leiomyosarcoma showing a cellular neoplasm

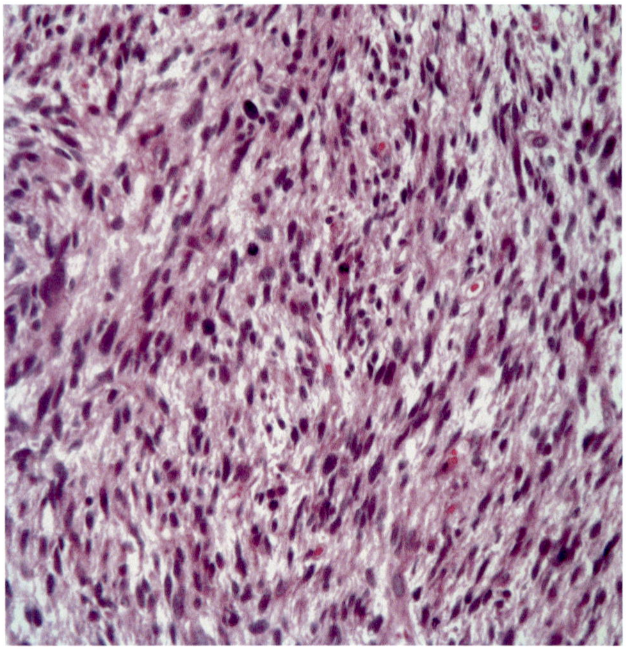

Fig. 12.77 Intermediate-grade leiomyosarcoma showing increase mitotic activity

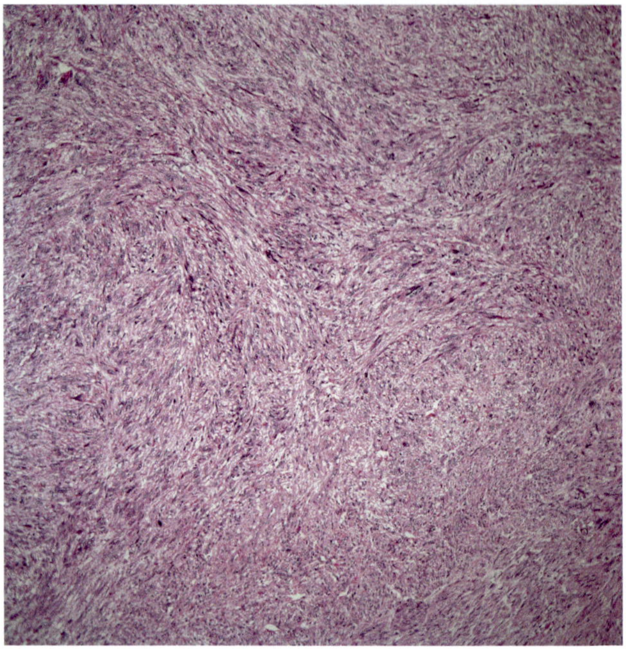

Fig. 12.78 Low power view of a high-grade leiomyosarcoma showing marked nuclear atypia

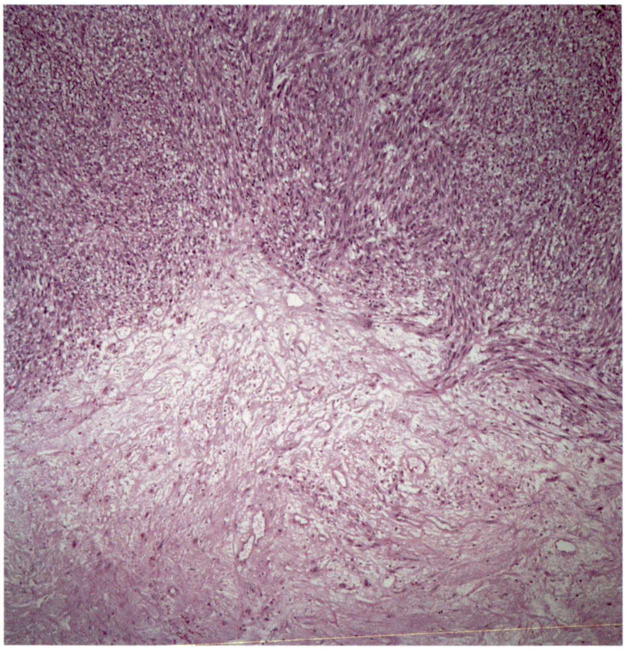

Fig. 12.79 High-grade leiomyosarcoma showing focal areas of infarction

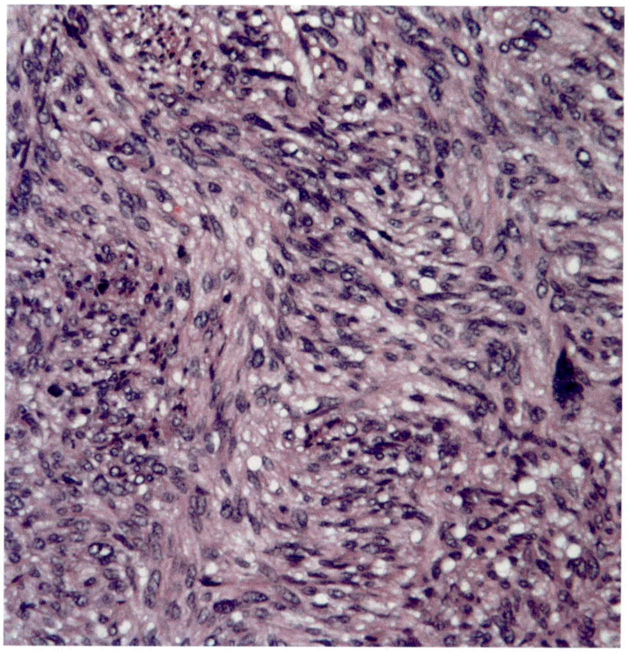

Fig. 12.80 High-grade leiomyosarcoma showing marked nuclear atypia

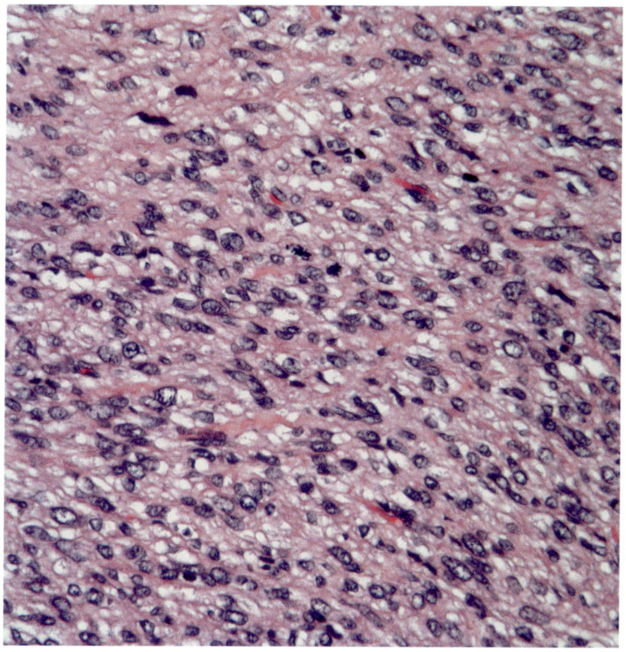

Fig. 12.81 High-grade leiomyosarcoma showing cellular atypia and mitotic activity

5/6, Bcl-2, CD34, CD31, S-100 protein, HMB-45, CD68, and TLE-1. In general, the diagnosis of leiomyosarcoma is not deferred to molecular studies unless the possibility of another sarcoma is being considered. The histopathologic features of the tumor coupled with the use of immunohistochemical muscle markers solve the majority of cases in which the suspicion for smooth muscle origin is considered.

Differential Diagnosis

The considerations in cases of mediastinal leiomyosarcomas are diverse and can vary from separating leiomyosarcomas from other types of sarcomas to separating the tumors from more common epithelial tumors such as spindle cell thymoma, spindle cell thymic carcinoma, or extension into the mediastinum by sarcomatoid carcinoma. In this regard, the use of immunohistochemical stains will lead generally to the right interpretation. For instance, thymic epithelial tumors are generally positive for keratin 5/6, which is negative in smooth muscle tumors. In the setting of a sarcomatoid carcinoma, the use of keratin antibodies and negative staining for muscle markers should be of aid in proper interpretation. Regarding the separation of leiomyosarcomas from other types of sarcomas, once again, the use of muscle markers in addition to different immunohistochemical stains which could potentially be used in other tumors – such as vascular markers (CD31 and CD34), or Bcl-2, TLE-1 which in cases of synovial sarcoma will also show staining for keratin and EMA – should help. In cases in which the histological features and immunohistochemical stains are still doubtful, the use of specific molecular analysis to rule out a specific sarcoma could be performed.

Rhabdomyosarcoma

Contrary to reported cases of leiomyoma or leiomyosarcoma, the existence of primary mediastinal rhabdomyosarcomas appears to be much less common. In addition, many cases that have been described in the literature either have been poorly documented or in today's classification of tumors may not necessarily be coded as rhabdomyosarcomas [1, 99–101]. In some instances, even if the classification of the tumor appears to be adequate, the specific pathological description of the tumor has not provided better insights regarding mediastinal rhabdomyosarcoma [102]. More difficult yet is the fact that rhabdomyosarcomas are common neoplasms associated with germ cell tumors, which usually will occur in the similar setting of young patients.

The only description that considered many of the issues associated with the diagnosis of mediastinal rhabdomyosarcomas is a report of four cases of these tumors arising in the anterior mediastinum [103]. The authors described three men and one woman between the ages of 19 and 27 years. Clinically, the patients presented with non-specific symp-

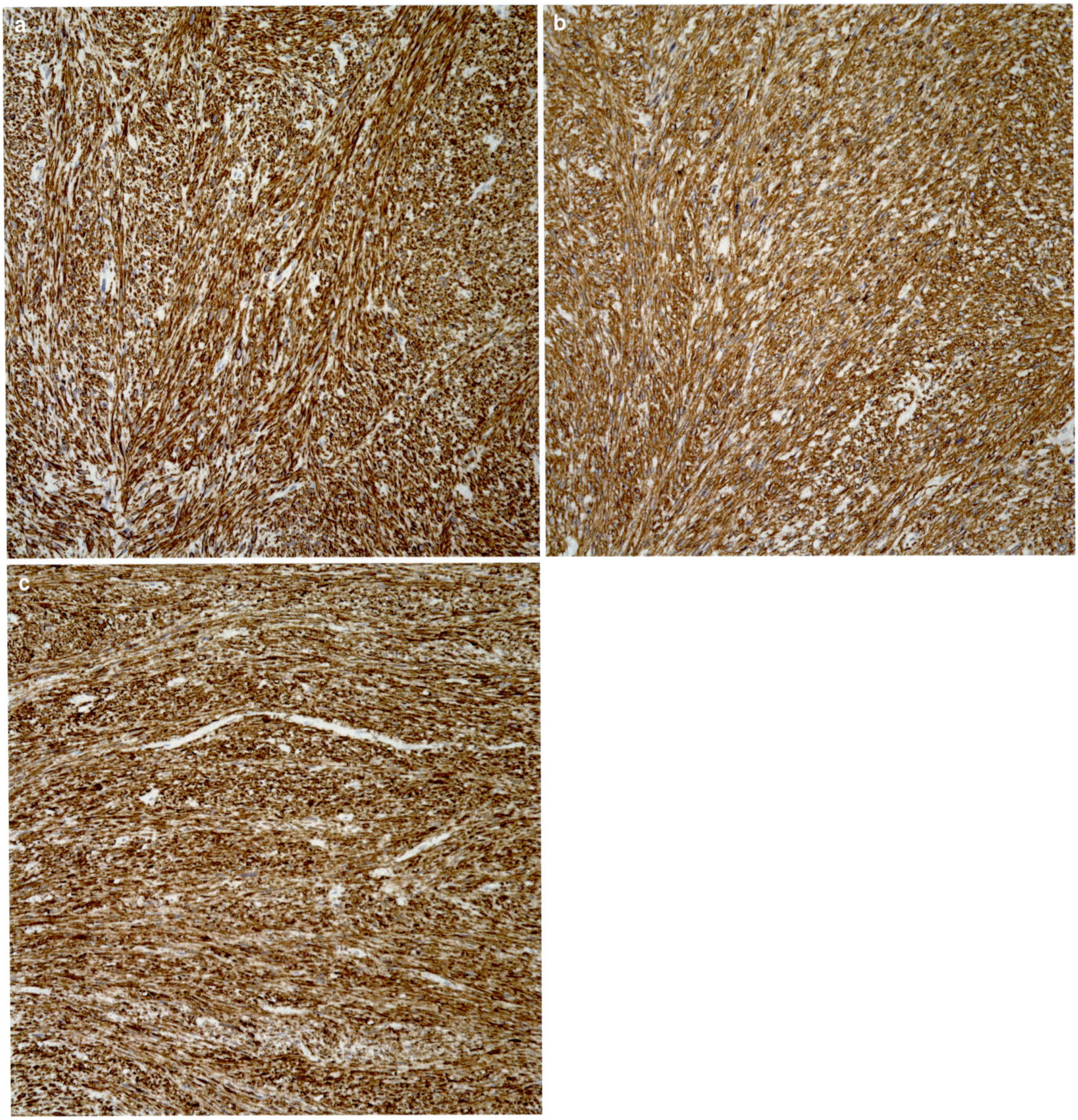

Fig. 12.82 (**a–c**) Leiomyosarcoma showing positive staining for (**a**) desmin, (**b**) smooth muscle actin, and (**c**) caldesmon

toms of cough, chest pain, dyspnea, and pleural effusion. Radiographically, the tumors appear to be infiltrative. All patients had metastatic disease within a period of 6 months after the initial diagnosis, and three of them were known to have died of tumor in that period of time. The authors concluded that mediastinal rhabdomyosarcomas are aggressive neoplasms, a diagnosis that should be carefully evaluated, making sure that the rhabdomyosarcoma is not a component of another neoplasm.

Pathological Features

Macroscopically, the tumors are ill defined, firm, and tan to gray in color. The cut surface is glistening and rubbery; areas of necrosis or hemorrhage may be present. The tumor size may vary from 4 to more than 10 cm in greatest diameter.

Histologically, similar to rhabdomyosarcomas in other areas, these tumors may show the full spectrum of differentiation, namely, alveolar, embryonal, and pleomorphic growth patterns. Thus, the tumors may show an alveolar, spindle cell, or pleomorphic cellular proliferation. The tumors may be arranged in monotonous small round blue cells, fascicles of spindle cells with focal myxoid changes, or showing atypical large, pleomorphic cellular proliferation with the presence of larger cells with round nuclei, prominent nucleoli, and ample eosinophilic cytoplasm. Areas of necrosis, mitoses, and hemorrhage may be seen in variable proportions (Figs. 12.83, 12.84, 12.85, 12.86, 12.87, and 12.88).

Immunohistochemical and Molecular Features

The use of immunohistochemical stains to aid in the diagnosis of rhabdomyosarcoma is important in separating these tumors from other high-grade sarcomas or primitive neuroectodermal tumors. In this setting, the use of muscle markers such as desmin, myoglobin, and Myo-D may prove useful in the diagnosis of rhabdomyosarcoma as these markers will show variable positive staining in tumors cells. Even though rhabdomyosarcomas may also express keratin staining in some cases, sarcomatoid carcinomas generally do not express muscle markers such as desmin, myoglobin, or Myo-D. Other stains – including S-100 protein, HMB-45, CD31, CD34, CD68, keratin 5/6, and STAT-6 – are negative in rhabdomyosarcomas.

Recent studies on molecular analysis for rhabdomyosarcomas in other sites have encountered that FOXO1 fusion-positive alveolar and MYOD1-mutant sclerosing are associated with unfavorable prognosis [104, 105]. Recently, Seki and coworkers [106] studied 60 cases of rhabdomyosarcoma and essentially divided specific subgroups: the alveolar histology often associated with PAX3/7 fusions and alterations in the cell cycle regulators while the embryonal histology often with CN alterations and/or allelic imbalances, FGFR4/RAS/AKT pathway mutations and PTEN mutations/methylation, and p53 inactivation.

Differential Diagnosis

Differential diagnosis will depend largely on the growth pattern of the rhabdomyosarcoma. However, because many of these tumors are seen in young patients, it is important to consider the so-called small round blue cell tumors such as primitive neuroectodermal tumor and neuroblastoma. In this setting, the use of muscle markers will lead to the correct interpretation. In rhabdomyosarcomas with more pleomorphic or spindle cell features, one would consider other types of high-grade or spindle cell sarcomas. Two additional important considerations include triton tumor and malignant schwannoma. In the former, the careful analysis of the neural component will lead to the correct interpretation, while in the latter the use of immunohistochemical stains for desmin, Myo-D, and myoglobin will prove useful. The use of a wide panel of immunohistochemical stains or the judicious use of molecular analysis should lead to the correct interpretation.

Fibroblastic, Myofibroblastic, and Fibrohistiocytic Tumors

This group of primary mediastinal neoplasms is rare and likely accounts for no more than 1% of all mesenchymal neoplasms of the mediastinum. However, it is important to mention that proper classification of these tumors may not be as simple as it may appear, mainly due to changes in the classification of previous and current soft tissue neoplasms. For instance, many tumors that in the past were more common, such as fibrosarcoma and hemangiopericytoma, can be reclassified in today's practice with the current immunohistochemical studies available under a different category, thus leaving only a small proportion of cases that actually may fulfill current criteria for this specific diagnosis. The tumors that will be included in this group are:

- Solitary fibrous tumor
- Inflammatory myofibroblastic tumor
- Angiomatoid fibrous histiocytoma
- Giant cell tumor
- Malignant fibrous histiocytoma

Solitary Fibrous Tumor

This tumor has particular affinity to occur in serosal membranes, specifically in the pleura [107]. However, the tumor has been described in numerous other locations including

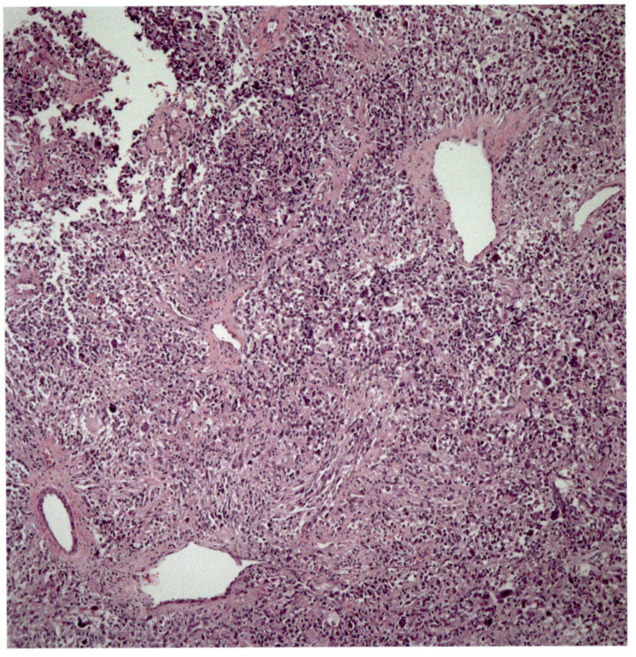

Fig. 12.83 Alveolar rhabdomyosarcoma showing a neoplastic cellular proliferation arranged in a subtle alveolar pattern

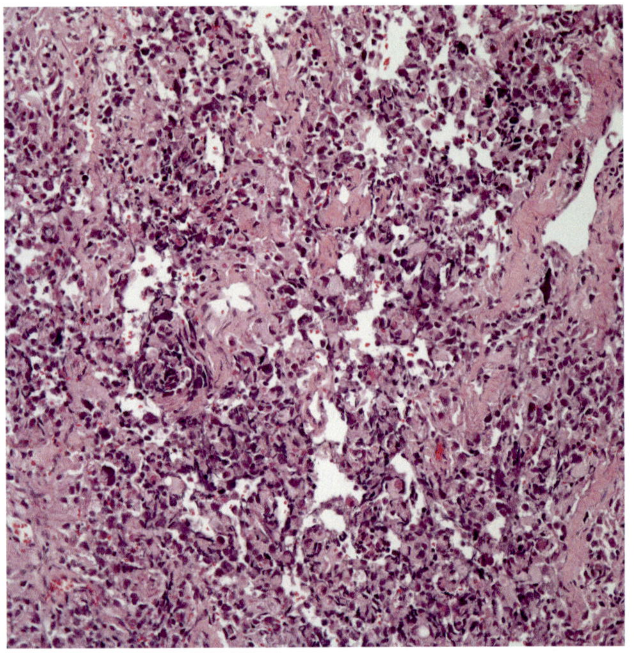

Fig. 12.84 Alveolar rhabdomyosarcoma showing a small round blue cell neoplastic cellular proliferation

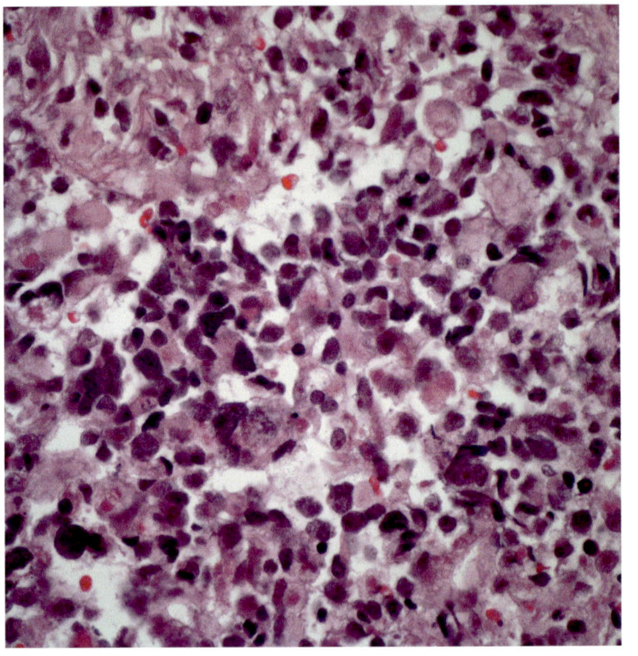

Fig. 12.85 Higher magnification of an alveolar rhabdomyosarcoma showing rhabdomyoblastic differentiation

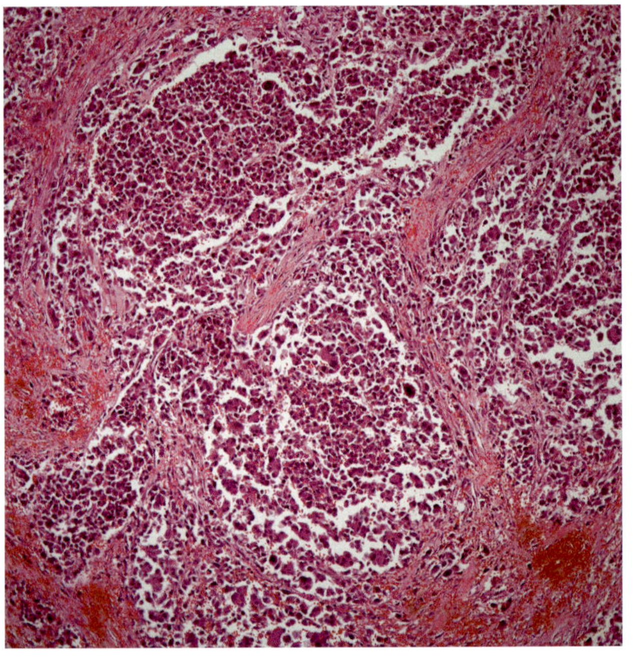

Fig. 12.86 Pleomorphic rhabdomyosarcoma showing prominent cellular atypia

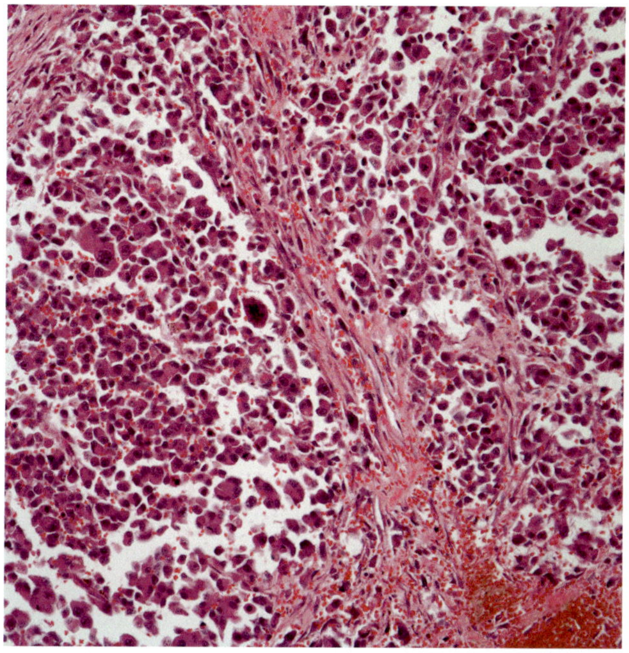

Fig. 12.87 Pleomorphic rhabdomyosarcoma showing cellular atypia and mitotic activity

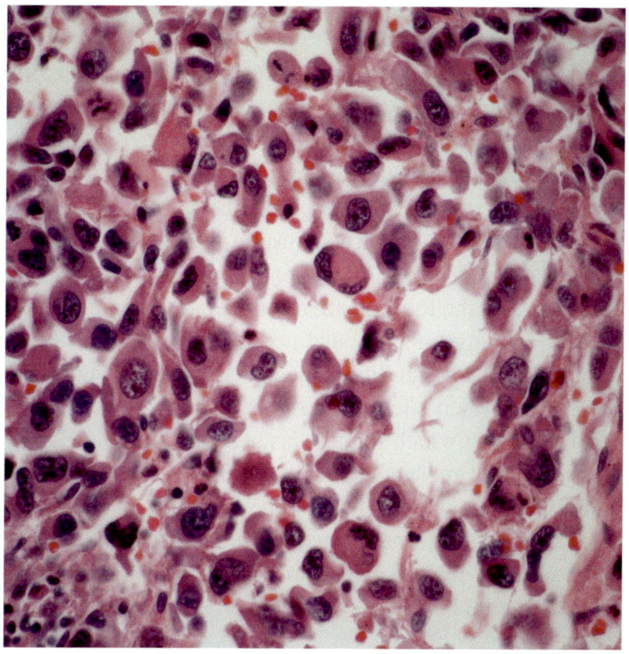

Fig. 12.88 Pleomorphic rhabdomyosarcoma showing rhabdomyoblastic differentiation

upper respiratory tract, peritoneum, liver, thyroid, and soft tissue. In the past, there have been numerous terms that have been employed to designate this neoplasm; these include sub-mesothelial fibroma, fibroma, localized mesothelioma, and localized fibrous tumor. Currently, the term solitary fibrous tumor is the one in use. In the description of 223 cases from the Armed Forces Institute of Pathology [107], the authors stated that common clinical finding for these patients included hypoglycemia, clubbing of the fingers, and pleural effusions. In addition, the authors stated that tumors attached by a pedicle had better prognosis regardless of the histology. Regarding histological features, the authors determined that the presence of necrosis, hemorrhage, and mitotic activity more than four mitoses per 10 hpf determined the separation between benign and malignant "localized" (fibrous) tumor. On the other hand, one aspect that is important to highlight is the spectrum of growth pattern that these tumors show whether in the serosal surfaces, viscera, or soft tissue. This particular issue was highlighted in a specific publication dealing with the numerous growth patterns that these tumor may show, which may include synovial sarcoma-like, neural-like, angiomatous-like, and hemangiopericytic, among others [108].

Credit to the initial description of solitary fibrous tumor in the mediastinum is given to Witkin and Rosai [109], who, in 1989, described 14 cases of this entity in the mediastinum. Clinically, the patients were eight men and six women between the ages of 27 and 70 years who presented with diverse symptomatology. Symptoms included cough, chest pain, and only one patient presented with hypoglycemia, clubbing of the fingers, and osteoarthropathy, while in three patients the tumor was identified on routine chest films. The histological features accounted for these tumors in the mediastinum mirror those described in similar tumors in the pleura. Since this original description, there have been sporadic case reports of solitary fibrous tumor in the mediastinum stressing histological or clinical features [110, 111]. Important to highlight is that, due to the heterogeneity that this tumor may show – including hemangiopericytic features – often the diagnosis of hemangiopericytoma has become intertwined with that of solitary fibrous tumor, and descriptions of hemangiopericytomas in the mediastinum have been reported [112]. In the series reported by Witkin and Rosai [109], the authors were able to provide meaningful follow-up in some cases, reporting that three patients had died of tumor within a period ranging from 4 months to

13 years. One patient was reported dead 9 years after initial diagnosis due possibly to complications of radiation therapy. Three patients were found alive with recurrence during a period of 3 months to 13 years after initial diagnosis, while four patients were found alive without evidence of disease in a period of 18 months to 13 years. The authors concluded that those tumors with frank sarcomatous areas are likely to behave more aggressively while larger tumors had higher risk of recurrence.

Pathological Features

Macroscopically, these tumors can reach very large size, and tumors in excess of 20 cm in greatest diameter have been described. The tumors are well circumscribed, lobulated and tan to gray in color. The cut surface is firm, slightly lobulated, and may show areas of hemorrhage and necrosis as well as cystic changes (Fig. 12.89). Cases in which the tumor appears to be attached to the thymus by a pedicle have been described. Even though the tumor may be arising in the mediastinum, in some cases it may be adherent to the pleura or invading superficially the lung parenchyma.

Histologically, the tumors may show different growth patterns; however, the tumor characteristically shows alternating hypo- and hypercellular areas (Fig. 12.90). The hypocellular areas show scant spindle cell proliferation and areas of hyalinization. Focal calcification or ossification may be seen in these areas. On the contrary, the hypercellular areas may show a solid spindle cell proliferation, which may acquire the so-called herringbone growth pattern. In other areas, the tumor cells are admixed with collagen and ectatic vessels. Areas composed of round "epithelioid" cells can also be seen. The tumor may show neural-like areas, angiomatoid-like areas and, in the hypercellular areas, a monophasic synovial sarcoma-like/fibrosarcoma-like growth patterns. It is the constellation of different growth pattern that should alert to the diagnosis of solitary fibrous tumor. Areas of hemorrhage and necrosis may be seen, and the mitotic activity is variable in these tumors, ranging from no mitotic activity to more than 10 per 10 hpf (Figs. 12.90, 12.91, 12.92, 12.93, 12.94, 12.95, 12.96, and 12.97).

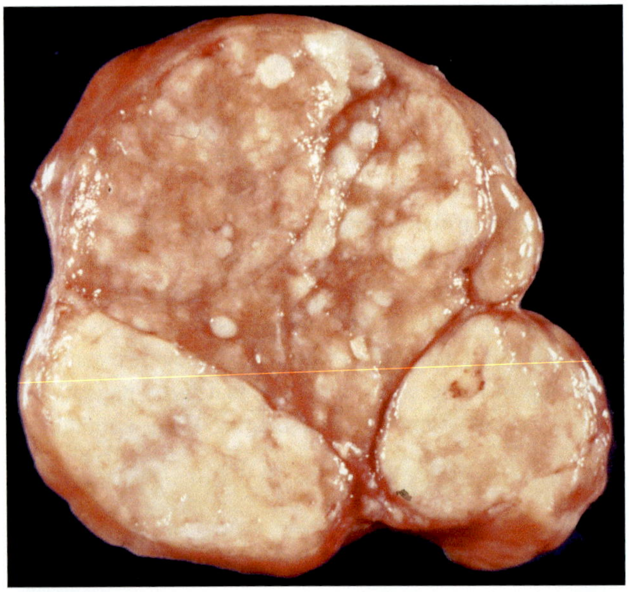

Fig. 12.89 Solitary fibrous tumor of the mediastinum showing a solid lobulated tumor mass

Immunohistochemical Features

The most important immunohistochemical stains in the diagnosis of solitary fibrous tumors include vimentin, Bcl-2, CD34, and STAT6 (Fig. 12.98a–c). The tumors may also show focal positive staining for smooth muscle actin, but in general they are negative for keratin, desmin, CD31, S-100 protein, and HMB-45. However, it is important to note that some of the stains that show positive staining in solitary fibrous tumor, such as vimentin and Bcl-2, may also be found positive in other tumors, such as synovial sarcoma, while CD34 being a vascular marker may also show positive staining in vascular tumors. STAT6 appears to be for the time being a more specific stain for solitary fibrous tumor.

Differential Diagnosis

Due to the heterogeneity that this tumor may show, the differential diagnosis may be wide but in the mediastinum will include more common tumoral conditions such as spindle cell thymoma, spindle cell thymic carcinoma, and monophasic synovial sarcoma. In this setting, the use of immunohistochemical stains – mainly the use of keratin 5/6 – will be helpful as the majority of thymomas are positive for this marker, while the focal positivity for keratin and EMA with positive staining for Bcl-2 and negative staining for STAT6 should raise the possibility of monophasic synovial sarcoma. In cases in which such diagnosis is a strong consideration and in cases in which immunohistochemistry is not definitive, the use of molecular studies for the specific translocation for synovial sarcoma should be investigated. If another type of spindle cell malignancy is being considered, then a wider panel of immunohistochemistry or specific molecular analysis should be considered.

Inflammatory Myofibroblastic Tumor

The occurrence of this tumor in the mediastinal location is rare. By far, these tumors are more common in intrapulmonary location. However, the tumor has ubiquitous distribution. Coffin and coworkers [113] presented their experience with 84 such cases in extrapulmonary location. The tumor distribution was in the upper respiratory tract, retroperitoneum,

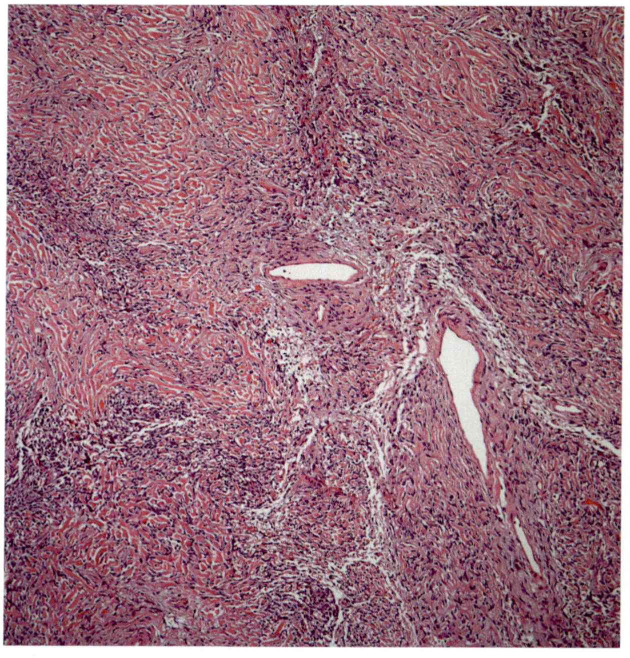

Fig. 12.90 Solitary fibrous tumor showing the classic features of spindle cell proliferation admixed with strands of collagen

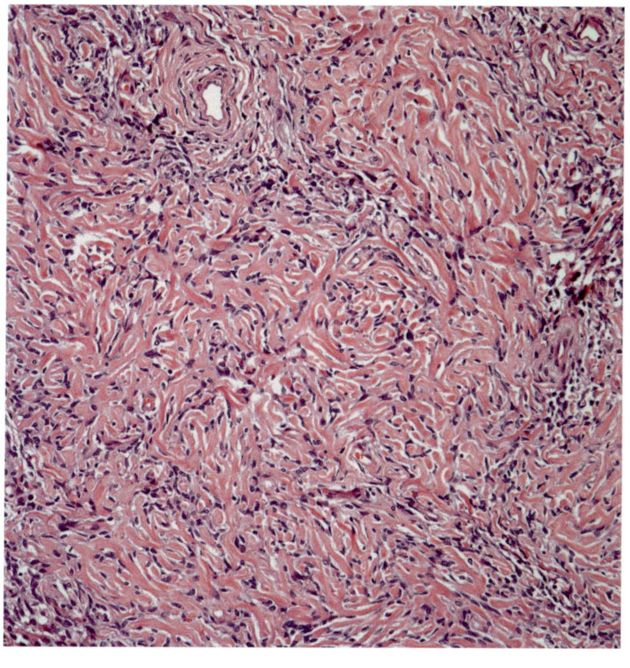

Fig. 12.91 Higher magnification of solitary fibrous tumors showing spindle cell proliferation admixed with collagen, note the absence of cellular atypia or mitotic activity

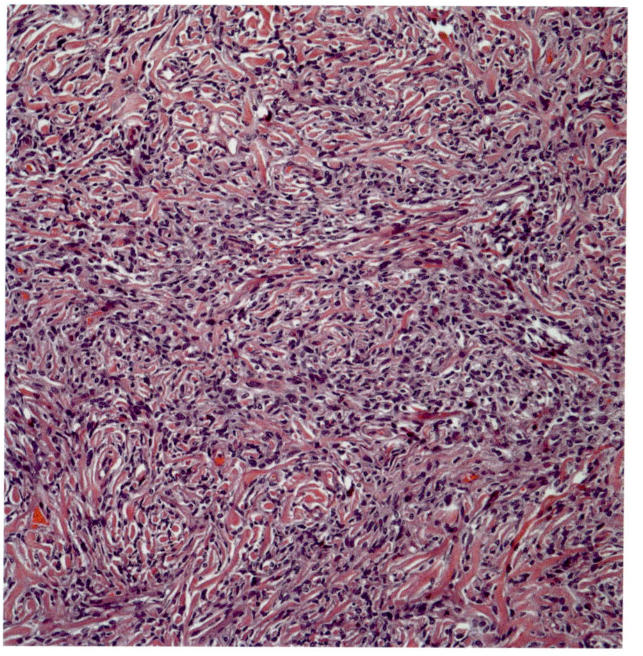

Fig. 12.92 Cellular areas of solitary fibrous tumor in which the collagen component is more subtle

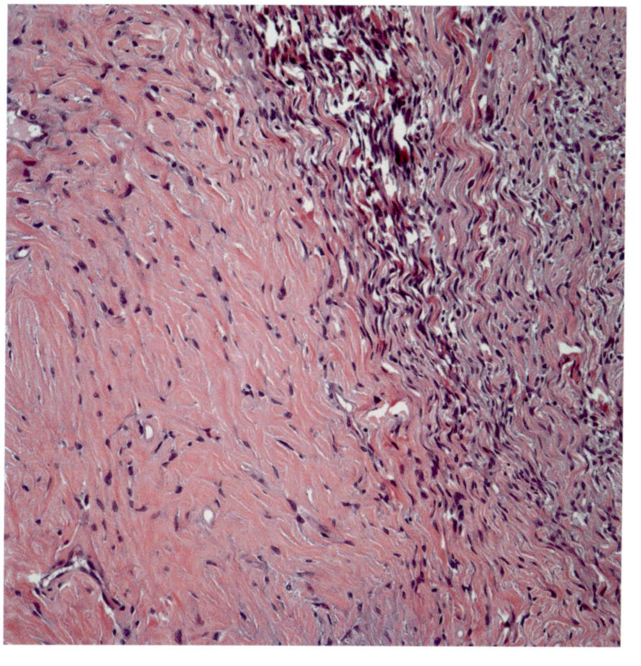

Fig. 12.93 Alternating hypo- and hypercellular areas in solitary fibrous tumor

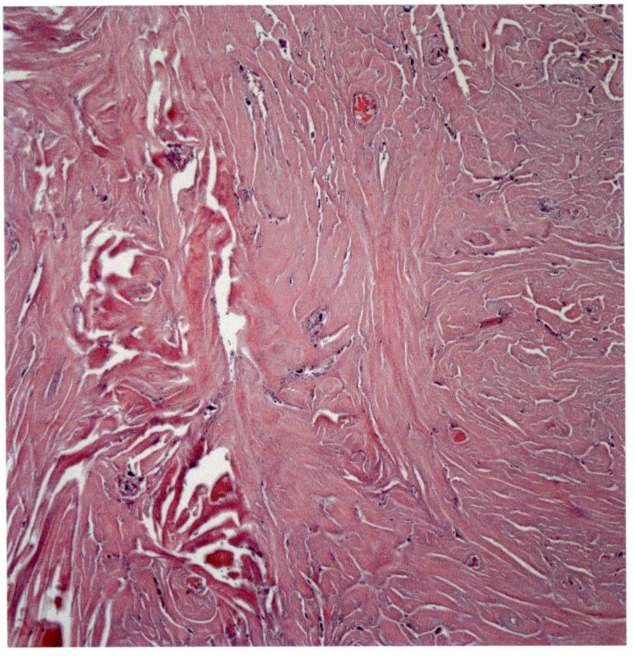

Fig. 12.94 Extensive hyalinization in solitary fibrous tumor

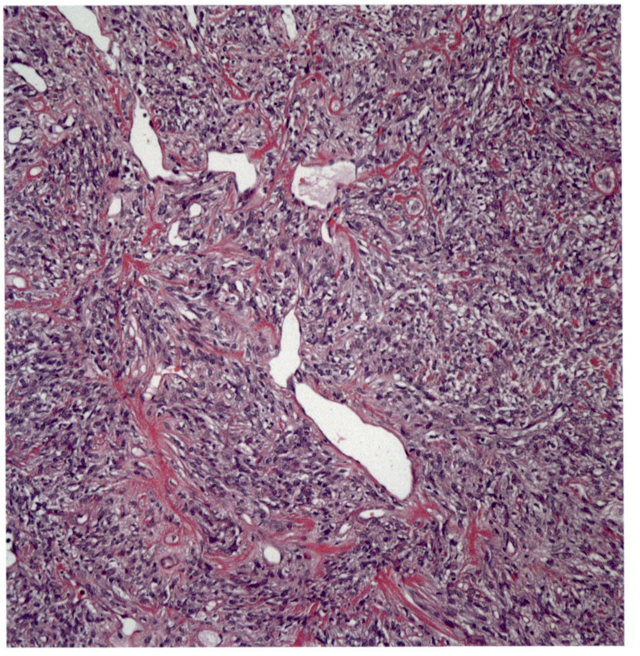

Fig. 12.96 Hypercellular areas in solitary fibrous tumor with a hemangiopericytic growth pattern

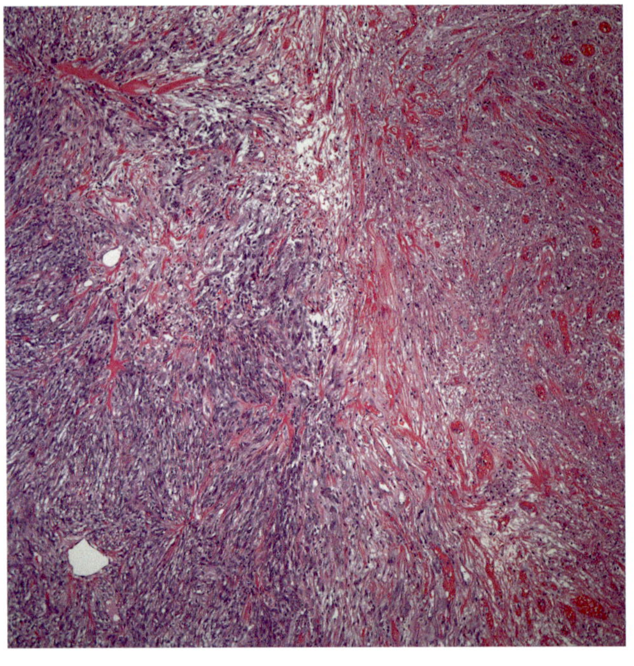

Fig. 12.95 Spindle cell component associated with areas of necrosis in solitary fibrous tumor, a feature associated with more aggressive behavior

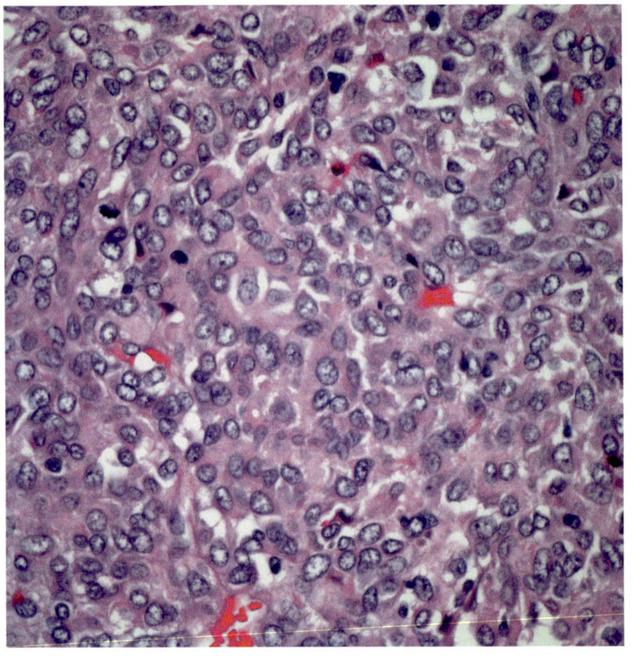

Fig. 12.97 Higher magnification shows mitotic activity, which is also another feature associated with aggressive behavior

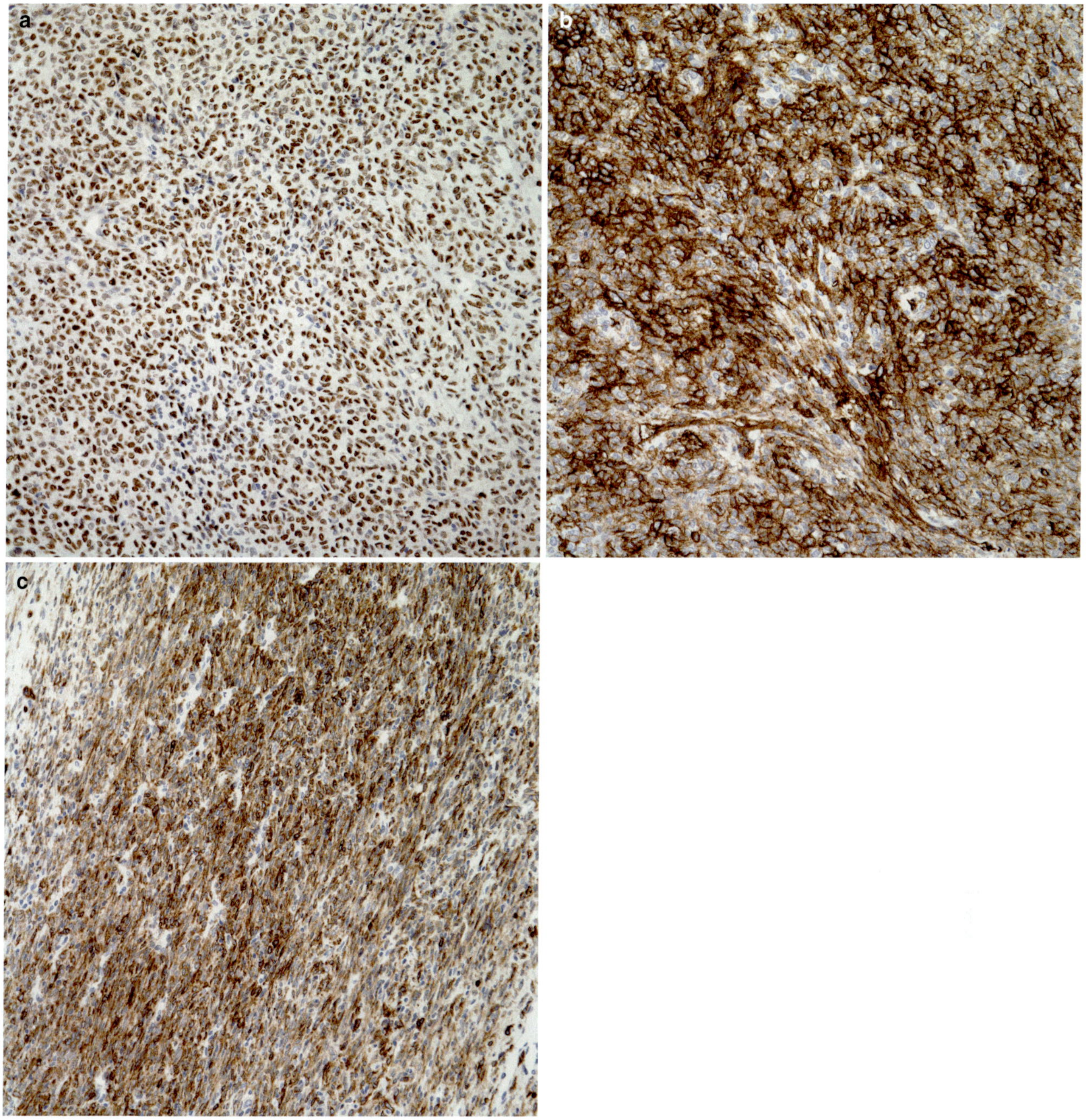

Fig. 12.98 (**a**) Immunohistochemical stain for STAT6 shows strong nuclear positivity, (**b**) CD34 shows strong positivity in tumor cells, (**c**) Bcl-2 shows also positive staining in tumor cells

abdomen, head and neck, pelvis, and extremities. The patients were 48 females and 36 males between the ages of 3 months and 46 years. The symptomatology was also diverse including pain, presence of a mass, fever, and weight loss. In addition, laboratory abnormalities – including anemia, thrombocytosis, polyclonal hypergammaglobulinemia, and elevated erythrocyte sedimentation rate – were noted. Clinical follow-up was provided in 53 patients, showing that 44 patients were alive with no evidence of disease and 4 patients were alive with tumor. Recurrence was documented in 13 patients who had one or more recurrences, ranging from 1 to 24 months after initial diagnosis. The occurrence of inflammatory myofibroblastic tumor in the mediastinum has been recorded mainly as case reports [114, 115]. Makimoto [114] reported a 59-year-old man with a posterior mediastinal tumor who underwent surgical resection of the tumor. No long-term follow-up was provided even though the postoperative was uneventful. Also, Chen and coworkers [115] described a 58-year-old woman with an anterior mediastinal tumor that was invading the sternum, pericardium, and pleura. In this patient, surgical resection was undertaken, and a follow-up of 6 months with no recurrence was provided.

Even though the occurrence of this tumor in the mediastinum is not common, it is likely that the behavior of the tumors will be similar to those tumors occurring in the lung or other extrapulmonary locations. Essentially, the tumor may be localized or invade adjacent structures. However, surgical resection appears to be the treatment of choice whenever possible. Recurrences are seen in some patients.

Pathological Features

Macroscopically, these tumors may be rather small or reach larger size, but usually in the mediastinum, the tumors are around 10 cm in greatest diameter. Even though the tumor appears to be relatively well circumscribed, it can involve adjacent structures such as pleura or pericardium, as it has been documented in some cases.

Histologically, the tumors are characterized by a spindle cellular proliferation with variable amounts of inflammatory cells, namely, plasma cells and lymphocytes. The spindle cellular proliferation is arranged in fascicles with a subtle storiform growth pattern. The spindle cells have an elongated nuclei, and mitotic activity is rare. The bundles of spindle cells are commonly admixed with variable amounts of plasma cells and lymphocytes (Figs. 12.99, 12.100, 12.101, 12.102, and 12.103). Although areas of necrosis are not common, in some cases focal necrotic foci may be seen. In addition, the tumor may show myxoid, collagenous, and solid cellular areas.

Immunohistochemical and Molecular Features

Inflammatory myofibroblastic tumors may show positive staining for smooth muscle actin, vimentin, calponin, and p53. The tumor is generally negative for desmin, caldesmon, CD34, STAT6, and keratin. In approximately 50% of the cases, ALK immunostain may show cytoplasmic positive staining.

In the case described by Makimoto and associates [114], the authors performed FISH analysis showing ALK gene rearrangement, characterized by the separation of the centromeric and telomeric probes on either side of the common ALK breakpoint. In the case described by Chen and associates [115], the tumor was reported to be negative for ALK immunostain.

Differential Diagnosis

The most important differential diagnosis will be with other spindle cell tumors of either epithelial or mesenchymal origin. However, in this setting, the use of immunohistochemical stain such as keratin 5/6 or muscle markers may help in separating this tumor from spindle cell thymoma or smooth muscle neoplasms. The use of other stains – such as Bcl-2, STAT, EMA, TLE1 – may be useful in evaluating the possibility of synovial sarcoma or solitary fibrous tumor.

Angiomatoid Fibrous Histiocytoma

The occurrence of this tumor in the mediastinum is rare and has been recorded only in general description of angiomatoid fibrous histiocytomas in different locations or as single case reports [116–118]. Clinically, the tumors have been described in adults with no specific symptoms. Diagnostic imaging has shown the presence of a mediastinal mass. However, it is important to highlight that the diagnosis of this particular tumor in a mediastinoscopic biopsy may pose significant problems in interpretation and in separating it from other more common mediastinal neoplasms. It is possible that a definitive diagnosis of this tumor in the mediastinal region may require complete surgical resection and a wide panel of immunohistochemical stains.

Surgical resection of the tumor appears to be the treatment of choice, and the clinical outcome for these patients may be similar to that of patients with tumors in the soft tissues.

Pathological Features

Macroscopically, the tumor has variable size and appears to be well circumscribed but not encapsulated. The cut surface of the tumor is rather smooth and glistening, light tan in color. Areas of necrosis are not common; however, the tumor may show some cystic changes and areas of hemorrhage.

Histologically, the tumor is characterized by the presence of a spindle cell proliferation arranged in fascicles with a subtle storiform pattern and variable component of inflammatory cells, namely, plasma cells and lymphocytes. The

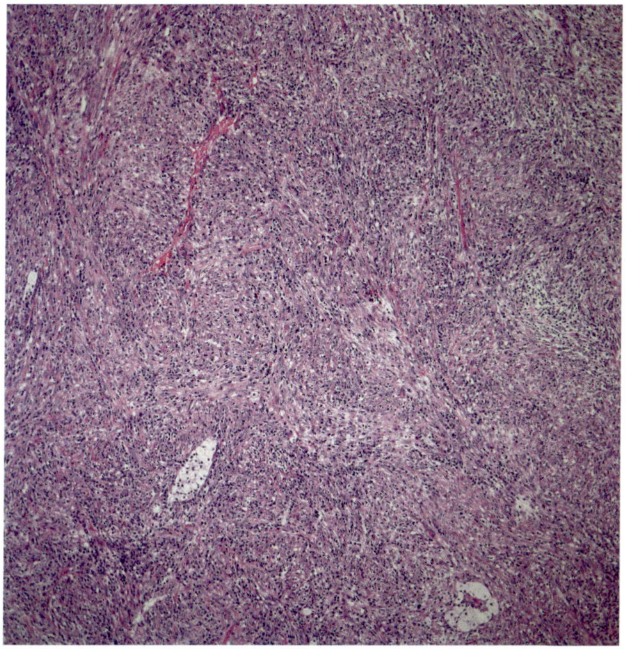

Fig. 12.99 Low power of an inflammatory myofibroblastic tumor showing a spindle cell proliferation

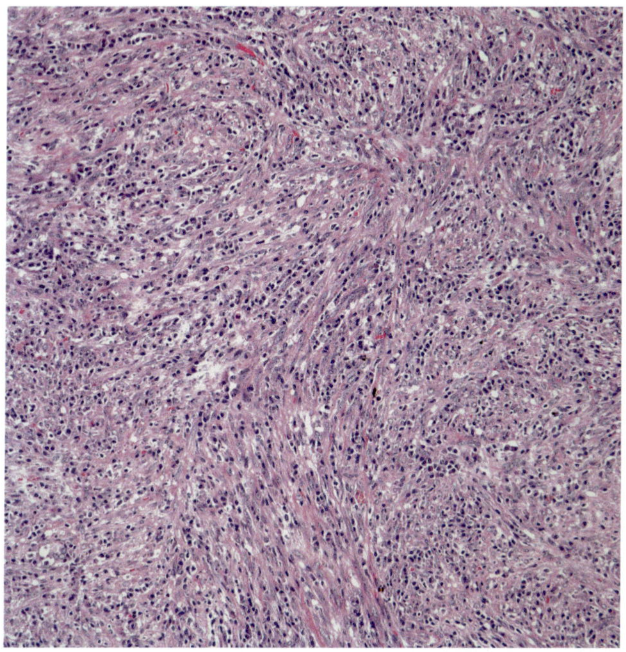

Fig. 12.100 Inflammatory myofibroblastic tumors showing a mixture of spindle cell and inflammatory component

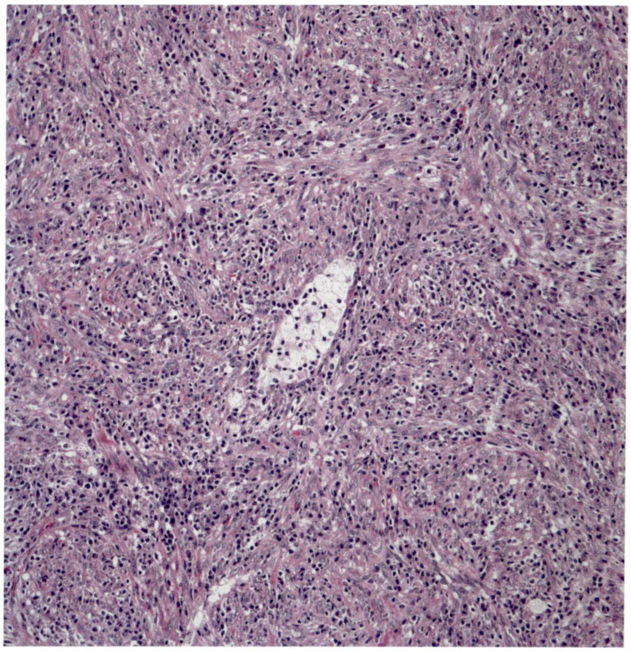

Fig. 12.101 Focal collections of foamy macrophages in an inflammatory myofibroblastic tumor

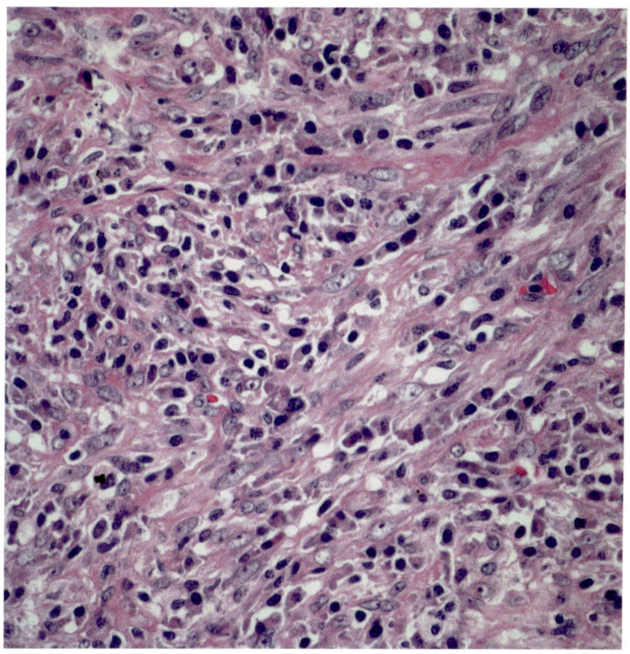

Fig. 12.102 Higher magnification of an inflammatory myofibroblastic tumor showing prominent plasma cell component

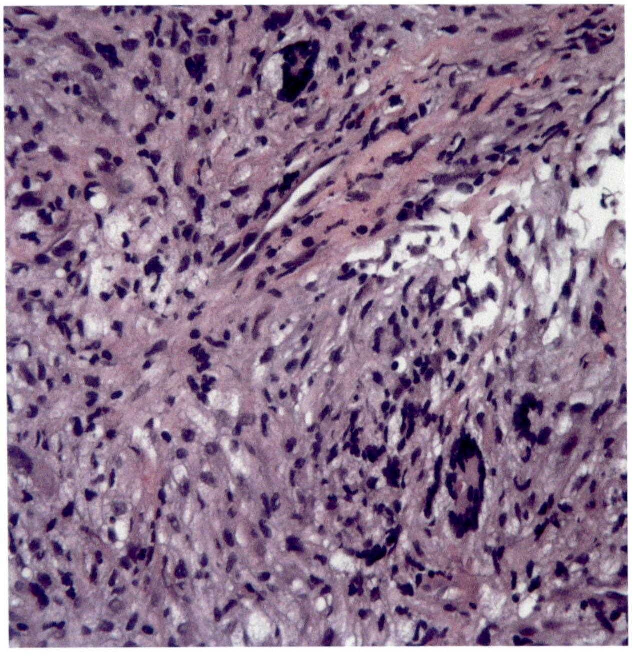

Fig. 12.103 Inflammatory myofibroblastic tumor showing focal areas with multinucleated giant cells

spindle cells have a plump nuclei, and mitotic activity is rare. Solid areas of spindle cell intermixed with inflammatory cells are commonly seen. In some areas, it is possible to identify the presence of an inflammatory infiltrate in the periphery of the tumor (Figs. 12.104, 12.105, 12.106, 12.107, 12.108, and 12.109). In focal areas, the presence of cystic and hemorrhagic areas may be seen.

Immunohistochemical Features

Essentially, this tumor is negative for epithelial, muscle, and neuroendocrine markers in addition to S-100 protein, HMB-45, and Melan A. However, the tumor shows positive staining for CD68 (Fig. 12.110) and low nuclear labeling for Ki-67.

Due to the rarity of this tumor in the mediastinum, there are no specific molecular studies to be done, but the results are likely to be similar to those reported in soft tissues.

Differential Diagnosis

Due to the rarity of this tumor in the mediastinum and the morphological features of the tumor, it is likely that it needs to be separated from other spindle cell tumors that are more common such as spindle cell thymoma. In this regard, the use of keratin 5/6 should be of help as most spindle cell thymoma are positive for this marker, while angiomatoid fibrous histiocytoma is negative. Other considerations will include dendritic reticulum cell sarcoma, synovial sarcoma, leiomyosarcoma, and solitary fibrous tumor. In this setting, a wider panel of immunohistochemical stains should lead to the correct interpretation or at least to rule out such possibilities.

Giant Cell Tumor

This particular tumor is included in this group of tumors in view of the possible relationship with other histiocytic tumors, and their affinity for having positive staining for histiocytic markers such as CD68.

The occurrence of the this tumor in the mediastinum is rare and originally reported by Fu and associates [119], with a description of two patients: a woman 30 years old and a young man of 18 years. Clinically, one patient presented with symptoms of paresthesia and pain in the right shoulder, while the other patient was asymptomatic, and the tumor was found during a routine chest film. Diagnostic imaging revealed that in both patients, the tumor was limited to the posterior mediastinal compartment. There was no previous history of tumor elsewhere in either patient. Surgical resection took place in both patients, and clinical follow-up from 8 to 108 months showed both patients alive with no evidence of recurrence or metastases.

Pathological Features

Macroscopically, the tumor may be of variable size, and in the cases described it has ranged from 2 to 8 cm in greatest diameter. Areas of necrosis and hemorrhage may be present, and for the most part, the tumor is firm and not encapsulated.

Histologically, the tumor is characterized by the presence of a dual population composed of mononuclear cells with round to oval nuclei and inconspicuous nucleoli and bland appearance. However, rare mitotic figures may be present in this component. The second component is composed of multinucleated giant cells of the osteoclast type. These multinucleated giant cells are intermixed without any specific pattern with the mononuclear component (Figs. 12.111 and 12.112). These multinucleated cells lack nuclear atypia and mitotic activity. Focal areas of calcifications and hemorrhage may be present in some cases.

Immunohistochemical Features

This tumor characteristically shows positive staining for CD68 and vimentin and negative for keratin, S-100 protein, desmin, smooth muscle actin, CD45, CD15, and other neuroendocrine markers.

Differential Diagnosis

The histology of giant cell tumors is rather straightforward. The most important interpretation would be ruling out the possibility of a metastasis from a tumor either from soft tissue or bone. Once that differential has been excluded, the interpretation should be made with ease. However, it is important to highlight that giant cell tumors are not mitotically active tumors, which should help in separating this tumor from another high-grade sarcoma, namely, malignant fibrous histiocytoma.

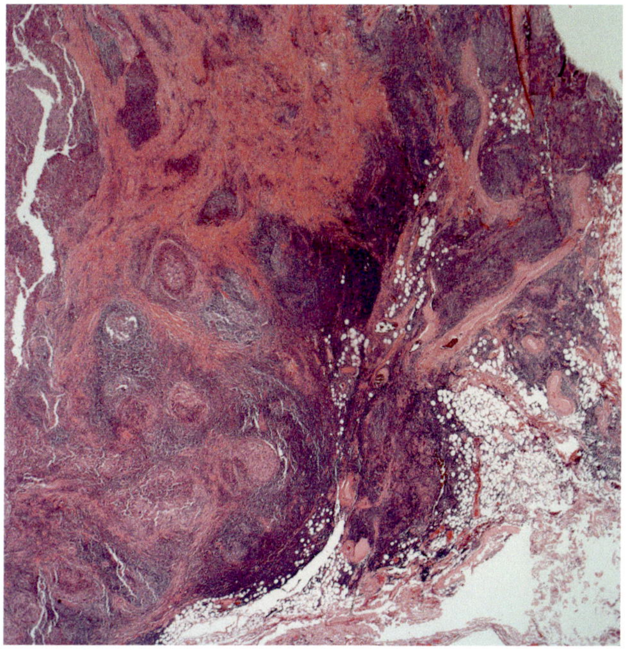

Fig. 12.104 Low-power magnification of angiomatoid fibrous histiocytoma showing a rim of thymic tissue

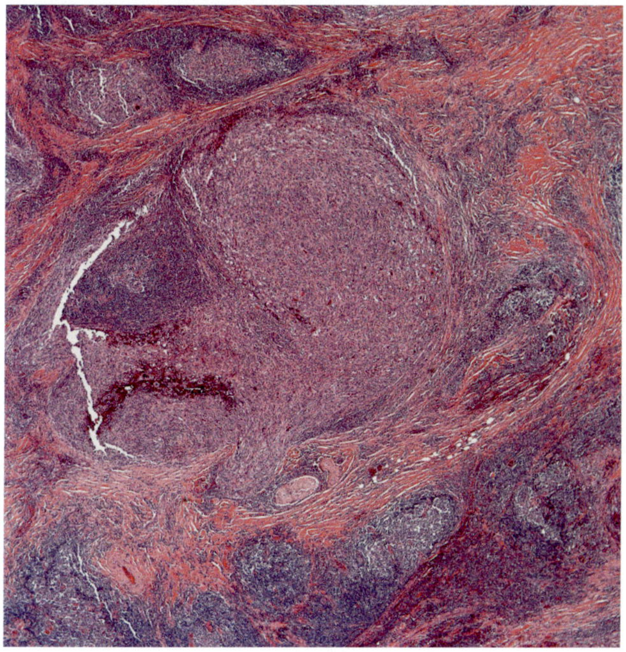

Fig. 12.105 Angiomatoid fibrous histiocytoma showing a lobular architecture

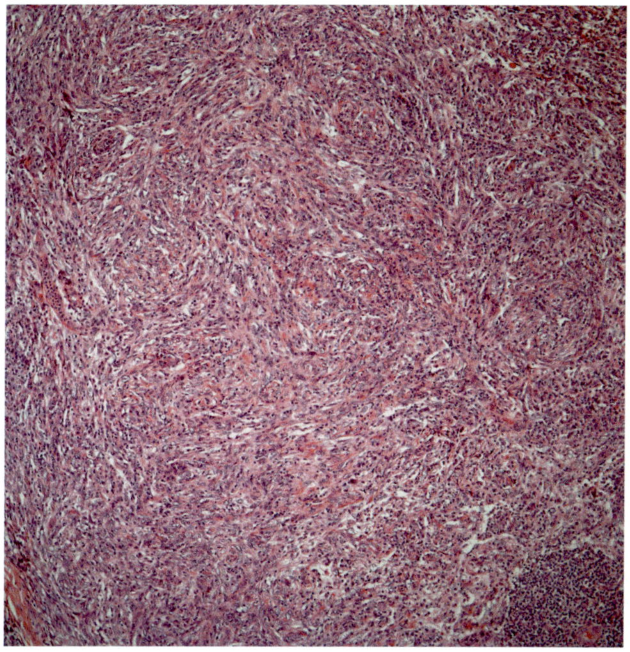

Fig. 12.106 Angiomatoid fibrous histiocytoma showing a spindle cell proliferation admixed with inflammatory cells

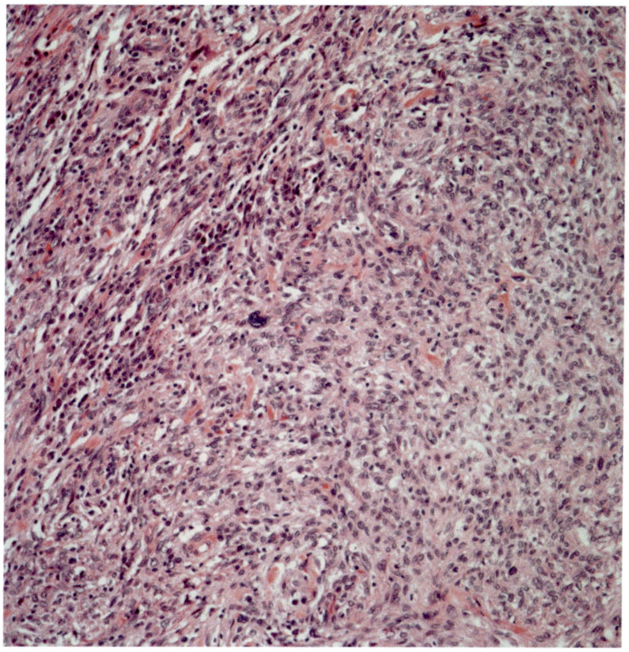

Fig. 12.107 Solid spindle cell proliferations with scattered atypical cells; note adjacent areas composed of plasma cells

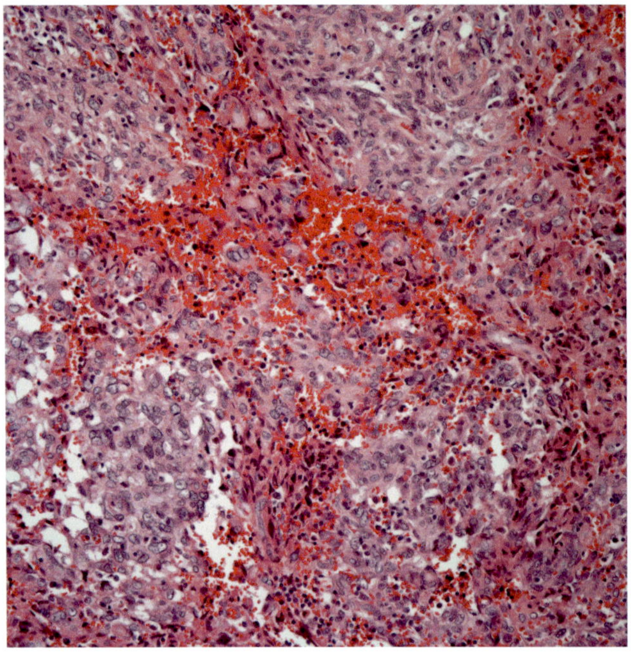

Fig. 12.108 Angiomatoid fibrous histiocytoma showing areas mimicking a vascular neoplasm

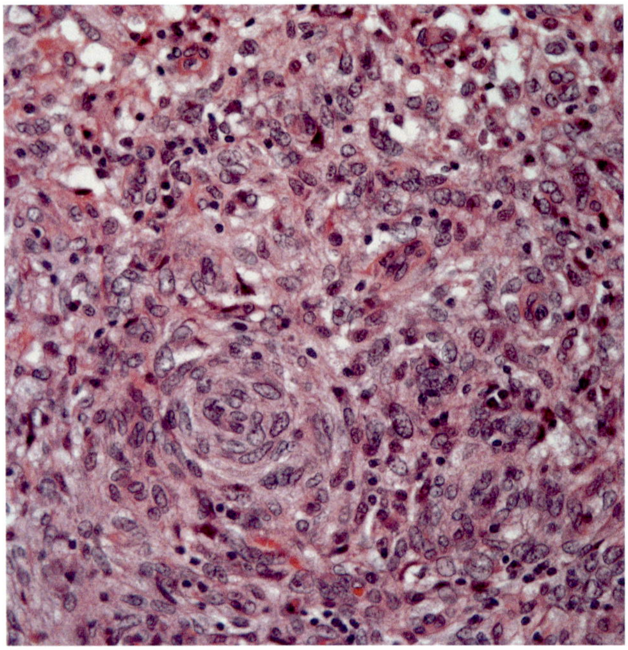

Fig. 12.109 High power magnification of an angiomatoid fibrous histiocytoma showing elongated cells with oval nuclei and in some with prominent nucleoli; note the absence of mitotic activity

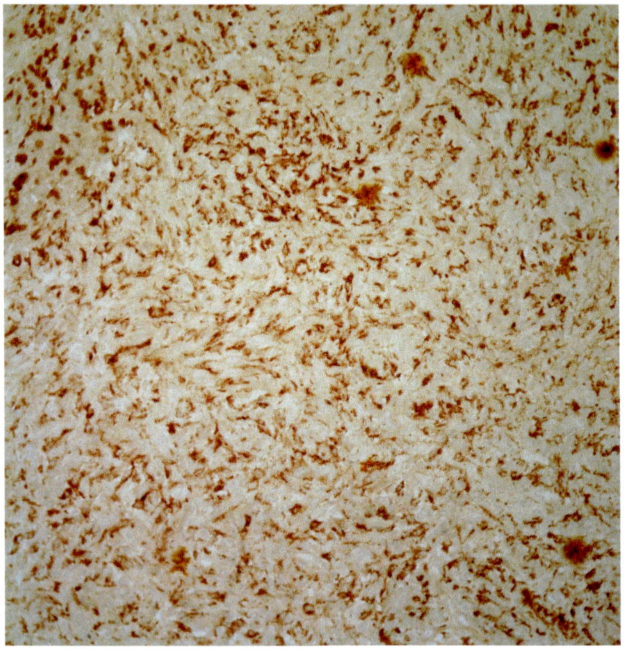

Fig. 12.110 Immunohistochemical stain for CD68 is strongly positive in the histiocytic component of angiomatoid fibrous histiocytoma

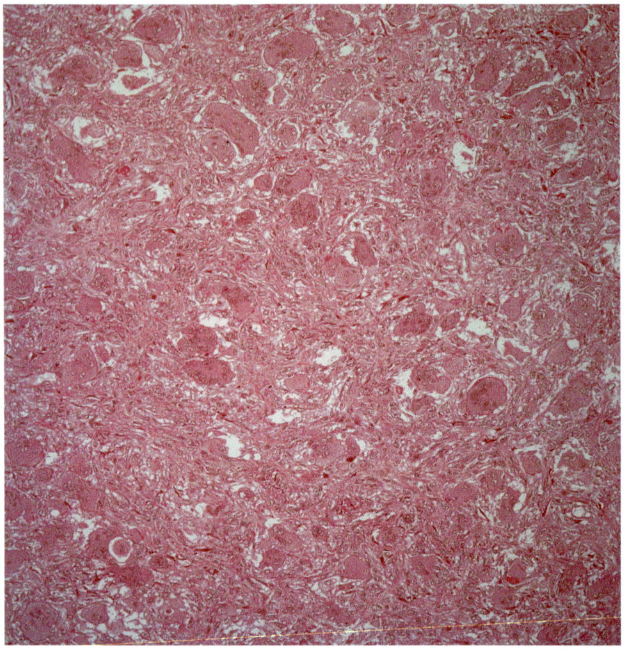

Fig. 12.111 Mediastinal giant cell tumor showing a dual population of mononuclear and multinucleated giant cells

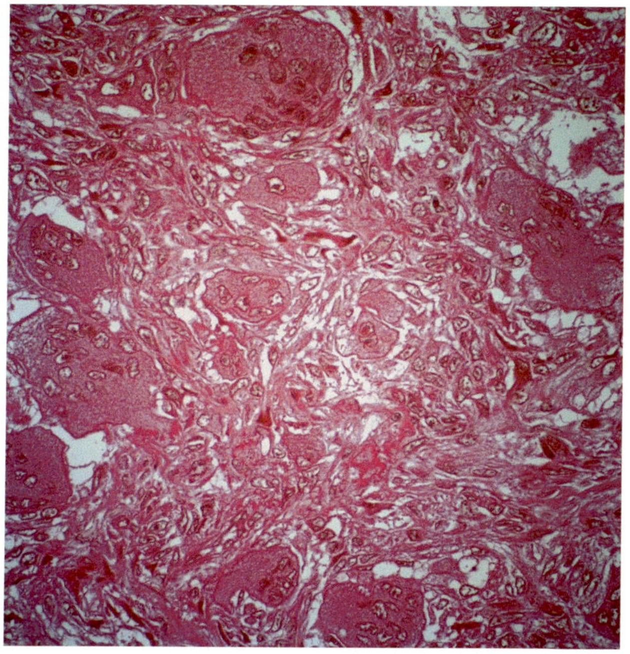

Fig. 12.112 Higher magnification of a mediastinal giant cell tumor showing absence of atypia and mitotic activity

Malignant Fibrous Histiocytoma

This is another tumor of unusual occurrence in the mediastinal compartment. Most of what is in the literature has been reported as single case reports [120, 121]. In general, primary mediastinal sarcomas are rare, and, in the current practice with the use of immunohistochemistry and molecular diagnostics, it is possible that the diagnosis of MFH is left for those tumors with the right histology and negative results for specific markers or molecular diagnostics. Thus, it is possible that tumors that in the past may have been considered as this type of sarcoma in today's nomenclature may correspond to a different category. On the other hand, in many cases, even though the histology is that of a high-grade sarcoma, the tendency is to code cases as high-grade sarcoma not otherwise specified. Therefore, the true incidence of cases that will fit as MFH in the mediastinum is rather unknown. In addition, it is important to properly document that the patient does not have any previous history of tumor elsewhere and that the tumor mass is in fact in the mediastinum and not in the lung or chest wall.

Nishida and associates [121] reported a case in a 72-year-old man as MFH developing from a "foreign body granuloma." The patient had a previous history of pulmonary tuberculosis and was found to have an anterior mediastinal mass. He died 18 months after initial diagnosis with recurrence. In a different case described by Imai and associates [120], the authors described a 63-year-old man with a history of acute coronary syndrome who was found to have an anterior mediastinal mass. The authors described the tumor as originating from the thymus in view of the presence of Hassall's corpuscles within the tumor. No clinical follow-up was provided in this case.

Pathological Features

Macroscopically, these tumors may have variable size with infiltrative borders; they are not encapsulated. The cut surface of the tumor is light tan to gray in color, and areas of necrosis and hemorrhage may be present. The tumor is firm, and focal mucoid areas may be seen.

Histologically, the tumor shows similar features as those described in soft tissue, essentially the features of a high-grade sarcoma (Figs. 12.113, 12.114, and 12.115), composed of spindle cells arranged in a storiform growth pattern. The cells have an elongated nuclei, eosinophilic cytoplasm; nuclear atypia and mitotic activity are easily identifiable. The presence of atypical mitotic figures is commonly seen. Some tumors may show prominent myxoid areas or be almost exclusively myxoid. Giant cells may be seen in some cases.

Immunohistochemical Features

This tumor also is characterized by showing negative staining for specific markers such as desmin, S-100 protein, CD34, STAT6, and CD31. Keratin may show focal positive staining in some cases. However, the tumor is usually positive for CD68 and vimentin. Ki-67 will label more than 50% of the nuclei.

Differential Diagnosis

The most important consideration is another high-grade sarcoma, either primary or metastatic to the mediastinum. In this setting, the use of a wide panel of immunohistochemical markers directed toward epithelial, muscle, neuroectodermal, or neuroendocrine neoplasm should lead in the correct interpretation, therefore leaving the diagnosis of MFH to tumors that do not show any specific differentiation and that have the right morphology.

Biphasic Neoplasms

This term as it is applied for this group of tumors essentially includes two malignant neoplasms: Synovial sarcoma and carcinosarcoma of the mediastinum. It is important to highlight that synovial sarcoma is included in this section even though in many cases the tumor does not show biphasic histology. These two neoplasms (synovial sarcoma and carcinosarcoma) in the thoracic cavity are much more common in intrapulmonary locations. In general, the occurrence of these tumors in the thoracic cavity is rare, and

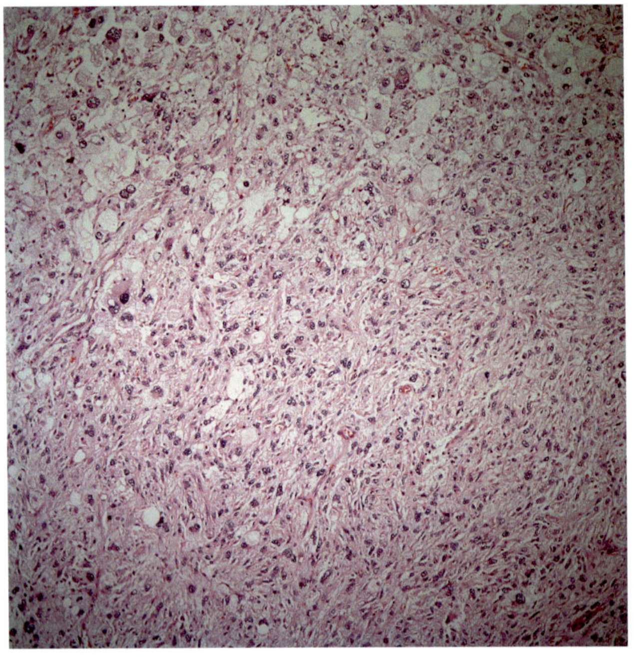

Fig. 12.113 High-grade sarcoma with features of MFH showing marked cellular atypia

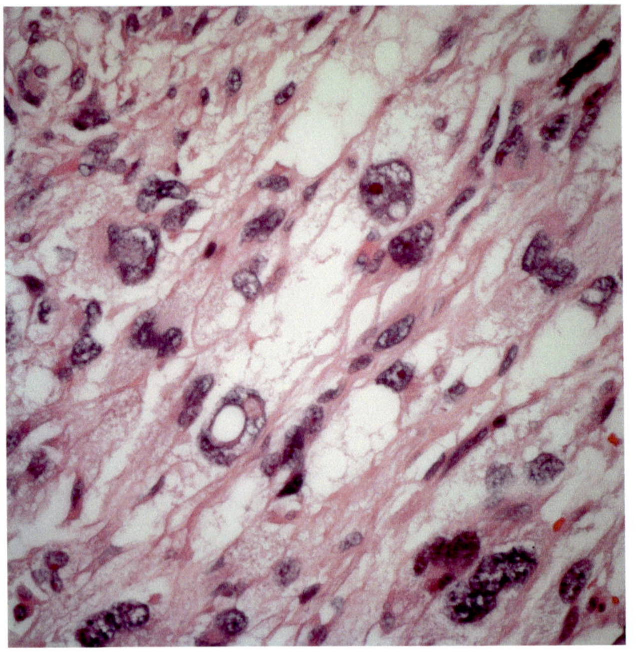

Fig. 12.115 Higher magnification showing marked nuclear atypia

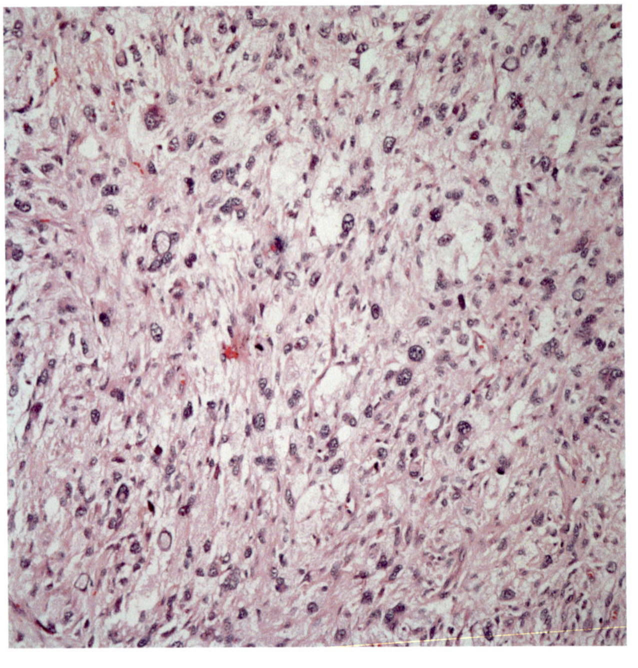

Fig. 12.114 The neoplastic cellular proliferation composed of medium-sized cells with oval nuclei and indistinct cell borders

most of what is known is based on single case reports, and in some instances on relatively large series of cases. Just the same as with other sarcomas of the mediastinum, it is essential that a good radiological evaluation be performed in order to determine that the tumor is in fact originating in the mediastinal compartment and not in the periphery of the lung or represents metastasis from an extrathoracic origin.

Synovial Sarcoma

The occurrence of synovial sarcoma as primary mediastinal neoplasm is rare, but it is more common than carcinosarcoma. The original description of this tumor in the mediastinum is credited to Witkin and associates [122], who, in 1989, described four patients with a biphasic tumor with features of synovial sarcoma. Clinically, the patients were four adult men between the ages of 40 and 73 years, who presented with diverse symptomatology including hoarseness, cough, dyspnea, and hemoptysis. All the patients had surgical resection; one patient had additional radiation therapy, and another patient had radiation and chemotherapy. Clinical follow-up information provided in three patients showed that they had died in a period of 10 months to 4 years. However, the largest series of synovial sarcomas of the mediastinum by Suster and Moran reported 15 such cases in this location [123]. The authors described ten male and five female patients between the ages of 3 and 83 years. Anatomically, nine tumors were located in the anterior mediastinum, while six tumors were located in the posterior mediastinal compartment. The symptomatology also depended on the location of the tumors, as, in those located in the posterior mediastinum, the patients presented with neck and back pain, while patients with tumors in the anterior mediastinum presented with chest pain, shortness of breath, and pleural effusions. All patients had surgery, and in some of the patients additional radiation therapy was documented. Unfortunately, meaningful follow-up was not available in the majority of patients, and in some patients, metastasis and recurrences were documented. However, it is important to highlight that the tumor not only can present as an anterior mediastinal tumor but it also can occur in the posterior compartment. In addition, important to highlight is that, even though in the original description by Witkin and associates [122] the authors emphasize the biphasic nature of these tumors, it seems that the biphasic histology is less frequent, as documented in the description of 15 cases [123] in which 10 of the tumors described corresponded to the monophasic variant of the tumor.

Outside of those two early publications, the report of mediastinal synovial sarcomas has been essentially of single case reports or by presenting these tumors in a group of sarcomas within the thoracic cavity [124–127]. For instance, in a recent publication of 26 synovial sarcomas in the thoracic cavity, the authors documented that the majority of tumors were either in the lung or pleura, with only a minority of cases in the mediastinum [125].

Pathological Features

Macroscopically, the tumor can vary in size from 5 cm to a large size of 20 cm in greatest dimension. Some tumors appear well circumscribed, while some other tumors appear to be ill defined with infiltrative borders, which could be seen infiltrating adjacent structures such as the pleura, lung, great vessels, or heart. The cut surface of these tumors is tan to gray in color, homogeneous with areas ranging from firm, friable to gelatinous consistency. Areas of hemorrhage, necrosis, and cystic changes can be seen in some cases.

Histologically, these tumors can display either monophasic of biphasic histological features. Biphasic tumors are characterized by a monotonous spindle cell proliferation admixed with an atypical glandular component (Fig. 12.116a–e). These two components may vary or be equal in proportion. The glandular component of the tumor may also vary in growth pattern and can show papillary, pseudopapillary, or glandular appearance. These areas are formed by a cuboidal or columnar epithelium with round to oval nuclei and inconspicuous nucleoli and moderate or abundant cytoplasm. The lumen of the glandular component may be filled with acellular material. The spindle cell component is composed of elongated cells with vesicular nuclei and scant cytoplasm. Mitotic activity may range between two and five mitoses per 10 hpf. Cystic changes, areas of necrosis, and hemorrhage may be seen in some cases. On the contrary, the monophasic variant of synovial sarcoma is characterized by the absence of the glandular or papillary epithelial component, and the tumors are essentially composed of an atypical spindle cell proliferation that may show different growth patterns including a herringbone, hemangiopericytic, or solid component. In this variant, it is also possible to identify cystic changes, myxoid areas, necrosis, and hemorrhage. Mitotic activity in this variant may also range from 2 to more than 10 × 10 hpf (Fig. 12.117a–e).

Immunohistochemical, Ultrastructural, and Molecular Features

The staining pattern of both variants – biphasic and monophasic – is somewhat different (Fig. 12.118a–e). Biphasic synovial sarcomas characteristically show strong positive staining in the epithelial areas for low and high molecular weight keratin as well as EMA. In addition, the spindle cell component of the tumor shows positive staining for vimentin, Bcl-2, and CD99 while focally positive for keratin and EMA. In the monophasic variant, the staining pattern is similar to that seen in the spindle cell component of the biphasic tumor. In addition, other stains that commonly are positive in the spindle cell component of the tumor include FLI-1 and TLE1. Other immunohistochemical markers – including desmin, smooth muscle actin, CD34, CD30, and CD31 – are usually negative.

Electron microscopy of these tumors, mainly in the spindle cell component, shows that the spindle cells contained scattered immature, desmosome-type cell junctions. The molecular features of these tumors have been well characterized as the tumor shows a balanced reciprocal translocation found in about 80% of the cases consisting of gene fusion product SYT-SSX chimeric RNA. The breakpoints of the translocation involved the fusion of SSY gene at 18q11 to either two homologous genes SSX1 and SSX2. It appears that the SSX1 gene is more commonly seen in the biphasic tumors, while the SSX2 is seen in the monophasic variant. It also appears that the SYT-SSX1 is more commonly associated with worse clinical outcome.

Differential Diagnosis

The most important differential diagnosis in synovial sarcoma will depend on the growth pattern observed. By far, the monophasic variant is the one that may pose problems in the diagnosis as it can be confused with other spindle cell tumors of the mediastinum. The most important considerations include spindle cell thymoma, spindle cell thymic carcinoma, leiomyosarcoma, and solitary fibrous tumor. In cases of primary thymic epithelial tumors, the use of keratin 5/6 may be of aid, as most thymic epithelial tumors are commonly positive for keratin 5/6, while monophasic synovial sarcoma is negative. In cases of leiomyosarcoma, the positive staining for muscle markers and negative staining for Bcl-2, TLE1,

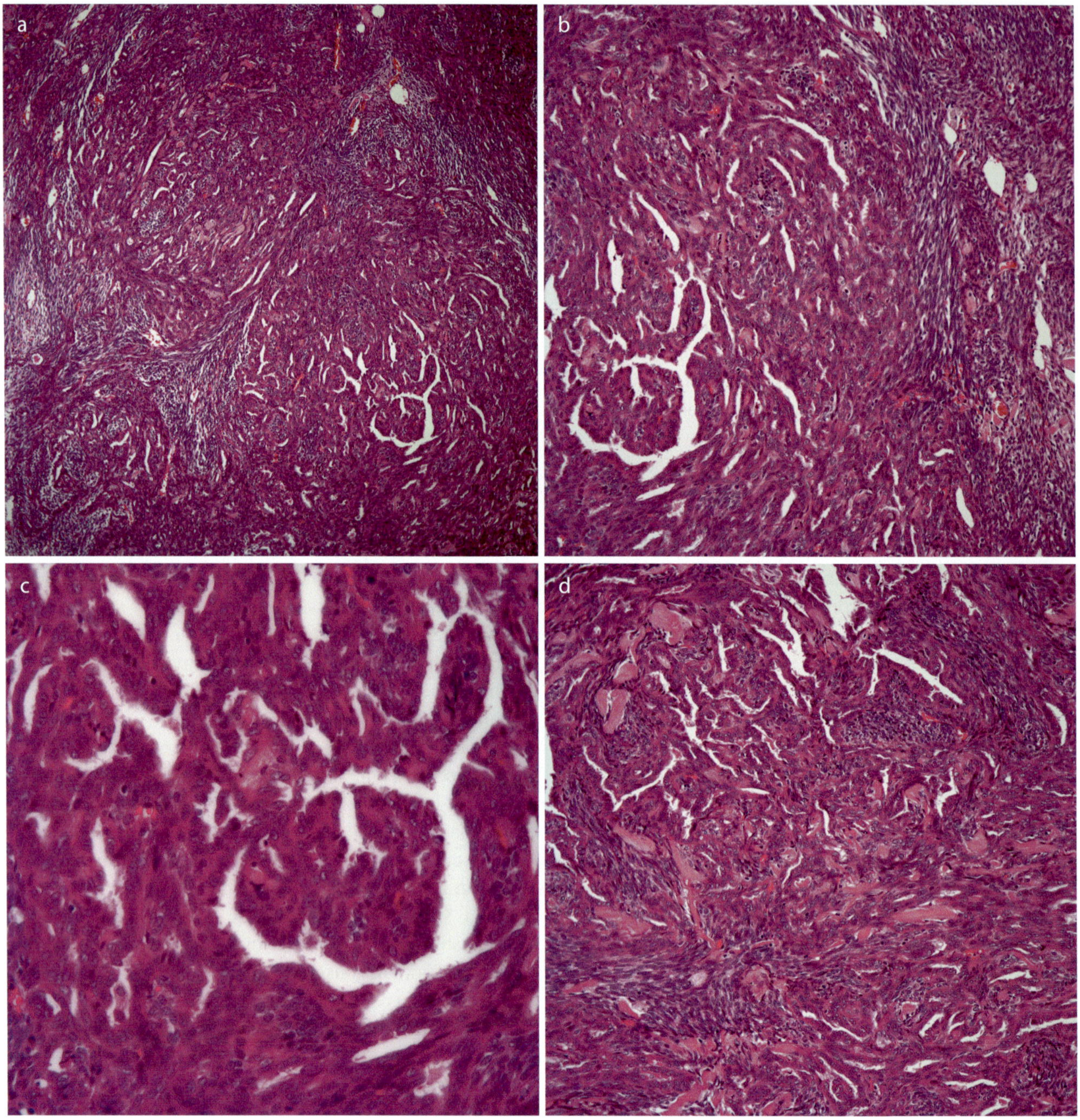

Fig. 12.116 (**a**) Biphasic synovial sarcoma showing prominent epithelial glandular component, (**b**) biphasic synovial sarcoma showing glandular and spindle cell component, (**c**) closer view of the glandular component of biphasic synovial sarcoma showing some papillary features, (**d**) glandular and spindle cell components admixed with collagenous areas

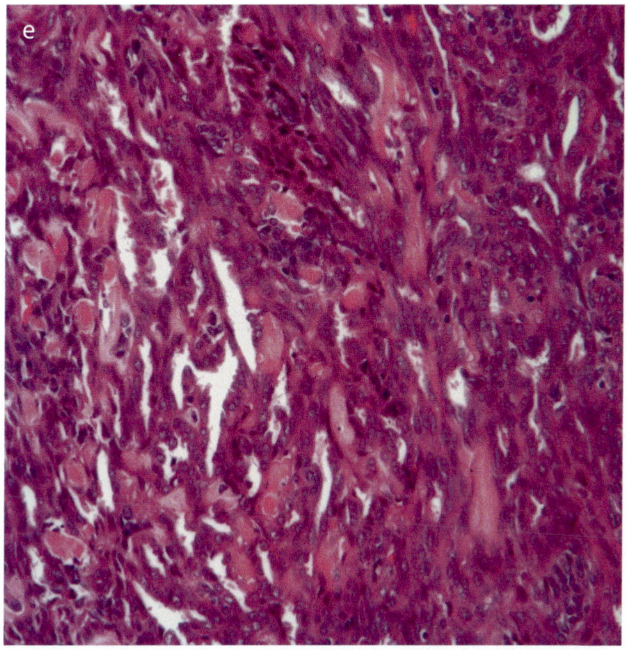

Fig. 12.116 (continued) (**e**) More subtle areas of the glandular component in biphasic synovial sarcoma

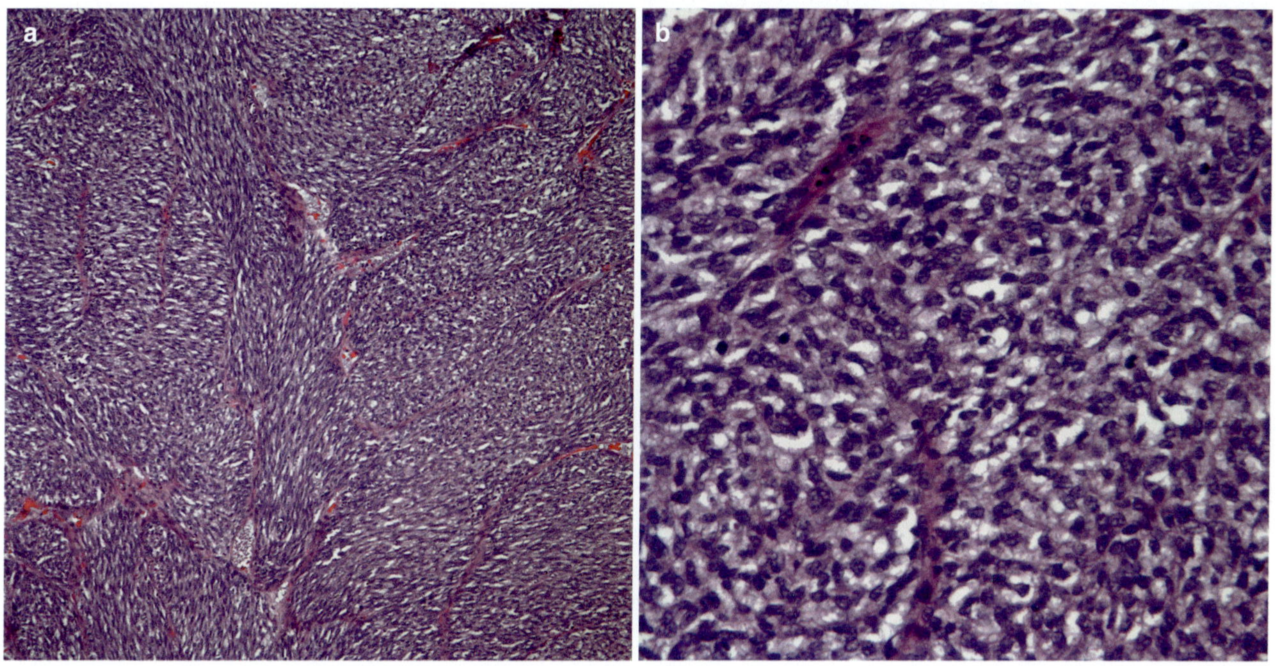

Fig. 12.117 (**a**) Monophasic synovial sarcoma with prominent solid spindle cell component, (**b**) higher magnification of the solid component showing mitotic activity

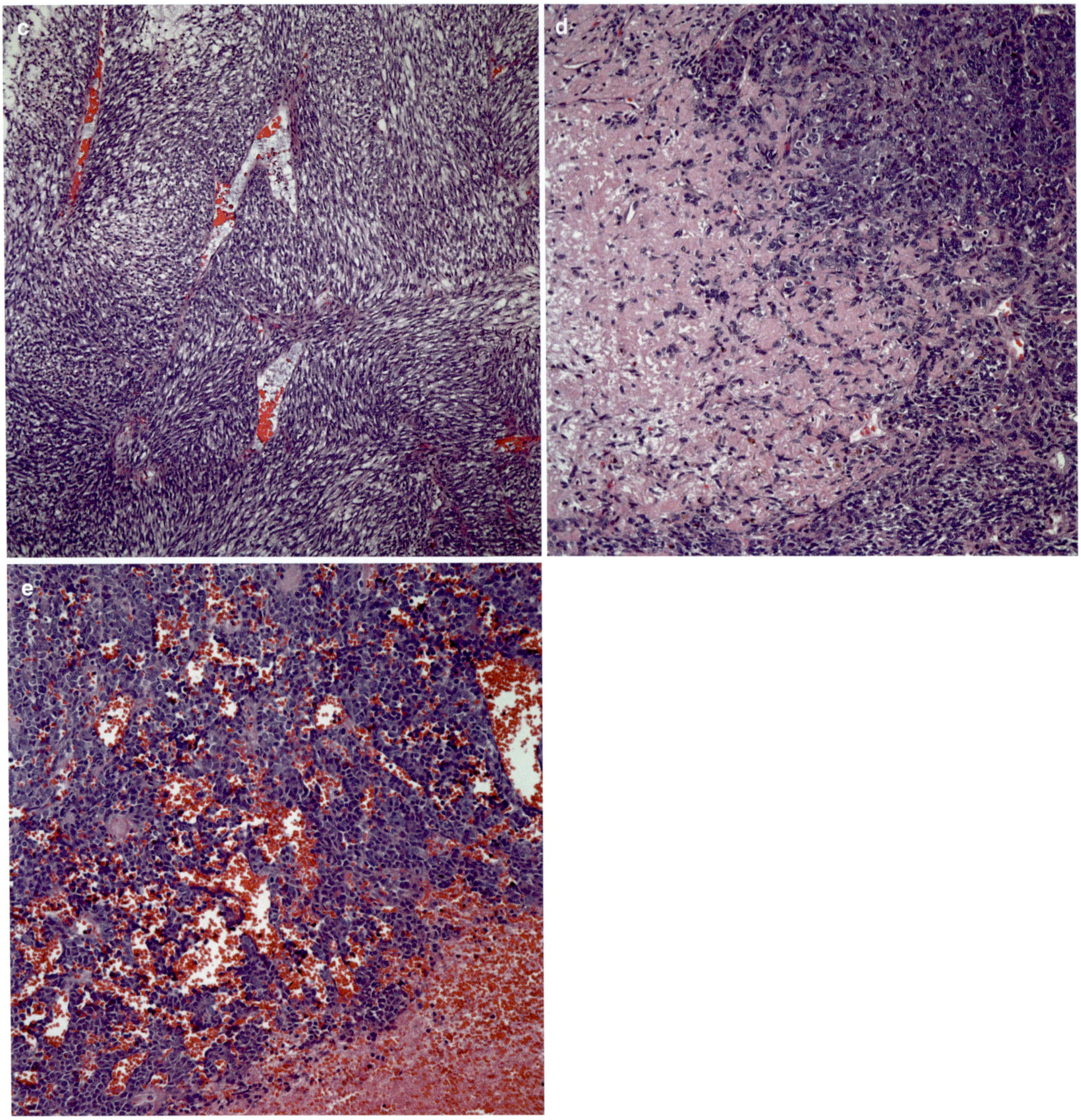

Fig. 12.117 (continued) (**c**) Areas with ectatic blood vessels and a subtle hemangiopericytic pattern, (**d**) areas of collagenization in monophasic synovial sarcoma, (**e**) areas of hemorrhage and clefts with red cells mimicking a malignant vascular neoplasm

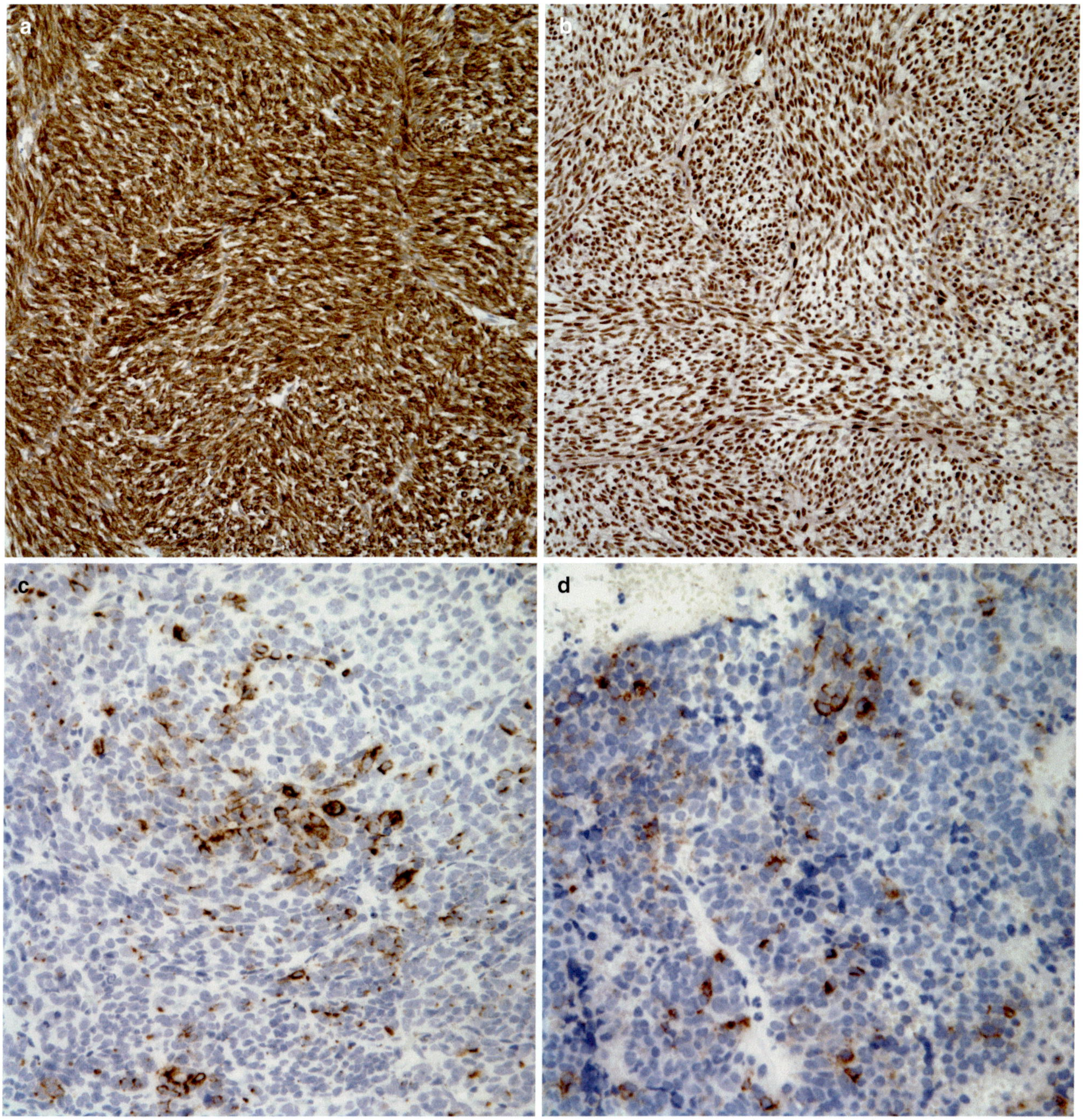

Fig. 12.118 (**a**) Strong positive staining with Bcl-2, (**b**) FL1 positive nuclear staining, (**c**) focal positive staining for keratin cocktail, (**d**) focal positive staining for EMA

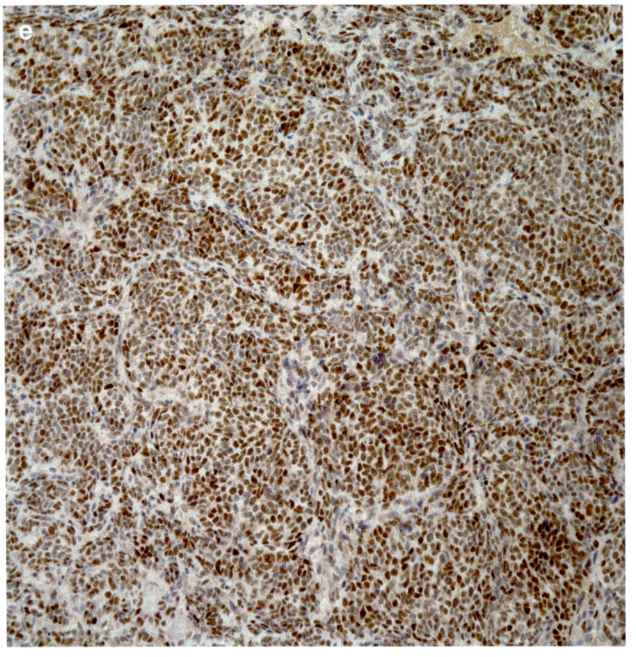

Fig. 12.118 (continued) (**e**) Strong nuclear positive staining for TLE1

or FLI-1 may be of aid. If the immunoprofile still raises question about the diagnosis, the molecular studies will ultimately define the tumor in the majority of cases. With solitary fibrous tumor, it is well known that the spectrum of growth patterns may be seen in SFT, and, in addition, both tumors may share some immunophenotypical features such as positive staining for Bcl-2 and CD99. However, the use of STAT6 will help in defining the specific entity, as monophasic synovial sarcomas are negative for STAT6. Once again, in difficult cases, the use of molecular techniques should lead to the correct interpretation.

In cases of biphasic histology, the tumor shows enough distinctive features to be able to make a correct interpretation. However, one possible consideration would be carcinosarcoma. In this latter possibility, however, it is essential to identify heterologous elements in order to properly categorize the tumor as carcinosarcoma. Since these tumors may also occur in the posterior mediastinum, the possibility of glandular schwannoma may also enter in the differential diagnosis. However, glandular schwannomas are likely to show negative staining for Bcl-2, keratin, EMA, FLI1, and TLE.

Carcinosarcoma

There are only a few reports of this tumor in the mediastinal compartment. However, it is important to properly define this tumor, as a tumor that must contain unequivocal areas of carcinoma and unequivocal areas of sarcoma. Interestingly, in the few cases in which the possibility or the interpretation has been that of carcinosarcoma, all the cases have shown the presence of rhabdomyoblastic differentiation [128–130], which to some extent is interesting as it is this specific component (rhabdomyomatous component) that has been shown to be present in some cases of thymoma and thymic carcinoma [131, 132].

The case described by Okudela and associates [130] is the most recent and the one that appears to be described in better detail. The authors documented an 83-year-old patient who had autoimmune hemolytic syndrome and who was discovered to have a large anterior mediastinal mass. A biopsy was obtained, which was interpreted as rhabdomyosarcoma. The patient subsequently died, and an autopsy was performed identifying a mediastinal tumor with invasion into the pleura/lung and metastasis to spleen.

Based on the few well-documented cases available, it is difficult to draw meaningful conclusions about carcinosarcomas in the mediastinum. However, it is logical to conclude that the clinical behavior of these tumors in the mediastinum may be similar to those tumors in other thoracic structures such as the lung. There is no specific treatment for carcinosarcomas, and possible complete surgical resection followed by additional medical therapy may be adequate as treatment.

Pathological Features

Macroscopically, these tumors may reach a large size in the mediastinal compartment. The tumors may be solid and friable, with areas of necrosis and hemorrhage. They may be ill defined with infiltrative border that may involve adjacent structures such as pleura or pericardium.

Histologically, as mentioned previously, it is essential to demonstrate unequivocal areas of carcinoma and sarcoma. In the cases described of this tumor, it appears the sarcomatous component has been that of rhabdomyosarcoma with the characteristic features as those seen in soft tissue tumors: spindle cell component with presence of rhabdomyoblasts. The epithelial component expected in a thymic tumor would most likely be squamous cell carcinoma (Fig. 12.119a, b).

Immunohistochemical Features

The epithelial component of the tumor would show positive staining for keratin low and high molecular weight in addition to keratin 5/6, p63, and p40. The sarcomatous component, namely, if it is rhabdomyosarcoma, would show positive staining for desmin, myoglobin, and MyoD. Other immunohistochemical stains may be of use only if the sarcomatous component is thought to represent a different type of sarcoma. Then, the use of a wider panel would be appropriate.

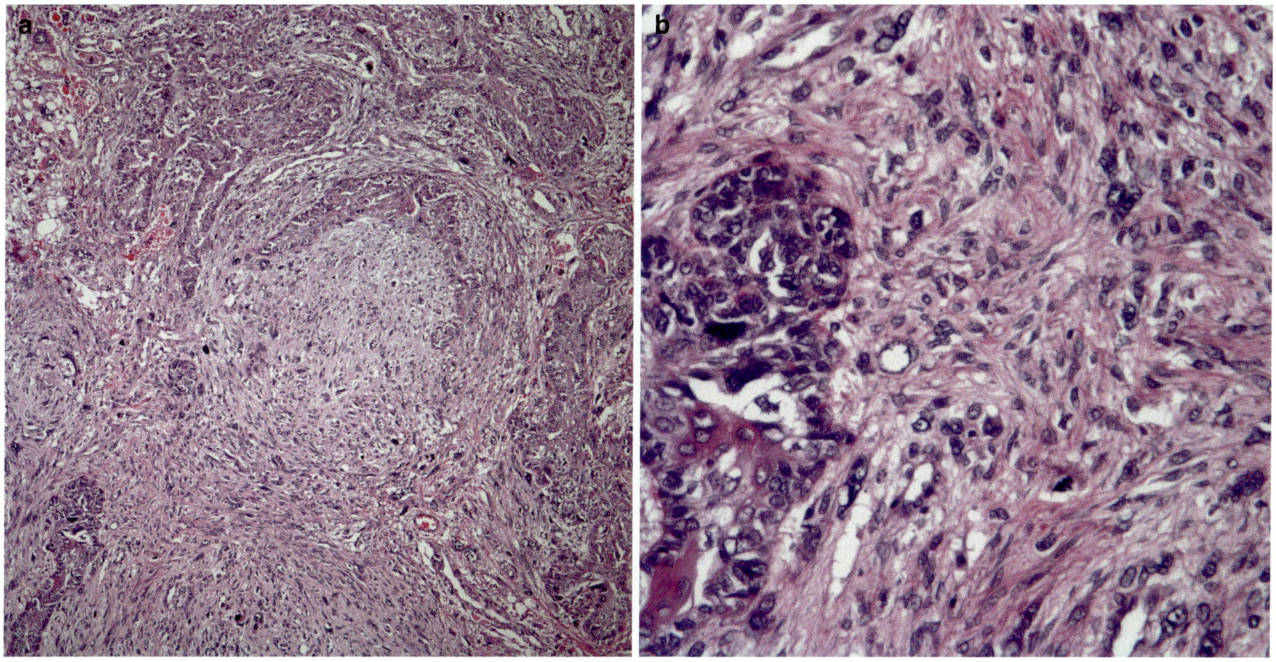

Fig. 12.119 (**a**) Low power view of a carcinosarcoma showing a biphasic neoplastic population – squamous cell carcinoma and a high-grade sarcoma, (**b**) closer magnification showing a prominent cellular atypia and mitotic activity in the sarcomatous (mesenchymal) component

Differential Diagnosis

The most important differential diagnosis for this tumor is either a thymoma or a thymic carcinoma with rhabdomyomatous differentiation. Either one of these tumors will have a different prognosis and different treatment options. In cases in which there is only a small mediastinoscopic biopsy available for interpretation, the sampling issue will likely lead to an interpretation of either sarcoma or carcinoma. The final interpretation would thus be in a resected tumor.

Cartilaginous Tumors

Essentially, the occurrence of cartilaginous tumors in the mediastinal compartment without involvement of bony structures is rather rare. In addition, such occurrence is more commonly reported when tumors are of the malignant type; thus, the number of cases reported as mediastinal chondrosarcomas is much more common than reports of benign cartilaginous tumors [133–138]. However, it is important to highlight that there has been documentation not only pathologically but also radiologically about the presence of cartilaginous lesions, either benign or malignant, in the anterior and posterior mediastinum

Many reports about different variants of mediastinal chondrosarcomas have been presented more often through single case reports. Chetty [133] reported a mesenchymal chondrosarcoma in a 25-year-old man who presented with dyspnea and who, on thoracic imaging, showed the presence of a posterior mediastinal mass. Surgical resection was performed, and the tumor was described as not being associated with the bone. Clinical follow-up in this patient showed recurrence and metastatic disease in both lungs 6 months after initial diagnosis. The largest series of malignant cartilaginous tumor of the mediastinum was reported in 1997 by Suster and Moran [139]. The authors described six patients: five women and one man between the ages of 11 and 63 years. Clinically, four patients presented with symptoms of backache, chest pain, dyspnea, and dysphagia. Two patients were asymptomatic, and the tumor was discovered during a routine radiographic film. In this description, the histopathological features of the tumors showed the spectrum that has been seen in these tumors when they occur in the bone. All the tumors were in the posterior mediastinum, and, radiologically, none of the tumors had any connection with bony structures. Surgical resection took place in all the cases, and in two patients postoperative radiation therapy was documented. Clinical follow-up in five patients showed local recurrence in two patients 3 and 7 years after initial diagnosis; one patient developed metastases and died of the tumor, and one patient was alive without evidence of recurrence 6 years after initial diagnosis. One additional patient was lost to follow-up; however, the patient was known to have bilateral pulmonary metastasis 10 months after initial diagnosis.

Based on the limited number of cases reported in the mediastinal compartment, it is difficult to draw meaningful conclusions regarding the clinical outcome in these patients; however, it appears that these tumors in the mediastinum can follow an aggressive course with metastatic disease. Complete surgical resection followed by additional therapy appears to be an appropriate approach in the treatment of these patients. However, it is highly important to properly document the absence of bone involvement in the evaluation of these tumors in order to properly designate them as originating in the mediastinal compartment.

Pathological Features

Macroscopically, the tumors appear to be well circumscribed and can range from 5 cm to more than 10 cm in greatest diameter (Fig. 12.120). The cut surface is lobulated and rubbery with focal areas of hemorrhage and calcifications. Areas of myxoid or gelatinous changes may be seen in some tumors.

Histologically, the tumor may show features of mesenchymal chondrosarcoma, myxoid chondrosarcoma, and high-grade chondrosarcoma (Fig. 12.121a–g). Mesenchymal chondrosarcomas are characterized by the presence of an atypical cellular proliferation composed of spindle or oval cells, which in some areas may contain chondroid matrix. The cellular proliferation is somewhat monotonous, with large vesicular nuclei and unevenly dispersed chromatin. Mitotic activity can be seen, but it is not increased and may range from one to two mitoses per 10 hpf. The tumor may have the presence of branching dilated vascular spaces, which impart a hemangiopericytic appearance. Some tumors may show the presence of mature cartilage or calcifications. Areas of hemorrhage can be seen; however, tumoral necrosis is not a common feature in these tumors. In myxoid chondrosarcoma, the tumors have a subtle lobulated appearance, and the neoplastic cellular proliferation is embedded in a chondromyxoid stroma. The cellular proliferation is composed of islands, short strands, or chords of round cells with hyperchromatic nuclei, some containing a centrally placed nucleoli and eosinophilic cytoplasm. Increased mitotic activity is not seen, and areas of hyaline matrix or calcifications are not present. In the high-grade chondrosarcoma, the

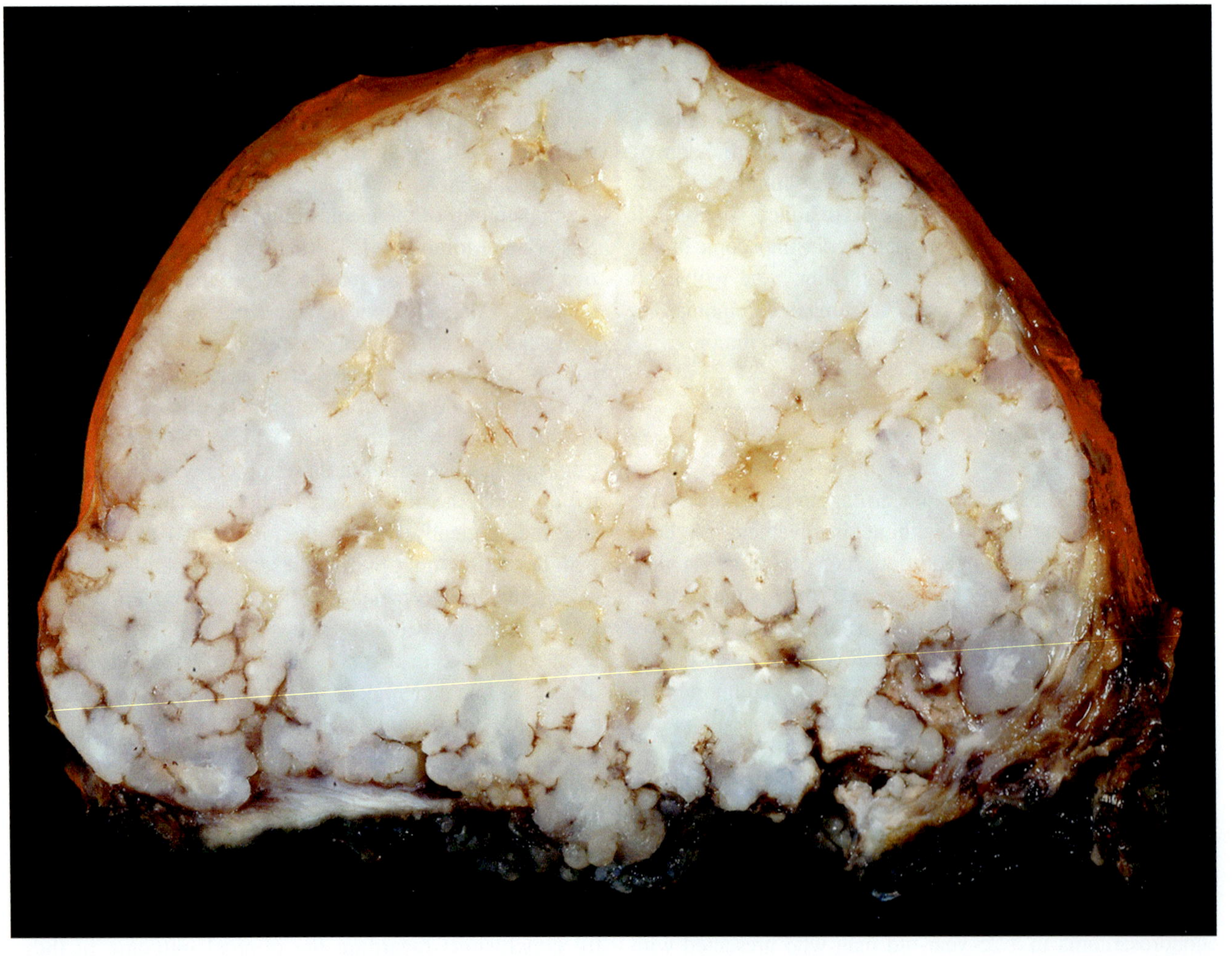

Fig. 12.120 Mediastinal chondrosarcoma; the tumors show slightly lobulated features

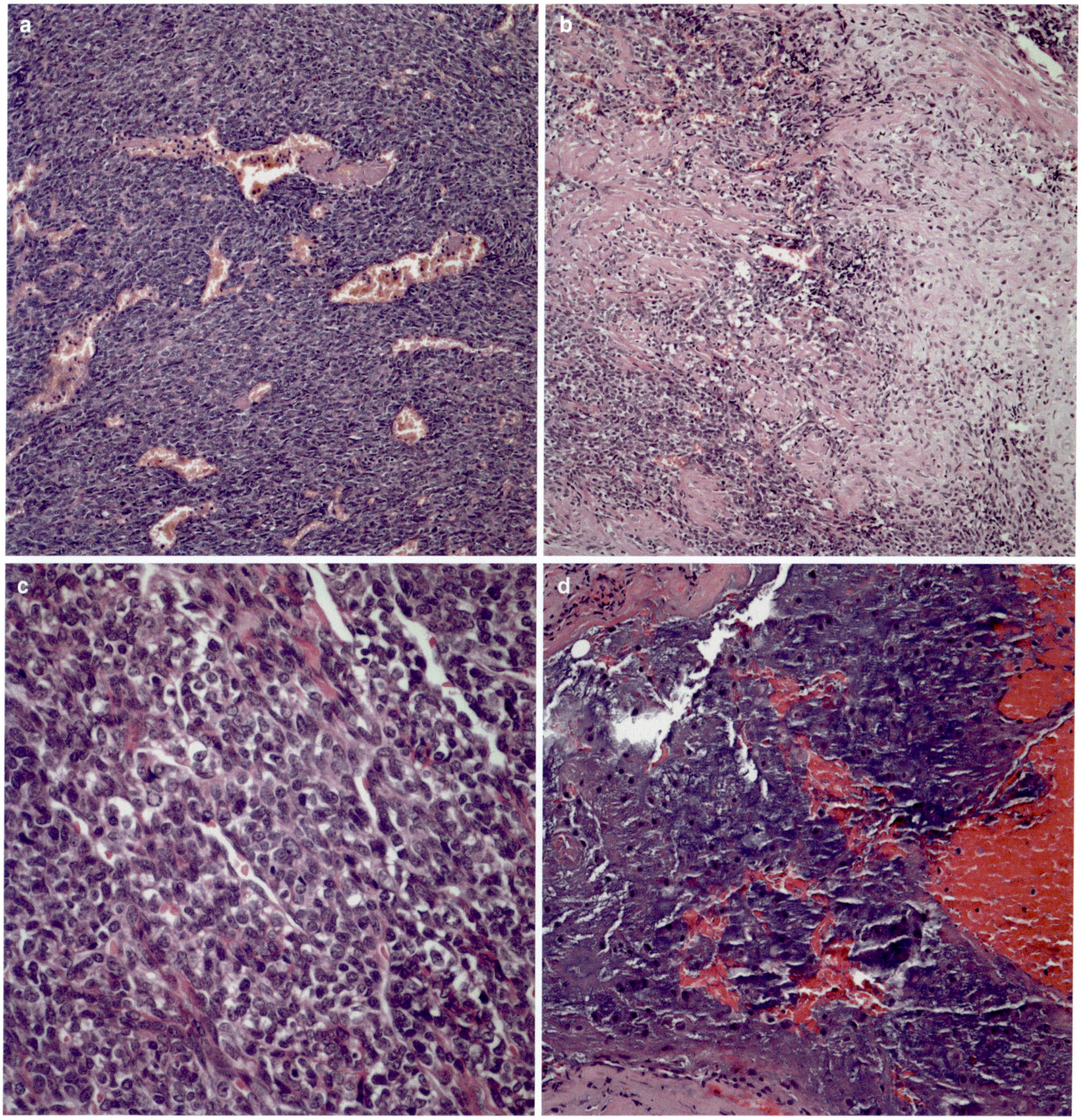

Fig. 12.121 (**a**) Mesenchymal chondrosarcoma showing a subtle hemangiopericytic growth pattern, (**b**) mesenchymal chondrosarcoma showing areas of more conventional chondrosarcoma, (**c**) higher magnification of a mesenchymal chondrosarcoma showing a small neoplastic cellular proliferation, (**d**) mediastinal chondrosarcoma showing more conventional areas of cartilaginous tumor

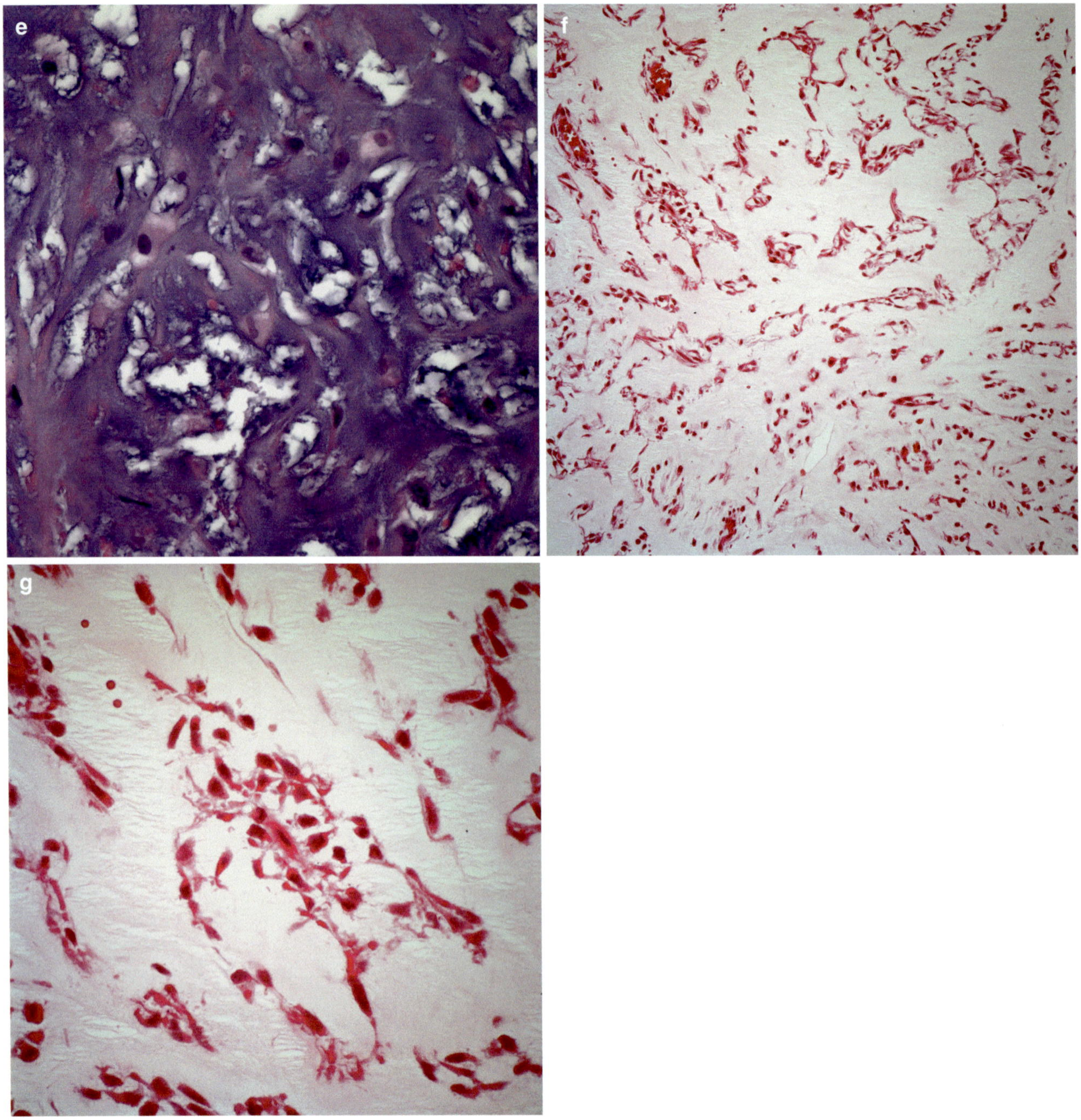

Fig. 12.121 (continued) (**e**) Higher magnification of a conventional mediastinal chondrosarcoma, (**f**) mediastinal myxoid chondrosarcoma, note the presence of abundant myxoid matrix, (**g**) higher magnification of the neoplastic cells embedded in a myxoid matrix

tumors also show a lobulated appearance with loose chondromyxoid areas separated by thin fibrovascular tissue.

Immunohistochemical Features

The use of immunohistochemical stains in the diagnosis of chondrosarcoma is rather limited. However, S-100 protein, vimentin, and SOX10 appear to be good cartilaginous markers but with variable staining patterns and intensity. These tumors are negative for keratin, EMA, CEA, desmin, smooth muscle actin, CD34, CD31, and STAT6.

Differential Diagnosis

The diagnosis of chondrosarcoma is not difficult. However, in cases of mesenchymal chondrosarcoma, the tumor may be confused with other tumors that may share some histopathological features. Those tumors will include solitary fibrous tumor and malignant schwannoma, and, in cases with prominent myxoid features, chordomas should be included in the differential diagnosis. However, the use of immunohistochemical stains – namely, STAT6 for solitary fibrous tumor and keratin for chordomas – will aid in diagnosis. In cases of malignant schwannoma, it may be a bit more difficult to rely only on immunohistochemical stains for the diagnosis as both tumors may show similar immunophenotypical features. However, the morphological features of both neoplasms should be more carefully analyzed.

Miscellaneous Tumors

In this particular section, two unusual neoplasms will be presented, which, although rare in the mediastinum, have been described as originating from the mediastinum. Needless to say, their occurrence in the mediastinum is not only difficult to explain, but in one of the tumors, one can only hypothesize a possible origin of the tumor. These two tumors are the following:

- Alveolar soft part sarcoma
- Chordoma

Alveolar Soft Part Sarcoma

Alveolar soft part sarcoma is an unusual neoplasm that more commonly occurs in younger individuals in the soft tissues of the extremities or in the head and neck areas. Since the original description by Christopherson and associates in 1952 [140], numerous reports have been presented in the literature, and, although it is more commonly seen in soft tissues, the tumor has also been described in other anatomic areas including female genital tract, pituitary gland, stomach, and retroperitoneum, among other sites.

In the mediastinum, there are only a few cases reported in the literature [141, 142]. In the original description of this tumor in the mediastinum [142], the authors described two male patients ages 22 and 23 years who presented with symptoms of chest pain. One tumor was in the anterior mediastinum, and one was in the posterior compartment. Surgical resection of the tumor was performed in both cases. Clinical follow-up showed that the patient with an anterior mediastinal tumor died 14 months after initial diagnosis, while the patient with the posterior mediastinal tumor was alive without recurrence or metastasis 14 years after initial diagnosis. Interestingly, in both patients, pulmonary metastases were discovered at the time of diagnosis; however, the authors stated that the bulk of the tumor was in the mediastinal compartment. More recently, Kameda and associates [141] described a 53-year-old man who had been diagnosed with a mediastinal alveolar soft part sarcoma 10 years previous to the development of metastatic disease to the lungs.

Based on the limited available literature on this tumor in the mediastinal compartment, it appears that the tumor may occur in either anterior or posterior compartment, the symptomatology is likely not specific, surgical resection appears an initial treatment, and the clinical course seems to be variable, as a long survival period in some of the cases has been reported.

Pathologic Features

The tumors may vary in size from 4 cm to 8 cm in greatest diameter. They are fleshy, light tan, and hemorrhagic. The tumors are not encapsulated.

Histologically, the morphological characteristics of the tumors are the predominant alveolar growth pattern with focal solid areas, nests of neoplastic cells separated by thin delicate fibrovascular tissue, and occasional dilated vascular spaces (Fig. 12.122a–e). The tumor cells are large, polygonal with abundant eosinophilic cytoplasm, and well-defined cell borders. The nuclei of the cells are eccentrically placed, large, vesicular, and with prominent nucleoli. Nuclear atypia is moderate, and mitotic activity is seen, but it is not increased. In some cases, it is possible to distinguish the presence of intracytoplasmic crystals (Fig. 12.123), which can be more apparent using periodic acid-Schiff histochemical stain.

Immunohistochemical Features

Essentially, the common markers used in diagnostic surgical pathology are negative in this tumor, namely, keratins, neuro-

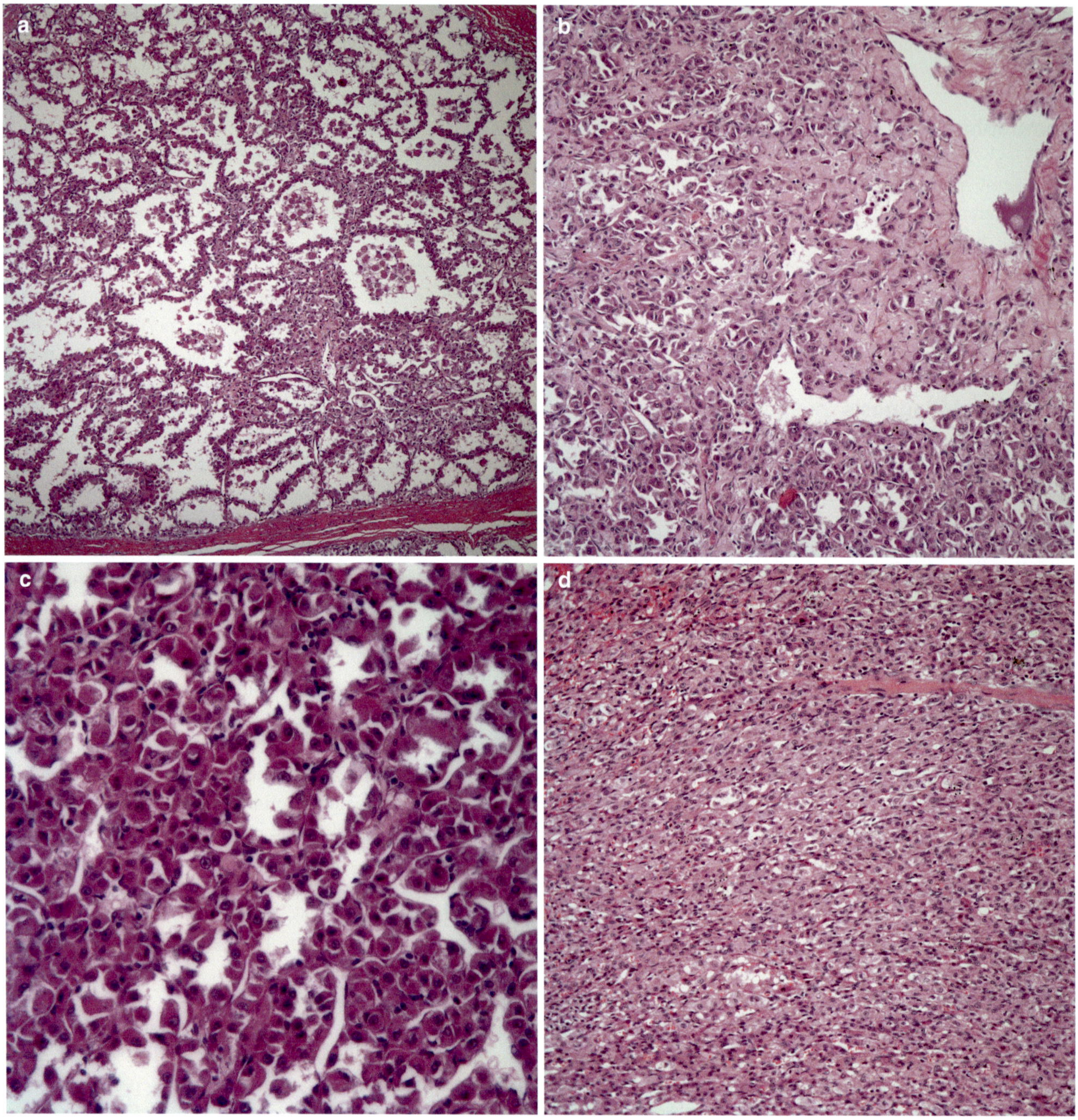

Fig. 12.122 (**a**) Low power of alveolar soft part sarcoma showing the typical alveolated growth pattern, (**b**) presence of dilated vascular structures in alveolar soft part sarcoma, (**c**) higher magnification showing larger cells with nuclear atypia and absence of mitotic activity, (**d**) alveolar soft part sarcoma showing a solid growth pattern

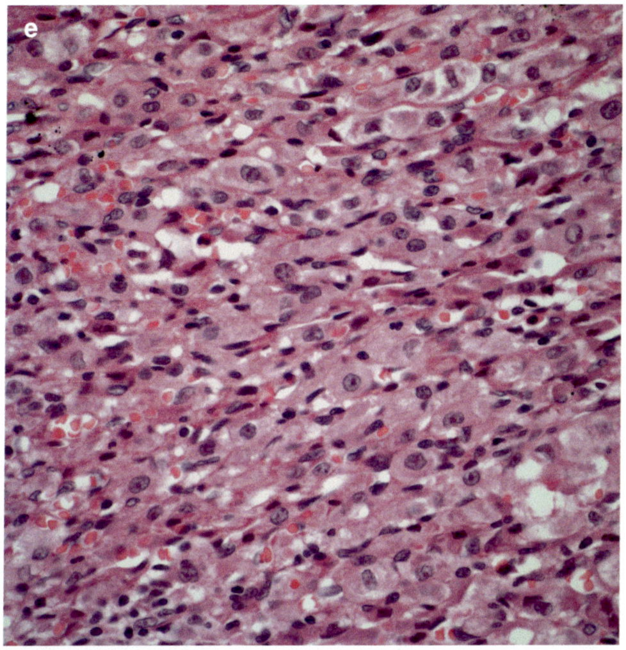

Fig. 12.122 (continued) (**e**) Higher magnification of a solid growth pattern of alveolar soft part sarcoma, note the absence of mitotic activity

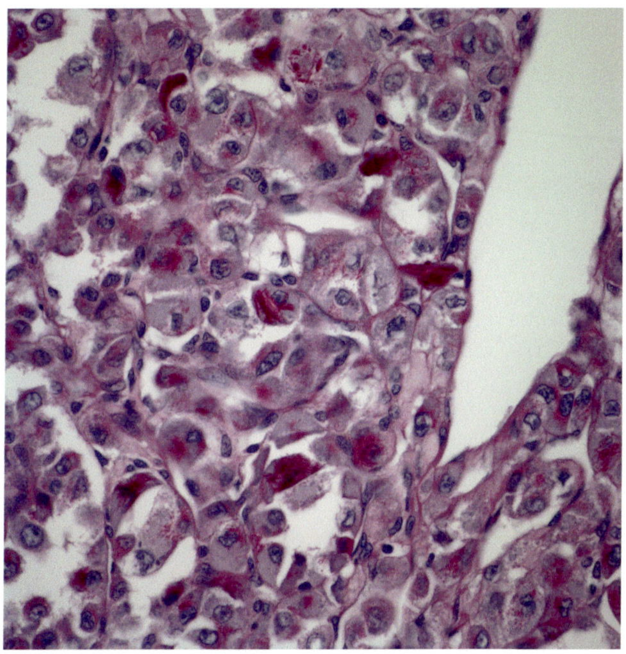

Fig. 12.123 Periodic acid-Schiff (PAS) stain in alveolar soft part sarcoma showing intracytoplasmic crystals

endocrine markers, and muscle markers. In some cases S-100 protein may show positive staining. Immunohistochemical staining for ASPL-TFE3 may be useful in cases in which the histology of the tumor raises other possibilities.

Differential Diagnosis

Although the morphology of the tumor is characteristic, in the mediastinum, the tumors that may be considered in the differential diagnosis would include paraganglioma, neuroendocrine carcinomas, and clear cell carcinoma of the thymus. In this setting, the use of neuroendocrine markers or epithelial markers should lead to the correct interpretation.

Chordoma

The occurrence of chordomas in the mediastinum is rare and difficult to explain, knowing that the origin of these tumors is from remnants of notochord, thus their predominance to occur in axial skeleton, particularly at the base of the skull and sacrococcygeal regions. However, the occurrence of such tumors within the mediastinal compartment without bone involvement has been reported previously in the literature [143–150], mainly as case reports. The tumors have been described in a wide range of ages without particular gender predilection. The largest series of these tumors by Suster and Moran reported six patients with posterior mediastinal tumors without bone involvement [151]. The patients were three males and three females between the ages of 8 and 65 years who presented with diverse symptomatology including dysphagia, chest pain, backache, and shortness of breath. Diagnostic imaging revealed a posterior mediastinal mass without involvement of the thoracic or dorsal spine. Complete or partial resection of the tumors was documented in all the cases, while the clinical follow-up showed that two patients had died with recurrences and metastases 1–3 years after initial diagnosis; two patients were alive without recurrence within a period of 16 months and 3 years. Two patients were lost to follow-up.

Pathological Features

Macroscopically, the tumors range in size from 8 to more than 10 cm in greatest diameter, are thinly encapsulated, well circumscribed, and at cut surface shows a soft, gelatinous consistency with areas of hemorrhage.

Histologically, the tumors may show a lobular growth pattern with the neoplastic cellular proliferation arranged in cords and strands of large tumor cells with abundant cytoplasm, large hyperchromatic nuclei, and inconspicuous nucleoli (Fig. 12.124a–c). The neoplastic cellular proliferation is embedded in a mucoid stroma. The presence of large cells with prominent bubbly vacuolated cytoplasm characteristic of physaliphorous cells is seen scattered throughout the tumor. Hemorrhagic areas as well as areas with collections of foamy macrophages, cholesterol cleft granulomas, and immature chondroid matrix may be seen in some cases. Areas composed of spindle cells with increased mitotic activity can be seen in some cases as well.

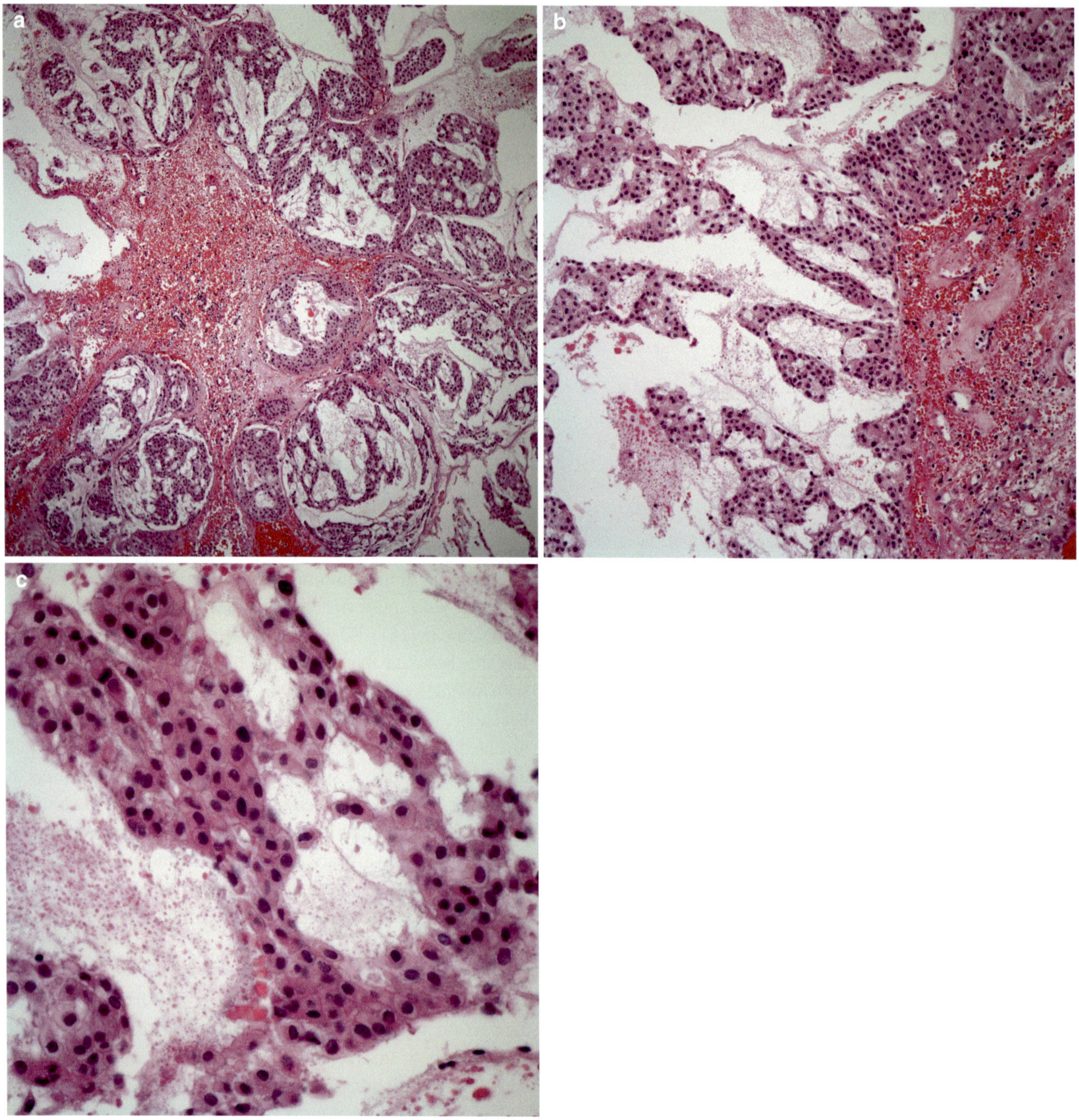

Fig. 12.124 (**a**) Low-power view of a mediastinal chordoma showing a neoplastic cellular proliferation embedded in a myxoid matrix, (**b**) mediastinal chordoma showing cords of neoplastic cells, (**c**) higher magnification showing polygonal cells with moderate nuclear atypia and scattered mitotic activity

Immunohistochemical Features

The characteristic immunoprofile of these tumors is the positive staining for keratin while negative for S-100 protein. Other immunostains – including muscle and neuroendocrine markers, CD31, CD34, HMB-45, CEA, and EMA – are generally negative in these tumors.

Differential Diagnosis

The most important differential diagnosis for chordomas is the separation of these tumors from extraskeletal myxoid chondrosarcomas. In that setting, the positive staining for keratin markers should lead to the correct interpretation. In the mediastinal location, the tumor may also be confused with unusual variants of thymoma or thymic carcinoma. However, the majority of thymic epithelial neoplasms – thymoma and thymic carcinoma – generally stain for markers commonly used for squamous cell carcinoma, such as keratin 5/6, p63, and p40, which, if used in conjunction, will likely lead to the correct interpretation.

References

1. Pachter MR, Lattes R. Mesenchymal tumors of the mediastinum. I. Tumors of fibrous tissue, adipose tissue, smooth muscle, and striated muscle. Cancer. 1963;16:74–94.
2. Swanson PE. Soft tissue neoplasms of the mediastinum. Semin Diagn Pathol. 1991;8:14–34.
3. De Bakker MA, Marx A, Mukai K, Strobel P. Mesenchymal tumours of the mediastinum –Part I. Virchows Arch. 2015;467: 487–500.
4. Lange L. Über ein Lipom des thymus. Zentralbl Allg Pathol. 1916;27:97.
5. Dew AW, Foot NC. Report of a large thymic tumor successfully removed by operation. J Thorac Surg. 1937;6:648–59.
6. Hall GFM. A case of thymolipoma. With observations on a possible relationship to intrathoracic lipomata. Br J Surg. 1949;36:321–4.
7. Toyama T, Mizuno T, Masaoka A, Shibata K, Yamakawa Y, Niwa H, et al. Pathogenesis of thymolipoma: report of three cases. Jpn J Surg. 1995;25:86–8.
8. Rieker RJ, Schirmacher P, Schnabel PA, Moser K, Hoffmann H, Dienemann H, et al. Thymolipoma. A report of nine cases, with emphasis on its association with myasthenia gravis. Surg Today. 2010;40:132–6.
9. Damadoglu E, Salturk C, Takir HB, Ertugrul M, Yilmaz A, Atasalihi A, et al. Mediastinal thymolipoma: an analysis of 10 cases. Respirology. 2007;12:924–7.
10. Otto HF, Lachenmayer L, Janzen RW, Janzen RW, Gürtler KF, Fischer K. Thymolipoma in association with myasthenia gravis. Cancer. 1982;50:1623.
11. Reintgen D, Fetter BF, Roses A, McCarty KS Jr. Thymolipoma in association with myasthenia gravis. Arch Pathol Lab Med. 1978;102:463.
12. Gunnells JC, Miller E, Jacoby WJ, May RL. Thymolipoma simulating cardiomegaly: opacification of the tumor by cineangiocardiography. Am Heart J. 1963;66:670.
13. Benton C, Gerard P. Thymolipoma in a patient with Graves' disease. J Thorac Surg. 1966;51:428.
14. Boetsch CH, Swoyer GB, Adams A, Walker JH. Lipothymoma. Report of two cases. J Dis Chest. 1966;50:539.
15. Levine S, Labiche H, Chandor S. Thymolipoma. Report of a case. 1968;98:875.
16. Barnes RDS, Gorman PO. Two cases of aplastic anemia associated with tumors of the thymus. J Clin Pathol. 1962;15:264.
17. Rosado-de-Christenson M, Pugatch RD, Moran CA, Galobardes J. Thymolipoma: Analysis of 27 cases. Radiology. 1994;193: 121–6.
18. Moran CA, Rosado-de-Christenson M, Suster S. Thymolipoma: clinicopathologic review of 33 cases. Mod Pathol. 1995;8:741–4.
19. Ajaz B, Tran TAN, Truong T, Manoucheri M. Thymolipoma with sebaceous differentiation: a hitherto unreported variant of thymolipoma. Int J Surg Pathol. 2013;21:526–30.
20. Kim YK, Shin N, Park WY, Park DY, Huh GY, Lee CH. Mediastinal thymolipoma with striated myoid cells: report of a peculiar case. Korean J Pathol. 2013;47:596–8.
21. Iseki M, Tsuda N, Kishikawa M, Shimada O, Hayashi T, Kawahara K, et al. Thymolipoma with striated myoid cells: histological, Immunohistochemical, and ultrastructural study. Am J Surg Pathol. 1990;14:395–8.
22. Gannon BR, Dexter DF, Petsikas D, Isotalo PA. Mediastinal thymolipoma: a rare occurrence with striated myoid cells. Tumori. 2007;93:198–200.
23. Moran CA, Zeren H, Koss MN. Thymofibrolipoma: a histological variant of thymolipoma. Arch Pathol Lab Med. 1994;118:281–2.
24. Weissferdt A, Moran CA. Lipomatous tumors of the anterior mediastinum with muscle differentiation: a clinicopathological and Immunohistochemical study of three cases. Vichows Arch. 2014;464:489–93.
25. Bertrand G, Bidabe MC, George P, Dubin P, Touzard C. Angiomyolipoma of the central mediastinum. An apparently undescribed entity. Ann Chir. 1984;38:679–81.
26. Candas F, Berber U, Yildizhan A, Yiyit N, Görür R, Işitmangil T. Anterior mediastinal angiomyolipoma. Ann Thorac Surg. 2013;95:1431–2.
27. Morita K, Shida Y, Shinozaki K, et al. Angiomyolipomas of the mediastinum and lung. J Thorac Imaging. 2012;27:W21–3.
28. Knight CS, Cerfolio RJ, Winokur TS. Angiomyolipoma of the anterior mediastinum. Ann Diagn Pathol. 2008;12:293–5.
29. Watts KA, Watts JR. Incidental discovery of an anterior mediastinal angiomyolipoma. J Thorac Imaging. 2007;22:180–1.
30. Amir AM, Zeebregts CJ, Mulder HJ. Anterior mediastinal presentation of a giant angiomyolipoma. Ann Thorac Surg. 2004;78:2161–3.
31. Fukuzawa J, Shimizu T, Sakai E, Ido A, Fujita Y, Tsuji T, et al. Case report of angiomyolipoma of the posterior upper mediastinum. Nihon Kyobu Shikkan Gakkai Zasshi. 1992;30:464–7.
32. Downes KA, Goldblum JR, Montgomery EA, Fisher C. Pleomorphic liposarcoma: a clinicopathologic analysis of 19 cases. Mod Pathol. 2001;14:179–84.
33. Alaggio R, Coffin CM, Weiss SW, Bridge JA, Issakov J, Oliveira AM, et al. Liposarcomas in young patients: a study of 82 cases occurring in patients younger than 22 years of age. Am J Surg Pathol. 2009;33:645–58.
34. Chen M, Yang J, Zhu L, Zhou C, Zhao H. Primary intrathoracic liposarcoma: a clinicopathologic study and prognostic analysis of 23 cases. J Cardiothorac Surg. 2014;9:119–26.
35. Razzuk MA, Ursckel HC, Race GJ, Kingsley WB, Paulson DL. Liposarcoma of the mediastinum: case report and review of the literature. J Thorac Cardiovasc Surg. 1971;61:819–26.
36. Schweistzer DL, Aguam AS. Primary liposarcoma of the mediastinum: report of a case and review of the literature. J Thorac Cardiovasc Surg. 1977;74:83–97.
37. Standerfer RJ, Armistead SH, Paneth M. Liposarcoma of the mediastinum: report of a two cases and review of the literature. Thorax. 1981;36:693–4.
38. Havlicek F, Rosai J. A sarcoma of the thymic stroma with features of liposarcoma. Am J Clin Pathol. 1984;82:217–24.

39. Dogan R, Kara M, Yazicioglu A, Onder S. Giant atypical lipomatous tumor of the mediastinum. Tuberkuloz ve Toraks Dergisi. 2008;56:100–3.
40. Klimstra DS, Moran CA, Periono G, Koss MN, Rosai J. Liposarcoma of the anterior mediastinum and thymus: a clinicopathologic study of 28 cases. Am J Surg Pathol. 1995;19:782–91.
41. Hahn HP, Fletcher CDM. Primary mediastinal liposarcoma: clinicopathologic analysis of 24 cases. Am J Surg Pathol. 2007;31:1868–74.
42. Boland JM, Colby TV, Folper AL. Liposarcomas of the mediastinum and thorax: a clinicopathologic and molecular cytogenetic study of 24 cases, emphasizing unusual and diverse histologic features. Am J Surg Pathol. 2012;36:1395–403.
43. Ortega P, Suster D, Falconieri G, Zambrano E, Moran CA, Morrison C, et al. Liposarcomas of the posterior mediastinum: clinicopathologic study of 18 cases. Mod Pathol. 2015;28:721–31.
44. Evans HL, Khurana KK, Kemp BL, Ayala AG. Heterologous elements in the dedifferentiated component of dedifferentiated liposarcoma. Am J Surg Pathol. 1994;18:1150–7.
45. Evan HL. Smooth muscle in atypical lipomatous tumors: a report of three cases. Am J Surg Pathol. 1990;14:714–8.
46. Suster S, Wong TY, Moran CA. Sarcomas with combined features of liposarcoma and leiomyosarcoma. Am J Surg Pathol. 1993;17:905–11.
47. Tallini G, Erlandson RA, Brennan MF, Woodruff JM. Divergent myosarcomatous differentiation in retroperitoneal liposarcoma. Am J Surg Pathol. 1993;17:546–56.
48. Shanks JH, Banerjee SS, Eyden BP. Focal rhabdomyosarcomatous differentiation in primary liposarcoma. J Clin Pathol. 1996;49:770–2.
49. Zamecnik M, Michal M, Sulc M. Atypical lipomatous tumors with smooth muscle differentiation: report of two cases. Pathology. 1999;31:425–7.
50. Gomez-Roman JJ, Val-Bernal JF. Lipoleiomyosarcoma of the mediastinum. Pathology. 1997;29:428–30.
51. Folpe AL, Weiss SW. Lipoleiomyosarcoma (well-differentiated liposarcoma with leiomyosarcomatous differentiation). Am J Surg Pathol. 2002;26:742–9.
52. Weissferdt A, Moran CA. Lipomatous tumors of the anterior mediastinum with smooth muscle differentiation: a clinicopathological and Immunohistochemical study of three cases. Virchows Arch. 2014;464:489–93.
53. Miettinen M, Enzinger FM. Epithelioid variant of pleomorphic liposarcoma: a study of 12 cases of a distinctive variant of high-grade liposarcoma. Mod Pathol. 1999;12:722–8.
54. Huang HY, Antonescu CR. Epithelioid variant of pleomorphic liposarcoma: a comparative Immunohistochemical and ultrastructural analysis of six cases with emphasis on overlapping features with epithelial malignancies. Ultrastruct Pathol. 2002;26:299–300.
55. Wang L, Ren W, Zhou X, Sheng W, Wang J. Pleomorphic liposarcoma: a clinicopathological, Immunohistochemical and molecular cytogenetics study of 32 additional cases. Pathol Int. 2013;63:523–31.
56. Doyle LA, Tao D, Marino-Enriquez A. STAT6 is amplified in a subset of dedifferentiated liposarcoma. Mod Pathol. 2014;27:1231–7.
57. Seybold WD, McDonald JR, Clagett OT, Harrington SW. Metastatic tumors of vascular origin. J Thorac Surg. 1949;18:503–7.
58. Pachter MR, Lattes R. Mesenchymal tumors of the mediastinum. II Tumors of blood vascular origin. Cancer. 1963;16:95–107.
59. Pachter MR, Lattes R. Mesenchymal tumors of the mediastinum. III Tumors of lymph vascular origin. 1963;16:108–17.
60. Hall ER, Blades B. Lymphangioma of the mediastinum. Dis Chest. 1957;XXXII:1–7.
61. Dische MR. Mediastinal lymphangioma with chylothorax in infancy. Report of a case and review of the literature. Am J Clin Pathol. 1968;49:392–7.
62. Sanes S, Macmanus JE, Scatchard N. Cystic lymphangioma of the mediastinum. J Thorac Surg. 1944:253–8.
63. Shennan T. Histologically non-malignant angioma with numerous metastases. J Pathol. 1914;19:139–54.
64. Davis JM, Mark GJ, Greene R. Benign blood vascular tumors of the mediastinum. Report of four cases and review of the literature. Radioloagy. 1978;126:581–7.
65. Leibovici D, Oner V. Hemangioma of the posterior mediastinum: review of the literature and report of a case. Am Rev Respir Dis. 1962;86:415–9.
66. Gindhart TD, Tucker WY, Choy SH. Cavernous hemangioma of the superior mediastinum: Report of a case with electron microscopy and computerized tomography. Am J Surg Pathol. 1979;3:353–61.
67. Coher AJ, Sbaschnig RJ, Hochholzer L, Lough FC, Albus RA. Mediastinal Hemangiomas. Ann Thorac Surg. 1987;43: 656–9.
68. John I, Folpe AL. Anastomosing hemangiomas arising in unusual locations: a clinicopathologic study of 17 soft tissue cases showing a predilection for the paraspinal region. Am J Surg Pathol. 2016;40:1084–9.
69. Moran CA, Suster S. Mediastinal hemangiomas: a study of 18 cases with emphasis on the spectrum of morphological features. Hum Pathol. 1995;26:416–21.
70. McAdams HP, Rosado-de-Christenson ML, Moran CA. Mediastinal hemangioma: radiographic and CT features in 14 patients. 1994;193(2):399–402.
71. Deyrup AT, Tighiouart M, Montag AG, Weiss SW. Epithelioid hemangioendothelioma of soft tissue: a proposal for risk stratification based on 49 cases. Am J Surg Pathol. 2008;32:924–7.
72. Anderson T, Zhang L, Hameed M, Rusch V, Travis WD, Antonescu CR. Thoracic epithelioid malignant vascular tumors: a clinicopathologic study of 52 cases with emphasis on pathologic grading and molecular studies of WWTR1-CAMTA1 fusions. Am J Surg Pathol. 2015;39:132–9.
73. Lamovec J, Sobel HJ, Zidar A, Jerman J. Epithelioid hemangioendothelioma of the anterior mediastinum with osteoclast-giant cells. Light microscopic, Immunohistochemical and electron microscopy study. Am J Clin Pathol. 1990;93:813–7.
74. Toursarkissian B, O'Connor WN, Dillon ML. Mediastinal epithelioid hemangioendothelioma. Ann Thorac Surg. 1990;49:680–5.
75. Weidner N. Atypical tumor of the mediastinum: epithelioid hemangioendothelioma containing metaplastic bone and osteoclast like giant cells. Ultrastruct Pathol. 1991;15:481–8.
76. Kumar A, Lopez YK, Arrossi AV, et al. Mediastinal epithelioid hemangioendothelioma. Am J Respir Crit Care Med. 2016;193:e7–8.
77. Li XM, Lin XY, Xu HT, Yu J-H, Wang L, Fan C-F, et al. Mediastinal epithelioid hemangioendothelioma with abundant spindle cells and osteoclast-like giant cells mimicking malignant fibrous histiocytoma. Diagn Pathol. 2013;8:103.
78. Suster S, Moran CA, Koss MN. Epithelioid hemangioendothelioma of the anterior mediastinum: Clinicopathologic, Immunohistochemical, and ultrastructural analysis of 12 cases. Am J Surg Pathol. 1994;18:871–81.
79. Weinreb I, Cunningham KS, Perez-Ordonez B, Hwang DM. CD10 is expressed in most epithelioid hemangioendotheliomas: a potential diagnostic pitfall. Arch Pathol Lab Med. 2009;133:1965–8.
80. Kardamakis D, Bouboulis N, Ravazoula P, Dimopoulos P, Dougenis D. Primary hemangiosarcoma of the mediastinum. Lung Cancer. 1996;16:81–6.
81. Gibbs AR, Johnson NF, Giddings JC, Powell DE, Jasani B. Primary angiosarcoma of the mediastinum: light and electron microscopic demonstration of factor VIII –related antigen in neoplastic cells. Hum Pathol. 1984;15:687–91.

82. Chen TJ, Chiou CC, Chen CH, Kuo TT, Hong HS. Metastasis of mediastinal epithelioid angiosarcoma to the finger. Am J Clin Dermatol. 2008;9:181–3.
83. Deyrup AT, Miettinen M, North PE, Khoury JD, Tighiouart M, Spunt SL, et al. Angiosarcomas arising in the viscera and soft tissue of children and young adults: a clinicopathologic study of 15 cases. Am J Surg Pathol. 2009;33:264–9.
84. Meis-Kindblom JM, Kindblom LG. Angiosarcoma of soft tissue: a study of 80 cases. Am J Surg Pathol. 1998;22:683–97.
85. Weissferdt A, Kalhor N, Suster S, Moran CA. Primary angiosarcomas of the anterior mediastinum: a clinicopathologic and immunohistochemical study of 9 cases. Hum Pathol. 2010;41:1711–7.
86. Domingue-Malagon H, Cano-Valdez AM, Moran CA, Suster S. Germ cell tumors with sarcomatous components: a clinicopathologic and Immunohistochemical study of 46 cases. Am J Surg Pathol. 2007;31:1356–62.
87. Luina Contreras A, Punar M, Tamboli P, Tu SM, Pisters L, Moran C, et al. Mediastinal germ cell tumors with angiosarcomatous component: a report of 12 cases. Hum Pathol. 2010;41:832–7.
88. Sunderrajan EV, Luger AM, Rosenholtz MJ, Maltby JD. Leiomyosarcoma in the mediastinum presenting as superior vena cava syndrome. Cancer. 1984;53:2553–6.
89. Weiss KS, Zidar BL, Wang S, Magovern GJ Sr, Raju RN, Lupetin AR, et al. Radiation-induced leiomyosarcoma of the great vessels presenting as superior vena cava syndrome. Cancer. 1987;60:1238–42.
90. Gupta S, Jindal SK, Vashist R, Singh H, Malik SK. Leiomyosarcoma of the mediastinum. Eur J Respir Dis. 1983;64:69–71.
91. Herlitzka AJ, Gale JW. Tumors and cyst of the mediastinum. Arch Surg. 1958;76:697–703.
92. Lincoln JCR. Leiomyosarcoma of the anterior mediastinum. Thorax. 1965;20:362–4.
93. Rasaretnam R, Panabokke RG. Leiomyosarcoma of the mediastinum. Br J Dis Chest. 1975;69:63–9.
94. Matsuoka H, Nishio W, Sakamoto T, Harada H, Sashikata T, Tsubota N. Mediastinal angioleiomyoma. Ann Thorac Surg. 2002;73:1653–4.
95. Ouadnouni Y, Achir A, Bekarsabein S, Bouchikh M, Smahi M, Msougar Y, et al. Primary mediastinal leiomyoma: a case report. Cases J. 2009;2:8555.
96. Baldo X, Sured C, Gimferrer JM, Belda J. Primary mediastinal leiomyoma: an angiographic study and embolization of the feeding vessels to improve the surgical approach. Eur J Cardiothorac Surg. 1997;11:574–6.
97. Vrtik M, Larbalestier RI, Cameron D, et al. Mediastinal angioleiomyoma. Ann Thorac Surg. 2002;73:1653–4.
98. Moran CA, Suster S, Perino G, et al. Malignant smooth muscle tumors presenting as mediastinal soft tissue masses. Cancer. 1994;74:2251–60.
99. Fox JP, Hospers CA. Solid teratoid tumors of the anterior mediastinum. Am J Cancer. 1936;28:273–90.
100. Horn RC, Enterline HT. Rhabdomyosarcoma: a clinicopathologic study and classification of 39 cases. Cancer. 1958;11:181–99.
101. Patton RB, Horn RC. Rhabdomyosarcoma: clinical and pathological features and comparison with human fetal and embryonal skeletal muscle. Surgery. 1962;52:572–84.
102. Crist WM, Raney RB, Newton W, Lawrence W, Tefft M, Foulkes MA. Intrathoracic soft tissue sarcomas in children. Cancer. 1982;50:598–604.
103. Suster S, Moran CA, Koss MN. Rhabdomyosarcomas of the anterior mediastinum: report of four cases unassociated with germ cell, teratomatous, or thymic carcinomatous components. Hum Pathol. 1994;25:349–56.
104. Allagio R, Zhang L, Sung YS, Huang SC, Chen CL, Bisogno G, et al. A molecular study of pediatric spindle and sclerosing rhabdomyosarcoma: identification of novel and recurrent VGLL2-related fusions in infantile cases. Am J Surg Pathol. 2016;40:224–35.
105. Owosho AA, Huang SCm Chen S, Kashikar S, Estilo CL, Wolden SL, et al. A clinicopathologic study of head and neck rhabdomyosarcomas showing FOXO1 fusion-positive alveolar and MYOD1-mutant sclerosing are associated with unfavorable outcome. Oral Oncol. 2016;61:89–7.
106. Seki M, Nishimura R, Yoshida K, Shimamura T, Shiraishi Y, Sato Y, et al. Integrated genetic and epigenetic analysis defines novel molecular subgroups in rhabdomyosarcoma. Nat Commun. 2015;6:7557.
107. England DM, Hochholzer L, McCarthy MJ. Localized benign and malignant fibrous tumors of the pleura: a clinicopathologic review of 223 cases. Am J Surg Pathol. 1989;13:640–58.
108. Moran CA, Suster S, Koss MN. The spectrum of histologic growth pattern in benign and malignant fibrous tumors of the pleura. Semin Diagn Pathol. 1992;9:169–80.
109. Witkin GB, Rosai J. Solitary fibrous tumor of the mediastinum: a report of 14 cases. Am J Surg Pathol. 1989;13:547–57.
110. Suehisa H, Yamashita M, Komori E, Sawada S, Teramoto N. Solitary fibrous tumor of the mediastinum. Gen Thorac Cardiovasc Surg. 2010;58:205–8.
111. De Raet J, Sacre R, Hoorens A, Fletcher C, Lamote J. Malignant giant solitary fibrous tumor of the mediastinum. J Thorac Oncol. 2008;3:1068–70.
112. Chnaris A, Barbetakis N, Efstathiou A, Fessatidis I. Primary mediastinal hemangiopericytoma Case Report. World J Surg Oncol. 2006;4:23–8.
113. Coffin CM, Watterson J, Priest JR, Dehner LP. Extrapulmonary inflammatory myofibroblastic tumor (inflammatory pseudotumor). A clinicopathologic and Immunohistochemical study of 84 cases. Am J Surg Pathol. 1995;19:859–72.
114. Makimoto Y, Nabeshima K, Iwasaki H, Ishiguro A, Miyoshi T, Shiraishi T, et al. Inflammatory myofibroblastic tumor of the posterior mediastinum: an older adult case with anaplastic lymphoma kinase abnormalities determined using immunohistochemistry and fluorescence in situ hybridization. Virchows Arch. 2005;446:451–5.
115. Chen CH, Lin RL, Liu HC, Chen CH, Hung TT, Huang WC. Inflammatory myofibroblastic tumor mimicking anterior mediastinal malignancy. Ann Thorac Surg. 2008;86:1362–4.
116. Chen G, Folpe AL, Colby TV, Sittampalam K, Patey M, Chen MG, et al. Angiomatoid fibrous histiocytoma: unusual sites and unusual morphology. Mod Pathol. 2011;24:1560–70.
117. Asakura S, Tezuka N, Inoue S, Kihara N, Fujino S. Angiomatoid fibrous histiocytoma in mediastinum. Ann Thorac Surg. 2001;72:283–5.
118. Seethala R, Moran CA. Angiomatoid fibrous histiocytoma of the mediastinum. Pathol Case Rev. 2006;11(5):222–5.
119. Fu K, Suster S, Moran CA. Primary mediastinal giant cell tumors: a clinicopathologic and Immunohistochemical study of two cases. Ann Diagn Pathol. 2002;6:100–5.
120. Imai K, Saito H, Minamiya Y, Hashimoto M, Kimura Y, Ogawa J. Malignant fibrous histiocytoma originating from thymus. Gen Thorac Cardiovasc Surg. 2008;56:606–9.
121. Nishida T, Nishiyama N, Kawata Y, Yamamoto T, Inoue K, Suehiro S. Mediastinal malignant fibrous histiocytoma developing from a foreign body granuloma. Jpn J Thorac Cardiovasc Surg. 2005;53:583–6.
122. Witkin GB, Miettinen M, Rosai J. A biphasic tumor of the mediastinum with features of synovial sarcoma: report of four cases. Am J Surg Pathol. 1989;13:490–9.
123. Suster S, Moran CA. Primary synovial sarcoma of the mediastinum: a clinicopathologic, Immunohistochemical, and ultrastructural study of 15 cases. Am J Surg Pathol. 2005;29: 569–78.

124. Ershad R, Rahim M, Davari H. Primary synovial sarcoma: a rare case report. Int J Surg Case Rep. 2016;27:169–71.
125. Lan T, Chen H, Xion B, Zhou T, Peng R, Chen M, et al. Primary pleuropulmonary and mediastinal synovial sarcoma: a clinicopathologic and molecular study of 26 genetically confirmed cases in the largest institution of southwest China. Diagn Pathol. 2016;11:62.
126. Kara HV, Javidfar J, D'Amico TA. Surgical excision of mediastinal synovial sarcoma with limited response to chemotherapy. Ann Thorac Surg. 2014;98:69–70.
127. Trupiano JK, Rice TW, Herzog K, Barr FG, Shipley J, Fisher C, et al. Mediastinal synovial sarcoma: report of two cases with molecular genetic analysis. Ann Thorac Surg. 2002;73:628–30.
128. Snover DC, Levine GD, Rosai J. Thymic carcinoma. Five distinct histological variants. Am J Surg Pathol. 1982;6:451–70.
129. Vilela DS, Valien JSS, Moran MAG, Garcia FI, Velasco JRR, et al. Thymic carcinosarcoma associated with a spindle cell thymoma. Histopathology. 1992;21:263–8.
130. Okudela K, Nakamura N, Sano J, Ito T, Kitamura H. Thymic carcinosarcoma consisting of squamous cell carcinoma and embryonal rhabdomyosarcomatous component. Pathol Res Pract. 2001;197:205–10.
131. Moran CA, Koss MN. Rhabdomyomatous thymoma. Am J Surg Pathol. 1993;17:633–6.
132. De Queiroga EM, Chikota H, Bacchi CE, Moran CA, Suster S. Rhabdomyomatous carcinoma of the thymus. Am J Surg Pathol. 2004;28:1245–50.
133. Chetty R. Extraskeletal mesenchymal chondrosarcoma of the mediastinum. Histopathology. 1990;17:261–78.
134. Montresor E, Abrescia E, Bertrand C, Piazzola E, Girardi C, Iacono C, et al. Mediastinal chondrosarcoma: Case report. Acta Chir Scand. 1990;156:733–6.
135. Pescarmona E, Rendina EA, Venuta F, Pisacane A, Baroni CD. Myxoid chondrosarcoma of the mediastinum. Appl Pathol. 1989;7:318–21.
136. Phillips GWL, Choong M. Case Report: chondrosarcoma presenting as an anterior mediastinal mass. Clin Radiol. 1991;43:63–4.
137. Widdowson DJ, Lewis-Jones HG. A large soft tissue chordoma arising in the posterior mediastinum. Clin Radiol. 1988;39:33–335.
138. Angulo-Hervias E, Lacasa CL, Crespo-Rodriguez AM, Romeo DY. Chondrosarcoma mesenquimal primario en el mediastino. Radiologia. 2007;49:358–61.
139. Suster S, Moran CA. Malignant cartilaginous tumors of the mediastinum: clinicopathological study of six cases presenting as extraskeletal soft tissue masses. Hum Pathol. 1997;28:588–94.
140. Christopherson WM, Foote FW, Stewart FW. Alveolar soft part sarcomas: structurally characteristic tumors of uncertain histogenesis. Cancer. 1952;5:100–11.
141. Kameda Y, Nishii T, Tsuboi M, Arai H, Inui K, Kaneko T, et al. Alveolar soft part sarcoma of the mediastinum: a case report. SAGE Open Med Case Rep. 2017;23(5):2050313.
142. Flieder D, Moran CA, Suster S. Primary alveolar soft part sarcoma of the mediastinum: a clinicopathological and Immunohistochemical study of two cases. Histopathology. 1997;31:469–73.
143. Crowe GG, Muldoon PB. Thoracic chordoma. Thorax. 1951;6:403–7.
144. Geukdjiian SA. Chordoma of the dorsal spine. Can J Surg. 1958;2:106–8.
145. Caputo PJ. Chordoma of the thoracic spine. Case report of a rare entity. Northwest Med. 1959;58:553–4.
146. Clemons RL, Blank RH, Hutchenson JB, Ruffolo EH. Chordoma presenting as posterior mediastinal mass. J Thorac Cardiovasc Surg. 1972;63:922–4.
147. Castellano GC, Johnston HW. Intrathoracic chordoma presenting as a posterior mediastinal tumor. Case Report. South Med J. 1975;68:109–12.
148. Maesen F, Baur C, Lamers J, Versteege C, Willighagen R. Chordoma of the thorax. Eur J Respir Dis. 1986;68:68–72.
149. Ahrendt MN, Wesselhoeft CW. Chordoma presenting as a posterior mediastinal mass in a pediatric patient. J Pediatr Surg. 1992;27:1515–8.
150. Matsubayashi J, Sato E, Nomura M, Kakihana M, Uchida O, Saji H, et al. A case of paravertebral mediastinal chordoma without bone destruction. Skelet Radiol. 2012;41:1641–4.
151. Suster S, Moran CA. Chordomas of the mediastinum: clinicopathologic, Immunohistochemical, and ultrastructural study of six cases presenting as posterior mediastinal masses. Hum Pathol. 1995;26:1354–62.

13 Lymphoproliferative Disorders

Introduction

Primary lymphoproliferative tumors of the mediastinum, similarly to their counterparts in the lymph nodes, have undergone significant changes over the last decade. These changes have been not only in terms of classification but also in terms of new approaches regarding their diagnosis. Needless to say, particularly in the mediastinum, the significant developments in our understanding of these tumors have modified older concepts and terms that may have created confusion in the literature. Terms such as granulomatous thymoma [1] have been correctly reinterpreted as Hodgkin's lymphoma and in turn have provided significant changes in the treatment and survival of these patients.

Even though there is vast information regarding lymphomas in general, in this chapter we will focus our discussion in those tumors occurring in the mediastinum. In addition, the chapter will be presented from the practical point of view for the practicing pathologist who may be called upon to interpret these lesions. In cases in which the utility of more advanced studies is needed, specific mention of it will be made. However, the chapter will focus more on the histopathological and immunohistochemical approach to mediastinal lymphoproliferative lesions. In addition, it is important to highlight that the focus will be on primary mediastinal lymphomas and not on the involvement of the mediastinum by lymphoma as a systemic disease. It has been stated that approximately 10–25% of patients with lymphoma (NHL) will develop mediastinal involvement, while such involvement by Hodgkin's lymphoma (HL) may be up to 60%. On the contrary, primary lymphomas of the mediastinum are relatively rare [2–8]. To this particular point, it is highly important to mention the work of Lichtenstein and colleagues [9], who in 1980 clearly outlined the difference between diseases presenting peripherally, associated with incidental abnormalities on the initial chest film, and diseases that present primarily within the mediastinum. In this latter presentation, the patient will seek medical attention due to an enlarged mediastinal mass. Therefore, this set the basis for what is now known as primary mediastinal lymphomas.

The lymphoproliferative disorders that will be presented in this chapter include:

- Non-Hodgkin's lymphoma
  - Large B-cell lymphoma/primary mediastinal B-cell lymphoma
  - Gray zone lymphoma
  - Anaplastic large cell lymphoma
  - MALT lymphoma
- Lymphoblastic lymphoma
- Hodgkin's lymphoma
- Dendritic cell tumors
- Plasmacytoma
- Castleman's disease
- Extramedullary hematopoiesis (as mediastinal tumor)

Non-Hodgkin's Lymphoma

General Considerations

In 1972, Benjamin and colleagues [10] reviewed the subject of primary lymphatic tumor of the mediastinum and extracted 36 primary tumors out of a series of 215 cases treated at a single institution between the years 1950–1969. These 36 tumors represented about 17% of the total of mediastinal tumors. The authors stated that these tumors are more prevalent in the younger age group, a minority of patients may be asymptomatic, and their tumor is discovered during a routine chest film, while in the symptomatic patients, common symptoms included cough, chest pain, and facial-cervical cyanosis with edema. Approximately two thirds of the tumors were in the anterior mediastinum. The authors encountered that the distribution of these tumors accounted for 15 patients with Hodgkin's lymphoma, 12 with reticulum cell sarcoma, 4 malignant lymphomas (lymphocytic type), and 4 angiomatous lymphoid hamartoma (today's

© Springer Nature Switzerland AG 2019

N. Kalhor, C. Moran, *Mediastinal Pathology*, https://doi.org/10.1007/978-3-319-98980-8_13

Castleman's disease). Also, Al-Naaman and colleagues [11] reviewed 28 cases of mediastinal tumors, encountering only 3 patients with lymphoproliferative lesions, which the authors designated as Hodgkin's lymphoma, lymphosarcoma, and reticulum cell sarcoma. Adkins and colleagues [12] reviewed their experience evaluating 38 patients with primary malignant mediastinal tumors of all types from which the authors identified 7 patients with lymphoproliferative diseases: six with Hodgkin's lymphoma and one with thymic lymphoblastic lymphoma. In 1999, Glick and La Quaglia [13] reviewed the subject of lymphomas of the mediastinum and stated that lymphomas are the most common cause of masses in the mediastinum in children, 50% of children with lymphoblastic lymphoma present with anterior mediastinal mass, and more than one third of all patients with non-Hodgkin's lymphoma (NHL) have their primary site in the mediastinum. The authors described three main subcategories for NHL: small non-cleaved, lymphoblastic, and large cell, the three of them being high grade. The undifferentiated tumors made up for 40–50% of childhood NHL, 30% of lymphoblastic lymphoma, and 15% large cell lymphoma. In a more complete and direct approach to mediastinal large cell lymphomas, Suster [14] presented a review of the subject emphasizing the existence of a group of tumors occurring in the anterior mediastinum and showing features of non-lymphoblastic/non-Hodgkin's large cell lymphomas, capable of adopting unusual morphological appearances, which collectively fall into the category of diffuse large cell lymphomas of the mediastinum. In addition, Suster [14] stated that a significant number of these tumors belong to a distinct type of lymphoproliferative process most likely arising from a native B-cell population in the thymus and described the different morphological growth patterns that these tumors may also show.

Already into this century, the number of reviews presented on the topic of mediastinal lymphomas has become a subject of increased interest. Petersdorf and Wood [15] reviewed the subject of lymphoproliferative disorders presenting as mediastinal tumors and stated that the most common types of non-Hodgkin's lymphomas involving the mediastinum included lymphoblastic lymphoma and large cell lymphoma. The authors also stated that the patients often present with symptoms attributable to the mediastinal mass compressing adjacent organs. On the other hand, Barth and colleagues [16] stated that mediastinal (thymic) large B-cell lymphoma has become a defined subtype of diffuse large B-cell lymphoma and that its histogenesis is not yet fully understood. More recently, reviews on this subject have addressed the subtyping of primary mediastinal large B-cell lymphoma as a subtype of diffuse large B-cell lymphoma as a tumor with distinct clinical and molecular features, many of which are similar to that of nodular sclerosis Hodgkin's lymphoma [17]. Others have emphasized the diagnosis and treatment of primary diffuse large cell lymphoma and have estimated that it represents approximately 2–4% of non-Hodgkin's lymphoma, and that it more often occurs in female patients, stressing that molecular analysis of those tumors shows that it represents a distinct entity [18, 19], while some have stated the overlapping morphological features between primary mediastinal B-cell lymphoma and Hodgkin's lymphoma [20] and the proper use of immunohistochemistry to sort out these two different lymphoproliferative disorders.

Demographics

Liu and colleagues [21], using the surveillance, epidemiology, and end results (SEER) databased during the years 2001–2012, evaluated the incidence and survival of patients with primary mediastinal B-cell lymphoma among major ethnic groups. The authors were able to identify 426 patients, which included 336 Caucasians, 46 blacks, and 44 others; the median age in these groups was 37, 36, and 37 years, respectively. Female patients had a higher incidence, with an incidence rate ratio of 1.4635 for all races combined (1.4938 for Caucasians, 1.12.02 for blacks, and 1.7303 for others). Interestingly, the female predominance was seen in Caucasians and others, while in the black population, male and female occurrence was similar. All races showed a unimodal pattern of age-distribution with incidence peak at age 30–39 years. In terms of overall survival (OS) according to race, the 5-year OS for Caucasians was 84.5%, for blacks 83.8%, and 69.9% for others. The authors also observed that OS significantly decreases in patients older than 60 years, advanced stage, or with medium poverty. In addition, the authors noted that radiation therapy significantly improved patient's survival in the period from 2001 to 2012, but this mode of therapy did not influence OS in primary mediastinal B-cell lymphomas diagnosed between 2006 and 2012. In a different study from a single institution, Maeshima and colleagues [22] analyzed the distribution of 76 cases malignant lymphomas of the anterior mediastinum between the years 1997 and 2016. The authors identified 283 patients with anterior mediastinal tumors of which 16% were primary mediastinal large B-cell lymphomas (PMBL) and 10% Hodgkin's lymphoma. Of the newly diagnosed lymphomas in 60 patients, PMBL was the most common with 46%. The authors also noted a female predominance under 40 years of age with 58% of the cases. Recently, Martelli and colleagues [23] reviewed the subject of primary mediastinal large B-cell lymphomas and acknowledged the only one population-based study in the incidence of PMLBC performed by Liu and colleagues [21] in which an annual rate of 0.4 per million was estimated. Important to highlight is the developing understanding in the diagnosis of PMBCL as a distinct entity from other types of diffuse large B-cell lymphoma [24], as these patients may respond better to some different treatment options.

Clinical Features

Over the last 30 years, there have been numerous clinicopathological correlations on the subject of primary B-cell lymphomas of the mediastinum, and over the years, there have been some gains, namely, in the immunohistochemical approach, molecular analysis, and the treatment options. In 1982, Trump and Mann [25] reported 11 cases of diffuse large cell and undifferentiated lymphomas, excluding Hodgkin's lymphoma and lymphoblastic lymphoma. The patients presented with large anterior mediastinal tumors; seven patients were women and 10 of the 11 patients were under 43 years of age. Clinically, the patients presented with non-specific findings including chest pain, cough, and dyspnea. Facial swelling was seen in two patients, and three patients had fever, weight loss, and night sweats. The authors subclassified these lymphomas as diffuse large cell ("histiocytic") and one undifferentiated non-Burkitt's type. Histologically, sclerosis was present in four cases. Nine patients died within 26 months after initial diagnosis. Levitt and coworkers [26], in an evaluation of 215 lymphoma patients between 1975 and 1979, identified 12 (6%) of these patients with mediastinal lymphomas. Eleven of these 12 patients had extensive contiguous extranodal disease with involvement of pericardium, sternum, chest wall, pulmonary parenchyma, and/or superior vena cava obstruction. Eight cases were classified as diffuse large cell lymphoma, and four tumors were not characterized as either B- or T-cell lymphomas. Even though the age of these patients ranged from 19 to 72 years, eight patients were younger than 30 years and six patients were women. The majority of these patients presented with non-specific symptoms. Yousem and coworkers [27] also reported their experience with 19 patients of which 17 were subclassified as diffuse large cell, one immunoblastic, and one follicular and diffuse. The patients were nine women and ten men between the ages of 15 and 74 years with a median age of 29 years. Histologically, approximately one third of these tumors showed sclerosis. In a histopathologic analysis of 20 primary mediastinal large cell lymphomas, Waldrom and coworkers [28] stated that varying degrees of sclerosis were observed in each one of the 20 cases studied. However, this latter issue of "sclerosis" was more specifically presented by Perrone and coworkers [29] in a retrospective study of 60 cases of mediastinal diffuse large cell lymphoma, which the authors designated as mediastinal large cell lymphoma with sclerosis. In this report by Perrone and coworkers [29], 43 patients were women and 17 were men; 85% of the patients were 35 years or younger. The authors encountered that the extrathoracic involvement was more commonly seen in the liver, lymph nodes, kidney, pancreas, gastrointestinal tract, and ovary. Twenty patients died of tumor with a median time of 16.5 months; however, the authors identified as unfavorable prognostic factors the following: younger than 25 years, extrathoracic involvement at presentation, and disease recurrence. On the other hand, favorable prognostic factors included response to initial therapy and marked tumor sclerosis. Also, Menestrina and coworkers [30], following Perrone's description [29], reported eight additional cases that the authors coded as mediastinal large cell lymphoma of B-cell type, with sclerosis. The patients in this report corresponded to five women and three men between the ages of 15 and 32 years (mean age: 25 years). On the other hand, Addis and Isaacson [31], in a description of 15 mediastinal lymphomas, placed more emphasis in the thymic origin of the lymphoma, as the authors demonstrated the B-cell origin with monotypic immunoglobulin production in two cases. Kirn and coworkers [32] evaluated 57 patients with large cell and immunoblastic lymphomas of the mediastinum; fifty six of the 57 patients presented with disease that was confined to sites above the diaphragm with bulky disease and intrathoracic infiltration. Thirty (53%) of the patients described were men and 27 women, with a median age of 30 years; 60% of the tumors were classified as diffuse large cell and 40% as immunoblastic. Histologically, the authors observed varying degrees of sclerosis in all the cases, but such change was not quantitated. Immunophenotyping was performed in 30 cases showing 80% B-cell phenotype and 20% T-cell phenotype. The overall 5-year survival was estimated at 50%. Abou and coworkers [33] also presented their experience with 43 primary mediastinal large B-cell lymphomas in 20 men and 23 women with a median age of 42 years. Only 9% of these patients had marrow involvement, and all these tumors were positive for CD20. Complete remission was observed in 63% of the patients, and the 5-year overall survival was 46%. The authors also compared this group of primary mediastinal lymphomas with 352 patients with non-mediastinal diffuse large B-cell lymphoma and concluded that there was no significant clinical difference between these two groups. However, the authors also noted that the younger age, female predominance, mediastinal location, and size of the mass may justify the recognition of PMBCL as a clinical syndrome. Hatem and coworkers [34] also evaluated 141 mediastinal large B-cell lymphomas and compared them with 916 non-mediastinal large B-cell lymphomas. The authors stated that the clinical features of PMBCL are rather homogenous and distinct from non-MLCL, occurring more often in young female patients (59%) with a mean age of 37 years in contrast to 42% and a mean age of 54 years for the non-MLCL. Also, important to highlight is that the authors identify two common patterns: (1) large cells with clear cytoplasm and (2) presence of fibrosis, which was marked in

25% of their cases. However, the authors did not consider that those histological features had an impact on prognosis. However, 79% of patients with PMBCL achieved a complete remission compared to 68% in the non-MLCL group. Interestingly, in a histomorphologic study of 109 cases of mediastinal B-cell lymphoma, Paulli and coworkers [35] stated that the term "diffuse large cell lymphoma" falls short of the broad morphological spectrum that this entity represents in the mediastinum, and they advise to further subclassify these tumors.

Even though the majority of mediastinal large B-cell lymphomas occurs in adults or young adults, the occurrence of similar tumor in the pediatric age group has been also described. Piira and coworkers [36] reported nine children ranging in age from 10 to 17 years. Histological classification of these lymphomas is three immunoblastic, three large cell multilobated, two large cell non-cleaved, and one large cell, clear cell. However, the authors stated that varying degrees of sclerosis were seen in all cases, and in immunophenotyping, all the tumors were B-cell lineage. The clinical follow-up presented showed that three children had died of disease within 8–19 months. Also, Carr and coworkers [37] reported four children, three boys and one girl ages 2–11 years. All children presented with superior vena cava syndrome due to their anterior mediastinal mass; histologically all showed features of diffuse large B-cell lymphoma with sclerosis and B-cell immunophenotype. Follow-up available in these children showed that one child died due to infections, and the others were alive 43 months post diagnosis.

In more recent years, primary mediastinal B-cell lymphoma (PMBCL) has been recognized as a distinct clinicopathologic entity that predominantly affects young adults, more commonly female patients. However, even though PMBCL is considered a subtype of diffuse B-cell lymphoma, some of the clinical, morphological, and biological features overlap with some of nodular sclerosing Hodgkin's lymphoma. These two tumoral conditions also share some features with mediastinal gray zone lymphoma, which has features between PMBCL and nodular sclerosing Hodgkin's lymphoma, and they are believed to represent a unique molecular entity [38]. PMBCL is believed to derive from thymic B-cells and possibly is on a pathobiologic spectrum of diseases with NSHL –CD15, CD30 positive and PMBCL –CD20 positive and in between mediastinal gray zone lymphoma with intermediate features between both of them. Some genomic studies in PMBCL and NSHL have identified Janus kinase/signal transducers and activators of transcription (JAK-STAT), signaling activation is a characteristic feature of both of these entities. In addition, more than 50% of PMBCL have genomic gains of chromosome 9p containing a locus for JAK2. Somatic mutations for SOCS1 have similar frequency in PMBCL and classic Hodgkin's lymphoma. Mutations in the gene PTPN1 also have been identified in about 20% of PMBCL and Hodgkin's lymphoma. However, it is considered that PMBCL and mediastinal gray zone lymphoma represent distinct clinicopathologic entities that have distinct management compared with other types of diffuse large B-cell lymphoma. Ahn and coworkers [39] recently reported 25 cases of PMBCL from a single center; the patients were 17 women and 8 men between the ages of 15 and 78 years (median age: 31 years), and all the patients presented with a mediastinal mass. Nineteen patients achieved complete remission, and 18 were alive after a follow-up ranging from 1 to 92 months (median, 43 months). Also, the occurrence of PMBCL in pregnancy has been described [40]. From the histological point of view, in a study of 137 PMBCL, the tumors show diffuse growth pattern with sclerosis, varying degrees of nuclear pleomorphism, and clear to basophilic cytoplasm. In addition, molecular studies performed in 40 of these cases showed that half of the cases displayed bcl-6 gene mutations and/or MUM1/1RF4 expression, thus supporting the concept that this tumor is derived from activated germinal centers or post-germinal center cells. One of the differences with other aggressive B-cell lymphomas is that PMBCL shows defective Ig production despite the expression of Oct-2, BOB.1, and PU.1 transcription factors and lack of IgV_H gene crippling mutations [41].

The clinical outcome of patients with thymic B-cell lymphomas has varied over the years. In 1997, Lazzarino and coworkers [42] reported 106 patients from a multicenter study and concluded that mediastinal B-cell lymphoma is an aggressive non-Hodgkin's lymphoma with a 3-year survival rate of 52% for all patients and 82% for responders. Zinzani and coworkers [43] in 1999 reported 50 patients with PMBCL with sclerosis and found that 43 patients (86%) achieved a complete response and 7 patients were nonresponders to treatment. Relapse-free survival rate was 93% at 96 months (median: 39 months); thus the authors concluded that MACOP-B (methotrexate, Adriamycin, cyclophosphamide, vincristine, prednisone, and bleomycin) plus radiation therapy is a useful first-line treatment. Todeschini and coworkers [44] reported long-term results from a retrospective multicenter experience in 138 patients treated with CHOP or MACOP-B/VACOP-B and encountered that complete remission was 51% with CHOP and 80% with MACOP-B/VACOP-B. Also, Broccoli and coworkers [45], in a report of 98 patients with PMBCL and two decades experience at a single center, concluded that MACOP could be considered a first-line treatment after 62% of their patients achieved complete response after MACOP-B with or without rituximab. The 17-year overall survival was estimated at 72%, while disease-free survival was estimated at 88%. However, Roth and associates [46] reported 156 patients – including children and adults – with PMBCL from 24 academic centers and stated that adjusted EPOCH (etoposide, doxorubicin, cyclophosphamide, vincristine, prednisone) chemotherapy and rituximab have become the standard of care for PMBCL. The 3-year overall survival was estimated at 95.4%. In a more focused study on PMBCL in children, Pillon and associates [47] reported 13 children between the ages of 12 and 18 years who were treated with high-dose methotrexate, cytarabine, and anti-CD20 and found that the 5-year overall survival was 91.7 with only one patient dying of progressive disease.

Pathological Features

At low magnification, remnants of thymic tissue may be seen (Figs. 13.1, 13.2, 13.3, and 13.4a–d), the tumor does not show specific pattern of growth, and the tumor shows more a diffuse distribution of the tumor cells. However, the tumor may also show different growth patterns, and the most often seen include the presence of varying degrees of sclerosis in what has been denominated large cell lymphoma with sclerosis. In these tumors, the presence of sclerosis may impart a subtle nested pattern in which the tumor cells are separated by or compartmentalized by the presence of fibrous bands of different thickness (Figs. 13.5, 13.6, 13.7, 13.8, 13.9, 13.10, and 13.11). In some tumors,

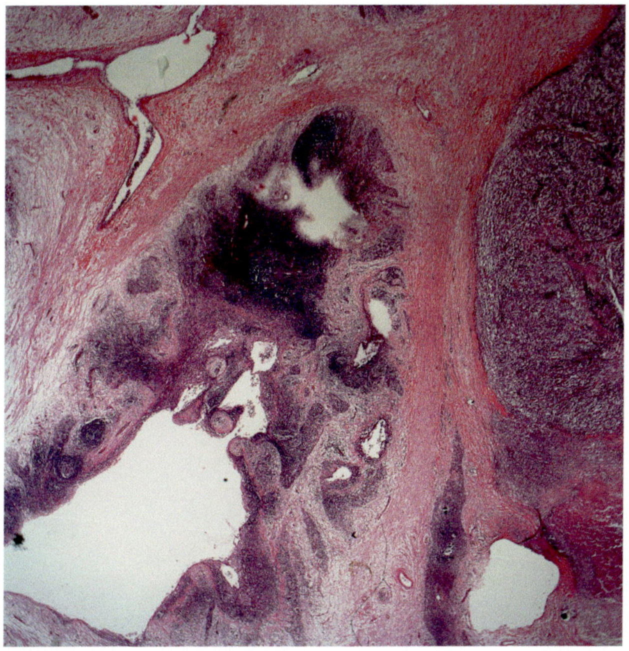

Fig. 13.2 Thymus with cystic changes with an adjacent B-cell lymphoma

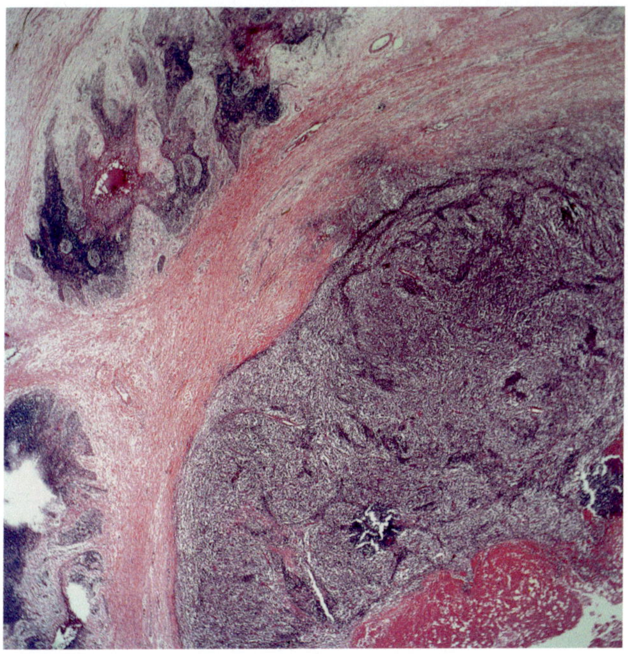

Fig. 13.1 Primary thymic B-cell lymphoma, note the presence of residual thymus in the periphery

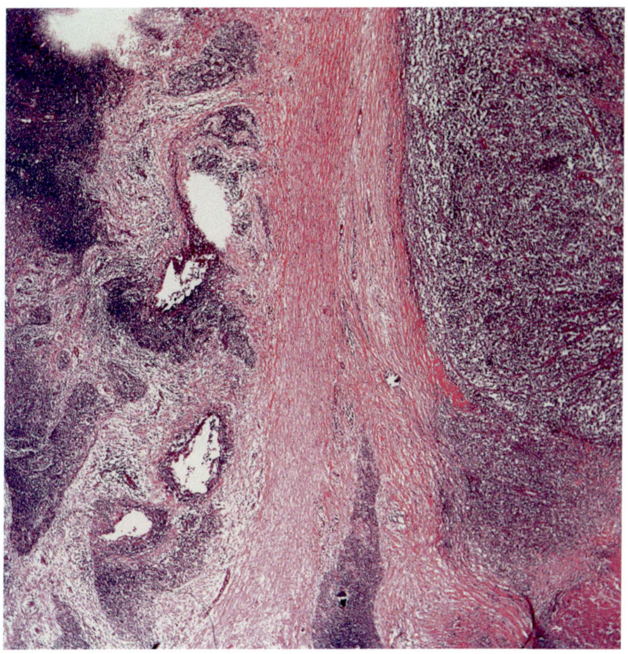

Fig. 13.3 Higher magnification of a thymic B-cell lymphoma with adjacent remnants of thymus

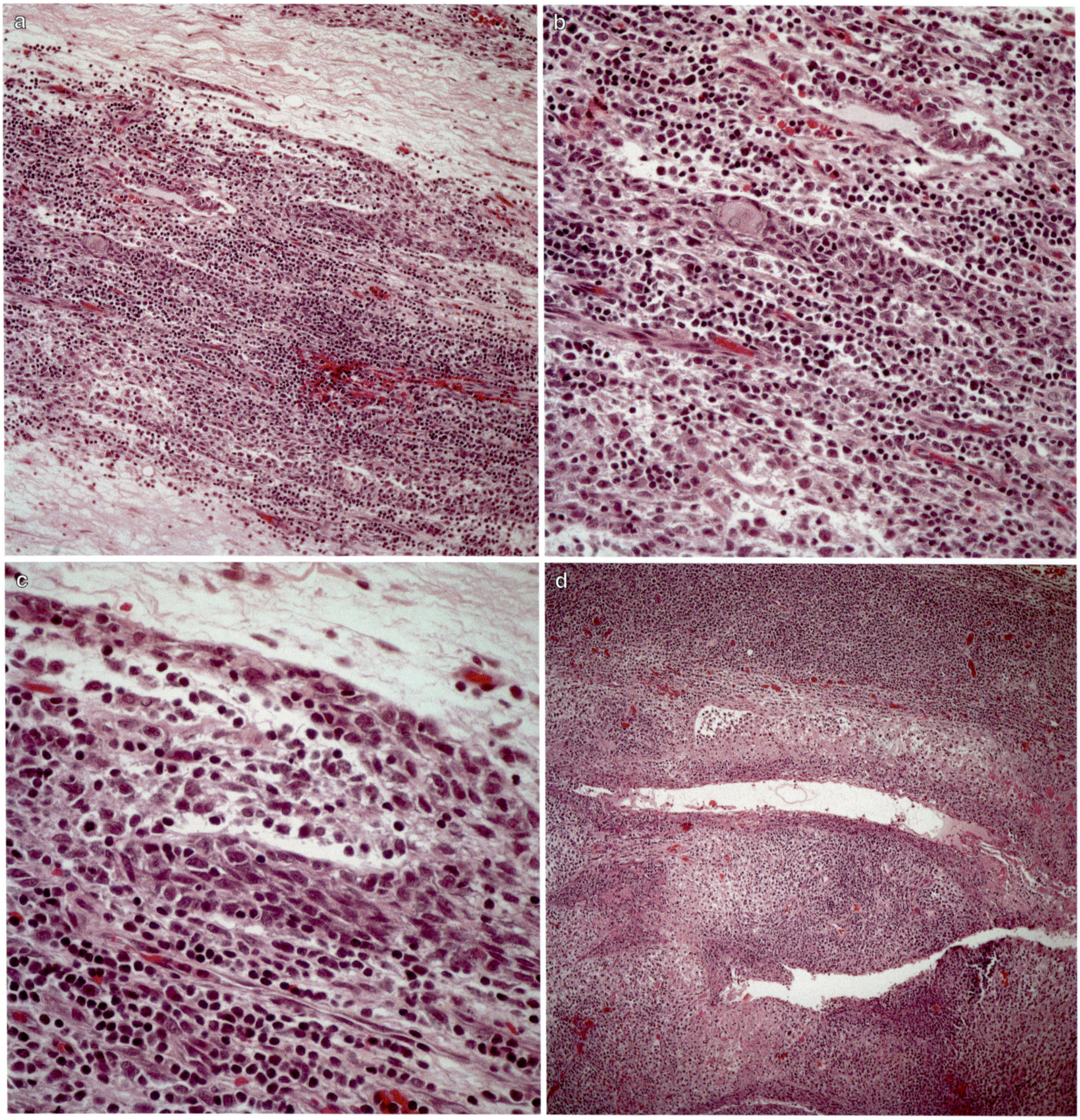

Fig. 13.4 (**a**) Low power view of a thymic B-cell lymphoma showing remnants of thymic epithelium and a Hassall corpuscle; (**b**) higher magnification showing the Hassall corpuscle admixed with lymphoma cells; (**c**) higher magnification contrasting the thymic epithelium and the lymphoma cells. (**d**) Cystic structure lined by squamous epithelium and adjacent large B-cell lymphoma

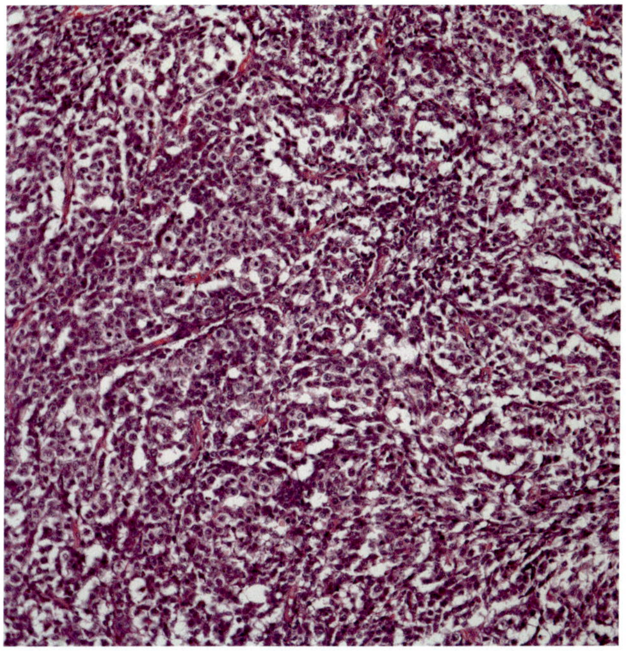

Fig. 13.5 Thymic B-cell lymphoma with more solid growth pattern

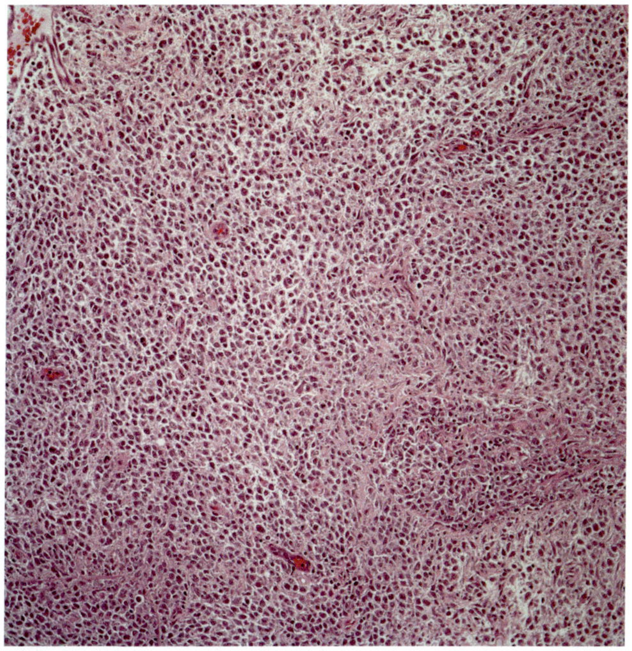

Fig. 13.7 Thymic B-cell lymphoma showing sheets of neoplastic cells

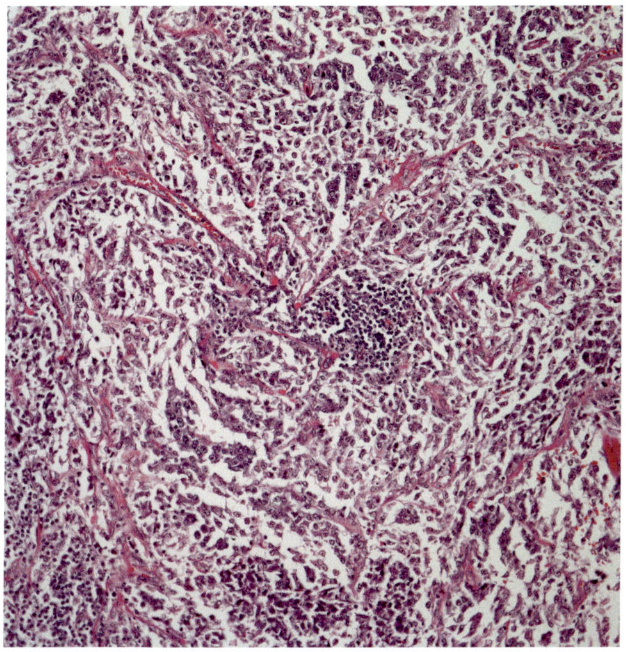

Fig. 13.6 Thymic B-cell lymphoma with only thin fibroconnective tissue and elongated vessels

the presence of sclerosis can be extensive, which can obscure the presence of the neoplastic cells (Figs. 13.11, 13.12, 13.13, 13.14, 13.15, 13.16, 13.17, 13.18, 13.19, and 13.20a, b). Areas of necrosis may be present in some tumors (Fig. 13.21a, b). One other common histological feature is the presence of clear cells. Such observation was originally described by Moller and associates [48] in a report of eight mediastinal tumors that occur in young adults, predominantly female patients. The cytologic feature of clear cells is often accompanied by the presence of sclerosis (Figs. 13.22a, b and 13.23a–e). At higher magnification, the histological characteristics of mediastinal large cell lymphoma are those of an atypical lymphoid proliferation composed of large round cells with dense chromatin and presence of nucleoli (Fig. 13.24a–c). On the other hand, the tumors may also show more cytologic atypia with presence of multinucleated cells or mononuclear cells with bizarre nuclei and Reed-Sternberg-like cells and yet demonstrate a B-cell lineage [49]. Other unusual features that may also be present in mediastinal B-cell lymphomas include signet ring cell and spindle cell appearance.

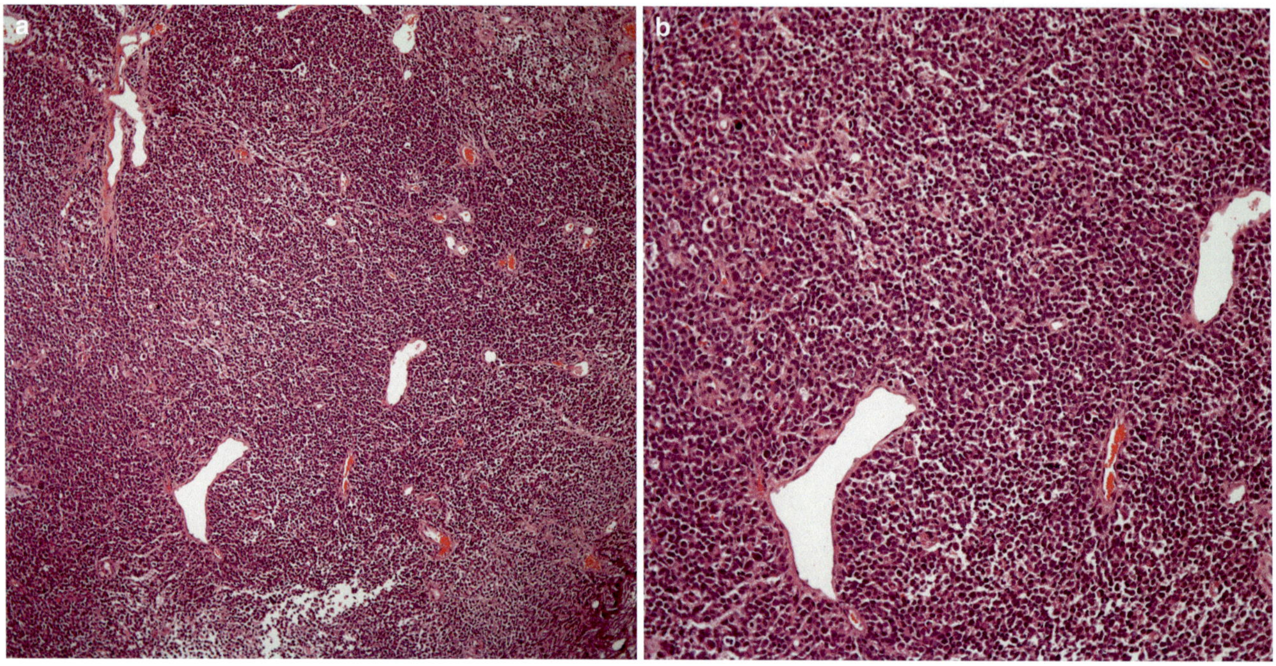

Fig. 13.8 (**a**) Thymic B-cell lymphoma with dilated vascular spaces. (**b**) Closer view showing larger cells with subtle plasmacytic changes and dilated vascular spaces

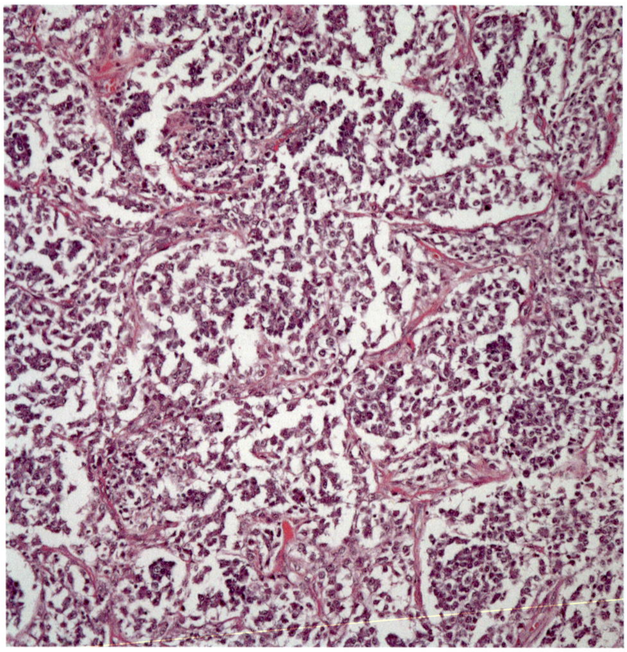

Fig. 13.9 Thymic B-cell lymphoma with subtle nested growth pattern; note the thick strands of fibroconnective tissue

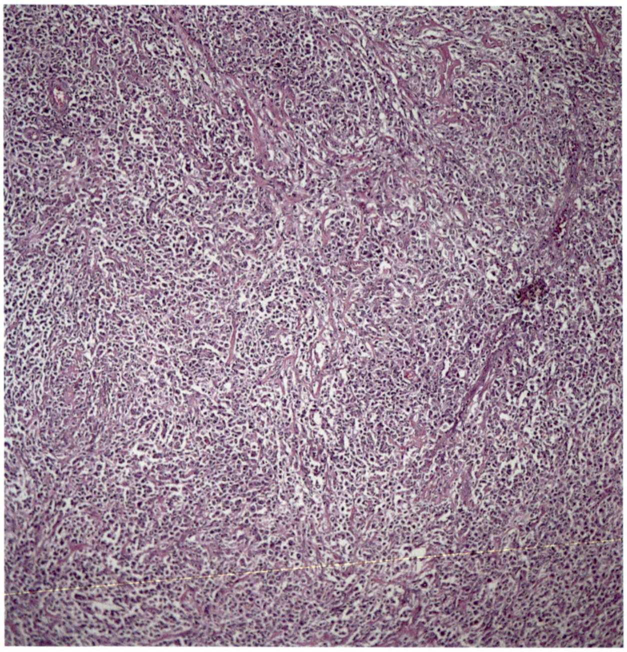

Fig. 13.10 Low power view of a thymic B-cell lymphoma showing discrete areas of fibrosis

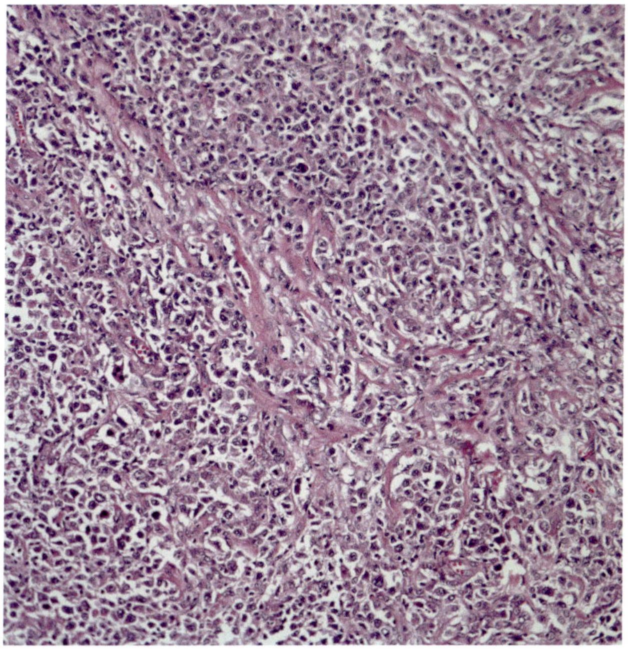

Fig. 13.11 Higher magnification of a thymic B-cell lymphoma showing areas of subtle fibrosis

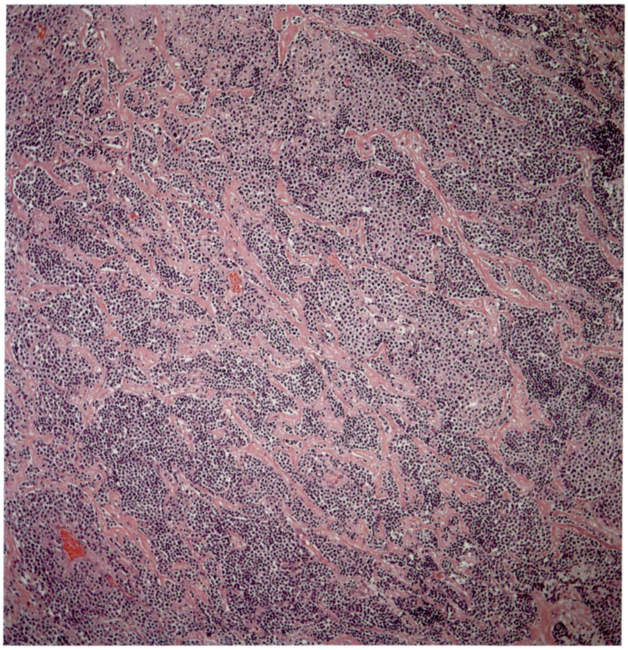

Fig. 13.12 Easily identifiable areas of fibrosis in this primary thymic B-cell lymphoma giving the appearance of nested growth pattern

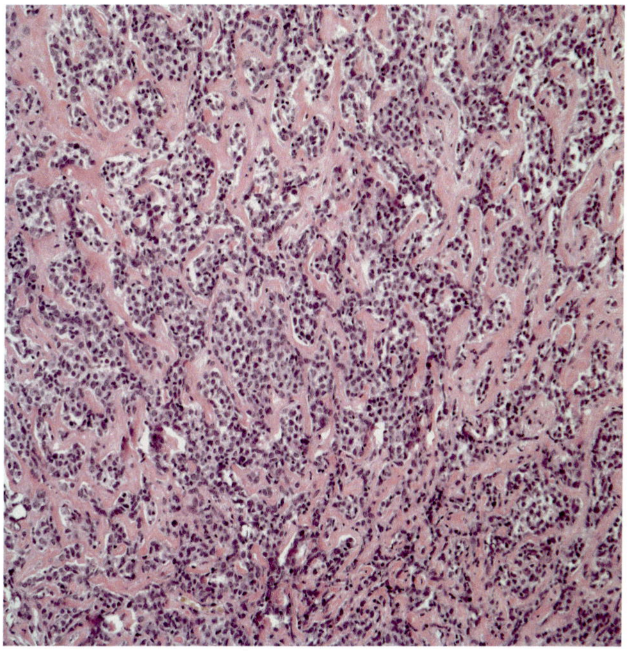

Fig. 13.13 Higher magnification showing lymphoma cells separated in small clusters by strands of fibroconnective tissue

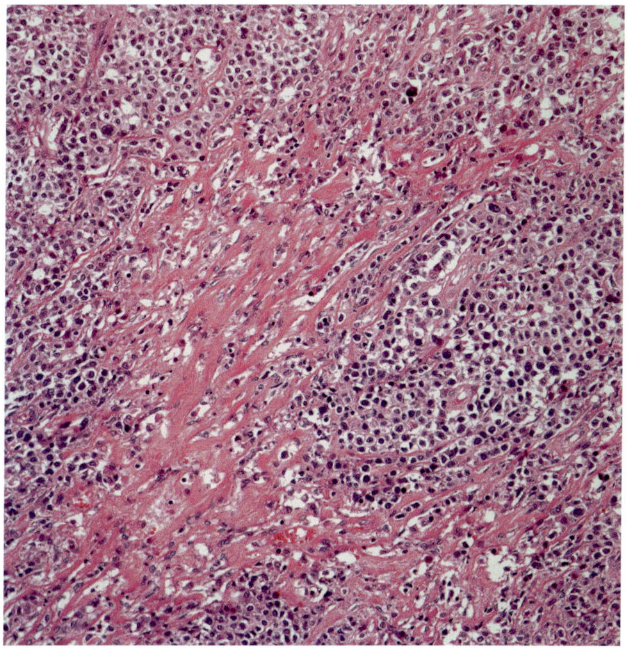

Fig. 13.14 Thymic B-cell lymphoma with more pronounced areas of fibrosis

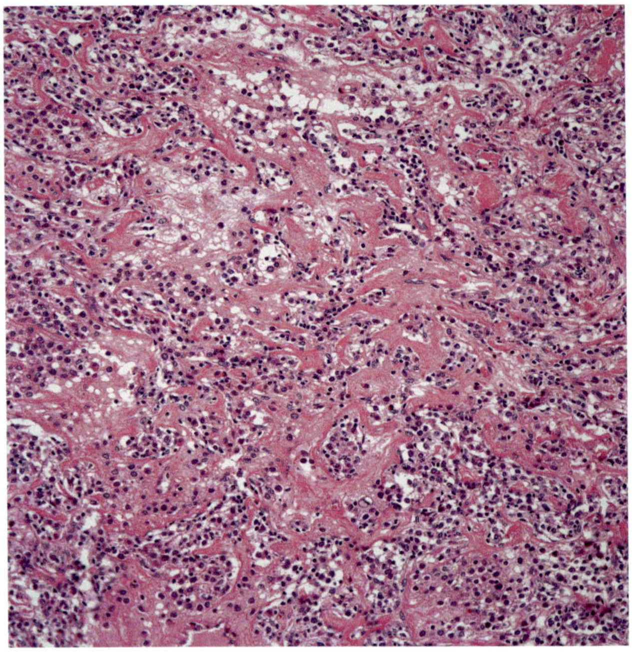

Fig. 13.15 More extensive areas of fibrosis in a primary thymic B-cell lymphoma

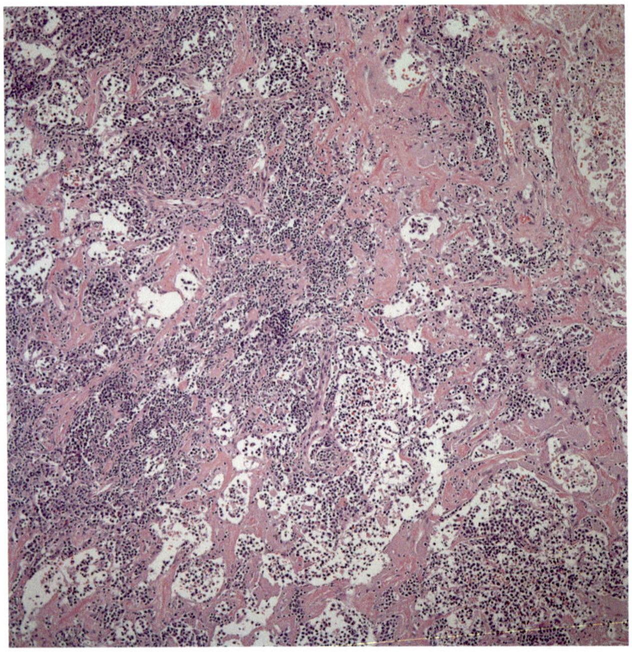

Fig. 13.16 Haphazard distribution of fibrosis and neoplastic cells in this thymic B-cell lymphoma

Immunohistochemical Features

The main thesis behind this group of tumors is the B-cell lineage that all these tumors exhibit. Essentially, all these tumors show positive staining for CD20. However, it has been observed that there are some differences in terms of the immunohistochemical staining pattern present in the diffuse large B-cell lymphoma and PMBCL. Although both of these tumors may show positive staining for CD45, CD20, CD79a, PAX-5, BOB-1, and OCT-2, PMBCL also shows positive staining for CD23 and negative for immunoglobulin, while diffuse large B-cell lymphoma is negative for CD23 and positive for immunoglobulin. Calaminici and associates [50] reported 24 PMBCL lymphomas, which were stained for CD23 and identify that approximately 70% of these tumors express this antibody, while about 15% of the non-mediastinal nodal diffuse large B-cell lymphoma may show such expression. In addition, it is important to highlight that PMBCL may also express CD30. Higgins and associates [51] evaluated 51 PMBCL with CD30 and identified 35 cases (69%) of these tumors staining for CD30. The staining was reported to range from strong membrane staining to rare individual cells. It is also important to highlight that PMBCL is negative for CD15, which may be of aid in difficult cases when compared to Hodgkin's lymphoma or gray zone lymphomas (Fig. 13.25a–g).

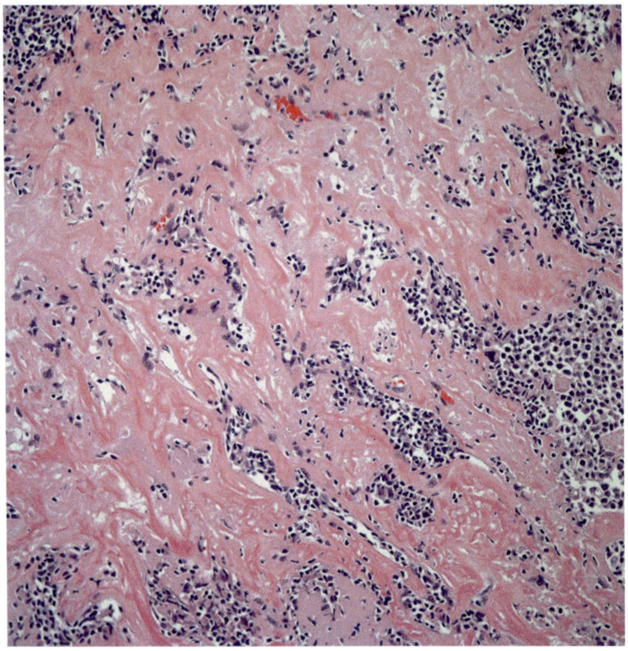

Fig. 13.17 Extensive fibrosis with still enough neoplastic cells

Molecular Features

Over the last few years, there have been important developments in the molecular features associated with PMBCL, which have led to the notion that PMBCL represents a distinct clinicopathological entity. For instance, genetic alterations – including 2p14 0 p16 gain involving the REL gene, 9p24 gain involving JAK2, PDL2, PDL1, SMARC2,

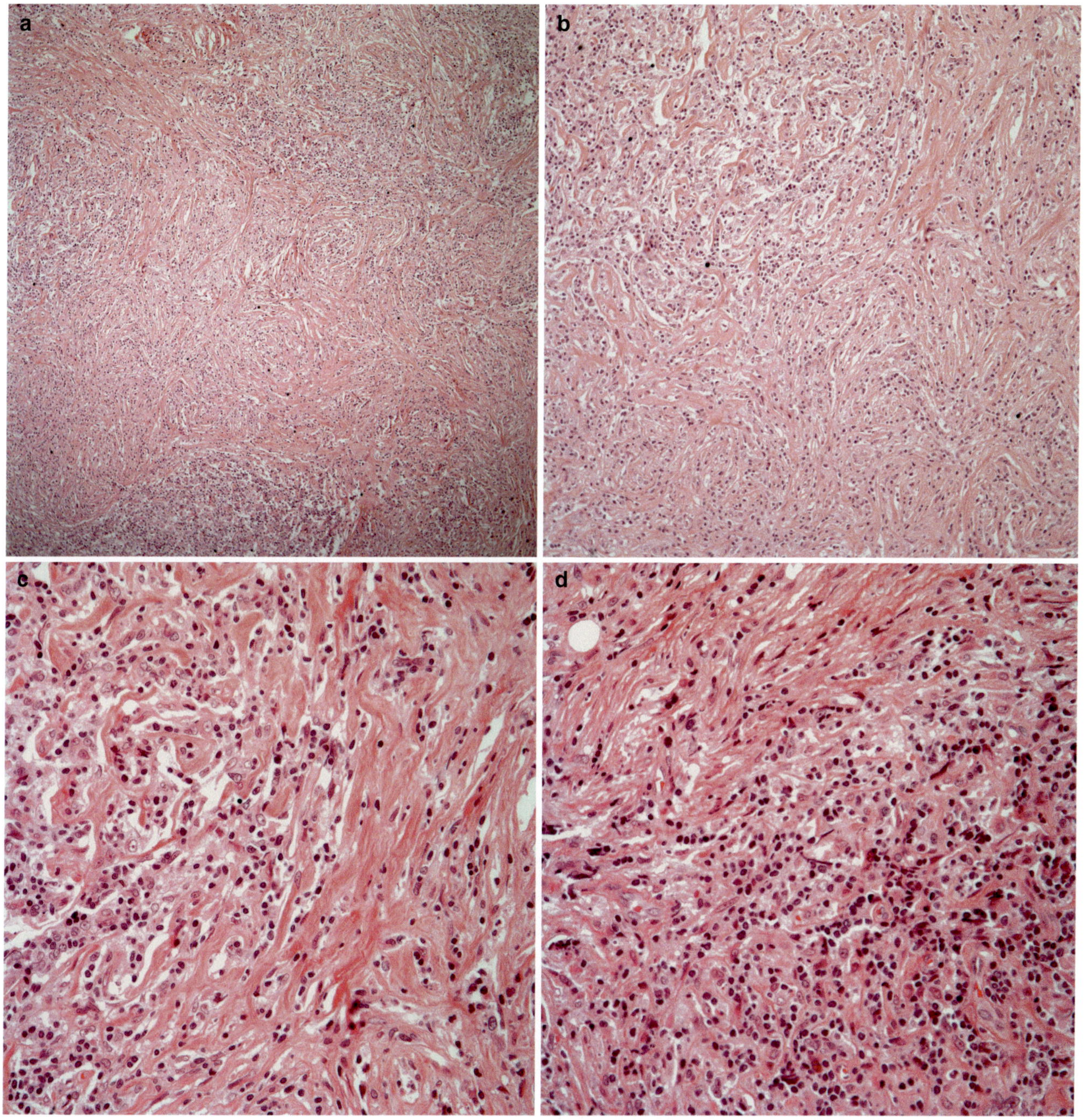

Fig. 13.18 (**a**) Low power view of a thymic B-cell lymphoma with areas of fibrosis mimicking a spindle cell neoplasm; (**b**) closer view show areas reminiscent of "ropy collagen" admixed with lymphoma cells; (**c**) higher magnification showing the lymphoid cells dissecting collagen; (**d**) neoplastic lymphoid cells admixed with fibrosis

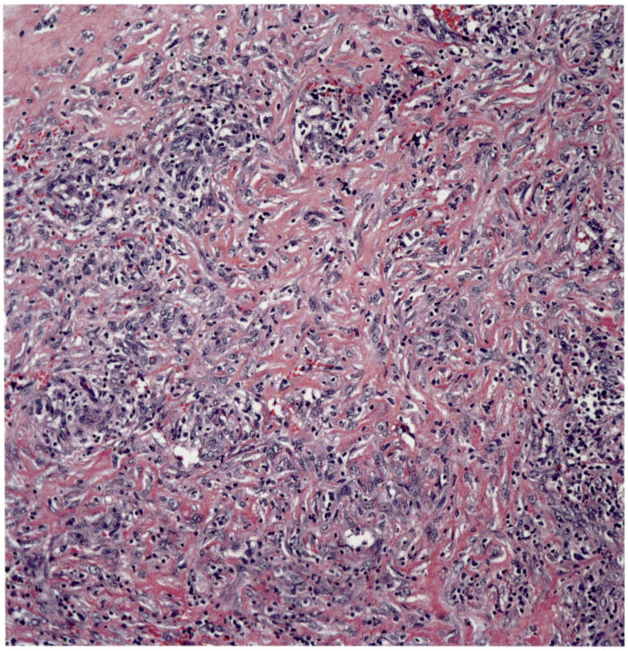

Fig. 13.19 Thymic B-cell lymphoma showing areas of spindle cell shaped cells

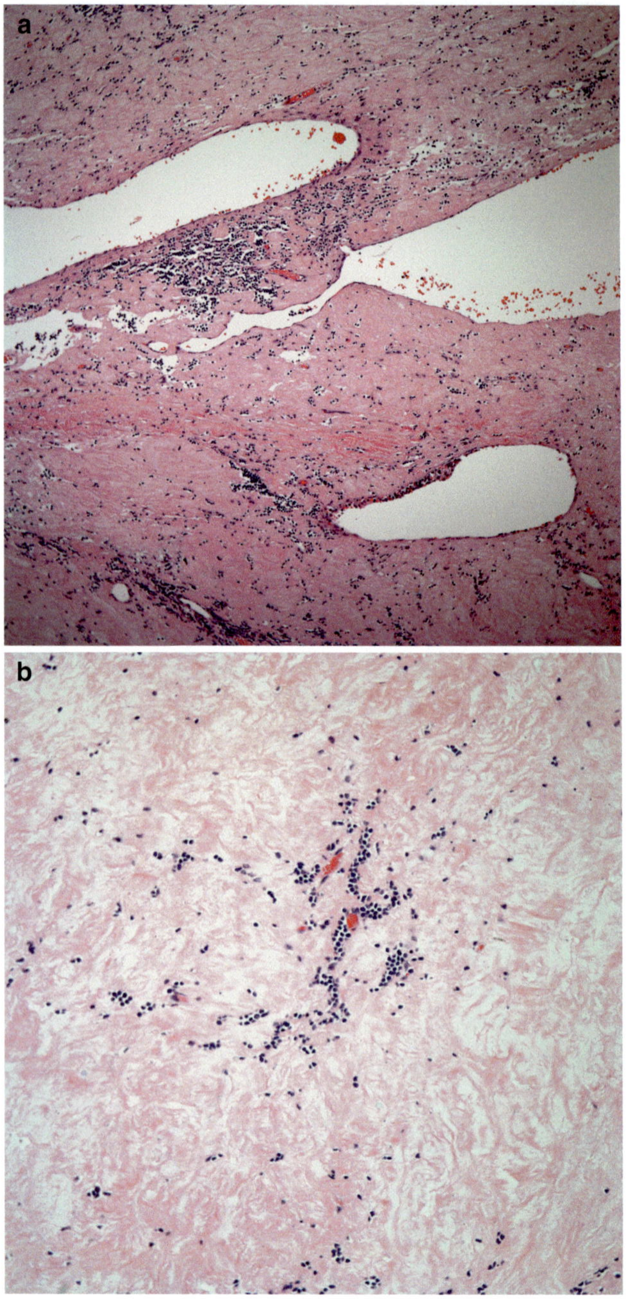

Fig. 13.20 (**a**) Extensive fibrosis with only clusters of neoplastic cells; (**b**) Focal cluster of lymphoma cells embedded in a collagenous stroma

JMJD2C, RANBP6 gene, 12q24 gain involving ELK3, EPS8, IFNG gene, 12q11-q13 involving IGF1 gene, and 16p13 rearrangements involving CIITA, SOCS1 gene – have been observed [17, 19]. In addition, Copie-Bergman and associates [52] reported the expression of the MAL (myelin and lymphocyte protein) gene by Northern blot and reverse transcription-polymerase chain reaction (RT-PCR) in 8 of 12 PMBCL, while 8 peripheral diffuse large B-cell lymphomas showed little or no MAL gene expression. Also, Tsang and associates [53] evaluated 16 PMBCL and encountered that bcl-1, bcl-2, ras genes, or EBV infections were not observed in any of the tumors evaluated. However, Pileri and associates [54], in a study of 45 PMBCL, identified that more than half of the cases will show BCL-6 gene mutations, which usually occurred along with functioning somatic IgV_H gene mutation and Bcl-6 and/or MUM1/IRF4 expression. Savage and associates [55] also identified that PMBCL has high levels of expression of inerleukin-13 (IL-13) receptor and downstream effectors of IL-13 signaling JAK2 and signal transducer and activator of transcription-1 (STAT1), tumor necrosis factor (TNF) family members, and TNF receptor-associated factor-1 (TRAF1). Thus, this supports the argument that these results identify a link between PMBCL and HL. In that regard, Rosenwald and associates [56] stated that over one third of the genes that were more highly expressed in PMBCL were also expressed in HL cells. The use of genomic hybridization and interphase cytogenetics have shown that gains in chromosomal material involving chromosomes 9p, 12q, and Xq, and also the amplification of the proto-oncogene REL have been identified in PMBCL [57]. More recently, Wang and Cook [58] reported that the use of PDCD1LG2 (PD-L2) RNA in situ hybridization is a sensitive specific and practical marker of primary mediastinal large B-cell lymphoma. The authors correlated the findings of immunohistochemistry (IHC) for CD274 (PD-L1) with CD274 RISH and PDCD1LG2 RISH and identified CD274 IHC in 25%, CD274 RISH in 44%, and PDCC1LG2 RISH in 72% of PMBCL.

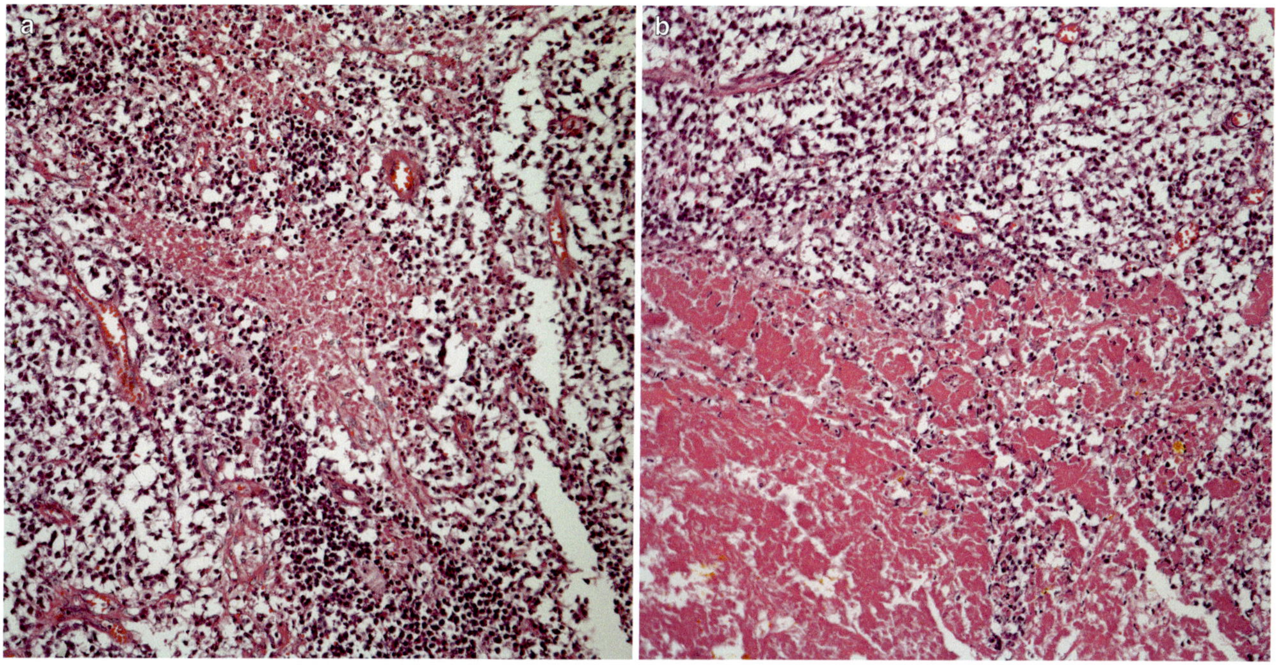

Fig. 13.21 (**a**) Thymic B-cell lymphoma showing focal areas of fibrinoid necrosis; (**b**) more extensive areas of infarcted necrosis

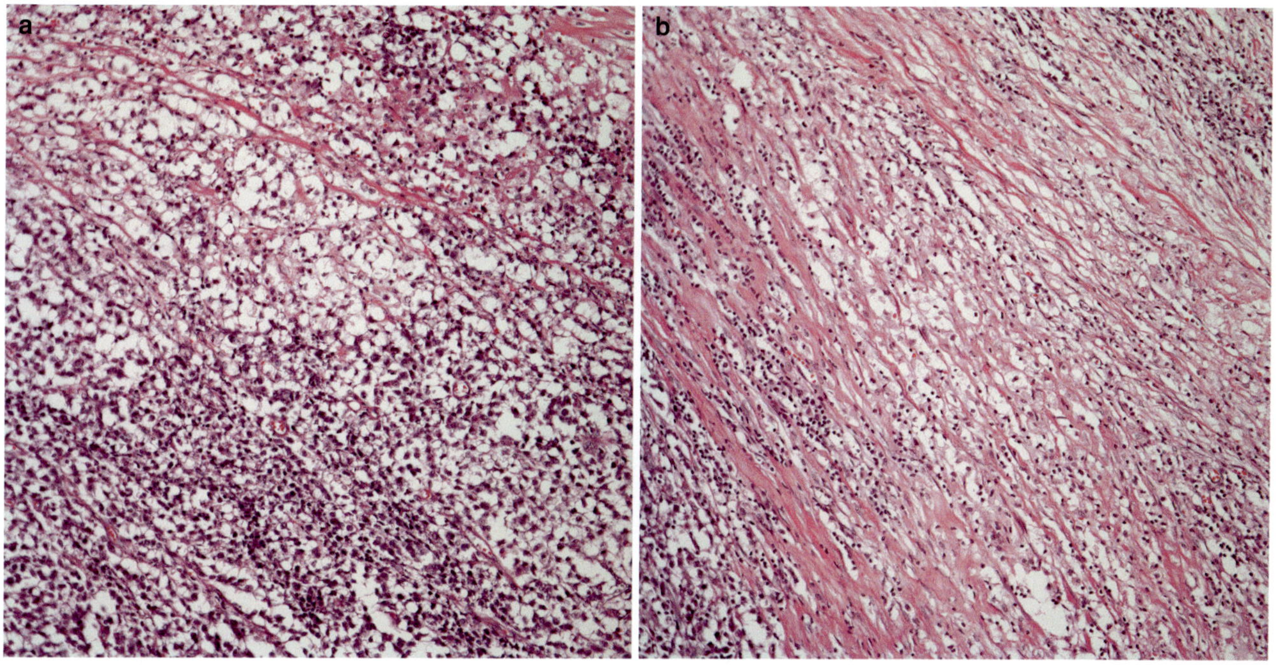

Fig. 13.22 (**a**) Thymic B-cell lymphoma with transitional conventional areas to clear cell areas; (**b**) clear cells dissecting areas of fibrosis

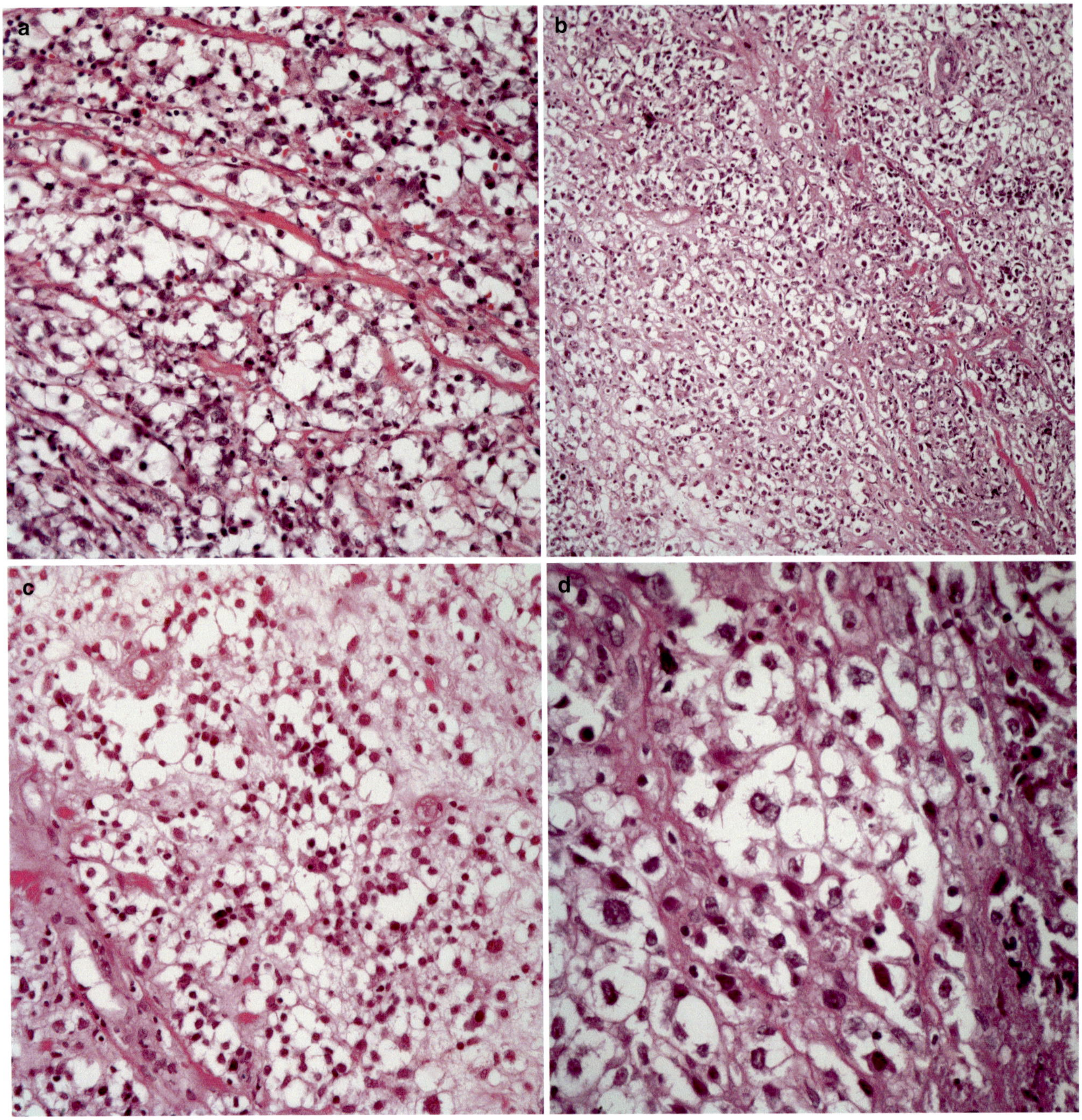

Fig. 13.23 (**a**) Clear cell lymphoma, note the cells separated by thick strands of fibroconnective tissue; (**b**) clear cell lymphoma with more subtle fibrosis; (**c**) higher magnification showing cells with clear cytoplasm and round nucleus; (**d**) clear cells with round to oval nucleus and some nucleoli

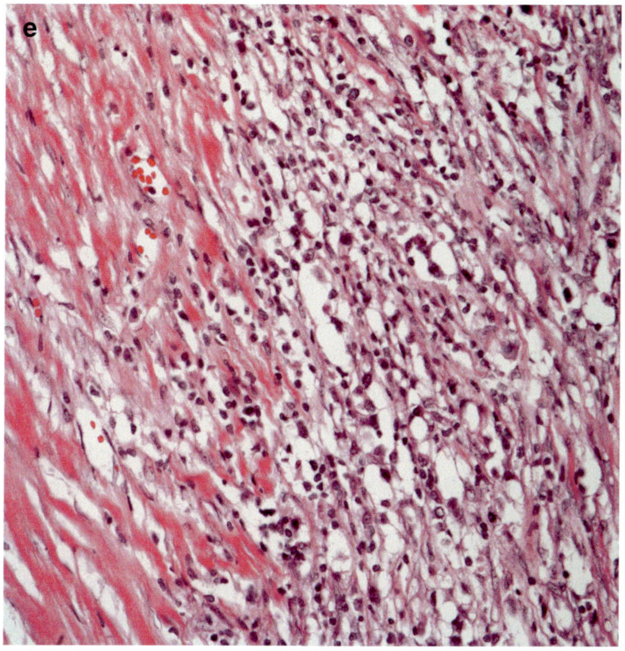

Fig. 13.23 (continued) (**e**) More extensive areas of fibrosis in a clear cell lymphoma

Mediastinal Gray Zone Lymphoma

This is an unusual primary lymphoma in the mediastinum and is defined as a tumor that shows overlapping features between PMBCL and classic HL. Although the existence of this tumor has become known for approximately 10 years, it is possible that such tumors have been described in a more descriptive manner in the past. For instance, descriptions of B-cell lymphomas under the term "pleomorphic" lymphomas [49], in which the description in some of these cases are of cells mimicking Reed-Sternberg cells, raise the possibility that the tumor has existed for some time, but it has only been acknowledged for the last 10 years. In addition, it is important to highlight that other authors have also reported the existence of large B-cell lymphomas in the mediastinum with Hodgkin's features. Garcia and associates [59] described six out of nine cases in young men presenting with mediastinal tumors. The histopathology described in those tumors was that of a polymorphous background, pleomorphic cytology, and the presence of Reed-Sternberg cells. Also, Gomez-

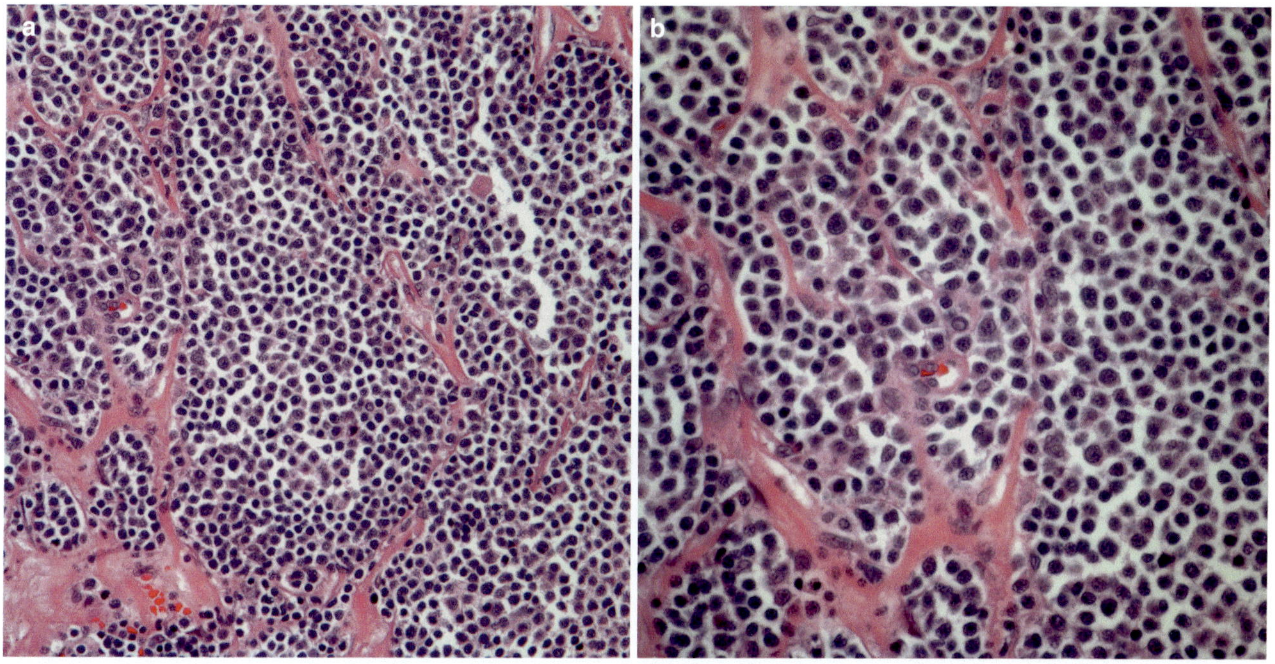

Fig. 13.24 (**a**) Thymic B-cell lymphoma showing a homogenous cellular proliferation separated by thin fibrocollagen; (**b**) higher magnification showing tumor cells with subtle plasmacytoid appearance

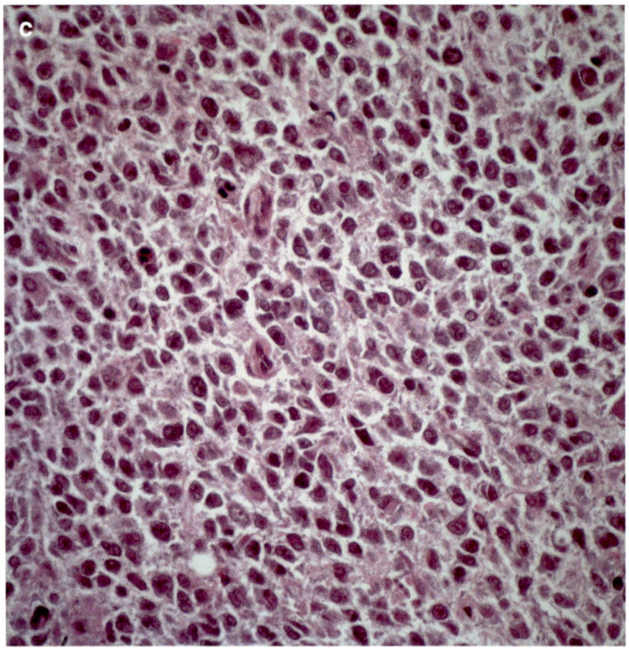

Fig. 13.24 (continued) (**c**) Medium to large cells with moderate amount of cytoplasm, irregular nucleus and some with nucleoli. Mitotic figures are present

Gelvez and Smith [60] have described Reed-Sternberg-like cells in otherwise non-Hodgkin's lymphoma. However, the largest study so far defining the entity of mediastinal gray zone lymphoma is credited to Traverse-Glehen and associates [61], who collected and reported 21 such cases in the mediastinum after a review of 20 years. The patients described were 10 men and 11 women between the ages of 13 and 62 years (median age: 31 years). The authors concluded that, based on the morphological features and immunophenotype present in these tumors, it is possible that this type of lymphoma represents the missing link between classic HL and PMBCL. Important to mention is that mediastinal gray zone lymphoma may also occur in children. Oschlies and associates [62], in a study of PMBCL, identified 4 out of 52 cases of PMBCL as mediastinal gray zone lymphoma in pediatric patients. Similar to the clinical presentation of PMBCL, mediastinal gray zone lymphoma also presents with an anterior mediastinal tumor. The most important issue is the management of these two tumoral conditions, and, to that extent, it appears that the most important issue is the separation of PMBCL and mediastinal gray zone lymphomas from other subtypes of diffuse large B-cell lymphomas,

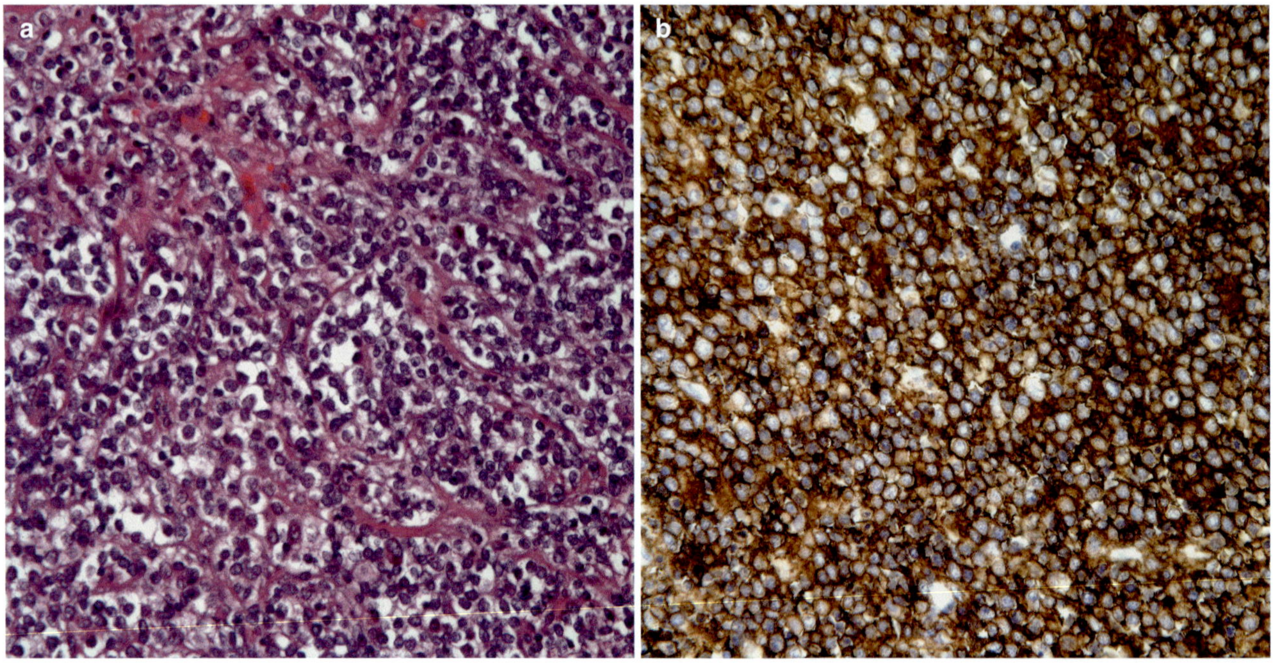

Fig. 13.25 (**a**) Higher magnification of thymic B-cell lymphoma with sclerosis; (**b**) CD20 immunohistochemical stain shows positive staining in tumor cells

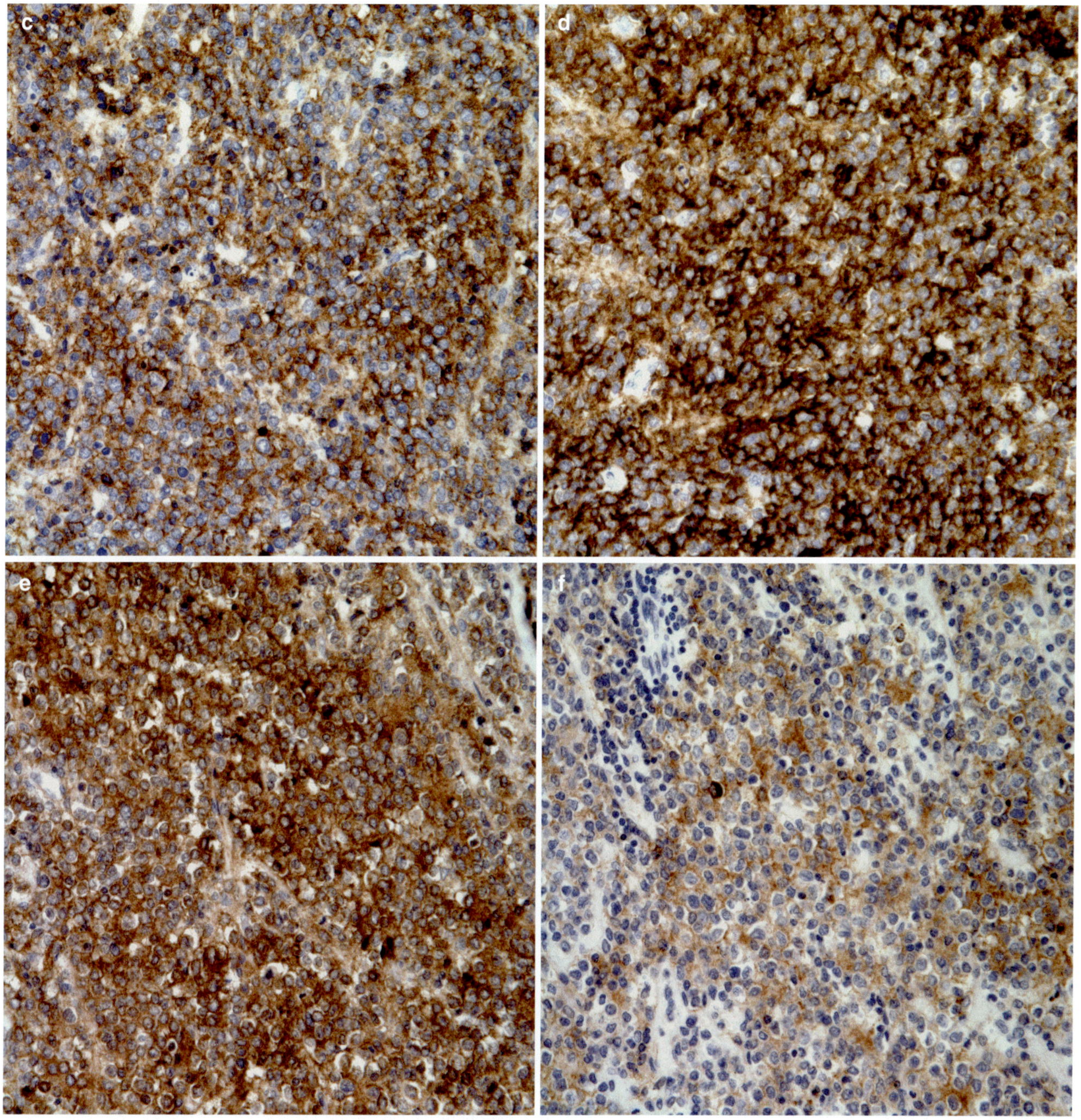

Fig. 13.25 (continued) (**c**) CD45 positive staining in tumor cells. (**d**) CD23 positive staining in tumor cells; (**e**) focal CD30 positive staining in tumor cells; note the staining in cytoplasm and membrane. (**f**) Focal weak positive staining in tumor cells for CD10

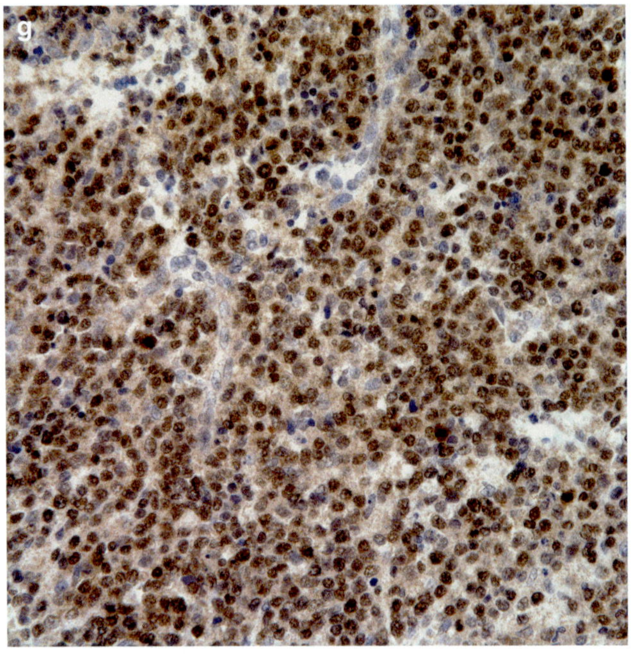

Fig. 13.25 (continued) (**g**) PAX5 positive staining in tumor cells

which may need a different approach [63]. In general terms, when mediastinal gray zone lymphoma (MGZL) is compared to PMBCL, it appears that MGZL is more common in the same age group with a median age of 35 years and has similar staging, but MGZL seems to be more common in men than women.

Pathological Features

The low power view of this tumor may show features either more in keeping with PMBCL or of classic HL. In the cases that appear to have the growth pattern of PMBCL, they are characterized by the presence of sheets of monomorphic large neoplastic cells with minimal inflammatory background (Fig. 13.26a–c). However, focal areas containing inflammatory cells including eosinophils can be seen in some cases. Areas of sclerosis may be present with areas of nodules containing cells resembling the lacunar cells of Reed-Sternberg. On the other hand, the tumor may show features more suggestive of NS-HL in which the tumor shows an inflammatory background including eosinophils and neutrophils.

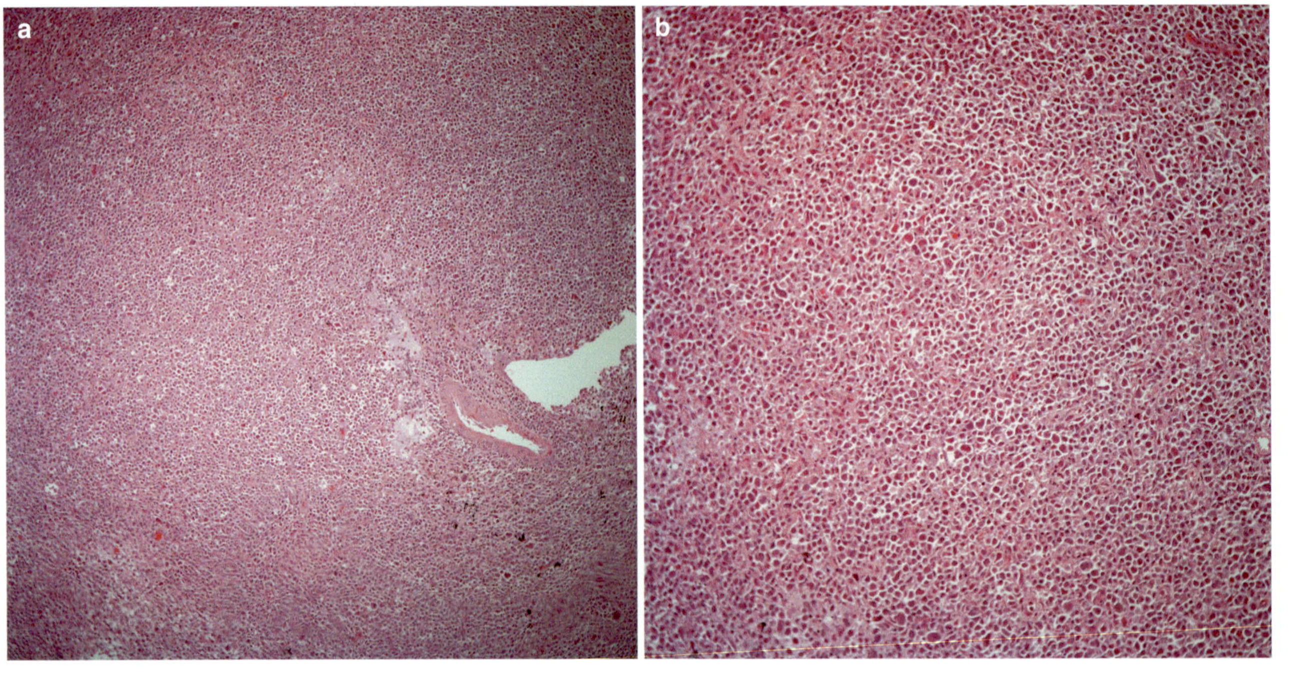

Fig. 13.26 (**a**) Low power view of a mediastinal gray zone lymphoma, which at low power appears to have the pattern of a B-cell lineage; (**b**) intermediate view showing a population of larger cells

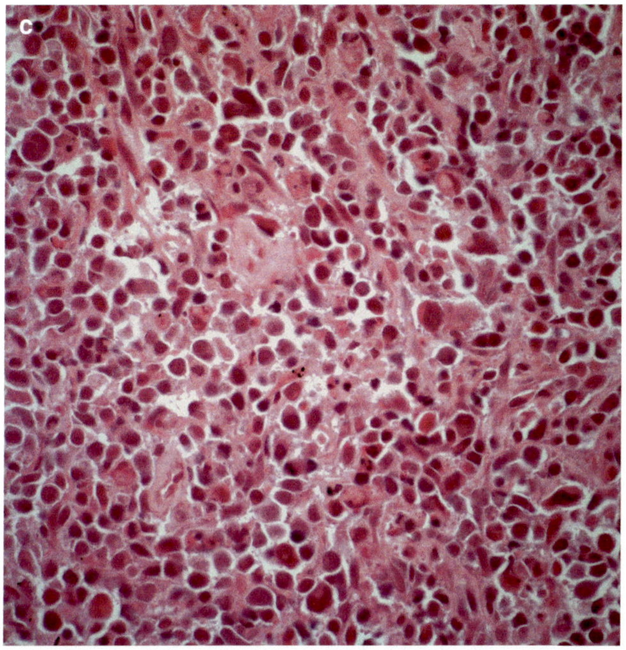

Fig. 13.26 (continued) (**c**) Reed-Sternberg-like cells

Immunohistochemical Features

In the cases described by Traverse and associates [61], the growth pattern in which the tumor shows features more in keeping with a PMBCL, the large cells present stained positively for Cd15 and CD30, while CD20 showed variable staining pattern, and, in a few cases, it was negative. On the contrary, in the growth pattern that resembles NS-HL, CD20 showed strong positive reaction, while CD30 and CD15 were positive in most of the cases but not all. In addition, PAX5, BOB.1, and Oct-2 were variable, but only one case resembling PMBCL was negative for both BOB.1 and Oct-2. The transcription factor PU.1 expression was expressed in seven of nine cases tested. MAL staining was performed in 13 cases showing nine cases positive. Other authors have expressed the value of CD23 expression as an additional marker in separating PMBCL from HL [64], while still others consider that such separation is best accomplished by using BOB.1, CD79a, and cyclin E [65]. However, both tumors – PMBCL and mediastinal gray zone lymphoma – may share positive staining for the following studies: CD45, CD30, CD15, CD20, CD79a, PAX5, BOB.1, OCT-2, and MAL expression. Immunoglobulin is commonly negative in both tumors, while CD23 seems to be the only marker that may show positive staining for PMBCL and negative in mediastinal gray zone lymphoma. It appears that CD23, while showing positive staining in PMBCL, will show negative staining in diffuse large B-cell lymphoma, classic HL, and mediastinal gray zone lymphoma.

Anaplastic Large Cell Lymphoma (ALCL)

This tumor is of unusual occurrence in the mediastinal region. It is possible that when it occurs, it may involve mediastinal lymph nodes rather than the thymus gland. A few well-documented cases have been reported in the literature [66, 67].

The clinical presentation of patients with ALCL is not different from those of other lymphomas in terms of revealing the presence of an anterior mediastinal mass. However, because this lymphoma shares some morphological and immunohistochemical features with other lymphomas including HL and PMBCL, it is important to properly assess the staining pattern of this tumor.

Histologically, the tumor is composed of large epithelioid cells with ample eosinophilic cytoplasm. However, the nuclei of the cells may show different shapes and forms including horseshoe-shaped, multinucleated, or large irregular nuclei with prominent nucleoli and vesicular chromatin (Fig. 13.27a–d). Contrary to NSHL, ALCL rarely shows an inflammatory background and extensive areas of fibrous bands separating the tumor in nodules.

Immunohistochemical stains play an important role in the diagnosis of ALCL. Common immunophenotype is that of CD30 positive and CD15 negative. In addition, the tumor may show positive staining in tumor cells for epithelial membrane antigen (EMA) and also for ALK-1. Regarding this latter stain, it is also known that not all ALCL are positive for ALK; however, positive staining for ALK in a difficult case in which HL is a consideration essentially rules out HL. In the case described by Gonin and associates [67], the tumor also showed positive staining for CD30, ALK-1, EMA, CD7, TiA1, granzyme B, and CD20, while negative for CD2, CD3, CD5, CD4, CD8, and CD79a.

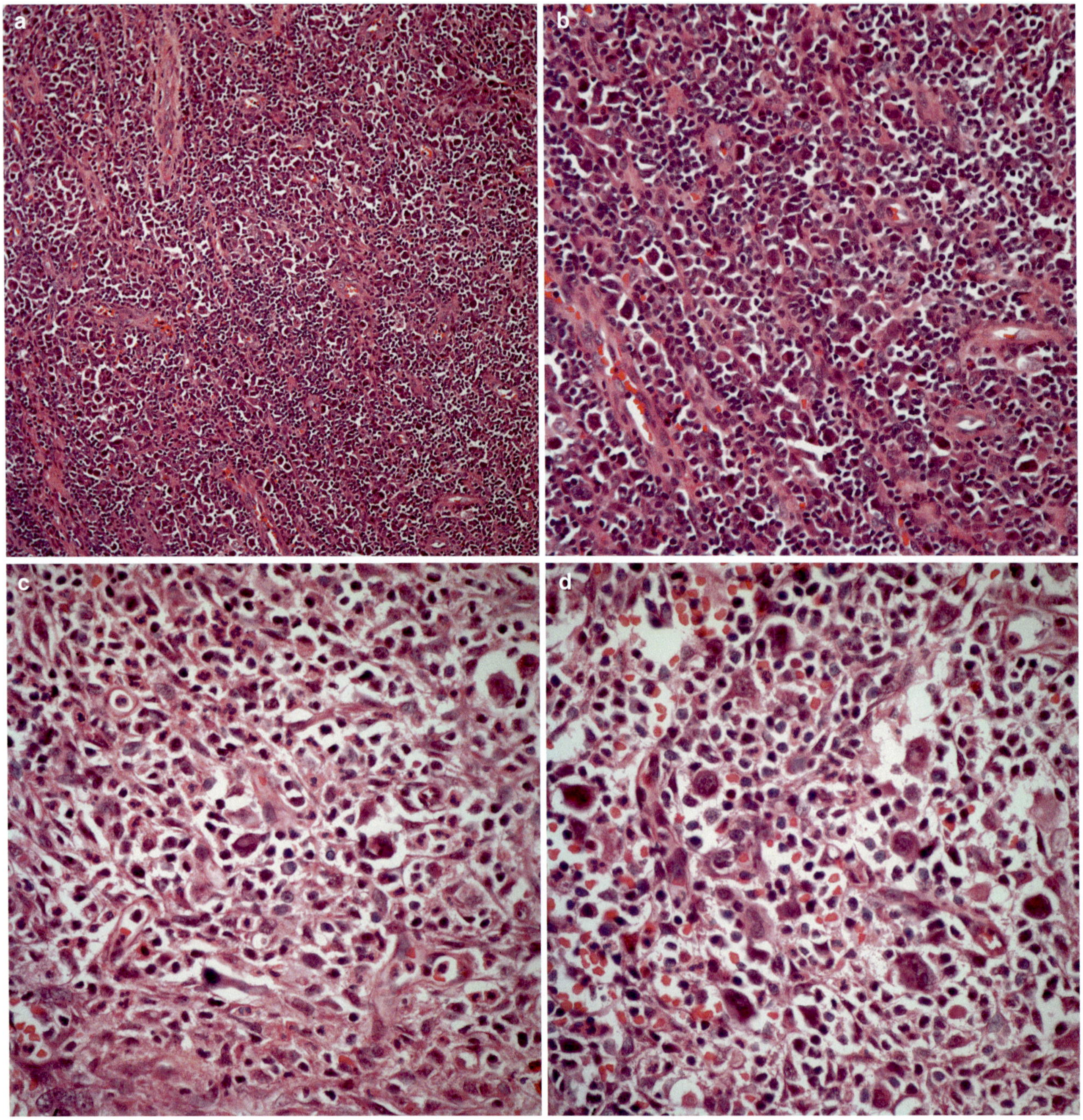

Fig. 13.27 (**a**) Low power view of a ALCL lymphoma showing larger cells; (**b**) numerous mono- and multinucleated large cells; (**c**) some large cells with a horseshoe-like appearance; (**d**) large cells with irregular nuclei and prominent nucleoli

Mucosa-Associated Lymphoid Tissue (MALT)-Lymphoma

Contrary to the occurrence of diffuse large B-cell lymphomas or Hodgkin's lymphoma, the occurrence of MALT-type lymphomas in the thymus is rare. Most of the existing literature is either in the form of single case reports of small series of cases [68–89]. In some small series of cases, the authors have assembled previously reported cases and added one or two of their own. Credit for the first description of this type of lymphoma is given to Isaacson and associates [68] who, in 1990, reported two cases of this type of lymphoma as an analogous tumor previously described in the gastrointestinal tract. Interestingly, in the two cases described by Isaacson [68], neither of the patients had a history of an autoimmune process or Sjogren's syndrome. One patient was a 50-year-old Caucasian man with a long history of petit mal, while the other patient was a 55-year-old Chinese woman hospitalized for cellulitis of the foot and who was otherwise asymptomatic. Both of these patients showed an anterior mediastinal mass, and, in both patients, surgical resection of the mass was performed. Also interesting is that none of the tumors was described as cystic. Following Isaacson description of this lymphoma, several other reports have been presented as single case reports in which the tumor has been described in association to clinical conditions, predominantly Sjogren's syndrome, rheumatoid arthritis, or other connective tissue disorders. One small series of such cases, presented by Lorsback and colleagues [90], described three patients with long-standing history of autoimmune disease. The patients were two women 54 and 36 years of age and a man aged 68 years. Imaging showed an anterior mediastinal mass in these patients, and their tumors were surgically resected. Also, important to note is that there is no mention in the description of whether the tumors were cystic or solid. More recently, we had the opportunity to study and report six patients with MALT type of lymphoma of the thymus [91]; the patients were six women between the ages of 48 and 59 years. Five of the women were Caucasian with one woman being of Asian background. Two of these patients had a history of Sjogren's syndrome, and one patient was being investigated for the possibility of an autoimmune process. However, three of the women did not have any history of an autoimmune process, and, in two of them, the anterior mediastinal mass was an incidental finding, while one patient presented with symptoms of chest pain and shortness of breath. All the patients were surgically treated with resection of the anterior mediastinal mass, and the resected mass was described as cystic or partially cystic in all the cases. Therefore, based on the available literature, MALT type of lymphoma is more commonly reported in middle-aged women with Asian background with a history of an autoimmune process or Sjogren's syndrome. Nevertheless, such clinical background may account for approximately 50% of the cases, thus leaving another 50% of the cases in which such a scenario is not present. It is important to highlight that MALT-type lymphoma has been described in men without a history of autoimmune disease, which may account for approximately 15–20% of all MALT-type of lymphomas of the thymus. Since an unequivocal diagnosis of this type of lymphoma has proven to be difficult in small biopsies of the mediastinum, it is commonly seen that the final diagnosis is done after complete surgical resection of the mediastinal mass. Also, important to highlight is the fact that, even though in many cases the tumor is confined to the mediastinum, in some cases, mediastinal lymph nodes may also be involved, while in other patients MALT lymphoma may also be present in other organs systems. The clinical follow-up in these patients is that of a low-grade malignancy, and, if the tumor is circumscribed to the thymus, complete surgical resection appears to be an adequate treatment. However, the tumor may involve lymph nodes and other organ systems, which, if associated with other autoimmune process, may alter the clinical outcome in these patients.

Pathological Features

Macroscopically, these tumors have been described as either solid or cystic tumors or a combination of both. The tumor sizes may vary from 2 to more than 5 cm in greatest dimension. The weight of these tumors, when that information is available, also varies from 30 to 50 grams.

Histologically, the low power view of these tumors is that of a solid or cystic tumor. In the cystic tumors, the low power is that of multiple cystic structures separated by extensive areas of lymphoid tissue (Fig. 13.28a, b). In some of these cystic structures, one can identify the presence of edematous fluid "colloid-like" filling the cystic structures (Fig. 13.29). The cysts are commonly lined by squamous or cuboidal epithelium without pseudoepitheliomatous hyperplasia. Within the lymphoid component, one can observe the presence of germinal centers and strands of thymic epithelium and the presence of cholesterol cleft granulomas. Hassall's corpuscles and calcifications may also be present within the lymphoid component (Fig. 13.30a–d). At higher magnification, an atypical lymphoid proliferation extends into the adipose tissue; however, the normal lobulation of the adipose tissue is preserved (Fig. 13.31a–d). The atypical lymphoid proliferation is composed of small lymphocytes with round nuclei and clear cytoplasm, characteristic of a monocytoid proliferation. In some cases, areas of plasmacytoid differentiation may be seen. MALT lymphomas commonly lack necrosis and hemorrhage and increase mitotic activity.

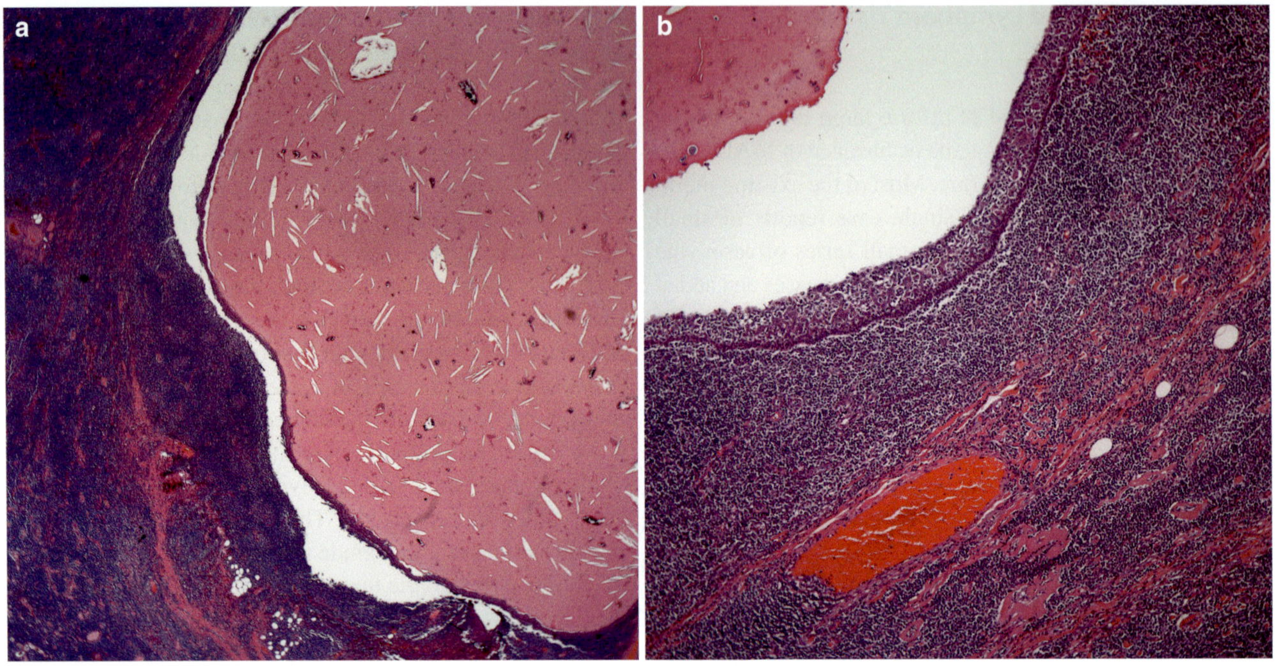

Fig. 13.28 (**a**) Low power view of a MALT lymphoma of the thymus showing a large cyst; (**b**) the cyst is lined by squamous epithelium and in the wall the atypical lymphoid proliferation

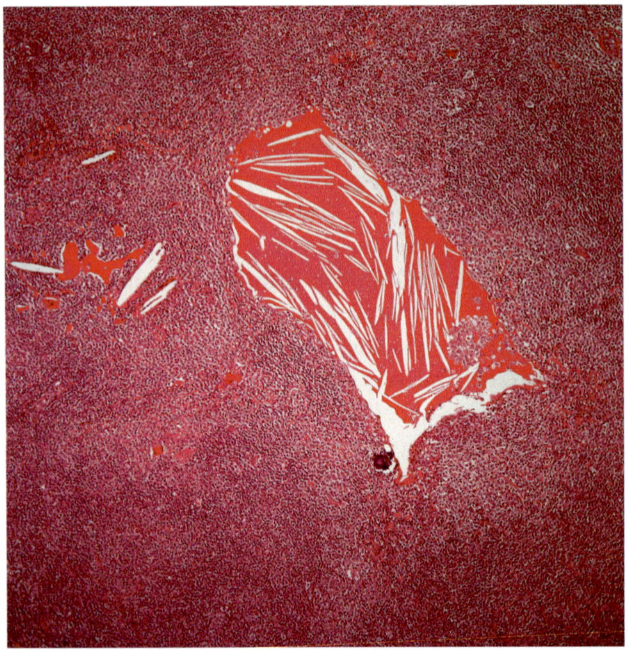

Fig. 13.29 Cystically dilated area filled with colloid-like material

Immunohistochemical studies are often used as an aid in the diagnosis. The tumor shows positive staining for CD20 (Fig. 13.32) and CD4, while keratin stains will highlight the epithelial component of the tumor. On the other hand, CD5 and CD10 are often negative, while in some cases kappa monocytic expression may be seen. In addition, most cases also express IgA phenotype.

Lymphoblastic Lymphoma

Credit for the first description of lymphoblastic lymphoma is given to Sternberg [92], who in 1916 described the first case of this entity. Later on, Cooke [93] identified the occurrence of this tumor as a mediastinal mass in children, and subsequently Smith and colleagues [94] determined that thymic lymphocytes were the origin of this tumor. However, the name of lymphoblastic lymphoma was coined by Barcos and Lukes [95] in 1975 by comparing this tumor to acute lymphoblastic leukemia (ALL), and a year later, Nathwani and colleagues [96] introduced the term diffuse lymphoblastic lymphoma. The common use of monoclonal antibodies in the evaluation of neoplasia in general and specifically in lymphoproliferative lesions has improved our understanding about these tumors and has helped to define certain tumoral conditions, which in turn has helped to improve treatment options [97]. Although there is abundant overlap between ALL and lymphoblastic lymphoma, it is considered that, if a patient presents with a bulky anterior mediastinal tumor with absent or minimal peripheral blood or bone marrow involvement, the word lymphoma is used in cases in which there is less than 25% bone marrow blasts. Although these two entities are considered under the umbrella of T-cell or B-cell lymphoblastic leukemia/lymphoma, some studies have identified possible molecular differences between T-lymphoblastic lymphoma and T-acute lymphoblastic leukemia. Gene expression profiling has shown overexpression of MML1 in T-lymphoblastic lymphoma and CD47 in T-acute lymphoblastic leukemia, while the

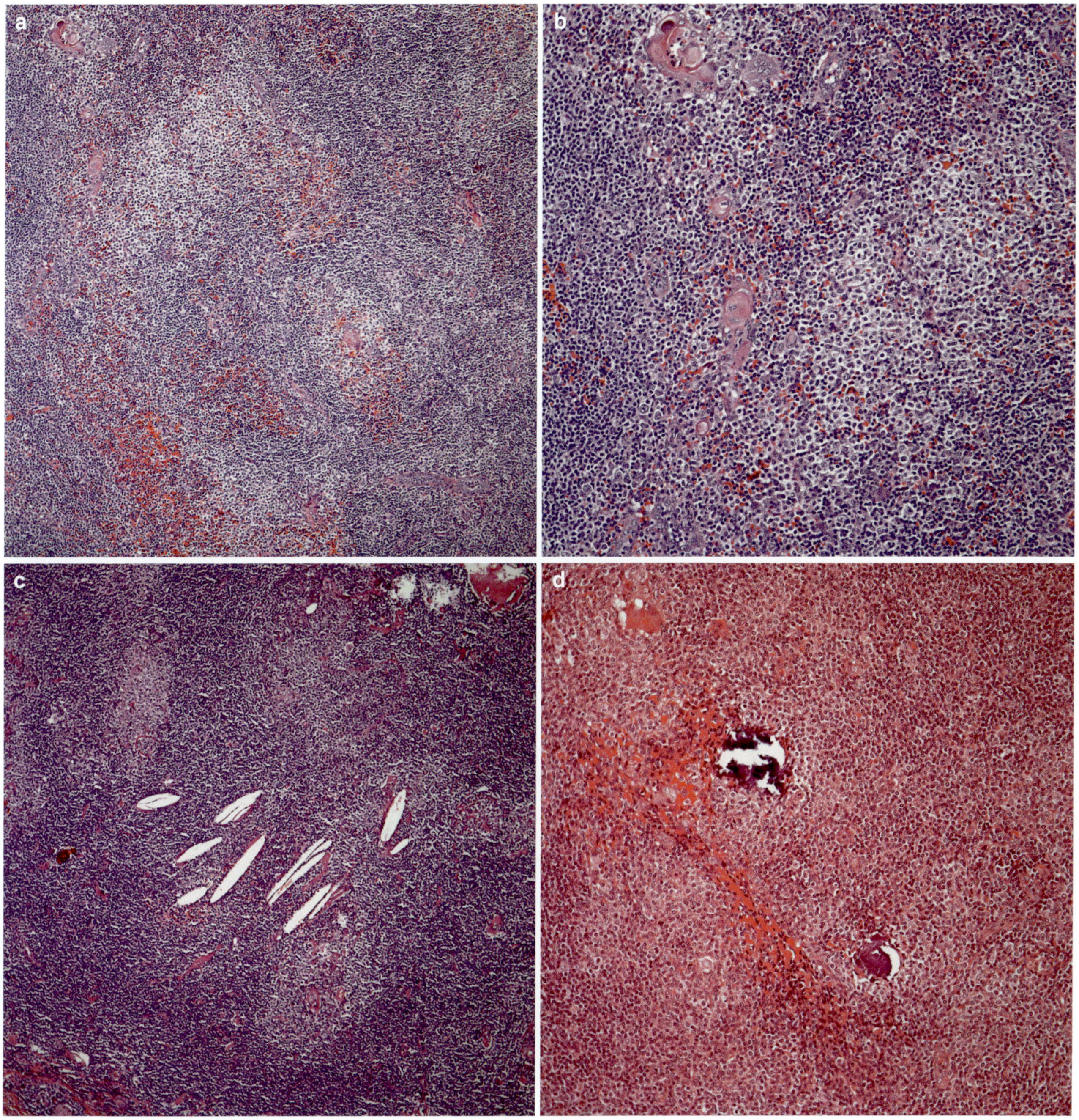

Fig. 13.30 (**a**) MALT lymphoma showing a few Hassall corpuscles; (**b**) Hassall corpuscles admixed with a monocytoid cellular proliferation; (**c**) presence of cholesterol clefts; (**d**) focal areas of calcifications

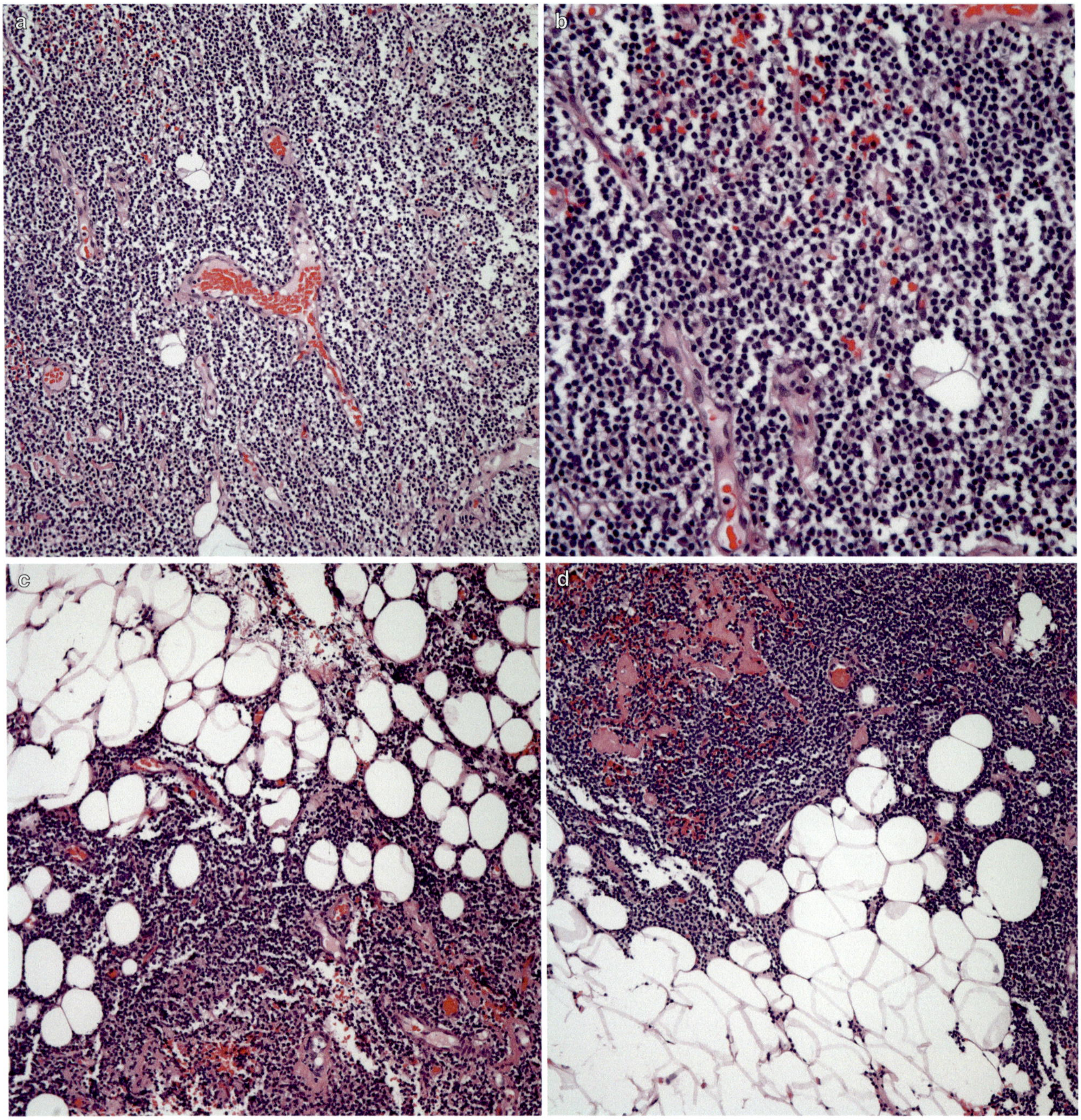

Fig. 13.31 (**a**) Monocytoid cellular proliferation with numerous ectatic blood vessels; (**b**) higher magnification of the monocytoid cellular proliferation composed of cells with clear cytoplasm and small round nuclei; (**c**) tumor infiltrates adipose tissue; (**d**) infiltration of the adipose tissue but with preservation of the adipose tissue

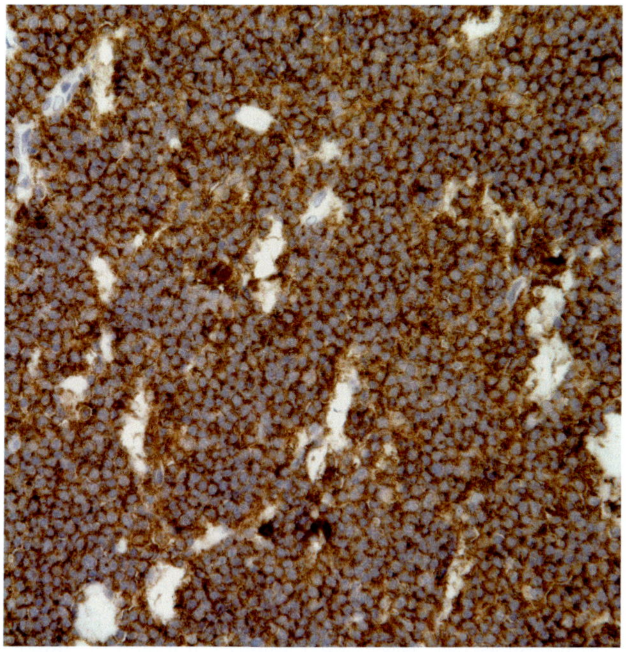

Fig. 13.32 Immunohistochemical stain for CD20 showing strong positive staining in tumor cells

immunophenotypes of both of these conditions is very much the same [98].

The tumor appears to be more common in children, with an estimated occurrence of 40% of all non-Hodgkin's lymphomas, while it represents approximately 3–4% in the adult population. Interestingly, peaks in the distribution of this tumor have been noted: one in the second decade of life with male predominance and another peak in patients older than 40 years. Even though B-cell lymphoblastic lymphoma accounts for approximately 10% of all lymphoblastic lymphomas, in a study of lymphoma survival patterns between the years 1975 and 2003, Han and colleagues [99] encountered that B-cell lymphoblastic lymphoma is more common in males than females, three times more often in Caucasians than blacks, with the highest incidence in Hispanics. T-lymphoblastic lymphoma accounts for approximately 85–90% of all lymphoblastic lymphomas. Despite the fact that chromosomal abnormalities have been described in lymphoblastic lymphoma, no specific oncogene has been specifically associated with the tumor. In addition, there is limited information regarding the cytogenetics of this tumor, and one of the most commonly reported abnormalities include the presence of an additional chromosome 21, a rare occurrence in acute lymphoblastic leukemia. In B-cell lymphoblastic lymphoma, the karyotype may be normal, hyperdiploidy, or show structural abnormalities without abnormal chromosome 21, while in T-cell lymphoblastic lymphoma, up to 70% of the cytogenetic abnormalities include the 14q11–13 region and chromosomes 9, 10, and 11. The karyotype in these tumors may show pseudodiploidy, hyperdiploidy, chromosomal deletions, and translocations in the 9q34 region [100, 101].

Portell and Sweetenham [102] addressed the topic of lymphoblastic lymphoma in the adult and estimated an incidence of 1–2% of all non-Hodgkin's lymphomas; they stated, even though lymphoblastic lymphoma is chemotherapy-sensitive with high initial response, relapses are common with conventional lymphoma regimens. The authors stated that the overall goal in the relapse setting is to consolidate with either an autologous or allogeneic bone marrow transplant. On the subject of lymphoblastic lymphoma of the adult, Gouill and colleagues [103] evaluated 92 patients retrospectively who were under 61 years of age. There was male predominance with 66% of the cases, median age of 31 years, bone marrow involvement in 22% of the patients, mediastinal involvement in 66% of the patients, and elevated LDH in 62% of the patients. Complete remission was observed in 71% of the patients at the end of the treatment, while 43% of the patients relapsed at a median time of 10 months. The 5-year overall survival was that of 32%, while the event-free survival was of 22%, after a median follow-up of 34 months. The authors concluded that the only favorable significant factor was young age. In a more recent review, Cortelazzo and colleagues [104] estimated 8% for lymphoblastic lymphoma among all lymphoid malignancies with a survival in the adult population of 86% and 90% for children (under 14 years) at 5 years. The authors also included as a risk factors ionizing radiation during childhood or young adulthood, HTLV-1, infants born with trisomy 21, and possibly benzene exposure. In a different study by Mlika and colleagues [105] on prognostic factors of lymphoblastic lymphomas of the mediastinum, the authors retrospectively studied 31 cases between the years 2000 and 2015. The multivariate analysis performed in this subset of patients encountered that gender was a relevant prognostic factor. Interestingly, age and stage were not statistically significant in this particular study. In addition, the authors estimated a global survival of 24 months.

Clinical Features

Patients commonly present with symptoms of cough, shortness of breath, and chest pain due to the large anterior mediastinal mass, which can reach sizes of over 10 cm in greatest diameter. Facial swelling and vascular obstruction leading to superior vena cava syndrome may also been seen [106]. Pericardial effusion, tracheal obstruction, and cardiac tamponade may also occur in some patients. In the six young adult patients (20–38 years of age) described by Schwartz and colleagues [107], three patients presented with cardiac tamponade and one patient with superior vena cava syndrome. In the majority of patients, involvement of the liver, spleen, and/or bone marrow is present at the time of diagnosis. Macon and colleagues [108] reported a case of lymphoblastic leukemia/lymphoma in a 64-year-old woman who presented with acute pulmonary edema secondary to heart failure and who had received radiation therapy for thymoma. The thymoma recurred, and, with this recurrence, the patient also had evidence of lymphoblastic leukemia/lymphoma involving mediastinal lymph nodes. Liu and colleagues [109] reported an interesting association of lymphoblastic lymphoma and myasthenia gravis in a 60-year-old man who developed an anterior mediastinal tumor. Also, Posner and colleagues [110] reported a 19-year-old young man who presented with dyspnea, chest pain, weight loss, and anterior mediastinal mass who, on evaluation, showed a T-cell lymphoblastic lymphoma. Twenty-five months after the initial diagnosis, the patient developed an acute nonlymphocytic leukemia.

Staging of the disease is important in order to assess prognosis; however, the system used for adults may be different than the one used for children. In adults, the Ann Arbor system is more commonly used, while for children the St Jude's Children's Research Hospital is more common. In this latter system, there is specific stage for all primary intrathoracic tumors (mediastinal, pleural, etc.) – Stage IIIB – while in the Ann Arbor, the occurrence of primary mediastinal mass may be staged as II (localized involvement of an extranodal site). However, it is important to highlight that the staging procedures for lymphoblastic lymphoma are similar to those of non-Hodgkin's lymphoma and generally include CT scans, evaluation of cerebrospinal fluid, bone marrow aspirate, and 18F-fluorodeoxyglucose positron emission tomography (18F-FDG-PET).

Despite the aggressive nature of this tumor, the prognosis has improved over the years, with a disease-free survival in children of approximately 70–90% and approximately 60–70% in adults. Even though localized disease in lymphoblastic lymphoma accounts for approximately 10% of the cases, it has been observed that late relapses occur with possible evolution to acute lymphoblastic leukemia [111, 112].

Pathological Features

The histological features of lymphoblastic lymphoma are similar to those seen in small round cell tumors. In some cases, the tumor may be seen infiltrating the thymus (Fig. 13.33a, b). Diffuse growth pattern composed of small to medium atypical lymphocytes with round to convoluted nuclei, fine chromatin, inconspicuous nucleoli, and scant cytoplasm. The tumor characteristically invades adipose tissue preserving the architecture of the fat cells (Fig. 13.34a–e). In some cases, the tumor may show a proliferation of small vessels (Fig. 13.35a, b). In unusual cases, lymphoblastic lymphoma may show extensive areas of fibrosis, which in some areas may mimic small cell carcinoma with areas of crush artifact (Fig. 13.36a–e). Mitotic activity is high, and the presence of macrophages gives the tumors the appearance of the so-called starry sky. Even though the distinction between lymphoblastic leukemia and lymphoma may be difficult, the presence of peripheral blood involvement or bone marrow involvement appears to be cut off discriminants for those two entities.

Approximately 80–90% of lymphoblastic lymphoma in the adult is of T-cell phenotype. However, cases of mediastinal lymphoblastic lymphoma with immature B-cell immunophenotype have also been described. Sander and coworkers [113] described a 19-year-old young man in whom the gene rearrangement analysis demonstrated that the neoplasm was B-cell lineage and the tumor cells expressed CD19, CD20, and CD22 while negative for T-cell markers and immunoglobulins. The authors interpreted their findings as an early stage of B-cell differentiation (pre-pre B-cell stage). Also, Manning and coworkers [114] reported a case of a 46-year-old man with a mediastinal mass, which the authors interpreted as mediastinal lymphoblastic lymphoma with non-lymphoblastic histological features in which the immunophenotype was that of thymocyte phenotype, but the DNA flow cytometric analysis showed a high S + G_2 M fraction of 29%.

In B-lymphoblastic lymphoma, the tumor cells are positive for CD19, CD79a, and CD22. In addition, they are also positive for CD10, CD24, PAX5, and TdT with variable expression of CD20 and CD34, while CD45 may be negative. In T-cell lymphoblastic lymphomas, the tumor cells are positive for TdT and may also express CD1a, CD2, CD3, CD4, CD5, CD7, CD8, CD10, CD99, and CD34 (Fig. 13.37a–d). Myeloid antigens such as CD13 and CD33 may be expressed in about 20–20% of the cases. There is no specific immunophenotype for T-cell lymphoblastic lymphoma, and it appears that the most common expressed antibodies may be CD2, CD5, and CD7.

Cytogenetic findings may prove to be difficult to distinguish lymphoblastic lymphoma from T-cell ALL as several karyotypic translocations are common to both entities, thus suggesting that these two tumoral conditions may represent different manifestations of the same disease. The most common chromosomal abnormalities in T-cell lymphoblastic lymphoma include 14q11–13. However, translocations such as t(9;17) (q34;q23) are limited to lymphoblastic lymphoma, and their presence is associated with poor prognosis. Unusual variants of lymphoblastic lymphoma include B-lineage lymphoblastic lymphoma, which expresses B-cell markers and TdT with absent surface immunoglobulin. Interestingly, B-cell lymphoblastic lymphoma rarely involves the mediastinum, and the tumor more commonly involves lymph nodes [115].

Most histopathological features, chromosomal and molecular abnormalities do not appear to correlate with prognosis. In adult individuals, tumor burden and advance stage may play a role in prognosis.

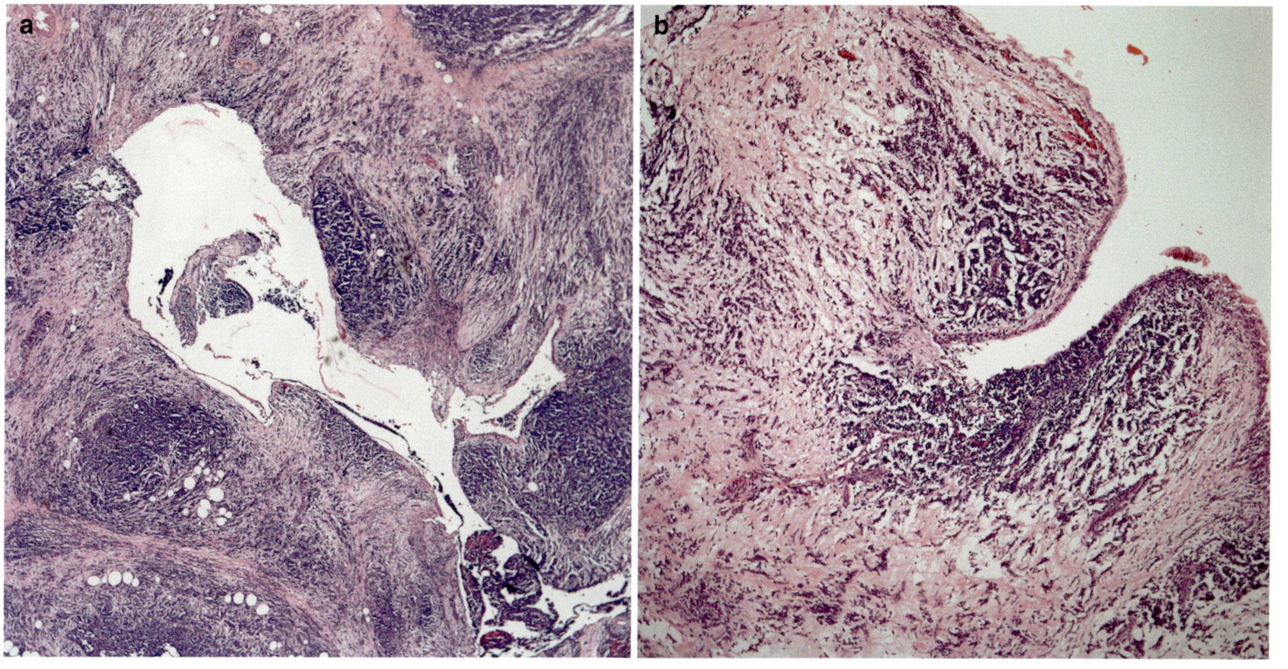

Fig. 13.33 (**a**) Lymphoblastic lymphoma involving thymus with cystic changes; (**b**) closer view of the thymic cystic structure lined by an attenuated cuboidal epithelium

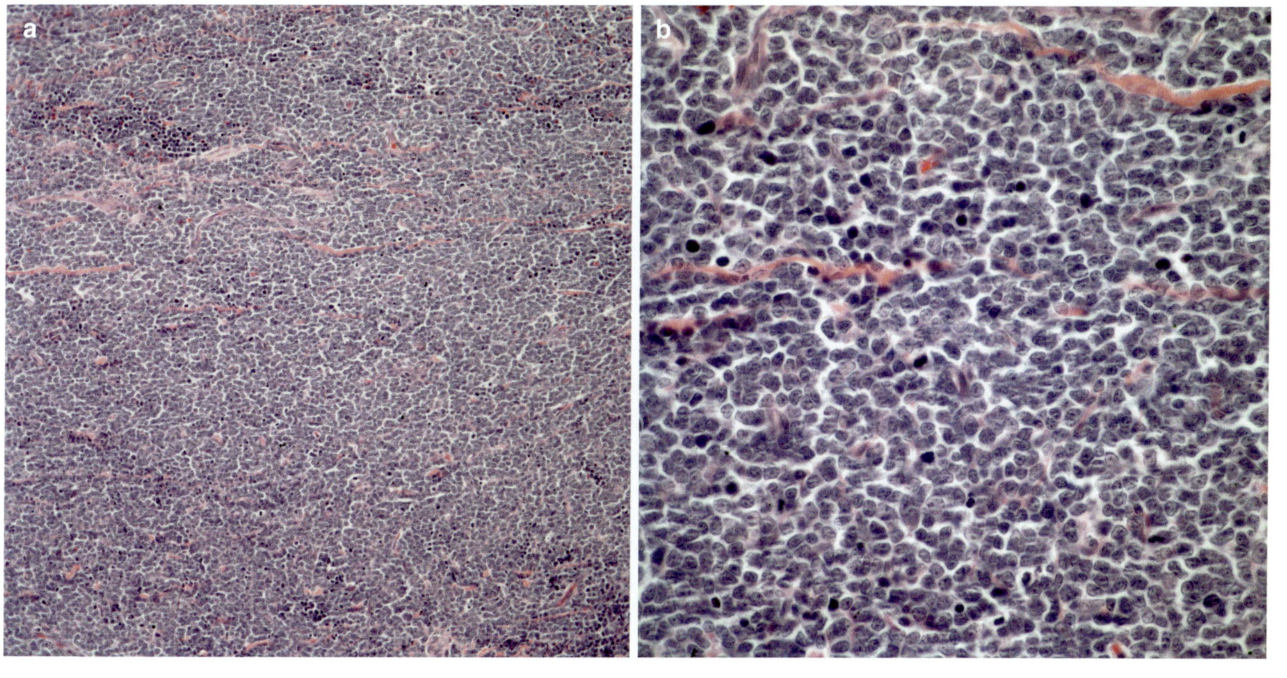

Fig. 13.34 (**a**) Lymphoblastic lymphoma showing sheets of neoplastic cells with little intervening stroma; (**b**) higher magnification showing round cells with irregular nuclei, inconspicuous nucleoli, and numerous mitotic figures

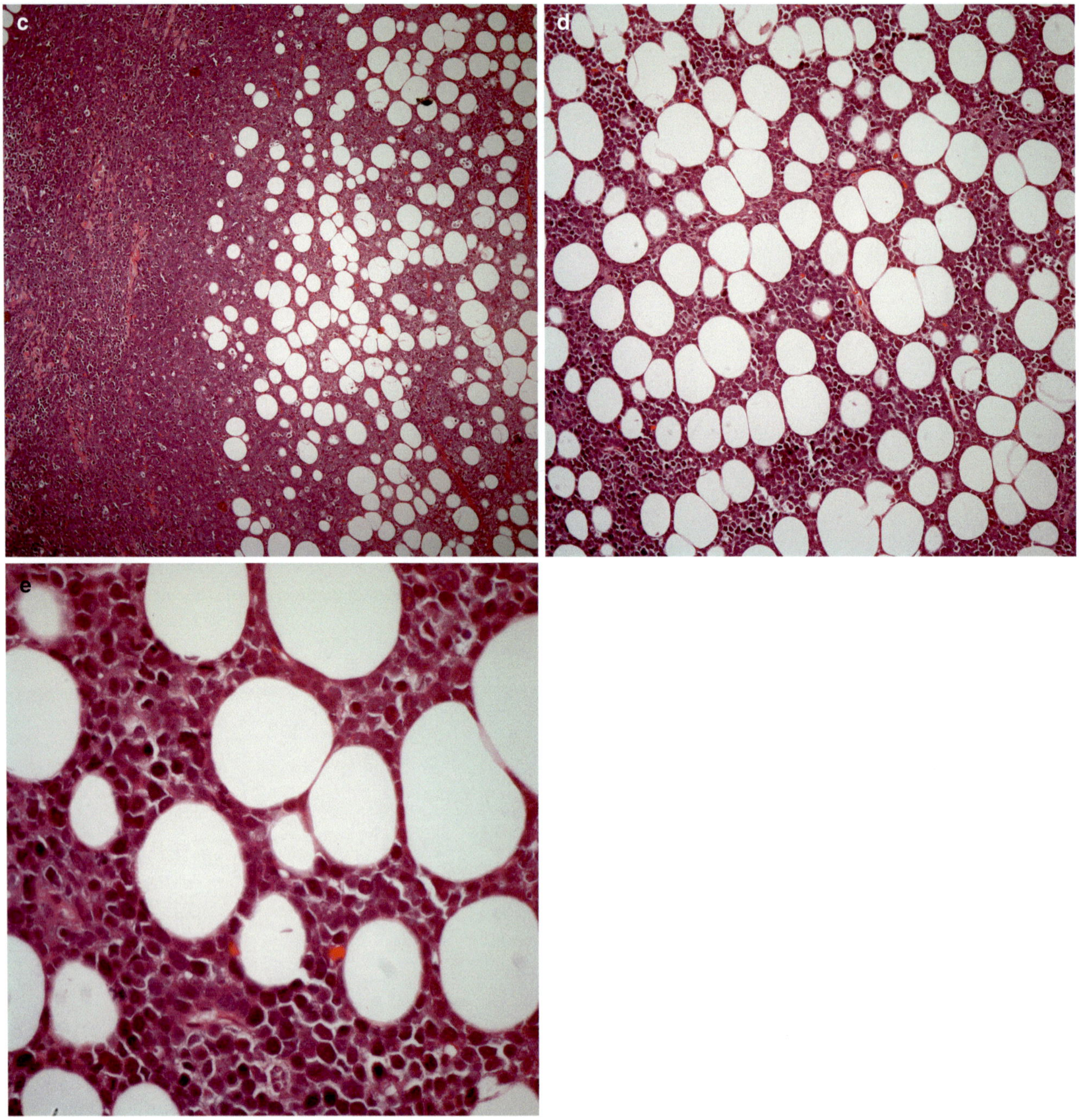

Fig. 13.34 (continued) (**c**) Lymphoblastic lymphoma invading adipose tissue. (**d**) Adipose tissue architecture is preserved. (**e**) Preserved adipose tissue infiltrated by lymphoblastic lymphoma

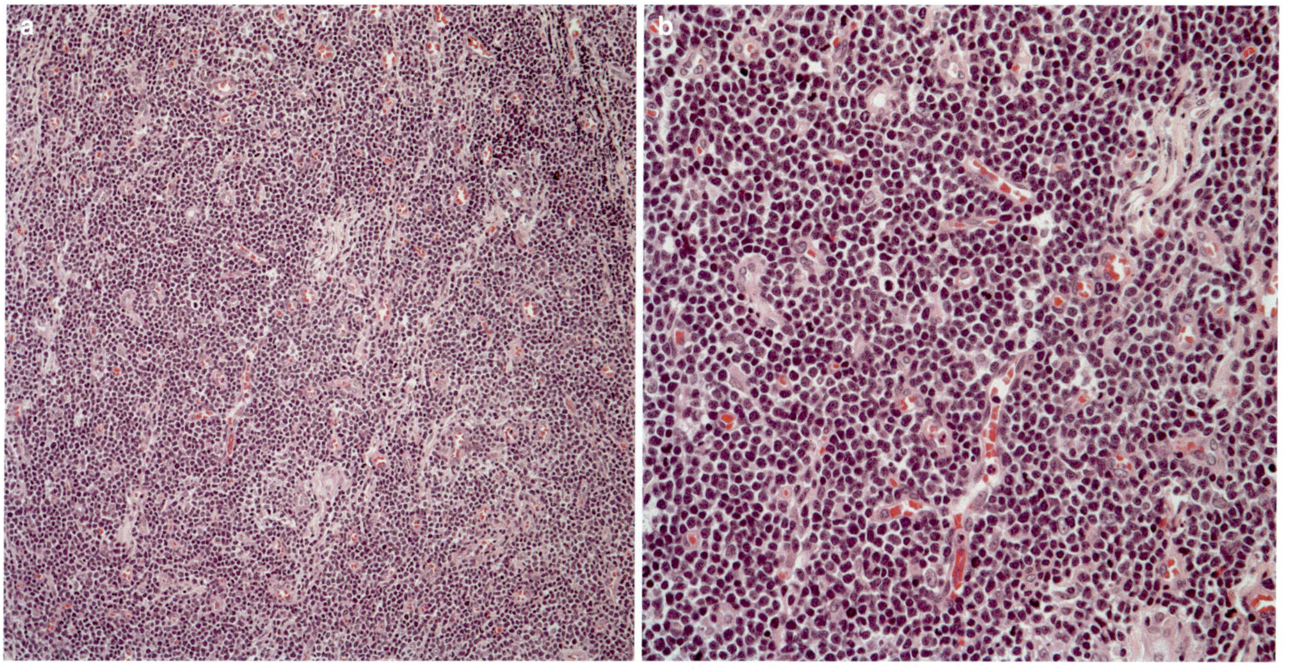

Fig. 13.35 (**a**) Lymphoblastic lymphoma showing a proliferation of numerous vessels; (**b**) higher magnification of the small vessels admixed with lymphoblastic lymphoma

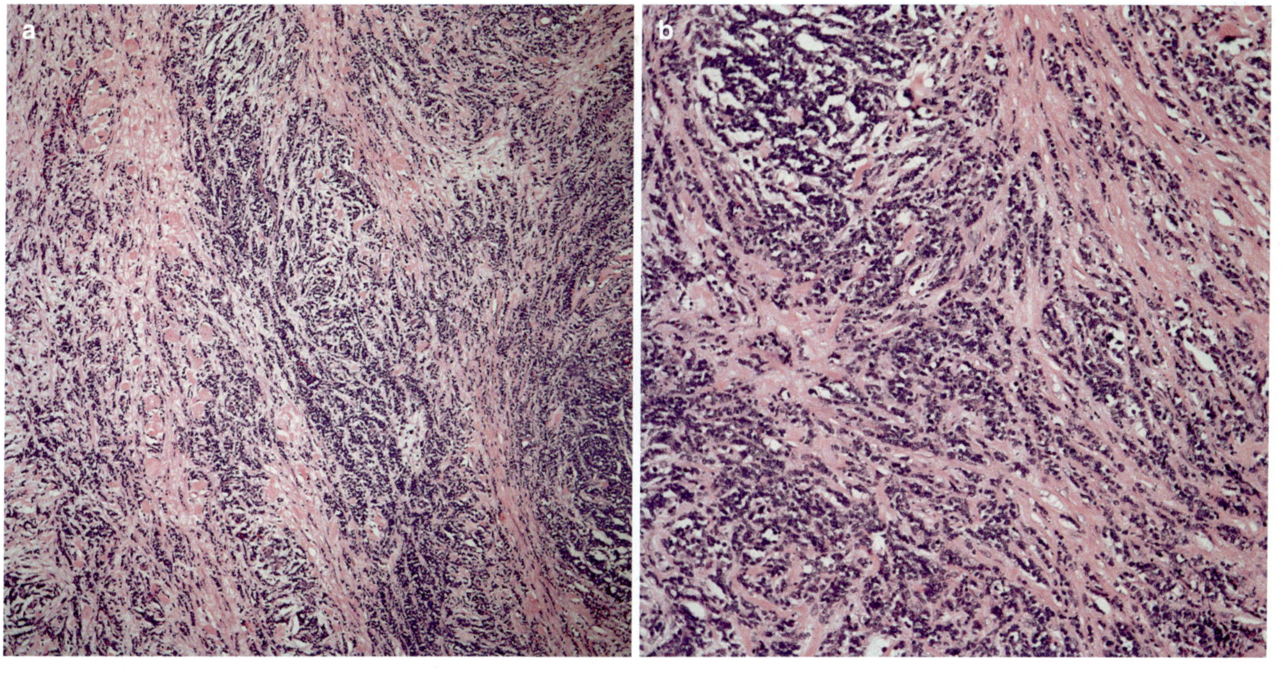

Fig. 13.36 (**a**) Lymphoblastic lymphoma with extensive areas of fibrosis; (**b**) lymphoma cells dissecting fibroconnective tissue

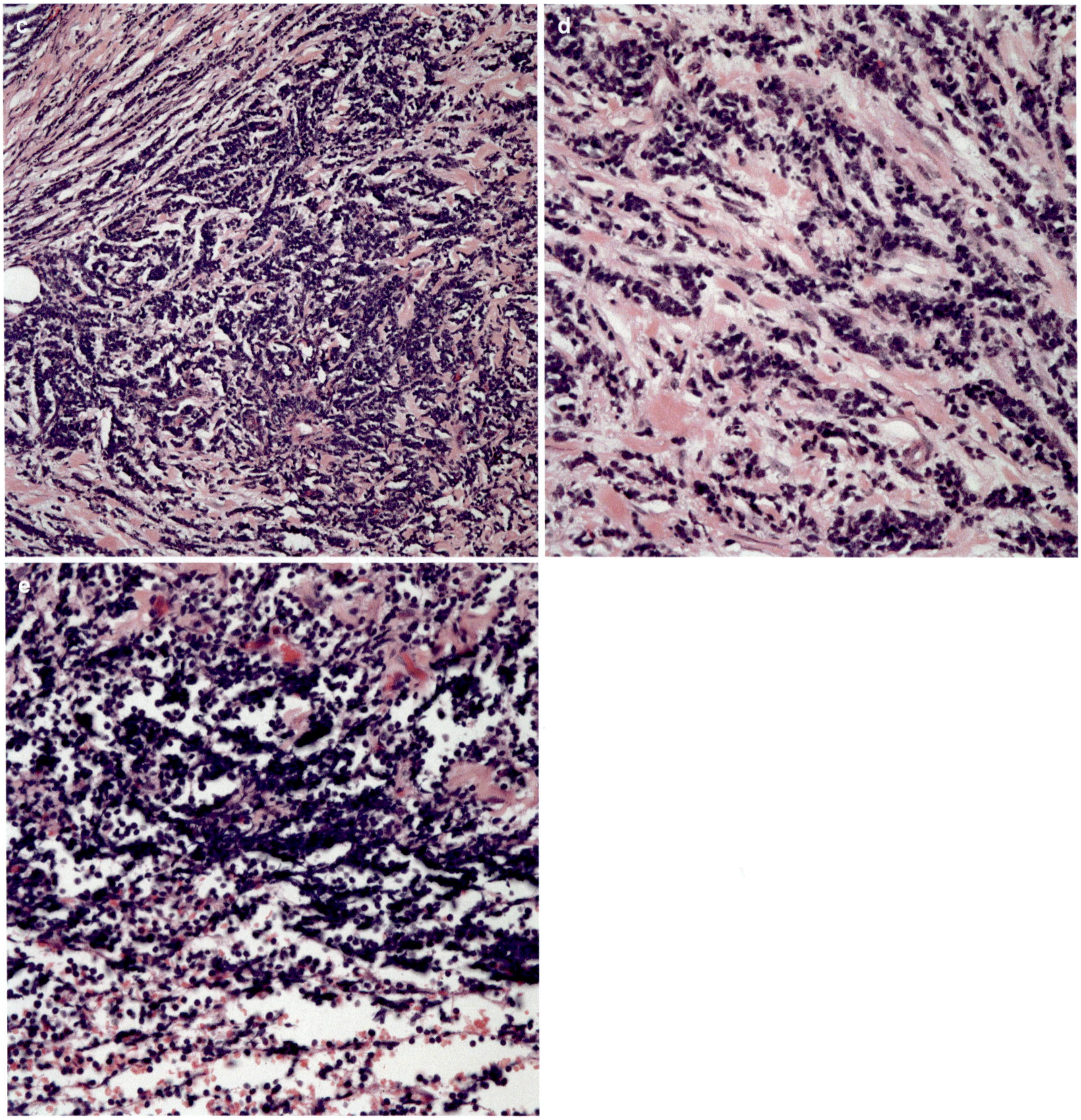

Fig. 13.36 (continued) (**c**) Haphazard distribution of the neoplastic cells infiltrating fibrous tissue; (**d**) lymphoblastic lymphoma mimicking small cell carcinoma; (**e**) lymphoblastic lymphoma with crush artifact

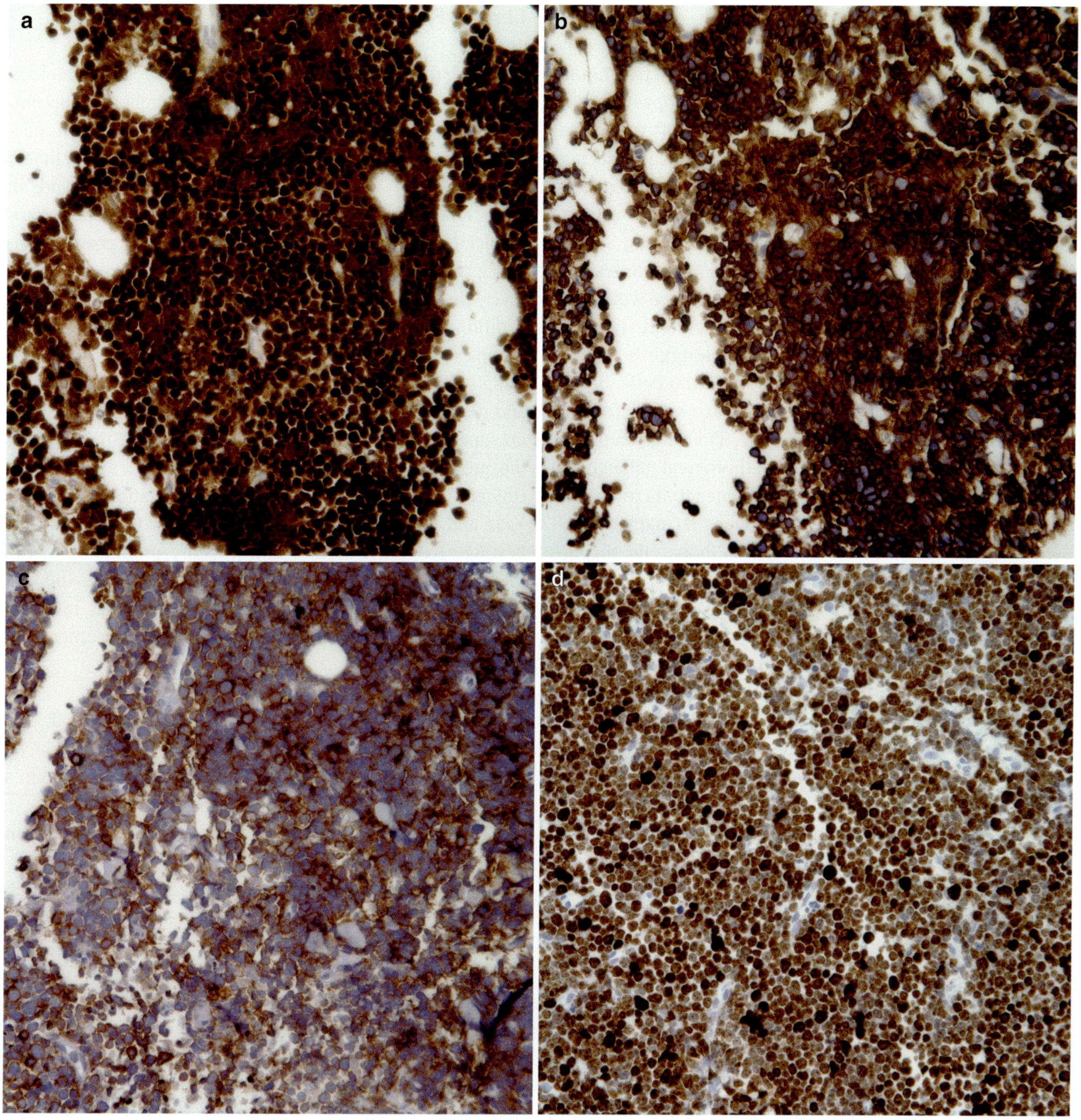

Fig. 13.37 (**a**) Positive staining for Tdt in lymphoblastic lymphoma; (**b**) CD3 positive staining in lymphoblastic lymphoma. (**c**) CD1a positive staining in lymphoblastic lymphoma; (**d**) Ki-67 labeling is high lymphoblastic lymphoma

Hodgkin's Lymphoma

Hodgkin's Lymphoma was originally described by Thomas Hodgkin in 1832 under "On Some Morbid Appearances of the Absorbent Glands and the Spleen" in an effort to separate this process from other more common diseases such as tuberculosis. Some of these original illustrations have been presented elsewhere [116]. However, Hodgkin's original observations were not appreciated until later when Samuel Wilks re-evaluated the material, provided more clinical and pathological description, and acknowledged the work done by Hodgkin [117]. Subsequently, Greenfield in 1878 described multinucleated giant cells in Hodgkin's disease, and, in 1898, Sternberg also identified similar cells, but his interpretation was that Hodgkin's disease was a form of tuberculosis [118]. However, in 1902, Dorothy Reed published a classic paper "On the pathological changes in Hodgkin's disease, with especial reference to its relation to tuberculosis" [119]. Thus, we have the name Reed-Sternberg cells. By the mid-1940s, even though the diagnosis of Hodgkin's disease appears to have some specific symptoms and signs to make the diagnosis on clinical grounds, it was advisable to obtain surgical material for histological evaluation in order to confirm the diagnosis [120]. Over the last five decades, the entity described as an inflammatory condition (thus the name Hodgkin's disease) has undergone significant changes not only in the diagnostic approach but also in its clinical course, immunohistochemical approach, molecular biology, treatment, and prognosis. In the mediastinum itself, terms such as granulomatous thymoma were abandoned for Hodgkin's disease and now by Hodgkin's lymphoma, which represents the most accurate interpretation for this process. More understanding of its biology and of the nuances in treatment options has changed the dynamics in how HL is approached. For instance, the use of radiation has been modified by chemotherapy, and the use of staging laparotomy has been modified by the use of clinical prognostic factors to determine who gets the benefit of whatever treatment option is available. In general terms, HL is less frequent than non-HL lymphomas in a proportion of 1:7, and it does not seem to have a special predilection for men or women [121]. However, a trend toward better survival over the last 10–20 years has been observed. Even though the cell of origin is not known, some factors that may be associated with HL include higher socioeconomic status and prior EBV infection (infectious mononucleosis) [122]. Nevertheless, in general, HL is rare in the thymus [123], but a type of lymphoma that needs separation from other non-Hodgkin's lymphomas as classic HL of the thymus has a good clinical outcome [8]. Large series of thymic classic Hodgkin's lymphoma are not numerous due to the rarity of this tumor in the thymus.

Clinical Features

Although there is emphasis on the different symptomatology of patients with HL, it is important to highlight that approximately 30–50% of patients with mediastinal classic HL may be asymptomatic. However, in general terms, the clinical presentation of Hodgkin's lymphoma is variable, and, in early reports in which clinical emphasis was more pronounced, patients will show lymphadenopathy, possible evidence of involvement of other organ systems (spleen, liver), fever, polymorphonuclear leukocytosis, and anemia [5]. In addition, it appears that patients were separated in three main groups: (1) localized lymphadenopathy, (2) generalized lymphadenopathy with or without involvement of the spleen, and (3) patients with constitutional symptoms with little or no superficial involvement of lymph nodes [120]. However, the presence of Hodgkin's lymphoma in the mediastinum (thymus) suffered from different interpretations. In 1969, Katz and Lattes [124] reported 24 cases with features suggesting Hodgkin's disease and possibly originating in the thymus. Interestingly, in this report, the authors did not include typical cases of Hodgkin's disease that involved mediastinal lymph nodes. The authors defined the criteria for inclusion as follows:

- Lesion apparently limited to the thymus gland. No demonstrable disease elsewhere.
- Low power may resemble nodular sclerosing Hodgkin's disease. Thymic epithelium present in nodular foci.
- "Reed-Sternberg" cells associated with or derived from thymic epithelium.
- Active participation of thymic epithelium with formation of squamoid sheets or cystic structures.

The follow-up provided by the authors in 17 patients showed that 10 were apparently free of disease 2–9 years after diagnosis, while 6 patients developed extrathoracic disease. The authors further stated that radiation therapy alone or with surgery, appeared to be a better treatment than surgery alone. The authors finally concluded that "granulomatous thymoma" is basically a "peculiar" manifestation of Hodgkin's disease, primarily involving the thymus. Also, in 1969, Fechner [125] reported three patients (two female patients between the ages of 21 and 31 years and one male patient age 18 years) who presented with mediastinal mass. At least in one of these cases, the mediastinal tumor appeared to show cystic changes. The author stated that the morphologic changes present were suggestive of nodular sclerosing Hodgkin's disease. In addition, the author stated that these tumors should be designated as "Hodgkin's disease of the thymus" and not granulomatous thymoma. In 1974, Keller and Castleman [126] reported 41 patients that the authors designated as Hodgkin's disease of the thymus gland.

However, in this report, the authors stated that half of the cases had involvement of the thymus and the other half had involvement of mediastinal lymph nodes. The patients with thymic involvement were younger and with male predominance. The 5-year survival was estimated at 79% with or without thymus involvement.

It is important to highlight that over the years, the histological type of Hodgkin's lymphoma has been associated with prognosis. In 1955, Smetana and Cohen correlated the histological classification of those years: paragranuloma, granuloma, and sarcoma with the mortality of those patients [127]. By 1966, Lukes and Butler [128], acknowledging the importance of histological types in relation to clinical stage and survival, subdivided Hodgkin's disease into lymphocytic and/or histiocytic (L&H) nodular, L&H diffuse, nodular sclerosis, mixed, diffuse fibrosis, and reticular. The authors noted that nodular sclerosis has remarkable high incidence in the mediastinum, exceeding all other types. In a study of 1659 patients with nodular sclerosing Hodgkin's disease, MacLennan and coworkers [129] reported that subdividing nodular sclerosing Hodgkin's disease may prove beneficial, as those with extensive areas of lymphocytic depletion or with numerous anaplastic Hodgkin's cells (Grade II NS) have poor response to initial therapy, increase relapse, and decrease survival, compared to other variants of NS-Hodgkin's (Grade I NS). In that regard, Ferry and coworkers [130] reported a study of 79 patients diagnosed with NS-HD (55 females and 24 male patients between the ages of 10 and 57 years (mean, 27 years); 58 cases were classified as NS grade I and 21 as grade II. The 5-year survival rate for NS grade I was 100% and for NS grade II 75%. The presence of B symptoms (night sweats, weight loss, fever) was significantly associated with risk of relapse after initial therapy. The authors concluded that histological classification of NS-HD appears clinically relevant. However, contrary to that experience, Hess and coworkers [131] reported 254 surgically staged patients with NS-HD with a median follow-up of 123 months. Of this group of patients, 221 were classified as grade I and 43 as grade II, no differences in distribution by age, number of sites, B symptoms, or extent of mediastinal disease were observed. The 15-year overall survival rates were 87% and 93% for grade I and grade II, respectively (not statistically significant). When the same group was analyzed by pathologic stage or by initial treatment, no differences were observed. Therefore, the authors concluded that histologic subclassification of NS-HD had no prognostic significance.

Regarding diagnostic imaging for Hodgkin's lymphoma, Heron and coworkers [132] evaluated the CT scans of 50 patients with evidence of thoracic disease who were examined for primary staging, and the authors identified that the thymus was enlarged in 15 patients (30%). Also, Priola [133] reported a case using chemical-shift magnetic resonance imaging to separate primary mediastinal Hodgkin's lymphoma from rebound thymic hyperplasia. However, in general, HL commonly shows widening of the mediastinum. Other laboratory findings that have been found to be associated with HL include anemia (normochromic/normocytic), hemolytic anemia, neutrophilia, eosinophilia, and leukocytosis. In advanced cases of HL, serum level of lactate dehydrogenase may be elevated.

On the other hand, many of the treatment decisions regarding HL are based on the stage of the tumor. The Ann Arbor staging classification is commonly followed for those decisions. Thus, a common staging for thymic HL is stage I_E, II, or II_E; more often the lymphoma is limited to the thymus gland. Other features that may affect prognosis in patients with mediastinal HL include large mediastinal mass, B symptoms, or unexplained anemia. However, the use of prognostic factors (International Prognostic Score) which include clinical, staging, and laboratory findings mainly in advanced HL appears to correlate with prognosis.

Pathological Features

Mediastinal HL may occur as an enlargement of mediastinal lymph nodes or by the presence of a tumor mass in the thymus gland. When the tumor is in the thymus, the tumors may show a solid configuration with a well-defined tumor mass (Fig. 13.38a). The cut surface may show slight nodularity, and it is firm and light tan in color. Areas of hemorrhage and necrosis are not common. However, often the tumor will show prominent cystic changes, which may mimic some of the changes observed in multilocular thymic cyst. In such cases, it is prudent to sample the tumor appropriately so that the risk of missing the diagnostic component is avoided. The tumors vary in size from a few centimeters to more than 10 cm in greatest diameter.

Histologically, the most common subtype of HL in the thymus is nodular sclerosis (NSHL). If the mass is solid, the tumor may be well circumscribed, and areas of residual thymic tissue may be present adjacent to the main tumor mass (Fig. 13.38b, c). On the contrary, if the lesion is cystic, the tumor may show areas reminiscent of multilocular thymic cyst (Fig. 13.39a–d). The low power view of this tumor is that of a nodular growth pattern separated by different thickness of collagen bands. Higher magnification of these different nodules shows the presence of an inflammatory infiltrate composed of plasma cells, eosinophils, small mature lymphocytes, and macrophages. Closer view of this infiltrate often shows the presence of large either mononuclear or multinucleated cells with oval nuclei and prominent nucleoli (Reed-Sternberg cells) (Fig. 13.40a–d). Often when the

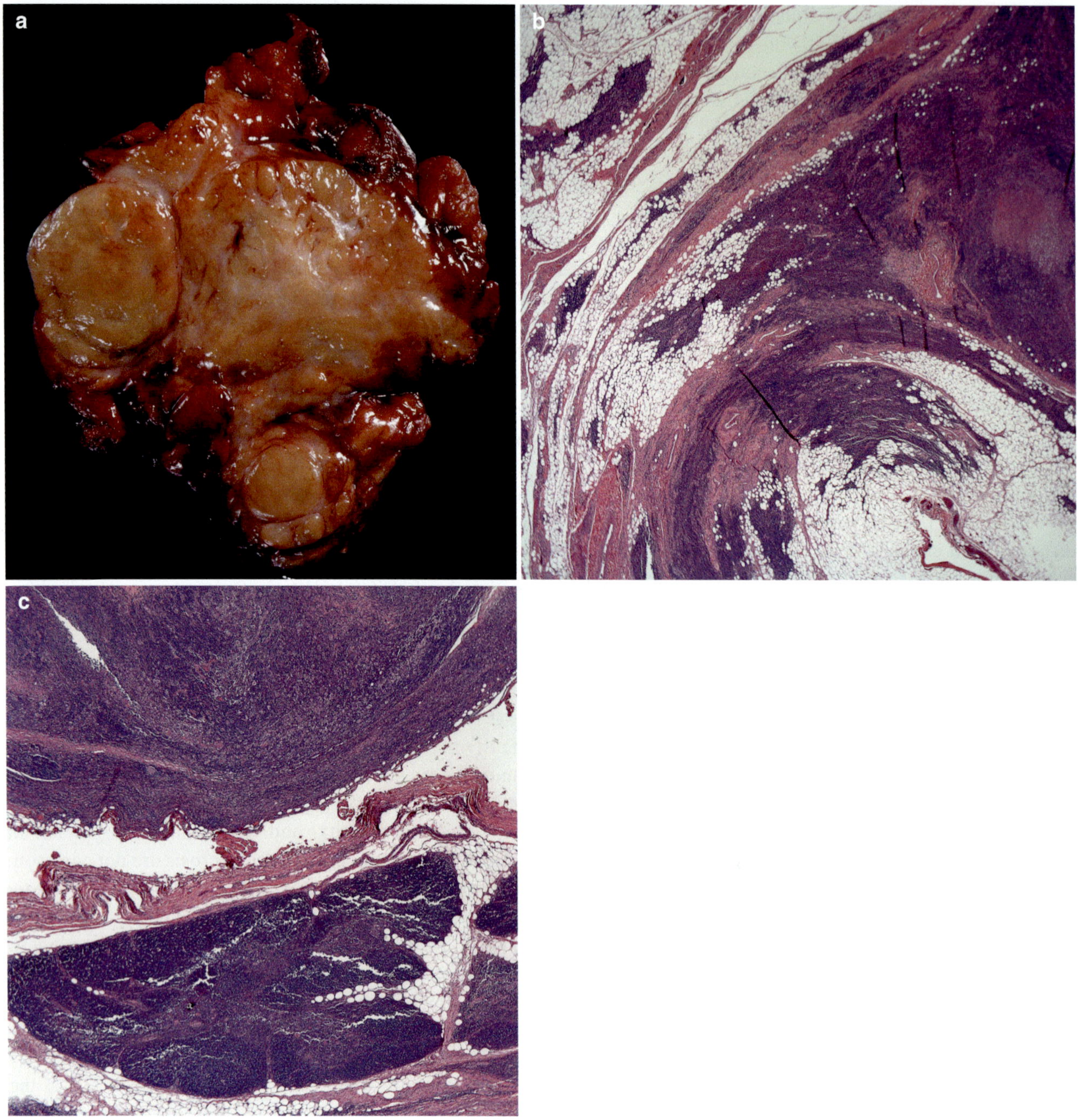

Fig. 13.38 (**a**) HL involving the thymus, note the nodular appearance of the tumor; (**b**) HL of the thymus; note the presence of thymic tissue in the periphery of the tumor mass; (**c**) HL with an adjacent portion of thymus

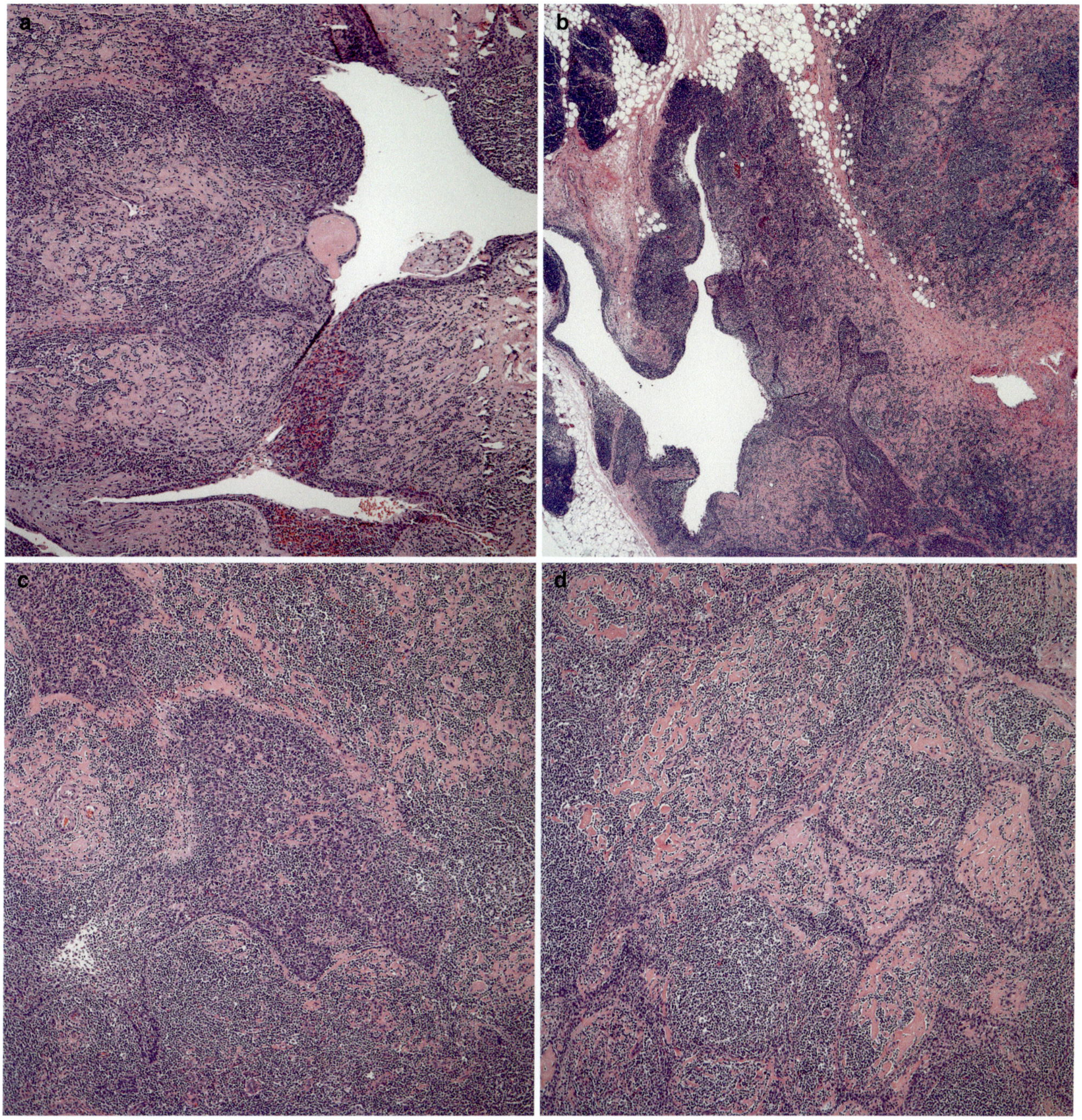

Fig. 13.39 (**a**) HL showing areas mimicking multilocular thymic cyst; (**b**) cystic areas adjacent to HL; (**c**, **d**) residual thymic epithelium in HL

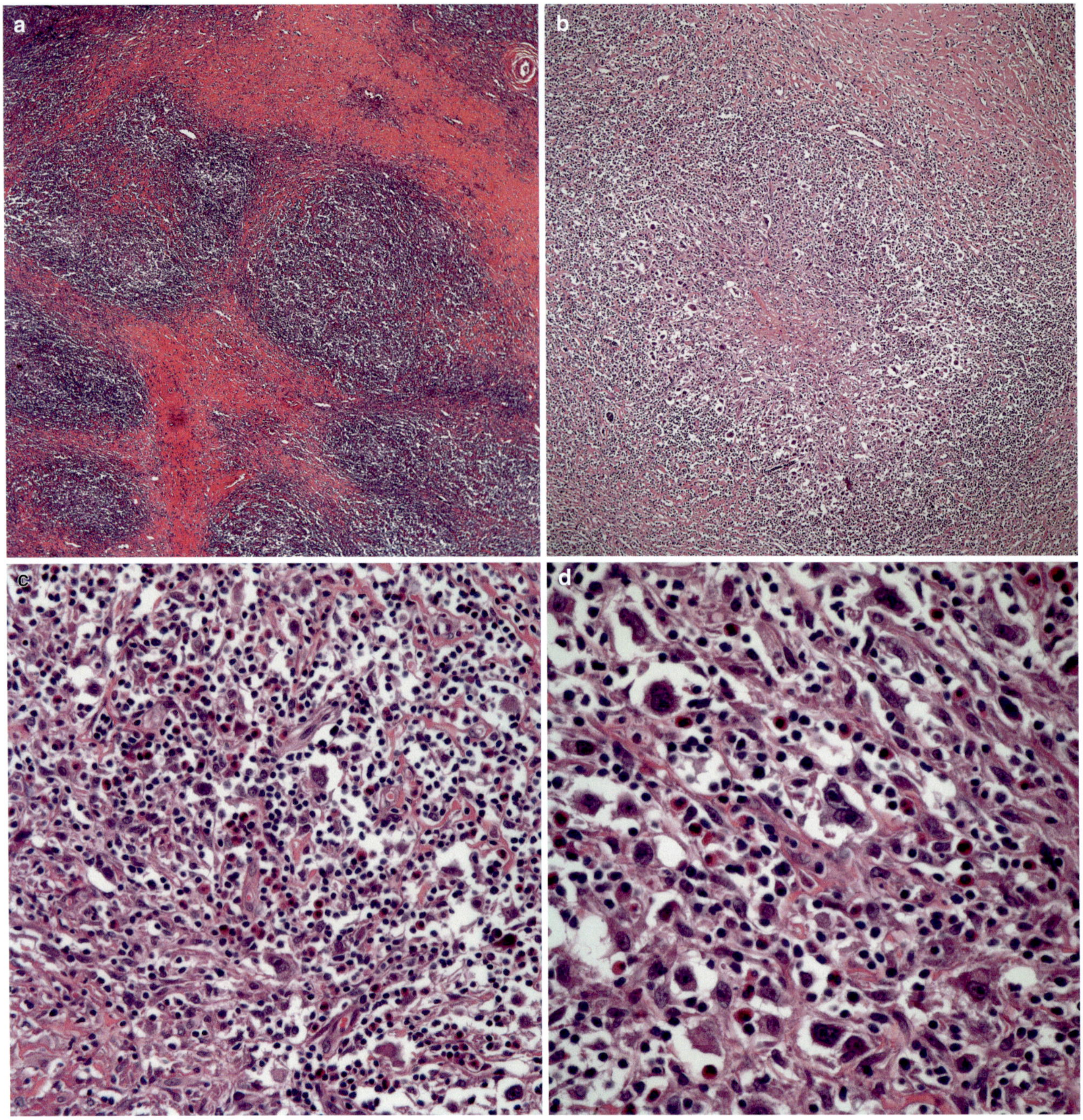

Fig. 13.40 (**a**) Low power view of NSHL; (**b**) nodule with inflammatory cells and numerous larger cells. (**c**) Reed-Sternberg cells admixed with inflammatory cells. (**d**) Higher magnification of Reed-Sternberg cells

tumor shows a solid growth pattern, one can identify remnants of thymic tissue in the periphery of the tumor or just strands of thymic epithelium merging with the tumor. In cases in which the tumor shows cystic component, the histological changes may show a wider array of histological features. The tumor in some areas may show conventional features of multilocular thymic cyst, namely, cystic structures lined by squamous epithelium, lymphoid hyperplasia, and cholesterol cleft granulomas. However, in the walls of the cysts, it is possible to identify an inflammatory infiltrate in which one can identify scattered Reed-Sternberg cells, which ultimately would lead to the correct interpretation. In some cases, areas of necrosis, spindle cell features, and abundant macrophages may be seen (Fig. 13.41a–d), while in other cases, granulomatous reaction may be present (Fig. 13.42a–c); however, Reed-Sternberg cells are still identifiable (Fig. 13.43a, b).

Immunohistochemical Features

The most common immunohistochemical stains used in the diagnosis of HL are CD15 and CD30, as those immunostains will stain the Reed-Sternberg cells (Fig. 13.44a, b). Other immunohistochemical stains – including CD45, surface immunoglobulins, CD3, and CD23 – are negative, while CD20 may be seen weakly and focally positive in about 20% of the HL. Schmid and coworkers [134] reported a study in which the authors use B-cell markers in cases of classic HL and identified that in 87% at least one B-cell marker (CD19, CD20, CD22, CD_w75, MB2) showed positive staining. On the other hand, the inflammatory background may show positive staining for CD3, CD20, and PAX5. Also, CD15 is commonly seen positive in inflammatory cells. Harris and coworkers [135] evaluated the use of CD163 and CD68 in cases of classical Hodgkin's lymphoma with macrophages and concluded that CD163 staining is lower than CD68 with less non-specific staining.

Molecular Features

Attempts to define the lineage of Hodgkin and Reed-Sternberg (HRS) cells have been done over the last 20–30 years. Kuppers and coworkers [136] have suggested that somatic mutations and intraclonal diversity in the V_H rearrangement indicate a germinal center B-cell origin and speculated that the HRS may originate from B-lineage at various stages of development. Further analysis by the same group in a larger number of cases led the authors to conclude that stop codon in some in-frame V gene rearrangements suggests that the HRS cell precursor resides inside germinal centers, and has acquired crippling mutations that prevent antigenic selection [137]. Even though the pathogenesis of HL is still a work in progress, some signaling pathways such as NF_kB pathway appear to be important in our understanding of HL [138]. Other pathways that appear to be important include JAK-STAT signaling pathway, REL gene amplification, NFKBIA point mutations/deletions, NFKBIE point mutations/deletions, TNFAIP3 point mutations/deletions, SOCS1 point mutations/deletions, TP53 point mutations/deletions, and MDM2 gains [139]. Some of these alterations, as it was pointed out earlier, may be shared with PMBCL and MGZL.

Follicular Dendritic Cell Sarcoma (FDCS)

These tumors are presumed to arise from benign follicular dendritic cells, which are located within lymphoid follicles. Credit for the first description of this tumor in the lymph nodes is given to Monda and coworkers [140], who reported four such cases in lymph nodes. However, the existence of this tumor in the mediastinum is of rare occurrence, with most of the cases reported being single case reports [141–145].

Le and coworkers [141] reported a single case of a 63-year-old man who presented with nonproductive cough, shortness of breath, and chest pain. Chest imaging showed the presence of a mediastinal mass. At thoracotomy, the patient was found to have a large posterior mediastinal mass that was inseparable from the right lower lobe of the lung. On histological examination, the diagnosis of FDCS arising in the background of Castleman's disease was made. Hu and coworkers [142] reported 3 cases in 3 female patients between the ages of 51 and 72 years. Diagnostic imaging showed the presence of a mediastinal mass, slightly lobulated, with speckled, strip-like, coarse or arborizing calcifications. In one of these cases, the tumor was arising in a background of Castleman's disease. Clinical follow-up in these patients showed that, despite chemotherapy, two patients died within 1 year after initial diagnosis. Viola and coworkers [143] reported seven intrathoracic cases, six of these cases in the mediastinum. Three cases were associated with Castleman's disease, while two cases in which high mitotic rate was present at histological examination recurred after resection. Hartert and coworkers [144] also reported a mediastinal FDCS in association with immature T-cell and myasthenia gravis, while Jiang and coworkers [145] reported another case with bone marrow involvement.

In general, the clinical course of FDCS is variable; however, recurrence and metastasis are common. Although there is no specific treatment for these patients, surgical resection followed by radiation and chemotherapy is commonly employed.

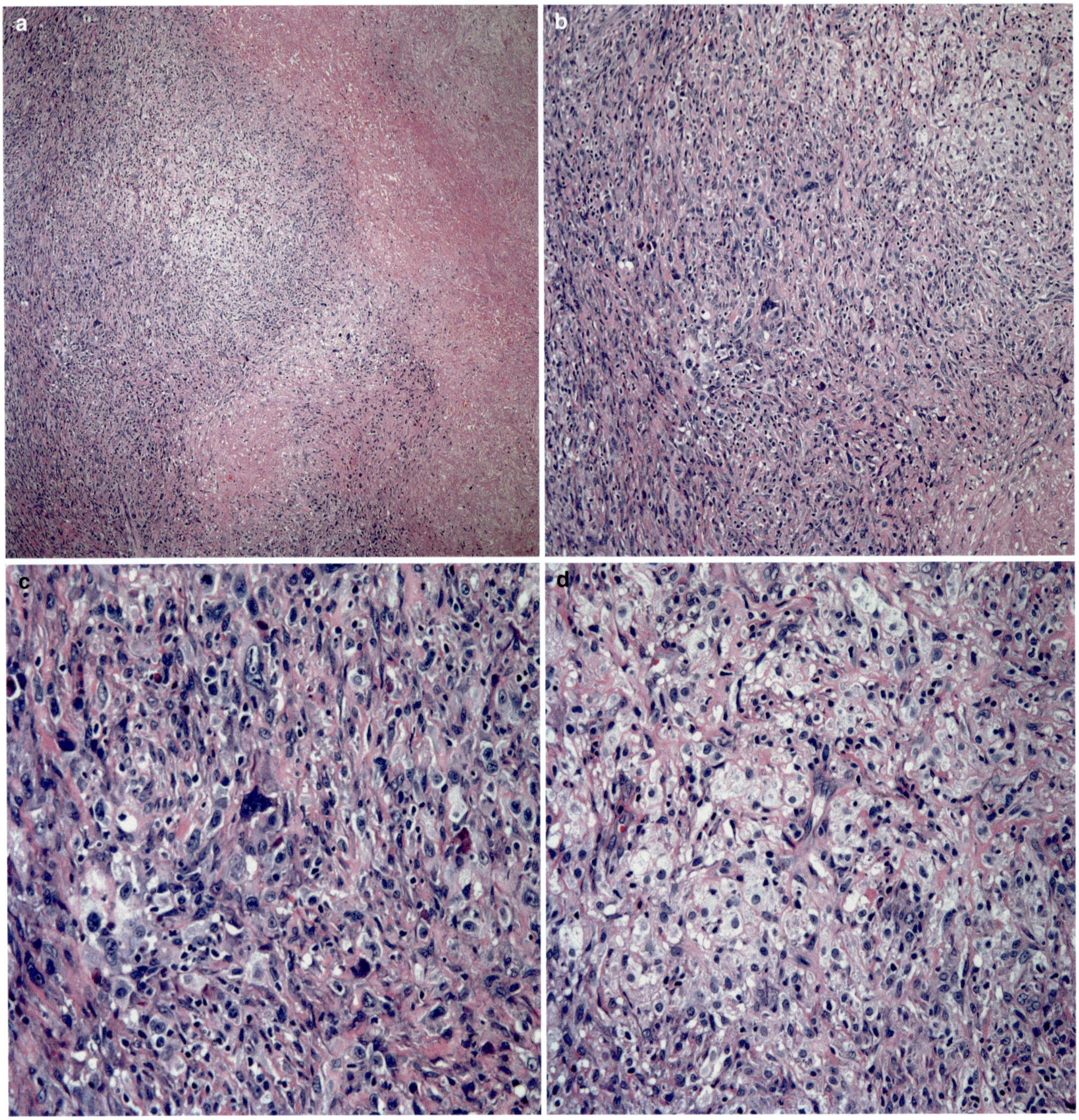

Fig. 13.41 (**a**) HL with areas of necrosis; (**b**) HL with spindle cell features; (**c**) spindle cell morphology and Reed-Sternberg cells; (**d**) HL with abundant macrophages

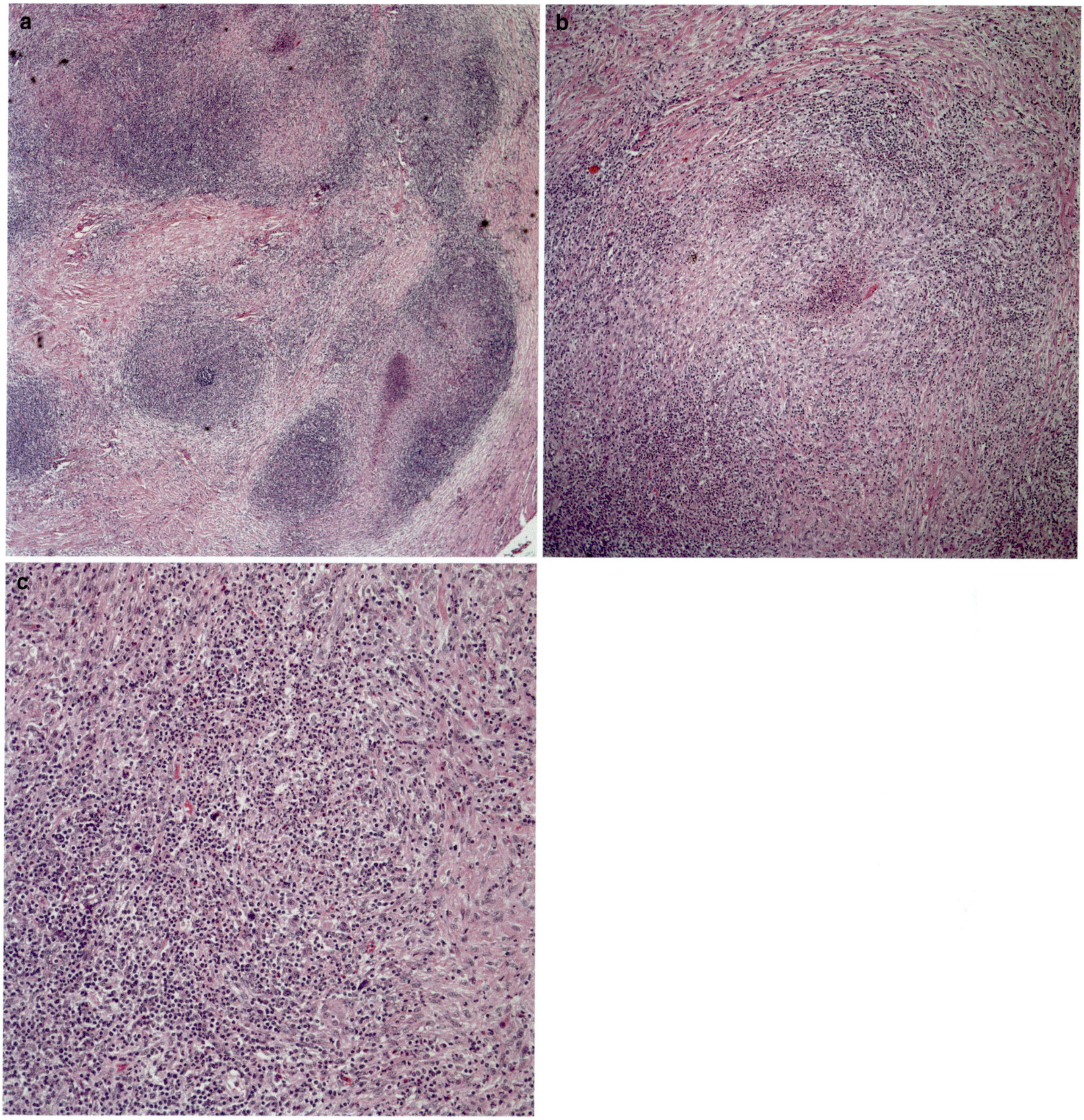

Fig. 13.42 (**a**) NSHL with true granulomatous reaction; (**b**) closer view of the granulomatous reaction; (**c**) areas of acute inflammatory cells

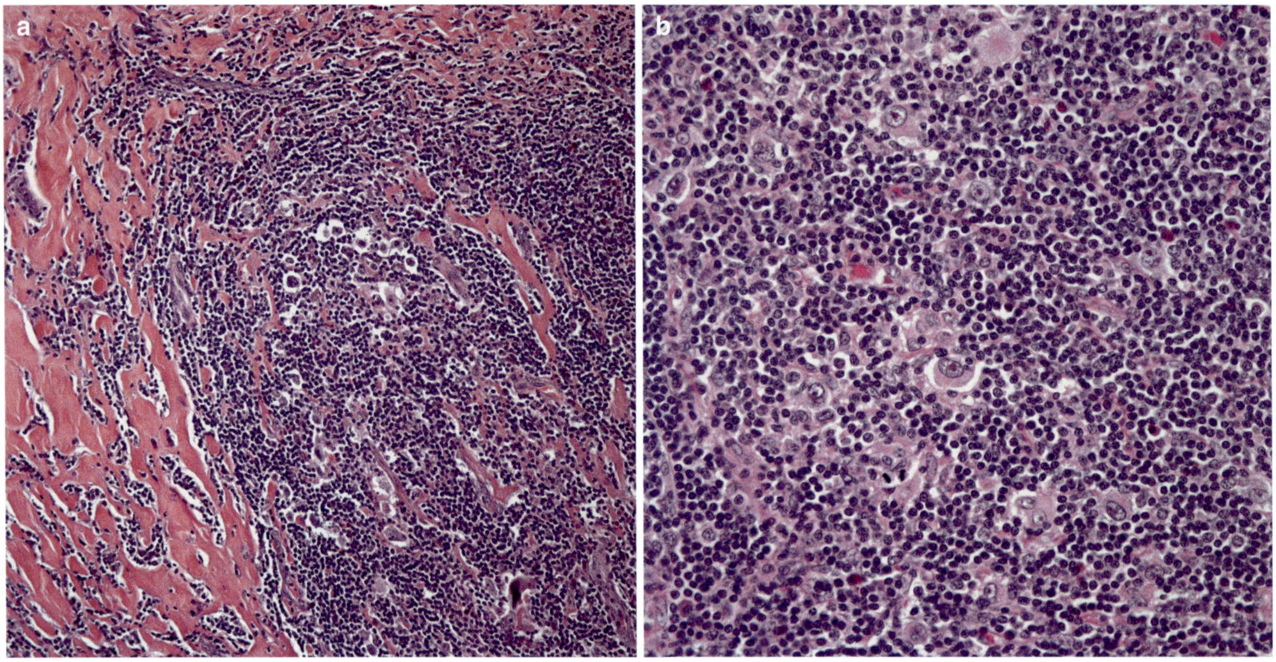

Fig. 13.43 (**a**) HL with areas of sclerosis and R-S cells; (**b**) closer view of the R-S cells

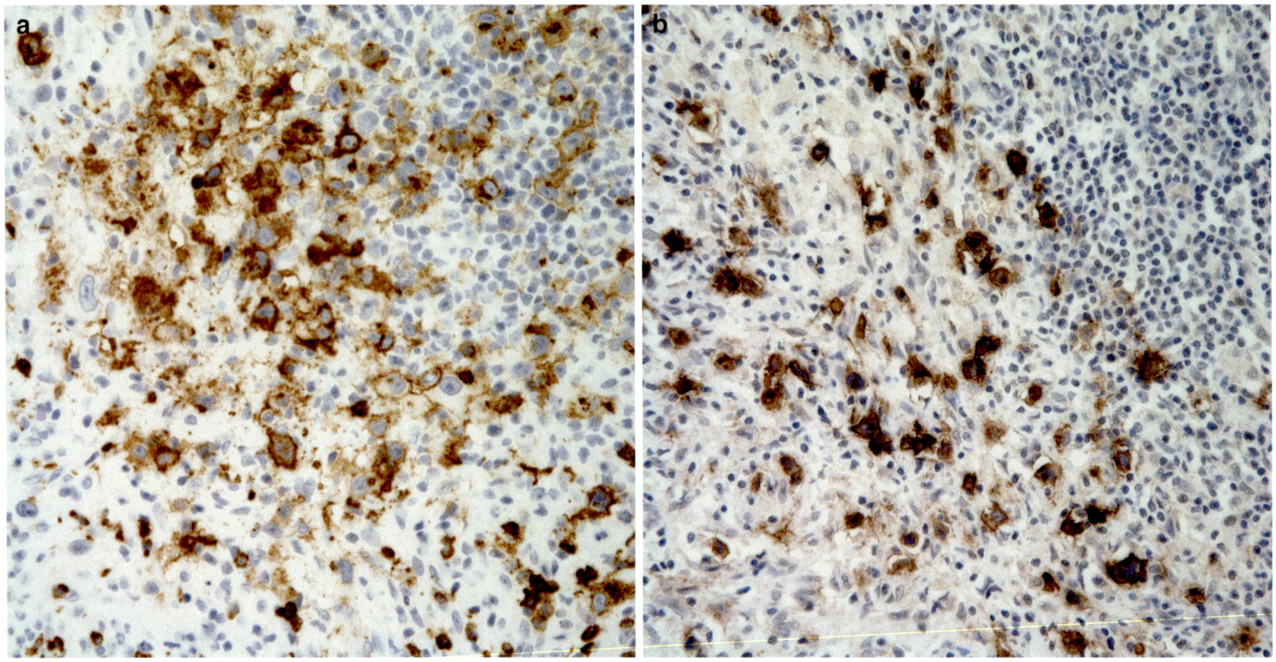

Fig. 13.44 (**a**) CD15 immunohistochemical stain showing positive staining; (**b**) CD30 immunohistochemical stain also showing positive staining

Pathological Features

The tumor masses can vary in size from a few centimeters to more than 10 cm in greatest diameter. Histologically, the tumor is characterized by the presence of a spindle cell proliferation that may show inflammatory changes (Fig. 13.45a–e) arranged in fascicles, concentric whorls, storiform, trabecular, or nodular growth pattern. In many cases, more than one growth pattern is present. Other unusual histological features that may be present in these tumors include myxoid, cystic, vascular, and pseudopapillary changes. Areas of sclerosis or the presence of lymphocytic component may be present. Higher magnification shows that the spindle cells show an elongated nuclei, and small nucleoli may be present in some cells. Areas of necrosis and hemorrhage are not common in these tumors. However, the mitotic activity is variable, but, in most cases, it is not high. In some cases the tumor may be arising from Castleman's disease (Fig. 13.46a–c) or may have prominent epithelioid features (Fig. 13.47a, b)

By immunohistochemistry, FDCS commonly expressed CD21, CD23, and CD35 (Fig. 13.48a, b). In addition, FDCS may also show positive staining for epithelial membrane antigen (EMA) vimentin, desmoplakin, and HLA-DR. Immunohistochemical stains for S-100 protein and CD68 have shown variable weak and focal positive staining. In cases in which there is a lymphocytic component, these cells may show positive staining for CD20 and CD3 but commonly negative for CD5.

Mediastinal Plasmacytoma

The occurrence of extramedullary plasmacytomas primarily presenting as mass is rare but has been well documented in the literature [146–152]. Ahmed and coworkers [149] described a 68-year-old woman with myasthenia gravis and anterior mediastinal mass. Subsequent studies revealed involvement of lymph nodes and gastrointestinal system. Lee and coworkers [150] reported an asymptomatic 64-year-old man who was found to have a posterior mediastinal mass on a routine chest film. Histological evaluation of the mass disclosed an IgG kappa type extramedullary plasmacytoma. The patient received radiation treatment. In the case described by Wheterbee and Dincer [151], the patient was a 70-year-old man who had a large mediastinal mass involving the right suprahilar area, hilar, and subcarinal areas, with significant mass effect to the esophagus, and numerous pleural-based nodules throughout the right lung. In the case described by Sato and coworkers [152], in a 31-year-old woman, the mass was located in the anterior mediastinum. Surgical resection was performed without radiation therapy, and, 2 years post-surgical resection, the patient remained alive. In our experience with two cases of extramedullary plasmacytomas [148], the patients were a man and a woman, ages 59 and 62, respectively, who presented with mediastinal mass, one in the anterior and one in the posterior mediastinum. Both patients went on to develop multiple myeloma 6 and 24 months after the initial diagnosis of mediastinal plasmacytoma. Surgical resection of the tumor was performed in both cases, and clinical follow-up showed that one patient had died 2 years after diagnosis and one patient had remained alive and well 4 years after surgical resection.

Pathological Features

Macroscopically, in the resected specimens, the tumor has varied in size from a few centimeters to more than 10 cm in greatest diameter. Some of these tumors have been described as well demarcated and slightly lobulated.

Microscopically, the low power view of these tumors shows an atypical homogeneous cellular proliferation, which may in some areas be separated by thick bands of fibroconnective tissue. The tumor cells also commonly invade surrounding adipose tissue and the areas of fibroconnective tissue separating the tumor in lobules. At higher magnification, it is easily identifiable the presence of an atypical proliferation of plasma cells, which in some areas may show the presence of Russell bodies. Multinucleated plasma cells are commonly identified as well as the presence of atypical plasma cells with bizarre nuclei (Fig. 13.49a–f). However, mitotic activity is either low or absent in these tumors. Necrotic and hemorrhagic areas are commonly absent in these neoplasms.

By immunohistochemistry, the plasma cells may show positive staining for CD138 and MUM1. EMA may also show positive staining in plasma cells. However, the most important studies would be the finding of a monoclonal light chain. In that respect, some cases of predominant λ light chain have been reported.

Castleman's Disease (CD)

In 1956, over the course of studying tumors of the thymus gland, Castleman, Iverson, and Menendez [153] identified 13 cases that had been previously classified as thymomas, and the authors considered that the histopathological changes present in these tumors were different enough to warrant a separation from thymoma. The patients were eight men and five women between the ages of 19 and 54 years. None of the patients had a history of myasthenia gravis, and some were asymptomatic, while others had non-specific symptoms of cough and dyspnea. Their mediastinal was discovered incidentally during a routine chest film. Anatomically, only a

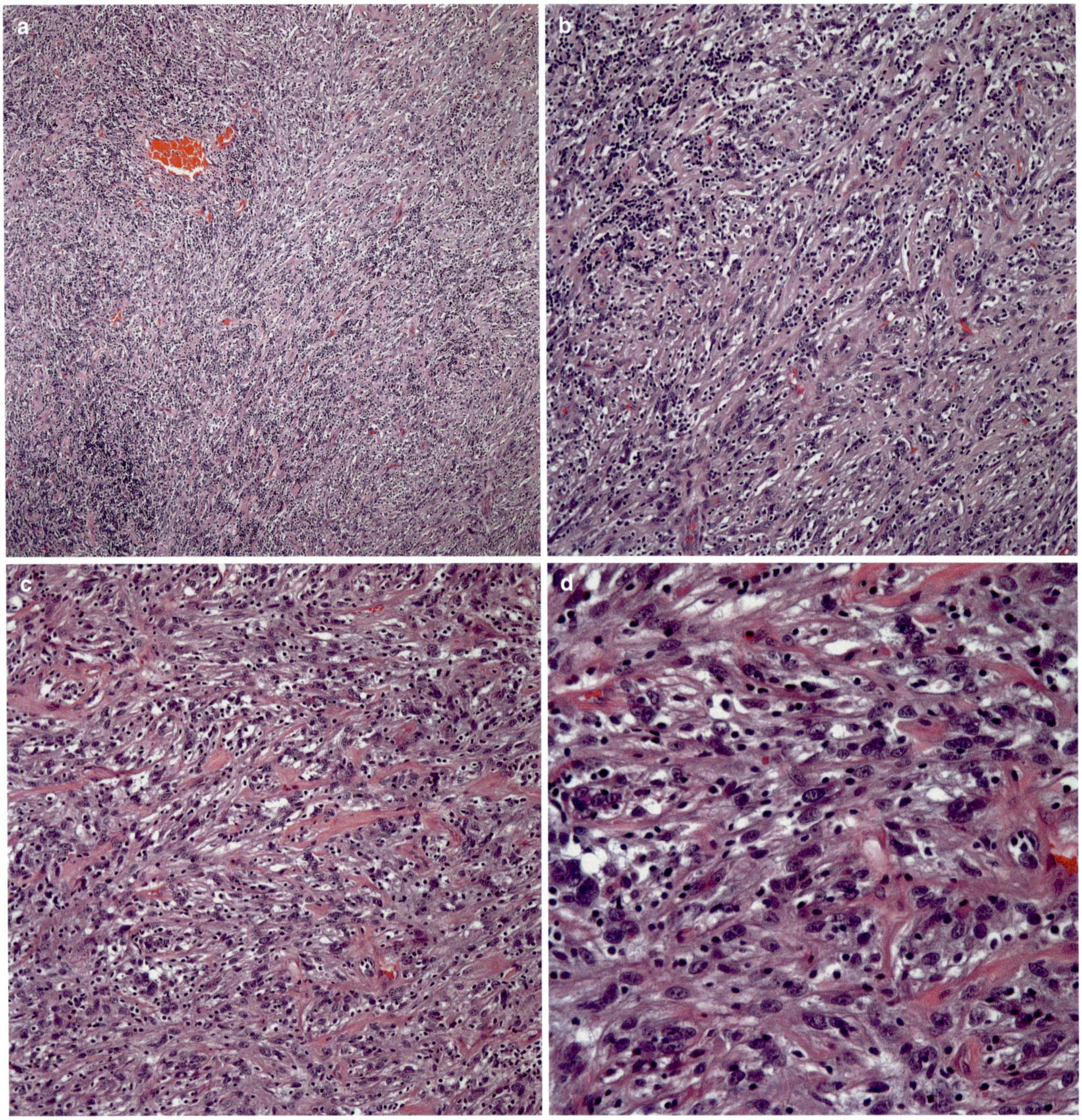

Fig. 13.45 (**a**) Follicular dendritic cell sarcoma (FDSC) showing spindle cells admixed with inflammatory cells; (**b**) elongated cells with fusiform nuclei and conspicuous nucleoli; (**c**) similar areas without inflammatory reaction; (**d**) Spindle cells with oval and fusiform nuclei; no mitotic activity is present

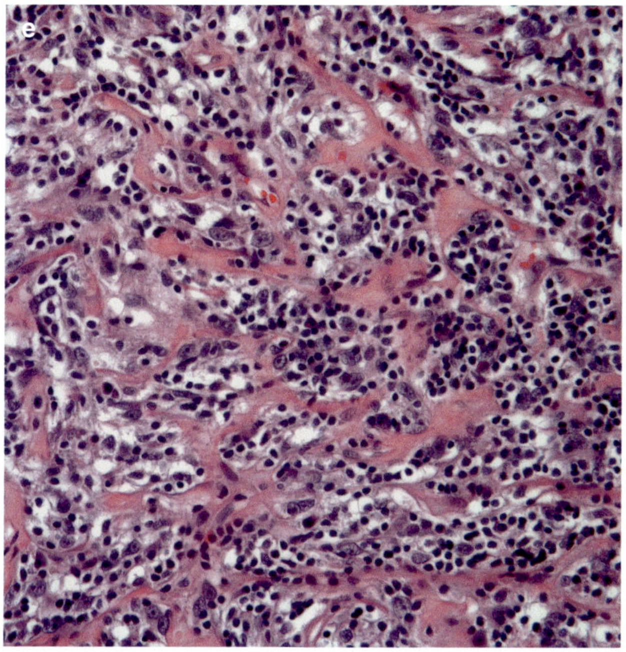

Fig. 13.45 (continued) (**e**) Higher magnification of the spindle cells admixed with inflammatory cells

couple of these lesions were in the mid-superior anterior mediastinum, and the majority of the lesions were lateral in the mediastinal compartment, in locations where one often finds lymph nodes. In one case, the lesion appeared to be in the posterior mediastinum. It is also important to highlight that the authors also noted that they had seen similar lesions in other anatomical locations including the costovertebral angle and the lower abdomen. Histologically, the most relevant morphological findings were those of germinal center formation and marked capillary proliferation. The authors interpreted these findings as benign hyperplastic lymph nodes not of thymic origin. Following this publication, others authors reported individual cases in different intrathoracic locations, some of them emphasizing the large size, while others emphasizing the posterior mediastinal location of the lesion [154–156]. Interestingly, Lattes and Pachter reported 12 cases of similar lesions; however, the authors interpreted the lesion as a possible hamartoma [157]. In 1972, Keller and coworkers [158] analyzed 81 cases of this newly described lesion and reviewed the literature identifying 183 cases up to

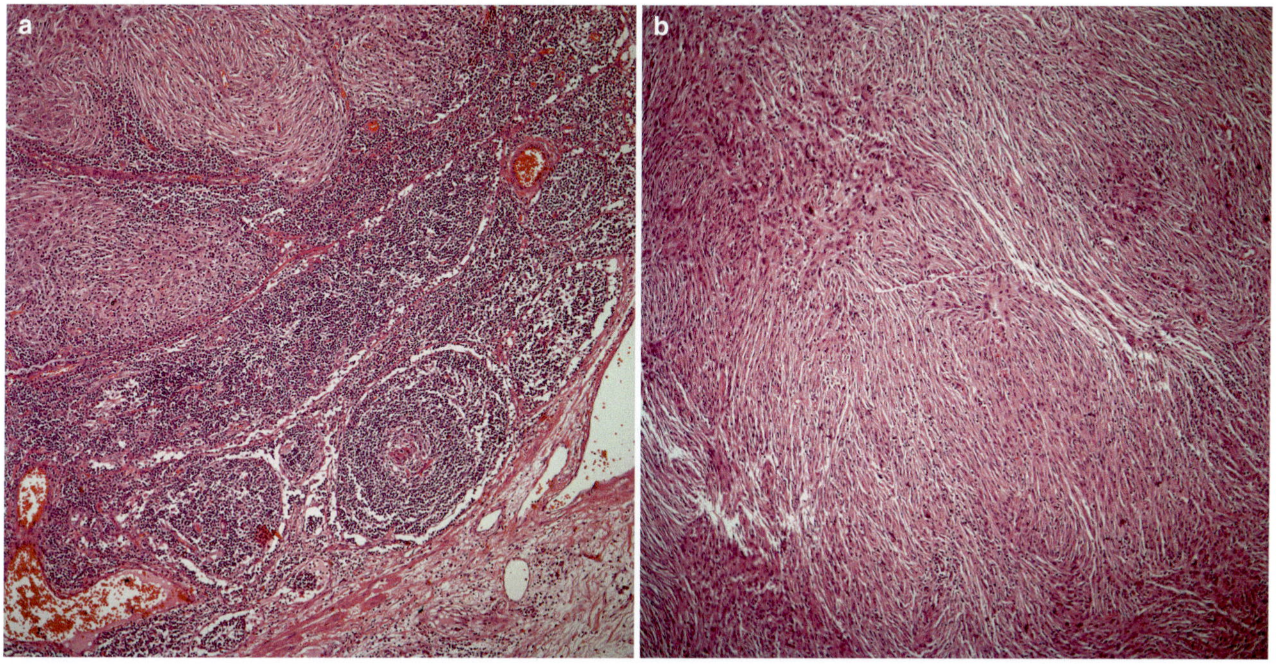

Fig. 13.46 (**a**) FDCS growing continuous to Castleman's disease; (**b**) prominent spindle cell proliferation

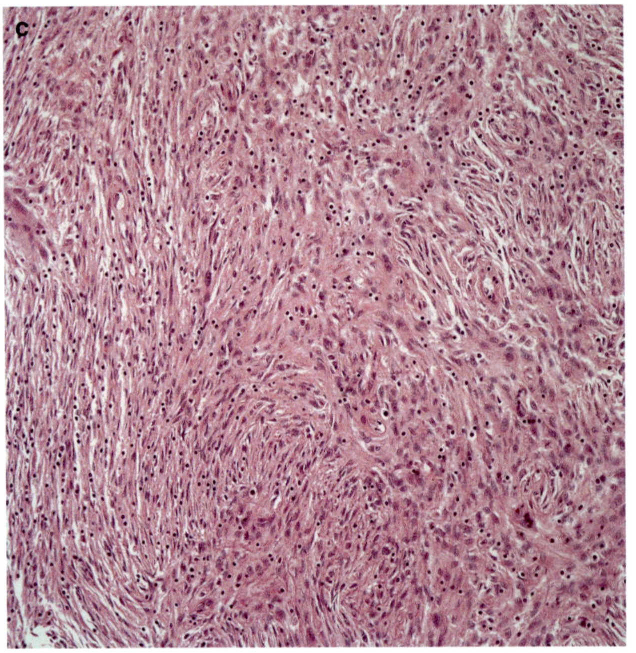

Fig. 13.46 (continued) (**c**) Spindle and epithelioid cells

1972, the majority of them (71%) in intrathoracic location. Keller and coworkers [158] identified a more ubiquitous distribution of this process with lesions in the pelvis, axilla, neck, and retroperitoneum. However, the majority of the lesions were in intrathoracic locations including intrapulmonary location. More importantly is that, in the process of analyzing these cases, the authors separated two distinct histopathological variants: the hyaline-vascular type characterized by interfollicular capillary proliferation and the plasma cell variant characterized by large follicles with intervening sheets of plasma cells. Clinically, symptoms of fever, anemia, and hyperglobulinemia were common, which led the authors to consider that this process was of possible infectious or inflammatory etiology. Meanwhile, descriptions of this process with more unusual clinical associations such as nephrotic syndrome, myelofibrosis, myasthenia gravis, lung carcinoma, presenting as a tracheal mass, and mimicking malignancy in the mediastinum have been reported, while others have continued describing cases in the anterior and posterior mediastinum [159–166]. Unusual features – such as intramediastinal lymph node spread in a mediastinal Castleman's disease,

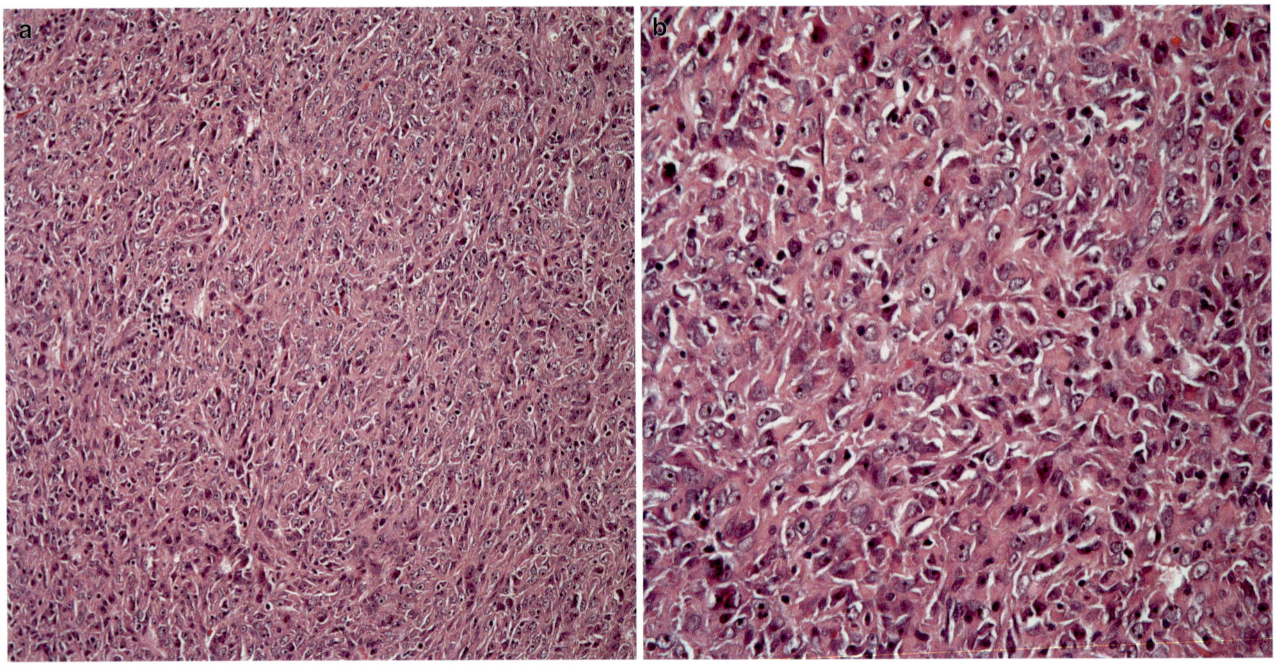

Fig. 13.47 (**a**) Prominent epithelioid cells in FDSC; (**b**) higher magnification of round to oval cells with prominent nucleoli

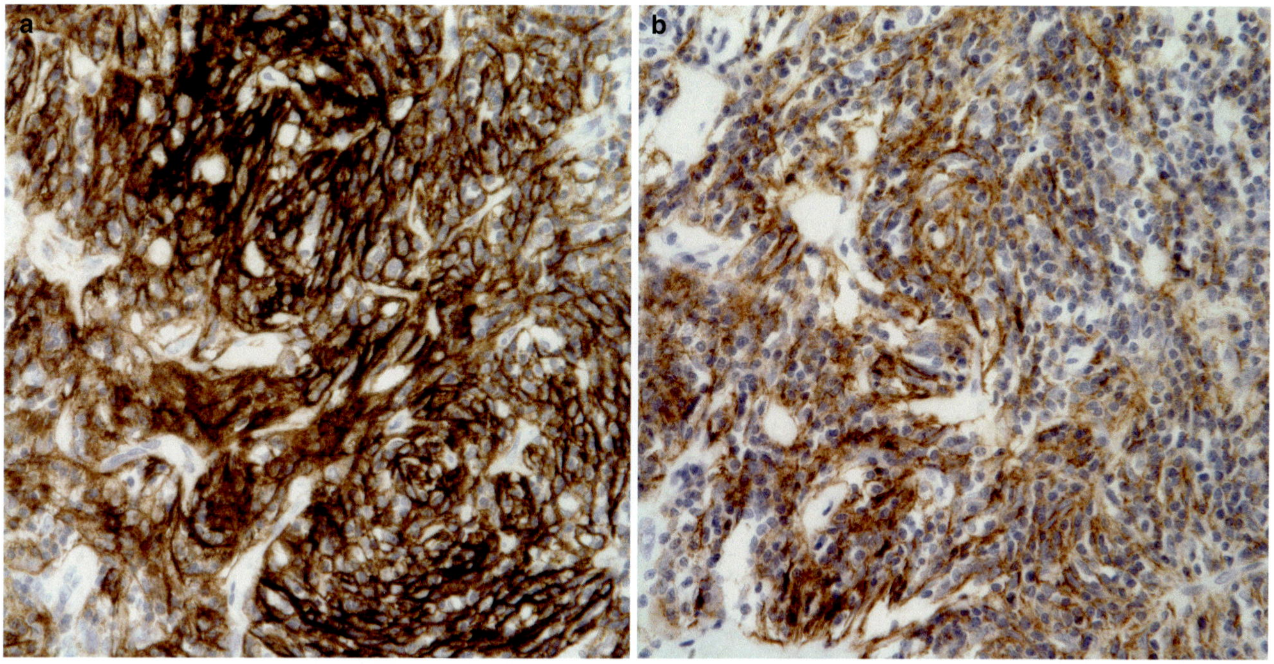

Fig. 13.48 (**a**) Positive immunohistochemical stain for CD21; (**b**) positive immunohistochemical stain for CD35

plasma cell variant, or unicentric mediastinal plasma cell type Castleman's disease – have been described [167, 168]. Others have emphasized different treatment options [167–172].

Currently, CD is classified depending on the number of regions of enlarged lymph nodes that show the characteristic features of CD; thus, unicentric CD involves a single enlarged lymph node, while multicentric CD involves multiple lymph nodes of different regions. In addition, multicentric CD is further categorized as idiopathic, associated with Kaposi sarcoma-associated herpesvirus (KSHV)/human herpesvirus-8 (HHV-8) infection, monoclonal plasma cells associated neuropathy, organomegaly, endocrinopathy, monoclonal plasma cell disorder, and skin changes (POEMS) syndrome (POEMS-associated multicentric CD), or TAFRO syndrome (thrombocytopenia, anasarca, myelofibrosis, renal dysfunction, and organomegaly). However, it is also important to highlight that multicentric CD can occur in patients with HHV-8-negative. On the contrary, unicentric CD is commonly asymptomatic, and its discovery is during a routine physician examination; usually surgical resection of the lymph node is curative. Possible etiologies for unicentric CD include infectious, reactive inflammatory, and neoplastic. The cell type responsible for its pathogenesis has not been clearly defined. In some patients with systemic symptoms but with unicentric CD, it is possible the interleukin-6 (IL-6) may be involved [173]. IL-6, which is a potent stimulus for the production of B-cells, is expressed in germinal centers of hyperplastic lymph nodes in multicentric CD. Such expression of viral IL-6 is unique to HHV-8 and is prominent in multicentric CD [174]. Regarding the diagnosis of HHV-8-negative idiopathic multicentric CD, recent criteria have been developed to properly diagnose those cases and include exclusion of all reactive, secondary mimics, which include autoimmune diseases and infection, presence of typical histopathological features in a lymph node biopsy and evidence of multicentric disease, and 2 of 11 minor criteria from clinical laboratory abnormality [175].

Although there is not an accurate estimate about the incidence of CD, it has been estimated that the occurrence of CD is approximately 21–25 per million person-years, which if

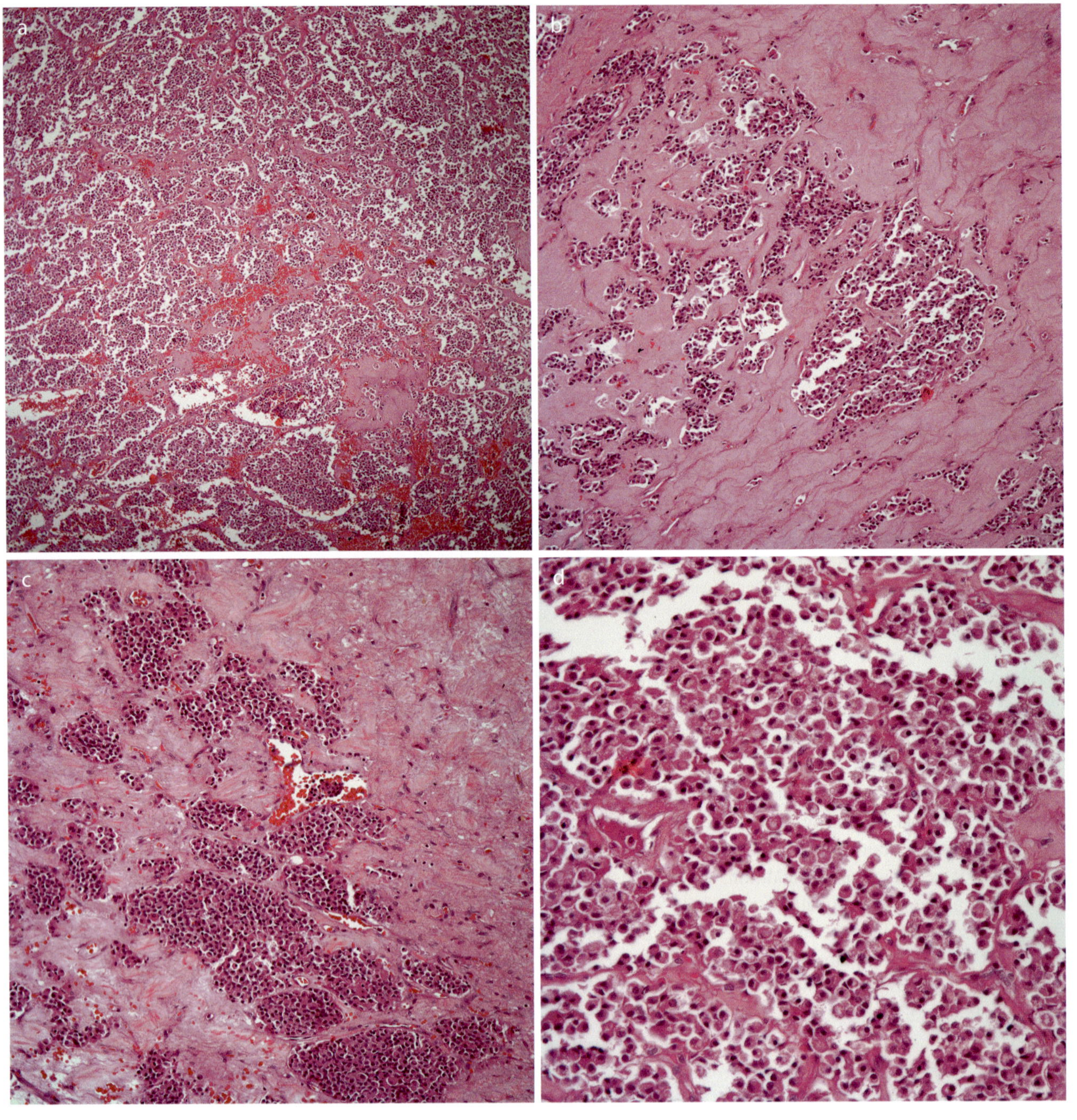

Fig. 13.49 (**a**) Low power of a mediastinal plasmacytoma; (**b**) atypical plasma cell proliferation with areas of fibrosis; (**c**) subtle areas with atypical plasma cells in a nested pattern; (**d**) large atypical plasma cell proliferation

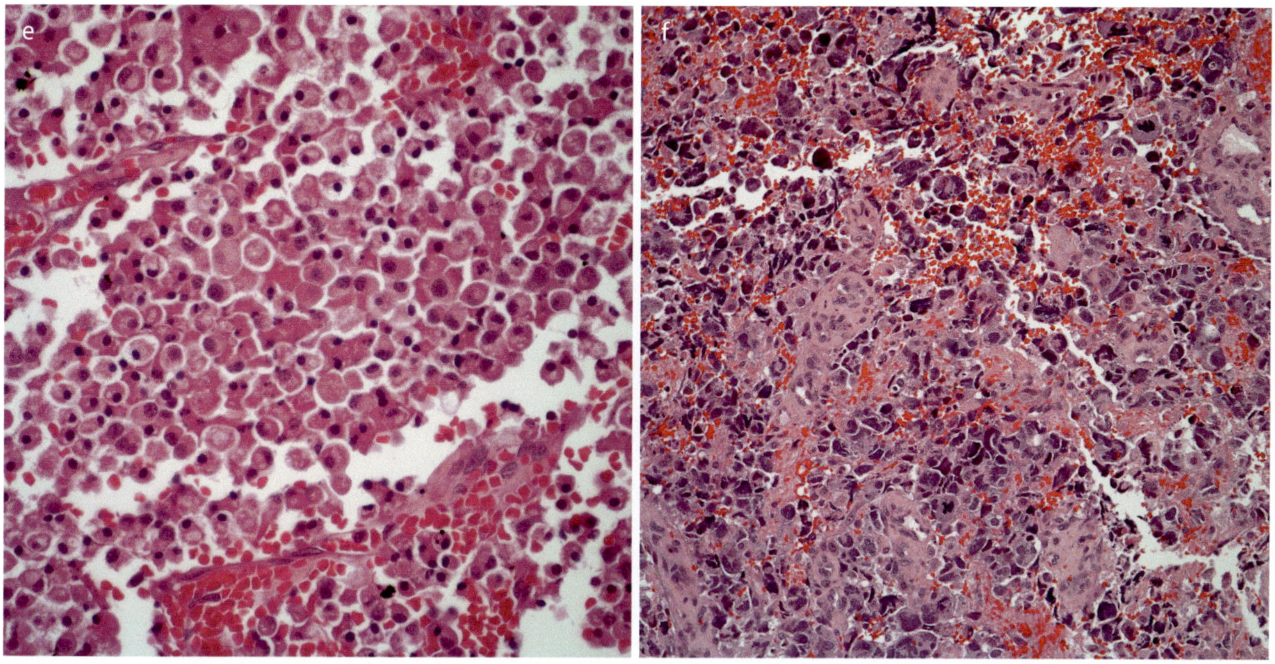

Fig. 13.49 (continued) (**e**) Higher magnification of plasma cell without cytologic atypia; (**f**) focal areas of prominent atypia and mitotic activity

taken face value will translate into an incidence in the USA at 4–5 thousand patients per year for patients 25 and older. On the other hand, the estimated incidence of unicentric CD is approximately 15 per million patients per year, while the incidence of multicentric CD is approximately 5 per million persons per year [176].

Regarding the treatment of CD, it may vary depending on the clinical presentation whether it is unicentric, multicentric, or idiopathic. In cases of idiopathic multicentric CD, the use of monoclonal antibodies targeting interleukin-6 signaling pathways is the frontline therapy. Rituximab is often used as initial therapy for more indolent idiopathic cases. Chemotherapy is usually reserved for relapse cases, while autologous stem cell transplantation is a consideration in patients with the POEMS syndrome [177].

Pathological Features

Essentially there are three subtypes of CD, which can present as mediastinal tumors: hyaline-vascular (Fig. 13.50a–e), which is the most common, plasma cell type (Fig. 13.51a–d), and mixed. The histological features of the hyaline-vascular type include the presence of lymphoid follicles with atrophic or regressed germinal centers with the presence of blood vessels penetrating the atrophic germinal center. The germinal centers are formed by residual follicular dendritic cells, which give the common histological features of "onionskin," prominent mantle zone containing small lymphocytes. In the plasma cell type, there is extensive presence of plasma cells in interfollicular areas, while the presence of germinal centers can be either hyperplastic or regressed. Plasma cell subtype is the most common variant of multicentric CD with approximately 75% of the cases, while representing 10–20% in unicentric CD [178]. The mixed type shows features of both of the hyaline-vascular and the plasma cell subtype, and it is more common in HHV-8-related multicentric CD. In some unusual cases, Castleman's disease may show extensive areas of hyalinization (Fig. 13.52a, b). Further laboratory analysis and imaging will depend on the type of CD diagnosed.

Immunohistochemical stains in the unicentric type hyaline-vascular CD show presence of B cells mainly in the expanded mantle zone; therefore, CD20 will show positive staining in those areas. IgD may also show positive staining in the mantle zone areas as well as CD5. In addition, CD21 (Fig. 13.53) and CD23 may show positive staining in the dendritic cells within follicles. In the plasma cell type, the immunohistochemical stains would show polytypic immunoglobulin light chain expression. In cases associated with HHV-8, in situ hybridization often identifies lambda light chain-restricted plasmablasts within the mantle zone.

Extramedullary Hematopoiesis (EMH)

Extramedullary hematopoiesis is observed in several other organs including the liver, lymph nodes, and the lung. However, the occurrence of EMH presenting as a mediastinal mass and mimicking a malignant neoplasm is rare but well recognized in the literature, and in some instance, such occurrence has been coded under different terminology,

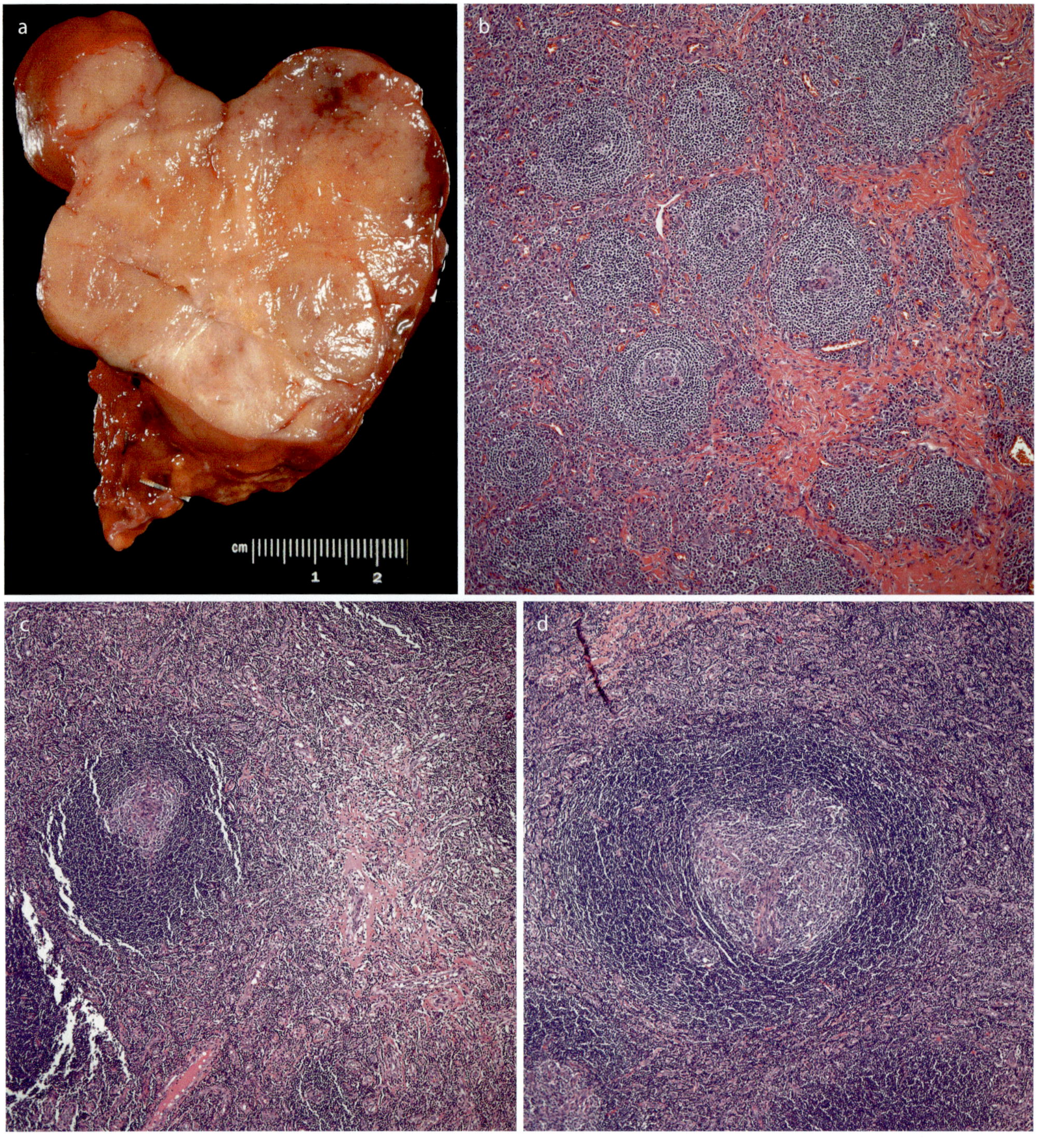

Fig. 13.50 (**a**) Well-circumscribed mediastinal mass, light tan with subtle nodularity; (**b**) Castleman's disease hyaline-vascular type showing numerous germinal centers; (**c**) germinal center adjacent to areas of vascular proliferation; (**d**) typical feature of the so-called onionskin and a small vessel piercing the germinal center

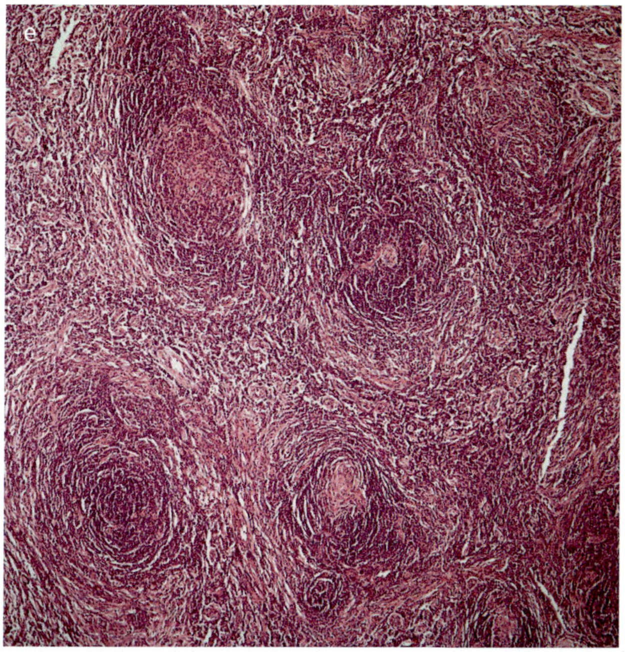

Fig. 13.50 (continued) (**e**) Castleman's disease showing germinal centers in different stages

which would include myelolipoma and erythroblastoma [179–191]. EMH occurs as a compensatory phenomenon in association with conditions that disturbed the normal function of the bone marrow. It is important to highlight that erythropoiesis may also occur in the normal thymus [192].

Although, the histological features likely do not pose a significant problem in the diagnosis, the clinical and radiological features of patients with mediastinal EMH may raise some concerns about the possibility of a malignant neoplasm. Clinically, EMH has been associated with different hematological disorders including thalassemia, unclassified anemias, chronic hemolytic anemia, and sickle-cell disease. In 1960, Knoblich [179] reviewed the current literature of intrathoracic extramedullary hematopoiesis and encountered seven cases of such occurrence from infants to adult individuals; however, interestingly all the cases reported at that time were postmortem findings. Subsequently, there have been numerous single case reports of such occurrence either in the anterior or posterior mediastinum, and most of these reports have been in adult individuals who have presented with a mediastinal mass. In our experience [191], we reported four cases of such occurrence with tumor masses occurring in the posterior mediastinum (Fig. 13.54). Even though three of those patients had an associated clinical history of a hematologic disorder, one patient was completely asymptomatic, and the mass was discovered during a routine chest image.

From the diagnostic point of view, the diagnosis of EMH in the mediastinum should not pose difficulties. EMH may be composed exclusively of hematologic cells of myeloid and erythroid lineage admixed with abundant megakaryocytes (Fig. 13.55a, b). However, in some cases, the presence of these elements may be associated with areas of adipose tissue (Fig. 13.56a–c) and fibroblastic proliferation (myelolipoma), which on limited biopsies may create some confusion as to the true nature of this process.

As it would be expected, surgical resection of the mediastinal mass is curative in these patients; however, the long-term follow-up is determined by the underlying hematologic disorder.

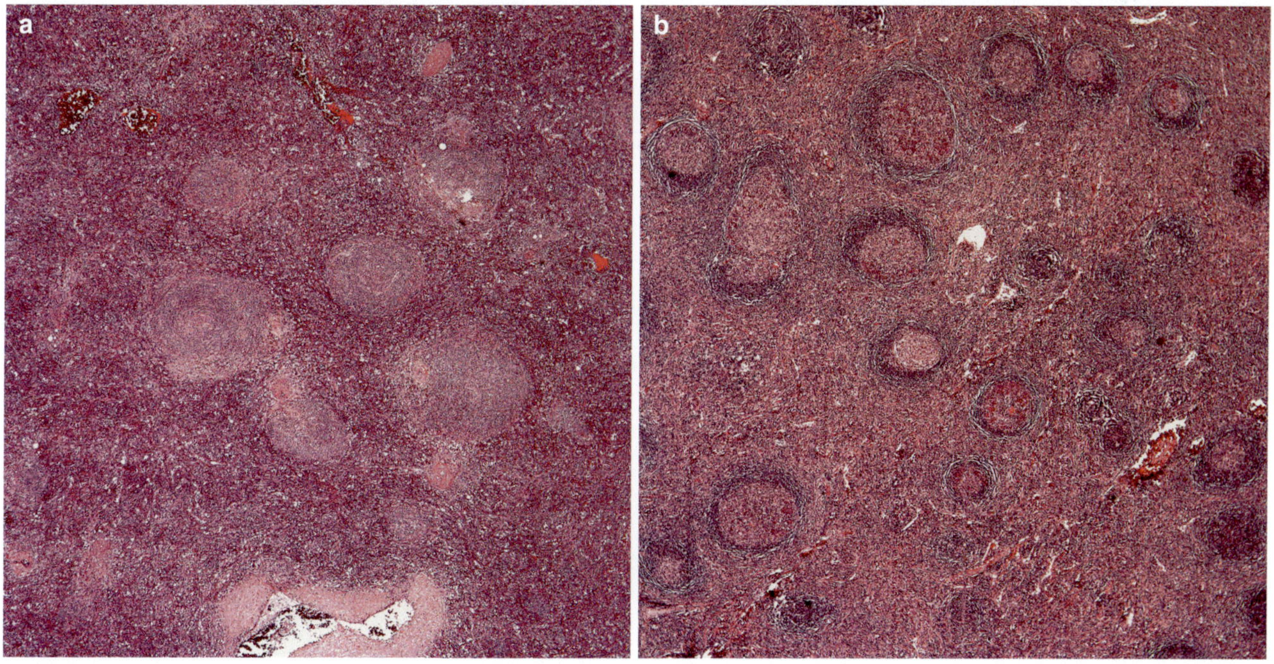

Fig. 13.51 (**a**) Low power view of Castleman's disease, plasma cell type; note the low power appearance of "spleen-like"; (**b**) numerous germinal centers separated by plasma cells

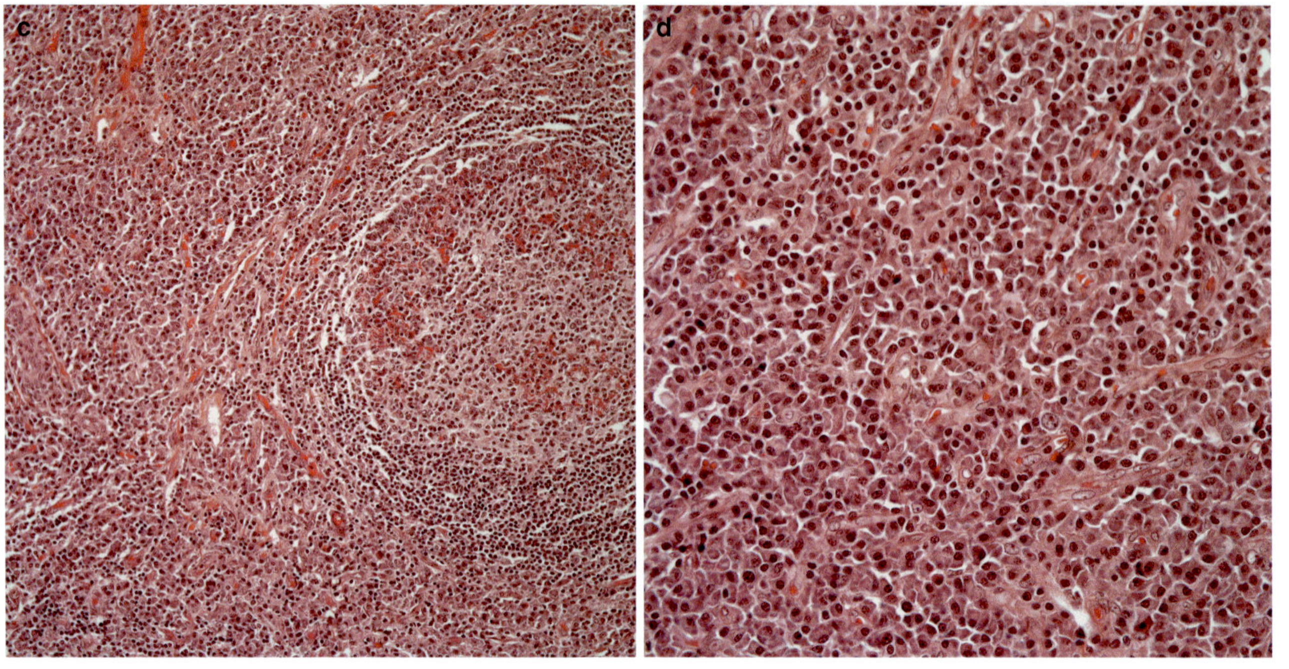

Fig. 13.51 (continued) (**c**) Extensive plasma cell component; (**d**) closer view at the mature plasma cells

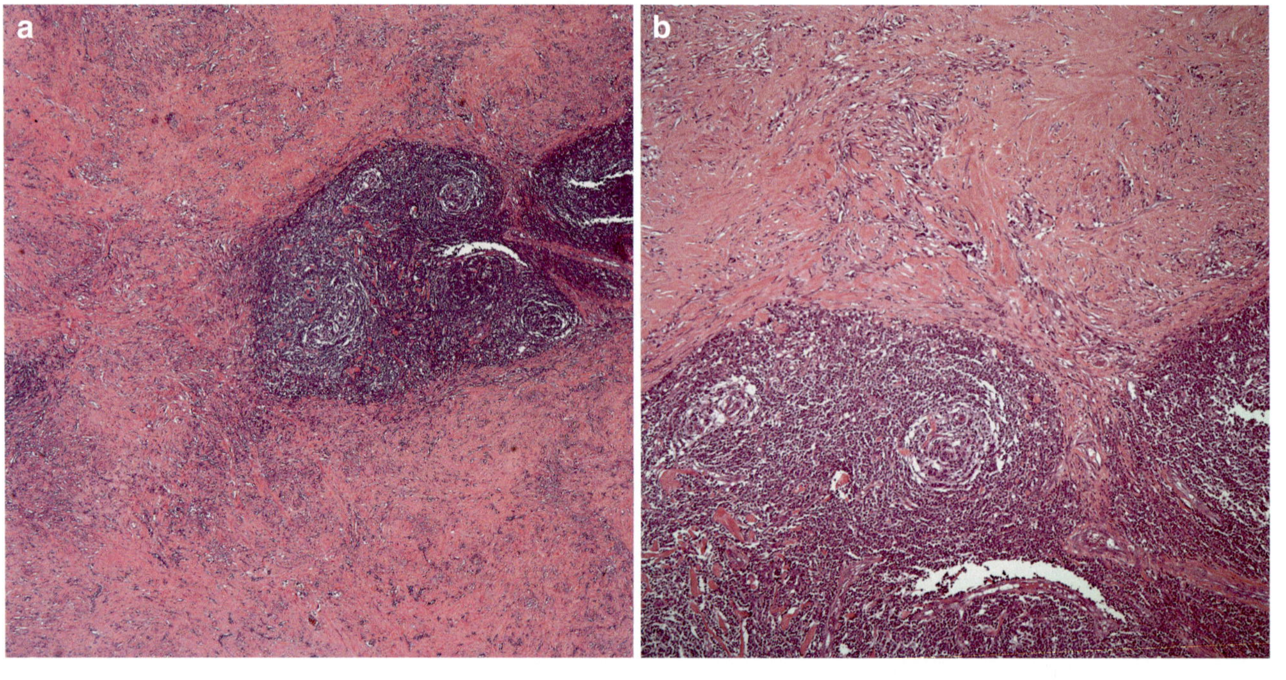

Fig. 13.52 (**a**) Castleman's disease with extensive fibrosis. (**b**) Closer view at the atrophic germinal center adjacent to fibrotic areas

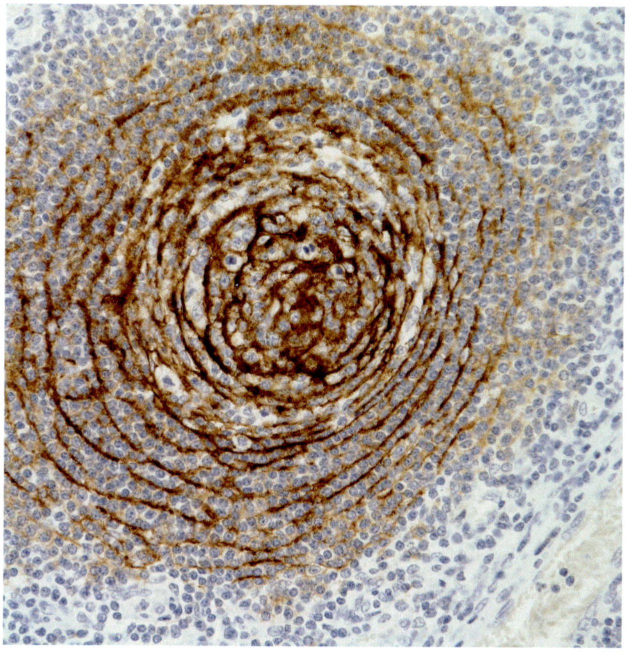

Fig. 13.53 Immunohistochemical stain for CD21 decorates the cells of a germinal center

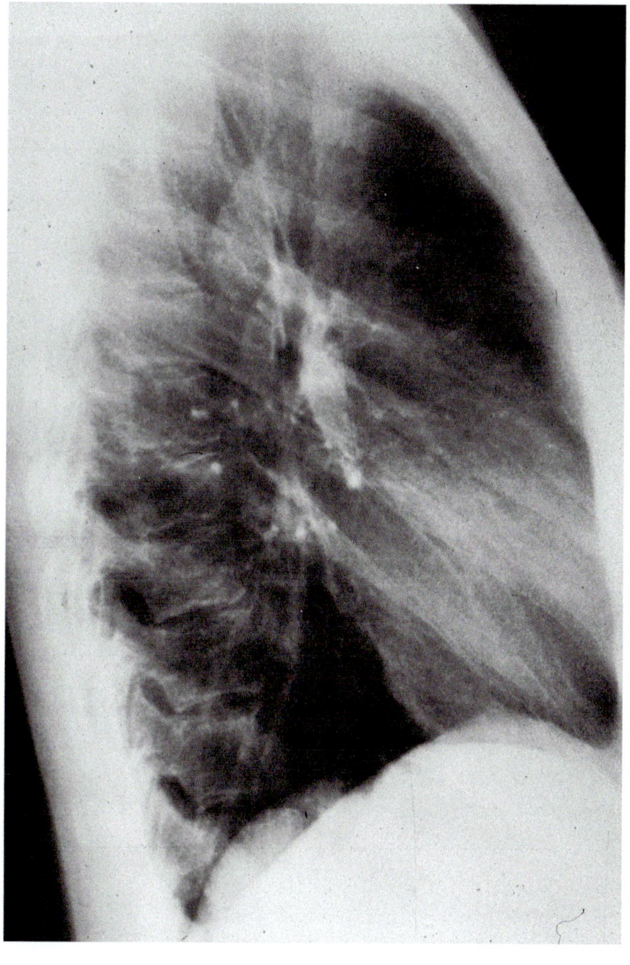

Fig. 13.54 Lateral view of a posterior mediastinal mass corresponding to extramedullary hematopoiesis (EMH)

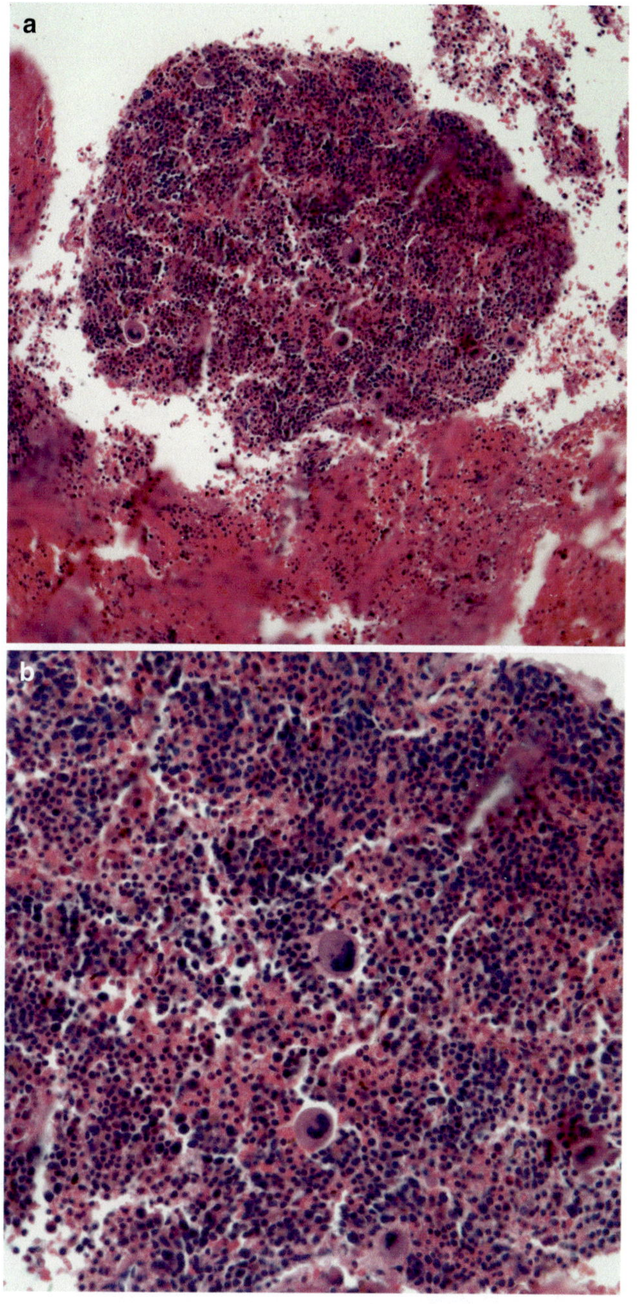

Fig. 13.55 (**a**) Mediastinal EMH showing normal elements including megakaryocytes; (**b**) higher magnification showing normal elements and megakaryocytes

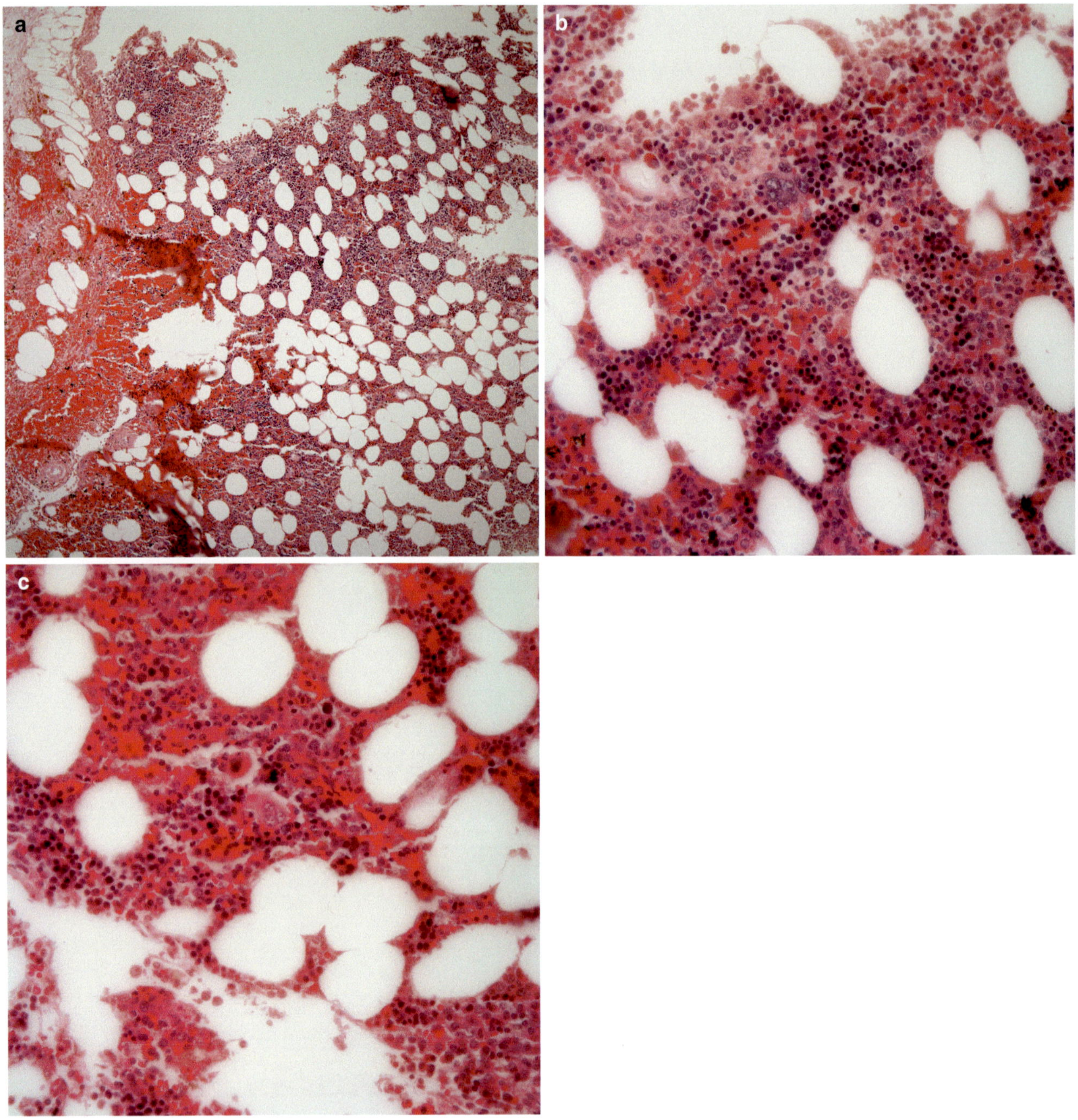

Fig. 13.56 (**a**) EMH showing normal elements and adipose tissue (myelolipoma); (**b**) adipose tissue and normal elements including megakaryocytes; (**c**) high power view of megakaryocytes

References

1. Remigio PA. Granulomatous thymoma associated with erythroid hyperplasia. Am J Clin Pathol. 1971;55:68–72.
2. Strickler JG, Kurtin PJ. Mediastinal lymphoma. Semin Diagn Pathol. 1991;8:2–13.
3. Jones SE, Fuks Z, Bull M, Kadin ME, Dorfman RF, Kaplan HS, et al. Non-Hodgkin's lymphomas. Clinicopathologic correlation of 405 cases. Cancer. 1973;31:806–23.
4. Chabner BA, Johnson RE, Young RC, Canellos GP, Hubbard SP, Johnson SK, et al. Sequential non-surgical and surgical staging of non-Hodgkin's lymphoma. Ann Intern Med. 1976;85:149–54.
5. Manoharan A, Pitney WR, Schonell ME, Bader LV. Intrathoracic manifestations in non-Hodgkin's lymphoma. Thorax. 1979;34:29–32.
6. Goffinet DR, Warnke R, Dunnick NR, Castellino R, Glatstein E, Nelsen TS, et al. Clinical and surgical (laparotomy) evaluation of patients with non-Hodgkin's lymphoma. Cancer Treat Rep. 1977;61:981–92.
7. Lukes RJ, Butler JJ, Hicks EB. Natural history of Hodgkin's disease as related to its pathological picture. Cancer. 1966;19:317–44.
8. Colby TV, Hoppe RT, Warnke RA. Hodgkin's disease: a clinicopathologic study of 659 cases. Cancer. 1981;49:1848–58.
9. Lichtenstein AK, Levine A, Taylor CR, Boswell W, Rossman S, Feinstein DI, et al. Primary mediastinal lymphoma in adults. Am J Med. 1980;68:509–14.
10. Benjamin SP, McCormack LJ, Effler DB, Groves LK. Primary lymphatic tumors of the mediastinum. Cancer. 1972;30:708–12.
11. Al-Naaman YD, Al-Ani M, Al-Omeri M. Primary mediastinal tumours. Thorax. 1974;29:475–81.
12. Adkins RB, Maples MD, Hainsworth JD. Primary malignant mediastinal tumors. Ann Thorac Surg. 1984;38:648–59.
13. Glick RD, La Quaglia MP. Lymphomas of the anterior mediastinum. Semin Pediatr Surg. 1999;8:69–77.
14. Suster S. Primary large cell lymphomas of the mediastinum. Semin Diagn Pathol. 1999;16:51–64.
15. Petersdorf SH, Wood DE. Lymphoproliferative disorders presenting as mediastinal neoplasms. Semin Thorac Cardiovasc Surg. 2000;12:290–300.
16. Barth TFE, Leithauser F, Joos S, Bentz M, Möller P. Mediastinal (thymic) large B-cell lymphoma: where do we stand? Lancet Oncol. 2002;3:229–34.
17. Faris JE, LaCasce AS. Primary mediastinal large B-cell lymphoma. Clin Adv Hematol Oncol. 2009;7:125–33.
18. Martelli M, di Rocco A, Russo E, Perrone S, Foà R. Primary mediastinal lymphoma: diagnosis and treatment options. Exp Rev Hematol. 2015;8(2):173–86.
19. Bhatt VR, Mourya R, Shrestha R, Armitage JO. Primary mediastinal large B-cell lymphoma. Cancer Treat Rev. 2015;41:476–85.
20. Aggarval R, Rao S, Dhawan S, Bhalla S, Kumar A, Chopra P. Primary mediastinal lymphomas, their morphological features and comparative evaluation. Lung India. 2017;34:19–24.
21. Liu PP, Wang KF, Xia Y, Bi XW, Sun P, Wang Y, et al. Racial patterns of patients with primary mediastinal large B-cell lymphoma. Medicine. 2016;95:27(e4054).
22. Maeshima AM, Taniguchi H, Suzuki T, Yuda S, Toyoda K, Yamauchi N, et al. Distribution of malignant lymphomas in the anterior mediastinum: a single institution study of 76 cases in Japan 1997-2016. Int J Hematol. 2017;106:675–80.
23. Martelli M, Ferreri A, Di Rocco A, Ansuinelli M, Johnson PWM. Primary mediastinal B-cell lymphoma. Crit Rev Oncol Hematol. 2017;113:318–27.
24. Zinzani PL, Piccaluga PP. Primary mediastinal DLBCL: evolving biologic understanding and therapeutic strategies. Curr Oncol Rep. 2011;13:407–15.
25. Trump DL, Mann RB. Diffuse large cell and undifferentiated lymphomas with prominent mediastinal involvement. A poor prognostic subset of patients with non-Hodgkin's lymphoma. Cancer. 1982;50:277–82.
26. Levitt LJ, Aisenberg AC, Harris NL, Linggood RM, Poppema S. Primary non-Hodgkin's lymphoma of the mediastinum. Cancer. 1982;50:2486–92.
27. Yousem SA, Weiss LM, Warnke RA. Primary mediastinal non-Hodgkin's lymphomas: a morphologic and immunologic study of 19 cases. Am J Clin Pathol. 1985;83:676–80.
28. Waldrom JA, Dohring EJ, Farber LR. Primary large cell lymphoma of the mediastinum: an analysis of 20 cases. Semin Diagn Pathol. 1985;2:282–95.
29. Perrone T, Frizzera G, Rosai J. Mediastinal diffuse large cell lymphoma with sclerosis. A clinicopathologic study of 60 cases. Am J Surg Pathol. 1986;10:176–91.
30. Menestrina F, Chilosi M, Bonetti F, Lestani M, Scarpa A, Novelli P, et al. Mediastinal large-cell lymphoma of B-type, with sclerosis: histopathological and immunohistochemical study of eight cases. Histopathology. 1986;10:589–600.
31. Addis BJ, Isaacson PG. Large cell lymphoma of the mediastinum: a B-cell tumour of probable thymic origin. Histopathology. 1986;10:379–90.
32. Kirn D, Mauch P, Shaffer K, Pinkus G, Shipp MA, Kaplan WD, et al. Large cell and immunoblastic lymphoma of the mediastinum: prognostic features and treatment outcome in 57 patients. J Clin Oncol. 1993;11:1336–43.
33. Abou-Elella AA, Weisenburger DD, Vose JM, Kollath JP, Lynch JC, Bast MA, et al. Primary mediastinal large B-cell lymphoma: a clinicopathologic study of 43 patients from the Nebraska lymphoma study group. J Clin Oncol. 1999;17:784–90.
34. Cazals-Hatem D, Lepage E, Brice P, Ferrant A, d'Agay MF, Baumelou E, et al. Primary mediastinal large B-cell lymphoma: a clinicopathologic study of 141 cases compared with 916 nonmediastinal large B-cell lymphoma, a GELA ("Groupe d'Etude des Lymphomes de l'Adulte"). Am J Surg Pathol. 1996;20:877–88.
35. Paulli M, Strater J, Gianelli U, Rousset M-T, Gambacorta M, Orlandi E, et al. Mediastinal B-cell lymphoma: a study of its histomorphologic spectrum based on 109 cases. Hum Pathol. 1999;30:178–87.
36. Piira T, Perkins SL, Anderson AT, Meadows AT, Chilcote RR, Kadin M, et al. Primary mediastinal large cell lymphoma in children: a report from the childrens cancer group. Pediatr Pathol Lab Med. 1995;15:561–70.
37. Carr TF, Lockwood L, Stevens RF, Morris-Jones PH, Lewis I, DaCosta PE, et al. Childhood B cell lymphomas arising in the mediastinum. J Clin Pathol. 1993;46:513–6.
38. Dunleavy K. Primary mediastinal B-cell lymphoma: biology and evolving therapeutic strategies. Hematology. 2017;2017:298–304.
39. Ahn HJ, Yoon DH, Kim S, Lee K, Kang E, Huh J, et al. Primary mediastinal large B-cell lymphoma: a single center experience in Korea. Blood Res. 2014;49:36–41.
40. Fiascone S, Datkhaeva I, Winer ES, Rizak T. Primary mediastinal large B-cell lymphoma in pregnancy. Leuk Lymphoma. 2016;57:240–3.
41. Pileri S, Zinzani PL, Gaidano G, Falini B, Gaulard P, Zucca E, et al. Pathobiology of primary mediastinal B-cell lymphoma. Leuk Lymphoma. 2003;44(supplement 3):S21–6.
42. Lazzarino M, Orlandi M, Paulli M, Sträter J, Klersy C, Gianelli U, et al. Treatment outcome and prognostic factors for primary mediastinal (thymic) B-cell lymphoma: a multicenter study of 106 patients. J Clin Oncol. 1997;15:1646–53.
43. Zinzani PL, Martelli M, Magagnoli M, Pescarmona E, Scaramucci L, Palombi F, et al. Treatment and clinical management of primary mediastinal large B-cell lymphoma with sclerosis: MACOP-B

regime and mediastinal radiotherapy monitored by [67]Gallium scan in 50 patients. Blood. 1999;94:3289–93.
44. Todeschini G, Secchi S, Morra E, Vitolo U, Orlandi E, Pasini F, et al. Primary mediastinal large B-cell lymphoma (PMBCL): long term results from a retrospective multicenter Italian experience in 138 patients treated with CHOP or MACOP-B/VACOP-B. Br J Cancer. 2004;90:372–6.
45. Broccoli A, Casadei B, Stefoni V, Pellegrini C, Quirini F, Tonialini L, et al. The treatment of primary mediastinal large B-cell lymphoma: a two decades monocentric experience with 98 patients. BMNC Cancer. 2017;17:276–83.
46. Giulino-Roth L, O'Donohue T, Chen Z, Bartlett NL, LaCasce A, Martin-Doyle W, et al. Outcomes of adults and children with primary mediastinal B-cell lymphoma treated with dose-adjusted EPOCH-R. Br J Haematol. 2017;179:739–47.
47. Pillon M, Carraro E, Mussolin L, Conter V, Tondo A, Aricò M, et al. Primary mediastinal large B-cell lymphoma: outcome of a series of pediatric patients treated with high-dose methotrexate and cytarabine plus anti-CD20. Pediatr Blood Cancer. 2018;65:e26855.
48. Moller P, Lammler B, Eberlein-Gonska M, Feichter GE, Hofmann WJ, Schmitteckert H, et al. Primary mediastinal clear cell lymphoma of B-cell type. Virchows Arch [Pathol Anat]. 1986;409:79–92.
49. Suster S, Moran CA. Pleomorphic large cell lymphoma of the mediastinum. Am J Surg Pathol. 1996;20:224–32.
50. Calaminici M, Piper K, Lee AM, Norton AJ. CD23 expression in mediastinal large B-cell lymphomas. Histopathology. 2004;45:619–24.
51. Higgins JP, Warnke RA. CD30 expression is common in mediastinal large B-cell lymphoma. Am J Clin Pathol. 1999;112:241–7.
52. Copie-Bergman C, Gaulard P, Maouche-Chretien L, Brière J, Haioun C, Alonso MA, et al. The MAL gene is expressed in primary mediastinal large B-cell lymphoma. Blood. 1999;94:3567–75.
53. Tsang P, Cesarman E, Chadburn A, Liu YF, Knowles DM. Molecular characterization of primary mediastinal B-cell lymphoma. Am J Pathol. 1996;148:2017–25.
54. Pileri SA, Gaidano G, Zinzani PL, Falini B, Gaulard P, Zucca E, et al. Primary mediastinal B-cell lymphoma: high frequency of BCL-6 mutations and consistent expression of the transcription factors OCT-2, BOB1, and PU.1 in the absence of immunoglobulins. Am J Pathol. 2003;162:243–53.
55. Savage KJ, Monti S, Kutok JL, Cattoretti G, Neuberg D, De Leval L, et al. The molecular signature of mediastinal large B-cell lymphoma differs from that of other diffuse large B-cell lymphomas and shares features with classical Hodgkin's lymphoma. Blood. 2003;102:3871–9.
56. Rosenwald A, Wright G, Leroy K, Yu X, Gaulard P, Gascoyne RD, et al. Molecular diagnosis of primary mediastinal B cell lymphoma identifies a clinically favorable subgroup of diffuse large B cell lymphoma related to Hodgkin lymphoma. J Exp Med. 2003;198:851–62.
57. Joos S, Joos MI, Ziegler S, Brüderlein S, du Manoir S, Bentz M, et al. Primary mediastinal (thymic) B-cell lymphoma is characterized by gains of chromosomal material including 9p and amplification of the REL gene. Blood. 1996;87:1571–8.
58. Wang Z, Cook JR. PDCD1LG2 (PD-L2) RNA in situ hybridization is a sensitive specific, and practical marker of primary mediastinal large B-cell lymphoma. Br J Haematol. 2018;181(4):564–6.
59. Garcia JF, Mollejo M, Fraga M, Forteza J, Muniesa JA, Pérez-Guillermo M, et al. Large B-cell lymphoma with hodgkin's features. Histopathology. 2005;47:101–10.
60. Gomez-Gelvez JC, Smith LB. Reed-Sternberg-like cells in non-Hodgkin's lymphoma. Arch Pathol Lab Med. 2015;139:1205–10.
61. Traverse-Glehen A, Pittaluga S, Gaulard P, Sorbara L, Alonso MA, Raffeld M, et al. Mediastinal gray zone lymphoma: the missing link between classic Hodgkin's lymphoma and mediastinal large B-cell lymphoma. Am J Surg Pathol. 2005;29:1141–421.
62. Oschlies I, Burkhardt B, Salaverria I, Rosenwald A, d'Amore ES, Szczepanowski M, et al. Clinical, pathological and genetic features of primary mediastinal large B-cell lymphoma and mediastinal gray zone lymphomas in children. Haematologica. 2011;96:262–8.
63. Dunleavy K. Management of primary mediastinal B-cell lymphoma and gray zone lymphoma. Oncology. 2017;6:499–501.
64. Salama M, Mariappan MR, Inamdar K, Tripp SR, Perkins SL. The value of CD23 expression as an additional marker in distinguishing mediastinal (thymic) large B-cell lymphoma from Hodgkin's lymphoma. Int J Surg Pathol. 2010;18:121–8.
65. Hoeller S, Zihler D, Zlobec I, Obermann EC, Pileri SA, Dirnhofer S, et al. BOB.1, CD79a, and cyclin E are the most appropriate markers to discriminate classical Hodgkin's lymphoma from primary mediastinal large B-cell lymphoma. Histopathology. 2010;56:217–28.
66. Etienne B, Guillaud PH, Loire R, Coiffier B, Berger F, Cordier JF. Aggressive primary mediastinal non-Hodgkin's lymphomas: a study of 29 cases. Eur Respir J. 1999;13:1133–8.
67. Gonin J, Kadiri H, Bensaci S, Le Tourneau A, Molina TJ, Diebold J, et al. Primary mediastinal anaplastic alk-2-positive large cell lymphoma of T/NK-cell type expressing CD20. Virchows Arch. 2007;450:355–8.
68. Isaacson PG, Chan JKC, Tang C, Addis BJ. Low-grade B-cell lymphoma of mucosa-associated lymphoid tissue arising in the thymus. A thymic lymphoma mimicking myoepithelial sialadenitis. Am J Surg. 1990;14:342–51.
69. Nagasaka T, Lai R, Harada T, Chen YY, Chen WG, Arber DA, et al. Coexisting thymic and gastric lymphomas of mucosa-associated lymphoid tissues in a patient with Sjogren's syndrome. Arch Pathol Lab Med. 2000;124:770–3.
70. Moriyama E, Yokose T, Kodama T, Matsuno Y, Hojo F, Takahashi K, et al. Low-grade B-cell lymphoma of mucosa-associated lymphoid tissue in the thymus of a patient with pulmonary amyloid nodules. Jpn J Clin Oncol. 2000;30:349–53.
71. Kamimura K, Nakamura N, Ishibashi T, Maruyam Y, Abe M. Somatic hypermutation of immunoglobulin heavy chain variable region genes in thymic marginal zone B-cell lymphoma of MALT type of a patient with Sjogren's syndrome. Histopathology. 2002;40:292–304.
72. Sunada K, Hasegawa Y, Kodama T, Anami Y, Satoh H, Ohtsuka M, et al. Thymic and pulmonary mucosa-associated lymphoid tissue lymphomas in a patient with Sjogren syndrome and literature review. Respirology. 2007;12:144–7.
73. Yamada S, Tadasu K, Mingyon M, Yoshiaki A, Noriko M. Mucosa-associated lymphoid tissue lymphoma of the thymus resected using combined thoracoscopic and transcervical approaches. Ann Thorac Surg. 2003;76:293–5.
74. Kim JM. Primary extranodal marginal zone B-cell lymphoma of mucosa associated lymphoid tissue type in the thymus of a patient with Sjogren's syndrome and rheumatoid arthritis. J Korean Med Sci. 2003;18:897–900.
75. Kuroki S, Nasu K, Murakami K, Hayashi T, Sekiguchi R, Nishida H, et al. Thymic MALT lymphoma MR imaging findings and their correlation with histopathological findings on four cases. J Clin Imaging. 2004;28:272–7.
76. Ortone N, Copie-Bergman C, Remy P, Delfau-Larue MH, Alonso MA, Mariette X, et al. Mucosa-associated lymphoid tissue lymphoma of the thymus: a case report with no evidence of MALT1 rearrangement. Virchows Arch. 2005;446:189–93.
77. Nakamura S, Koshikawa T, Kaba S, Tokoro Y, Suchi T, Kurita S. Imprint cytology of low-grade B-cell lymphoma of mucosa-associated lymphoid tisdsue arising in the thymus: a case report. Diagn Cytopathol. 1993;9:665–7.

78. Takagi N, Nakamura S, Yamamoto K, Kunishima K, Takagi I, Suyama M, et al. Malignant lymphoma of mucosa-associated lymphoid tissue arising in the thymus of a patient with Sjogren's syndrome. Cancer. 1992;69:1347–55.
79. Parrens M, Dubus P, Danjoux M, Jougon J, Brousset P, Velly JF, et al. Mucosa-associated lymphoid tissue of the thymus. Hyperplasia vs lymphoma. Am J Clin Pathol. 2002;117:51–6.
80. Inagaki H, Chan JKC, Ng JWM, Okabe M, Yoshino T, Okamoto M, et al. Primary thymic extranodal marginal zone B-cell lymphoma of mucosa associated lymphoid tissue type exhibits distinctive clinicopathological and molecular features. Am J Pathol. 2002;160:1435–43.
81. Shimizu K, Ishii G, Nagai K, Yokose T, Ishizawa K, Tamaru J, et al. Extranodal marginal zone B-cell lymphoma of mucosa-associated lymphoid tissue (MALT lymphoma) in the thymus: report of four cases. Jpn J Clin Oncol. 2005;35:412–6.
82. Sunohara M, Hara K, Osamura K, Tashiro N, Shibuya H, Nakahara K, et al. Mucosa associated lymphoid tissue (MALT) lymphoma of the thymus with trisomy 18. Intern Med. 2009;48:2025–32.
83. Kitai R, Sasaki M, Sato K, Kubota T, Takeuchi H, Imamura Y. Thymic mucosa-associated lymphoid tissue lymphoma associated with bilateral orbital pseudotumor. Gen Thorac Cardiovasc Surg. 2009;57:566–9.
84. Sakamoto T, Yamashita K, Mizumoto C. MALT lymphoma of the thymus with Sjogren's syndrome: biphasic changes in serological abnormalities over a 4-year period following thymectomy. Int J Hematol. 2009;89:709–13.
85. Maeda A, Hayama M, Nakata M, Masaki H, Tanemoto K. Mucosa associated lymphoid tissue lymphoma in the thymus of a patient with systemic lupus erythematosus. Gen Thorac Cardiovasc Surg. 2008;56:288–91.
86. Kinoshita N, Ashizawa K, Abe K, Yamasaki N, Nakamura A, Tagawa T, et al. Mucosa-associated lymphoid tissue lymphoma of the thymus associated with Sjogren's syndrome: report of a case. Surg Today. 2008;38:436–9.
87. Harigae H, Ichinohasama R, Miura I, Kameoka J, Meguro K, Miyamura K, et al. Primary marginal zone lymphoma of the thymus accompanied by chromosomal anomaly 46,X,dup(X) (p11p22). Cancer Genet Cytogenet. 2002;133:142–7.
88. Yamasaki S, Matsushita H, Tanimura S, Nakatani T, Hara S, Endo Y, et al. B-cell lymphoma of mucosa-associated lymphoid tissue of the thymus: a report of two cases with a background of Sjogren's syndrome and monoclonal gammopathy. Hum Pathol. 1998;29:1021–4.
89. McCluggage WG, McManus K, Qureshi R, McAleer S, Wotherspoon AC. Low-grade B-cell lymphoma of mucosa associated lymphoid tissue (MALT) of thymus. Hum Pathol. 2000;31:255–9.
90. Lorsbach RB, Pinkus GS, Shahsafaei A, Dorfman DM. Primary marginal zone lymphoma of the thymus. Am J Clin Pathol. 2000;113:784–91.
91. Weissferdt A, Moran CA. Primary MALT-type lymphoma of the thymus: a clinicopathological and immunohistochemical study of six cases. Lung. 2011;189:461–6.
92. Sternberg C. Leukosarcomatose and myeloblastenleukaamie. Beitr Pathol. 1916;61:75.
93. Cooke JV. Mediastinal tumor in acute leukemia. A clinical and roentgenologic study. Am J Dis Child. 1932;44:1153.
94. Smith JL, Clein GP, Barker CR, Collins RD. Characterisation of malignant mediastinal lymphoid neoplasm (Sternberg sarcoma) as thymic in origin. Lancet. 1973;1:74.
95. Barcos MGP, Lukes RJ. Malignant lymphoma of the convoluted lymphocytes. A new entity of possible T-cell type. In: Sinks L, Godden J, editors. Conflicts in childhood Cancer: an evaluation of current management. New York: Liss; 1975. p. 147.
96. Nathwani BN, Kim H, Rappaport H. Malignant lymphoma, lymphoblastic: a clinicopathologic study of 95 patients. Cancer. 1976;48:2347.
97. Borowitz MJ, Falletta JM. Leukemias and lymphomas of thymic differentiation. Clin Lab Med. 1988;8:119–34.
98. Cortelazzo S, Ponzoni M, Ferreri AJM, Hoelzer D. Lymphoblastic lymphoma. Crit Rev Oncol Hematol. 2011;79:330–43.
99. Han X, Kilfoy B, Zheng T, Holford TR, Zhu C, Zhu Y, et al. Lymphoma survival patterns by WHO subtype in the United States, 1973-2003. Cancer Causes Control. 2008;19:841–58.
100. Swerdlow SH, Campo E, Harris N, Jaffe ES, Pileri SA, Stein H, et al. WHO classification of tumours of hematopoietic and lymphoid tissues. Lyon: IARC; 2008.
101. Bassan R, Maino E, Cortelazzo S. Lymphoblastic lymphoma: an updated review on biology, diagnosis, and treatment. Eur J Haematol. 2015;96:447–60.
102. Portell CA, Sweetenham JW. Adult lymphoblastic lymphoma. Cancer J. 2012;18:432–8.
103. Le Gouill S, Lepretre S, Briere J, Morel P, Bouabdallah R, Raffoux E, et al. Adult lymphoblastic lymphoma: a retrospective analysis of 92 patients under 61 years included in the LNH87/93 trials. Leukemioa. 2003;17:2220–4.
104. Cortelazzo S, Ferreri A, Hoelzer D, Ponzoni M. Lymphoblastic lymphoma. Crit Rev Oncol Hematol. 2017;113:304–17.
105. Mlika M, Khanfir D, Mansouri R, El-Mezni F. Multivariate analysis of prognostic factors of lymphoblastic lymphomas of the mediastinum. Ann Hematol. 2016;95:1731–2.
106. Thomas DA, Kantarjian HM. Lymphoblastic lymphoma. Hematol Oncol Clin North Am. 2001;15:51–95.
107. Schwartz EE, Conroy JF, Bonner H. Mediastinal involvement in adults with lymphoblastic lymphoma. Acta Radiol. 1987;28:403–7.
108. Macon WR, Rynalski TH, Swedlow SH, Cousar JB. T-cell lymphoblastic leukemia/lymphoma presenting in a recurrent thymoma. Mod Pathol. 1991;4:524–8.
109. Liu KL, Herbrecht R, Tranchant C, Gasser B, Warter JM, Wihlm JM, et al. Malignant thymic lymphoblastic lymphoma and myasthenia gravis: an exceptional association. Nouv Rev Fr Hematol. 1992;34:221–3.
110. Posner MR, Said J, Pinkus GS, Nadler LM, Hardy R, Flatow F, et al. T-cell lymphoblastic lymphoma with subsequent acute non-lymphocytic leukemia. Cancer. 1982;50:118–24.
111. Hvizdala EV, Berard C, Callihan T, Falletta J, Sabio H, Shuster JJ, et al. Lymphoblastic lymphoma in children –a randomized trial comparing LSA2 L2 with the A-COP+ therapeutic regime: a pediatric oncology group study. J Clin Oncol. 1988;6:26–33.
112. Patte C, Kalifa C, Flamant F, Hartmann O, Brugières L, Valteau-Couanet D, et al. Results of the LMT81 protocol, a modified LSA2L2 protocol with high dose methotrexate, on 84 children with non-B-cell (lymphoblastic) lymphoma. Med Pediatr Oncol. 1992;20:105–13.
113. Sander CA, Jaffe ES, Gebhardt FC, Yano T, Medeiros LJ. Mediastinal lymphoblastic lymphoma with an immature B-cell immunophenotype. Am J Surg Pathol. 1992;16:300–5.
114. Manning JT, Pugh WC, El-Naggar A, Ordonez NG. Mediastinal lymphoblastic lymphoma with non-lymphoblastic histologic features. Mod Pathol. 1994;7:59–63.
115. Sweetenham JW. Lymphoblastic lymphoma in adults. Curr Hematol Malig Rep. 2006;1:241–7.
116. Dawson PJ. The original illustrations of Hodgkin's disease. Ann Diagn Pathol. 1999;3:386–93.
117. Aisenberg AC. Historical review. Br J Haematol. 2000; 109:466–76.
118. Dawson PJ. Whatever happened to Dorothy reed? Ann Diagn Pathol. 2003;7:195–203.
119. Reed DM. On the pathological changes in Hodgkin's disease, with especial reference to its relation to tuberculosis. Johns Hopkins Rep. 1902;10:113–96.
120. Jackson H, Parker F. Hodgkin's disease.VI. Clinical diagnosis. NEJM. 1946;234:37–41.

121. Tsang RW, Hodgson DC, Crump M. Hodgkin's lymphoma. Curr Probl Cancer 2006;30:107–58.
122. Hjalgrim H, Askling J, Rostgaard K, Hamilton-Dutoit S, Frisch M, Zhang J-S, et al. Characteristics of Hodgkin's lymphoma after infectious mononucleosis. NEJM. 2003;349:1324–32.
123. Piña-Oviedo S, Moran CA. Primary mediastinal classical Hodgkin's lymphoma. Adv Anat Pathol. 2016;23(5):285–309.
124. Katz A, Lattes R. Granulomatous thymoma or Hodgkin's disease of the thymus. Cancer. 1969;23:1–15.
125. Fechner RE. Hodgkin's disease of the thymus. Cancer. 1969;1:16–23.
126. Keller AR, Castleman B. Hodgkin's disease of the thymus gland. Cancer. 1974;33:1615–23.
127. Smetana HF, Cohen BM. Mortality in relation to histologic type of Hodgkin's disease. Blood. 1956;11:211–24.
128. Lukes RJ, Butler JJ. The pathology and nomenclature of Hodgkin's disease. Cancer Res. 1966;26:1063–81.
129. MacLennan KA, Bennett MH, Tu A, Hudson BV, Easterling MJ, Hudson GV, et al. Relatioship of histopathologic features to survival and relapse in nodular sclerosing Hodgkin's disease. A study of 1659 patients. Cancer. 1989;64:1686–93.
130. Ferry JA, Linggood RM, Convery KM, Efird JT, Eliseo R, Harris NL. Hodgkin's disease, nodular sclerosis type. Implications of histologic subclassification. Cancer. 1993;71:457–63.
131. Hess JL, Bodis S, Pinkus G, Silver B, Mauch P. Histopathologic grading of nodular sclerosis Hodgkin's disease. Lack of prognosticd significance in 254 surgically staged patients. Cancer. 1994;74:708–14.
132. Heron CW, Husband JE, Williams MP. Hodgkin disease: CT of the thymus. Radiology. 1988;167:647–51.
133. Priola AM, Priola SM. Primary mediastinal Hodgkin lymphoma and rebound thymic hyperplasia: differentiation with chemical-shift magnetic resonance imaging after treatment. Int J Haematol. 2009;90:8–10.
134. Schmid C, Pan L, Diss T, Isaacson PG. Expression of B-cell antigens by Hodgkin's and reed-Sternberg cells. Am J Pathol. 1991;139:701–7.
135. Harris JA, Jain S, Ren Q, Zarineh A, Liu C, Ibrahim S. CD163 versus CD68 in tumor associated macrophages of classical Hodgkin's lymphoma. Diagn Pathol. 2012;7:12–7.
136. Kupper R, Rajewsky K, Zhao M, Simons G, Laumann R, Fischer R, et al. Hodgkin disease: Hodgkin and reed-Sternberg cells picked from histological sections show clonal immunoglobulin gene rearrangements and appear to be derived from B-cells at various stages of development. Proc Natl Acad Sci. 1994;91:10962–6.
137. Kanzler H, Kuppers R, Hansmann ML, Rajewsky K. Hodgkin and reed-Sternberg cells in Hodgkin's disease represents the outgrowth of a dominant tumor clone derived from (crippled) germinal center B cells. J Exp Med. 1996;184:1495–505.
138. Kuppers R, Hansmann ML. The Hodgkin and Reed/Sternberg cell. Int J Biochem Cell Biol. 2005;37:511–7.
139. Kuppers R. The biology of Hodgkin's lymphoma. Nat Rev Cancer. 2009;9:15–27. https://doi.org/10.1038/nrc2542.
140. Monda L, Warnke R, Rosai J. A primary lymph node malignancy with features suggestive of dendritic reticulum cell differentiation. A report of 4 cases. Am J Pathol. 1986;122:562–72.
141. Le BE, Korst RJ, Taskin M. Right pneumonectomy for resection of a posterior mediastinal follicular dendritic cell sarcoma arising from Castleman's disease. Ann Thorac Surg. 2014;97:e101–3.
142. Hu J, Dong D, Jiang Z, Hu H. Clinicopathological characgteristics of mediastinal follicular dendritic cell sarcoma: report of three cases. J Cardiothorac Surg. 2016;11:56–9.
143. Viola P, Vroobel KM, Devaraj A, Jordan S, Ladas G, Dusmet M, et al. Follicualr dendritic cell tumour/sarcoma: a commonly misdiagnosed tumour in the thorax. Histopathology. 2016;69:752–61.
144. Hartert M, Strobel P, Dahm M, Nix W, Marx A, Vahl CF. A follicular dendritic cell sarcoma of the mediastinum with immature T-cells and association with myasthenia gravis. Am J Surg Pathol. 2010;34:742–5.
145. Jiang L, Admirand JH, Moran CA, Ford RJ, Bueso-Ramos CE. Mediastinal follicular dendritic cell sarcoma with involving bone marrow: a case report and review of the literature. Ann Diagn Pathol. 2006;10:357–62.
146. Gupta RM, Roy DC, Gupta IM, Khanna S. Extramedullary plasmacytoma IgG type I presenting as mediastinal syndrome. Br J Dis Chest. 1974;68:65.
147. Arbona GL, Loyd TV, Lucas J. Mediastinal extramedullary plasmacytoma. South Med J. 1981;73:670.
148. Moran CA, Suster S, Fishback NF, Koss MN. Extramedullary plasmacytoma presenting as mediastinal masses: clinicopartho-logic study of two cases preceding the onset of multiple myeloma. Mod Pathol. 1995;8:257–9.
149. Ahmed R, Marchbank AJ, Nicholson AG, Wotherspoon AC, Ladas GP. Extramedullary plasmacytoma presenting with myasthenia gravis and mediastinal mass. Ann Thorac Surg. 2000;70:1390–2.
150. Lee SY, Kim JH, Shin JS, Shin C, In KH, Kang KH, et al. A case of extramedullary plasmacytoma arising from the posterior mediastinum. Korean J Intern Med. 2005;20:173–6.
151. Wetherbe ER, Dincer HE. IgG myeloma presenting as a large mediastinal mass and pleural effusion. J Bronchology Interv Pulmonol. 2012;19:65–7.
152. Sato K, Fumimoto S, Fukada T, Chihashi Y, Ochi K, Satomi H, et al. Extramedullary plasmacytoma arising from the anterior mediastinum. Ann Thorac Surg. 2017;103:e393–5.
153. Castleman B, Iverson L, Menendez VP. Localized mediastinal lymph node hyperplasia resembling thymoma. Cancer. 1956;9:822–30.
154. Inada K, Kawai K, Katsumura T, Nakano A. Giant lymph node hyperplasia if mediastinum: case report with review of literature. Am Rev Resp Dis. 1959;79:232–7.
155. Katz I, Dziadiw R. Localized mediastinal lymph node hyperplasia: report of case with roentgen findings simulating porterior mediastinal neurofibroma. Am J Roentgenol Radium Ther Nucl Med. 1960;84:206–12.
156. Wolfel DA, Antonius JI, Cowley A. Posterior mediastinal lymph node hyperplasia. Am J Roentgenol. 1964;91:120–4.
157. Lattes R, Pachter M. Benign lymphoid masses of probable hamatomatous nature: analysis of 12 cases. Cancer. 1962;15:197–214.
158. Keller AR, Hochholzer L, Castleman B. Hyaline-vascular and plasma cell types of giant lymph node hyperplasia of the mediastinum and other locations. Cancer. 1972;29:670–83.
159. Karcher DS, Pearson CE, Butler WM, Hurwitz MA, Cassell PF. Giant lymph node hyperplasia involving the thymus with associated nephrotic syndrome and myelofibrosis. Am J Clin Pathol. 1982;77:100–4.
160. Regal MAH, Aljehani YM, Bousbalt H. Primary mediastinal Castleman's disease. Rare Tumors. 2010;2:e11.
161. Shah S, Shah S. Posterior mediastinal Castleman's disease: a case report. Indian J Surg Oncol. 2010;1:343–5.
162. Ishikawa K, Kato T, Aragaki M, Ohbuchi T, Kimura S, Matsui Y, et al. A case of Castleman's disease with myasthenia gravis. Ann Thorac Cardiovasc Surg. 2014;20(supplement):585–8.
163. Kim CH, Jeong JS, Kim SR, Choe YH, Park HS, Lee YC. Coexistence of mediastinal Caatleman's disease with spindle cell carcinoma of the lung. Am J Respir Crit Care Med. 2017;196:652–4.
164. Yu JY, Oh IJ, Kim KS, Kim YI, Lim SC, Kim YC, et al. Castleman's disease presenting as a tracheal mass. Ann Thorac Surg. 2014;97:1798–800.

165. Hussein H, Khawar M, Cherry M, Youness H. Castleman's disease presenting as a mediastinal mass: mimicker of malignancy. Am J Med. 2016;129:e67–8.
166. Paci M, Valli R, Renconi S, Sgarbi G. Mediastinal Castleman's disease mimicking thoracic paravertebral schwannoma. Interact Cardiovasc Thorac Surg. 2011;13:346–7.
167. Aoki M, Otsuka T, Yanagi M, Yokomakura N, Nagata T, Nakamura Y, et al. A case of resected plasma cell type of Castleman's disease with intramediastinal lymph node spread. Ann Thorac Cardiovasc Surg. 2014;20(supplement):682–5.
168. Nistor C, Davidescu M, Giuche A, Bluoss C, Motaş N, Motaş C, et al. A rare case of unicentric plasma cell type Castleman's disease in the mediastinum. Pneumologia. 2010;59:32–5.
169. Haro A, Kuramitsu E, Fukuyama Y. Complete resection of unicentric Castleman disease in the superior mediastinum: a case report. Int J Surg Case Rep. 2016;25:44–7.
170. Slater B, Nordin AB, Allen CE, Elghetany MT, Heinle JS, Kim ES. Resection of mediastinal Castleman's disease: a case report. Pediatr Hematol Oncol. 2013;30:554–6.
171. Lorenz JM, Zangan SM, Leef JA. Mediastinal Castleman's disease: embolization without surgery. J Vasc Interv Radiol. 2009;20:1393–4.
172. Hountis P, Dedeilias P, Douzinas M. The management of Castleman's disease of the mediastinum: a case report. Cases J. 2008;1:330.
173. Fajgenbaum DC, Shilling D. Castleman disease pathogenesis. Hematol Oncol N Am. 2018;32:11–21.
174. Parravinci C, Coprbellino M, Pauli M, Magrini U, Lazzarino M, Moore PS, et al. Expression of a virus-derived cytokine, KSHV vL-6, in HIV seronegative Castleman's disease. Am J Pathol. 1997;151:1517–22.
175. Wu D, Lim MS, Jaffe ES. Pathology of Castleman disease. Hematol Oncol Clin N Am. 2018;32:37–52.
176. Simpson D. Epidemiology of Castleman disease. Hematol Oncol Clin N Am. 2018;32:1–10.
177. Van Rhee F, Greenway A, Stone K. Treatment of idiopathic Castleman disease. Hematol Oncol Clin N Am. 2018;32:89–106.
178. Szalat R, Munshi NC. Diagnosis of Castleman disease. Hematol Oncol Clin N Am. 2018;32:53–64.
179. Knoblich R. Extramedullary hematopoiesis presenting as intrathoracic tumors. Report of a case in a patient with thalassemia minor. Cancer. 1960;13:462–8.
180. Da Costa JL, Loh YS, Hanam E. Extramedullary hemopoiesis with multiple tumor-simulating mediastinal masses in hemoglobin E-thalasemia disease. Chest. 1974;65:210–2.
181. Cantinella FP, Boyd AD, Spencer FC. Intrathoracic extramedullary hematopoiesis simulating anterior mediastinal tumor. J Thorac Cardiovasc Surg. 1985;89:580–4.
182. Verani R, Olson J, Moake JL. Intrathoracic extramedullary hematopoiesis. Report of a case in a patient with sickle-cell disease –beta-thalasemia. Am J Clin Pathol. 1980;73:133–7.
183. Krag D, Reich S. Heteropic marrow (myelolipoma) of the mediastinum. Chest. 1972;61:514.
184. Covey GW. Erythroblastosis: report of a cases presenting erythroblastic tumor in thoracic cavity. Am J Pathol. 1935;11:551.
185. Hanford RB, Schneider GP, McCarthy JD. Massive thoracic extramedullary hematopoiesis. N Engl J Med. 1960;263:120.
186. Andras C, Lassen KP, Holaday WJ. Tumor simulating intrathoracic extramedullary hematopoiesis. Ann Thorac Surg. 1970;10:75.
187. Condon WB, Safarik LR, Elzi EP. Extramedullary hematopoiesis simulating intra-thoracic tumor. Arch Surg. 1965;90:643.
188. Foster JBT. Primary thoracic myelolipoma: case report. AMA Arch Pathol. 1958;65:295.
189. Varizi M, Sadeghipour A, Pazooki A, Shoolami LZ. Primary mediastinal myelolipoma. Ann Thorac Surg. 2008;85:1805–6.
190. Loh CK, Alcorta C, McElhinney J. Extramedullary hematopoiesis simulating posterior mediastinal tumors. Ann Thorac Surg. 1996;61:1003–5.
191. Moran CA, Suster S, Fishback N, Koss MN. Extramedullary hematopoiesis presenting as posterior mediastinal mass: a study of four cases. Mod Pathol. 1995;8:249–51.
192. Albert S, Wolf PL, Pryjma I, Vasquez J. Erythropoiesis in the human thymus. Am J Clin Pathol. 1966;45:460–4.

Index

© Springer Nature Switzerland AG 2019
N. Kalhor, C. Moran, *Mediastinal Pathology*, https://doi.org/10.1007/978-3-319-98980-8